Pelvic Cancer Surgery

Hitendra R.H. Patel • Tim Mould
Jean V. Joseph • Conor P. Delaney
Editors

Pelvic Cancer Surgery

Modern Breakthroughs and Future Advances

Springer

Editors
Hitendra R.H. Patel MRCS, PhD, FRCS(Urol), FRCS(Eng)
Urology
University Hospital of North Norway
Tromsø
Norway

Jean V. Joseph MD, MDA, MBA
Laparoscopic and Robotic Surgery
University of Rochester Medical Center
Rochester
New York
USA

Tim Mould
University College London Hospital
London
United Kingdom

Conor P. Delaney
Colorectal Surgery
University Hospitals Case
Medical Center
Cleveland
Ohio
USA

ISBN 978-1-4471-4257-7 ISBN 978-1-4471-4258-4 (eBook)
DOI 10.1007/978-1-4471-4258-4
Springer London Heidelberg New York Dordrecht

Library of Congress Control Number: 2015932098

Printed on acid-free paper

Springer is part of Springer Science+Business Media (www.springer.com)

To my incredibly supportive and loving family Venita, Maanya and Ishaan – HP

To my loving and supportive family, Mette, Livy and Dan – TM

To my wonderful and supportive family, Johann, Julian and Xavier – JJ

To my wife Clare, for her continuing love, guidance and support – CD

To all the writers, contributors, and their families for being generous with their time to complete this manuscript, advancing the field, for the betterment of all.

Acknowledgment

We would like to thank all the people who are a part of our extended team that allows us to excel to the very highest standards in the pursuit of high quality surgery. Without them we could not help patients.

Contents

Contributors

Nadeem R. Abu-Rustum, MD, FACOG, FACS Gynecology Service, Department of Surgery, Memorial Sloan Kettering Cancer Center, New York, NY, USA

Jean-Philippe Adam, MD Colorectal Surgery, Sainte-Andre Hospital, Bordeaux University Hospital, Bordeaux, France

Vineet Agrawal, MD, FRCSEd (Urol), FEBU Department of Urology, University of Rochester Medical Center, Rochester, NY, USA

Sonsoles Alonso, MD Department of Gynecologic Oncology, MD Anderson Cancer Center, Madrid, Spain

Knut Magne Augestad, MD, PhD Department of Gastrointestinal Surgery, Norwegian National Centre of Telemedicine and Integrated Care, University Hospital North Norway (UNN – Tromsø), Tromsø, Norway

Riccardo Autorino, MD, PhD, FEBU Urology Institute, University Hospitals Case Western Reserve University, Cleveland, OH, USA

Gopal Badlani, MD Department of Urology, Wake Forest University Baptist Medical Center, Winston Salem, NC, USA

Susana Banerjee, MA, MBBS, MRCP, PhD Department of Medicine, Royal Marsden NHS Foundation Trust, London & Sutton, UK

Etai Bogen, MD Department of Gastrointestinal Surgery, Norwegian National Centre of Telemedicine and Integrated Care, University Hospital North Norway (UNN – Tromsø), Tromsø, Norway

Gregory B. Boustead, MBChB, MMed, FCS(SA), FRCS(Urol) Consultant Urological Surgeon & Clinical Director, Herts & South Bedsfordshire Urological Cancer Centre, Lister Hospital, Stevenage, UK

Gina Brown, MBBS, MD, FRCR Department of Radiology, Royal Marsden Hospital, Sutton, Surrey, UK

Lill-Tove Busund, MD, PhD Department of Clinical Pathology, University Hospital of Northern Norway, Institute of Medical Biology, University of Tromsø, Tromsø, Norway

Hartwig Büttner, MD, FECSM Medical Department, Men's Health ACE (Australia, Canada, Europe), Lilly Deutschland GmbH, Bad Homburg v.d.H, Germany

Riccardo Garruto Campanile, MD Department of Gynaecologic Oncology, Oxford University Hospital, Oxford, Oxfordshire, UK

Francesco Carli, MD, MPhil Department of Anesthesia, McGill University Health Centre, Montreal, QC, Canada

Erik P. Castle, MD Department of Urology, Mayo Clinic, Phoenix, AZ, USA

Yannick Cerantola, MD Department of Urology, University Hospital Lausanne (CHUV), Lausanne, Switzerland

Manish Chand, MBBS, BSc, MRCS Department of Radiology, Royal Marsden Hospital, Sutton, Surrey, UK

George J. Chang, MD, MS Department of Surgical Oncology, University of Texas MD Anderson Cancer Center, Houston, TX, USA

Scott M. Cheney, MD Department of Urology, Mayo Clinic, Phoenix, AZ, USA

Dennis S. Chi, MD Gynecology Service, Pelvic Reconstructive Surgery, Department of Surgery, Memorial Sloan Kettering Cancer Center, New York, NY, USA

Kelly A. Chiles, MD, MSc Male Reproductive Medicine and Microsurgery, Department of Urology, Weill Cornell Medical College, New York, NY, USA

Luis M. Chiva, MD, PhD Department of Gynecologic Oncology, MD Anderson Cancer Center, Madrid, Spain

James M. Church, MD, MBChB, MMedSci, FRACS Department of Colorectal Surgery, Digestive Disease Institute, Cleveland Clinic, Cleveland, OH, USA

Stefano Cianci, MD Department of Gynaecologic Oncology, Oxford University Hospital, Oxford, Oxfordshire, UK

David Cibula, MD, PhD Department of Obstetrics and Gynecology, Gynecologic Oncology Center, General University Hospital, First Medical School, Charles University, Prague, Czech Republic

Manuel Ferreira Coelho, MD Department of Urology, Hospital Prof. Doutor Fernando Fonseca, EPE, Amadora, Portugal

Lance J. Coetzee, MD Consultant Urological Surgeon, Pretoria Urology Hospital, Pretoria, South Africa

Janet Colli, MD Department of Urology, Tulane University School of Medicine, New Orleans, LA, USA

Daniel M. de Bruin, MSc, PhD Department of Urology, Academic Medical Center, Amsterdam, The Netherlands

Mia DeBarros, MD Department of General Surgery, Madigan Army Medical Center, Fort Lewis, WA, USA

Jean J.M.C.H. de la Rosette, PhD Department of Urology, Academic Medical Center, Amsterdam, The Netherlands

Quentin Denost, MD Colorectal Surgery, Sainte-Andre Hospital, Bordeaux University Hospital, Bordeaux, France

Nandita M. deSouza, MR, FRCP, FRCR CRUK/EPSRC Cancer Imaging Centre, Institute of Cancer Research, Royal Marsden Hospital, Sutton, Surrey, UK

João Real Dias, MD Department of Urology, Hospital CUF Descobertas, Lisboa, Portugal

Anja Dietel, MD, PhD Department of Urology, University of Leipzig, Leipzig, Germany

Antonino Ditto, MD Department of Gynecologic Oncology, National Cancer Institute of Milan, Milan, Italy

Craig F. Donatucci, MD Department of Men's Health, Eli Lilly and Company, Indianapolis, IN, USA

Eric J. Dozois, MD Department of Colon and Rectal Surgery, Mayo Clinic, Rochester, MN, USA

John A. Dumot, DO, FASGE Division of Gastroenterology and Hepatology, Case Western Reserve University, University Hospitals of Cleveland, Cleveland, OH, USA

Digestive Health Institute, Ahuja Medical Center, Beachwood, OH, USA

Patricia J. Eifel, MD Department of Radiation Oncology, MD Anderson Cancer Center, Houston, TX, USA

Eric L. Eisenhauer, MD Gynecologic Oncology, Department of Obstetrics and Gynecology, University of Cincinnati College of Medicine, Cincinnati, OH, USA

Gemma K.D. Eminowicz, MBChB, MRCP, MSc, FRCR Department of Oncology, University College London Hospital, London, UK

Giorgio Fachechi, MD Department of Gynaecologic Oncology, Oxford University Hospital, Oxford, Oxfordshire, UK

James E. Ferguson, MD Division of Urology, Department of Surgery, University of North Carolina, Chapel Hill, NC, USA

Fernando Ferrito, MD Department of Urology, Hospital Prof. Doutor Fernando Fonseca, EPE, Amadora, Portugal

Simon Fleming, MBBS Lond., MRCS (Eng), M.Sc (Dist), MAcadMEd, MFSTEd, AFHEA ST4 Trauma and Orthopaedics Registrar, NE Thames, Percivall Pott, London, UK

Michael J. Flynn, MD Department of Oncology, University College London, London, UK

Veerabhadram Garimella, MD, FRCS Department of Colorectal Surgery, University Hospital of North Midlands, Staffordshire, UK

Aleksandra Gentry-Maharaj, PhD Department of Women's Cancer, Gynaecological Cancer Research Centre, University College London, Institute for Women's Health, London, UK

Ioannis Georgiopoulos, MD Department of Urology, University of Patras, Patras, Greece

C. Blake Gilks, MD, FRCPC Department of Pathology and Laboratory Medicine, Vancouver General Hospital, Vancouver, BC, Canada

Francisco Carrasquinho Gomes, MD Department of Urology, Hospital Prof. Doutor Fernando Fonseca, EPE, Amadora, Portugal

Michael A. Gorin, MD James Buchanan Brady Urological Institute, Johns Hopkins University School of Medicine, Baltimore, MD, USA

Bruno Graça, MD Department of Urology, Hospital Prof. Doutor Fernando Fonseca, EPE, Amadora, Portugal

James S.A. Green, MBBS, LLM, FRCS (Urol) Department of Urology, Whipps Cross University Hospital, Barts Health NHS Trust, London, UK

Department of Health and Social Care, London Southbank University, London, UK

Kumar Gubbala, Department of Gynaecologic Oncology, Oxford University Hospital, Oxford, Oxfordshire, UK

Angelita Habr-Gama, MD, PhD Department of Colorectal Surgery, Angelita and Joaquim Gama Institute, São Paulo, Brazil

Ayshea Hameeduddin, MBBS, BA, MSc Department of Imaging, Bart's Cancer Centre, St. Bartholomew's Hospital, London, UK

Richard E. Hautmann, MD, MD hon Department of Urology, University of Ulm, Neu-Ulm, Germany

Richard J. Heald, CBE, MChir, FRCS Department of Surgery, Pelican Cancer Foundation, Basingstoke, Hampshire, UK

Michael Höckel, MD, PhD Department of Gynecology, Women's and Children's Center, University of Leipzig, Leipzig, Germany

Martin Hubner, PhD Department of Visceral Surgery, Lausanne University Hospital (CHUV), Lausanne, Switzerland

Tracy L. Hull, MD Department of Colon and Rectal Surgery, Cleveland Clinic, Cleveland, OH, USA

Terence Jackson, MD Department of General Surgery, University Hospital Case Medical Center, Case Western Reserve University, Cleveland, OH, USA

Rozh T. Jalil, MBChB, MRCS, MD Department of Urology, Healtherwood and Wexham Park Hospital NHS Trust, Slough, Berkshire, UK

Ahmed Z. Janjua, FCS, FRCSI, FRCSI (GENSURG) Department of Surgery, Hampshire Hospitals Foundation Trust, Basingstoke, Hampshire, UK

Jean V. Joseph, MD, MDA, MBA Section of Laparoscopic and Robotic Surgery, University of Rochester Medical Center, Rochester, NY, USA

Matias Jurado, Department of Gynecology, University of Navarre, Pamplona, Spain

Panagiotis S. Kallidonis, MD, PhD(Urol), MSc(Clin Pharma) Department of Urology, University of Patras, Rion, Patras, Greece

Jatinderpal Kalsi, PhD Department of Women's Cancer, Gynaecological Cancer Research Centre, University College London, Institute for Women's Health, London, UK

Burzeen E. Karanjawala, MD Department of General Surgery, University of Texas Medical School at Houston, Houston, TX, USA

Robin H. Kennedy, MB BS, MS, FRCS Department of Surgery, St. Mark's Hospital, Middlesex, UK

Shelize S. Khakoo, MBChB, BSc, MRCP Department of Medicine, Royal Marsden NHS Foundation Trust, Sutton, London, UK

Cherry E. Koh, MBBS(Hons), MS(Col Surg), FRACS Royal Prince Alfred Hospital, Camperdown, NSW, Australia

Surgical Outcomes Research Centre (SOuRCe), Camperdown, NSW, Australia

Discipline of Surgery, University of Sydney, Newtown, NSW, Australia

Stavros Kontogiannis, MD Department of Urology, University of Patras, Rion, Patras, Greece

Rebecca Kristeleit, MD, PhD Department of Oncology, University College London, London, UK

Iason Kyriazis, MD Department of Urology, University of Patras, Rion, Patras, Greece

Benjamin W. Lamb, MBBS, MA, MRCS, PhD Department of Urology, University College Hospital, UCLH NHS Foundation Trust, London, UK

Department of Surgery and Cancer, Imperial College London, London, UK

Fernando Lapuente, MD Department of Gynecologic Oncology, MD Anderson Cancer Center, Madrid, Spain

Kristoffer Lassen, MD, PhD Department of GI/HPB Surgery, University Hospital Northern Norway, Tromsø, Norway

Evangelos N. Liatsikos, MD, PhD Department of Urology, University of Patras, Rion, Patras, Greece

Rolv-Ole Lindsetmo, MD The National Advisory Unit on Incontinence and Pelvic Floor Health of Norway, University Hospital of North Norway, Tromsø, Norway

Department of Clinical Medicine, Faculty of Health Sciences, University of Tromsø, Tromsø, Norway

Domenica Lorusso, MD Department of Gynecologic Oncology, National Cancer Institute of Milan, Milan, Italy

Steven M. Lucas, MD Department of Urology, Wayne State University School of Medicine, Detroit, MI, USA

Patricio Bernardo Lynn, MD Department of Colorectal Surgery, Angelita and Joaquim Gama Institute, São Paulo, Brazil

Hugh Mackenzie, MBBS, BSc, MRCS Department of Surgery and Cancer, Imperial College London, London, UK

Haider Mahdi, MD Women's Health Institute/Gynaecologic Oncology Division, Cleveland Clinic Health System, Cleveland, OH, USA

Hooman Soleymani Majd, MD, MRCOG Department of Gynaecologic Oncology, Churchill Hospital, Oxford University Hospitals NHS Trust, Oxford, Oxfordshire, UK

Fabio Martinelli, MD Department of Gynecologic Oncology, National Cancer Institute of Milan, Milan, Italy

Mary McCormack, BSc, MSc, PhD, MBBS, FRCR Department of Oncology, University College London Hospital, London, UK

Patrick McKenzie, MD Department of Urology, Wake Forest University, Winston-Salem, NC, USA

Alan S. McNeill, BM BS, FRCS(Eng, Ed), FRCS(Urol) Department of Urology, Western General Hospital, Edinburgh, UK

Nelya Melnitchouk, MD Department of Surgery, Memorial Sloan Kettering Cancer Center, New York, NY, USA

Usha Menon, MBBS, MD(Res), FRCOG Department of Women's Cancer, Gynaecological Cancer Research Centre, University College London, Institute for Women's Health, London, UK

Amit Merchea, MD Department of Colon and Rectal Surgery, Mayo Clinic, Jacksonville, FL, USA

Minh Do Hoang, MD, PhD Department of Urology, University of Leipzig, Leipzig, Germany

Danilo Miskovic, PhD, MD, FRCS The John Goligher Colorectal Unit, St. James University Hospital, University of Leeds, Leeds, West Yorkshire, UK

John R.T. Monson, MD, FRCS(Ire,Ed,Eng,Glas), FACS Division of Colorectal Surgery, Department of Surgery, University of Rochester Medical Center, Rochester, NY, USA

Department of Colorectal SurgeryUniversity of Rochester Medical Center, Rochester, NY, USA

Brendan J. Moran, FRCSI, MCh, FRCS Department of Surgery, Hampshire Hospitals Foundation Trust, Basingstoke, Hampshire, UK

John P. Mulhall, MD, FECSM Male Sexual and Reproductive Medicine Program, Memorial Sloan Kettering Cancer Center, New York, NY, USA

Berrend G. Muller, MD, PhD Department of Urology, Academic Medical Center, Amsterdam, The Netherlands

Stig Müller, MD, PhD Department of Surgery, Institute of Clinical Medicine, University of Oslo, Oslo, Norway

Department of Urology, Akershus University Hospital, Lorenskog, Norway

Jeffrey K. Mullins, MD James Buchanan Brady Urological Institute, Johns Hopkins University School of Medicine, Baltimore, MD, USA

Jochen Neuhaus, MD, PhD Department of Urology, University of Leipzig, Leipzig, Germany

Tamim Mohammad Niazi, MD Department of Radiation Oncology, Jewish General Hospital, Montreal, QC, Canada

Stig Norderval, MD, PhD The National Advisory Unit on Incontinence and Pelvic Floor Health, University Hospital of North Norway, Tromsø, Norway

Department of Clinical Medicine, Faculty of Health Sciences, University of Tromsø, Tromsø, Norway

Mathew Oommen, MD Department of Urology, Tulane University School of Medicine, New Orleans, LA, USA

Anup Patel, BSc, MBBS, MS, FRCS(Urol) Department of Urology, Royal London Hospital at Barts Health NHS Trust, London, UK

Bijendra Patel, MS, FRCS(Ed), FRCS(Gen Surg) Barts and The Royal London Hospital, Barts Cancer Institute, Queen Mary University of London, London, UK

Hitendra R.H. Patel, MRCS, PhD, FRCS(Urol), FRCS(Eng) Department of Urology, University Hospital North Norway, Tromsø, Norway

Christian P. Pavlovich, MD James Buchanan Brady Urological Institute, Johns Hopkins University School of Medicine, Baltimore, MD, USA

Rodrigo Oliva Perez, MD, PhD Colorectal Surgery Division, Department of Gastroenterology, Angelita and Joaquim Gama Institute, University of São Paulo School of Medicine, São Paulo, Brazil

Beata M.E. Persson, MD, FEBU Department of Urology, Őrebro University Hospital, Őrebro, Sweden

Philip M. Pierorazio, MD James Buchanan Brady Urological Institute, Johns Hopkins University School of Medicine, Baltimore, MD, USA

Raj S. Pruthi, MD Division of Urology, Department of Surgery, University of North Carolina, Chapel Hill, NC, USA

Abhay Rane, MS, FRCS(Urol) Department of Urology, East Surrey Hospital, Redhill, UK

Francesco Raspagliesi, MD Department of Gynecologic Oncology, National Cancer Institute of Milan, Milan, Italy

Eleanor R. Ray, MBBCh, BSc, MS, FRCS(Urol) Department of Urology, University College Hospital London, London, UK

Elin H. Richardsen, MD, PhD Department of Clinical Pathology, University Hospital of Northern Norway, Tromsø, Norway

Lukas Rob, MD, PhD Department of Obstetrics and Gynecology, 2nd Medical Faculty, Charles University, Prague, Czech Republic

Peter G. Rose, MD Women's Health Institute/Gynaecologic Oncology Division, Cleveland Clinic Health System, Cleveland, OH, USA

Adam N. Rosenthal, PhD, MRCOG Department of Women's Health, University College London Hospitals NHS Foundation Trust & Department of Women's Cancer, UCL EGA Institute for Women's Health, London, UK

Eric Rullier, MD Colorectal Surgery, Sainte-Andre Hospital, Bordeaux University Hospital, Bordeaux, France

Dinesh Samarasekera, MD, FRCSC Glickman Urologic and Kidney Institute, Cleveland Clinic, Cleveland, OH, USA

Pedro Bargão Santos, MD Department of Urology, Hospital Prof. Doutor Fernando Fonseca, EPE, Amadora, Portugal

Department of Urology, Hospital CUF Descobertas, Lisboa, Portugal

Somita Sarkar, MB ChB, MRCS Department of Urology, Whipps Cross University Hospital, Barts Health NHS Trust, London, UK

Department of Surgery and Cancer, University Imperial College London, London, UK

Thilo Schwalenberg, MD, PhD Department of Urology, University of Leipzig, Leipzig, Germany

Anthony J. Senagore, MD, MS, MBA Department of Surgery, University Hospitals/Case Western Reserve University, Cleveland, OH, USA

Nick Sevdalis, BSc, MSc, PhD Department of Surgery and Cancer, Imperial College London, London, UK

John H. Shepherd, FRCS, FRCOG, FACOG Department of Gynaecological Oncology, The Royal Marsden Hospital, London, England, UK

Emily S. Shepherd, MBBS, BMedSci, DRCOG Department of Obstetrics and Gynaecology, St Mary's Hospital Imperial College NHS Trust, London, UK

Lucy E. Side, MD, MB, BCh Department of Women's Cancer, UCL EGA Institute for Women's Health & North East Thames Regional Genetics Service, Great Ormond Street Hospital, London, UK

Christopher Thomas Siegel MD, PhD Department of Surgery, Division of Hepatobiliary and Transplant Surgery, Liver Center of Excellence, UH Digestive Health Institute, Cleveland, OH, USA

Department of SurgeryUniversity Hospital Case Medical Center, Case Western Reserve University, Cleveland, OH, USA

Michael J. Solomon, MB, BAO, MSc(Clin Epid), FRACS Royal Prince Alfred Hospital, Camperdown, NSW, Australia

Surgical Outcomes Research Centre (SOuRCe), Camperdown, NSW, Australia

Discipline of Surgery, University of Sydney, Newtown, NSW, Australia

Tayana Soukup, BSc, MSc Department of Surgery and Cancer, Imperial College London, London, UK

Mona Stedenfeldt, BSc(Hons), MSc, PhD The National Advisory Unit on Incontinence and Pelvic Floor Health of Norway, University Hospital of North Norway, Tromsø, Norway

Scott R. Steele, MD Department of Surgery, Madigan Healthcare System, Tacoma, WA, USA

Colon and Rectal Surgery, Madigan Army Medical Center, Tacoma, WA, USA

Jens-Uwe Stolzenburg, MD, PhD, FRCS (Ed), FRCS (Eng) Department of Urology, University of Leipzig, Leipzig, Germany

Cath Taylor, PhD Florence Nightingale Faculty of Nursing and Midwifery, Kings College London, London, UK

Peter Tenke, MD, PhD Department of Urology, Jahn Ferenc South Pest Hospital, Budapest, Hungary

Raju Thomas, MD, FACS, MHA Department of Urology, Tulane University School of Medicine, New Orleans, LA, USA

Roberto Tozzi, MD, PhD Department of Gynaecologic Oncology, Oxford Cancer Centre, Oxford University Hospital, Oxford, UK

Department of Gynaecologic Oncology, Oxford University Hospital, Oxford, Oxfordshire, UK

Michael A. Valente, DO, FACS, FASCRS Department of Colon and Rectal Surgery, Cleveland Clinic, Cleveland, OH, USA

Massimo Valerio, MD Department of Urology, University Hospital Lausanne (CHUV), Lausanne, Switzerland

Willemien van den Bos PhD Department of Urology, Academic Medical Center, Amsterdam, The Netherlands

Charles Vincent, PhD Department of Experimental Psychology, University of Oxford, Oxford, UK

Té Vuong, MD Department of Radiation Oncology, Jewish General Hospital, Montreal, QC, Canada

Anita Wale, BM, BS Department of Radiology, The Royal Marsden Hospital NHS Foundation Trust, Sutton, Surrey, UK

Martin R. Weiser, MD Colorectal Service, Department of Surgery, Memorial Sloan Kettering Cancer Center and Weill Cornell Medical College, New York, NY, USA

Ian D. White, MBBS Surgery B, Meir General Hospital, Kfar Saba, Israel

Michael E. Woods, MD Division of Urology, Department of Surgery, University of North Carolina, Chapel Hill, NC, USA

Part I

Training and Environment for Pelvic Surgery

1 Improving Multidisciplinary Team Working in Pelvic Oncology

Somita Sarkar, Benjamin W. Lamb, Rozh T. Jalil, Cath Taylor, Tayana Soukup, Charles Vincent, Nick Sevdalis, and James S.A. Green

1.1 Introduction

Multidisciplinary teams (MDTs) and MDT meetings to decide treatment options are increasingly becoming the gold standard of care for patients with cancer across the world and in the UK the delivery of cancer care by MDTs has increased from 20 % in 1996 to over 80 % by 2006 [1]. At their best, MDTs can provide a means of bettering decision-making, coordination and communication between healthcare professionals. Recent evidence has even suggested that the benefits of multidisciplinary working in cancer care can also improve patient outcomes [2]. However, some clinicians are unsatisfied at the time and resources taken up with MDT meetings, without seeing significant improvement in patient care.

In 1995, MDT working was introduced in the UK following evidence of variation in the quality of cancer services [1]. In particular there was evidence of discrepancies in access to specialist care, shortfalls in cancer services, a fragmented system of referral to and between specialists, as well as inconsistencies in the frequency of individual treatments, the caseload for particular doctors, and most importantly variation in patient survival. Healthcare professionals worked in teams, but there was little standardization of the organization of services or operating processes, and referrals were made on an ad hoc basis. In the 1990s evidence started to emerge about the benefits of treating patients with a multidisciplinary team approach, rather than treatment by individual clinicians [3]. Furthermore, studies had found

S. Sarkar, MBChB, MRCS
Department of Urology, University Whipps Cross University Hospital, Barts Health NHS Trust, London, UK

Department of Surgery and Cancer, University Imperial College London, London, UK

B.W. Lamb, MBBS, MA, MRCS, PhD (✉)
Department of Urology, University College Hospital, UCLH NHS Foundation Trust, London, UK

Department of Surgery and Cancer, Imperial College London, London, UK
e-mail: Benjamin.lamb@imperial.ac.uk

R.T. Jalil, MBChB, MRCS, MD
Department of Urology, Healtherwood and Wexham Park Hospital NHS Trust, Slough, Berkshire, UK

C. Taylor, PhD
Florence Nightingale Faculty of Nursing and Midwifery, Kings College London, London, UK

T. Soukup, BSc, MSc
Department of Surgery and Cancer, Imperial College London, London, UK

C. Vincent, PhD
Department of Experimental Psychology, University of Oxford, Oxford, UK

N. Sevdalis, BSc, MSc, PhD
Department of Surgery and Cancer, Imperial College London, London, UK

J.S.A. Green, MBBS, LLM, FRCS (Urol)
Department of Urology, Whipps Cross University Hospital, Barts Health NHS Trust, London, UK

Department of Health and Social Care, London Southbank University, London, UK

H.R.H. Patel et al. (eds.), *Pelvic Cancer Surgery: Modern Breakthroughs and Future Advances*, DOI 10.1007/978-1-4471-4258-4_1, that patients' surgical outcomes improved when surgeons with higher numbers of cases treated them, and in centers that carried out higher volumes of cases [4]. It was this evidence that the Chief Medical Officers for England and Wales drew on in the Calman-Hine report in 1995 to recommend that cancer care should be delivered by MDTs at specialist cancer centers arranged into site-specific cancer networks [5].

1.2 "A Systems Approach" to MDT Meetings

Recently, the process of decision-making in MDT meetings has been studied scientifically. Over the last 5 years, our team has undertaken a program of research to apply qualitative and quantitative methodologies from existing research in team performance in healthcare, to scientifically measure and improve the quality of teamwork and decision-making in Urology MDT meetings.

Outside of cancer care there has recently been increasing interest and an expanding evidence base on the description, assessment and improvement of non-technical skills in healthcare, in particular in team working across a diverse range of specialties. The majority of this work has been translated from research in other industries that share the need for reliability with high reliance on human interaction. These industries, including commercial aviation and the military also share the potential for disastrous consequences when communication fails or team leadership is inadequate. The application of this work to healthcare has suggested that factors including the environment, team factors, and an individual's non-technical skills all affect clinical outcomes [6]. Non-technical skills have been grouped into behavioral and cognitive skills. Behavioral skills refer to skills such as teamwork and leadership. Cognitive skills include situational awareness (the awareness of the surgeon to what is happening in the operating room) and decision-making. Decision-making includes the choices the surgeon makes i.e. when to operate, as well as judgements e.g. of risk and are based on the surgeon's experience and personal beliefs. Consideration of these factors alongside traditional indicators of performance such as technical skills and patient factors has given rise to a new 'systems

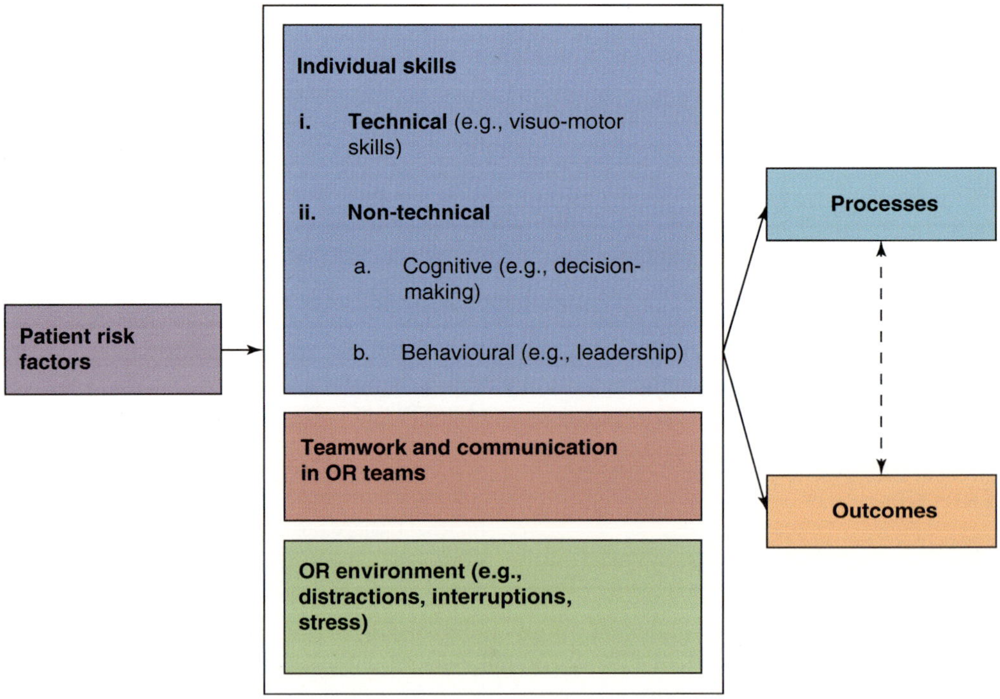

Fig. 1.1 The systems approach to surgical performance (Adapted from Undre et al. [6])

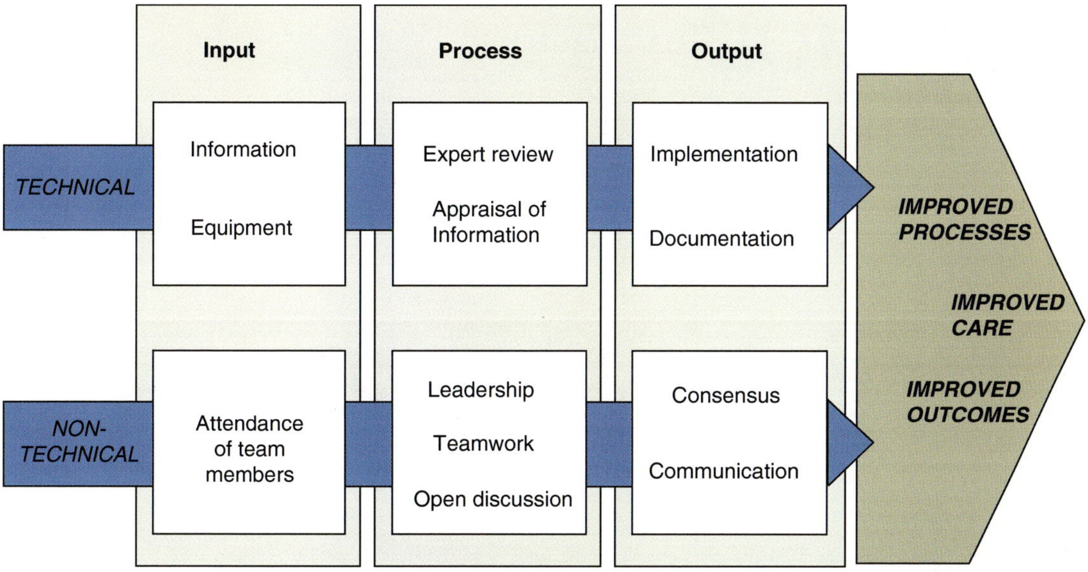

Fig. 1.2 A systems approach to decision-making in MDT meetings. 'Technical' refers to organizational factors and clinical skills. 'Non-technical' refers to team skills (Adapted from Lamb et al. [8])

approach' to performance in healthcare (Fig. 1.1). Within healthcare, research on team skills was pioneered in surgery and anesthesia and has since been adapted to other many other specialities including emergency medicine. Work to improve team performance has been achieved using a variety of qualitative and quantitative methodologies that has led to the development of robust, validated tools for team assessment and feedback and simulation-based training. A significant portion of this research has been carried out in urological surgery [7].

The evidence for decision-making in MDT meetings covers many different aspects of the MDT meeting across a range of specialities [8]. Several studies have found that MDTs make a difference to the outcome of care management decisions, compared with the decisions of individual clinicians. However, decisions in MDT meetings cannot always be reached, often due to the lack of clinical information. Furthermore, MDT decisions are not always implemented, because information relating to the patients' clinical state or their comorbid conditions is sometimes insufficient. In particular, patient's preferences are not taken into account when such decisions are made. Studies suggest that high-quality, feasible decisions also require support from good leadership, protected time for team-members to prepare prior to the meeting and adequate organizational facilities. The roles played by different team members within the MDT are varied, with typically lower importance placed on the input of nurses, who have skills in understanding patient's psychosocial issues and choices for treatment.

This array of factors that can potentially impede the quality of decision-making is complex and difficult to understand as a whole. In order to better understand and assess decision-making in MDT meetings we took the systems approach as described above and applied it to the evidence for decision-making in MDT meetings [8]. By applying this approach we were able to develop a model of the factors that affect decision-making (Fig. 1.2). This model has provided a useful framework that we have used to systematically study the quality of teamwork and decision-making in MDT meetings.

1.3 Assessing Decision-Making in MDT Meetings

With a better understanding of MDT decision-making and the aspects that are important to high quality performance, we set out to construct a

MDT-*MODe*

*M*etric for the *O*bservation of *De*cision-making

			Information						Discussion								OUTCOME	
#	Site	point	Hx	X-ray	Path	Psy/soc/	comorbid	Patient view	Chair	Surg	Phys	Oncolo	Nurse	Radiolo	Histopath	MDTC	Y/D/N	Free text
1																		
2																		
3																		
4																		
5																		

History	5	Fluent, comprehensive case history	Psycho-social	5	Comprehensive first-hand knowledge of patients' personal circumstances, social and psychological issues.
	3	Partial case history		3	Vague first-hand knowledge or good second-hand knowledge of personal circumstances, social and psychological issues.
	1	No patient case history		1	No knowledge of personal circumstances, social and psychological issues.
x-ray	5	Radiological images	Co-morbidity	5	Comprehensive first-hand knowledge of past medical history and performance status
	3	Radiological information from a report/ account		3	Vague first-hand knowledge, or good second-hand knowledge of past medical history or performance status
	1	No provision of radiological information		1	No knowledge of past medical history or performance status
Pathology	5	Histopathological information from pathologist	Patient's views	5	Comprehensive first-hand knowledge of patient's wishes or opinions regarding treatment
	3	Histopathological information from a report/account		3	Vague first-hand knowledge, or good second-hand knowledge of patient's wishes or opinions regarding treatment
	1	No provision of Histopathological information		1	No knowledge of patient's wishes or opinions regarding treatment
Chair	5	Good leadership enhanced team discussion and decision making	Members	5	Clear contribution of speciality.
	3	Leadership neither enhanced or impeded team discussion and decision making		3	Contribution inarticulate or vague
	1	Poor/inadequate leadership impeded team discussion and decision making		1	No contribution
Point	Pre Rx	Pre treatment	Decision	Y	Clear treatment decision
	Post Rx	Post treatment		N	No decision/ Decision deferred
	R	Recurrence/surveillance			

Fig. 1.3 Figure displaying MDT-*MODe* used to score behaviors during MDT meetings—including information provision and team-member contribution. Observed behaviors are compared to and scored against examples of behaviors of varying quality (Copyright 2013 Imperial College London. Accessed from http://www1.imperial.ac.uk/medicine/about/institutes/patientsafetyservicequality/cpssq_publications/resources_tools/mdt/)

tool for the scientific assessment of MDT decision-making. In order to improve something, you first must be able to measure it. Using the principles of the observational assessment of team working from other areas of healthcare and other industries, along with evidence from the literature and our own research, we developed an observational tool, MDT-*MODe* to assess behaviors and information presentation in MDT meetings (Fig. 1.3). MDT-*MODe* was tested for inter-rater reliability, assessors' learning curves, and cross-validated against MDT members' own self-assessment. Presentation of a patient's case history, radiological, and pathological information, information on psychosocial aspects and the patient's comorbidities and their own views were assessed, as well as ratings of the MDT Chair's effectiveness, and contribution to decision-making of the different MDT members, including urologists, oncologists, radiologists, pathologists, Clinical Nurse Specialists and MDT Coordinators. Whether a treatment decision was reached for each case, meeting characteristics including the number and profession of team members in attendance, number of cases discussed per meeting and start and end times of the meeting were also recorded.

This assessment tool was piloted with eight MDTs over 500 cases. Good reliability and learning curves were obtained in the assessment of MDT performance (median reliability coefficient = 0.71) [9]. Positive correlations were found between observational and self- assessments of MDTs (Spearman's Rho = 0.66–0.91; Ps < 0.05)—thus

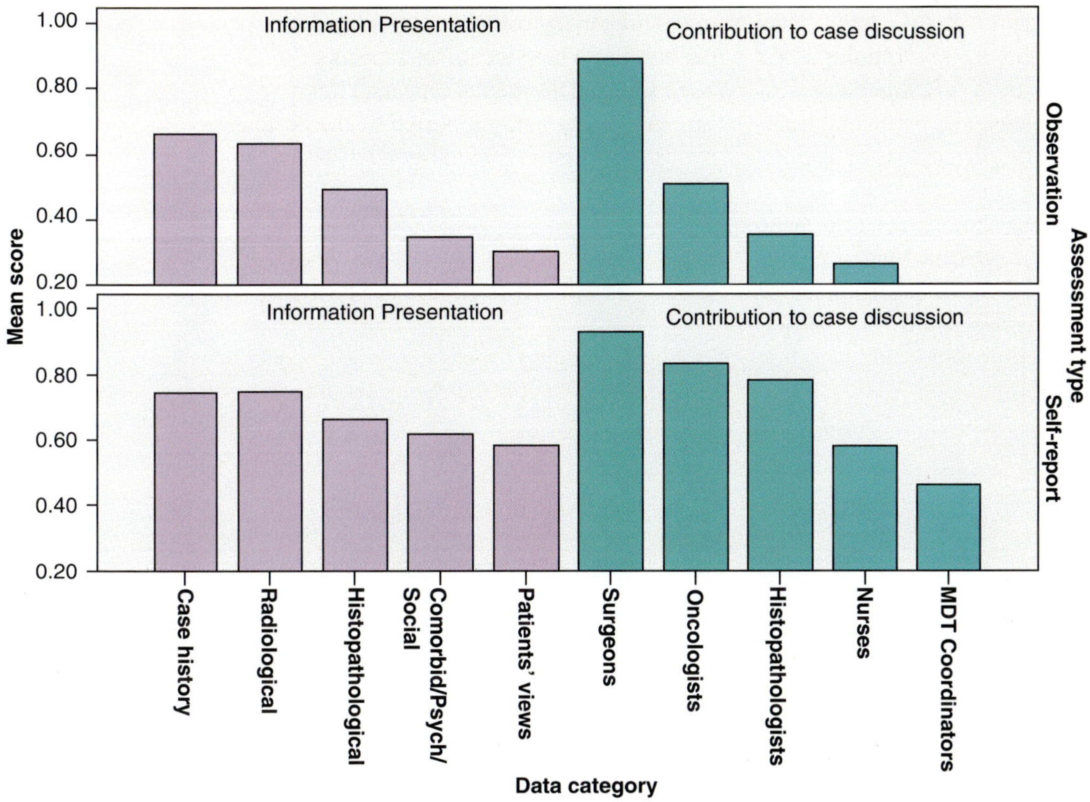

Fig. 1.4 Bar graphs displaying mean scores for information presentation and contribution to case discussion in MDT meetings for observational and self-report data (From Lamb et al. [10])

showing validity [10]. The lack of standardization in MDT meetings was apparent during the study leading to variability in the information presented, case discussion between the team members and team decision-making. The observers found that information was presented in a haphazard manner and discussions did not always include all team members. The overall pattern of results suggested that bio-medical information is more comprehensively presented than patient-centered information, and urologists dominated the case discussion and inadvertently, other MDT members often had little overt involvement in team decision-making (Fig. 1.4). Treatment decisions were reached in 85 % of cases. Cases towards the end of meetings were associated with lower rates of decision-making, information quality and team working ($r=-0.15$ to -0.37). Increased numbers of cases per meeting and team-members in attendance were associated with better information and team working ($r=0.29$–0.43). More time per case was associated with improved team working ($r=0.16$). A positive correlation was found between the ability to reach decisions and improved information and team working ($r=0.36$–0.54) (all $P \leq 0.001$) [11].

1.4 MDT Meeting Checklist

Equipped with tools to objectively and reliably measure the quality of decision-making in urology MDT meetings, we conducted a prospective longitudinal study over a 16-month period which evaluated decision-making for 1421 urological cancer patients treated at large cancer center in London [12]. Interventions to improve the MDT processes were introduced in stages including the development of a checklist, MDT-*QuIC* (Fig. 1.5), MDT team training, and simple written guidance to team-members. We found significant improvement over the course of the study:

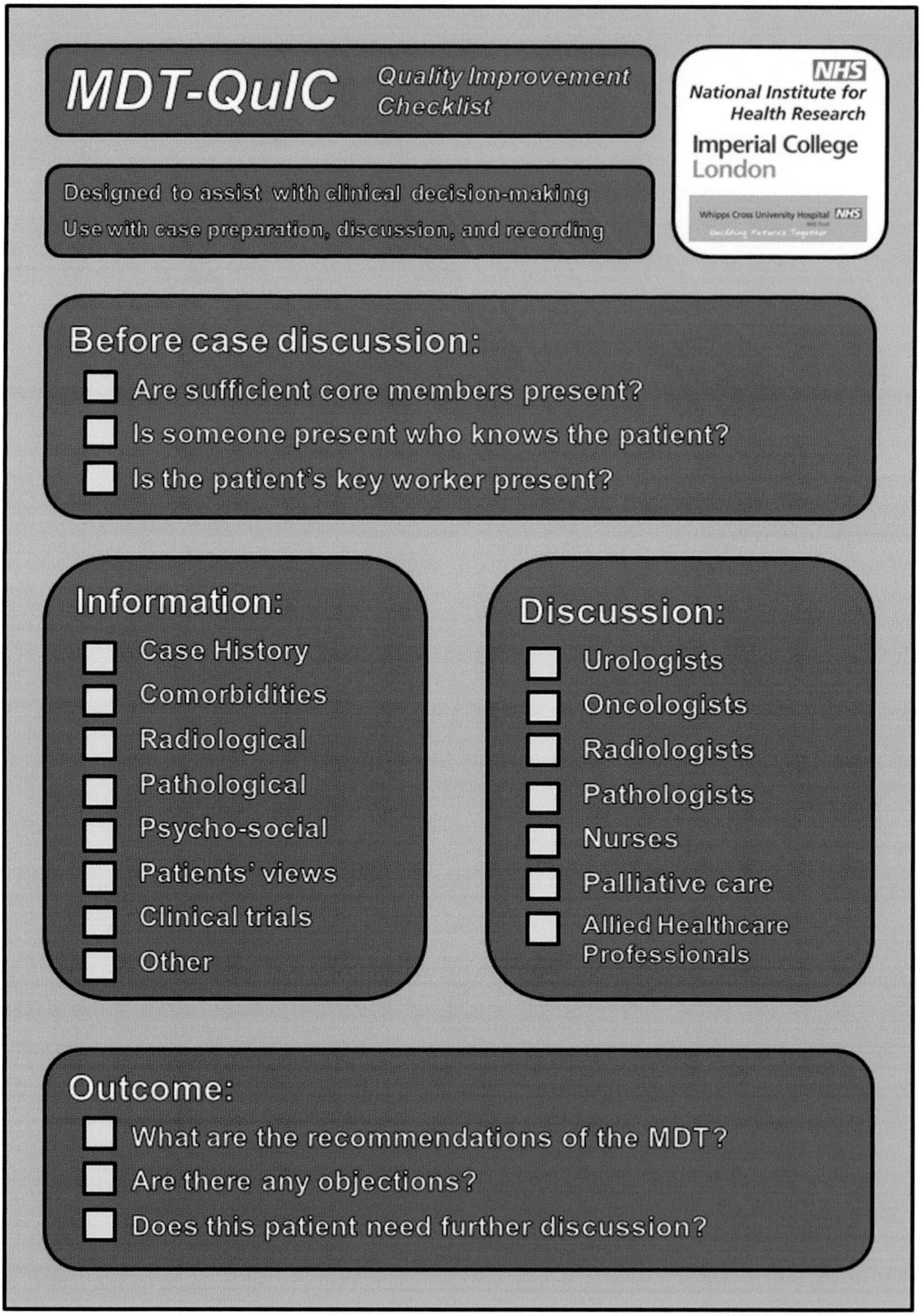

Fig. 1.5 Figure displaying MDT-*QuIC*, a checklist designed to improve MDT decision-making (Copyright 2013 Imperial College London. Accessed from http://www1.imperial.ac.uk/medicine/about/institutes/patient-safetyservicequality/cpssq_publications/resources_tools/mdt/)

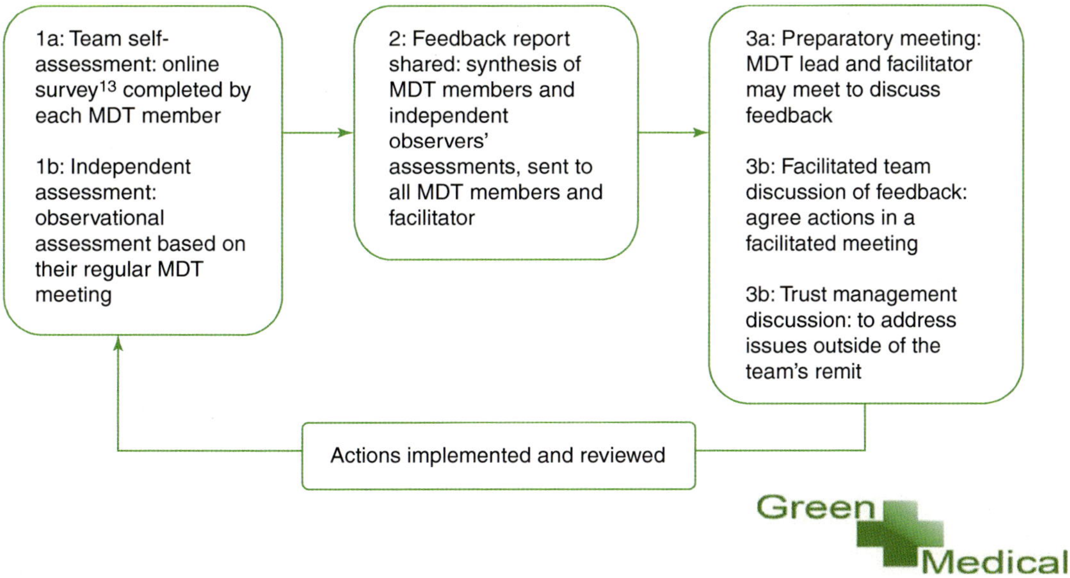

Fig. 1.6 Figure displaying MDT FIT, a program for structured assessment and feedback for the self-improvement of cancer multidisciplinary teams. (Copyright 2013 Greencross Medical Ltd. Accessed from http://www.nhsiq.nhs.uk/improvement-programmes/long-term-conditions-and-integrated-care/mdt-fit-tool.aspx)

the MDT's ability to reach a decision rose 13 %, quality of information presentation at the MDT meeting showed a 29 % increase, and quality of team working within the MDT improved by 14 %. The MDT's ability to reach a treatment decision was related to the quality of available information and the quality of the team working within the MDT. Across the study period, the top three barriers to the teams' ability to decide on a treatment plan were inappropriate patient referrals, inadequate radiological information and inadequate pathological information. This study suggested that both the decision-making ability and also the levels of team working and information quality within the MDT meeting is variable and could be improved using a combination of simple, evidence-based interventions.

1.5 Multidisciplinary Teamworking; Assessment and Feedback

Our team also developed a self assessment tool that facilitates anonymized team member self-assessment of teamworking across the whole pathway (not just focusing on MDT meetings) [13]. This latter tool is a component of an evidence-based team improvement intervention called MDT-FIT (Feedback for Improving Team working) (Fig 1.6). Based upon input and testing with over 100 MDTs, it is an assessment tool and feedback process that provides teams with the space to reflect on how they function as a team and prioritize actions for improving the team as a whole and improving future patient care. A further study was carried to assess how urology MDTs compared to breast, colorectal, lung MDTs. Our results show significant differences between tumor types with regards to the quality of information exchange and quality of contribution from individual MDT members as well as the meeting characteristics. The four tumors differed in the number of core members present ($H(3) = 12.23$, $p < 0.01$), number of cases reviewed per meeting ($H(3) = 17.38$, $p < 0.001$) and average time spent per case ($H(3) = 31.77$ $p < 0.001$). Urology had the most members present (mdn = 12). In terms of case volumes, urology had the highest case volumes (mdn = 42). Average time per case was the lowest for urology (median = 2 min 46 s) [14].

Taken together, the current findings add to our understanding of the decision-making processes across MDTs. This shows that differences between MDTs are tumor-specific, i.e., each MDT meeting is characterized by a specific pattern of strengths and weaknesses. As a result, these findings have practical implications for future clinical practice in that, firstly, each MDT may need to assess these strengths and weaknesses and design organizational strategies of improvement along with team training for members to enhance their contribution towards decision-making. As previous research in the area suggests, systems for evaluating effectiveness of teams and methods to monitor performance, team working and outcome are required to ensure high quality care for patients [15]. Secondly, the large variability across MDTs discovered by this study may reflect sheer diversity of the management of the tumors themselves. Therefore, tumor specific factors, especially in urology, may have a differential impact on the way the MDT is run and as a result affect the decision-making processes. This raises the notion for tumor-specific guidelines and intervention for MDTs.

1.6 Standardization of Information and Improving Decision Making

Although we have found that comprehensive information is both desirable and necessary for good decision-making, we have consistently found that information relating to patients' disease is of higher quality than patient-centered information. The introduction of minimum data sets for radiological and pathological information, comorbidities and patients' views and circumstances might ensure that all cases have the foundations necessary to make suitable clinical decisions. Given that patients do not attend the MDT meeting, the question of how best to bring patient preferences and values into decision-making is a complex one. Findings from our focus groups suggests that patients value nurses as the team member with whom they can relate to and who can act as their advocate. This suggests that MDT members should encourage more participation from the nurses in the discussions.

It may not be sufficient to ensure that team members make use of information presented at the meeting or contribute to the discussion. Standardising the format of case discussions helps to ensure that all the required information is presented and relevant team members contribute-giving MDT members who are less inclined to input an obligation to contribute. Working in a more structured way may aid the meetings to run more efficiently by defining what should be prepared before meetings and eliminating what is not relevant. An intervention such as our checklist, MDT-*QuIC* may be one way of standardising case discussion. Following on from this, our finding of a negative association between cases towards the end of meetings and the ability to reach a decision suggests that more consideration should be given to structuring the whole MDT meeting and prioritizing cases. It may be reasonable to order cases discussed at MDT meetings such that more difficult cases get discussed first in order to increase the chances of a higher quality discussion. Findings from our interview study of urology MDT members, suggested that all cases did not need to be discussed in full at the meeting [16]. Instead a protocol-driven treatment plan could be used so that the MDT registered cases but time could be given to more complex discussions.

There are also circumstances in which case discussions should not proceed. Personal knowledge of patients is required for decisions that are clinically appropriate and acceptable to patients, therefore discussion of a patient should not proceed without the presence of a team member who has met the patient in addition to minimum datasets for clinical and personal information necessary for the discussion. Our focus group participants stated they would rather their case was deferred if there was no one present at the discussion who knew the patient personally. At present, pressure to manage patients within time restrictions means that medical and nursing team members may have little time to discuss their investigations, medical or social background, or treatment preferences with patients. The need for prompt investigation and diagnosis must be balanced against the need for thorough and usable information gathering, which may require some healthcare providers to change the format of their pre- MDT services.

Conclusion

MDT working in cancer care has been around for almost 20 years, and evidence is now emerging of benefits to healthcare professionals and their patients. Overall, the idea of MDT working is popular among patients, clinicians and policy makers and is being considered as a model for other areas of complex decision-making outside cancer care. However, if not done to standards of high quality, MDT working can be onerous to healthcare services and of little value to patients. With an increasing body of evidence for how MDTs functions, and how they can be conducted effectively, it may be time to look objectively at how it can be delivered in an efficient and sustainable way for the years ahead.

Key Points

- Multidisciplinary team working is becoming the gold standard of cancer care delivery
- MDTs can provide a means of bettering decision-making, coordination and communication between healthcare professionals
- Work to improve healthcare teams has been achieved using scientific methods
- Evidence is emerging on how MDTs work, and how meetings can be conducted effectively
- There should be a 'systems approach' to MDT working
- Simple, evidence-based interventions exist to measure and improve the clinical decision-making process in MDT meetings
- Good teamworking between MDT members leads to better MDT discussion
- High quality teamworking and decision making by MDTs can lead to better outcomes for patients

References

1. Griffith C, Turner J. United Kingdom National Health Service, Cancer Services Collaborative "Improvement Partnership", Redesign of Cancer Services: a National Approach. Eur J Surg Oncol. 2004;30 Suppl 1:1–86.
2. Kesson EM, Allardice GM, George WD, Burns HJ, Morrison DS. Effects of multidisciplinary team working on breast cancer survival: retrospective, comparative, interventional cohort study of 13 722 women. BMJ. 2012;344:e2718.
3. Junior E, Hole D, Gillis C. Management of ovarian cancer: referral to a multidisciplinary team matters. Br J Cancer. 1994;70(2):363–70.
4. Gillis CR, Hole DJ. Survival outcome of care by specialist surgeons in breast cancer: a study of 3786 patients in the west of Scotland. BMJ. 1996; 312(7024):145–8.
5. Calman D, K. H. A policy framework for commissioning cancer services: a report by the Expert Advisory Group on Cancer to the Chief Medical Officers of England and Wales. Accessed online from http://webarchive.nationalarchives.gov.uk/20080814090336/dh.gov.uk/en/Publicationsandstatistics/Publications/PublicationsPolicyAndGuidance/DH_4071083
6. Undre S, Arora S, Sevdalis N. Surgical performance, human error and patient safety in urological surgery. Br J Med Surg Urol. 2009;2(1):2–10.
7. Undre S, Sevdalis N, Healey AN, Darzi A, Vincent CA. Observational teamwork assessment for surgery (OTAS): refinement and application in urological surgery. World J Surg. 2007;31(7):1373–81.
8. Lamb B, Green JS, Vincent C, Sevdalis N. Decision making in surgical oncology. Surg Oncol. 2011;20(3): 163–8.
9. Lamb BW, Wong HW, Vincent C, Green JS, Sevdalis N. Teamwork and team performance in multidisciplinary cancer teams: development and evaluation of an observational assessment tool. BMJ Qual Saf. 2011;20(10):849–56.
10. Lamb BW, Sevdalis N, Mostafid H, Vincent C, Green JS. Quality improvement in multidisciplinary cancer teams: an investigation of teamwork and clinical decision-making and cross-validation of assessments. Ann Surg Oncol. 2011;18(13):3535–43.
11. Lamb BW, Sevdalis N, Benn J, Vincent C, Green JS. Multidisciplinary cancer team meeting structure and treatment decisions: a prospective correlational study. Ann Surg Oncol. 2012;20(3);715–22.
12. Lamb BW, Green JS, Benn J, Brown KF, Vincent CA, Sevdalis N. Improving decision making in multidisciplinary tumor boards: prospective longitudinal evaluation of a multicomponent intervention for 1,421 patients. J Am Coll Surg. 2013;217(3):412–20.
13. Taylor C, Brown K, Sevdalis N, Lamb B, Green JSA. Developing and testing TEAM (Team Evaluation and Assessment Measure) a tool for team self-assessment of cancer MDT performance. Ann Surg Oncol. 2012;19(13):4019–27.

14. Sarkar S, Arora S, Soukup T, Lamb BW, Shah S, Green JSA, et al. A multi-centre study evaluating performance of multidisciplinary teams: urology vs the top cancer killers. Eur Urol Suppl. 2014;13(1):e878–ea.
15. Blazeby JM, Wilson L, Metcalfe C, Nicklin J, English R, Donovan JL. Analysis of clinical decision-making in multi-disciplinary cancer teams. Ann Oncol. 2006; 17(3):457–60.
16. Sarkar S, Arora S, Lamb BW, Green JS, Sevdalis N, Darzi A. Case review in urology multidisciplinary team meetings: what members think of its functioning. J Clin Urol. 2014 [Epub ahead of print].

Setting Up Simulation Training for Pelvic Surgery

2

Stig Müller and Hitendra R.H. Patel

2.1 Minimal Invasive Surgery and Clinical Training

Since the introduction of minimal invasive surgery, many surgeons have implemented laparoscopic and robot-assisted technique in a wide range of surgical specialties. The immediate and obvious benefits of the conversion to minimal invasive technique are improved vision, especially in pelvic surgery, and reduced blood loss, postoperative pain and length of stay. Over the past few years, there is a growing body of evidence in favor of minimal invasive surgery. Laparoscopic technique leads to a fourfold risk reduction of small bowel obstruction after abdominal surgery within 5 years after the index surgery [1]. As for colonic surgery, laparoscopic technique is associated with less bleeding and fewer thromboembolic complications in high risk patients [2], lower morbidity, shorter length of stay, lower hospital charges [3] and even lower mortality [4]. As a result of this overwhelming evidence, the conversion to minimal invasive surgery should no longer be optional.

However, the change of practice towards minimal invasive surgery is a challenge due to a number of reasons. Most importantly, surgeons needs to be trained properly. The transition to laparoscopic surgery must not compromise outcome. Also, all personnel involved in the patient's clinical pathway need to support and acknowledge the change of practice. This is of particular importance where several surgeons work together in a department.

In principle, the clinical pathway of a surgical patient is affected by four different factors (Fig. 2.1). The WHO-checklist for surgical safety was introduced as a means to improve team communication and to avoid preventable human error. The initial success [6] has led to a worldwide implementation. With regards to the other factors affecting the patient in the surgical pathway, patient factors are partly given by the patient's disease profile or comorbidities. Patient selection criteria for surgery are used to minimize potential adverse effects of patient factors. Surgeon factors i.e. whether the surgeon is competent to perform the procedure undoubtedly affects outcome. However in most countries, there are to date no certification systems with regards to specific procedures or the use of specific techniques such as robotic systems. A general qualification as a specialist in a surgical specialty does not necessarily account for competence in these fields. This problem can be met by a systematic training program that includes simulation training and modular training in the clinical setting.

S. Müller, MD, PhD (✉)
Department of Surgery, Institute of Clinical Medicine, University of Oslo, Oslo, Norway

Department of Urology, Akershus University Hospital, Lorenskog, Norway
e-mail: stig.mueller@ahus.no

H.R.H. Patel, MRCS, PhD, FRCS(Urol), FRCS(Eng)
Department of Urology, University Hospital North Norway, Tromsø, Norway

H.R.H. Patel et al. (eds.), *Pelvic Cancer Surgery: Modern Breakthroughs and Future Advances*,
DOI 10.1007/978-1-4471-4258-4_2, © Springer-Verlag London 2015

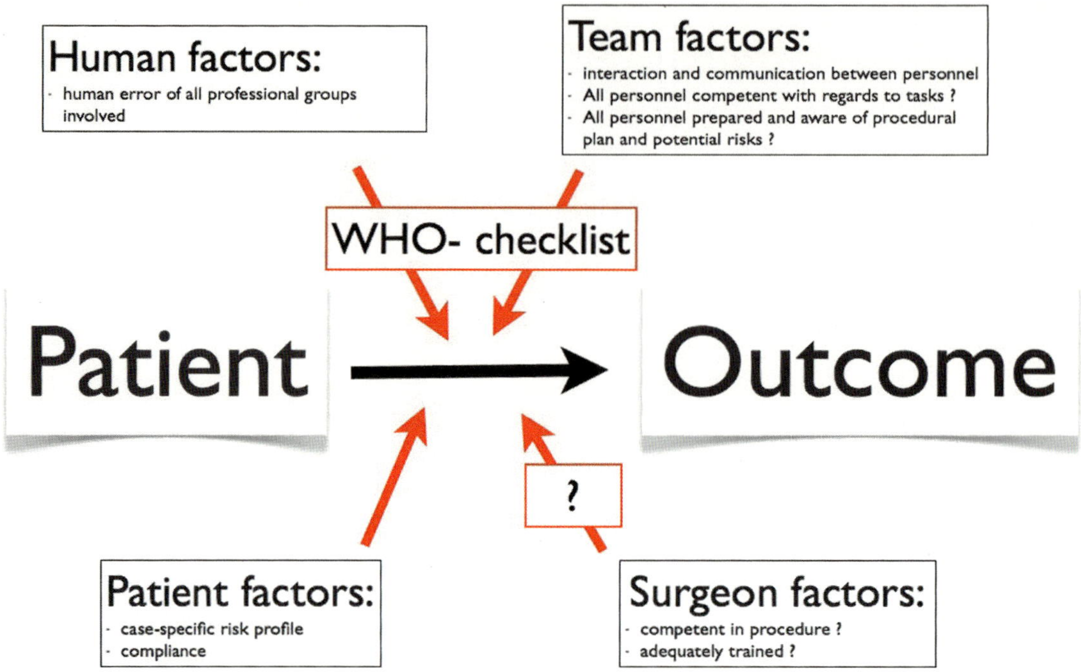

Fig. 2.1 Factors affecting the clinical pathway of a surgical patient. The WHO checklist for surgical safety is a means to ensure Human and Team factors. A quality control for surgeon factors is challenging but can be achieved by step-wise, modular training systems (Adapted from Patel and Joseph [5])

Surgical training is currently challenged by working hour directives and high quality standards. The traditional "master-apprentice" model cannot meet the demands of high quality, increasingly complex procedures and the need for new surgeons. Simulation training is effective and a means to shorten learning curves in laparoscopic surgery [7]. Simulation training is often divided into basic skills training, advanced skills training and laparoscopic team training (Fig. 2.2). Basic and advanced skills training is preferably done in box trainers and/or Virtual Reality (VR) simulators. Both are proven effective for the training of spatial skills and eye-hand coordination [7]. Box trainers are cheap and versatile, VR simulators include the advantage of objective assessment and progress reports, repeatability and standardization of the tasks [8]. Training curricula using VR simulators for standard procedures e.g. laparoscopic cholecystectomy have been shown to shorten learning curves and improve technical proficiency compared to standard training [9,10]. These training programs generally consist of an initial basic skills training followed by procedure related tasks.

Laparoscopic pelvic surgery has early on been considered technically challenging due to limited work space, complex anatomy and in many cases the need for reconstruction, i.e. suturing. Attempts have been made to classify the level of difficulty of laparoscopic procedures in order to improve training [11]. In a traditional master-apprentice surgical training model, a sequential allocation of procedures by the degree of difficulty would be reasonable but is time-consuming, inefficient and impracticable. Also, the level of difficulty of a procedure basically refers to the difficulty of learning the necessary skills to perform the procedure. Thus, simulation in surgical training attenuates long and challenging curricula for advanced laparoscopic surgery, in particular pelvic surgery.

In complex laparoscopic surgery, learning curves are often considered to be a measure of how many procedures a trainee has to attend/perform in order to become competent. However, the sole number of procedures does not reflect the level of difficulty of the case or if the procedure was successful. Performing a minimum number of procedures does not necessarily lead to competence. In

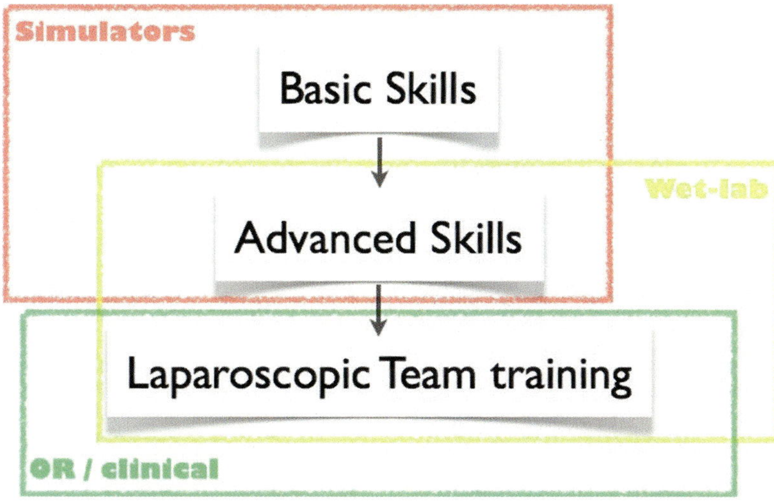

Fig. 2.2 The three steps of laparoscopic training. Basic and advanced skills are trained in simulators. Advanced skills can also be trained in animal models/wel-lab. Laparoscopic team training is usually done in a clinical setting but is also possible in a wet-lab

many European countries, this system of a minimum number of different procedures is used in the accreditation of surgeons. Even though this quality control appears better than no specified requirements at all, it is possible to differentiate the factors that determine whether a single procedure is a "rookie" or "expert" case. For instance in prostate cancer prostatectomy, prostate size, clinical tumor stage, histological tumor burden and pelvic comorbidity are factors that complicate the procedure and increase the level of difficulty. A preoperative assessment of surgical risk factors increases the preparedness of the trainee.

Laparoscopic pelvic surgery usually involves many steps and reconstruction towards the end of the procedure. Performing a complete procedure is oftentimes overwhelming for a trainee. Breaking down the procedure into steps and subtasks is in this respect beneficial. The trainee can perform single subtasks or steps of the operation that have been assigned different levels of difficulty. As the clinical training progresses, the trainee performs steps with gradually increasing level of difficulty. The easier steps are then done by another trainee or the mentor, so that the trainee can focus on a defined task. This training concept is known as modular training and has been validated for e.g. laparoscopic radical prostatectomy. Interestingly, the modular approach in training shortens the learning curve significantly without compromising outcome [12,13].

Another underestimated asset to surgical training is self-observership and assessment. Laparoscopic procedures should in principle be recorded for documentation and the self-assessment of the trainee—preferably together with a mentor—improves training. Such debriefs can be done straight after the procedures or later. The self-observation and assessment shortens the learning curve and is highly motivating for trainees. However, dedicated mentors and time for debriefs must be provided to implement this concept. The principle of self-assessment is widely used in e.g. aviation and athletics and has been shown to improve training in a simulated environment. Laparoscopic suturing skills in surgical trainees improve significantly by video self-assessment mirroring the training effect of a larger volume [14]. This training effect is also applicable to single steps or complete procedures and the debrief sessions utilize this effect.

In addition to self-assessment, athletes have long used mental training to improve preparedness and focus and ultimately improve their performance. Interestingly, mental training can also be utilized in simulation training. In a recent study by Eldred-Evans et al. [15] and colleagues, medical students performed two basic laparoscopic tasks in a box trainer and VR Simulator. They were randomized to either box training, box training supplemented by a VR simulator session, box training supplemented by mental training or VRS training supplemented by mental training. Mental training consisted of one session of 30 min. The tasks, e.g. cutting a circle, were divided into 12 sub-steps, so-called nodal points. The mental training session focused on mental visualization of these nodal points. All participants were assessed after the intervention, both in a box trainer and a VR simulator. The combination of box training and mental training lead to the highest scores with regards to precision, accuracy and overall performance when assessed in a box trainer. In the VR simulator assessment, the combination of box training and VR simulator performed best followed by box training and mental training. The group that did not receive any box training had the lowest scores with regards to speed, precision, accuracy and performance compared to the other groups regardless if assessed in a box trainer or VR simulator. The study shows that mental training as a supplement to box training improves laparoscopic skills compared to box training alone. Interestingly, this enhancing effect does not seem to apply to VRS training. One reason might be that mental training enhances the sensory experience acquired in the box trainer. The VRS trained group might lack these due to limited haptic feedback of the system. Also, mental training alone cannot replace conventional training. In a study with similar design, a group of novices merely received mental training and the post-training assessment could not match the effect of box or VRS training [16].

In both studies, skills acquired in box training were transferable to VRS assessment while not all skills acquired in VRS training were reproducible at box trainer assessment. This shows that box trainers still are the mainstay for basic skills training.

Mental training amends basic skill training in a simulated setting and the implementation has great potential. However, the principle can already be utilized in clinical training. In modular training, the trainee performs a number of predefined steps of an operation and the focus on particular tasks increases the trainee's preparedness. This can be formalized by a short, preoperative briefing where technical aspects of the steps are repeated. This mental rehearsal improves performance [17] and is supported by the postoperative debrief session including video assessment.

2.2 How to Set Up Simulation Training for Pelvic Training

Simulation training for any surgical specialty that involves laparoscopic technique should start with basic skills training. This should be organized as a systematic, structured program with defined tasks and certification of the participants. A certification of basic skills is recommended since not all candidates will acquire the necessary skills within a given number of training sessions [18]. Next, more advanced and procedure-related simulation tasks are trained. There are numerous models for e.g. prostatectomy [19] and gynecological surgery [20]. The clinical training can start simultaneously. Specific tasks e.g. anastomotic suture in prostatectomy are practiced in a simulated setting (Fig. 2.3).

2.3 Robotic Surgery

In robot-assisted laparoscopic surgery, the same challenges in training apply as in conventional laparoscopic surgery. In addition, the robotic equipment itself requires training. The latest models of the da Vinci® system feature a simulation system for both basic and more procedure-related skills. After a wide implementation globally, one has recognized the need for validated training models and a certification process. In Europe, the Robotic Urology Section of the European Association of Urology is currently discussing a certification for robotic urology. The modular training model is just as applicable in robotic surgery as in conventional laparoscopic surgery.

However, surgical proficiency is not all about technical skills as F.C. Spencer, the former President of the American College of Surgeons, stated in 1978: A skillfully performed operation is 75 % decision making and only 25 % dexterity [21]. The cognitive and social skills of experienced

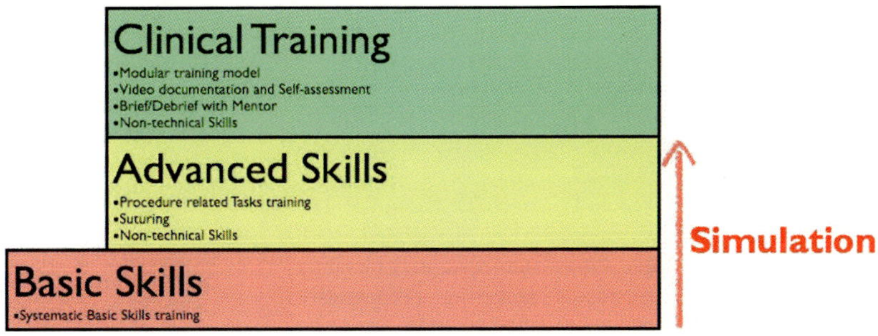

Fig. 2.3 Training model for laparoscopic pelvic surgery. Simulation facilitates basic and advanced skills training

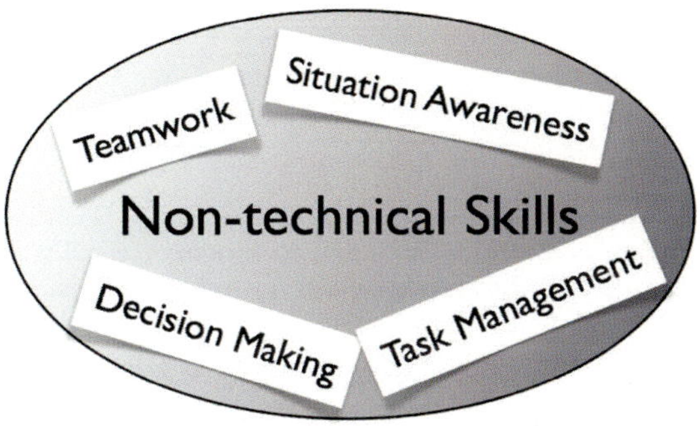

Fig. 2.4 The four main components of non-technical skills

professionals have been named non-technical skills (NTS) and these are not necessarily acquired with experience. The importance of NTS have long been recognized in high-risk industries like aviation. Specific NTS training programs have become a fundamental part of e.g. flight crew and maintenance personnel training [5]. Undoubtedly, NTS have a significant impact on the surgical patient's pathway and modern training programs should therefore implement NTS training. Simulated crisis scenarios for instance can be used for NTS training. In the clinical setting, NTS qualities like decision making, situation awareness, teamwork and task management can be addressed during the brief/debrief as well as during surgery (Fig. 2.4).

In conclusion, simulation training is fundamental for laparoscopic pelvic surgery. Moreover, simulation training should be an essential part of a structured, stepwise training program. Modular training models should be applied in clinical training since learning curves are shortened without compromising outcome. Finally, the implementation of NTS training in surgical training will result in more proficient surgeons and ultimately, better patient outcome.

Key Points

- The implementation of minimal invasive surgery is no longer optional
- The surgical pathway of patients is affected by several factors e.g. whether the surgeon is adequately trained
- There is a need for certification of skills, especially when high-tech devices are involved as in robotic surgery
- Simulation training is an effective method to improve surgical skills
- Skills acquired in simulation are transferable to clinical procedures
- Box trainers are efficient for training basic skills and versatile for procedure related training
- Virtual Reality simulators have the advantage of reproducibility, standardization of tasks and advanced measurements of performance
- Non-technical skills are important in surgical training and trainable in simulated environment
- Simulation is an integral part of surgical training for pelvic surgery
- New concepts like mental training, techniques that increase preparedness and self-assessment improve the quality of surgical training

References

1. Angenete E, Jacobsson A, Gellerstedt M, Haglind E. Effect of laparoscopy on the risk of small-bowel obstruction: a population-based register study. Arch Surg. 2012;147(4):359–65.
2. Sulu B, Aytac E, Stocchi L, Vogel JD, Kiran RP. The minimally invasive approach is associated with reduced perioperative thromboembolic and bleeding complications for patients receiving preoperative chronic oral anticoagulant therapy who undergo colorectal surgery. Surg Endosc. 2013;27(4):1339–45.
3. Masoomi H, Buchberg B, Nguyen B, Tung V, Stamos MJ, Mills S. Outcomes of laparoscopic versus open colectomy in elective surgery for diverticulitis. World J Surg. 2011;35(9):2143–8.
4. Trastulli S, Cirocchi R, Desiderio J, Guarino S, Santoro A, Parisi A, et al. Systematic review and meta-analysis of randomized clinical trials comparing single-incision versus conventional laparoscopic cholecystectomy. Br J Surg. 2013;100(2):191–208.
5. Patel HRH, Joseph JV. Simulation training in laparoscopy and robotic surgery. London: Springer; 2012.
6. Haynes AB, Weiser TG, Berry WR, Lipsitz SR, Breizat AH, Dellinger EP, et al. A surgical safety checklist to reduce morbidity and mortality in a global population. N Engl J Med. 2009;360(5):491–9.
7. Zendejas B, Brydges R, Hamstra SJ, Cook DA. State of the evidence on simulation-based training for laparoscopic surgery: a systematic review. Ann Surg. 2013;257(4):586–93.
8. Patel HRH, Patel BP. Virtual reality surgical simulation in training. Expert Rev Anticancer. 2012;12(4):417–20.
9. Palter VN, Orzech N, Reznick RK, Grantcharov TP. Validation of a structured training and assessment curriculum for technical skill acquisition in minimally invasive surgery: a randomized controlled trial. Ann Surg. 2013;257(2):224–30.
10. Ahlberg G, Enochsson L, Gallagher AG, Hedman L, Hogman C, McClusky 3rd DA, et al. Proficiency-based virtual reality training significantly reduces the error rate for residents during their first 10 laparoscopic cholecystectomies. Am J Surg. 2007;193(6):797–804.
11. Guillonneau B, Abbou CC, Doublet JD, Gaston R, Janetschek G, Mandressi A, et al. Proposal for a "European scoring system for laparoscopic operations in urology". Eur Urol. 2001;40(1):2–6; discussion 7.
12. Stolzenburg JU, Rabenalt R, Do M, Horn LC, Liatsikos EN. Modular training for residents with no prior experience with open pelvic surgery in endoscopic extraperitoneal radical prostatectomy. Eur Urol. 2006;49(3):491–8.
13. Ganzer R, Rabenalt R, Truss MC, Papadoukakis S, Do M, Blana A, et al. Evaluation of complications in endoscopic extraperitoneal radical prostatectomy in a modular training programme: a multicentre experience. World J Urol. 2008;26(6):587–93.
14. Jamshidi R, LaMasters T, Eisenberg D, Duh QY, Curet M. Video self-assessment augments development of videoscopic suturing skill. J Am Coll Surg. 2009;209(5):622–5.
15. Eldred-Evans D, Grange P, Cheang A, Yamamoto H, Ayis S, Mulla M, et al. Using the mind as a simulator: a randomized controlled trial of mental training. J Surg Educ. 2013;70(4):544–51.
16. Mulla M, Sharma D, Moghul M, Kailani O, Dockery J, Ayis S, et al. Learning basic laparoscopic skills: a randomized controlled study comparing box trainer, virtual reality simulator, and mental training. J Surg Educ. 2012;69(2):190–5.
17. Arora S, Aggarwal R, Sirimanna P, Moran A, Grantcharov T, Kneebone R, et al. Mental practice enhances surgical technical skills: a randomized controlled study. Ann Surg. 2011;253(2):265–70.
18. Grantcharov TP, Funch-Jensen P. Can everyone achieve proficiency with the laparoscopic technique? Learning curve patterns in technical skills acquisition. Am J Surg. 2009;197(4):447–9.
19. Laguna MP, Arce-Alcazar A, Mochtar CA, Van Velthoven R, Peltier A, de la Rosette JJ. Construct validity of the chicken model in the simulation of laparoscopic radical prostatectomy suture. J Endourol. 2006;20(1):69–73.
20. Arden D, Hacker MR, Jones DB, Awtrey CS. Description and validation of the Pelv-Sim: a training model designed to improve gynecologic minimally invasive suturing skills. J Minim Invasive Gynecol. 2008;15(6):707–11.
21. Spencer FC. Teaching and measuring surgical techniques—the technical evaluation of competence. Bull Am Coll Surg. 1978;63:9–12.

3 Pelvic Virtual Reality Systems

Simon S. Fleming and Bijendra Patel

3.1 Introduction

The role of simulation techniques for teaching technical skills is well established. Skills acquired on simulator can shorten learning curve. As surgeons gain expertise, their skills become automated. This blend of psychomotor and cognitive skills is essential for surgical mastery.

Most training by simulation curriculum offer psychomotor skills teaching based on instructional material on the basic elements and procedural steps of an operation thus making it difficult to achieve "expertise" in s simulated environment in absence of cognitive skills learning. Experts teaching complex knowledge unintentionally leave out significant proportion of information trainees need to learn. This results in trainee learning by "trial and error."

A simulation center that is driven by the curriculum needs of participants is most likely to be successful. A defined and well-rounded curriculum encompassing both psychomotor and cognitive skills necessary for learning complex pelvic surgery is necessary. Unfortunately advances in teaching cognitive skills are lagging behind teaching psychomotor skills. Cognitive skills are still widely learned by trial and error resulting in only partial skills acquisition of a complex operative procedure in a simulated environment.

It is essential for every surgical educators involved in setting up simulation training for pelvic surgery to develop a curriculum incorporating both relative contribution of task (motor skills) to concept (thought process) required for mastery in pelvic surgery. There is a need for a cognitive task analysis model for pelvis surgery to be developed to complement the practical skills teaching using simulation technology.

It is also important to accurately define the outcome of the curriculum in other word a proficiency based curriculum with validated objective assessment. VR simulators provide an excellent platform for being able to measure matrix.

3.2 Design of a Successful Curriculum

It is vital to have a robust curriculum if a simulation-training program is to be successful. It is often said that aims are like strategy, objectives are like tactics, which very much fits in with the concept that aims are related to the teaching of a topic whereas objectives are far more related to that which you hope the student might learn [1]. Many trainers are still used to having the vaguest of aims and even more vague outcomes.

S.S. Fleming, MBBS Lond., MRCS (Eng), M.Sc (Dist), MAcadMEd, MFSTEd, AFHEA (✉)
ST4 Trauma and Orthopaedics Registrar, NE Thames, Percivall Pott, London, UK
e-mail: simonsfleming@doctors.org.uk

B. Patel, MS, FRCS(Ed), FRCS(Gen Surg)
Barts and The Royal London Hospital, Barts Cancer Institute, Queen Mary University of London, London, UK

H.R.H. Patel et al. (eds.), *Pelvic Cancer Surgery: Modern Breakthroughs and Future Advances*, DOI 10.1007/978-1-4471-4258-4_3,

Both aims and outcomes must be meaningful not only to the staff, so they might be used as an assessment tool or guide but also meaningful to the student, as a guide for effective and directed learning.

When designing a simulation-training curriculum keep the following "terms" in mind. This is because, as simulation requires the teaching of both a clinical skill and clinical reasoning, it requires our learning objectives to cover all of Blooms six (cognitive) levels of cognitive ability, these being

- Knowledge
- Comprehension
- Application
- Analysis
- Synthesis
- Evaluation [2].

There then begins the three stages of curriculum design.

1. **Cognitive stage**—understanding the theory behind the procedure
2. **Psychomotor stage**—translating theory into performance with task repeated and practiced, movements become smoother and more efficient (task fragmentation)
3. **Automated stage**—In which subject can perform task fluidly and competently without thinking of how to do it

It is suggested here that a simulation training curriculum for pelvic surgery should contain clear and well described learning objectives for developing following key skills

1. Generic Skills (Laparoscopic, robotic and endoscopic skills)
   - Eye-hand coordination
   - Depth perception using a video image
   - Laparoscopic orientation
   - Bimanual skills—Laparoscopic instrument manipulation
2. Specific Skills
   - Laparoscopic suturing
   - Safe and accurate use of Electrocautery
   - Safe Clipping and cutting
3. Procedure Skills
   - Cystoscopy
   - Ureteroscopy
   - TURP
   - PCNL

Once one has a clearly documented curriculum, the training program itself can be designed and this relies on;

1. Sound curriculum with defined proficiency criteria's for learning both psychomotor and cognitive skills
2. Simulation center equipped with both low fidelity and high fidelity virtual reality and robotic simulator
3. Expert supervision and feedback

3.3 Educational Offerings

A comprehensive education institutes should have resources to offer various educational and research opportunities including, but not limited to the following;

1. Short courses
2. Mini-fellowships
3. Diploma/PG Certificate/Masters in Surgical Skills
4. New procedure training modules
5. Perceptorship
6. Telementoring
7. Evaluations and Assessments
8. Research and validation studies

3.4 Models and Simulators

There are available in the wider world a huge variety of simulators, each offering its own benefits and disadvantages.

When considering setting up a simulation service, one should consider the needs of those you intend to educate and then look at the different types of simulator, choosing that which suits your needs best.

Simulators can be broadly classified into two areas and then four types Below are examples of simulators one can use for each area, though this list is of course, not exhaustive.

3.5 Psychomotor Skills

1. Anatomy models—Torso Simulator
2. Box Trainer

(a) Basic Laparoscopy Trainer
(b) Bristol TURP Trainer
(c) Uro-Scopic Trainer
3. Virtual reality simulator—Simbionix
4. Robotic Simulator

3.6 Cognitive Skills

(a) Integrated simulator—The Mock Operating Theater—Instructor-driven simulator
(b) Model-driven simulator

3.7 Anatomy Models

When your students first begin their education, it is wise to have an appropriate model (Fig. 3.1) for learning applied clinical anatomy and allowing for clear demonstration of how they will be expected to orientate their laparoscope. It is much easier to use a model to explain 3-D positioning than with a 2D diagram.

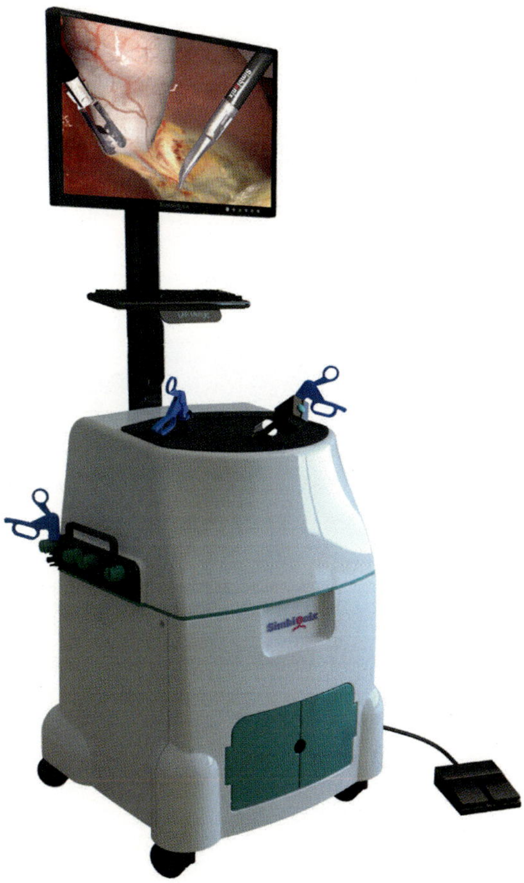

Fig. 3.1 Torso simulator (From www.chiropractictools.com/pelvis_model.php)

After the basic sciences have been mastered, the student can move on to develop their psychomotor skills, beginning with a basic box trainer and moving onto the virtual reality and robotic simulator, all of which have been shown to have huge educational value [3–5].

3.8 Box Trainer

Learning of pelvic surgery should start with achieving proficiency in technical skills required in basic laparoscopic surgery using box trainer and validated curriculum of fundamentals of laparoscopic surgery (FLS). The FLS program may be effectively used to teach and assess both cognitive and technical skill aspects related to laparoscopic surgery. The simulated laparoscopic manipulation includes instrument navigation, coordination and cutting or knot-tying. It is wise to begin with the most basic of box trainers (Fig. 3.2), as if one considers simulation to be "the act of mimicking a real object, event or process by assuming its appearance or outward qualities" [6], then a box trainer is absolutely the place to start to 'mimic' laparoscopic surgery.

Once simple psychomotor skills such as triangulation and camera handling have been mastered, the simulation student could move on to a more Task specific box trainer. There are many versatile models (Figs. 3.3 and 3.4), which provide a range of techniques and procedural skills to be acquired over time. The anatomically and spatially realistic constraints found in this type of box trainer means that the student progresses their skills in line with the curriculum objectives that you will have set. For example, on the TURP trainer (Fig. 3.3), the student might begin with simply learning how to manage fluids during a TURP and can progress to resection of the prostate.

The uro-scopic trainer is a versatile model that provides for a range of urological endoscopic techniques and procedures to be acquired in line with a trainees clinical progression these skills include the following;

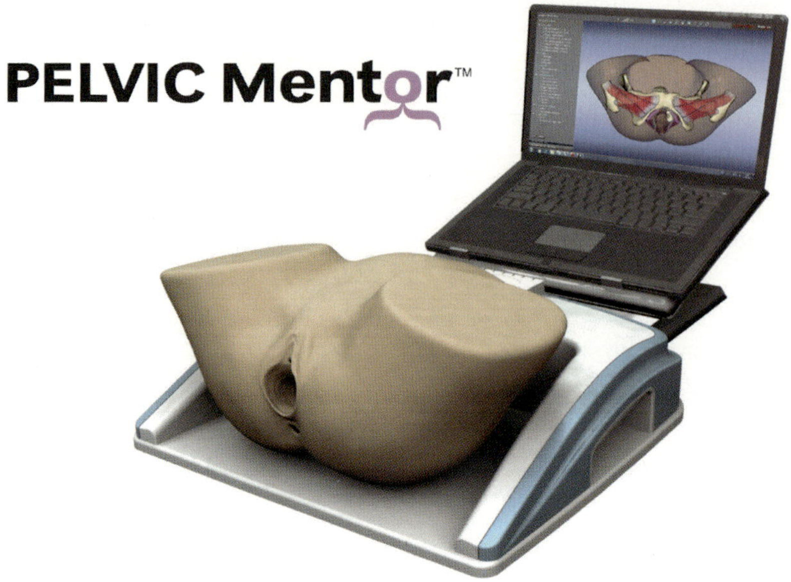

Fig. 3.2 Basic box trainer (From http://limbsandthings.com/uk/products/category/urology)

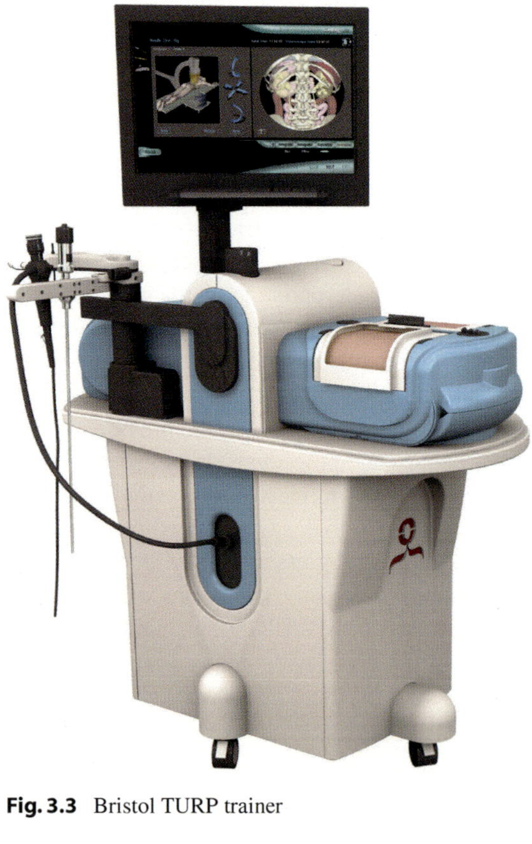

Fig. 3.3 Bristol TURP trainer

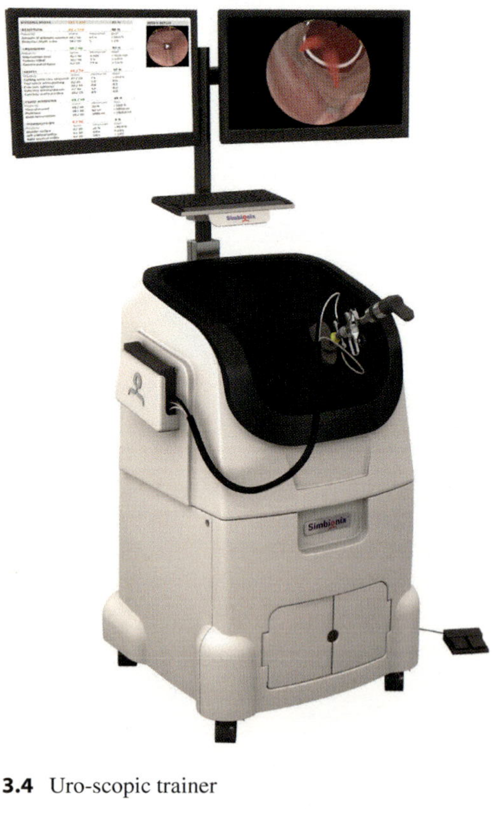

Fig. 3.4 Uro-scopic trainer

- Fluid management
- Insertion, manipulation and removal of instruments
- Urethroscopy and Cystoscopy
- Stent and guidewire insertion
- Lithotripsy
- Stone retrieval

3.9 Virtual Reality Simulator

Box trainers have their place however; a certain suspension of disbelief is required by the student in order for them to be truly effective. However, with the use of virtual reality technology the more complex procedures, along with the equally complex anatomy, can be brought to life for each student. It is through looking towards other professional areas such as airline pilots or even piano players that it was discovered that, to become what the lay person might consider an "expert," requires 10,000 h or 10 years of practice [7] and that to maintain this level of skill requires our students not to simply be "in the job" but in fact a new concept in surgical training—deliberate practice [8–10]. The implication is that having spent hours and hours on a box trainer, mastering basic skills, there needs to be a way on which our students can spend similar amounts of time mastering more complex procedures—from beginning to end. The answer—virtual reality.

The Mentor System by Simbionix (Fig. 3.5) is one such system, with the following possible

1. LAP Mentor™.
2. URO Mentor™,
3. VirtaMed TURPSim
4. PELVIC Mentor

These ergonomically designed systems allow for real-time simulation, using the same inputs the student can expect to find in an operating theater. Equally, when practicing those essential skills in your simulation center, many of these units give haptic feedback (vibration, resistance and the same) to make the experience even more lifelike.

Each system has basic modules, with psychomotor skills tested, just as with the basic box trainer. However, these units then go on to offer anatomical, physiological, technical and surgical training, second to none. It is through the acquisition of a comprehensive set of pelvic surgical skills that a student can become not only safe but confident to perform these procedures on an actual patient.

The Lap Mentor unit allows the students to develop both basic and advanced laparoscopic skills including full procedure training with the potential for challenges such as variation in anatomy and bleeding. The URO mentor allows for everything from cystoscopes and ureteroscopes to cutting strictures and fluoroscopy/C-arm control.

The PELVIC Mentor is more aimed towards pelvic floor reconstruction with an emphasis on transvaginal mesh procedures. This system was the first to train surgeons for pelvic floor repair, using its hybrid mannequin/3D visualization system.

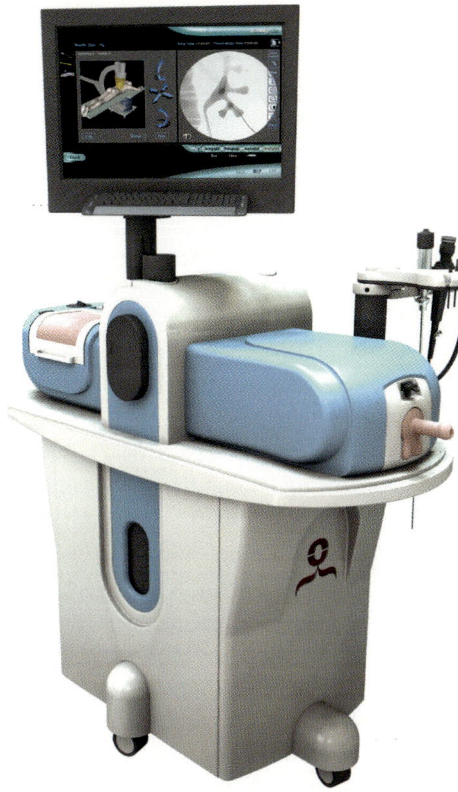

Fig. 3.5 Simbionix – PELVIC mentor™ (From http://simbionix.com/simulators/pelvic-mentor)

The presence of virtual reality simulators means that the student can progress onto more advanced simulators as their skills advance, so that, for example, once they have mastered the Bristol TURP trainer, they can progress onto advanced training.

3.10 Virtamed Turpsim

The VirtaMed TURPSim, has been called "The Most Advanced Training Simulator for TURP Procedures and BPH Treatment" [11] Once the student has mastered the basics of TURPs, this system allows for revisiting these skills in a more high fidelity fashion, as well as managing complications, again, while not having to wait for a real patient, with a real complication. As with all of the previously mentioned systems, the skills begin at a basic level and progress until mastery of all skills is eventually achieved.

Of note, though you will have set up your own comprehensive curriculum, many VR systems also come with their own "in built" training curriculum, with modules that must be mastered before moving onto the next. Your younger surgeons will feel more like they are playing a computer game, having to finish one level before they can progress onto the next. This means, that with the use of this and a box trainer, they will find themselves more comfortable with:

- Heavy bleeding
- Capsule perforation
- Verumontanum or sphincter resection
- Fluid overload

However, as any educator will know, a curriculum is really of no use without assessment. All VR trainers have, in some form or another, built in tools for both feedback and assessment.

Objective Feedback Reports

The Mentor systems all allow for objective performance assessment as well as allowing the supervisor to set their own standards for things such as economy of movements or complications handling. These feedback reports are always available to both your students and yourself, so that reflection and improvement is always possible. Another feature is that all this data can be used not only for individual development but also for research and statistical analysis.

The most advanced pelvic surgeons are now performing da Vinci surgery—and so, as the skill set required for pelvic surgeons grows, so the availability of simulation equipment grows.

3.11 Training for Da Vinci® Surgery

The robotic surgery simulator made by Simbionix has instruments designed to replicate the motions of the human hand, just as with a "real" da Vinci unit. For even greater realism, the Suturing Module can be used on the genuine *da Vinci* console, which means your students will not only become confident with the skills but the equipment required in robotic surgery.

All of the afore-mentioned equipment means that a surgeon in training can develop psychomotor, procedural skills in an interactive and "active learning" fashion. They will be forced to respond to a multitude of situations which can include procedure selection or the decision to proceed/abort a procedure as well as the extent of their dissection, manipulation, suturing and even which components they wish to use.

3.12 Cognitive Knowledge and Clinical Judgement

A seamless blend of psychomotor and cognitive skills is essential for surgical skills mastery. A defined and well-rounded curriculum encompassing both psychomotor and cognitive skills is necessary for learning complex pelvic surgery. Contents should be developed and validated by panels of experts to teach and test aspects of pelvic surgery. The contents should also include suggested reading material, clinical scenarios the learner may confront and computer based multiple choice questions as well as (critical) review of operative videos.

Many of the clinical judgement skills learned in this way can be tested further in another simulation environment, that of the Integrated Simulator, sometimes referred to as the Mock Operating Theater.

Integrated Simulator: The Mock Operating Theater

The next step in a simulation is to leave the simulation room! In the end, each student is very aware that he or she is stood in casual clothes, "playing" with a virtual reality simulator. After a certain period, the cognitive and affective skills of your trainee will need to be tested and improved [12, 13]. The operating room is a dynamic work environment in which effective cognitive functioning and decision making are vital to safe delivery of care and thus to a trainee's learning. Thus one can build a Mock Operating theater. These can be from the most basic, a room with an anesthetic machine, a bed and a model to the fully immersive, realistic training environments, that certain units and companies can provide. The fully immersive environments, which use both instructor driven and model driven simulation are the best for practicing cognitive and judgment skills [14]. By using instructors (an instructor is present to feed information to the trainee) as well as models, either virtual reality, simulation models or Human Patient Simulators (a real person using prosthetics and makeup/special effects) a student can develop cognitive skills required to become an expert surgeon, such as open communication, adaptive response, and the use of a shared mental model [15].

3.13 Resources and Facilities

None of the previous mentioned facilities are possible without the resources, space and funding to run such a service. With this in mind the American College of Surgeon (ACS) developed their accreditation requirement for simulation centers.

ACS has established specific criteria for learners, curriculum, personnel and resources required for centers seeking ACS accreditation AS Comprehensive Education Institutes (Level I) or Basic Education Institutes (Level II). Detailed discussion of application process for obtaining accreditation is beyond the scope of this book; a brief summary is outlined below.

There are three major components (called "standards") to the accreditation of both Level I and II centers

- Standard 1 : refers to learner
- Standard 2: encompasses the curriculum
- Standard 3: covers technology support, facilities and resources

Level I and II criteria share similarities in term of the curriculum principles (standard 2), but differ significantly in terms of space and personnel (standard 3)

The ACS goes on to clarify

- Level 1 Skills Center

  - Accommodate 20 trainees for hands-on training at any given time
  - Provide education to at least three different learner groups (surgeons, trainees, medical students, nurses and allied health professionals)
  - Have exclusive use of no less than 1, 200 sq.ft, and in addition 4,000 sq.ft shared space available for conference rooms, storage, vivarium, teleconferencing facilities and offices.

- Level 2 Skills Center

  - Accommodate six to ten trainees for hands-on training at any given time
  - Provide education to at least one learner group in addition to surgeons
  - Minimum 800–1,000 sq.ft area housed within a defined geographic area with signage for easy identification
  - Offer walk-in education opportunities
  - Teleconferencing facilities

Table 3.1 is author's suggestion on number of simulators required for setting up simulation training for pelvic surgery.

Table 3.1 Resources for a level 1 and 2 simulation center

Resources required	Level 1	Level 2
Skills lab space	1,200 Sq Ft	800 Sq Ft
Number of simulator stations	10	5
(i) Advanced simulators	2	1
(ii) Intermediate simulators	4	2
(iii) Basic simulator	4	2
Tutor to trainee ration	Preferred 1:3 Minimum 1:4	Preferred 1:3 Minimum 1:4

3.14 Finance

No educator is naive enough to think that anything can be achieved without funding and so it is wise to have a realistic idea of both your income and outgoings. Some of this will vary depending on what facilities, resources and equipment your unit already has. It may seem like charging for courses is a great money-spinner however, there are major expenses and as such other sources of income should be sought as well; grants, sponsorship and more creative sources of funding will help with both start-up and maintenance (Table 3.2).

Table 3.2 Example of possible incomes and expenses for a simulation center

Income	Expense
1. Income from courses	1. Space rent and space renovation cost
2. University and government grants	2. Salary (a) Institute director and teaching staff salary (b) Business manager and accountant (c) Simulators technician salary (d) Course co-ordinator/administrator
3. Industry sponsorship	3. Equipment's (a) High fidelity—virtual reality simulators (b) Low fidelity—intermediate and basic simulators (c) Synthetic models for simulation (d) Suturing set/instruments (e) Sutures and disposables
4. Private investor's	4. Guest lecturer and external examiner costs
5. Bank loan	5. Equipment maintenance and service contract 6. Overhead cost 7. Furniture 8. Audiovisual—live AV link 9. Office supplies 10. Internet access/computer hardware/software/networking 11. IT support—web site designing and maintaining 12. Marketing/advertising cost 13. Interest on loan 14. Conference cost—traveling/registration/accommodation 15. Lab spaces hire cost 16. Staff and students awards/prizes 17. Miscellaneous

3.15 Summary

Surgical training is generally considered to be modeled on a four-stage approach;

1. Demonstration of the skill at normal speed with little or no explanation
2. Repetition of the skill with full explanation, encouraging the trainee to ask questions and be generally inquisitive
3. Skills performed for a third time by the demonstrator, but this time the trainee prompts each action and in turn is quizzed by the demonstrator, who also corrects any errors made by the trainee. This step is often repeated numerous times out of necessity as one can progress to the fourth step until this is near perfect.
4. The trainee now carries out the skill under close supervision, describing each step before it is taken [16].

A leading exponent of simulation training has himself noted this issue and said "simulators are only of value within the context of a total educational curriculum, and the technology must support the training goals [17]. However, a well organized and set up simulation center allows the fulfillment of all of the above four stages, with no risk to patients and allowing for these to be performed over and over again, at both the trainer and trainee's leisure.

With proper planning at every level, a simulation center can be the best training resource available to a surgical training scheme.

Yet we must be always be mindful and as Kneebone states, "*Above all, simulation must take its place as one component of a larger picture, supporting and supported by research, technology, clinical practice, professionalism and education*" [18].

Key Points

- No risk to patients as errors can occur safely
- Management of routine events and procedures can be practiced and improved
- Realistic setting
- Scenarios can be created to provide (time) flexible and specific learning opportunities
- Training is easily reproducible
- Learning is experiential, participatory and enjoyable
- Immediate feedback is possible
- Significant set up costs
- Risk that the technology over shadows educational principles
- No need to wait for a pelvic case to "come along" that is safe to use for education purposes

References

1. http://www.nottingham.ac.uk/medical-school/tips/aims_objectives.html. Accessed 13 Nov 2010.
2. Bloom BS. Taxonomy of educational objectives, handbook 1; the cognitive domain. New York: David Mcay; 1979.
3. Cuschieri A, Szabo Z. Chapter 4: Intracorporeal knots in endoscopic surgery. In: Cuschieri A, Szabo Z, editors. Tissue approximation in endoscopic surgery. Oxford: ISIS Medical Media; 1995. p. 42–67.
4. Szabo Z, Hunter J, Berci G, Sackier J, Cuschieri A. Analysis of surgical movements during suturing in laparoscopy. Endosc Surg Allied Technol. 1994;2:55–61.
5. Larsson A. Intracorporeal suturing and knot tying in surgical simulation. Stud Health Technol Inform. 2001;81:2662–71.
6. Gorman PJ, Meier AH, Krummel TM. Simulation and virtual reality in surgical education. Real or unreal? Arch Surg. 1999;134:1203–8.
7. Small S. Thoughts on patient safety education and the role of simulation. Virtual Mentor. 2004;6:3.
8. Gaba D. Anaesthesiology as a model for patient safety in health care. BMJ. 2000;320:785–8.
9. Ericsson KA. The acquisition of expert performance: an introduction to some of the issues. In: Ericsson KA, editor. The road to excellence: the acquisition of expert performance in the arts and sciences, sports and games. Mahwah: Lawrence Erlbaum Associates; 1996. p. 1–50.
10. Ericsson KA, Krampe RT, Tesch-Romer C. The role of deliberate practice in the acquisition of expert performance. Psychol Rev. 1993;100:363–406.
11. TURP Simulator http://simbionix.com/simulators/virtamed-turpsim/.
12. Peters JH, Fried GM, Swanstrom LL, Soper NJ, Sillin LF, Schirmer B, Hoffman K. Development and

validation of a comprehensive program of education and assessment of the basic fundamentals of laparoscopic surgery. Surgery. 2004;135(1):21–7.
13. Powers KA, Rehrig ST, Irias N, Albano HA, Malinow A, Jones SB, Moorman DW, Pawlowski JB, Jones DB. Simulated laparoscopic operating room crisis: an approach to enhance the surgical team performance. Surg Endosc. 2008;22:885–900.
14. Beaubien JM, Baker DP. The use of simulation for training teamwork skills in health care: how low can you go? Qual Saf Health Care. 2004;13:51–6.
15. Entin EE, Serfaty D. Adaptive team coordination. Hum Factors. 1999;41:312–25.
16. Peyton JWR. Teaching and learning in medical practice. Rickmansworth: Manticore Europe; 1998. p. 174–7.
17. Satava RM. Surgical education and surgical simulation. World J Surg. 2001;25:1484–9.
18. Kneebone J. Simulation in surgical training: educational issues and practical implications. Blackwell Med Educ. 2003;37:267–77.
19. Satava RM. Accomplishments and challenges of surgical simulation. Surg Endosc. 2001;15:232–41.

Telemedicine as a Quality Improvement Facilitator in Pelvic Cancer Surgery

4

Knut Magne Augestad, Etai Bogen, and Hitendra R.H. Patel

4.1 Introduction

Sixty years ago Dr. Gershon-Cohen began to send x-rays using facsimiles over a distance of 28 miles by using simple telephone services to transmit the images. In 1962, DeBakey pioneered the field of telemedicine with the first videoconferencing (VC) demonstration of open-heart surgery to be transmitted overseas by satellite, allowing medical staff in Geneva to view an aortic valve replacement being performed at The Methodist Hospital in Houston, Texas [1]. Another early example of long-distance use of telemedicine was in 1967 in Boston, when a medical station at Logan International Airport was linked to Massachusetts General Hospital in downtown Boston using a two-way microwave audio-video link [2]. Since the 1960s, there has been substantial development in the use of telemedicine among medical personnel, including surgeons [3]. In recent years, the cost of telemedicine equipment has become less expensive and advanced technical skills are not required to operate such systems. Therefore, new applications of telemedicine in surgery are emerging in trauma and emergency medicine, for postoperative follow-up of patients, education of surgeons, multidisciplinary team meetings, and in surgical telementoring. Surgical telementoring, a process during which an experienced surgeon remotely guides another surgeon through a procedure using a telecommunication system, offers a viable option for facilitating the transfer of knowledge and skills, as it cost-effectively expands the mentor pool and in- creases experienced surgeons' availability to assist in educating other surgeons (Fig. 4.1). In this chapter, we will focus on how telemedicine and emerging videoconferencing technology can be used to improve surgical education and to meet the increasing demand for surgeons.

4.2 Telemedicine and the Surgical Workforce

Surgical telementoring might be a way to meet societies need for new surgeons. The length of time it takes to train surgeons, the anticipated decrease in hours worked by surgeons in younger generations, and the potential decreases in graduate medical education funding suggest that there may be an insufficient surgeon workforce to meet population needs. Surgeons are often sparsely geographically distributed, and with a predicted shortage of surgeons distance education might become increasingly important. Existing

Mobile Medical Mentor Group (M3)

K.M. Augestad, MD, PhD (✉) • E. Bogen, MD
Department of Gastrointestinal Surgery, Norwegian National Centre of Telemedicine and Integrated Care, University Hospital North Norway (UNN – Tromsø), Tromsø, Norway
e-mail: knut.magne.augestad@telemed.no

H.R.H. Patel, MRCS, PhD, FRCS(Urol), FRCS(Eng)
Department of Urology, University Hospital North Norway, Tromsø, Norway

H.R.H. Patel et al. (eds.), *Pelvic Cancer Surgery: Modern Breakthroughs and Future Advances*,
DOI 10.1007/978-1-4471-4258-4_4,

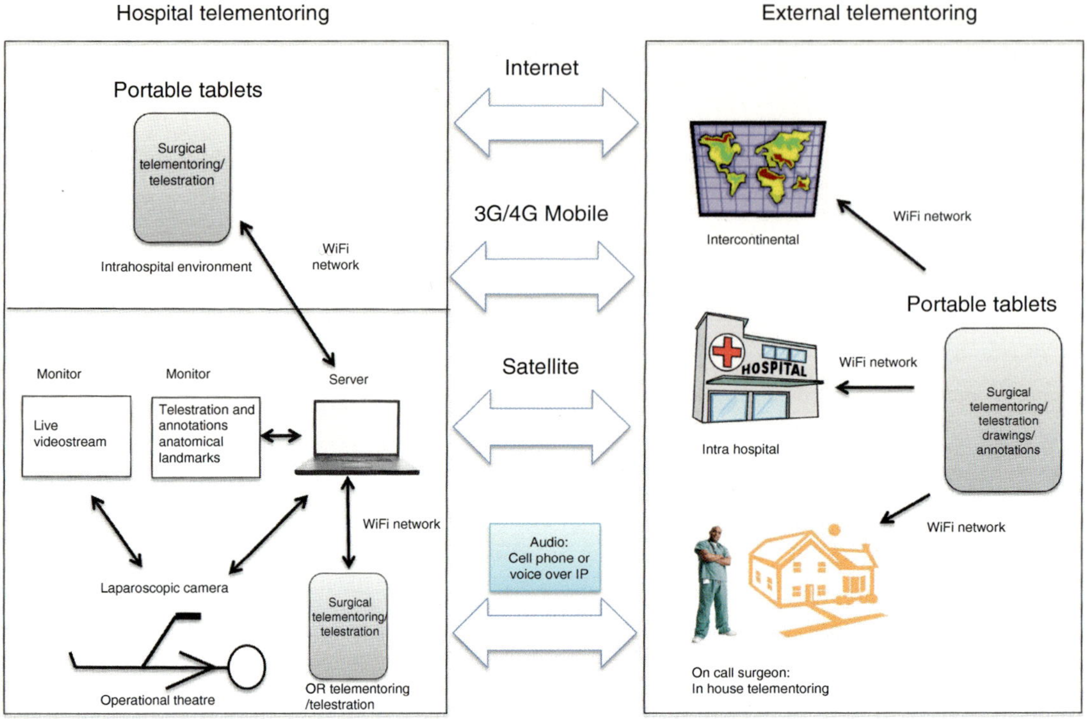

Fig. 4.1 Suggested architecture of a distributed mobile surgical telementoring system

maldistribution patterns are likely to be exacerbated, leading to delayed or lost access to time-sensitive surgical procedures, particularly in rural areas [4]. Forecasts show that overall surgeon supply will decrease 18 % during the period form 2009 to 2028 with declines in all specialties except colorectal, pediatric, neurological surgery, and vascular surgery. Model simulations suggest that none of the proposed changes to increase graduate medical education currently under consideration will be sufficient to offset declines [4]. Recently, an estimate was made that by 2030, there would be a 9 % shortage in the general surgical workforce, with greater shortages in other surgical specialties [4, 5]. In 2009, there were only 3.18 urologists per 100,000 habitants in the US, which is a 30-year low. Mirroring this nationwide lack of urologists, a recent survey of the academic urologic workforce predicts that over 369 faculty positions need to be filled out in the next 5 years, suggesting that the shortage of academic urologists is more severe than that of other specialities [6]. Unless the rate at which general and urological surgeons are trained increases, the number of surgeons per population will continue to decline [7]. The imminent nature of reductions in surgical workforce supply, combined with increased utilization that will result from a changing and growing population (and potentially from insurance expansion or some form of coverage reform), suggests that proactive actions to graduate medical education training numbers, new models of care, and extending surgical productivity are needed. Without making these changes, there is a risk that there will be access issues—particularly in rural communities—as increasing numbers of surgeons retire. Thus, there is a significant need to increase the rate and volume of surgical education. In our opinion, tele-mentoring and telemedicine may be used as tools to enhance surgical education to meet the increasing surgical demand [3].

4.3 Tele-mentoring in Surgery

Reported results of mentoring are improved surgical practice, education, treatment and postoperative care and telementoring is described as a natural fit in surgery. Mentoring using videoconferencing technology has gained increasing popularity in all

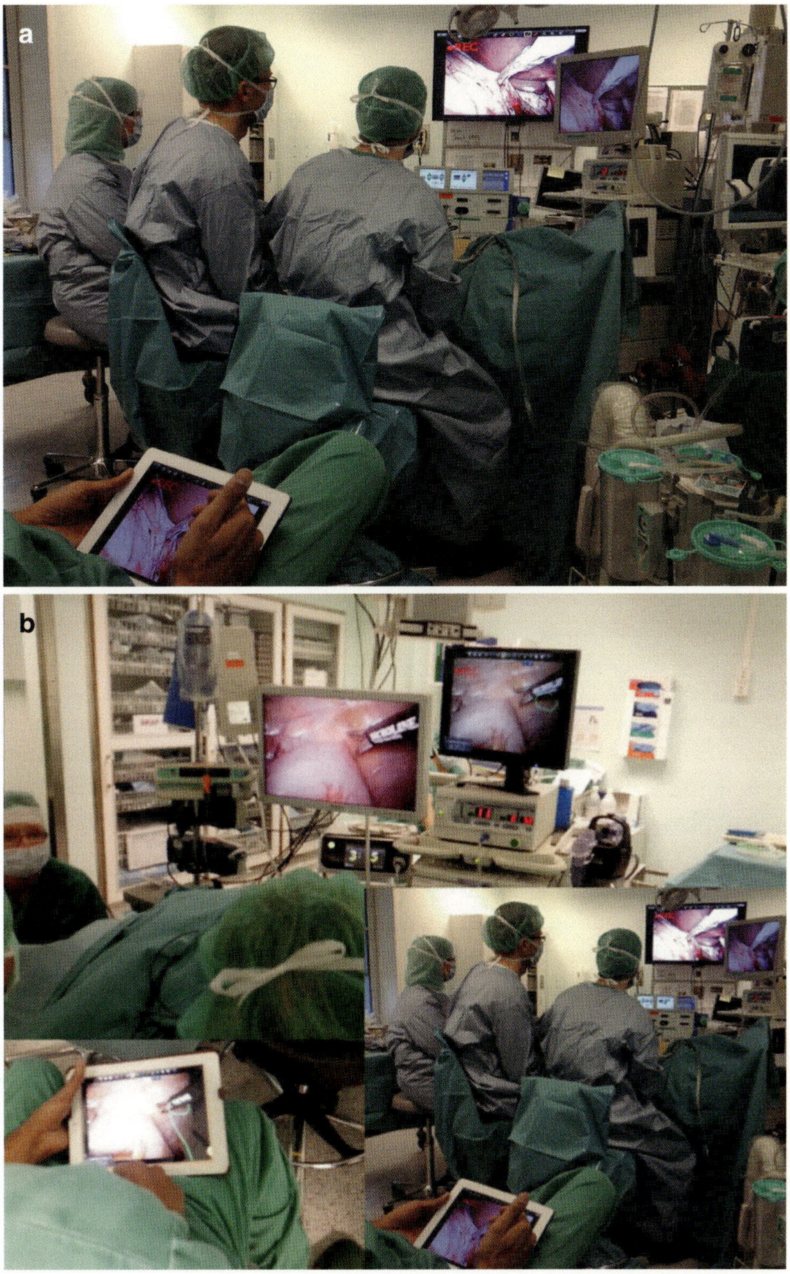

Fig. 4.2 On-site telementoring on: (**a**) Partial nephrectomy and (**b**) Adrenalectomy surgeries. We have developed a unique, low cost telementoring system at the Department of Urology—University Hospital North Norway (UNN)

fields of medicine, especially in education of medical personnel [3, 8–11]. Solutions have been demonstrated for laparoscopic surgery and in combination with robotic surgery [12–14]. More recently, mobile solutions for surgical telementoring have been demonstrated (Fig. 4.2) [15].

Recent developments in information technology have led to a renewed interest in the potential of telemedicine to provide new collaborative solutions. Recently a national US research initiative was launched; The American Medical Foundation for Peer Review and Education has brought together several specialty surgical societies to determine whether telementoring is an effective way for physicians to learn new skills and improve old ones [16]. Telementoring has been shown to be successful in training residents. A 2010 study in the Journal of the American College of Surgeons reported that eight general surgery residents operating on animal cadavers while telementored achieved higher

Table 4.1 Assessment tool of surgical performance (global operative assessment of laparoscopic skill)

Description	1 point	3 point	5 point
Knowledge of anatomy	Gaps in knowledge of anatomy prevented smooth flows of operation	Basic understanding of anatomy allowed smooth progression of procedure	Excellent understanding of anatomy allowed rapid progression from one step to the next
Preventions of complications	Poor knowledge of critical steps to avoid complications	Aware of several critical steps to avoid complications	Aware of most critical steps to avoid complications
Tissue handling	Frequently used unnecessary force on tissue or caused damage by inappropriate use of instruments	Careful handling of tissue but occasionally caused damage	Consistently handled tissue appropriately with minimal damage to tissue
Time and motion	Many unnecessary moves	Efficient time and motion but some unnecessary moves	Clear economy of movement and maximum efficiency
Flow of operation	Frequently stopped operating and seemed unsure of next move	Demonstrated some forward planning with reasonable progression of procedure	Obviously planned course of operation with effortless flow from one move to the next
Principles of operation	Poor knowledge of laparoscopic surgery	Displayed partial knowledge of laparoscopic surgery	Have excellent knowledge of laparoscopic surgery
Knowledge and use of equipment	Poor knowledge of what, how and when to use equipment	Basic understanding of purpose and use of instruments and tools	Used and manipulated surgical instruments with clear understanding of their purpose
Overall performance	Very poor	Competent	Clearly superior

From Vassiliou et al. [25]
This assessment tool is among the most common educational assessment tool in surgical telementoring

overall mean performance scores when compared with completing the same operations without the telerobotic proctoring. The residents also said they felt more competent when they were telementored [17].

Safety issues during surgical telementoring has been debated. Recently, Augestad et al. reported a 5 % complication rate during 433 telementored surgical procedures [18]. This means that the safety during surgical telementoring is similar to that reported in onsite mentoring. Recently, a meta-analysis supports evidence that trainees can obtain similar clinical results to expert surgeons in laparoscopic colorectal surgery if supervised by an experienced trainer [10]. Two surveys of laparoscopic telementoring were included in this review, showing no significant difference in conversion, anastomotic leak or mortality compared to on site mentoring [19, 20]. Similar results were also shown by Panait et al. [21]. One study reports decreased operation time of telementoring compared to physical presence [22]. In contrast Schlachta's surveys revealed an increased operating time, but a significant decrease in hospital days [19, 23]. Most studies were not randomized, this makes it difficult to estimate significance of the survey. There is no evidence in included studies of increased cost-effectiveness of surgical telementoring, for instance reduced transfers between hospitals or other terms of resource utilization. Telementoring as a tool for education between different levels of healthcare has been described by different surgical specialties. Demartines et al. assessed telemedicine in surgical education and patient care [24]. Participant satisfaction was high and the opportunity to discuss case management were significantly improved. However, there are insufficient proof of the educational benefits of surgical telementoring. In a recent review of 34 trials of surgical telementoring, eight surveys (23 %) had an educational assessment as primary outcome [18]. Surgical performance was evaluated by recognition of anatomical landmarks, the "Global Operative Assessment of Laparoscopic Skills" (Table 4.1) [25], or measurement of task performance (grasping, cutting, clip applying, suturing, economy of movement). All surveys report an expert-novice mentor situation. Two surveys included simulation, three surveys robotics (remote camera control or grasper). All reviewed surveys report a positive outcome of telementoring on surgical education (Table 4.2).

Table 4.2 Surveys assessing educational outcomes of surgical telementoring

Educational aspects		Specifications (n = 8)
Mentored participants	Medical students	63
	Surgical residents	24
	General Surgeons	53
Procedures		Laparoscopic cholecystectomy
		Bovine surgery
		Endoscopic procedures
		Open thyroidectomy
		Laparoscopic inguinal hernia n
Educational assessment tool		Global operative assessment of laparoscopic skills
		Global rating scale
		Recognition anatomical landmarks
		Task performance (navigation, clip applying, grasping, suturing, economy of movement)
Simulators		2
Robotics		3
Stationary VC units		6
Mobile VC units		2
Enhanced surgical performance		8

From Augestad et al. [18]; used with permission
Eight (23 %) of thirty-four reviewed surveys reported a primary outcome focusing on surgical education. All of these surveys report improved surgical performance
VC videoconferencing

4.4 Telemedicine in Multidisciplinary Teams (MDTs)

Bringing together multiple experts to focus as a group on a single patient is now a formidable organizational and logistical challenge. With telemedicine, discussion of a series of patients among a broad range of experts is possible across vast distances, resulting in a level of consultation at a cost otherwise not possible. MDTs should improve coordination, communication, and decision-making between health-care team members and patients, and hopefully produce more positive outcomes. VC as a tool to improve communication between different levels of health care has been described from different surgical sub-specialities [26]. However, bringing together multiple experts to focus on a single patient is a logistical challenge. With videoconferencing and telementoring, discussion of a series of patients among a broad range of experts is possible across vast distances (Fig. 4.3). Kunkler et al. performed a trial where it was shown that multidisciplinary team meetings by videoconferencing was cost-effective and have similar clinical effectiveness to standard 'in-person' meetings [27]. Norum et al. published a study demonstrating the feasibility of VC for clinical and educational support between specialists at the University Hospital of North Norway and colleagues at the oncology and palliative care unit of the Nordland Hospital in Bodø, 300 miles apart. VC was a success in the education and clinical case discussion with the remote oncologists in Bodø. During a 12-month period, 32 VCs were performed, the study demonstrated that telemedicine can be used to incorporate a remote palliative care unit into a university department [28].

Dickson-Witmer et al. recently published a study of a VC network to discuss prospective patient management issues. Information was shared on a weekly basis with discussion of treatment decisions and diagnostic procedures. The VC led to an increase in National Cancer Institute treatment and accrual to cancer control clinical trials [29, 30]. Kunkler et al. have proposed a comprehensive methodology to assess the clinical and economic effectiveness of VC in MDTs [30]. This methodology was later tested in a randomized breast cancer trial where 473 MDT patient discussions in two district general hospitals were cluster randomized to the intervention of telemedicine linkage to breast specialists in a cancer center or to the control group of 'in-person' meetings. VC was cost-effective and MDTs have similar clinical effectiveness to standard 'in-person' meetings [27]. There is a shortage of surgeons in the UK. MDT meetings supported by telemedicine were therefore introduced, the telemedicine meetings saved over 3 working weeks of thoracic surgical time during the year [31]. MDT meetings are

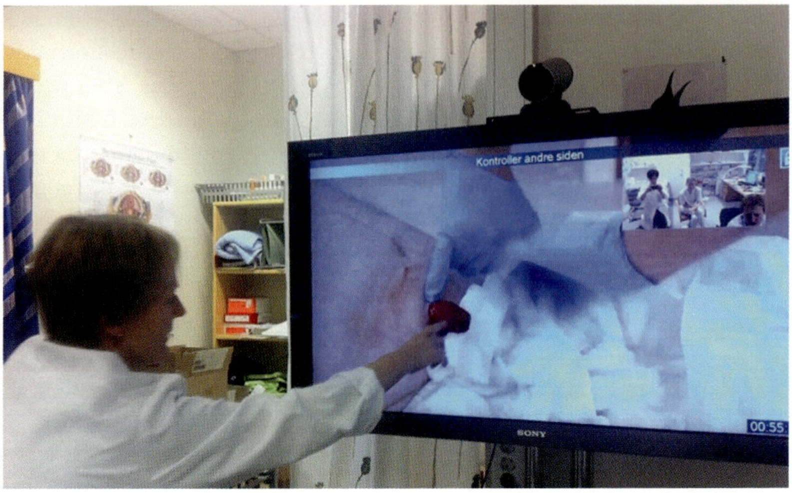

Fig. 4.3 A multidisciplinary team conference examining a patient with stoma problems. The patient is located in a district medical center 5 h drive from the University Hospital North Norway

used for establishing diagnoses, for tumor, node, and metastasis (TNM) classification. In a Swedish study, telemedicine was introduced to link the regional hospital to two of the three district general hospitals. The conclusion was that costs could be saved by carrying out MDT meetings by means of telemedicine instead of face-to-face meetings [32]. A recent report on cancer services in Wales recommended an integrated cancer service with VC as a clinical tool. Regular MDT meetings reduced the need for patients to travel. They also increased access to expert opinion and reduced the delay in implementing treatment [33].

4.5 Technology Issues in Telemedicine

One major aspect in achieving adoption of new technology is the experience of the mentors and trainees, however user acceptance of current technology is lacking. Some studies focus on the mentors and trainees satisfaction with the technological solution used for telementoring. Furthermore, no evidence from systematic studies therefore exists on what picture resolution is required to achieve high-perceived video resolution quality among mentors and trainees. In the evaluation of perceived audio quality high perceived quality is reported in 60 % of the studies [18]. Another important user aspect is experienced delay. Few studies (35 %) report measured delay and very few reports how the delay was measured (both ways vs. only one way). We used an acceptance criterion of 250 ms, one way, 500 ms both ways, based on our experience with video conferencing [18]. From a clinical perspective aspects like video encoding and video resolution in telementoring solutions is important. Video encoding affects for instance how nuances in color of the intestines get represented in the video signal. Picture resolution affects what anatomical landmarks that may be identified with a high degree of certainty. It is therefore surprising that these two aspects are the least reported; only three studies report the video resolution used and at the same time provides an evaluation of perceived picture quality. A video resolution of 768 × 492 and higher is perceived to give high perceived video quality, while 320 × 240 and lower is evaluated to provide medium perceived picture quality. The most reported technical feature is telestration (44 %) and we believe this feature is mandatory for all telementoring solutions [18].

The current focus on mobile devices as cell phones and tablet PC's (Ipad) opens a new dimension. There has been renewed interest in mobile telemedicine solutions owing to new and emerging mobile technology such as third and fourth generation of mobile device communication (3G and 4G), increased usability of mobile phones and internet-enabled mobile devices.

Videoconferencing has been used in multiple settings during the past decades, however most of these systems have been stationary units. A mobile videoconference solution will bring new and important aspects to this technology, as surgeons can easily transport and use the system in multiple settings [15]. We believe that mobile videoconference solutions based on tablet PC technology have a potential to positively impact surgical practice, but further research is needed (Fig. 4.1).

4.6 Future Telementor Research

Technological barriers of videoconferencing and telemedicine have been substantially reduced and high quality commercial solutions for telementoring and videoconferencing are easy accessible. There is therefore decreased need for surveys focusing on technical aspects and future trials of surgical telementoring should focus on:

- *Education of surgeons*: How can videoconferencing and telementoring contribute to a more cost-effective surgical education?
- *Patient safety*: Is telementoring a safe method to educate new or inexperienced surgeons or does complication rates increase when surgical education is not performed hands on?
- *Telementoring and simulation*: How can telementoring be combined with simulators, robotics and mobile platforms for educational and clinical purposes?
- *Licensure and liability problems*: Telementoring are often performed across organizational borders. How shall organizational issues like licensure, credentialing, hospital finances, legal matters and potential malpractice be dealt with?

4.7 Summary

Surgery is a visual speciality where live pictures provide detailed information about anatomical landmarks, giving the mentor instant information about the patient's normal anatomy and pathological structures. Based upon this instant information the mentor can give advice to the operating surgeon and immediately correct his or her surgical actions. Telementoring is well suited to overcome geographical barriers and is suitable for surgical education. The technological barriers of surgical telementoring have decreased during recent years, and high quality videoconference equipment is accessible on a commercial basis. However, implementation of telemedicine and videoconference is slower than expected within the surgical community. The complication and conversion rate of surgical telementoring is similar when compared to onsite mentoring. To meet the increasing demand for general surgeons, surgical telementoring for educational purposes should be further explored and evaluated. New surgical telementor surveys should have a clearly defined research objective, assessing clinical and educational aspects in a systematic manner.

Acknowledgements: Mobile Medical Mentor (M3) Project Group Knut Magne Augestad, MD, Ph.D (Research Leader Department of Research and Innovation, Norwegian Centre for Telemedicine and Integrated Care and Department of Gastrointestinal Surgery, University Hospital North Norway, Tromsø, Norway), Andrius Budrionis, MSc (Research Fellow, Tromsø Telemedicine Laboratory, Norwegian Centre for Telemedicine and Integrated Care, Tromsø, Norway), Etai Bogen, MD (Research fellow, Department of Gastrointestinal Surgery, Norwegian Centre for Telemedicine and Integrated Care, Tromsø, Norway), Johan Gustav Bellika MSc, Ph.D (Associate Professor, Norwegian Centre for Telemedicine and Integrated Care, Tromsø, Norway), Rolv- Ole Lindsetmo MD, MPh, PhD (Professor and Chief, Department of Gastrointestinal Surgery, University Hospital North Norway, Tromsø, Norway), Gunnar Hartvigsen PhD (Professor, Department of Computer Science, Faculty of Science, University of Tromsø, Norway), Per Hasvold MSc (Research Fellow, Norwegian Centre for Telemedicine and Integrated Care, Tromsø, Norway), Stig Muller MD, PhD (Consultant, Department of Surgery, University Hospital North Norway, Tromsø; Norway), Hiten Patel MD, PhD (Professor, Department of Surgery, Section of Laparoscopic Urology, University Hospital North Norway, Tromsø, Norway), Conor Delaney MD, Ph.D (Professor of Surgical Education and Chief Division of Colorectal Surgery, University Hospitals Case Medical Center, Cleveland, OH, USA), Alexander Horsch PhD (Professor Institute for Medical Statistics and Epidemiology, University of Technology, Munich, Germany), Kim Mortensen MD, PhD (Consultant,

Key Points

- Solutions have been existing for decades.
- Commercial low cost solutions exist.
- The surgical workforce will decrease substantially in all specialities.
- Surgical telementoring might be a way to meet societies need for new surgeons, by improving surgical education.
- Telementoring is described as a natural fit in surgery.
- Telementoring improves surgical practice, education, and treatment.
- Telementoring trials are needed to further explore the impact in surgical education
- Telemedicine improve coordination, communication, and decision-making for multi-disciplinary teams.
- Video and audio quality vary in the existing systems; delay of voice might cause communication problems.
- Further assessment of the role of telemedicine in education and its effects on patient safety are needed.

Department of Surgery, University Hospital North Norway, Tromsø Norway), Sture Pettersen MSc (CEO Tromsø Telemedicine Laboratory, Norwegian Centre for Telemedicine and Integrated Care, Tromsø, Norway).

Disclosures Mr. Budrionis was financially supported by a grant from HST Helse Nord. Dr. Augestad and Dr. Bogen have no financial disclosures.

References

1. DeBakey ME. Telemedicine has now come of age. Telemed J. 1995;1:3.
2. Murphy R, Bird K. Telediagnosis: a new community health resource. Observations on the feasibility of telediagnosis based on 1000 patient transactions. Am J Publ Health (NY). 1974;64:113–9.
3. Augestad KM, Lindsetmo RO. Overcoming distance: video-conferencing as a clinical and educational tool among surgeons. World J Surg. 2009;33:1356–65.
4. Fraher EP, Knapton A, Sheldon GF, Meyer A, Ricketts TC. Projecting surgeon supply using a dynamic model. Ann Surg. 2013;257:867–72.
5. Etzioni DA, Finlayson SR, Ricketts TC, Lynge DC, Dimick JB. Getting the science right on the surgeon workforce issue. Arc Surg. 2011;146(4):1–4.
6. Gonzalez C, McKenna P. Challenges facing academic urology training programs: an impending crisis. Urology. 2013;81:475–9.
7. Jarvis-Selinger S, Chan E, Payne R, Plohman K, Ho K. Clinical telehealth across the disciplines: lessons learned. Telemed J E Health. 2008;14:720–5. Audio, transactions of the IRE professional group on 2008.
8. Lavrentyev V, Seay A, Rafiq A, Justis D, Merrell RC. A surgical telemedicine clinic in a correctional setting. Telemed e Health. 2008;14:385–8.
9. Doarn C. The power of video conferencing in surgical practice and education. World J Surg. 2009;33:1366–7.
10. Miskovic D, Wyles SM, Ni M, Darzi AW, Hanna GB. Systematic review on mentoring and simulation in laparoscopic colorectal surgery. Ann Surg. 2010;252: 1–9.
11. Doarn C. Telemedicine in tomorrow's operating room: a natural fit. Surg Innov. 2003;10:121–6.
12. Eadie L, Seifalian A, Davidson B. Telemedicine in surgery. Br J Surg. 2003;90:647–58.
13. Agarwal R, Levinson A, Allaf M, Makarov D, Nason A, Su L. The RoboConsultant: telementoring and remote presence in the operating room during minimally invasive urologic surgeries using a novel mobile robotic interface. Urology. 2007;70:970–4.
14. Challacombe B, Wheatstone S. Telementoring and telerobotics in urological surgery. Curr Urol Rep. 2010;11:22–8.
15. Parker A, Rubinfeld I, Azuh O. What ring tone should be used for patient safety? Early results with a blackberry-based telementoring safety solution. AJS. 2010;199:336–41.
16. Wood D. No surgeon should operate alone: how telementoring could change operations. Telemed e-Health. 2011;17:150–2.
17. Rothenberg SS, Yoder S, Kay S, Ponsky T. Initial experience with surgical telementoring in pediatric laparoscopic surgery using remote presence technology. J Laparoendosc Adv Surg Tech. 2011;19:S219–22.
18. Augestad K, Bellika JG, Budrionis A, Chomutare T, Lindsetmo RO, Patel H, Delaney CP. Surgical telementoring in knowledge translation—clinical outcomes and educational benefits: a comprehensive review. Surg Innov. 2013;20:276–84.
19. Schlachta CM, Kent SA, Lefebvre KL, McCune ML, Jayaraman S. A model for longitudinal mentoring and telementoring of laparoscopic colon surgery. Surg Endosc. 2008;23:1634–8.
20. Sebajang H, Trudeau P, Dougall A, Hegge S, McKinley C, Anvari M. The role of telementoring and telerobotic assistance in the provision of laparoscopic colorectal surgery in rural areas. Surg Endosc. 2006;20:1389–93.

21. Panait L, Rafiq A, Tomulescu V. Telementoring versus on-site mentoring in virtual reality-based surgical training. Surg Endosc. 2005;20:113–8.
22. Ereso A, Garcia P, Tseng E. Live transference of surgical subspecialty skills using telerobotic proctoring to remote general surgeons. ACS. 2010;211:400–11.
23. Schlachta C, Lefebvre K, Sorsdahl A, Jayaraman S. Mentoring and telementoring leads to effective incorporation of laparoscopic colon surgery. Surg Endosc. 2009;24:841–4.
24. Desmartines N. An evaluation of telemedicine in surgery. Ann Surg. 2000;135:849–53.
25. Vassiliou M, Feldman L, Andrew CG. A global assessment tool for evaluation of intraoperative laparoscopic skills. AJS. 2005;190:7–7.
26. Kitamura C. How effective is video consultation in clinical oncology? A systematic review. Curr Oncol. 2010;17:17.
27. Kunkler I, Prescott R, Lee R. TELEMAM: a cluster randomised trial to assess the use of telemedicine in multi-disciplinary breast cancer decision making. Eur J Cancer. 2007;43:2506–14.
28. Norum J, Pedersen S, Størmer J. Prioritization of telemedicine services for large scale implementation in Norway. J Telemed Telecare. 2007;13:185–92.
29. Dickson-Witmer D, Petrelli N, Witmer D. A statewide community cancer center videoconferencing program. Ann Surg Oncol. 2008;15:3058–64.
30. Kunkler I, Fielding RG, Brebner J. A comprehensive approach for evaluating telemedicine-delivered multidisciplinary breast cancer meetings in southern Scotland. J Telemed Telecare. 2005;11 Suppl 1: 71–3.
31. Go P, Payne J, Satava R, Rosser J. Teleconferencing bridges two oceans and shrinks the surgical world. Surg Endosc. 1996;10:105–6.
32. Stalfors J, Bjorholt I, Westin T. A cost analysis of participation via personal attendance versus telemedicine at a head and neck oncology multidisciplinary team meeting. J Telemed Telecare. 2005;11:205–10.
33. Axford A, Askill C, Jones A. Virtual multidisciplinary teams for cancer care. J Telemed Telecare. 2002; 8 Suppl 2:3–4.

Enhanced Recovery After Surgery for Pelvic Cancer

5

Yannick Cerantola, Massimo Valerio, Martin Hubner, Kristoffer Lassen, Francesco Carli, Beata M.E. Persson, and Hitendra R.H. Patel

5.1 Introduction

Enhanced Recovery After Surgery (ERAS) is a multimodal standardized perioperative care pathway built on evidence-based treatments and designed to reduce surgical stress and maintain physiological function. ERAS aims at achieving early recovery for patients undergoing major surgery [1]. It has been shown to decrease the occurrence of negative surgical outcomes such as morbidity and prolonged length of stay [2]. First developed for colonic surgery, ERAS protocols have been modified and successfully applied to many other specialties including pancreatic [3], gynecological [4, 5], vascular [6], thoracic [7], pediatric [8] and orthopedic [9] surgery as well as urology [10–12]. The goal of this chapter is to highlight the basics of ERAS care pathways and to give an overview of their application to pelvic cancer surgery, in particular for rectal, uterine, ovarian, prostate and bladder surgery.

Y. Cerantola, MD (✉) • M. Valerio, MD
Department of Urology, University Hospital Lausanne (CHUV), Lausanne, Switzerland
e-mail: yannick.cerantola@chuv.ch

M. Hubner, PhD
Department of Visceral Surgery, Lausanne University Hospital (CHUV), Lausanne, Switzerland

K. Lassen, MD, PhD
Department of GI/HPB Surgery, University Hospital Northern Norway, Tromsø, Norway

F. Carli, MD, MPhil
Department of Anesthesia, McGill University Health Centre, Montreal, QC, Canada

B.M.E. Persson, MD, FEBU
Department of Urology, Őrebro University Hospital, Őrebro, Sweden

H.R.H. Patel, MRCS, PhD, FRCS(Urol), FRCS(Eng)
Department of Urology, University Hospital Northern Norway, Tromsø, Norway

5.2 Background

Patho-physiology

Despite steady improvement of anesthetic and surgical technique in different fields over the years, postoperative complications remain one of the major drawbacks of surgery, for the patient, but also for the surgeon and the care team. Assuming no anesthetic or surgical failure occurs, one of the main pathogenic factors leading to postoperative morbidity is the so-called surgical stress response. The progressive understanding of the physiological basis of postoperative stress response has lead to the development of interdisciplinary teams, incorporating surgeons, anesthesiologists and nursing staff among others (Table 5.1), aiming to minimize surgical stress response.

Already in 1984, Bessey et al. demonstrated the causality relation between stress hormones

H.R.H. Patel et al. (eds.), *Pelvic Cancer Surgery: Modern Breakthroughs and Future Advances*,
DOI 10.1007/978-1-4471-4258-4_5,

Table 5.1 ERAS represents a multimodal approach to perioperative care

ERAS items	Surgeon	Anesthesiologist	Nursing staff / dietician / stoma specialist
Counseling and education	Involved	Involved	Involved
Medical optimization		Involved	
No oral mechanical bowel preparation	Involved		Involved
Carbohydrates loading	Involved		Involved
Avoid preoperative fasting	Involved	Involved	Involved
Avoid long-lasting preanasthesia medication		Involved	
Epidural analgesia		Involved	
Minimally invasive approach	Involved		
Avoid resection site drainage	Involved		
Antimicrobial prophylaxis and skin preparation	Involved	Involved	
Standard anesthetic protocol		Involved	
Perioperative fluid management		Involved	
Preventing intraoperative hypothermia		Involved	
Thrombosis prophylaxis	Involved		
Nasogastric intubation	Involved	Involved	
Avoid prolonged urinary drainage	Involved		
Prevention of postoperative ileus	Involved		
Prevention of PONV	Involved		Involved
Postoperative analgesia	Involved	Involved	Involved
Early mobilization			Involved
Early oral diet	Involved		Involved
Audit	Involved	Involved	Involved

The key players and their involvements are displayed below. Items which concern mainly preoperative care are highlighted in green. Items which concern mainly intra-operative care are highlighted in yellow. Items which concern mainly post-operative care are highlighted in blue

and systemic response by testing infusion of catecholamines and cortisol in healthy volunteers [13]. The authors observed that this artificial endocrine imbalance induced a systemic stress response, similar to what it is observed after low to intermediate injuries. Nowadays, it has been clarified that surgery induces a complex cascade resulting in inflammatory response, immune suppression, altered metabolism with hypercatabolism which lead to impaired wound healing and multi-organ failure [14]. The mediators of this endocrine-metabolic stress response are cytokines, arachidonic acid, nitric oxide and free oxygen radicals [15]. While the mechanisms mentioned above have been extensively studied, to date, no single intervention has been shown to eliminate postoperative morbidity and mortality. Thus, multimodal combined interventions may lead to a reduction of the undesirable effects of surgery with improved recovery and consequently reduced postoperative morbidity and overall costs.

5.3 Development of ERAS

Considering that the immediate challenge to improving the quality of surgical care is not discovering new knowledge, but rather to integrate what we already know [16], the concept "fast track" was introduced in the 1990 [17]. It was demonstrated that by applying evidence-based perioperative principles to patients undergoing open colonic surgery, the post-operative complication rate was halved and length of hospital stay was brought down to 2–3 days [18]. The initial items were complemented over the years by a multitude of perioperative measures with proven or probable impact on the surgical stress response. The current protocol consists of over 20 elements (Table 5.1). This multimodal perioperative care pathway was first propagated and further developed in northern Europe and Great Britain. In order to standardized practice and draw recommendation, the ERAS study group was created in 2001 and soon discovered that there were a variety of traditions in use in different units. There was also a great discrepancy between the actual practices and what was already known to be best practice, based on the literature [19]. This prompted the group to examine the process of change from tradition to best-practice.

ERAS represents a paradigm shift in perioperative care in two ways. First, it re-examines traditional practices, replacing them with evidence-based best practices when necessary. Second, it is comprehensive in its scope, covering all areas of the patient's journey through the surgical process.

Since its creation, the ERAS Society has published recommendations for the use of ERAS protocols in colonic [20], rectal [21] and pancreatic surgery [3]. Several randomized controlled trials have been undertaken and included in two meta-analysis which demonstrate the significant and reproducible benefits of applying ERAS protocols to colorectal patients [22, 23].

5.4 ERAS Pathways Applied to Rectal Surgery

As already emphasized, standardization of perioperative care relying mostly on evidence-based measures reduces complications by 50 % and hospital stay by 2.5 days [23]. Moreover, ERAS programs have proven highly cost-effective [24]. The ERAS study group initially published comprehensive guidelines which did not differentiate between colon and rectal surgery, although there are important differences between the respective procedures and patient collectives [20, 25]. Later, dedicated recommendations were agreed on for "rectal/pelvic surgery" [21].

At first sight, rectal guidelines are very similar to those for colon surgery (Table 5.2). Obviously, these are general measures to reduce surgical stress response and prevention of postoperative ileus, such as optimized fluid management, no pre-operative sedation, carbohydrate loading, early mobilization and early oral intake. However, distinct differences have been underlined that could also be extrapolated for other pelvic surgeries mentioned in this chapter. Examples include dedicated pre-operative counseling for potential ostomy carriers, bowel preparation for low resections, acceptance of intrapelvic drains and prolonged urinary drainage. However, many items remain subject to debate, since no definitive evidence exists. This is especially true for perioperative pain management. Indeed, epidural analgesia—the backbone of opioid-sparing strategies—is questioned more and more in laparoscopic but also in open surgeries. Emerging

Table 5.2 Summary of the main ERAS items and their modifications when applied to pelvic cancer surgery

ERAS items	Colonic surgery	Rectal surgery	Urology	Gynecology
Preoperative counseling and education	Surgical details, hospital stay and discharge criteria in oral and written form; stoma education; patient's expectations	Idem	Idem	Idem
Oral mechanical bowel preparation	Can be safely omitted	Might be needed when diverting ileostomy is planned and for total mesorectal excision	Can be safely omitted	Can be safely omitted
Preoperative carbohydrates loading	Should be administered to all non-diabetic patients	Idem	Idem	Idem
Preoperative fasting	Clear fluids until 2 h, solids until 6 h before induction of anesthesia	Idem	Idem	Idem
Epidural analgesia	Opioid-sparing thoracic epidural analgesia in open surgery, level T9–11, duration: 72 h	Idem	Idem	Idem
Minimally invasive approach	At most feasible; in trial setting Long term oncological results awaited	Not recommended outside of a trial	Cystectomy: not recommended outside of a trial Prostatectomy: robotic approach seems beneficial	Conflicting results
Resection site drainage	Perianastomotic and/or pelvic drain can be omitted	Should not be used routinely	Cystectomy: no evidence for avoidance of drainage Prostatectomy: drain can be safely removed at day 1	No evidence for avoidance of drainage
Perioperative fluid management	Goal-directed to optimize cardiac output and organ perfusion	Idem	Idem	Idem
Nasogastric intubation	Not indicated postoperatively	Idem	Idem	Idem
Urinary drainage	Transurethral bladder catheter for 1–2 days, independently of epidural anesthesia	Can be safely removed at day 1 if low risk of urinary retention	Cystectomy: optimal duration of ureteral stenting unknown Prostatectomy: urethral catheter usually removed between day 5–10	Can be safely removed at day 1
Prevention of postoperative ileus	Multimodal approach Gum chewing and oral magnesium	Multimodal approach Gum chewing and oral magnesium	Multimodal approach Gum chewing and oral magnesium	Multimodal approach
Postoperative analgesia	Multimodal postoperative analgesia should include thoracic epidural analgesia	Idem	Idem	Idem

(continued)

Table 5.2 (continued)

ERAS items	Colonic surgery	Rectal surgery	Urology	Gynecology
Early mobilization	2 h out of bed POD 0 6 h out of bed POD 1	Idem	Idem	Idem
Early oral diet	Normal diet starting 4 h after surgery	Idem	Idem	Idem
Audit	Routine audit of outcomes, cost-effectiveness, compliance and changes in protocol	Idem	Idem	Idem

Colonic surgery is considered as the reference. Items that are considered as "standard of care" such as preoperative medical optimization, thrombosis prophylaxis, antimicrobial prophylaxis and skin preparation, standard anesthetic protocol, preventing intraoperative hypothermia and prevention of nausea and vomiting are not displayed in the table

alternatives include intrathecal analgesia, regional blocks and IV lidocaine [26]. Another open debate is the management of intra- and early postoperative fluids. While two randomized studies showed little benefit of sophisticated Doppler-guided fluid regimes [27, 28], the situation might be very different for major rectal, urological and gynecological procedures with longer duration and higher fluid shifts. In any event, the current protocols will be continuously developed and adapted according to the current evidence in order to keep ERAS as dynamic as possible and not to fall in "new dogmas"!

5.5 ERAS Pathways Applied to Gynecological Surgery

One cohort study investigated the effects of an adapted ERAS protocol in patients operated for ovarian cancer [4]. The protocol included avoidance of bowel preparation and nasogastric decompression combined with the use of epidural analgesia, PONV prophylaxis, laxatives, and early oral nutrition and ambulation. The ERAS protocol was applied to 69 patients, which were compared with 72 historical controls receiving standard care. ERAS patients showed a reduced hospital stay (5 vs. 6 days; $P<0.05$)) and a reduced morbidity (2 vs. 14 %; ($P<0.01$)). The readmission rate was not increased, thus clearly favoring an ERAS care.

As far as uterine cancer surgery is concern, different ERAS protocols have been investigated. One randomized study applied a modified ERAS protocol, including no use of sedatives for premedication, pre-emptive anti-emetic therapy, intravenous fluid restriction, analgesics based on non-opioids, early enteral nutrition and mobilization, and standard criteria for discharge, to 162 women undergoing hysterectomy. The type of anesthesia, general vs. spinal, did not significantly impact on the LOS. Bowel recovery time was shorter in the spinal anesthesia group, but vomiting was more frequent [29]. Intrathecally administered morphine combined with a low-dose mode of total intravenous anesthesia allows for a shorter LOS, when compared to patient-controlled analgesia, although no difference were shown with respect to morbidity [30]. Results concerning potential benefits of a minimally invasive approach are somehow conflicting [31–34].

5.6 ERAS Pathways Applied to Urology

Bladder Cancer

Despite standardization of the surgical technique, improved anesthesia protocols and perioperative care, radical cystectomy with bladder reconstruction is still considered as the most significant surgical challenge in urology [35]. Indeed, morbidity after open radical cystectomy with bilateral pelvic lymph node dissection and urinary diversion or bladder reconstruction mounts up to 30–64 % [36, 37]. Cystectomy patients may therefore be ideal candidates for an ERAS pathway as the potential for reduction of surgical stress and complications is very high.

However, ERAS guidelines issued from colonic surgery [25] might not be applied identically to bladder cancer patients as the surgical procedure itself differs widely (small bowel anastomosis, risk of renal insufficiency in obstructive bladder tumors, urine within the peritoneal cavity during and after surgery, both extra- and intraperitoneal access, longer operative time, increased risk of blood loss). Moreover, colorectal ERAS items such as urinary and abdominal drains might not be applicable to cystectomy patients. Nevertheless, modified ERAS protocols have been investigated and are described below.

Maffezzini et al. applied a modified ERAS protocol complying with 6 of the 22 classic ERAS items (no oral mechanical bowel preparation, epidural analgesia, antimicrobial prophylaxis, standard anesthetic protocol, preventing intraoperative hypothermia, early nasogastric tube removal) to 71 patients undergoing radical cystectomy. When compared to 40 historical retrospective patients, those in the study group showed a reduced mean time to normal diet (from 7 to 4 days) and a shorter LOS (from 22 to 15 days). Morbidity did not differ significantly between the two groups [38]. Another retrospective study compared 56 consecutive patients undergoing open radical cystectomy with standard perioperative care to 56 patients after implementation of an enhanced recovery program including 7 of 22 items (no bowel preparation, no preoperative fasting, epidural analgesia, PONV prophylaxis, early oral nutrition, early mobilization, early removal of abdominal drain) [10]. Morbidity and time to first bowel movement did not differ between the two groups. LOS was significantly reduced (from 17 to 13 days) in the enhanced recovery group. Pruthi et al. published their experience of enhance recovery programs after cystectomy [12]. Two-hundred and sixty-two retrospective patients were compared to the most recent consecutive 100 patients. The protocol included 9 of 22 ERAS items (preoperative information, deep vein thrombosis prophylaxis, antibiotics prophylaxis, early removal of nasogastric tube, early oral nutrition, early mobilization, prevention of PONV, prevention of ileus, postoperative analgesia). However, due to inconsistent protocol throughout time and methodological flaws, no comparison of these two cohorts is possible. Donat et al. combined early nasogastric tube removal with metoclopramide in 27 prospectively included patients undergoing cystectomy and compared them with 54 controls receiving no metoclopramide and in which nasogastric tube was removed only after return of normal bowel function. Complication rate and LOS was similar in both groups. The study group showed earlier return to normal bowel sounds and tolerance to liquid and solid food. By combining thoracic epidural analgesia, early nasogastric tube removal, early oral nutrition and mobilization in 15 prospective patients, Brodner et al. showed a reduction of the time to first defecation, with no difference with regards to morbidity or LOS when compared to 15 patients undergoing a standard care plan [39].

In summary, several studies have been undertaken to evaluate the role of some kind of ERAS care pathways on outcomes after radical cystectomy. All found significant benefits in either postoperative morbidity, return to bowel function or LOS. Unfortunately, none of these studies applied a full ERAS protocol, but rather implemented from 3 to 9 of the 22 classic ERAS items. Therefore, the real benefits of a full ERAS pathway applied to cystectomy patients remain unknown, but might be higher than the ones reported when partial ERAS protocols are applied.

Prostate Cancer

Multimodal ERAS protocols have been applied to patients undergoing radical prostatectomy. One RCT included 50 patients undergoing laparoscopic radical prostatectomy randomized between standard care ($n=25$) or ERAS pathway ($n=25$). Despite the small sample size, the ERAS group showed a significant reduction in postoperative complication rate (24 vs 56 %, $p=0.02$) and a shorter LOS (3.6 vs 6.7 days, $p<0.001$) [40]. However, it should be highlighted that the protocol used in this study included only ten items suggested by the ERAS society, and that a minimal invasive laparoscopic approach was used also in the control group. As a consequence, the effect of ERAS pathways on postoperative outcome is likely to be underestimated in this study.

Some unimodal ERAS interventions have been evaluated in radical prostatectomy. For instance, a meta-analysis showed a decrease in complications rate and in LOS when a minimally invasive approach was used, as compared to an open approach [41]. In addition, based on a comparative series including 560 patients, the avoidance of pelvic drainage does not seem to increase the complication rate, and might decrease LOS and bowel recovery [42]. Interestingly, the use of thoracic epidural anesthesia, which represents one of the central elements of ERAS, has been shown to reduce intraoperative blood loss, time to return of bowel function [43] and even recurrence rate [44]. The effect of other single ERAS interventions, which may have an important role in enhanced recovery after radical prostatectomy have not been extensively studied in terms of complications rate, LOS or recovery of bowel motility.

There is an urgent need for high-quality studies evaluating the use of fast-track intervention compared to standard care in order to validate the studies mentioned above, in order to extend the possible benefit of such strategies in non-ERAS adherent centers.

5.7 Summary/Conclusions

Enhanced Recovery After Surgery (ERAS) is standard of care in colon surgery. ERAS allows for a reduction of morbidity, as well as length of hospital stay and total costs. While the ERAS protocol used in colon surgery stands as a reference, there is overwhelming evidence for the use of ERAS pathways for rectum surgery, which integrate important specific changes. There can be no doubt that ERAS principles have to be applied also in other major pelvic surgeries, such as cystectomy, radical prostatectomy and hysterectomy. However, there is clearly a need for careful adaptation of the many ERAS items for the different types of surgeries. This process mandates a prospective audit that can best be performed by a centralized multi-center data base.

While the body of evidence for the use of ERAS protocols in pelvic cancer surgery increases rapidly, some drawbacks remain. For instance, most of the studies are of poor quality, either underpowered or retrospective. Initial results of ERAS randomized studies have been criticized by some surgeons, arguing that the improved outcome was mainly due to the so-called Hawthorne effect [21]. It is therefore mandatory to measure clinical outcome in a standardized manner to provide the highest and most reliable evidence. Of note, beneficial outcomes from randomized studies have also been reproduced in large prospective observational studies [45], thus arguing against a possible Hawthorne effect. Application of evidence-based recommendations is traditionally slow. This seems to be a particular problem of ERAS pathways, which challenge long-standing dogmas [46]. This is worrisome as adherence to the protocol is clearly correlated with improved outcomes [47, 48]. Also, the compliance to the protocol is of major importance and often requires an initial increase of workload at implementation, which might be considered as a drawback by the surgeon. Finally, there is a need for standardization and adaptation of protocols tailored to the surgical specifics of the respective specialty. Such protocols are not yet widely available. Prospective auditing is more likely to prove efficiency than more randomized trials, which might nowadays be considered unethical. Moreover, being a highly complex intervention, ERAS protocols are not particularly well suited for randomized design [49].

Multicenter, prospective studies using a centralized database will certainly help in answering open questions such as the optimal perioperative nutritional support, the need, type and duration of pelvic and urinary catheterization, the real benefits of full ERAS protocols on morbidity, mortality, LOS, readmission rate and costs.

Future development of ERAS will focus on maintaining the concept as dynamic as possible, by objectively evaluating and including new evidence from clinical experiences and thus eliminate some items and add new ones to this multimodal concept.

References

1. Kehlet H, Wilmore DW. Evidence-based surgical care and the evolution of fast-track surgery. Ann Surg. 2008;248(2):189–98.
2. Varadhan KK, Neal KR, Dejong CH, Fearon KC, Ljungqvist O, Lobo DN. The enhanced recovery after surgery (ERAS) pathway for patients undergoing major elective open colorectal surgery: a meta-analysis of randomized controlled trials. Clin Nutr. 2011;29(4):434–40.
3. Lassen K, Coolsen MM, Slim K, Carli F, de Aguilar-Nascimento JE, Schafer M, et al. Guidelines for perioperative care for pancreaticoduodenectomy: Enhanced Recovery After Surgery (ERAS((R))) society recommendations. World J Surg. 2012;31:817.
4. Marx C, Rasmussen T, Jakobsen DH, Ottosen C, Lundvall L, Ottesen B, et al. The effect of accelerated rehabilitation on recovery after surgery for ovarian malignancy. Acta Obstet Gynecol Scand. 2006;85(4):488–92.
5. Arsalani-Zadeh R, ElFadl D, Yassin N, MacFie J. Evidence-based review of enhancing postoperative recovery after breast surgery. Br J Surg. 2011;98(2): 181–96.
6. Muehling B, Schelzig H, Steffen P, Meierhenrich R, Sunder-Plassmann L, Orend KH. A prospective randomized trial comparing traditional and fast-track patient care in elective open infrarenal aneurysm repair. World J Surg. 2009;33(3):577–85.
7. Das-Neves-Pereira JC, Bagan P, Coimbra-Israel AP, Grimaillof-Junior A, Cesar-Lopez G, Milanez-de-Campos JR, et al. Fast-track rehabilitation for lung cancer lobectomy: a five-year experience. Eur J Cardiothorac Surg. 2009;36(2):383–91; discussion 391–2.
8. Reismann M, Dingemann J, Wolters M, Laupichler B, Suempelmann R, Ure BM. Fast-track concepts in routine pediatric surgery: a prospective study in 436 infants and children. Langenbeck's Arch Surg/Deutsche Gesellschaft fur Chirurgie. 2009;394(3):529–33.
9. Husted H, Jensen CM, Solgaard S, Kehlet H. Reduced length of stay following hip and knee arthroplasty in Denmark 2000–2009: from research to implementation. Arch Orthop Traumatol Surg. 2012;132(1): 101–4.
10. Arumainayagam N, McGrath J, Jefferson KP, Gillatt DA. Introduction of an enhanced recovery protocol for radical cystectomy. BJU Int. 2008;101(6):698–701.
11. Maffezzini M, Gerbi G, Campodonico F, Parodi D. A multimodal perioperative plan for radical cystectomy and urinary intestinal diversion: effects, limits and complications of early artificial nutrition. J Urol. 2006;176(3):945–8; discussion 948–9.
12. Pruthi RS, Nielsen M, Smith A, Nix J, Schultz H, Wallen EM. Fast track program in patients undergoing radical cystectomy: results in 362 consecutive patients. J Am Coll Surg. 2010;210(1):93–9.
13. Bessey PQ, Watters JM, Aoki TT, Wilmore DW. Combined hormonal infusion simulates the metabolic response to injury. Ann Surg. 1984;200(3):264–81.
14. Kehlet H, Dahl JB. Anaesthesia, surgery, and challenges in postoperative recovery. Lancet. 2003;362(9399):1921–8.
15. Kehlet H. Multimodal approach to control postoperative pathophysiology and rehabilitation. Br J Anaesth. 1997;78(5):606–17.
16. Urbach DR, Baxter NN. Reducing variation in surgical care. BMJ (Clinical research ed). 2005;330(7505):1401–2.
17. Bardram L, Funch-Jensen P, Jensen P, Crawford ME, Kehlet H. Recovery after laparoscopic colonic surgery with epidural analgesia, and early oral nutrition and mobilisation. Lancet. 1995;345(8952):763–4.
18. Andersen J, Hjort-Jakobsen D, Christiansen PS, Kehlet H. Readmission rates after a planned hospital stay of 2 versus 3 days in fast-track colonic surgery. Br J Surg. 2007;94(7):890–3.
19. Lassen K, Hannemann P, Ljungqvist O, Fearon K, Dejong CH, von Meyenfeldt MF, et al. Patterns in current perioperative practice: survey of colorectal surgeons in five northern European countries. BMJ (Clinical research ed). 2005;330(7505):1420–1.
20. Gustafsson UO, Scott MJ, Schwenk W, Demartines N, Roulin D, Francis N, et al. Guidelines for perioperative care in elective colonic surgery: Enhanced Recovery After Surgery (ERAS((R))) society recommendations. World J Surg. 2012;31(6):783–800.
21. Nygren J, Thacker J, Carli F, Fearon KC, Norderval S, Lobo DN, et al. Guidelines for perioperative care in elective rectal/pelvic surgery: Enhanced Recovery After Surgery (ERAS((R))) society recommendations. World J Surg. 2012;31(6):801–16.
22. Adamina M, Kehlet H, Tomlinson GA, Senagore AJ, Delaney CP. Enhanced recovery pathways optimize health outcomes and resource utilization: a meta-analysis of randomized controlled trials in colorectal surgery. Surgery. 2011;149(6):830–40.
23. Varadhan KK, Neal KR, Dejong CH, Fearon KC, Ljungqvist O, Lobo DN. The enhanced recovery after surgery (ERAS) pathway for patients undergoing major elective open colorectal surgery: a meta-analysis of randomized controlled trials. Clin Nutr (Edinb Scotl). 2010;29(4):434–40.
24. Sammour T, Zargar-Shoshtari K, Bhat A, Kahokehr A, Hill AG. A programme of Enhanced Recovery After Surgery (ERAS) is a cost-effective intervention in elective colonic surgery. N Z Med J. 2010; 123(1319):61–70.
25. Lassen K, Soop M, Nygren J, Cox PB, Hendry PO, Spies C, et al. Consensus review of optimal perioperative care in colorectal surgery: Enhanced Recovery After Surgery (ERAS) Group recommendations. Arch Surg. 2009;144(10):961–9.

26. Levy BF, Scott MJ, Fawcett W, Fry C, Rockall TA. Randomized clinical trial of epidural, spinal or patient-controlled analgesia for patients undergoing laparoscopic colorectal surgery. Br J Surg. 2011; 98(8):1068–78.
27. Brandstrup B, Svendsen PE, Rasmussen M, Belhage B, Rodt SA, Hansen B, et al. Which goal for fluid therapy during colorectal surgery is followed by the best outcome: near-maximal stroke volume or zero fluid balance? Br J Anaesth. 2011;109(2):191–9.
28. Srinivasa S, Taylor MH, Singh PP, Yu TC, Soop M, Hill AG. Randomized clinical trial of goal-directed fluid therapy within an enhanced recovery protocol for elective colectomy. Br J Surg. 2013;100(1):66–74.
29. Borendal Wodlin N, Nilsson L, Kjolhede P. The impact of mode of anaesthesia on postoperative recovery from fast-track abdominal hysterectomy: a randomised clinical trial. BJOG. 2011;118(3): 299–308.
30. Kroon UB, Radstrom M, Hjelthe C, Dahlin C, Kroon L. Fast-track hysterectomy: a randomised, controlled study. Eur J Obstet Gynecol Reprod Biol. 2010;151(2):203–7.
31. Moller C, Kehlet H, Friland SG, Schouenborg LO, Lund C, Ottesen B. Fast track hysterectomy. Eur J Obstet Gynecol Reprod Biol. 2001;98(1):18–22.
32. DeNardis SA, Holloway RW, Bigsby GE, Pikaart DP, Ahmad S, Finkler NJ. Robotically assisted laparoscopic hysterectomy versus total abdominal hysterectomy and lymphadenectomy for endometrial cancer. Gynecol Oncol. 2008;111(3):412–7.
33. Sharma R, Bailey J, Anderson R, Murdoch J. Laparoscopically assisted radical vaginal hysterectomy (Coelio-Schauta): a comparison with open Wertheim/Meigs hysterectomy. Int J Gynecol Cancer. 2006;16(5):1927–32.
34. Uccella S, Laterza R, Ciravolo G, Volpi E, Franchi M, Zefiro F, et al. A comparison of urinary complications following total laparoscopic radical hysterectomy and laparoscopic pelvic lymphadenectomy to open abdominal surgery. Gynecol Oncol. 2007;107(1 Suppl 1): S147–9.
35. Hautmann RE, Abol-Enein H, Davidsson T, Gudjonsson S, Hautmann SH, Holm HV, et al. ICUD-EAU International Consultation on Bladder Cancer 2012: urinary diversion. Eur Urol. 2012;63:67.
36. Hollenbeck BK, Miller DC, Taub D, Dunn RL, Khuri SF, Henderson WG, et al. Identifying risk factors for potentially avoidable complications following radical cystectomy. J Urol. 2005;174(4 Pt 1):1231–7; discussion 1237.
37. Shabsigh A, Korets R, Vora KC, Brooks CM, Cronin AM, Savage C, et al. Defining early morbidity of radical cystectomy for patients with bladder cancer using a standardized reporting methodology. Eur Urol. 2009;55(1):164–74.
38. Maffezzini M, Gerbi G, Campodonico F, Parodi D. Multimodal perioperative plan for radical cystectomy and intestinal urinary diversion. I. Effect on recovery of intestinal function and occurrence of complications. Urology. 2007;69(6):1107–11.
39. Brodner G, Van Aken H, Hertle L, Fobker M, Von Eckardstein A, Goeters C, et al. Multimodal perioperative management—combining thoracic epidural analgesia, forced mobilization, and oral nutrition—reduces hormonal and metabolic stress and improves convalescence after major urologic surgery. Anesth Analg. 2001;92(6):1594–600.
40. Gralla O, Haas F, Knoll N, Hadzidiakos D, Tullmann M, Romer A, et al. Fast-track surgery in laparoscopic radical prostatectomy: basic principles. World J Urol. 2007;25(2):185–91.
41. Novara G, Ficarra V, Rosen RC, Artibani W, Costello A, Eastham JA, et al. Systematic review and meta-analysis of perioperative outcomes and complications after robot-assisted radical prostatectomy. Eur Urol. 2012;62(3):431–52.
42. Sharma S, Kim HL, Mohler JL. Routine pelvic drainage not required after open or robotic radical prostatectomy. Urology. 2007;69(2):330–3.
43. Stevens RA, Mikat-Stevens M, Flanigan R, Waters WB, Furry P, Sheikh T, et al. Does the choice of anesthetic technique affect the recovery of bowel function after radical prostatectomy? Urology. 1998;52(2): 213–8.
44. Biki B, Mascha E, Moriarty DC, Fitzpatrick JM, Sessler DI, Buggy DJ. Anesthetic technique for radical prostatectomy surgery affects cancer recurrence: a retrospective analysis. Anesthesiology. 2008;109(2): 180–7.
45. Ahmed J, Khan S, Lim M, Chandrasekaran TV, Macfie J. Enhanced recovery after surgery protocols—compliance and variations in practice during routine colorectal surgery. Colorectal Dis. 2012;14(9): 1045–51.
46. Kehlet H, Buchler MW, Beart Jr RW, Billingham RP, Williamson R. Care after colonic operation—is it evidence-based? Results from a multinational survey in Europe and the United States. J Am Coll Surg. 2006;202(1):45–54.
47. Gustafsson UO, Hausel J, Thorell A, Ljungqvist O, Soop M, Nygren J. Adherence to the enhanced recovery after surgery protocol and outcomes after colorectal cancer surgery. Arch Surg. 2011;146(5):571–7.
48. Maessen J, Dejong CH, Hausel J, Nygren J, Lassen K, Andersen J, et al. A protocol is not enough to implement an enhanced recovery programme for colorectal resection. Br J Surg. 2007;94(2):224–31.
49. Craig P, Dieppe P, Macintyre S, Michie S, Nazareth I, Petticrew M. Developing and evaluating complex interventions: the new Medical Research Council guidance. BMJ (Clinical research ed). 2008;337:a1655.

Dealing with Pelvic Dysfunction: Multi and Interdisciplinary Team Approach

6

Mona Stedenfeldt, Rolv-Ole Lindsetmo, and Stig Norderval

6.1 Introduction

Despite improvement in surgical technique emphasizing the importance of nerve sparing dissection, dysfunction of pelvic organs appears frequently after pelvic cancer surgery. The addition of pre- or postoperative radiation therapy may further affect pelvic function negatively, with symptoms occurring months to years after surgery. Furthermore, the aging population has led to an increase in old patients fit for surgery, but where the effect of general aging makes postoperative pelvic dysfunction more likely to occur. The most common complaints are impaired sexual function, urinary retention or incontinence, anal incontinence, obstructed defecation or pelvic floor pain. Although there has been an increasing focus on these side effects following successful cancer treatment, many patients seem unprepared when affected, and the knowledge among general practitioners and specialists about possible treatment options is often sparse. Furthermore, many patients experience multiple dysfunctions, and a multidisciplinary approach is advisable before treatment attempts are initiated. Pelvic cancer surgery also carries a substantial risk of surgical complications as deep infections or abscesses, fistulas and anastomotic leaks frequently needing reoperations. This will further increase the risk for later pelvic dysfunction.

The nature and symptoms of pelvic dysfunctions are closely related to the resected organ. However, the pelvic innervation might be damaged from the cancer itself but also from the cancer surgery independent of the specialist involved.

The aim of this chapter is to provide information about the specter of common pelvic dysfunctions following the various procedures, and to discuss the importance of a multidisciplinary approach to patients experiencing pelvic dysfunction after surgery for pelvic cancer.

Resection of pelvic organs is associated with postoperative pelvic dysfunction, with the degree of problems in part being dependent on the procedure performed, technique used, and the stage of the cancer. When radiotherapy is used as part of the treatment, pelvic floor dysfunction is more likely to occur than after surgery alone.

Dysfunctions After Gynecological Pelvic Cancer Procedures

Conventional radical hysterectomy (RH) is followed by bladder dysfunction and bowel dysfunction like

M. Stedenfeldt, BSc (Hons), MSc, PhD (✉)
The National Advisory Unit on Incontinence and Pelvic Floor Health of Norway, University Hospital of North Norway, Tromsø, Norway
e-mail: mona.stedenfeldt@gmail.com

R.-O. Lindsetmo, MD, PhD • S. Norderval, MD, PhD
The National Advisory Unit on Incontinence and Pelvic Floor Health of Norway, University Hospital of North Norway, Tromsø, Norway

Department of Clinical Medicine, Faculty of Health Sciences, University of Tromsø, Tromsø, Norway

H.R.H. Patel et al. (eds.), *Pelvic Cancer Surgery: Modern Breakthroughs and Future Advances*,
DOI 10.1007/978-1-4471-4258-4_6, © Springer-Verlag London 2015

constipation, obstructed defecation, urgency or incontinence in at least 25 % of the women [1]. Furthermore, RH with pelvic lymphadenectomy for early- stage cervical carcinoma has a negative impact on sexual function compared with matched control groups [2, 3]. At 2 years after surgery reduced sexual interest, lack of lubrication, a bothersome feeling of a too small vagina during intercourse, senselessness around the labia, dyspareunia, and sexual dissatisfaction is significantly more common in the treatment group. Concomitant radiotherapy does not seem to be associated with a worsened outcome than after surgery alone [3]. Because of the substantial impact on sexual, bladder and rectal function there has been an increased focus on RH with nerve sparing technique [1], which is shown to significantly reduce the incidence of these dysfunctions [4].

Dysfunctions After Urological Pelvic Cancer Procedures

Open radical prostatectomy leads to urinary incontinence in about 10 % of the patients, and erectile dysfunction is experienced by at least 30 % [5]. With the introduction of laparoscopic technique, and more recently robotic-assisted laparoscopic procedure, there has been an increased focus on the ability to perform more precise dissection with potential reduction of incontinence and erectile dysfunction after prostatectomy. While the superiority of robotic-assisted prostatectomy is questioned in recent reviews [5], meta-analysis conclude that robotic-assisted procedure reduces the incidence of erectile dysfunction and incontinence, with similar resection margins as compared to open surgery [6–8].

Radical cystectomy with creation of ileal pouch and reconstruction of lower urinary tract is followed by daytime and nighttime incontinence in about 10–40 and 30–60 % respectively [9–11]. Voiding dysfunction with the need for self-catheterization appears in 20–40 %, more common among women [11]. Erectile dysfunction is as common as after prostatectomy alone, while 20 % of the patients experience persistent diarrhea [10].

Dysfunctions After Colorectal Pelvic Cancer Procedures

Low anterior rectal resection (LAR) for rectal cancer implies dissection in the mesorectal plane. Although care is taken to preserve the inferior hypogastric nerves, postoperative pelvic dysfunction is common. About 25–80 % of the patients experience low anterior resection syndrome (LARS), with symptoms such as urgency, frequent bowel movements, fragmented defecation and incontinence [12]. LARS is more likely to occur after total mesorectal excision than after partial mesorectal excision, and more frequent in patients treated with radiotherapy preoperatively than after surgery alone [13]. Bladder dysfunction resulting in urinary frequency or weak stream is seen in up to 30 % of the patients and more than 40 % of the male experience erectile dysfunction while 25 % of the women report substantial decreased sexual function [14]. While bladder dysfunction following LAR tends to improve over time, sexual dysfunction seems to increase with time. Laparoscopic rectal resection is so far not superior to open surgery, especially not for resections extending below the anterior peritoneal reflection [14]. Abdominoperineal rectal resection (APR) carries the same risk for bladder and sexual dysfunction as LAR with total mesorectal excision.

6.2 Extended Pelvic Cancer Procedures

In addition to the procedures mentioned above, some patients undergo extended resections with removal of several pelvic organs due to tumor invasion. Examples are resection of the posterior vaginal wall in addition to APR, resection of the seminal vesicles and/or prostate capsule for a T4 rectal cancer, or complete removal of several pelvic organs. Such extended resections, sometimes with the need for reconstruction by a plastic surgeon, further increase the likelihood for postoperative pelvic dysfunction to occur.

Pelvic Pain After Surgery for Pelvic Cancer

In addition to the dysfunctions mentioned above, some patients develop de novo chronic pelvic pain after surgery. The etiology is multifactorial, with premorbid history, nerve injury caused by surgery alone, by concomitant chemoradiotherapy or a combination of these two, development of perineural fibrosis, or muscular dysfunction as some of the factors. While infrequent after prostatectomy [15], de novo chronic pelvic pain is experienced by 5–15 % of women after hysterectomy [16, 17]. After abdominoperineal rectal resection up to half of the patients experience chronic pain, depending on the extent of the perineal excision performed [18].

6.3 The Multi and Interdisciplinary Approach to Patients with Pelvic Dysfunction

As mentioned most common complaints after pelvic cancer surgery are impaired sexual function, urinary retention or incontinence, anal incontinence, obstructed defecation or pelvic floor pain. The negative consequences of these health problems might include psychological morbidity, poor self–image, impaired social function and sexual avoidance or aversion [19–23]. Thus, appropriate care addressing all pelvic floor dysfunctions is important in order to obtain optimal result, aiming to improve the individual patient's daily life. Traditionally these health problems have been addressed by separate disciplines such as gynecologists, urologists, colorectal surgeons, physiotherapists, and occasionally neurologists, based on the presumably affected anatomical pelvic structure exemplified by Fig. 6.1. If there has been any collaboration between the disciplines it has often been in a sporadic and non-systematic manner. This would be unproblematic if the health problems had one facet only. However, more often than not, this is not the situation. As mentioned above, these patients have frequently several interconnected pelvic floor dysfunctions after the cancer treatment.

There is a common agreement that many problems or challenges in society cannot be solved appropriately without an interdisciplinary, or at least a multidisciplinary approach [24]. This is also most likely true in medicine. Complex patient problems have multiple facets, each of a particular concern to one medical speciality or health care discipline. In other words, on one hand a number of challenges will most likely be insufficiently solved by one speciality or discipline only. On the other hand, a number of complex problems or challenges will not be satisfactory solved without the presence of the

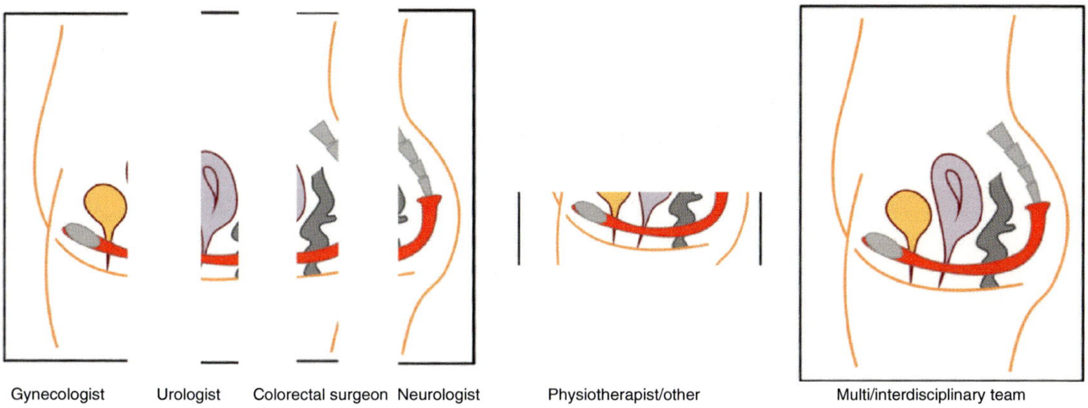

Fig. 6.1 An illustration of how traditional approaches to pelvic floor dysfunctions have been segmented according to disciplines and pelvic compartments

relatively narrow and specialized competence each medical speciality or health care discipline provide.

Multidisciplinary approach is never the less a challenge where hope often tends to triumph over experience, and this can easily stop the process of establishing a successful team. The important question is: why is it so?

The word discipline originates from the Latin word disciplus, which means obedient pupil and follower. The characteristics of a single speciality or discipline is specific structure and system of knowledge, language, and culture, reproduced by training [25], and disciplined thinking explicitly or implicitly " . . . omits or ignores a great many other possible causes and explanations—it would not be disciplined if it did not" [26]. This is also true for medical specialities, which is not just part of a particular medical subject matter, but also a system of rules, reproduced by schooling, training and practice. Medical specialities are evolved by many factors but also by:

- Developing language in form of expressions, theories, and concepts belonging to their field
- Identifying and isolating the patients main problem
- Identifying the main cause and effect relationship

Multidisciplinary teamwork is defined as: coupling of contributors from several disciplines to enlighten a common challenge. The different disciplines are working next to each other and there is no disciplinary integration, but the different contributors can inspire and develop the single disciplines contributors [25].

In addition to contribution from different disciplines there are real scientific integrations of the different contributions, theoretically and/or methodologically in interdisciplinary teamwork [25, 26]. In other words, multidisciplinary and especially interdisciplinary teamwork possesses a challenge since it somewhat contradicts the construct of a discipline. Optimal care of pelvic floor dysfunction after treatment of pelvic cancer will sometimes require a multidisciplinary approach, whereas other times the superb appropriate approach is interdisciplinary.

Due to the challenging nature of multi/interdisciplinary work it is necessary with some core structures for the team to work within to establish a good functioning pelvic floor team. This requires steady coordination and focus from someone having a principal responsibility to see the processes of the teambuilding through and to follow-up thereafter.

The Team

Who should be part of the team? In a team caring for patients with pelvic floor dysfunctions there should ideally be a gynecologist, urologist, colorectal surgeon, specialized nurse physiotherapist, radiologist and psychologist involved. However, sometimes there might not be enough resources to establish such a grand team. A vital success criterion, regardless of how many disciplines there is access to, is the motivation of each team member. A team is better off with four motivated members that have acknowledged and are willing to cooperate within the concept of multi/interdisciplinary work, instead of nine unmotivated uncooperative members.

Patient Care Lines

It is essential to establish consensus of the patient care lines that includes all steps to the final clinical audit. This is the frame of the clinical care production, i.e. investigations and treatments, involving the multi/interdisciplinary team. It is however important to understand that it is not only a "check-mark" system. While the system should ensure that investigation and/or treatment paths are followed, the multi/interdisciplinary thinking should also identify patients that show signs indicating that a more tailored and personalized path is necessary (Fig. 6.2).

Multi/Interdisciplinary Meetings

This is the arena for which the patients with complicated problems are discussed by the team.

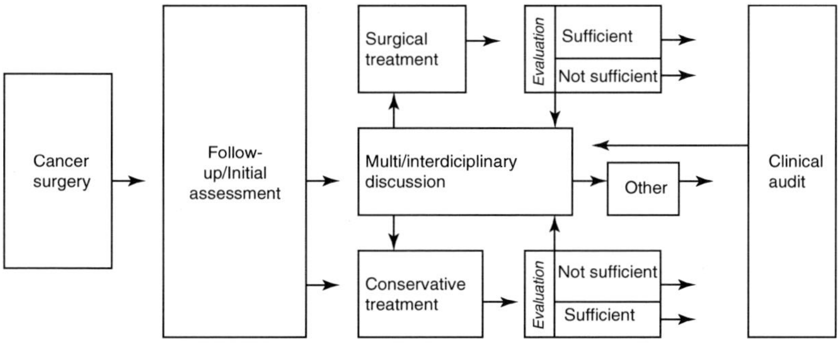

Fig. 6.2 An example of patient care lines with a multi/interdisciplinary approach for patients after cancer surgery

There are several purposes of multi/interdisciplinary meetings. First and foremost it is to achieve a common consensus based on the insight and knowledge generated from the whole group. Second, it is a learning arena for the team, expanding their knowledge by gaining knowledge from the other disciplines, and thirdly, this is where the process is audited. When the patient is discharged, the team should be presented an overview of the decisions, the investigations and treatments and the final outcome. It is advisable to have one person coordinating the meetings. The coordinator is responsible for:

- Calling the meeting with the appropriate team members (sometimes additional disciplines than the core team are needed)
- Preparing the cases for discussion
- Ensure that the patients get appointments according to the decided plan
- Follow-up with a written discharge plan when the patient is finished
- Present the final result to the group

Common Language, Evaluation: And Scoring-Tools

Each discipline usually has its own sets of tools evaluating the relatively narrow field of the discipline. To create a functional environment where clinical findings can be shared and evaluated by all members of the team, it has to be consensus of what type of scoring/evaluation tools to use for sharing, evaluating and comparing results within the group. If a system for clinical audit is established it is advisable to use validated scorings tool so that the data can be used for publications as well. Locally developed or not validated systems like incontinence diaries may be used additionally. Table 6.1 [27–36] shows an overview of relevant scoring tools.

Defining Responsibilities for Each Member of the Team

In all type of teamwork, there is a potential risk of destructive group dynamics: some not doing their share of work, some doing a vast amount of work, some that are very visible and others that are more or less invisible. These are dynamics that might cause a dysfunctional group. All members should be aware of their responsibility within the team, and the team manager should be able to address these issues and ensure a "healthy" group dynamic.

Creating Organizational Changes Where It Is Necessary and Possible

To allow a multi/interdisciplinary practice there might be necessary with organizational changes. As for example, if the patient is scheduled to see both physiotherapist and a nutritionist, the system should allow the patient to see them both in 1 day. To organize relevant outpatient clinics on the same day will also allow team members to naturally work closely in the clinical setting.

Table 6.1 Some relevant scoring tools for assessment of pelvic dysfunctions

Scoring tool	Reference
Anal incontinence	
St. Mark's score	Vaizey et al. [27]
Wexner incontinence score	Jorge and Wexner [28]
ICIQ-B	Cotterill et al. [29]
Low anterior resection syndrome	
LARS-score	Emmertsen and Laurberg [30]
Constipation	
KESS	Knowles et al. [31]
Wexner constipation score	Agachan et al. [32]
Obstructed defecation	
Obstructed defecation syndrome score	Renzi et al. [33]
Stress urinary incontinence	
ICIQ_UI_SF	Abrams et al. [34]
Roos screening test	Roos and Thakar [35]
Sexual dysfunction (men)	
IIEF-5	Rosen et al. [36]
Pain	
VAS-scale	

Clinical Audit

System for clinical audit is essential to evaluate the work and the processes. It is however a challenge to create a system that are crossing disciplines since the whole hospital organization is more often than not based on disciplines. Thus patient journal systems, management, traditional patient flow and care lines follow these rather rigid and straight-line structures. Because of this it is even more important to strive toward a good audit system to evaluate the result and resource used.

In addition, it is also important to acknowledge the importance of social skills in such work:

- Openness, trust and mutual respect is perhaps easier said than done but essential when highly skilled people shall collaborate and give good results
- There is not one discipline "owning" the problem, nor the solution.
- Interested in, and understanding of the nature of each speciality and health care discipline involved.

Conclusion

The most common dysfunctions or complaints following pelvic cancer surgery are impaired sexual function, urinary retention, urinary incontinence, anal incontinence, obstructed defecation and pelvic floor pain. When present, a multidisciplinary approach is important as many patients will experience dysfunctions and complaints involving several of the pelvic compartments after treatment for pelvic cancer.

Key Points

- Pelvic dysfunctions are common after surgical treatment for pelvic cancer
- Many patients experience post-surgical dysfunctions from more than one pelvic organ
- In general, laparoscopic technique does not seem to be superior to open in order to prevent pelvic dysfunctions following pelvic cancer surgery, while robotic surgery may show beneficial for some procedures.
- It is essential for health carers involved in the treatment of these patients to know about the natural course of the various dysfunctions in order to address further investigation and treatment appropriately.
- The negative consequences of the possible squeals after pelvic cancer surgery are many and affects the patents' average daily living if not addressed appropriately and multidisciplinary.
- Multidisciplinary teamwork is defined as coupling of contributors from several disciplines to enlighten a common challenge. Interdisciplinary teamwork is where real scientific integrations of the different contributions develop both theoretically and/or methodologically.
- Due to the challenging nature of multi/interdisciplinary work it is necessary with core structures to work within to establish a well functioning pelvic floor team.

- The purposes of multi/interdisciplinary meetings are to achieve a common consensus based on the insight and knowledge generated from the whole group, to establish a learning arena for the team, to gain knowledge from the other disciplines, and thirdly and to audit the process.
- There has to be consensus of what type of scoring/evaluation tools the group should use for sharing, evaluating and comparing clinical results within the multi/inter disciplinary setting.
- System for multi/inter disciplinary clinical audit is essential to evaluate the work and the processes ensuring quality care

References

1. Rob L, Halaska M, Robova H. Nerve-sparing and individually tailored surgery for cervical cancer. Lancet Oncol. 2010;11(3):292–301.
2. Jensen PT, Groenvold M, Klee MC, Thranov I, Petersen MA, Machin D. Early-stage cervical carcinoma, radical hysterectomy, and sexual function. A longitudinal study. Cancer. 2004;100(1):97–106.
3. Pieterse QD, Maas CP, ter Kuile MM, Lowik M, van Eijkeren MA, Trimbos JB, Kenter GG. An observational longitudinal study to evaluate miction, defecation, and sexual function after radical hysterectomy with pelvic lymphadenectomy for early-stage cervical cancer. Int J Gynecol Cancer. 2006;16(3):1119–29.
4. Cibula D, Velechovska P, Sláma J, Fischerova D, Pinkavova I, Pavlista D, Dundr P, Hill M, Freitag P, Zikan M. Late morbidity following nerve-sparing radical hysterectomy. Gynecol Oncol. 2010;116(3):506–11.
5. Boorjian SA, Eastham JA, Graefen M, Guillonneau B, Karnes RJ, Moul JW, Schaeffer EM, Stief C, Zorn KC. A critical analysis of the long-term impact of radical prostatectomy on cancer control and function outcomes. Eur Urol. 2012;61(4):664–75.
6. Ficarra V, Novara G, Rosen RC, Artibani W, Carroll PR, Costello A, Menon M, Montorsi F, Patel VR, Stolzenburg JU, Van der Poel H, Wilson TG, Zattoni F, Mottrie A. Systematic review and meta-analysis of studies reporting urinary continence recovery after robot-assisted radical prostatectomy. Eur Urol. 2012;62(3):405–17.
7. Ficarra V, Novara G, Ahlering TE, Costello A, Eastham JA, Graefen M, Guazzoni G, Menon M, Mottrie A, Patel VR, Van der Poel H, Rosen RC, Tewari AK, Wilson TG, Zattoni F, Montorsi F. Systematic review and meta-analysis of studies reporting potency rates after robot-assisted radical prostatectomy. Eur Urol. 2012;62(3):418–30.
8. Novara G, Ficarra V, Mocellin S, Ahlering TE, Carroll PR, Graefen M, Guazzoni G, Menon M, Patel VR, Shariat SF, Tewari AK, Van Poppel H, Zattoni F, Montorsi F, Mottrie A, Rosen RC, Wilson TG. Systematic review and meta-analysis of studies reporting oncologic outcome after robot-assisted radical prostatectomy. Eur Urol. 2012;62(3):382–404.
9. Joniau S, Benijts J, Van Kampen M, De Waele M, Ooms J, Van Cleynenbreugel B, Van Poppel H. Clinical experience with the N-shaped ileal neobladder: assessment of complications, voiding patterns, and quality of life in our series of 58 patients. Eur Urol. 2005;47(5):666–72.
10. Mottet N, Castagnola C, Rischmann P, Deixonne M, Guyot M, Coloby P, Mangin P. Quality of life after cystectomy: French national survey conducted by the French Association of Urology (AFU), the French Federation of Stoma Patients (FSF) and the French Association of Enterostomy Patients (AFET) in patients with ileal conduit urinary diversion or orthotopic neobladder. Prog Urol. 2008;18(5):292–8.
11. Stein JP, Dunn MD, Quek ML, Miranda G, Skinner DG. The orthotopic T pouch ileal neobladder: experience with 209 patients. J Urol. 2004;172(2):584–7.
12. Ziv Y, Zbar A, Bar-Shavit Y, Igov I. Low anterior resection syndrome (LARS): cause and effect and reconstructive considerations. Tech Coloproctol. 2013;17(2):151–62.
13. Bregendahl S, Emmertsen KJ, Lous J, Laurberg S. Bowel dysfunction after low anterior resection with and without neoadjuvant therapy for rectal cancer: a population-based cross-sectional study. Colorectal Dis. 2013;15(9):1130–9. doi:10.1111/codi.12244. Forthcomming.
14. Jayne DG, Brown JM, Thorpe H, Walker J, Quirke P, Guillou PJ. Bladder and sexual function following resection for rectal cancer in a randomized clinical trial of laparoscopic versus open technique. Br J Surg. 2005;92(9):1124–32.
15. Sall M, Madsen FA, Rhodes PR, Jønler M, Messing EM, Bruskewitz RC. Pelvic pain following radical retropubic prostatectomy: a prospective study. Urology. 1997;49(4):575–9.
16. Brandsborg B, Nikolajsen L, Hansen CT, Kehlet H, Jensen TS. Risk factors for chronic pain after hysterectomy: a nationwide questionnaire and database study. Anesthesiology. 2007;106(5):1003–12.
17. VanDenKerkhof EG, Hopman WM, Goldstein DH, Wilson RA, Towheed TE, Lam M, Harrison MB, Reitsma ML, Johnston SL, Medd JD, Gilron I. Impact of perioperative pain intensity, pain qualities, and opioid use onchronic pain after surgery: a prospective cohort study. Reg Anesth Pain Med. 2012;37(1):19–27.

18. Han JG, Wang ZJ, Wei GH, Gao ZG, Yang Y, Zhao BC. Randomized clinical trial of conventional versus cylindrical abdominoperineal resection for locally advanced lower rectal cancer. Am J Surg. 2012;204(3):274–82.
19. Goldberg RP, Kwon C, Gandhi S, Atkuru LV, Sand PK. Urinary incontinence after multiple gestation and delivery: impact on quality of life. Int Urogynecol J Pelvic Floor Dysfunct. 2005;16(5):334–6.
20. Madoff RD, Parker SC, Varma MG, Lowry AC. Feacal incontinence in adults. The Lancet. 2004;364(9434):621–32.
21. Jha S, Thakar R. Female sexual dysfunction. Eur J Obstet Gynecol Reprod Biol. 2010;153(2):117–23. doi:10.1016/j.ejogrb.2010.06.010.
22. Albaugh J, Hacker ED. Measurement of quality of life in men with prostate cancer. Clin J Oncol Nurs. 2008;12(1):81–6.
23. Sanda MG, Dunn RL, Michalski J, Sandler HM, Northouse L, Hembroff L, Lin X, Greenfield TK, Litwin MS, Saigal CS, Mahadevan A, Klein E, Kibel A, Pisters LL, Kuban D, Kaplan I, Wood D, Ciezki J, Shah N, Wei JT. Quality of life and satisfaction with outcome among prostate-cancer survivors. N Engl J Med. 2008;358(12):1250–61.
24. Dryzek JS. Discursive democracy: politics, policy and political science. Cambridge: Cambridge University Press; 1990.
25. Nyseth T, Jentoft S, Førde A, Bærenholdt JO, editors. Borderline of disciplines. [I disiplinens grenseland. Tverrfaglighet I teori og praksis]. Bergen: Fagbokforlaget; 2007.
26. Smelser NJ. Interdiciplinary in theory and practice. In: Camic C, Joas H, editors. The dialogical turn: new roles for sociology in the postdisciplinary age. Lanham, MD: Rowman & Littlefield, 2004, pp. 43–64.
27. Vaizey CJ, Carapeti E, Cahill JA, Kamm MA. Prospective comparison of faecal incontinence grading systems. Gut. 1999;44(1):77–80.
28. Jorge JM, Wexner SD. Etiology and management of fecal incontinence. Dis Colon Rectum. 1993;36(1):77–97.
29. Cotterill N, Norton C, Avery KN, Abrams P, Donovan JL. A patient-centered approach to developing a comprehensive symptom and quality of life assessment of anal incontinence. Dis Colon Rectum. 2008;51(1):82–7.
30. Emmertsen KJ, Laurberg S. Low anterior resection syndrome score: development and validation of a symptom-based scoring system for bowel dysfunction after low anterior resection for rectal cancer. Ann Surg. 2012;255(5):922–8. doi:10.1097/SLA.0b013e31824f1c21.
31. Knowles CH, Eccersley AJ, Scott SM, Walker SM, Reeves B, Lunniss PJ. Linear discriminant analysis of symptoms in patients with chronic constipation: validation of a new scoring system (KESS). Dis Colon Rectum. 2000;43(10):1419–26.
32. Agachan F, Chen T, Pfeifer J, Reissman P, Wexner SD. A constipation scoring system to simplify evaluation and management of constipated patients. Dis Colon Rectum. 1996;39(6):681–5.
33. Renzi A, Brillantino A, Di Sarno G, d'Aniello F. Five-item score for obstructed defecation syndrome: study of validation. Surg Innov. 2013;20(2):119–25. doi:10.1177/1553350612446354.
34. Abrams P, Avery K, Gardener N, Donovan J, ICIQ Advisory Board. The International Consultation on Incontinence Modular Questionnaire: www.iciq.net. J Urol. 2006;175:1063–6.
35. Roos AM, Sultan AH, Thakar R. Sexual problems in the gynecology clinic: are we making a mountain out of a molehill? Int Urogynecol J. 2012;23(2):145–52. doi:10.1007/s00192-011-1516-y.
36. Rosen RC, Cappelleri JC, Smith MD, Lipsky J, Peña BM. Development and evaluation of an abridged, 5-item version of the International Index of Erectile Function (IIEF-5) as a diagnostic tool for erectile dysfunction. Int J Impot Res. 1999;11(6):319–26.

Part II

Urologic

7 Anatomy of the Pelvis

Panagiotis S. Kallidonis, Evangelos N. Liatsikos,
Stavros Kontogiannis, Jochen Neuhaus,
Iason Kyriazis, Thilo Schwalenberg,
and Jens-Uwe Stolzenburg

7.1 Introduction

The field of pelvic anatomy is extensive and the intention of the current chapter is to provide a brief summary of the general pelvic anatomy, with special focus on recently obtained anatomical evidence. Specifically, the neuroanatomy of the pelvis has been extensively investigated recently since it is important to the performance of pelvic surgery. The neuroanatomy plays a significant role in the two major complications that affect patients' quality of life post-operatively: erectile dysfunction and urinary incontinence. The trifecta (cancer free surgery, erectile function and urinary continence preservation) is the desired outcome after each procedure [1]. As a result, the current chapter reviews the latest findings in the field of pelvic neuroanatomy. In addition, the so-called "neurovascular bundle" and the external sphincter mechanism are particularly discussed.

It is important to mention that the knowledge of neuroanatomy is useful not only to the urologic surgeons but also to surgeons of the rectum and gynecologists. These surgeons face the same issues while performing pelvic. Erectile dysfunction after a mesorectal resection and bladder dysfunction after an extended radical hysterectomy is not uncommon [2, 3]. The adequate knowledge of the traditional anatomy of the pelvis and the current findings on the neuroanatomy of the pelvis set the background for procedures with lower complication rates.

7.2 Anterior Abdominal Wall

Five tissue-anatomical lines serve as landmarks of the posterior aspect of the abdominal wall during the performance surgery. The first is the median umbilical ligament in the midline, which connects the urinary bladder with the umbilicus. From an embryological point of view, it is formed by the obliterated urachus of the fetus [4]. The two embryological umbilical arteries become the two medial umbilical ligaments, which are both formed laterally to the midline. The spaces between these lines are called the supra-vesical fossa and they are located where the superior vesical artery is normally identified in radical cystectomy. The other two lines on the posterior abdominal wall are the lateral umbilical ligaments or folds, which are situated more laterally than the medial umbilical ligaments. Under and

P.S. Kallidonis, MD, PhD(Urol), MSc(Clin Pharma) (✉)
E.N. Liatsikos, MD, PhD • S. Kontogiannis, MD
I. Kyriazis, MD
Department of Urology, University of Patras, Rion, Patras, Greece
e-mail: pkallidonis@yahoo.com

J. Neuhaus, MD, PhD • T. Schwalenberg, MD, PhD
J.-U. Stolzenburg, MD, PhD, FRCS (Ed), FRCS (Eng)
Department of Urology, University of Leipzig, Leipzig, Germany

H.R.H. Patel et al. (eds.), *Pelvic Cancer Surgery: Modern Breakthroughs and Future Advances*,
DOI 10.1007/978-1-4471-4258-4_7, © Springer-Verlag London 2015

lateral to the umbilical folds lie the inferior epigastric vessels, which derive from the external iliac vessels just before the inguinal ligament. The inferior epigastric vessels demarcate the direct from the indirect inguinal hernia. The inguinal rings and the external iliac vessels are also useful for the orientation in the pelvis. Another feature of surgical interest is the lacunar ligament, which connects the inguinal ligament to the superior pubic ramus. The lacunar ligament is the caudal end of the pelvic lymphadenectomy during radical prostatectomy or cystectomy [5].

7.3 Male Pelvis

In comparison with the female pelvis, the male pelvis is narrower and contains the rectum, the vas deferens, the seminal vesicles, the prostate, the ureters and the urinary bladder. The parietal peritoneum covers the upper part of the urinary bladder and the anterior part of the rectum and forms the recto-vesical space (the space of Douglas in the case of the female pelvis). The space beneath the peritoneum and between the bladder and the pubis is called the Retzius' space. One of the pelvic fascias is the endopelvic fascia which represents the visceral layer of the pelvic fascia. The puboprostatic ligaments are formed by the fusion of the endopelvic fascia and the prostatic fascia (fascial envelope of the prostate). Between the rectum and the prostate lies the Denonvilliers' fascia which is created by the deepening of the two layers of the peritoneum down to the pelvic floor. The possibility of separating the two layers during radical prostatectomy is questionable [6, 7].

7.4 Female Pelvis

The female pelvis is wider than the male one and contains the urinary bladder, the distal ureters, the rectum, the ovaries, the oviducts, the uterus and the vagina. The uterus is located between the urinary bladder and the rectum and the vagina between the urethra and the perineum. The peritoneum covers the upper part of the urinary bladder, the uterus and the anterior part of the upper two thirds of the rectum. It therefore creates two spaces, the recto-uterine space (Pouch of Douglas) and the utero-vesical peritoneal space. Two ligaments are associated with the uterus: the broad ligaments and the round ligaments of the uterus. Parts of the distal third of the ureters along with uterine arteries and veins are included in the broad ligament. The iatrogenic injury of the ureter represents a major complication of gynecologic surgery [8].

7.5 Pelvic Floor

The pelvic diaphragm is made by the levator ani muscle and the ischiococcygeus muscle. The levator ani muscle is made of the puborectal muscle, the iliooccygeus muscle and pubococcygeus muscle. The opening for the anus and the urethra for both males and females and the vagina for the females is shaped by the levator ani. The main innervation is derived from the sacral plexus, while the pudendal nerve plays some role in the innervation of the pudendal muscle. In females, the intact pelvic diaphragm musculature (including the urethral sphincter) is important for urinary continence and the understanding of their relationship may propose new methods for the management of urinary incontinence [9].

7.6 The Urinary Bladder

The layers of the urinary bladder wall are: the mucosa layer with transitional epithelial cells, the muscle layer with three layers of muscle fibers, and surrounding adipose and connective tissue. The bladder neck and the trigone have only two muscle layers. The lymph node drainage of the urinary bladder is made by the external, internal and common iliac lymph nodes and the lymph nodes of the obturator fossa.

The nervous system of the lower urinary tract is quite complex. Both somatic and autonomic components participate in bladder storage and emptying phase [10]. The inferior hypogastric plexus provides the bladder with autonomic nerve fibers. The sympathetic fibers result in the filling of the bladder by inhibiting the detrusor muscle and contracting the smooth portion of the external sphincter ("Musculus sphincter urethrae glaber") which provides continence during the bladder storage [11, 12]. The pudendal nerve stimulation (S2–S4) contracts the striated external sphincter ("Musculus sphincter urethrae transversostriatus") which provides continence during sudden increase in intra-abdominal pressure (i.e. cough, laugh) and is called guarding or continence reflex [10, 13]. The parasympathetic fibers (emerging from the S2–S4) induce the contraction of the detrusor.

7.7 The Prostate

The prostatic gland includes the prostatic urethra with a length of approximately 3 cm. The endoscopic classification of the prostatic lobes into lateral and middle lobe has been replaced by the histopathological classification of central, peripheral, transitional and anterior fibromuscular zone [14]. The blood supply of the prostate derives from the inferior vesical and the middle rectal artery as well as some smaller vessels that perforate the gland directly. An additional pudendal artery can be found in nearly a quarter of the patients [15].

The prostatic venous plexus or dorsal venous plexus of the prostate (Santorini's plexus) communicates with the venous plexus of the bladder and the dorsal veins of the penis. The lymphatic drainage of the prostate and bladder is received by the internal, external and common iliac lymph nodes as well as the obturator fossa lymph nodes.

7.8 The Neuroanatomy of the Pelvis

The Pelvic Plexus

The neuroanatomy of the pelvis is still a point of interest for researchers in urology, rectal surgery and gynecology. The preservation of erectile function, urinary continence and the bladder function plays a major role in patients' quality of life. As seen in Fig. 7.1, the sympathetic fibers derive from T10–12 and L1–2. In addition, the sacral parasympathetic fibers emerge as pelvic splanchnic nerves as clearly illustrated in Fig. 7.2. The pelvic plexus (also called inferior hypogas-

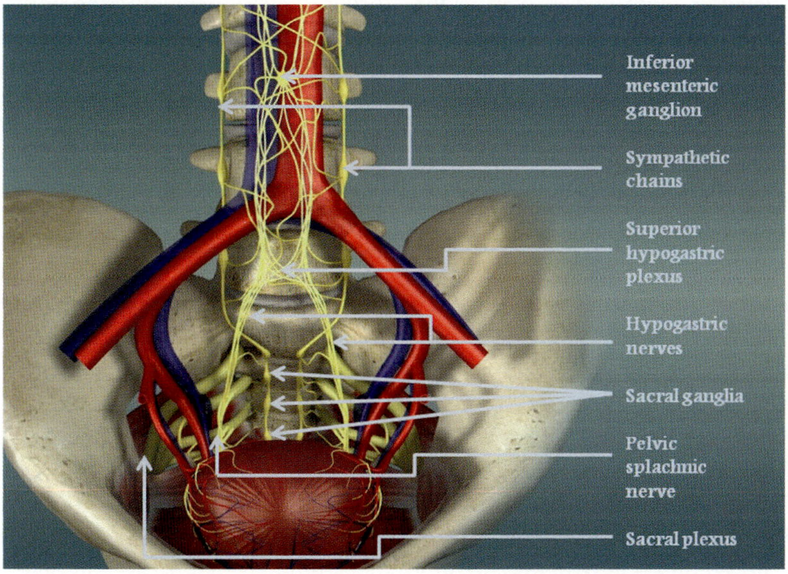

Fig. 7.1 Sympathetic and parasympathetic nervous fibers of the pelvis (Copyright © 2007; Jens-Uwe Stolzenburg and Moonsoft)

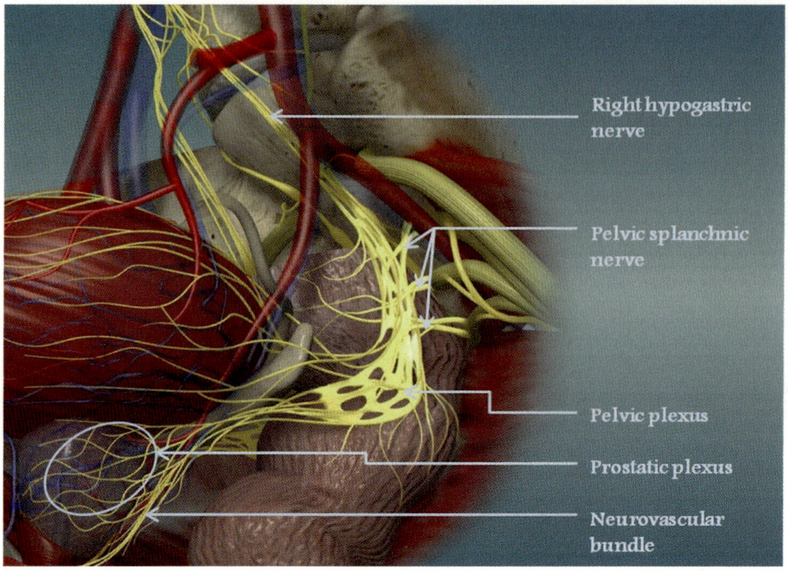

Fig. 7.2 Nerves of the pelvis (Copyright: Moonsoft and Stolzenburg (2007))

tric plexus) provides autonomic innervations of the pelvic viscera. The pelvic plexus can be defined as an aggregation of nerve fibers and ganglion cells that are distributed between the pelvic wall and the pelvic viscera. It is responsible for the autonomic innervation of the pelvic organs and the external genitalia. The nerves are derived from the superior hypogastric plexus, as well as the sacral sympathetic chain and also from the parasympathetic pelvic splanchnic nerves. It is located between the seminal vesicles and the ureters dorsally and the prostate and the rectum antero-laterally (Figs. 7.1 and 7.2). This region is at risk of injury in radical cystectomy, anti-reflux ureteral surgery and rectal surgery [16].

The Neurovascular Bundles

The cavernosal nerves, which contain branches of the autonomic nervous system, are responsible for the erectile function. The location of the large percentage of these autonomic nerve fibers is postero-laterally to the prostate, postero-laterally to the sphincter of the urethra and antero-laterally also to the rectum. These fibers can only be recognized by the accompanying vascular structures and are called neurovascular bundles (NVBs). The course of the NVBs is depicted in Fig. 7.3.

It is really interesting that the first surgeons who described erectile dysfunction after pelvic surgery were general surgeons that performed surgery to the rectum [17]. Surgeons performing resections of the rectum are following the Denonvilliers' fascia for the ventral dissection in order to avoid damaging the urinary and erectile function [18]. Walsh and Donker were the first to describe the NVBs and described the surgical technique to preserve these anatomical structures [19]. Each NVB is considered as the structure that contains the autonomic fibers to innervate the corpora cavernosa. It is situated between the lateral pelvic fascia and prostatic fascia (Fig. 7.4). It extends postero-laterally to the prostatic gland. There have been some recent studies showing some variations. A fan-like distribution is found in several cases, rather than a distinct location of the bundle [20, 21]. The further understanding of the pelvic fascias and the location of the NVBs has motivated surgeons to develop new techniques of nerve preservation [22–25] (Fig. 7.5). During the interfascial prostatectomy, the neurovascular bundle is preserved by incising the endopelvic fascia and the periprostatic fascia is excised along with the prostate.

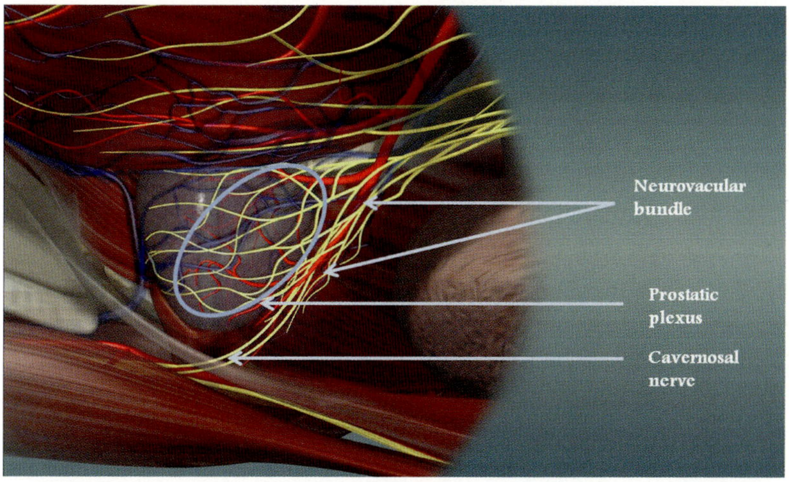

Fig. 7.3 The course of nerves and vessels around the prostate (Copyright © 2007; Jens-Uwe Stolzenburg and Moonsoft)

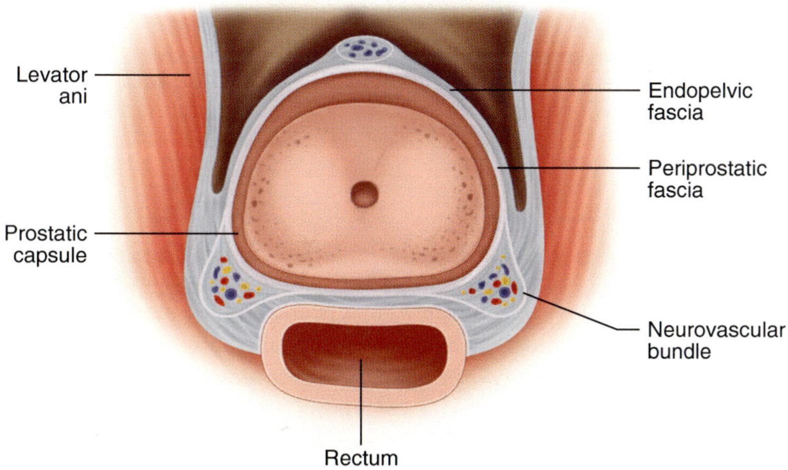

Fig. 7.4 The anatomical landmarks for the preservation of the neurovascular bundles

In the intrafascial technique, the dissection is performed right on the capsule of the prostate and the periprostatic fascia is not excised with the surgical specimen.

An accurate description of the NVB was investigated recently, dividing the NVB in three sections: the anterior section which supplies the cavernosal nerves, the lateral section which supplies the levator ani and the posterolateral section that supplies the rectum [26, 27]. This anatomic segmentation can lead to different surgical approaches in the future, such us partial preservation of the bundle or grafting [16].

Although, the NVBs are considered to carry the nerve fibers for erectile function and their excision results in erectile dysfunction, only a small portion of the patients who undergo non-nerve sparing radical prostatectomy have erectile function postoperatively. A possible explanation is that there is some additional autonomic nerve fibers that innervate the cavernosal body or that there are anastomotic bridges between the pudendal nerves and the cavernosal nerves [28, 29].

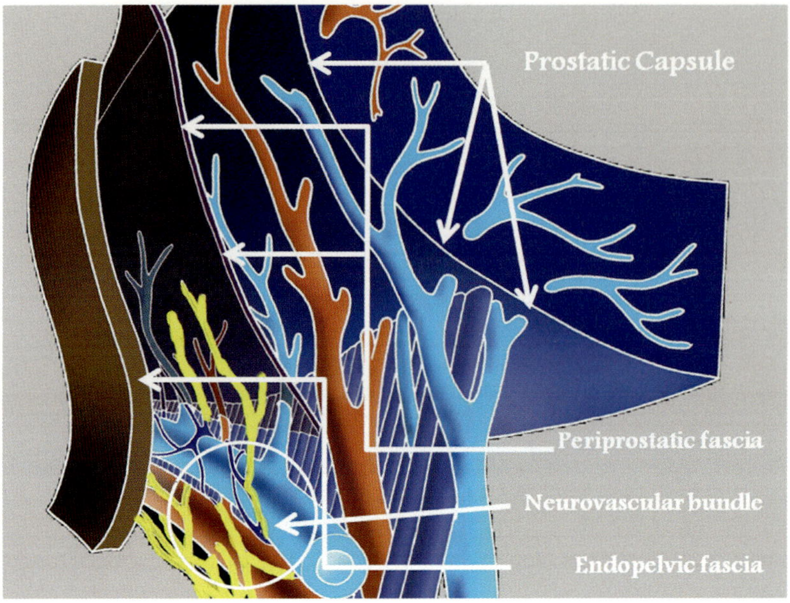

Fig. 7.5 The prostatic fascias and the neurovascular bundle. The dissection for interfascial nerve preservation takes place between the pelvic fascia and the periprostatic fascia. Thus, the periprostatic fascia is excised with the specimen. The intrafascial dissection takes place between the periprostatic fascia and the capsule of the prostate. The prostate with the capsule is only removed. The neurovascular bundles remain intact in both dissections

The Cavernosal and Pudendal Nerves

The course of the cavernosal nerves is depicted in Fig. 7.6. They are located at a few millimeters from the prostatic capsule at the 5 and 7 o'clock positions. The medial branches supply nerve fibers to the external urethral sphincter, while the lateral branches supply the corpora cavernosa. The course of the pudendal nerves is seen in Fig. 7.7. It is a somatosensory nerve that innervates the bulbospongiosus muscle, the ischiocavernosus muscle and the striated component of the external urethral sphincter. This nerve is often injured during vaginal delivery or pelvic bone fractures [16].

The External Urinary Sphincter

The autonomic innervation of the urethral sphincter is not well defined. Nerve fibers are supplied by the NVBs, while other branches derive from the pudendal nerves [30]. It seems that the urethral sphincter in males, unlike to females, is independent of the muscle tone of the pelvic floor [31]. The distance of the point where the pudendal nerves enter the muscle differs from 3 to 13 mm [32]. The external sphincter has two parts: the external striated segment and the internal smooth muscle segment. For the first segment, the term "rhabdosphincter" is widely used. The posterior part of the striated muscle is interrupted by a tendinous median dorsal raphe [33]. The reconstruction of this dorsal raphe of the posterior rhabdosphincter may increase the early recovery of continence after radical prostatectomy [34, 35]. The internal segment of the sphincter can be divided also to a layer with the muscle fibers oriented in a circumferential plane and another in the longitudinal plane [31]. Continence should probably be attributed to the contraction of external sphincter with the smooth

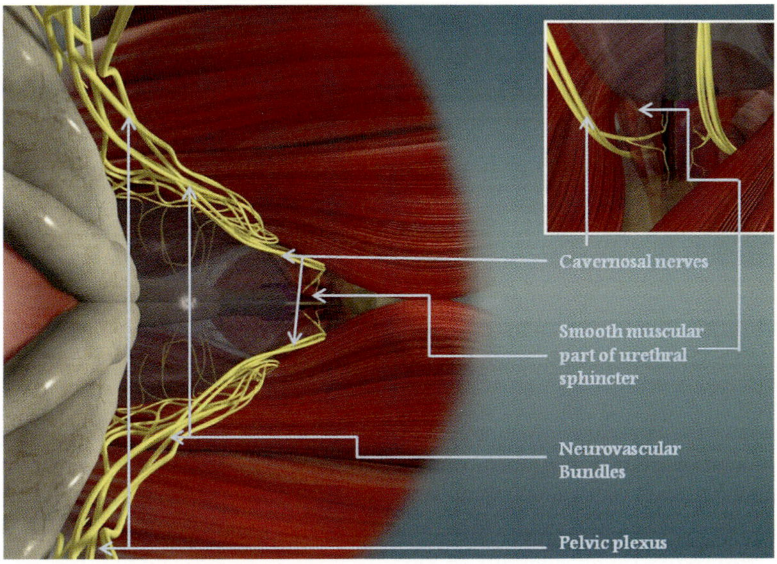

Fig. 7.6 The course of the nerve fibers towards the corpora cavernosa (Copyright © 2007; Jens-Uwe Stolzenburg and Moonsoft)

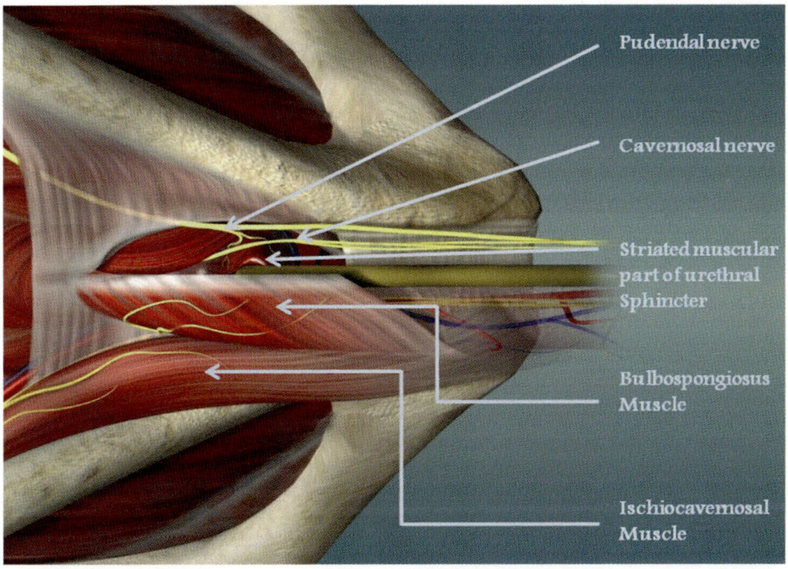

Fig. 7.7 The pudendal nerve and its motor branches to pelvic muscles (Copyright © 2007; Jens-Uwe Stolzenburg and Moonsoft)

component to provide "basic" continence and the striated component to provide continence during "stress conditions" such as coughing. In addition, the sphincteric system is supported by the surrounding musculofascial structures of the pelvic diaphragm [12, 36, 27].

Conclusion

The development of radical pelvic surgery led to the further investigation of the pelvic anatomy, in an attempt to prevent the several complications of pelvic procedures. Special interest has been shown to the neuroanatomy of the pelvis, as the autonomic nervous system plays a significant role in the bladder, rectum and erectile function as well as urinary continence. A major breakthrough was the description of the NVBs [9]. The nerve-sparing technique significantly improved the recovery of erectile function. Several refinements of surgical technique have been presented in the recent years in an attempt to achieve earlier recovery of urinary continence. All these techniques are based on the recent knowledge on the anatomy of the pelvis. Further investigations are needed for the complete depiction of the structural and functional anatomy of the pelvis and improvement the surgical techniques.

Key Points

- The anatomy of the pelvis is important not only to urologists but also to gynecologists and general surgeons. A multidisciplinary concept of pelvic surgery is of fundamental importance.
- The five tissue lines of the umbilical ligaments are the anatomical landmarks for orientation during laparoscopic procedures in the pelvis.
- The inguinal rings, external iliac and epigastric vessels are also additional landmarks. The inferior epigastric vessels demarcate direct from indirect inguinal hernia.
- The male pelvis is narrower than the female pelvis.
- The pelvic plexus is prone to injury in radical cystectomy, antireflux ureteral surgery and rectal surgery.
- The nerve fibers of the cavernosal nerves are mainly supplied by the neurovascular bundles which are located posterolaterally to the prostate.
- The interfascial technique of nerve-sparing includes the periprostatic fascia in the excision, while the intrafascial technique preserves the periprostatic fascia.
- An anatomical segmentation has been presented recently. This may lead to partial preservation of the neurovascular bundles in the future.
- The external urethral sphincter seems to be independent of the pelvic floor muscle tone in the male.
- The external urethral sphincter has one outer striated muscle segment and one inner smooth muscle segment.

References

1. Xylinas E, Durand X, Ploussard G, Campeggi A, Allory Y, Vordos D, Hoznek A, Abbou CC, de la Taille A, Salomon L. Evaluation of combined oncologic and functional outcomes after robotic-assisted laparoscopic extraperitoneal radical prostatectomy: trifecta rate of achieving continence, potency and cancer control. Urol Oncol. 2013;31(1):99–103.
2. Kauff DW, Kempski O, Huppert S, Koch KP, Hoffmann KP, Lang H, Kneist W. Total mesorectal excision—does the choice of dissection technique have an impact on pelvic autonomic nerve preservation? J Gastrointest Surg. 2012;16(6):1218–24.
3. Chen C, Li W, Li F, Liu P, Zhou J, Lu L, Su G, Li X, Guo Y, Huang L. Classical and nerve-sparing radical hysterectomy: an evaluation of the nerve trauma in cardinal ligament. Gynecol Oncol. 2012;125(1): 245–51.
4. Sulak O, Cankara N, Malas MA, Cetin E, Desdicioglu K. Anatomical development of the normal urachus during the fetal period. Saudi Med J. 2008;29(1): 30–5.
5. Heidenreich A, Ohlmann CH, Polyakov S. Anatomical extent of pelvic lymphadenectomy in patients undergoing radical prostatectomy. Eur Urol. 2007;52(1): 29–37.
6. Church JM, Raudkivi PJ, Hill GL. The surgical anatomy of the rectum—a review with particular relevance to the hazards of rectal mobilisation. Int J Colorectal Dis. 1987;2(3):158–66.
7. Boileau MA. Exposure of puboprostatic ligaments and dorsal vein complex during radical retropubic prostatectomy. Urol Clin North Am. 1990;17(1): 47–8.

8. Abboudi H, Ahmed K, Royle J, Khan MS, Dasgupta P, N'Dow J. Ureteric injury: a challenging condition to diagnose and manage. Nat Rev Urol. 2013; 10(2):108–15.
9. Jung J, Ahn HK, Huh Y. Clinical and functional anatomy of the urethral sphincter. Int Neurourol J. 2012;16(3):102–6.
10. Holstege G. Micturition and the soul. J Comp Neurol. 2005;493(1):15–20.
11. Dorschner W, Stolzenburg JU, Neuhaus J. Structure and function of the bladder neck. Adv Anat Embryol Cell Biol. 2001;159(III–XII):1–109.
12. Schwalenberg T, Neuhaus J, Dartsch M, Weissenfels P, Löffler S, Stolzenburg JU. Functional anatomy of the male continence mechanism. Urologe A. 2010;49(4):472–80.
13. Chancellor MB, Perkin H, Yoshimura N. Recent advances in the neurophysiology of stress urinary incontinence. Scand J Urol Nephrol. 2005;39(1):21–4.
14. Selman SH. The McNeal prostate: a review. Urology. 2011;78(6):1224–8.
15. Park BJ, Sung DJ, Kim MJ, Cho SB, Kim YH, Chung KB, Kang SH, Cheon J. The incidence and anatomy of accessory pudendal arteries as depicted on multidetector-row CT angiography: clinical implications of preoperative evaluation for laparoscopic and robot-assisted radical prostatectomy. Korean J Radiol. 2009;10(6):587–95.
16. Schwalenberg T, Neuhaus J, Liatsikos E, Winkler M, Löffler S, Stolzenburg JU. Neuroanatomy of the male pelvis in respect to radical prostatectomy including three-dimensional visualization. BJU Int. 2010;105(1):21–7.
17. Davis LP, Jelenko C. Sexual function after abdominoperineal resection. South Med J. 1975;68(4):422–6.
18. Clausen N, Wolloscheck T, Konerding MA. How to optimize autonomic nerve preservation in total mesorectal excision: clinical topography and morphology of pelvic nerves and fasciae. World J Surg. 2008;32(8):1768–75.
19. Walsh PC, Donker PJ. Impotence following radical prostatectomy: insight into etiology and prevention. J Urol. 1982;128(3):492–7.
20. Walz J, Burnett AL, Costello AJ, Eastham JA, Graefen M, Guillonneau B, Menon M, Montorsi F, Myers RP, Rocco B, Villers A. A critical analysis of the current knowledge of surgical anatomy related to optimization of cancer control and preservation of continence and erection in candidates for radical prostatectomy. Eur Urol. 2010;57(2):179–92.
21. Kiyoshima K, Yokomizo A, Yoshida T, Tomita K, Yonemasu H, Nakamura M, Oda Y, Naito S, Hasegawa Y. Anatomical features of periprostatic tissue and its surroundings: a histological analysis of 79 radical retropubic prostatectomy specimens. Jpn J Clin Oncol. 2004;34(8):463–8.
22. Ghani KR, Trinh Q-D, Menon M. Vattikuti Institute prostatectomy-technique in 2012. J Endourol. 2012;26(12):1558–65.
23. Chabert CC, Merrilees DA, Neill MG, Eden CG. Curtain dissection of the lateral prostatic fascia and potency after laparoscopic radical prostatectomy: a veil of mystery. BJU Int. 2008;101(10):1285–8.
24. Stolzenburg JU, Schwalenberg T, Horn L-C, Neuhaus J, Constantinides C, Liatsikos EN. Anatomical landmarks of radical prostatecomy. Eur Urol. 2007;51(3):629–39.
25. Stolzenburg JU, Kallidonis P, Minh D, Dietel A, Häfner T, Dimitriou D, Al-Aown A, Kyriazis I, Liatsikos EN. Endoscopic extraperitoneal radical prostatectomy: evolution of the technique and experience with 2400 cases. J Endourol. 2009;23(9): 1467–72.
26. Costello AJ, Brooks M, Cole OJ. Anatomical studies of the neurovascular bundle and cavernosal nerves. BJU Int. 2004;94(7):1071–6.
27. Walsh PC. Anatomical studies of the neurovascular bundle and cavernosal nerves. J Urol. 2005;174(2):566.
28. Akita K, Sakamoto H, Sato T. Origins and courses of the nervous branches to the male urethral sphincter. Surg Radiol Anat Sra. 2003;25(5–6):387–92.
29. Breza J, Aboseif SR, Orvis BR, Lue TF, Tanagho EA. Detailed anatomy of penile neurovascular structures: surgical significance. J Urol. 1989;141(2): 437–43.
30. Strasser H, Bartsch G. Anatomy and innervation of the rhabdosphincter of the male urethra. Semin Urol Oncol. 2000;18(1):2–8.
31. Dorschner W, Biesold M, Schmidt F, Stolzenburg JU. The dispute about the external sphincter and the urogenital diaphragm. J Urol. 1999;162(6): 1942–5.
32. Narayan P, Konety B, Aslam K, Aboseif S, Blumenfeld W, Tanagho E. Neuroanatomy of the external urethral sphincter: implications for urinary continence preservation during radical prostate surgery. J Urol. 1995;153(2):337–41.
33. Rocco F, Carmignani L, Acquati P, Gadda F, Dell'Orto P, Rocco B, Casellato S, Gazzano G, Consonni D. Early continence recovery after open radical prostatectomy with restoration of the posterior aspect of the rhabdosphincter. Eur Urol. 2007;52(2):376–83.
34. Rocco F, Carmignani L, Acquati P, Gadda F, Dell'Orto P, Rocco B, Bozzini G, Gazzano G, Morabito A. Restoration of posterior aspect of rhabdosphincter shortens continence time after radical retropubic prostatectomy. J Urol. 2006;175(6):2201–6.
35. Menon M, Muhletaler F, Campos M, Peabody JO. Assessment of early continence after reconstruction of the periprostatic tissues in patients undergoing computer assisted (robotic) prostatectomy: results of a 2 group parallel randomized controlled trial. J Urol. 2008;180(3):1018–23.
36. Burnett AL, Mostwin JL. In situ anatomical study of the male urethral sphincteric complex: relevance to continence preservation following major pelvic surgery. J Urol. 1998;160(4):1301–6.

Pelvic Lymphadenectomy for Prostate and Bladder Cancer

8

Christian P. Pavlovich, Michael A. Gorin, Philip M. Pierorazio, and Jeffrey K. Mullins

8.1 Introduction

Pelvic lymph node dissection (PLND) has been a part of radical prostatectomy (RP) for prostate cancer since the modern retropubic surgical approach was popularized in the 1980s. Prior to this, and even in some cases today, PLND was used as a staging procedure before RP. PLND has also been an essential component of radical cystectomy (RC) for bladder cancer since the inception of that operation. Its roles as an adjunct to primary organ extirpation for the surgical treatment of both prostate and bladder cancer include providing more accurate staging information, as well as increasing the likelihood of cure in cases of N1 disease. Its application in cases with gross and/or bulky prostate or bladder cancer-related adenopathy is not recommended; such disease is generally neither cured nor ameliorated in any appreciable way by PLND, and it is also riskier in such disease states. While it is clear that the data favor performing a PLND in most prostate and bladder cancer patients going to surgery, controversy currently exists regarding the role of extended-template PLNDs for patients at increased risk of nodal metastasis due to adverse clinicopathologic features associated with their prostate or bladder cancer.

Over the last few decades, there has been a marked downward stage migration of prostate cancer but little comparable downward stage migration for bladder cancer in the United States. These changes are largely due to the advent of prostate-specific antigen (PSA) testing and the more widespread prostate cancer screening of the last two decades. For prostate cancer, many surgical series from the United States have come to consist predominantly of patients with nonpalpable cancers of low-moderate grade and PSA levels well under 10. Whether these patients benefit from PLND at all is unclear and data suggest otherwise. Conversely, men with intermediate-to-high risk prostate cancer appear more likely to benefit from PLND, both prognostically and perhaps even therapeutically. As the pendulum now shifts away from screening, more advanced disease states will likely present and continue to require RP with concomitant PLND. For bladder cancer, the story is somewhat different, and PLND has and is likely to remain integral to RC for the foreseeable future. The controversy here is over the extent of the lymphadenectomy and not on whether one is necessary or beneficial.

In this chapter we plan to review the indications, benefits and complications/risks of PLND associated with RP and RC for prostate and bladder cancer respectively, discuss limited and extended templates, and present data from new imaging modalities that may allow for better

C.P. Pavlovich, MD (✉) • M.A. Gorin, MD
P.M. Pierorazio, MD • J.K. Mullins, MD
James Buchanan Brady Urological Institute, Johns Hopkins University School of Medicine, Baltimore, MD, USA
e-mail: cpavlov2@jhmi.edu

H.R.H. Patel et al. (eds.), *Pelvic Cancer Surgery: Modern Breakthroughs and Future Advances*,
DOI 10.1007/978-1-4471-4258-4_8,

patient selection for PLND and perhaps for targeted lymphadenectomy as the data matures.

8.2 PLND for Prostate Cancer

Who Needs a PLND?

True pathologic lymph node status remains unknown in the vast majority of contemporary men presenting with clinically localized prostate cancer because of the inability of standard imaging to accurately predict lymph node involvement (LNI). Conventional CT and MR are generally unreliable in predicting pathologic lymph node status, either for the detection of small metastatic deposits (<1–1.5 cm) or for detecting pathologic enlargement, as enlarged pelvic LNs do not reliably indicate the presence of metastasis [1]. Whereas there exist extremely promising modalities, such as superparamagnetic nanoparticle-MRI lymphography [2, 3], these are not currently FDA-approved in the United States and do not appear ready for routine use in any case. Because of the current limitations regarding imaging and LN status determination, pelvic lymphadenectomy has been and still remains the gold standard for detecting LNI in prostate cancer. Whereas historically, all patients underwent PLND at the time of RP, both the necessity of a PLND and its extent have more recently come under scrutiny.

Various preoperative staging nomograms have been designed to predict LNI and thus identify patients that may most benefit from PLND. The predictive ability of any nomogram is limited by the data used to create it, which, for predicting LN status, includes the data obtained from either a series of patients generally treated with limited-template PLND, or from more rare series where extended PLND is the norm. Using such nomograms and other available data, expert panels from the AUA, NCCN and EAU have created guidelines suggesting in whom PLND should be performed. The ultimate goals of these guidelines/nomograms are to help predict who is at risk of LNI, and to potentially predict who might derive a therapeutic benefit from lymphadenectomy. The NCCN recently updated their guidelines on the treatment of prostate cancer to include a recommendation that any man with a 2 % or greater chance of LNI undergo PLND, and furthermore the NCCN recommends that if PLND is to be performed that it should be extended [4]. Their rationale is that extended PLND detects metastases twice as often as PLND based on more limited templates and therefore is more likely to cure patients with occult nodal disease, most of whom are at greater than 2 % of predicted LNI by current nomograms. Conversely, data from both the Cleveland Clinic and CaPSURE suggest that omitting a limited template PLND from men at low risk of LNI does not compromise 5–10 year biochemical free recurrence [5, 6].

Most nomograms [7–11] including the well-known Partin tables [11] and Memorial Sloan-Kettering (MSK) nomograms [7], predict pathologic stage using preoperative clinical stage, biopsy Gleason score, preoperative PSA, and were derived using pathologic data from RP and limited PLND templates. Select nomograms have been created specifically with an intent to predict LNI, and have included more detailed information from preoperative biopsies, such as number of positive cores, and, in some cases, have been based on data from more extended lymphadenectomy [7–10]. The Partin tables were updated in 2007 and again in 2013 to more accurately reflect the general stage shift toward less advanced cancers [11]. The 2007 update demonstrated an accuracy of 0.89 in predicting pathologic stage in a large population (n = 5,730) where 1 % had positive LNs. Subsequently, a 2010 external validation of these tables examined the predictive ability of the tables in 11,185 men selected from the National Cancer Institute Surveillance, Epidemiology and End Results database who underwent RP. They found the area under the curve was 0.77 in predicting LNI in this expanded multi-center population [12]. Haese et al. applied the Hamburg nomogram for predicting LNI to a similar dataset from Johns Hopkins, and externally validated their predictive model in that fashion [13]. Cagiannos et al. at Memorial Sloan-Kettering developed a similar predictive nomogram more specifically targeting

Table 8.1 Different predictions from three nomograms that are commonly used to predict risk of positive lymph nodes

Nomogram (PLND type) used to derive % risk of finding positive LNs at RP	Low risk patient: cT1c, PSA 2.5, Gleason 3+3, 3/12 positive cores (%)	Intermed. Risk patient : cT2b, PSA 11, Gleason 3+4, 6/12 positive cores (%)	High risk patient: cT2b, PSA 15, Gleason 4+4, 8/12 positive cores (%)
Partin (standard PLND)	0	9	20
MSK (standard PLND)	1.1	6.4	14
Briganti (extended PLND)	<2.5	7.5	45

LNI that was based on limited PLND data from multiple institutions [7]. Their predictive accuracy was 0.78 based on 5,510 patients and a 3.7 % rate of LNI.

Briganti et al. have created one of the few nomograms based on ePLND, and have argued that the probability of correctly identifying those with LNI is in part dependent on the number of nodes sampled, a finding replicated in current versions of the online MSK nomogram [14]. An update of the Briganti nomogram using a population of 588 patients who all underwent extended PLND resulted in a nomogram demonstrating a predictive accuracy after bootstrap of 87.6 % for LNI [7]. The parameters used in the final nomogram were PSA, primary and secondary Gleason grade, clinical stage, and percentage of positive cores from the initial prostate needle biopsy. Percentage of positive cores was the greatest predictor of LNI. As this nomogram was based on an extended PLND series it may well be the most accurate operationally in determining true risk of LNI and is recommended for use when deciding whether or not to perform PLND.

For comparison's sake, the results from representative nomograms are summarized below using a sample patient representing each of the low, intermediate and high risk categories from the D'Amico classification system [15]. The predictive percentage of patients with LNI using the Partin tables, MSK and Briganti nomograms, respectively, for patients categorized using the D'Amico risk stratification are tabulated below for a 60 year old man with varying risk states of newly diagnosed prostate cancer (Table 8.1).

The nomograms are relatively consistent in men with low to intermediate-risk disease, but they are not in high risk disease states. The significantly higher LNI predictions using the Briganti nomogram are likely, in part, due to the ePLND data used to generate it since the probability of finding additional positive nodes increases as more nodes are sampled. The question to be asked for such patients is, at what point do the complications associated with an extensive node dissection outweigh any potential benefits? And what is an extended template PLND for prostate cancer?

Templates

The lymphatic drainage of the prostate has been well-described and confirmed by classic-era scintigraphic studies. More recently Cellini et al. demonstrated ascending, lateral, and posterior ducts which drain into external iliac nodes, internal iliac and obturator nodes, and sub-aortic sacral nodes, respectively [16]. Mattei at al. demonstrated that one third of the landing sites would be resected by a limited PLND and two thirds would be resected by an extended PLND [17]. Despite this detailed understanding, quite a bit of research has gone into determining which of these nodal groups, if any, represents the primary landing site for metastatic prostate cancer. In a study of metastatic cancer deposits from a cohort of 88 relatively high-risk men with pN+ disease after RP and extended pelvic lymphadenectomy, the most common site for metastasis (60 %) was the obturator fossa [18]. Overall however, 58 % had deposits in the internal iliac (hypogastric) and 36 % in the external iliac nodal areas, while 19 % had positive nodes in the hypogastric distribution alone. This broad spread of lymphatic metastases mirrors the broad drainage of lymph from the prostate gland, as nuclear medicine mapping studies have confirmed [17, 19].

In order to assess for nodal disease and perhaps achieve prostate cancer cure, several templates for PLND have been described. There is no value in performing PLND unilaterally for prostate cancer as drainage from the prostate is not limited to one side. A limited bilateral PLND can be considered the removal of the node-bearing tissue below the external iliac vein, out to the pelvic sidewall, bounded inferiorly by the obturator nerve, and medially by the bladder, collectively known as the *external iliac and obturator nodes*. A more standard PLND would consist of this dissection and in addition, all node-bearing tissue in the obturator fossa, deep to the obturator nerve and as proximal as feasible under the external iliac vein (the *obturator nodes*), although this template still consists of a limited sampling of nodes that drain the prostate. Finally, an extended PLND includes both of the above plus all fibro-fatty tissue surrounding the internal iliac vessels up to their insertion at the common iliac bifurcations (the *hypogastric or internal iliac nodes*); some surgeons even include the additional removal of sub-aortic and pre-sacral nodes in their definitions of ePLND. While the latter description is perhaps the most extensive in the literature, ePLND is most commonly considered to be a node dissection that involves the removal of all node-bearing tissue from an area bounded by the external iliac vein anteriorly, the pelvic sidewall laterally, the bladder wall medially, the floor of the pelvis posteriorly, Cooper's ligament distally, and the internal iliac artery proximally. There appears to be little indication and potential morbidity to resecting lymph nodes lateral to the external iliac vessels for prostate cancer.

Benefits

There is likely a diagnostic and prognostic benefit to PLND in terms of disease staging. It has become clear that as more nodes that are harvested, more positive nodes are found [14, 20–23]. In a cadaveric study, Weingartner et al. compared nodal counts in cadavers without prostate cancer subjected to PLND to actual counts resected during radical prostatectomy (RP) + PLND [1]. Their data support the notion that while there exists great heterogeneity in terms of LN number between patients, there exist, on average, some 20–25 nodes in the standard/limited template area if all nodes are carefully counted. Estimates of LN counts necessary for optimal staging accuracy have ranged from 20 to as high as 28 [1, 14]. The current literature supports what makes intuitive sense—that more extensive dissections result in an increasing LN yield, and that an increasing nodal yield detects higher rates LNI. Caveats regarding nodal yield are that (1) unless pathologists are focused on reporting lymph node counts, accuracy of number may not be a priority, (2) greater nodal yields have been noted when PLND are sent as separate packets (external iliac, obturator, etc.) vs. en bloc in the bladder cancer literature [24, 25], and (3) there is significant inter-patient variability of nodal count irrespective of cancer status [1].

There may also be therapeutic benefits to PLND in prostate cancer. Briganti et al. showed that patients with two or fewer positive LN on final pathology had significantly better outcomes at 15 years compared to those with more than two positive LN [26]. Daneshmand et al. similarly found that a positive node density of <20 % improved disease progression rates and survival [27]. Palapattu et al. found that 52 % of men with a positive node density of <15 %, Gleason score 7 or less, and negative seminal vesicle invasion remained free of BCF at 5 years [28]. Finally, several large series of patients with positive LN at RP as well as the well-known Messing study cohort have shown biochemical recurrence-free survivals of 14–20 % over the long-term in the absence of any adjuvant therapy [10, 22, 28, 29, 38, 39]. Keeping in mind the landing zone studies, it is likely that only those whose positive nodes all lie within the surgical dissection region truly benefit from a PLND.

If a low burden of nodal disease portends a good prognosis after PLND, then PLND might improve prostate cancer outcomes even in patients that were pN0 on routine pathologic analysis. If we are missing a significant number of occult nodes as suggested by Pagliarulo et al. from USC then the number of nodes removed and the extent of lymphadenectomy might improve outcomes in node negative patients [30]. This group carefully re-examined 3,914 "negative" nodes by immunohistochemistry in

274 pT3 patients, and found that 13.3 % of 180 patients originally defined as N0 harbored occult LN metastasis. These patients had significantly poorer survival rates than patients who were truly LN negative, and had outcomes comparable to men who had LNI on initial pathology. Overall however, it remains controversial whether the removal of nodes deemed negative actually reduces PSA recurrence. Studies of increasing lymph node yield in pN0 patients, a surrogate for extensiveness of PLND, remain conflicting, with reports indicating both an improvement as well as no effect on prostate cancer oncologic outcomes [22, 31]. Recent data from Murphy and colleagues appears to corroborate that LN yield is not a predictor of BCF in pN0 patients, even when the patients were stratified into high- and low-risk groups [32].

8.3 PLND for Bladder Cancer

Who Needs a PLND?

There is currently little debate on the utility of PLND at the time of RC for bladder cancer. Pathologic stage remains the most important prognostic factor after RC with patients harboring lymphatic metastases having a particularly poor prognosis [33]. Considering that up to 25 % of patients with muscle-invasive bladder cancer will have lymph node metastases at the time of RC, an appropriate PLND provides valuable prognostic information [33, 34]. Furthermore, numerous reports have suggested that patients with limited lymph node metastases may derive a therapeutic benefit from PLND [35–38]. For these prognostic and therapeutic reasons, a PLND should be considered a standard part of RC for all cases of invasive bladder cancer.

Templates

Although the need for PLND during RC is accepted, the extent of the dissection has been extensively debated. Initial attempts at describing an adequate PLND focused on number of lymph nodes removed. In fact, an overall survival advantage has been demonstrated in N0 and N+ patients having increasing numbers of nodes removed during PLND [36, 39, 40]. This has led to numerous studies suggesting nodal count cut-offs as surrogates for an adequate PLND. However, these cut-offs range widely, from 8 to 22 nodes, and no consensus has been reached concerning an appropriate nodal count for PLND [36, 39–41]. This is understood to be because nodal counts are influenced as much by surgical technique as by specimen submitting and processing practices and pathologic techniques for counting nodes [42, 43], which has led Koppie et al. to conclude that "no evidence was found that a minimum number of lymph nodes is sufficient for optimizing bladder cancer outcomes when a limited or extended pelvic LN dissection is performed during RC" [44]. Therefore, attention has been turned to better defining anatomic boundaries for an appropriate PLND.

An extended PLND including removal of the fibrofatty tissue surrounding the external iliac vessels, obturator fossa, hypogastric vessels, and common iliac vessels to the level of the ureter is currently the most accepted PLND template. Dhar et al. compared outcomes of patients undergoing RC and limited PLND versus RC and extended PLND and demonstrated an improvement in recurrence-free and overall survival in patients undergoing the more extended PLND [45]. Furthermore, Technetium-based mapping studies have demonstrated that 92 % of primary lymph nodes draining the bladder are below the uretero-iliac junction [46]. Additionally, surgical series have routinely demonstrated that ≤13 % of N+ patients will have positive nodes above the uretero-iliac junction, with no patients having isolated metastatic disease at this level (skip lesions) [47, 48]. Most importantly, studies have failed to demonstrate any survival benefit for removing LN's outside the true pelvis [49, 50].

Despite these data, surgical series demonstrating that detection of LN metastases is increased with removal of more lymphatic tissue have led some to suggest increasingly extended PLND templates [51]. Super-extended PLND includes all tissue removed in an extended PLND plus the fibrofatty tissue surrounding the common iliac vessels, the aorta/IVC distal to the inferior mesenteric vein, and presacral tissue. Although this technique has been safely performed with modest increases in operative times, oncologic benefits to super-extended PLND have not been demonstrated [49, 50, 52]. In a recent head-to-head comparison of extended and super-extended PLND, patients undergoing a more extensive PLND had more nodes removed and more metastatic disease discovered. However, and most importantly, there was no stage-stratified 5-year survival advantage in patients undergoing super-extended PLND [50]. SWOG trial S1011 is ongoing and will likely shed important insight into the appropriate level of dissection during PLND for bladder cancer. At present, the preponderance of data suggest that an extended PLND, as previously described, should be a routine part of RC.

Benefits

As with prostate cancer, PLND for bladder cancer has important staging and therapeutic benefits. With regards to staging, an accurate pathologic stage after RC is the most important prognostic factor. Stein et al. demonstrated significantly worse survival in N+ patients compared to N0 stratified by local tumor stage [33], confirming in a larger series the data from Skinner who reported a 35 % recurrence-free survival in patients harboring lymph node metastases at the time of RC [53]. This information is important not only for patient counseling but also for adjuvant systemic therapy considerations.

In addition to improved staging, PLND may indeed serve a therapeutic role in select patients. In fact, long-term survival has been described in patients with a limited burden of metastatic disease [35–38]. These patients typically have metastases involving 1 node located within the true pelvis with no evidence of extranodal spread. These observations led to the introduction of the concept of lymph node density (LND), defined as the number of positive nodes divided by the total number of nodes removed. Stein et al. demonstrated that patients in patients with N+ bladder cancer, those with a LND <20 % had a recurrence-free and overall survival advantage [35]. These observations strongly support the therapeutic role of PLND in select patients.

8.4 Risks and Complications of PLND

The benefits of performing a PLND must be weighed against the potential risks of developing a complication. Major complications of PLND include lymphocele formation, deep venous thrombosis (DVT), vascular, neurologic and ureteral injury, and lower extremity edema. Among these, lymphocele formation is the most common, occurring symptomatically in up to 10 % of cases [54]. Patients who go on to develop a lymphocele typically present within the first month of surgery and experience a wide range of symptoms including pain, abdominal fullness, constipation, urinary urgency and frequency, symptoms of a DVT or related pulmonary embolism, fever, and leukocytosis. Commonly these patients lack associated physical exam findings and the diagnosis is only made with pelvic ultrasound or cross-sectional imaging. Treatment for a lymphocele depends on the clinical context but often can be managed expectantly or with percutaneous drainage.

Risk factors for the development of a lymphocele include the extent of PLND [55–57] and subcutaneous heparin administration for DVT prophylaxis [58, 59]. Of note, classically it was felt that the risk of lymphocele was lower among patients undergoing a transabdominal versus extraperitoneal operation, as it was felt that the transabdominal approach allowed for a larger surface area for the reabsorption of lymphatic fluid. This, however, appears to not be the case as a not insignificant number of patients undergoing laparoscopic or robotic surgery still experience this complication [60]. Regardless of surgical approach, this risk of a lymphocele can minimized through meticulous use of surgical clips and the avoidance of subcutaneous heparin. When heparin administration is recommended by current guidelines, injection in the upper extremities is advised [61, 62].

One complication of a PLND directly related to the development of a lymphocele is venous thromboembolism. This complication is felt to arise due to the compressive effects of a lymphocele on the deep veins of the pelvis and lower extremities, thus resulting in a DVT. In a meta-analysis by Eifler et al. [63], the authors found that undergoing a PLND at the time of RP was associated with an approximately two-fold increased risk of developing venous thromboembolism. Consistent with this finding, one prospective study in which patients underwent an extended PLND on one side of the pelvis and a limited PLND on the contralateral side, found an increased rate of lymphocele and DVTs on the side of the extended template dissection [56].

Other less common complications of a PLND include vascular, neurologic and ureteral injury as well as the development of lower extremity edema. In terms of neurologic injury, structures at risk during a PLND include the obturator, gentiofemoral and femoral nerves. Of these, injury to the obturator nerve is most common and can be avoided by intraoperative visualization and careful clip placement. Most nerve injuries are recognized postoperatively with the development of pain, weakness or paresthesia. Fortunately serious injuries are rare and most can be managed with physical therapy and neuroleptic pain medications. Like neurologic injuries, vascular and ureteral injuries are also rare. These, however, are commonly identified intraoperatively and repaired at the time of recognition without any postoperative sequelae. One last uncommon complication of PLND is lower extremity lymphedema. Risk factors for this complication include extent of PLND and history of radiation therapy. Management options include the use of compressive stockings and exercise to promote fluid return from the lower extremities.

Key Points

- PLND should not be performed in all men with prostate cancer undergoing radical prostatectomy
- PLND should be limited to men with a nomogram risk of 2–2.5 % or greater of having lymph node involvement in prostate cancer
- PLND for prostate cancer, when performed, should be a thorough standard or extended dissection, and not a limited template dissection
- The main nodal fields to resect in prostate cancer cases are the external iliac, obturator and internal iliac nodal beds
- There is therapeutic value to PLND in cases of limited nodal involvement and low lymph node density (<15 %)
- PLND should be performed in all cases of bladder cancer undergoing radical cystectomy, as it has both prognostic and apparent therapeutic benefit
- Extended template PLND, but not super-extended template PLND, is appropriate in most radical cystectomy cases
- Removal of the fibrofatty tissue surrounding the external iliac vessels, obturator fossa, hypogastric vessels, and common iliac vessels to the level of the ureter is currently the most accepted extended PLND template for bladder cancer patients
- Complications of PLND increase as the extent of the lymphadenectomy increases
- Serious complications associated with PLND are rare but can be life-threatening, and include venous thromboembolism, major neural, ureteral, and/or vascular injury, lymphocele, and lower extremity edema.

References

1. Weingartner K, Ramaswamy A, Bittinger A, Gerharz EW, Voge D, Riedmiller H. Anatomical basis for pelvic lymphadenectomy in prostate cancer: results of an autopsy study and implications for the clinic. J Urol. 1996;156(6):1969–71.
2. Harisinghani MG, Barentsz J, Hahn PF, Deserno WM, Tabatabaei S, van de Kaa CH, et al. Noninvasive detection of clinically occult lymph-node metastases in prostate cancer. N Engl J Med. 2003;348(25):2491–9.
3. Heesakkers RA, Jager GJ, Hovels AM, de Hoop B, van den Bosch HC, Raat F, et al. Prostate cancer: detection of lymph node metastases outside the routine surgical area with ferumoxtran-10-enhanced MR imaging. Radiology. 2009;251(2):408–14.
4. National Comprehensive Cancer Network. Prostate Cancer (Version 2.2013). http://www.nccn.org/professionals/physician_gls/PDF/prostate.pdf. Accessed August 1, 2013.
5. Weight CJ, Reuther AM, Gunn PW, Zippe CR, Dhar NB, Klein EA. Limited pelvic lymph node dissection does not improve biochemical relapse-free survival at 10 years after radical prostatectomy in patients with low-risk prostate cancer. Urology. 2008;71(1):141–5.
6. Berglund RK, Sadetsky N, DuChane J, Carroll PR, Klein EA. Limited pelvic lymph node dissection at the time of radical prostatectomy does not affect 5-year failure rates for low, intermediate and high risk prostate cancer: results from CaPSURE. J Urol. 2007;177(2):526–9; discussion 529–30.
7. Cagiannos I, Karakiewicz P, Eastham JA, Ohori M, Rabbani F, Gerigk C, et al. A preoperative nomogram identifying decreased risk of positive pelvic lymph nodes in patients with prostate cancer. J Urol. 2003;170(5):1798–803.
8. Bluestein DL, Bostwick DG, Bergstralh EJ, Oesterling JE. Eliminating the need for bilateral pelvic lymphadenectomy in select patients with prostate cancer. J Urol. 1994;151(5):1315–20.
9. Briganti A, Karakiewicz PI, Chun FK, Gallina A, Salonia A, Zanni G, et al. Percentage of positive biopsy cores can improve the ability to predict lymph node invasion in patients undergoing radical prostatectomy and extended pelvic lymph node dissection. Eur Urol. 2007;51(6):1573–81.
10. Briganti A, Larcher A, Abdollah F, Capitanio U, Gallina A, Suardi N, Bianchi M, Sun M, Freschi M, Salonia A, Karakiewicz PI, Rigatti P, Montorsi F. Updated nomogram predicting lymph node invasion in patients with prostate cancer undergoing extended pelvic lymph node dissection: the essential importance of percentage of positive cores. Eur Urol. 2012;61(3):480–7.
11. Eifler JB, Feng Z, Lin BM, Partin MT, Humphreys EB, Han M, Epstein JI, Walsh PC, Trock BJ, Partin AW. An updated prostate cancer staging nomogram (Partin tables) based on cases from 2006 to 2011. BJU Int. 2013;111(1):22–9.
12. Yu JB, Makarov DV, Sharma R, Peschel RE, Partin AW, Gross CP. Validation of the partin nomogram for prostate cancer in a national sample. J Urol. 2010;183(1):105–11.
13. Haese A, Epstein JI, Huland H, Partin AW. Validation of a biopsy-based pathologic algorithm for predicting lymph node metastases in patients with clinically localized prostate carcinoma. Cancer. 2002;95(5):1016–21.
14. Briganti A, Chun FK, Salonia A, Gallina A, Zanni G, Scattoni V, et al. Critical assessment of ideal nodal yield at pelvic lymphadenectomy to accurately diagnose prostate cancer nodal metastasis in patients undergoing radical retropubic prostatectomy. Urology. 2007;69(1):147–51.
15. D'Amico AV, Whittington R, Malkowicz SB, Schultz D, Blank K, Broderick GA, et al. Biochemical outcome after radical prostatectomy, external beam radiation therapy, or interstitial radiation therapy for clinically localized prostate cancer. JAMA. 1998;280(11):969–74.
16. Cellini N, Luzi S, Mantini G, Mattiucci GC, Morganti AG, Digesu C, et al. Lymphatic drainage and CTV in carcinoma of the prostate. Rays. 2003;28(3):337–41.
17. Mattei A, Fuechsel FG, Bhatta Dhar N, Warncke SH, Thalmann GN, Krause T, et al. The template of the primary lymphatic landing sites of the prostate should be revisited: results of a multimodality mapping study. Eur Urol. 2008;53(1):118–25.
18. Bader P, Burkhard FC, Markwalder R, Studer UE. Is a limited lymph node dissection an adequate staging procedure for prostate cancer? J Urol. 2002;168(2):514–8; discussion 8.
19. Weckermann D, Dorn R, Trefz M, Wagner T, Wawroschek F, Harzmann R. Sentinel lymph node dissection for prostate cancer: experience with more than 1,000 patients. J Urol. 2007;177(3):916–20.
20. Allaf ME, Palapattu GS, Trock BJ, Carter HB, Walsh PC. Anatomical extent of lymph node dissection: impact on men with clinically localized prostate cancer. J Urol. 2004;172(5 Pt 1):1840–4.
21. Touijer K, Rabbani F, Otero JR, Secin FP, Eastham JA, Scardino PT, et al. Standard versus limited pelvic lymph node dissection for prostate cancer in patients with a predicted probability of nodal metastasis greater than 1 %. J Urol. 2007;178(1):120–4.
22. Masterson TA, Bianco Jr FJ, Vickers AJ, DiBlasio CJ, Fearn PA, Rabbani F, et al. The association between total and positive lymph node counts, and disease progression in clinically localized prostate cancer. J Urol. 2006;175(4):1320–4; discussion 1324–5.
23. Heidenreich A, Varga Z, Von Knobloch R. Extended pelvic lymphadenectomy in patients undergoing radical prostatectomy: high incidence of lymph node metastasis. J Urol. 2002;167(4):1681–6.
24. Bochner BH, Herr HW, Reuter VE. Impact of separate versus en bloc pelvic lymph node dissection on the number of lymph nodes retrieved in cystectomy specimens. J Urol. 2001;166(6):2295–6.

25. Stein JP, Penson DF, Cai J, Miranda G, Skinner EC, Dunn MA, et al. Radical cystectomy with extended lymphadenectomy: evaluating separate package versus en bloc submission for node positive bladder cancer. J Urol. 2007;177(3):876–81; discussion 881–2.
26. Briganti A, Karnes JR, Da Pozzo LF, Cozzarini C, Gallina A, Suardi N, et al. Two positive nodes represent a significant cut-off value for cancer specific survival in patients with node positive prostate cancer. A new proposal based on a two-institution experience on 703 consecutive N+ patients treated with radical prostatectomy, extended pelvic lymph node dissection and adjuvant therapy. Eur Urol. 2009;55(2):261–70.
27. Daneshmand S, Quek ML, Stein JP, Lieskovsky G, Cai J, Pinski J, et al. Prognosis of patients with lymph node positive prostate cancer following radical prostatectomy: long-term results. J Urol. 2004;172(6 Pt 1):2252–5.
28. Palapattu GS, Allaf ME, Trock BJ, Epstein JI, Walsh PC. Prostate specific antigen progression in men with lymph node metastases following radical prostatectomy: results of long-term followup. J Urol. 2004;172(5 Pt 1):1860–4.
29. Messing EM, Manola J, Yao J, Kiernan M, Crawford D, Wilding G, et al. Immediate versus deferred androgen deprivation treatment in patients with node-positive prostate cancer after radical prostatectomy and pelvic lymphadenectomy. Lancet Oncol. 2006;7(6):472–9.
30. Pagliarulo V, Hawes D, Brands FH, Groshen S, Cai J, Stein JP, et al. Detection of occult lymph node metastases in locally advanced node-negative prostate cancer. J Clin Oncol. 2006;24(18):2735–42.
31. DiMarco DS, Zincke H, Sebo TJ, Slezak J, Bergstralh EJ. Blute ML The extent of lymphadenectomy for pTXNO prostate cancer does not affect prostate cancer outcome in the prostate specific antigen era. J Urol. 2005;173(4):1121–5.
32. Murphy AM, Berkman DS, Desai M, Benson MC, McKiernan JM, Badani KK. The number of negative pelvic lymph nodes removed does not affect the risk of biochemical failure after radical prostatectomy. BJU Int. 2010;105(2):176–9.
33. Stein JP, Lieskovsky G, Cote R, Groshen S, Feng AC, Boyd S, Skinner E, Bochner B, Thangathurai D, Mikhail M, Raghavan D, Skinner DG. Radical cystectomy in the treatment of invasive bladder cancer: long-term results in 1,054 patients. J Clin Oncol. 2001;19(3):666–75.
34. Poulsen AL, Horn T, Steven K. Radical cystectomy: extending the limits of pelvic lymph node dissection improves survival for patients with bladder cancer confined to the bladder wall. J Urol. 1998;160(6 Pt 1):2015–9; discussion 2020.
35. Stein JP, Cai J, Groshen S, Skinner DG. Risk factors for patients with pelvic lymph node metastases following radical cystectomy with en bloc pelvic lymphadenectomy: concept of lymph node density. J Urol. 2003;170(1):35–41.
36. Herr HW, Bochner BH, Dalbagni G, Donat SM, Reuter VE, Bajorin DF. Impact of the number of lymph nodes retrieved on outcome in patients with muscle invasive bladder cancer. J Urol. 2002;167(3):1295–8.
37. Tarin TV, Power NE, Ehdaie B, Sfakianos JP, Silberstein JL, Savage CJ, Sjoberg D, Dalbagni G, Bochner BH. Lymph node-positive bladder cancer treated with radical cystectomy and lymphadenectomy: effect of the level of node positivity. Eur Urol. 2012;61(5):1025–30.
38. May M, Herrmann E, Bolenz C, Tiemann A, Brookman-May S, Fritsche HM, Burger M, Buchner A, Gratzke C, Wülfing C, Trojan L, Ellinger J, Tilki D, Gilfrich C, Höfner T, Roigas J, Zacharias M, Gunia S, Wieland WF, Hohenfellner M, Michel MS, Haferkamp A, Müller SC, Stief CG, Bastian PJ. Lymph node density affects cancer-specific survival in patients with lymph node-positive urothelial bladder cancer following radical cystectomy. Eur Urol. 2011;59(5):712–8.
39. May M, Herrmann E, Bolenz C, Brookman-May S, Tiemann A, Moritz R, Fritsche HM, Burger M, Trojan L, Michel MS, Wülfing C, Müller SC, Ellinger J, Buchner A, Stief CG, Tilki D, Wieland WF, Gilfrich C, Höfner T, Hohenfellner M, Haferkamp A, Roigas J, Zacharias M, Bastian PJ. Association between the number of dissected lymph nodes during pelvic lymphadenectomy and cancer-specific survival in patients with lymph node-negative urothelial carcinoma of the bladder undergoing radical cystectomy. Ann Surg Oncol. 2011;18(7):2018–25.
40. Leissner J, Hohenfellner R, Thüroff JW, Wolf HK. Lymphadenectomy in patients with transitional cell carcinoma of the urinary bladder; significance for staging and prognosis. BJU Int. 2000;85(7):817–23.
41. Herr HW, Faulkner JR, Grossman HB, Natale RB, deVere White R, Sarosdy MF, Crawford ED. Surgical factors influence bladder cancer outcomes: a cooperative group report. J Clin Oncol. 2004;22(14):2781–9.
42. Bochner BH, Cho D, Herr HW, Donat M, Kattan MW, Dalbagni G. Prospectively packaged lymph node dissections with radical cystectomy: evaluation of node count variability and node mapping. J Urol. 2004;172(4 Pt 1):1286–90.
43. Parkash V, Bifulco C, Feinn R, Concato J, Jain D. To count and how to count, that is the question: interobserver and intraobserver variability among pathologists in lymph node counting. Am J Clin Pathol. 2010;134(1):42–9.
44. Koppie TM, Vickers AJ, Vora K, Dalbagni G, Bochner BH. Standardization of pelvic lymphadenectomy performed at radical cystectomy: can we establish a minimum number of lymph nodes that should be removed? Cancer. 2006;107(10):2368–74.
45. Dhar NB, Klein EA, Reuther AM, Thalmann GN, Madersbacher S, Studer UE. Outcome after radical cystectomy with limited or extended pelvic lymph node dissection. J Urol. 2008;179(3):873–8. doi:10.1016/j.jur0.2007.10.076; discussion 878, Epub 2008 Jan 25.

46. Roth B, Wissmeyer MP, Zehnder P, Birkhäuser FD, Thalmann GN, Krause TM, Studer UE. A new multimodality technique accurately maps the primary lymphatic landing sites of the bladder. Eur Urol. 2010;57(2):205–11.
47. Leissner J, Ghoneim MA, Abol-Enein H, Thüroff JW, Franzaring L, Fisch M, Schulze H, Managadze G, Allhoff EP, el-Baz MA, Kastendieck H, Buhtz P, Kropf S, Hohenfellner R, Wolf HK. Extended radical lymphadenectomy in patients with urothelial bladder cancer: results of a prospective multicenter study. J Urol. 2004;171(1):139–44.
48. Miocinovic R, Gong MC, Ghoneim IA, Fergany AF, Hansel DE, Stephenson AJ. Presacral and retroperitoneal lymph node involvement in urothelial bladder cancer: results of a prospective mapping study. J Urol. 2011;186(4):1269–73.
49. Steven K, Poulsen AL. Radical cystectomy and extended pelvic lymphadenectomy: survival of patients with lymph node metastasis above the bifurcation of the common iliac vessels treated with surgery only. J Urol. 2007;178(4 Pt 1):1218–23; discussion 1223–4.
50. Zehnder P, Studer UE, Skinner EC, Dorin RP, Cai J, Roth B, Miranda G, Birkhäuser F, Stein J, Burkhard FC, Daneshmand S, Thalmann GN, Gill IS, Skinner DG. Super extended versus extended pelvic lymph node dissection in patients undergoing radical cystectomy for bladder cancer: a comparative study. J Urol. 2011;186(4):1261–8.
51. Capitanio U, Suardi N, Shariat SF, Lotan Y, Palapattu GS, Bastian PJ, Gupta A, Vazina A, Schoenberg M, Lerner SP, Sagalowsky AI, Karakiewicz PI. Assessing the minimum number of lymph nodes needed at radical cystectomy in patients with bladder cancer. BJU Int. 2009;103(10):1359–62. doi:10.1111/j.1464–410X.2008.08212.x. Epub 2008 Dec 8.
52. Brössner C, Pycha A, Toth A, Mian C, Kuber W. Does extended lymphadenectomy increase the morbidity of radical cystectomy? BJU Int. 2004;93(1):64–6.
53. Skinner DG. Management of invasive bladder cancer: a meticulous pelvic node dissection can make a difference. J Urol. 1982;128(1):34–6.
54. Ball MW, Gorin MA, Allaf ME. Reducing morbidity of pelvic and retroperitoneal lymphadenectomy. Curr Urol Rep. 2013;14:488–95.
55. Musch M, Klevecka V, Roggenbuck U, Kroepfl D. Complications of pelvic lymphadenectomy in 1,380 patients undergoing radical retropubic prostatectomy between 1993 and 2006. J Urol. 2008;179(3):923–8; discussion 928–9.
56. Clark T, Parekh DJ, Cookson MS, Chang SS, Smith Jr ER, Wells N, Smith Jr J. Randomized prospective evaluation of extended versus limited lymph node dissection in patients with clinically localized prostate cancer. J Urol. 2003;169(1):145–7; discussion 147–8.
57. Briganti A, Chun FK, Salonia A, Suardi N, Gallina A, Da Pozzo LF, Roscigno M, Zanni G, Valiquette L, Rigatti P, Montorsi F, Karakiewicz PI. Complications and other surgical outcomes associated with extended pelvic lymphadenectomy in men with localized prostate cancer. Eur Urol. 2006;50(5):1006–13. Epub 2006 Aug 31.
58. Catalona WJ, Kadmon D, Crane DB. Effect of minidose heparin on lymphocele formation following extraperitoneal pelvic lymphadenectomy. J Urol. 1980;123(6):890–2.
59. Gotto GT, Yunis LH, Guillonneau B, Touijer K, Eastham JA, Scardino PT, Rabbani F. Predictors of symptomatic lymphocele after radical prostatectomy and bilateral pelvic lymph node dissection. Int J Urol. 2011;18:291–6.
60. Novara G, Ficarra V, Rosen RC, Artibani W, Costello A, Eastham JA, Graefen M, Guazzoni G, Shariat SF, Stolzenburg JU, Van Poppel H, Zattoni F, Montorsi F, Mottrie A, Wilson TG. Systematic review and meta-analysis of perioperative outcomes and complications after robot-assisted radical prostatectomy. Eur Urol. 2012;62(3):431–52.
61. Forrest JB, Clemens JQ, Finamore P, Leveillee R, Lippert M, Pisters L, Touijer K, Whitmore K, American Urological Association. AUA Best Practice Statement for the prevention of deep vein thrombosis in patients undergoing urologic surgery. J Urol. 2009;181(3):1170–7.
62. Geerts WH, Bergqvist D, Pineo GF, Heit JA, Samama CM, Lassen MR, Colwell CW, American College of Chest Physicians. Prevention of venous thromboembolism: American college of chest physicians evidence-based clinical practice guidelines (8th edition). Chest. 2008;133(6 Suppl):381S–453.
63. Eifler JB, Levinson AW, Hyndman ME, Trock BJ, Pavlovich CP. Pelvic lymph node dissection is associated with symptomatic venous thromboembolism risk during laparoscopic radical prostatectomy. J Urol. 2011;185(5):1661–5.

9 Prostate and Bladder Carcinomas: Histology, Immunohistochemistry, Genetic Biomarkers

Elin H. Richardsen and Lill-Tove Busund

9.1 Introduction

PCa is a major health problem and among different types of cancer, only lung cancer kills more men each year [1]. Nearly two thirds are diagnosed in men aged 65 or older, and it is rare before age 40. The average age at the time of diagnosis is about 67 [2]. Asian-American men and Hispanic men have incidence rates lower than non-Hispanic white persons [3, 4]. The incidence is approximately 60 % higher and mortality rates are two-fold higher in black men than in white men [4, 5]. The cause of PCa is unknown, but the best known risk factors are age, ethnicity, and family history.

PCa is a heterogeneous disease, and from a molecular based point of view the histopathology of PCa is proposed to have different steps until development of invasive PCa (Fig. 9.1) [6, 7]. Today, researchers put a large effort in analyzing the molecular history of PCa, to identify groups of men at high risk of developing PCa who would benefit from more intensive screening or from chemoprevention trials, to discriminate indolent versus aggressive disease, and to improve screening techniques, and improve therapeutic strategies.

The different PCa tumors have varying growth rates and malignant potential for causing death. Screening for PCa should ideally target only tumors that would cause clinically important disease, but currently availably prognostic markers can only distinguish a small number of men having excellent prognosis [8]. However, they cannot say anything about the prognosis of those in the middle category (Gleason grades 3+4 vs. 4+3), which includes most of the men with PCa [9, 10]. Treatment decision is usually based on PSA levels and histopathological findings in biopsies, i.e., Gleason score.

PSA measurements have significant influence on diagnosis, treatment strategies and follow-up of PCa patients; however the specificity of total serum PSA is limited to treatment strategies especially for patients with low PSA serum levels (less than 4.0 ng/ml) [11–16] The specificity of PSA screening is lower among men with large prostate glands, including older men with benign prostatic hyperplasia (BPH) [17] The discrepancy between PCa diagnoses and PCa deaths indicates that probably most cancers detected by screening are clinically unimportant. Appropriate target that will detect the cancers causing clinical symptoms and death (i.e., Gleason score ≥7) has yet to be defined.

E.H. Richardsen, MD, PhD (✉)
Department of Clinical Pathology, University Hospital of Northern Norway, Tromsø, Norway
e-mail: elin.richardsen@unn.no; elin-r@live.no

L.-T. Busund, MD, PhD
Department of Clinical Pathology, University Hospital of Northern Norway, Institute of Medical Biology, University of Tromsø, Tromsø, Norway

H.R.H. Patel et al. (eds.), *Pelvic Cancer Surgery: Modern Breakthroughs and Future Advances*,
DOI 10.1007/978-1-4471-4258-4_9,

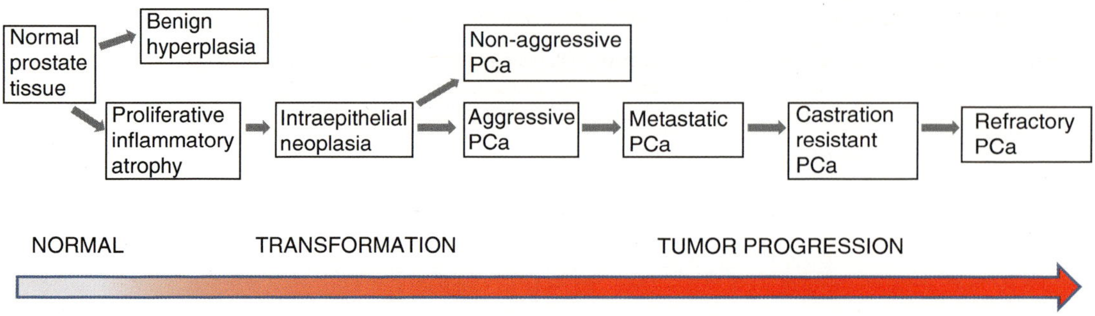

Fig. 9.1 The multistage process of prostate cancer development and tumor progression. *PCa* prostate cancer

9.2 Histological Diagnoses of Prostate Cancer

Specimen Preparation

Radical prostatectomy (RP) specimens are usually transported in buffered 4 % formaline saline, occasionally, fresh tissue is harvested in the laboratories for research reasons. However, is has been pointed out that the specimens should be placed in fixative as soon as possible, because of alteration in protein, DNA or RNA confirmation that must be satisfactory for the preservation of microscopic and IHC features [18]. The histological diagnosis of PCa is based on formalin fixed and paraffin embedded tissue. The initial diagnosis is based on needle biopsies, usually four or more biopsies from each patient. Prognosis after RP relies, in part, on accurate characterization of a number of histological features, including the status of the surgical margin, extra prostatic tumor growth, Gleason grade, tumor volume and whether tumor extends into the seminal vesicles and/or is metastatic to regional lymph nodes. The 2009 International Society of Urological Pathology Consensus Conference in Boston made recommendations regarding the standardization of pathology reporting of RP specimens [19, 20]. The use of whole mounts of sections from RP specimens has the advantage of displaying the whole architecture of the prostate and the location of tumor areas. Of most importance is assessment of free resection margins, therefore painting the surfaces gives more precise information about the margins [19, 20]. Separate histological examination of both apex and base should be prepared by cutting sagittal sections of the conus (Fig. 9.2) [19]. Histological examination of tumor tissues in prostatic apex and base predicts outcome [21].

Positive lymphatic involvement is generally considered as a poor prognostic indicator and has impact on treatment options [22]. Identifying lymphatic involvement requires accurate nodal staging. Some laboratories report enhanced retrieval of lymph nodes using Glacial acetic acid, ethanol, distilled water, and formaldehyde (GEWF), compared to formalin fixed specimens [23].

9.3 Microscopic Diagnoses

The Gleason Grading System

The Gleason grading system is so far the most commonly used system for histological characterization of prostate cancer, and it's the most powerful predictor of outcome for PCa patients [23]. Gleason grading depends solely on architectural patterns of the tumor. The grade is defined as the sum of the two most common grade patterns and reported as the Gleason score. Both the primary (predominant) and the secondary (second most prevalent) architectural patterns are identified and assigned a number from 1 to 5, were 1 being the most differentiated and 5 the least differentiated pattern [23]. Since the introduction of the Gleason grading system more than four decades ago many aspects of prostate cancer have changed, including PSA testing, transrectal

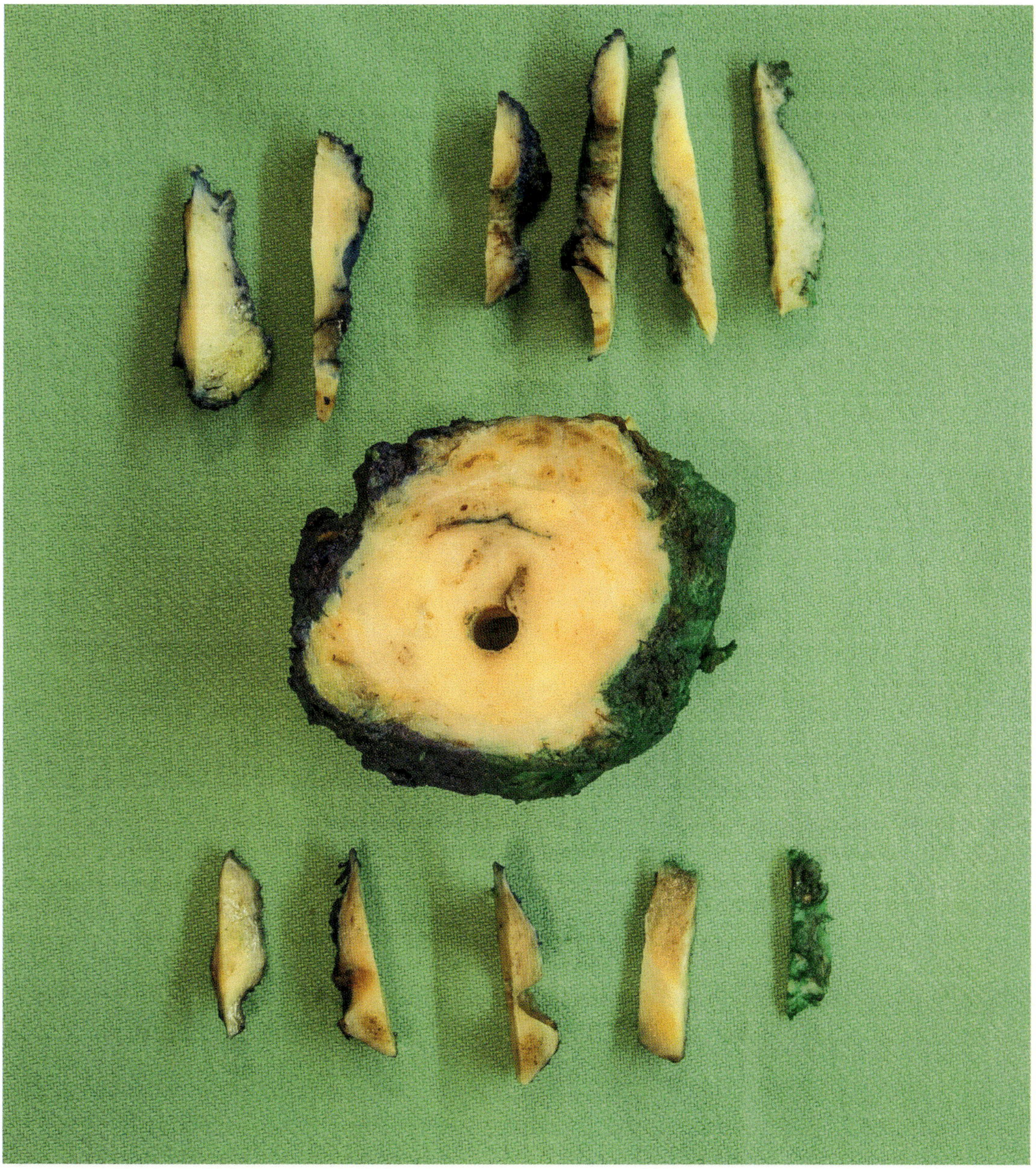

Fig. 9.2 Whole-mount tissue section of prostate (*center*) with sagittal sectioning of the base (*top*) and apex (*below*). For orientation and with regard to surgical reception margins, the prostate is inked *blue* to the right, *green* to the left and *black* at the posterior surgical margin

ultrasound guided prostate needle biopsies with sampling and immunohistochemistry for identification of basal cells. These techniques have changed the classification of prostate cancer and led to identification of new prostate cancer variants. Gleason grading system was updated in 2005 by experts in urological pathology at a consensus conference held by the International Society of Urological Pathology (ISUP). This has resulted in a more accurate grading system in both needle biopsies and RPs [24–27]. This modified system has also led to a better correlation between pathological stage, rate of positive margins, and biochemical recurrence with

Table 9.1 Gleason score comparison

Original Gleason system	2005 ISUP modified Gleason system
A diagnosis of GS <4 possible NB	GS of NB specimens <4 rarely, if ever made
Cribriform glands with rounded and smooth contours as well as with an irregular outer border are diagnosed as Gleason pattern 3	Most cribriform patterns with only rare cribriform lesions would satisfy the diagnostic criteria for cribriform pattern 3
The same GS is used for NB and RP specimens	Different GS used for NB and RP specimens
High-grade tumor of small quantity (<5 %) on NB should be excluded based on GS (5% threshold rule)	Different GS used for NB and RP specimens
High-grade tumor of small quantity (<5%) on NB should be excluded based on GS (<5 % threshold rule)	High-grade tumor of any quantity on NB should be include within the GS
Tumors on NB should be graded by listing the primary and secondary patterns, i.e., excluding tertiary patterns	For the tertiary pattern on NB specimens, both the primary pattern and the highest grade should be recorded
The GS of RP specimens should be assigned based on the primary and secondary patterns	For RP specimens, the pathologist should assign the GS based on the primary and secondary patterns; a comment should be added on the tertiary pattern
Separate or overall scoring to assess all grades of NB specimens	When NB specimens show different grads in separate cores, individual GS should be assigned to these cores (separate scoring)
The grade of the largest portion should be assigned, even if the second largest portion is of higher grade	When RP specimens show different grades in separate tumor nodules, a separate GS should be assigned to each of the dominant tumor nodules

Abbreviations: *GS* Gleason score, *NB* needle biopsy, *RP* radical prostatectomy

Gleason scores. Still, Gleason score is the only independent predictor of metastatic disease [28]. The main differences between the original system and the 2005 ISUP Modified Gleason grading system are summarized in Table 9.1 [24, 26, 27, 29].

PTNM-Classification

The pTNM-classification is currently under revision. Within category pT2 PCa, a wide variation in tumor extent may be seen, which varies from single microscopic lesions to large volume multifocal tumors, often involving both sides of the prostate. This heterogeneity of tumor volume of pT2 prostate cancers and the potential impact on prognostic assessment has resulted in attempts to subcategorize organ-confined tumors. In TNM 2002, pT2 was substaged in pT2a (tumor involves one half of one lobe or less), pT2b (tumor involves more than half of one lobe, but not both lobes), and pT2c (tumor involves both lobes). In the TNM 2010 staging, the pathological substaging of pT2 prostate cancers has been retained, although the prognostic value of this has been questioned.

The 2009 ISUP consensus conference in Boston made recommendations that the standardization of T2 substaging should be optional. Although, there was an overall agreement that the current pT2 substaging should not be used, there was no consensus what sort of substaging should replace it [30–33].

9.4 Immunohistochemistry (IHC)

IHC is widely used for diagnosing PCa in difficult cases. Awareness of the many pitfalls in prostate IHC is essential to avoid serious misdiagnosis i.e., identifying IHC staining as positive or negative. However, in the majority of cases haematoxylin-Eosin stained sections are sufficient for diagnosing cancer. The IHC diagnosis of PCa largely depends on panels of markers because no absolutely specific and sensitive marker has yet been discovered. Such panels usually include at least one basal cell-specific marker; high molecular-weight cytokeratin (HMWCK), or p63, and the prostate cancer-specific marker; alpha-methyl-CoA-Racemase (AMACR, antibody clone P504S). HMWCK or P63 is expressed in almost all normal basal cells of prostate with continuous intact circumferential immunostaining in most glands. However, HMWCK positivity is typically discontinuous in a variety of benign lesions such as post atrophic hyperplasia and atypical adenomatous hyperplasia, whereas in PCa with the loss of basal cells, these markers are negative. Almost all PCa of low and intermediate grade are negative for p63, while normal or hyperplastic prostatic gland, show strong and diffuse p63 expression. AMACR is usually overexpressed in PCa with strong coarsely granular staining and more accentuated along the luminal border. However, strong expression of AMACR can also be found in high grade prostatic intraepithelial neoplasia (HGPIN) lesions, but weak expression may be found in benign glands, and should not be interpreted as positive staining.

9.5 Role of Genetic Markers in Prostate Cancer

The huge advances in genotyping and gene sequencing technologies has potential to aid disease screening, improve prognostic discrimination and prediction of response to treatment.

PSA

Early detection of PCa through PSA screening has resulted in detection of men with PCa at earlier stages and with lower Gleason grade, but has also contributed to concerns about overdiagnosis and overtreatment of clinically insignificant disease. As a single test serum PSA has limitations, because some men with very low serum levels of PSA (<4.0 ng/ml) will develop prostate cancer (~15 %) [13], and men with benign conditions including BPH, prostatitis and medical intervention frequently elevate serum PSA. This makes serum PSA more sensitive than specific for PCa. However serum PSA is of great value in disease monitoring of existing cancer and for identification of recurrent disease after treatment. Among men undergoing radical prostatectomy, the persistence of undetectable serum levels of PSA can be used to confirm absence of recurrent disease.

Tumor Specific Autoantibodies, AMACR

In order to react against a tumor, the immune system must have antigens that are recognized as foreign. A number of alterations in gene expression occur in cells during tumorigenesis. Tumorigenesis may lead to expression of new antigens or alteration in existing antigens that are found in normal cells. These antigens may include membrane receptors, regulators of cell cycle and apoptosis, or molecules involved in signal transduction pathways. In PCa, AMACR, is a mitochondrial and peroxisomal enzyme that is involved in bile acid biosynthesis and beta-oxidation of branched-chain fatty acids. AMACR is overexpressed in PCa epithelium, making it a specific marker for cancer cells within the prostate gland. Furthermore, overexpression of AMACR is found in premalignant lesions like HGPIN, may increase PIN, may increase the risk of PCa. I addition, genome-wide scans for linkage in hereditary PCa families suggest that the chromosomal region for AMACR (5p13) is the location of a PCa susceptibility gene. Also, experimental studies have shown that loss of AMACR expression slows the growth of some PCa cell lines. As a biomarker AMACR is of important value in PCa.

9.6 Bladder Cancer

Histologically, most urinary bladder cancers (UC) are transitional cell carcinomas (TCC), but approximately 10 % includes squamous cell carcinoma and adenocarcinomas, both rising from the inner lining of the bladder probably because of chronic irritation and inflammation. A minor portion is small cell carcinoma and sarcoma. UC is one of the most common malignancies among men in Western countries (ratio worldwide is about 3.5:1 compared to women) [13]. Except for Japan, the highest incidence is observed in developed countries. Northern Africa and western Asia is also included among high risk areas, the latter is probably related to presence of urinary schistosomiasis (well-known to be associated with high risk of bladder cancer). Cigarette smoking is the predominant risk factor, followed by a small group with occupational exposure to aromatic amines and other industrial chemicals. Also a genetic predisposition is a considerable factor [34, 35]. The clinical behavior of the disease is heterogeneous, ranging from tumors with low malignant potential to highly malignant muscle-infiltrating tumors. Despite refined histology based classification systems, it is difficult to predict individual prognosis or response to therapy. For instance, one third of patients with T1 tumors remain recurrence-free after BCG treatment, while one third die from the disease. Classification schemes for bladder tumors, especially for TCC, which represents the vast majority of cases, have evolved over the past decades, and will continue to change as information regarding genomics and proteomics accumulates. Current prognostic parameters such as grade, stage, multifocality of carcinomas, and lymph node status cannot with certainty predict the long term outcome of bladder cancer.

Staging of bladder cancer

The prognosis and treatment decisions are mainly based on pathological criteria, and proper staging is highly dependent on good quality biopsies. Approximately 70 % of these tumors are papillary and confined to the urothelial mucosa (stage Ta) or to lamina propria (T1), whereas, the remaining invade the muscle (T2), the perivesical fat (T3) or surrounding organs (T4) (Fig. 9.3). Favorable prognostic factors for superficial TCC at stage Ta, compared to stage

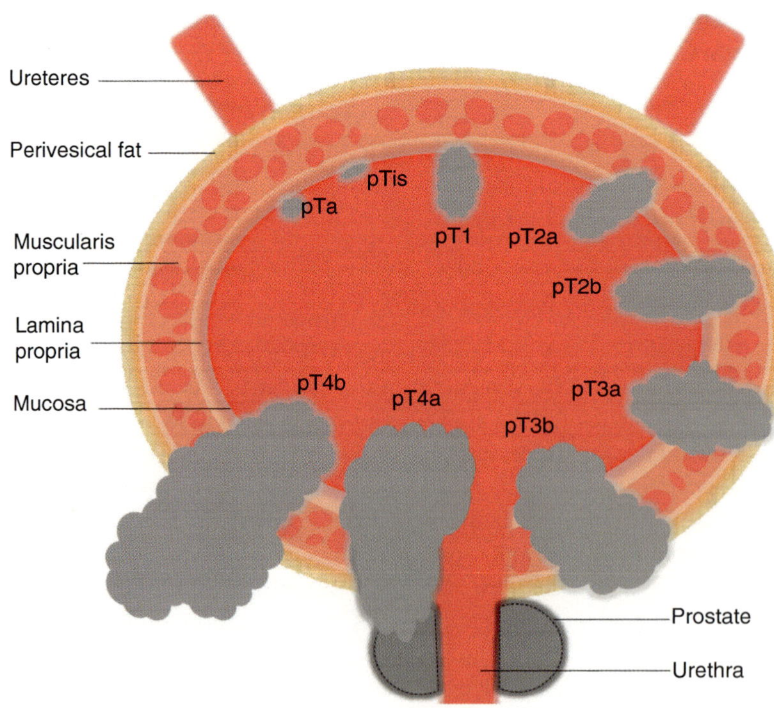

Fig. 9.3 Bladder cancer staging

T1 are: low grade and no dysplasia, whereas high grade, tumor multiplicity, tumor size greater than 5 cm, and vascular invasion increase the risk for tumor progression.

Histological Diagnoses of Bladder Cancer

Specimen Preparation

Among the established methods for detecting and confirming bladder cancer are bimanual palpation, cystoscopy with or without random or selected-site biopsies and urinary cytology.

In clinical routine, mainly formalin-fixed and paraffin-embedded tissue has been preserved, and by using light microscope, the histologic diagnoses are done according to World Health Organization (WHO)/International Society of Urological Pathology (ISUP) [36].

Urinary cytopathology is especially useful for detection and monitoring of patients with epithelial tumors, but this approach is best applied to high-grade tumors, where nearly all of the features are detectable in these specimens. This means that nearly all aggressive tumors can be detected in adequately sampled bladders. This method is less useful for the detection and monitoring of very low-grade tumors, because most of these tumors lack feature of malignancy [36].

Microscopic Diagnoses and Classification

TCC (urothelial carcinoma) can rise anywhere in the bladder. They are defined according to their histologic characteristics and so far, histologic examination is the most specific method for assessing these lesions [37]. The pattern of growth may be exophytic or endophytic or a combination of both. When histologically exophytic, the tumor may adopt a papillary configuration with a fibrovascular core, or a solid nodular appearance. The latter may result in clusters of tumor cells in the lamina propria. Stromal invasion of TCC proceed in two stages: invasion of the lamina propria and invasion of the muscle layer. The detection of muscle invasion is of great consequence, because of the influence on therapy and prognosis. Histological diagnose of early bladder cancer (superficial TCC) or non-muscle invasive bladder cancer, which includes papilloma (benign lesions), papillary urothelial neoplasms with low malignant potential (PUNLMP), Low grade papillary carcinomas CIS (TIS/CIS), is virtually never confused with high grade carcinomas. PUNLMP have many features in common with normal epithelium and the histologic feature of the cells on the stalks is preserved and the nuclear feature are only slightly abnormal [38]. Lacking significant nuclear pleomorphic appearance, PUNLMP cells are difficult to recognize in urinary samples. However, this entity is considered as neoplastic because they tend to recur in the same site, and if left untreated, they can grow and dedifferentiate into aggressive cancers. Urothelial carcinoma, low grade, is a predominantly papillary urothelial neoplasm which resembling PUNLMP features. Histologically, the superficial layer is preserved, and the cells are uniform in size and evenly distributed. The orientation of the nuclei are often normal, but are rounded and slightly pleomorphic. There distinction of PUNLMP from low grade carcinomas may be difficult. However, the cells of low grade carcinoma are smaller and more densely arranged on the fibrovascular stalks, than the cells of PUNLMP, and at high magnification, there is a slight degree of nuclear pleomorphism and the nuclear chromatin is finely granular and evenly distributed. Immunohistochemical analyses are unlikely to be helpful in the differential diagnosis. The tumor cells are typically uniform, but densely packed in tissue sections. The tumor cells have indistinct borders, little or no cytoplasm, and the nuclear are pleomorphic, and the nuclear borders are irregular with coarse and uneven chromatin structure. Almost all invasive urothelial neoplasms are high grade, at least there is a focus of invasion, whether the invasion is confined to the lamina propria or muscularis propria. Mitoses are common and may be abnormal. Differential diagnostic problems are not a large problem, but may raise when high TCC involve prostatic duct or when prostatic carcinomas have invaded the bladder base. However, there are histological differences between high grade TCC and prostate cancer cells. Of importance is to diagnose patients whom superficial tumors are less differentiated, large, multiple, or associated with CIS in other areas of the bladder mucosa. These patients are at great risk for recurrence and the development of invasive cancers. IHC is overall of limited value when reactions for cytokeratins (7 and 20), carcinoembryonic antigens (CEA)125, 34β[beta]E12, and thrombomodulin are not specific. However, cytokeratins (CK20, CK7), tumor suppressor gene (p53) and the proliferation marker, Ki67 is widely used, because the majority of urothelial carcinomas are CK7+/CK20/CEA125-. The expression of CK20 is restricted to superficial 'umbrella' cells and occasional in the intermediate cells in benign and reactive urothelium, and also in severe inflammation. In dysplasia and CIS there is usually a complete or at least focal loss of this cellular reaction in all layers of the urothelium [39]. CK20/CK7 positivity may be useful when both were positive, supporting the diagnose of urothelial cancer. However, if only one marker was positive, or both negative, these markers have limited usefulness for distinguish these carcinomas. Expression of p53 has also been associated with an adverse prognosis for patients with invasive bladder cancer. Retrospective studies have shown that presence of nuclear p53 is an independent predictor for recurrence among patients with T-1-T3 tumors [40–43].

Role of Genetic Markers in Bladder Cancer

The main trend recent years have been screening with cDNA array-based platforms. Many proteins have been suggested as candidate cancer biomarkers based on results from gene-expression analysis. Despite the fact that this kind of platforms offers a potential to simultaneously study a broad range of genes at transcript level, this is not a fully successful method, because there is not carried out information according to the inter- and intra-tumoral cell location of a marker. In bladder cancer diagnostics it is of importance to use methods describing the heterogeneity within a tumor rather than an average estimate. However, bladder cancer is a multifactorial disease whose initiation and progression involve a complex network of genes and pathways. It is likely that no single marker will be sufficient for prognosis but a combination of markers from several genes or pathways may be required.

9.7 Nucleic Acid Biomarkers

Methylated DNA

Cancer is a disease initiated and driven by the clonal evolution of cells transformed by genetic and epigenetic alterations, which can occur as either inherited (germline) mutations or acquired (somatic) mutation of key genes. Methylation, an epigenic alteration (promoter methylation), can be used as targets for detection of tumor cells in clinical specimens, such as tissue biopsies or body fluids (serum, urine).

There is a known correlation between DNA Methylation and aberrant gene regulation involved in the predisposition, initiation, and progression of cancer. Detection of DNA methylation changes often occur at an early stage in cancer and other disease, which makes DNA methylation biomarkers ideal targets for the early detection and appropriate treatment of many diseases. One highly promising molecular biomarker is DNA methylation. This enzymatic addition of a methyl group at the 5-position of the cytosine in a CpG (cytosine-guanine) dinucleotide is a normal process within cells. In cancer, despite a global hypomethylation, one observes hypermethylation in regions of the genome described as CpG islands [4, 43] These islands are present in almost half of all genes and are frequently promoter-associated [44]. The common occurrence of DNA hypermethylation in all types of cancer makes it an ideal biomarker, one that has been extensively investigated. An advantage of DNA methylation over protein-based markers is that it is readily amplifiable and easily detectable using PCR-based approaches. In addition, contrary to cancer-specific mutations, which could occur anywhere in a gene, cancer-specific DNA hypermethylation occurs in defined regions, usually in or near the promoter of genes. In cancer cells, this often involves DNA methylation silencing of protective genes such as tumor suppressors. Expression in normal cells suppresses tumor formation, but by methylation it is silenced which enables tumor formation and cancer progression. The assessment of epigenic events is therefore one of the most promising method for identifying marker candidates for early detection of cancer. Circulating tumor-related free methylated DNA in blood and urine of cancer patients have already been assessed for their clinical utility.

DNA methylation in prostate cancer

The natural history of the development of PCa is highly variable. Since many PCa patients present with advanced disease, and some present with nonspecific elevation of PSA without cancer, early detection with high specificity and sensitivity is considered to be the most important approach to reduce mortality and unwanted tension of men with high PSA. It is evident that DNA methylation alterations in PCa and in bladder cancer are highly prevalent and constitute a crucial factor in the development and progression of the disease. The DNA hyper- and hypo-methylation events associated with PCa initiation that were identified from the beginning of 1990s and up today are already explored as biomarkers for improved detection of PCa. The results are promising. Suzuki et al. [45] detected seven genes (*BIK*, *BNIP3*, *cFLIP*, *TMS1*, *DcR1*, *DcR2*, *CDKN2A*) to be fully or partially methylated in several PCa cells, and others have revealed the methylation status of eight other genes including *RARB2*, *GSTP1*, *FLNC*, *EFS*, *ECRG4*, *PITX2*, *PDLIM4* and *KCNMA1* [46], and there is a lot of other genes under current investigation.

DNA methylation in bladder cancer

Regarding bladder cancer, recent studies have revealed several genetic and biological alterations with an extensive repertoire of candidate genes and pathways that have been implicated in TCC development and progression. These include anti-apoptotic genes, cell cycle regulators, various immune, nuclear, and proliferative markers, and cellular growth factors [47]. However, DNA methylation studies integrating genetic, epigenetic, and expression changes will definitely provide a clearer picture of prostate cancer initiation and progression.

Several genome-wide technologies are available and have been utilized to examine the extent of DNA methylation in discovery-based studies involving several physiological and disease states. Although early in the process, aberrant DNA methylation is gaining strength in the fields of cancer risk assessment, diagnosis and therapy monitoring in different cancer types. Nevertheless, it is expected that elucidating the functional consequences of DNA methylation changes will present major challenges for research for quite some time yet.

MicroRNAs (miRNA)s

miRNAs are small, noncoding RNAs with important functions in development, cell differentiation, and regulation of cell cycle and apoptosis. miRNA expression is deregulated in cancer by a variety of chromosomal rearrangements (amplification, deletion, mutation, epigenetic silencing), promoter methylation and regulation of transcription. A single miRNA can target hundreds of mRNAs, and alterations in miRNAs are known to disrupt the expression of several mRNAs and proteins. Several studies have shown that miRNAs are involved in the initiation and progression of cancer. miRNAs are found in all nucleated cells represent about 1 % of the genome and it is believed that 60 % of all human genes are monitored by miRNAs [48]. The purpose of identifying miRNA genes is to reveal their function. Since miRNAs often serve their roles by interacting with other molecules, series of algorithms are being established to find target molecules for miRNAs. Some miRNAs as biomarkers are able to trace the tissue of origin of cancers of unknown primary origin [48]. Microarray analysis allows for parallel analysis of large numbers of miRNAs and can be used to detect the presence and/or regulation of a wide range of defined miRNAs. The initial step in miRNA microarray profiling is the purification of RNA or miRNAs from cells or tissue. Many protocols have been developed for the extraction of high-quality RNA using various kits and reagents, however, it is of importance to know that the detection of miRNAs by microarray analysis, appropriate probe design is critical and unlike profiling of miRNAs by using microarray analysis, deep sequencing measures absolute abundance and, because it is not limited by array content, allows for the discovery of novel miRNAs that have eluded previous cloning and standard sequencing efforts.

miRNAs in prostate cancer

miRNAs in PCa tissue might be promising biomarkers for detection of cancer, prognosis, biochemical recurrence, Gleason grade, PSA and other clinico-pathological parameters. Even circulating serum levels of miRNAs are found to correlate with risk, aggressiveness, staging and disease outcome. Because of contradictory results, there is several limitations to overcome before miRNAs can replace conventional biomarkers such as PSA. However, the differential miRNA profile affords a solid basis for further functional analyses of miRNAs in PCa. Quantifying promoter methylation of putative tumor-suppressor genes in circulating free DNA is a rapidly growing research topic for early cancer detection. However, in the PCa field, none of the reported biomarkers has reached clinical application, mainly because of the small numbers of PCa's and matched control specimens analyzed.

miRNAs in bladder cancer

Genome-wide profiling of miRNA expression patterns in TCC by deep sequencing studies has revealed that miRNAs were aberrantly expressed in TCC compared to normal epithelium, suggesting that they might play roles as oncogenes or tumor suppressor genes in the development or progression of TCC. However, as for PCa, several studies using miRNA microarrays with different, sometimes limited probes to profile the miRNA expression, the results has not always indicated consistent results. It is likely that no single biological marker will be sufficient for prognosis, but rather a combination of markers from several genes or pathways may be required. Therefore, it is most important to understand the underlying biological mechanisms as well as the potential gene-gene and gene-environment interactions.

9.8 Summary

The detection and characterization of PSA in the late 1980s, especially in the terms of PCa screening, has led to the diagnosis of many potentially indolent cancers. Aggressive treatment of these cancers has caused significant morbidity without clinical benefit in many cases. Tumor staging, Gleason score and serum levels of PSA are up today, the most important prognostic factors. However, they cannot perfectly predict which patients are at risk for development more aggressive cancers. Future research should focus on validating existing biomarkers, finding novel biomarkers, and approaches for combining biomarkers for identification of those men who will have an indolent or aggressive PCa and those who will have therapeutic resistance. It is of incredible value to continue focusing on risk factors, molecular characterization in early and later stage of PCa, hormone refractory PCa, the multiclonal origins of the multifocality of PCa, acquired or somatic defective genes and hormones involved.

Despite the use of clinical and pathological factors, the ability to assess patient prognosis is

Key Points

- Early detection of PCa significantly reduces PCa-related mortality and the risk of developing metastatic and advanced PCa.
- Treatment decision of PCa is usually made based on PSA levels and histopathological findings at biopsies.
- PSA measurements have significant influence for diagnosis, treatment strategies and follow-up of PCa patients; however the specificity of total serum PSA is limited to treatment strategies especially for patients with low PSA serum levels (less than 4.0 ng/ml).
- The use of whole mounts of sections from RP specimens has the advantage of displaying the whole architecture of the prostate and the location of tumor areas.
- The IHC diagnosis of PCa largely depends on panels of markers because no absolutely specific and sensitive marker has yet been discovered.
- Several germline genetic risk variants have been established for prostate cancer incidence, a key question is whether they are also related to survival.
- The prognosis and treatment decisions of TCC are mainly based on pathological criteria, and proper staging is highly dependent on good quality biopsies. TCC are defined according to the histologic characteristics and so far, histologic examination is the most specific method for assessing these lesions.
- Current prognostic parameters such as grade, stage, multifocality of carcinomas, and lymph node status cannot with certainty predict the long term outcome of bladder cancer.
- The biomarkers for TCC that have been suggested lack sufficient predictive power, at the moment there is no reliable test for bladder cancer.
- Testing for blood in the urine is not a useful screening test for the general population because of the low specificity.

not satisfactory. With reliable diagnostic tests for progression, suitable treatments could be tailored to every patient. This has led to a huge effort to find reliable biomarkers to predict progression in patients with TCC. These potential markers include genetic alteration, methylation patterns, cell adhesion molecules, proteases, growth factors and a lot of other molecular markers. However, the biomarkers that have been suggested lack sufficient predictive power, at the moment there is no reliable test for bladder cancer. Testing for blood in the urine is not a useful screening test for the general population because of the low specificity.

There is a need to improve existing methods for the diagnosis of PCa and TCC to identify the patients at risk for developing these diseases, as well as identify the tumors that will progress and have an aggressive behavior.

In conclusion, given the current rapid development of large-scale genome screening and sequencing techniques, including proteomics and natotechnology, it is likely that in the coming years we will see a comprehensive elucidation of DNA methylation alterations in PCa and TCC. This will provide further candidates for biomarker development and further insights into these diseases pathogenesis, and thereby identification of new targets for treatment and therapeutic intervention.

References

1. Cancer of the Prostate—SEER Stat Fact Sheets. 2011. Retrieved from surveillance epidemiology and end results: http://seer.cancer.gov/statfacts/html/prost.html
2. American Cancer Society. Cancer facts & figures 2013. Atlanta: American Cancer Society; 2013.
3. U.S. Cancer Statistics Working Group. United States cancer statistics: 1999–2007 incidence and mortality web-based report. Atlanta: U.S. Department of Health and Human Services, Centers for Disease Control and Prevention and National Cancer Institute; 2010.
4. Ben-Shlomo Y, Evans S, Ibrahim F, et al. The risk of prostate cancer amongst black men in the United Kingdom: the PROCESS cohort study. Eur Urol. 2008;53(1):99–105.
5. Ferlay J, Shin HR, Bray F, et al. GLOBOCAN 2008 v1.2, cancer incidence and mortality worldwide: IARC CancerBase no. 10 [Internet]. Lyon: International Agency for Research on Cancer; 2010.

6. De Marzo AM, Marchi VL, Epstein JI, Nelson WG. Proliferative inflammatory atrophy of the prostate: implications for prostatic carcinogenesis. Am J Pathol. 1999;155(6):1985–92.
7. Palapattu GS, Sutcliffe S, Bastian PJ, Platz EA, De Marzo AM, Isaacs WB, Nelson WG. Prostate carcinogenesis and inflammation: emerging insights. Carcinogenesis. 2005;26(7):1170–81.
8. Epstein JI, Allsbrook Jr WC, Amin MB, Egevad LL, ISUP Grading Committee. The 2005 International Society of Urological Pathology (ISUP) consensus conference on Gleason grading of prostatic carcinoma. Am J Surg Pathol. 2005;29(9):1228–42.
9. Fine SW, Epstein JI. A contemporary study correlating prostate needle biopsy and radical prostatectomy Gleason score. J Urol. 2008;179(4):1335–8.
10. Fine SW, Amin MB, Berney DM, Bjartell A, Egevad L, Epstein JI, Humphrey PA, et al. A contemporary update on pathology reporting for prostate cancer: biopsy and radical prostatectomy specimens. Eur Urol. 2012;62(1):20–39.
11. Brawer MK, Cheli CD, Neaman IE, Goldblatt J, Smith C, Schwartz MK, et al. Complexed prostate specific antigen provides significant enhancement of specificity compared with total prostate specific antigen for detecting prostate cancer. J Urol. 2000;163(5):1476–80.
12. Catalona WJ, Smith DS, Ornstein DK. Prostate cancer detection in men with serum PSA concentrations of 2.6 to 4.0 ng/mL and benign prostate examination. Enhancement of specificity with free PSA measurements. JAMA. 1997;277(18):1452–5.
13. Thompson IM, Pauler DK, Goodman PJ, Tangen CM, Lucia MS, Parnes HL, et al. Prevalence of prostate cancer among men with a prostate-specific antigen level < or =4.0 ng per milliliter. N Engl J Med. 2004;350(22):2239–46.
14. Partin AW, Catalona WJ, Finlay JA, Darte C, Tindall DJ, Young CY, et al. Use of human glandular kallikrein 2 for the detection of prostate cancer: preliminary analysis. Urology. 1999;54(5):839–45.
15. Catalona WJ, Partin AW, Finlay JA, Chan DW, Rittenhouse HG, Wolfert RL, Woodrum DL. Use of percentage of free prostate-specific antigen to identify men at high risk of prostate cancer when PSA levels are 2.51 to 4 ng/mL and digital rectal examination is not suspicious for prostate cancer: an alternative model. Urology. 1999;54(2):220–4.
16. Babaian RJ, Fritsche H, Ayala A, Bhadkamkar V, Johnston DA, Naccarato W, Zhang Z. Performance of a neural network in detecting prostate cancer in the prostate-specific antigen reflex range of 2.5 to 4.0 ng/mL. Urology. 2000;56(6):1000–6.
17. Han M, Partin AW, Piantadosi S, Epstein JI, Walsh PC. Era specific biochemical recurrence-free survival following radical prostatectomy for clinically localized prostate cancer. J Urol. 2001;166(2):416–9.
18. Oesterling JE, Jacobsen SJ, Chute CG, et al. Serum prostate-specific antigen in a community-based population of healthy men. Establishment of age-specific reference ranges. JAMA. 1993;270:860–4.
19. Best S, Sawers Y, FU VX, et al. Integrity of prostatic tissue for molecular analysis after robotic-assisted laparoscopic and open prostatectomy. Urology. 2007;70:328–32.
20. Saratunga H, Montironi R, True L, Epstein JI, Griffiths DF, Humphrey PA, The ISUP Prostate Cancer Group, et al. International Society of Urological Pathology (ISUP) consensus conference on handling and staging of radical prostatectomy specimens. Working group 1: specimen handling. Mod Pathol. 2011;24:6–15.
21. Bostwic DG, Montironi R. Evaluating radical prostatectomy specimens: therapeutic and prognostic importance. Virchows Arch. 1997;430:1–16.
22. Chuang AY, Epstein JI. Positive surgical margins in areas of capsular incision in otherwise organ-confined disease at radical prostatectomy; histologic features and pitfalls. Am J Surg Pathol. 2008;32:1201–6.
23. Palapattu GS, Allaf ME, Trock BJ, Epstein JI, Walsh PC. Prostate specific antigen progression in men with lymph node metastases following radical prostatectomy: results of long-term followup. J Urol. 2004;172:1860–4.
24. Gleason DF. Classification of prostatic carcinomas. Cancer Chemother Rep. 1966;50:125–8.
25. Epstein JI, Allsbrook Jr WC, Amin MB, Egevad LL. The 2005 International Society of Urological Pathology (ISUP) consensus conference on Gleason grading in prostatic carcinoma. Am J Surg Pathol. 2005;29:1228–42.
26. Brimo F, Montironi R, Egevad L, et al. Contemporary grading for prostate cancer: implication for patient care. Eur Urol. 2012;63:892–901.
27. Egevad L, Ahmad AS, Algaba F, et al. Standardization of gleason grading among 337 European pathologists. Histopathology. 2013;62:247–56.
28. Egevad L, Mazzucchelli R, Montironi R. Implications of the International Society of Urological Pathology modified Gleason system. Arch Pathol Lab Med. 2012;136:426–34.
29. Dong F, Wang C, Farris AB, WU S, Lee H, Olumi AF, et al. Impact on the clinical outcome of prostate cancer by the 2005 International Society of Urological Pathology modified Gleason grading system. Am J Surg Pathol. 2012;36:838–43.
30. Epstein JI. An update of the Gleason grading system. J Urol. 2010;2:433–40.
31. van der Kwast TH, Amin MB, Billis A, Epstein JI, Griffiths D, Humphrey PA, ISUP Prostate Cancer Group, et al. International society of urological pathology consensus conference on handling and staging of radical prostatectomy specimens. Working group 2: T2 substaging and prostate cancer volume. Mod Pathol. 2011;24(1):16–25.
32. Egevad L, Srigley JR, Delahunt B. International Society of Urological Pathology (ISUP) Consensus conference on handling and staging of radical prostatectomy specimens. Working group 2: T2 substaging and prostate cancer volume. Adv Anat Pathol. 2011;18(4):301–5.

33. Samaratunga H, Montironi R, True L, et al. International Society of Urological Pathology (ISUP) consensus conference on handling and staging of radical prostatectomy specimens. Working group 1: specimen handling. Mod Pathol. 2011;24(1):6–15.
34. Parkin M, Pisani P. Estimates of worldwide incidence of 25 major cancers in 1990. Int J Cancer. 1999;80:827–41.
35. Pelucchi C, Bosetti C, Negri E, et al. Mechanisms of disease: the epidemiology of bladder cancer. Nat Clin Pract Urol. 2006;3:327–40.
36. Epstein JI, Amin MB, Reuter VR, Mostofi FK. The World Health Organization. International Society of Urological Pathology concensus classification of urothelial (transitional) neoplasms of the urinary bladder. Bladder Consensus Committee. Am J Surg Pathol. 1998;22:1435–48.
37. Habuchi T, Marberger M, Droller MJ, Hemstreet 3rd GP, Grossman HB, Schalken JA, et al. Prognostic markers for bladder cancer: International Consensus Panel on bladder tumor markers. VB Urol. 2005;66(6 Suppl 1):64–74.
38. Koss LG. Diagnostic cytology and its histopathologic base, vol. 2. 4th ed. Philadelphia: J.B. Lippincott; 1992. p. 890–933.
39. Murphy WM, Takezawa K, Maruniak NA. Interobserver discrepancy using the 1998 World Health Organization/International Society of Urologic Pathology classification of urothelial neoplasms: practical choices for patient care. J Urol. 2002;168(3):968–72.
40. Harnden P, Allam A, Joyce AD, Patel A, Selby P, Southgate J. Cytokeratin 20 as an objective marker of urothelial dysplasia. Br J Urol. 1996;78:870–5.
41. Esrig D, Spruck 3rd CH, Nichols PW, Chaiwun B, Steven K, Groshen S, et al. Accumulating of nuclear p53 and tumor progression in bladder cancer. N Engl J Med. 1993;331(19):1259–64.
42. Lipponen PK. Over-expression of p53 nuclear oncoprotein in transitional-cell bladder cancer and its prognostic value. Int J Cancer. 1993;53(3):365–70.
43. Rideout 3rd WM, Eversole-Cire P, Spruck 3rd CH, Hustad CM, Coetzee GA, Gonzales FA, Jones PA. Progressive increases in the methylation status and heterochromatinization of the myoD CpG island during oncogenic transformation. Mol Cell Biol. 1994;14:6143–52.
44. Takai D, Jones PA. The CpG island searcher: a new WWW resource. In Silico Biol. 2003;3: 235–40.
45. Suzuki MM, Bird A. DNA methylation landscapes: provocative insights from epigenomics. Nat Rev Genet. 2008;9:465–76.
46. Murphy TM, Sullivan L, Lane C, O'Connor L, Barrett C, Hollywood D, et al. In silico analysis and DHPLC screening strategy identifies novel apoptotic gene targets of aberrant promoter hypermethylation in prostate cancer. Prostate. 2011;71:1–17.
47. Lintula S, Hotakainen K. Developing biomarkers for improved diagnosis and treatment outcome monitoring of bladder cancer. Expert Opin Biol Ther. 2010;10:1169–80.
48. Rosenfeld N, Aharonov R, Meiri E, Rosenwald S, Spector Y, et al. MicroRNAs accurately identify cancer tissue origin. Nat Biotechnol. 2008;26(4): 462–9.

Minimally Invasive Therapies for Pelvic Urological Cancer

10

Willemien van den Bos, Berrend G. Muller, Daniel M. de Bruin, and Jean J.M.C.H. de la Rosette

10.1 Introduction

During the past decade, a variety of ablation techniques have been introduced for the treatment of localized prostate cancer. These techniques include brachytherapy, cryotherapy, high-intensity focused ultrasound (HIFU), laser ablation therapy, radiofrequency ablation, irreversible electroporation (IRE) and photodynamic therapy (PDT). The first three modalities have emerged as alternative therapeutic options in patients with clinically localized prostate cancer by the European Urology Association and American Urological Association. The others are still considered experimental [1].

Because of increased detection of early stage local prostate cancer lesions, focal therapy fulfills a more significant role as a less invasive procedure in the management of the disease [2]. This increased detection rate is partially due to intensified PSA testing on one hand and improved imaging technologies on the other hand [3, 4]. The patients with high volume low risk and intermediate risk prostate cancer with localized disease are the best candidates for focal treatment. Especially when it contains unilateral disease and clinical stage ≤cT2a [5] (More details in Table 10.1). Focal treatment enables better tissue preservation, decreased morbidity and is potentially applicable in 50–66 % of men with prostate cancer [6, 7]. The different treatment scenarios are ultra-focal, hemi-ablation or whole-gland therapy, based on the localization and multifocality of the tumors (Fig. 10.1). The minimally invasive nature of these techniques usually results in a short hospital stay with a better side effect profile and less impact on quality of life, resulting in an increased popularity [8, 9]. Nevertheless, since the available diagnostic modalities are still not yet conclusive, it is important to take into account that small insignificant lesions can be kept undetected and therefore untreated. In this chapter, the principles of each focal modality as well as information on application and outcome are provided to help understanding the different techniques (Table 10.2).

Table 10.1 Ideal candidates for focal therapy [67]

Serum PSA	PSA <15 ng/ml PSA >15 ng/ml should be counselled with caution
Clinical stage	T1c–T2a
Pathology	Gleason score 3 + 3 Gleason score 3 + 4
Life expectancy	>10 years
Clinical stage	Any; except in case of HIFU: <40 mL

W. van den Bos, PhD • B.G. Muller, MD, PhD
D.M. de Bruin, MSc, PhD
J.J.M.C.H.de la Rosette, PhD (✉)
Department of Urology, Academic Medical Center, Amsterdam, The Netherlands
e-mail: j.j.delarosette@amc.uva.nl

H.R.H. Patel et al. (eds.), *Pelvic Cancer Surgery: Modern Breakthroughs and Future Advances*,
DOI 10.1007/978-1-4471-4258-4_10, © Springer-Verlag London 2015

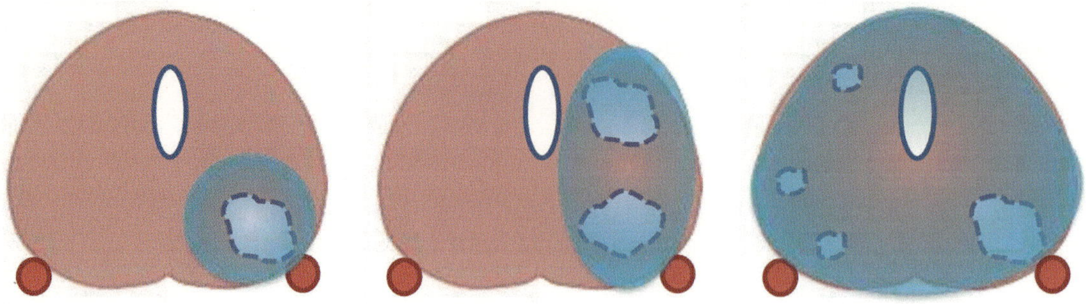

Fig. 10.1 Treatment scenarios

10.2 Thermal Ablations

Laser Ablation Therapy

Principles

Laser ablation therapy uses near infrared (NIR) light from a neodymium-yttrium-aluminum-garnet laser. It reaches the tissue of the prostate by laser fibers through a transperineal approach. The technique is based on the photo-thermal effect. This thermal action results from the absorption of NIR light by tissue chromophores, which is converted into heat in a very short time [10]. This effect depends on the intensity of light and the concentration of available tissue chromophores. Temperatures above 60 °C cause rapid coagulative necrosis in the targeted tissue followed by instant cell death. But also at lower hyperthermic temperatures (>42 °C) irreversible cell death is also achieved with prolongation of the procedure [11, 12]. Figure 10.2 shows the mechanisms of the thermal ablation techniques.

Application and Outcome

Besides the destruction of cells by the photo-thermal effect, a reaction can be observed in the reduction of blood perfusion. It is therefore possible to observe the delineation between viable and nonviable tissue with contrast-enhanced ultrasonography (CEUS) [13]. Until now, all studies about laser ablation are phase I clinical trials or contain small cohorts with a maximum of 12 patients [14]. This study of Lindner et al. showed on biopsies after 6 months post-treatment 67 % was free of tumor in the targeted area and 50 % was free of disease. Side effects according to this technique included perineal discomfort, hematospermia, dysuria and fatigue [13–15]. Further research is needed to demonstrate the long-term effectiveness.

Cryotherapy

Principles

Cryotherapy induces cell death by freezing. In the past, urinary incontinence, urethral sloughing and recto-urethral fistula were common side effects and a mortality rate of 1.9 % was reported [16]. More recently, the technique has changed and improved using multiprobe-devices, guided by advanced imaging techniques. Cryotherapy is

Table 10.2 Overview of techniques with indications, contra-indications, advantages and disadvantages

	Indications	Contra-indications	Advantages	Disadvantages
Brachytherapy	Stage T1b to T2a	Recent TURP High IPSS Worse flowmetry Prostate gland volume >50 mL Previous pelvic irradiation	Outcomes equal to radical approach Widely available Little interruption of daily life	Chronic urinary morbidity in 20 %
Cryotherapy	Stage T1 to T3 Unfit for surgery Life expectancy <10 years	Prostate gland volume >40 mL	Real time monitoring with TRUS and MRI Short hospital stay (1–4 days) Less side-effects than radical prostatectomy	Cold sink effect High post-operatively erectile dysfunction (47–100 %) [66] Intraprostatic needles insertion required High costs
HIFU	Stage T1-T2	Anterior tumor or tumor located near apex or midline	No intraprostatic needles required Short hospital stay Minimal rectal injury	Heat sink effect Time-consuming (10 g prostate/h) High costs
Radiofrequency ablation	Clinically localized cancer; not further specified	Not described	RFA can be performed with IV sedation in an outpatient setting	Heat sink effect Few data about efficacy
Laser ablation therapy	Clinically localized cancer: not further specified	Not described	MRI-guidance possible Erectile function preservation Short hospital stay	Heat sink effect Few data about efficacy
Irreversible electroporation	Clinically localized cancer: not further specified	Not described	No heat sink issues Real-time CT/US imaging Nerves and vessel-sparing	Intraprostatic electrodes required No data about efficacy
Photodynamic therapy	Clinically localized cancer: not further specified	Not described	Photosensitizer possible selective for malign cells Short hospital stay	Intraprostatic fibers Oxygen-dependency in hypoxic tumors Technique only reviewed after failure of radio- or brachytherapy

either used as primary treatment (partial or whole-gland) or as salvage treatment. It contains different mechanisms in destroying tumor tissue, including 'Freeze rupture,' a cellular response to freezing, which induces cell death known as necrosis and apoptosis [17]. Direct cell damage occurs when cell metabolism fails as a result of temperature drop. When temperature decreases until −20 °C, extracellular water crystallizes and causes a retraction of water out of the system. This results in a hyperosmotic extracellular environment followed by the extraction of water from the cells and end up in denaturation and electrolyte disturbances [18]. All parts of the

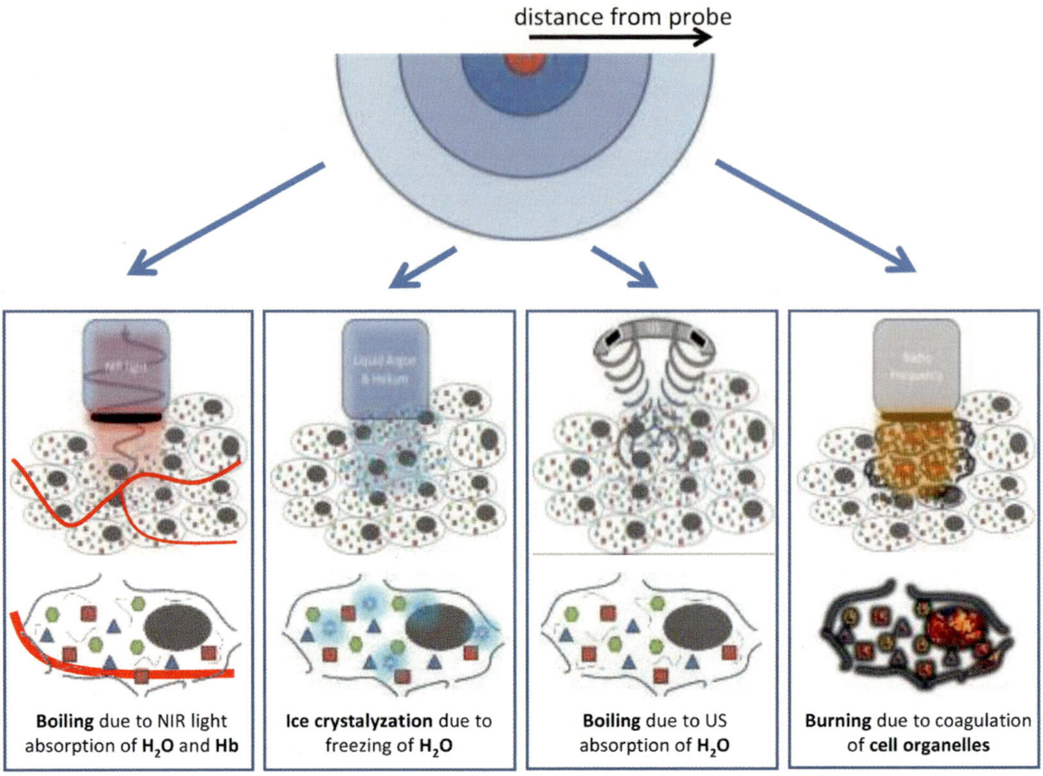

Fig. 10.2 Therapies based on hyper- and hypothermal ablation. From *left* to *right*: laser ablation therapy, cryotherapy, HIFU, radiofrequency ablation

freeze-thaw cycle can cause tissue damage. But the coldest tissue temperature is the main factor in generating cell death. It is also important that the cooling rate is as fast as possible. The optimal duration of freezing are unknown, but long lasting freezing increases tissue injury. Thawing rate is a prime destructive cause and it should be as slow as possible, thereby repetition of the freeze-thaw cycle is an important factor in effective therapy [19]. Furthermore, freezing until at least −40 °C is recommended since this causes intracellular ice crystal formation which is a severe threat to cell viability and nearly always lethal [20, 21]. Depending on the multifocality and extension of the tumor, the choice has to be made between whole or partial-gland cryoablation (See Fig. 10.2).

Application and Outcome

Cryotherapy is an option for low-, intermediate-, and high-risk patients [17]. The freezing is obtained by introducing transrectal ultrasound (TRUS) -guided needles using a transperineal approach. Limiting factor is the volume of the gland; the larger the prostate, the more difficult to achieve a uniformly cold temperature by pubic arch interference. Advantage is the ability of real-time visualization of the formed ice-ball by TRUS or Magnetic Resonance Imaging (MRI). Short-term complications are urinary retention because of gland swelling. Penile and scrotal swelling can occur, but are mostly self-limiting. Long-term morbidity differs between partial-gland and whole-gland treatment. A report from the National Cryo On-Line Database (COLD) Registry shows a high percentage of complete urinary continence (98.4 %) [22]. Erectile dysfunction ranged from 49 to 93 % at 1 year [23, 24]. Here for, cryoablation is considered as a treatment option in men who are not concerned with erectile function. Biochemical disease-free survival is diversely ranged along patients-cohorts. The 5-year biochemical disease-free survival rates for low-, intermediate-, and high-risk cases range from 65 to 92, 69 to 89, and 48 to 89 %, respectively [17, 24]. Another study (n = 60) shows biopsy proven recurrence found in up to 23 % of the patients after 15.2 months, mostly found in the untreated hemi-gland [25].

High-Intensity Focused Ultrasound

Principles

High-intensity focused ultrasound (HIFU) has seen several applications in tissue since the 1950s. Madersbacher et al. [26] stated in 1995 the value of HIFU in treating prostate cancer, leading to several clinical studies. HIFU uses focused ultrasound (US) to destroy tissue based on two principles; hyperthermia and cavitation. When the US beam is focused transrectally at a specific depth inside the prostate, the high-energy instigates heats above the denaturation-temperature of proteins inducing cell death. Besides, the US beam can interact with aqueous micro-bubbles in the sonicated area, leading to coagulative necrosis [27–29]. Two companies are providing HIFU devices: Ablatherm and Sonablate (See Fig. 10.2).

Application and Outcome

HIFU is used as both a primary treatment and as a salvage treatment. Best candidates for HIFU are patients with T1c-T3 tumors smaller than 40 mL that are not suitable for radical approach. Contra-indication is the absence or an inaccessible rectum since the technique applies a transrectal approach. Also, major calcifications larger than 1.0 cm have negative influence on treatment [30, 31]. The advantage of this procedure over other focal therapies is the ability to destroy cells over a distance from the US probe without being invasive. Most common complications of HIFU therapy are urinary retention (<1–20 %) caused by edematous prostate tissue, urinary tract infections (1.8–47.9 %) and incontinence (<1–34.3 %). Erectile dysfunction is reported in 20.0–81.6 %, which in less compared to other modalities. The incidence of recto-urethral fistulas (<2 %) has decreased with the improvement of devices and treatment procedures. Most complications are transient or treatable. Less common complications are urethral or bladder neck stenosis, urethral stricture, chronic perineal pain, infravesical obstruction, epididymitis and prostatitis [32, 33]. Cordeiro et al. [32] reviewed the outcome of 31 HIFU studies and stated that negative biopsy rates (mostly taken after 3–6 months) ranged from 35 to 95 %. Percentage of patients with a PSA nadir of 0.5 ng/mL ranged from 61 to 91 %. The 5-year biochemical disease-free rate (according to Phoenix criteria) was 72 %; 84 % for low-risk patients, 64 % for intermediate-risk patients and 45 % for high-risk patients [31].

Radiofrequency Ablation

Principles

This technique uses radiofrequency energy to ablate tissue. Through transperineal needles the monopolar electrodes can be inserted which are able to reach 50 W with a frequency of 460 kHz. It causes an irreversible destruction of tissue by hyperthermia of approximately 100 °C. Hyperthermia occurs by gradually raising the power. For 5 min this heat has to be maintained. This results in coagulative necrosis of the targeted tissue [34]. During this treatment, the urethra and rectum were cooled by cold saline. The procedure has been assessed as feasible, safe and reproducible in prostate cancer [35, 36] (see Fig. 10.2).

Application and Outcome

Radiofrequency ablation has been investigated in two different groups of patients. Firstly in patients with clinically localized prostate cancer; this showed no complications [35, 36]. Shariat et al. [37] treated patients after failed radiation and patients unfit for surgery. This study showed transient side effects as macrohematuria in 19 %, bladder spasms and dysuria in 9 %. At 12 months after RITA, 50 % of patients with sufficient follow-up had no residual cancer on repeat systematic 12-core biopsy cores and 67 % were cancer-free in biopsy cores sampled from the RITA-treated areas. No long-term outcomes have been reported in literature.

10.3 Non-thermal Ablations

Irreversible Electroporation

Principles

Bio-electrics is an interesting new area of medicine combining pulsed high-voltage engineering and cell biology [38–40]. Pulsating current alters the transmembrane potential of biological cells. If the duration of the applied electrical pulses is below the charging time of the outer cell membrane (approximately 100 ns for mammalian cells), there is interaction of the electric field with subcellular structures. Cell survival is inversely proportional to the electric field generated and by manipulating the pulse duration, the electric field intensity, and the number of pulses, it is possible to alter the effects on the target cells. The pulsed electric fields increase the permeability of the cell membrane by a process known as electroporation, a process that can be reversible or irreversible depending on the combination of the variables above [41]. Reversible electroporation temporarily makes the cell membrane more permeable [42]. The cell can survive this insult [43], and it has been employed in electro chemotherapy, to facilitate the uptake of chemotherapeutic agents into cells [42, 44], and gene therapy. Irreversible electroporation results in the permanent permeabilization of the cell membrane, which disrupts cell homeostasis and leads to cell death [42, 43]. In vitro, it has commercial application and has been used by the food industry to sterilize and pre-process food since 1961 [41]; it can also be used to sterilize water, because the process destroys bacteria and yeasts. In vivo, the irreversibly permeabilized cells are left in situ and are removed by the immune system [44] (See Fig. 10.3).

Applications and Outcome

IRE has been shown to effectively ablate tumor cells in vitro, in small and large animal experiments [43, 45, 46] and in a recent safety study on the IRE of focal liver, kidney and lung tumors [47, 48]. There are two main factors driving research into IRE as a treatment modality. First, tumor ablation experiments in animals and humans have shown that connective tissue structure is preserved and there is no damage to associated blood vessels, neural tissue, or other vital structures [43, 46, 49]. Second, IRE may ablate below the thermal damage threshold of 50 °C and there is no "heat sink" effect, a factor that decreases the effectiveness of other ablation therapies such as RFA near major vessels [44, 50–52]. It is anticipated that the preservation of surrounding tissue will reduce treatment-induced side effects inherent in current prostate cancer therapies.

Brachytherapy

Principles

Brachytherapy is broadly used in the management of localized prostate cancer. Brachytherapy is the delivery of radiation by radionuclides using sealed sources, placed close to the target. Guided by TRUS, hollow needles are placed inside the prostate. Radioactive seeds are injected through these needles for permanent implantation. This precise source placement enables high dose delivery within the tumor, avoiding structures as urethra, neurovascular bundle or rectum to be irradiated and accurate doses at the margins [53, 54] (See Fig. 10.3).

Application and Outcome

Brachytherapy can be considered in patients with clinically localized Stage 1–2 prostate cancer without metastases. The average overall-survival after whole-gland brachytherapy is equivalent to options as active surveillance, radical prostatectomy (RP) or external beam radiotherapy (EBRT). Therefore, the patients have to be given the choice of treatment [55]. Biggest advantage of brachytherapy is the minor interruption of

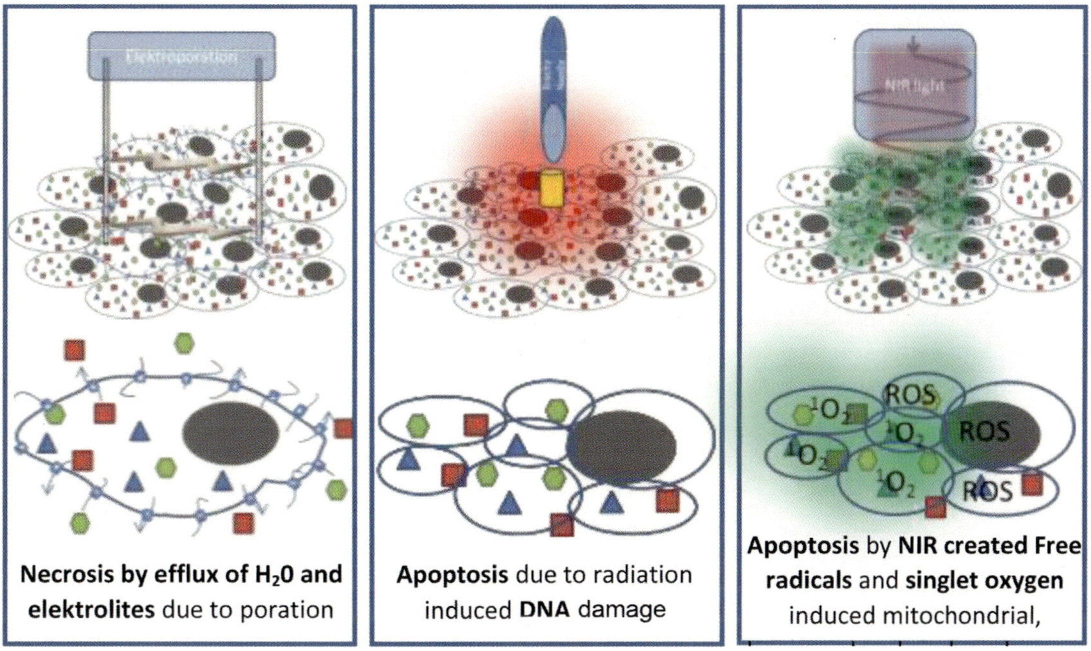

Fig. 10.3 Therapies based on non-thermal ablation method. From *left* to *right*: irreversible electroporation, brachytherapy, photodynamic therapy

daily life of the patient with a hospital-stay of 1–2 days. Recently focal application of brachytherapy has been investigated in treatment of prostate cancer. Until now only primary outcome parameter is adverse events because of the short follow-up time [56].

The most common side effect is urethritis, which is treated with alpha-blockers and non-steroidal anti-inflammatory drugs. Also, proctitis occurs frequently. Therefore, antibiotic prophylaxis is regularly prescribed after implantation [57]. After the procedure, about 15 % of the patients develop temporary acute urinary retention due to edema, which can be solved by catheterization. Fifteen-year biochemical control is 85.9, 79.9, and 62.2 % for low, intermediate, and high-risk patients, respectively treated with whole-gland brachytherapy [58]. Two focal brachytherapy studies are recently undertaken, concerning hemi-gland and ultra-focal procedures with the most important parameter of occurred adverse events [56, 59]. A consensus has been made about patient selection for ultra-focal brachytherapy by Langley et al. [60].

Photodynamic Therapy

Principles

Photodynamic therapy (PDT) was initially described at the start of the twentieth century [61, 62]. The technology is based on the interaction of a photosensitive agent (PS), which is administered systemically (intravenously or orally), with light brought to the tissue by a laser fiber, and oxygen that is present in the tissue. The absorption of a photon leads to a chain reaction inducing the release of a singlet oxygen and antioxidant enzymes. This singlet oxygen can directly kill tumor cells by induction of necrosis and apoptosis, or cause destruction of tumor vasculature, producing an acute inflammatory response that attracts leucocytes, such as dendritic cells and neutrophils [63]. Accomplishment of PDT requires intraprostatic laser fiber placement. This is achieved through transperineal approach using a brachytherapy template under TRUS guidance. After fiber placement, interstitial illumination must be conducted in a darkened room to prevent cutaneous photosensitization (See Fig. 10.3).

Application and Outcome

Arumainayagan et al. and Azzouzi et al. recently presented two studies including 40 and 85 patients [64, 65]. In both Padeliporfin is used as photosensitizer. Arumainayagan performed hemi-ablation and near whole gland with transperineal approach. MRI showed visible necrosis areas and only in two patients a side effect (recatherization) occurred. Azzouzi et al. achieved hemiablations that led to 87 % necrosis in the treated lobe. Side effects as prostatitis, hematuria and strictures occurred. Until now, no articles are published with data on biochemical control or other outcomes.

Key Points

- Focal therapy in prostate cancer is gaining popularity.
- Focal therapy can be used in patients with clinically localized cancer.
- Brachytherapy is the delivery of radiation by radionuclides using sealed sources, placed close to the target.
- Cryotherapy creates direct cell damage when cell metabolism fails as a result of temperature drop.
- HIFU causes high-energy which instigates heat above the denaturation-temperature of proteins inducing cell death.
- Laser ablation therapy causes thermal damage by the absorption of NIR light.
- Radiofrequency ablation provides irreversible destruction of tissue by hyperthermia.
- Photodynamic therapy is based on the interaction of a photosensitive agent with light, brought to the tissue by a laser fiber, and oxygen that is present in the tissue. This combination causes tissue damage.
- Irreversible electroporation provides pulsed electric fields, which increase the permeability of the cell membrane, followed by cell necrosis.

References

1. Heidenreich A, Bastian PJ, Bellmunt J, et al. EAU guidelines on prostate cancer. Part 1: Screening, diagnosis, and local treatment with curative intent-update 2013. Eur Urol. 2014;65(1):124–37. doi: 10.1016/j.eururo.2013.09.046.
2. Cooperberg MR, Lubeck DP, Meng MV, Mehta SS, Carroll PR. The changing face of low-risk prostate cancer: trends in clinical presentation and primary management. J Clin Oncol. 2004;22(11):2141–9.
3. Bott SR, Henderson A, McLarty E, Langley SE. A brachytherapy template approach to standardize saturation prostatic biopsy. BJU Int. 2004; 93(4):629–30.
4. Dickinson L, Ahmed HU, Allen C, Barentsz JO, Carey B, Futterer JJ, et al. Magnetic resonance imaging for the detection, localisation, and characterisation of prostate cancer: recommendations from a European consensus meeting. Eur Urol. 2011;59(4):477–94.
5. de la Rosette J, Ahmed H, Barentsz J, Johansen TB, Brausi M, Emberton M, et al. Focal therapy in prostate cancer-report from a consensus panel. J Endourol. 2010;24(5):775–80.
6. Karavitakis M, Winkler M, Abel P, Livni N, Beckley I, Ahmed HU. Histological characteristics of the index lesion in whole-mount radical prostatectomy specimens: implications for focal therapy. Prostate Cancer Prostatic Dis. 2011;14(1):46–52.
7. Bott SR, Ahmed HU, Hindley RG, Abdul-Rahman A, Freeman A, Emberton M. The index lesion and focal therapy: an analysis of the pathological characteristics of prostate cancer. BJU Int. 2010;106(11):1607–11.
8. Polascik TJ, Mouraviev V. Focal therapy for prostate cancer. Curr Opin Urol. 2008;18(3):269–74.
9. Barqawi AB, Crawford ED. The current use and future trends of focal surgical therapy in the management of localized prostate cancer. Cancer J. 2007;13(5):313–7.
10. Mordon SR, Wassmer B, Reynaud JP, Zemmouri J. Mathematical modeling of laser lipolysis. Biomed Eng Online. 2008;7:10.
11. Sapareto SA, Dewey WC. Thermal dose determination in cancer therapy. Int J Radiat Oncol Biol Phys. 1984;10(6):787–800.
12. Lindner U, Lawrentschuk N, Trachtenberg J. Focal laser ablation for localized prostate cancer. J Endourol. 2010;24(5):791–7.
13. Atri M, Gertner MR, Haider MA, Weersink RA, Trachtenberg J. Contrast-enhanced ultrasonography for real-time monitoring of interstitial laser thermal therapy in the focal treatment of prostate cancer. Can Urol Assoc J. 2009;3(2):125–30.
14. Lindner U, Weersink RA, Haider MA, Gertner MR, Davidson SR, Atri M, et al. Image guided photothermal focal therapy for localized prostate cancer: phase I trial. J Urol. 2009;182(4):1371–7.
15. Amin Z, Lees WR, Bown SG. Technical note: interstitial laser photocoagulation for the treatment of prostatic cancer. Br J Radiol. 1993;66(791):1044–7.

16. Merrick GS, Wallner KE, Butler WM. Prostate cryotherapy: more questions than answers. Urology. 2005;66(1):9–15.
17. Babaian RJ, Donnelly B, Bahn D, Baust JG, Dineen M, Ellis D, et al. Best practice statement on cryosurgery for the treatment of localized prostate cancer. J Urol. 2008;180(5):1993–2004.
18. Levy D, Avallone A, Jones JS. Current state of urological cryosurgery: prostate and kidney. BJU Int. 2010;105(5):590–600.
19. Gage AA, Baust J. Mechanisms of tissue injury in cryosurgery. Cryobiology. 1998;37(3):171–86.
20. Mazur P. Freezing of living cells: mechanisms and implications. Am J Physiol. 1984;247(3 Pt 1):C125–42.
21. Mazur P, Rall WF, Leibo SP. Kinetics of water loss and the likelihood of intracellular freezing in mouse ova. Influence of the method of calculating the temperature dependence of water permeability. Cell Biophys. 1984;6(3):197–213.
22. Ward JF, Jones JS. Focal cryotherapy for localized prostate cancer: a report from the national Cryo On-Line Database (COLD) Registry. BJU Int. 2012;109(11):1648–54.
23. Bahn DK, Lee F, Badalament R, Kumar A, Greski J, Chernick M. Targeted cryoablation of the prostate: 7-year outcomes in the primary treatment of prostate cancer. Urology. 2002;60(2 Suppl 1):3–11.
24. Donnelly BJ, Saliken JC, Ernst DS, Ali-Ridha N, Brasher PM, Robinson JW, et al. Prospective trial of cryosurgical ablation of the prostate: five-year results. Urology. 2002;60(4):645–9.
25. Ellis DS, Manny Jr TB, Rewcastle JC. Focal cryosurgery followed by penile rehabilitation as primary treatment for localized prostate cancer: initial results. Urology. 2007;70(6 Suppl):9–15.
26. Madersbacher S, Pedevilla M, Vingers L, Susani M, Marberger M. Effect of high-intensity focused ultrasound on human prostate cancer in vivo. Cancer Res. 1995;55(15):3346–51.
27. Crouzet S, Murat FJ, Pasticier G, Cassier P, Chapelon JY, Gelet A. High intensity focused ultrasound (HIFU) for prostate cancer: current clinical status, outcomes and future perspectives. Int J Hyperthermia. 2010;26(8):796–803.
28. Susani M, Madersbacher S, Kratzik C, Vingers L, Marberger M. Morphology of tissue destruction induced by focused ultrasound. Eur Urol. 1993;23 Suppl 1:34–8.
29. Stride EP, Coussios CC. Cavitation and contrast: the use of bubbles in ultrasound imaging and therapy. Proc Inst Mech Eng H. 2010;224(2):171–91.
30. Crouzet S, Rebillard X, Chevallier D, Rischmann P, Pasticier G, Garcia G, et al. Multicentric oncologic outcomes of high-intensity focused ultrasound for localized prostate cancer in 803 patients. Eur Urol. 2010;58(4):559–66.
31. Uchida T, Shoji S, Nakano M, Hongo S, Nitta M, Murota A, et al. Transrectal high-intensity focused ultrasound for the treatment of localized prostate cancer: eight-year experience. Int J Urol. 2009;16(11):881–6.
32. Cordeiro ER, Cathelineau X, Thuroff S, Marberger M, Crouzet S, de la Rosette JJ. High-intensity focused ultrasound (HIFU) for definitive treatment of prostate cancer. BJU Int. 2012;110(9):1228–42.
33. Uchida T, Nakano M, Hongo S, Shoji S, Nagata Y, Satoh T, et al. High-intensity focused ultrasound therapy for prostate cancer. Int J Urol. 2012; 19(3):187–201.
34. Cheng HL, Haider MA, Dill-Macky MJ, Sweet JM, Trachtenberg J, Gertner MR. MRI and contrast-enhanced ultrasound monitoring of prostate microwave focal thermal therapy: an in vivo canine study. J Magn Reson Imaging. 2008;28(1):136–43.
35. Zlotta AR, Djavan B, Matos C, Noel JC, Peny MO, Silverman DE, et al. Percutaneous transperineal radiofrequency ablation of prostate tumour: safety, feasibility and pathological effects on human prostate cancer. Br J Urol. 1998;81(2):265–75.
36. Djavan B, Susani M, Shariat S, Zlotta AR, Silverman DE, Schulman CC, et al. Transperineal radiofrequency interstitial tumor ablation (RITA) of the prostate. Tech Urol. 1998;4(2):103–9.
37. Shariat SF, Raptidis G, Masatoschi M, Bergamaschi F, Slawin KM. Pilot study of radiofrequency interstitial tumor ablation (RITA) for the treatment of radio-recurrent prostate cancer. Prostate. 2005;65(3):260–7.
38. Rubinsky B. Irreversible electroporation in medicine. Technol Cancer Res Treat. 2007;6(4):255–60.
39. Onik G, Mikus P, Rubinsky B. Irreversible electroporation: implications for prostate ablation. Technol Cancer Res Treat. 2007;6(4):295–300.
40. Maor E, Ivorra A, Leor J, Rubinsky B. The effect of irreversible electroporation on blood vessels. Technol Cancer Res Treat. 2007;6(4):307–12.
41. Al-Sakere B, Andre F, Bernat C, Connault E, Opolon P, Davalos RV, et al. Tumor ablation with irreversible electroporation. PLoS ONE. 2007;2(11):e1135.
42. Thomson KR, Cheung W, Ellis SJ, Federman D, Kavnoudias H, Loader-Oliver D, et al. Investigation of the safety of irreversible electroporation in humans. J Vasc Interv Radiol. 2011;22(5):611–21.
43. Ball C, Thomson KR, Kavnoudias H. Irreversible electroporation: a new challenge in "out of operating theater" anesthesia. Anesth Analg. 2010;110(5):1305–9.
44. Davalos RV, Mir IL, Rubinsky B. Tissue ablation with irreversible electroporation. Ann Biomed Eng. 2005;33(2):223–31.
45. Garner AL, Chen G, Chen N, Sridhara V, Kolb JF, Swanson RJ, et al. Ultrashort electric pulse induced changes in cellular dielectric properties. Biochem Biophys Res Commun. 2007;362(1):139–44.
46. Altunc S. Subnanosecond pulsed-power generated electric fields for cancer treatment. IEEE Nucl Plasma Sci Soc News. 2009;34:2012.
47. Miller L, Leor J, Rubinsky B. Cancer cells ablation with irreversible electroporation. Technol Cancer Res Treat. 2005;4(6):699–705.
48. Rubinsky B, Onik G, Mikus P. Irreversible electroporation: a new ablation modality—clinical implications. Technol Cancer Res Treat. 2007;6(1):37–48.

49. Joshi RP, Schoenbach KH. Bioelectric effects of intense ultrashort pulses. Crit Rev Biomed Eng. 2010;38(3):255–304.
50. Schoenbach KH. The effect of intense subnanosecond electrical pulses on biological cells. Eng Med. 2008;36:414–22. 2012.
51. Bertacchini C, Margotti PM, Bergamini E, Lodi A, Ronchetti M, Cadossi R. Design of an irreversible electroporation system for clinical use. Technol Cancer Res Treat. 2007;6(4):313–20.
52. Faroja M, Ahmed M, Appelbaum L, Ben-David E, Moussa M, Sosna J, et al. Irreversible electroporation ablation: is all the damage nonthermal? Radiology. 2013;266(2):462–70.
53. Nag S, Ciezki JP, Cormack R, Doggett S, DeWyngaert K, Edmundson GK, et al. Intraoperative planning and evaluation of permanent prostate brachytherapy: report of the American Brachytherapy Society. Int J Radiat Oncol Biol Phys. 2001;51(5):1422–30.
54. Zelefsky MJ, Yamada Y, Marion C, Sim S, Cohen G, Ben-Porat L, et al. Improved conformality and decreased toxicity with intraoperative computer-optimized transperineal ultrasound-guided prostate brachytherapy. Int J Radiat Oncol Biol Phys. 2003;55(4):956–63.
55. Hall JD, Boyd JC, Lippert MC, Theodorescu D. Why patients choose prostatectomy or brachytherapy for localized prostate cancer: results of a descriptive survey. Urology. 2003;61(2):402–7.
56. Cosset JM, Wakil G, Pierrat N, Cathelineau X, Marchand V, Vallancien G. Focal brachytherapy for prostate cancer: a pilot study. Radiother Oncol. 2011;99 Suppl 1:S283.
57. Buyyounouski MK, Davis BJ, Prestidge BR, Shanahan TG, Stock RG, Grimm PD, et al. A survey of current clinical practice in permanent and temporary prostate brachytherapy: 2010 update. Brachytherapy. 2012;11(4):299–305.
58. Sylvester JE, Grimm PD, Wong J, Galbreath RW, Merrick G, Blasko JC. Fifteen-year biochemical relapse-free survival, cause-specific survival, and overall survival following I (125) prostate brachytherapy in clinically localized prostate cancer: Seattle experience. Int J Radiat Oncol Biol Phys. 2011;81(2):376–81.
59. http://clinicaltrials.gov/show/NCT01354951. 2013. Ref Type: Online Source
60. Langley S, Ahmed HU, Al-Qaisieh B, Bostwick D, Dickinson L, Veiga FG, et al. Report of a consensus meeting on focal low dose rate brachytherapy for prostate cancer. BJU Int. 2012;109 Suppl 1:7–16.
61. Wilson BC, Patterson MS, Lilge L. Implicit and explicit dosimetry in photodynamic therapy: a new paradigm. Lasers Med Sci. 1997;12(3):182–99.
62. Zeng H, Korbelik M, McLean DI, MacAulay C, Lui H. Monitoring photoproduct formation and photobleaching by fluorescence spectroscopy has the potential to improve PDT dosimetry with a verteporfin-like photosensitizer. Photochem Photobiol. 2002;75(4):398–405.
63. Tyrrell JS, Campbell SM, Curnow A. The relationship between protoporphyrin IX photobleaching during real-time dermatological methyl-aminolevulinate photodynamic therapy (MAL-PDT) and subsequent clinical outcome. Lasers Surg Med. 2010;42(7):613–9.
64. Arumainayagam N, Moore CM, Ahmed HU, Emberton M. Photodynamic therapy for focal ablation of the prostate. World J Urol. 2010;28(5):571–6.
65. Azzouzi A-R, Emberton M. Results of Tookad soluble vascular targeted photodynamic therapy (VTP) for low risk localized prostate cancer. Washington, DC: AUA 2011.
66. van den Bos W, Muller BG, Ahmed H, Bangma CH, Barret E, Crouzet S, et al. Focal Therapy in Prostate Cancer: International Multidisciplinary Consensus on Trial Design. Eur. Urol., pp. 2–7, Jan 2014.
67. Shelley M, Wilt TJ, Coles B, Mason MD. Cryotherapy for localised prostate cancer. Cochrane Database Syst Rev. 2007;(3):CD005010.

Radical Retropubic Prostatectomy

11

Pedro Bargão Santos, Bruno Graça, Manuel Ferreira Coelho, Fernando Ferrito, João Real Dias, Francisco Carrasquinho Gomes, and Hitendra R.H. Patel

11.1 Introduction

The technique for performing RRP has improved considerably since Millin first introduced the retropubic approach in 1945 [1]. The morbidity of RRP, since described by Reiner and Walsh in 1979, has also decreased dramatically due to technical improvements [2] and better understanding of periprostatic anatomy [3]. RRP still remains the gold standard which other techniques are compared to. Some laparoscopic and robotic surgeons claim that only reproduce in their surgeries the open technique. The authors of this chapter describe the state of the art of the open technique and its advances.

11.2 Essential Instruments

RRP requires only a few special but essential instruments. A fiberoptic headlight (Fig. 11.1) is fundamental because most of the procedure is performed underneath the pubis where visualization could be very difficult. A 2.5–2.9× power-loupes (Fig. 11.1) are mandatory during all the procedure, allowing the minuteness of gestures to find the appropriate planes and to make a very careful dissection. A standard Balfour retractor or a designed self-retractor with a Richardson type blade (Fig. 11.2) is important to stabilize the operative field, providing cranial and posterior retraction of the bladder and peritoneum. Other essential instruments are bipolar coagulation forceps, Metzenbaum scissors and small, fine and regular right-angled forceps.

11.3 Position

The patient is placed in supine position, with the pubis centered over the break of the table, flexed, to elevate the pelvis and facilitate exposure. A 25–30° Trendelenburg position also improves vision and reduce blood loss on the venous dorsal complex approach [4].

P.B. Santos, MD (✉)
Department of Urology, Hospital Prof. Doutor Fernando Fonseca, EPE, Amadora, Portugal

Department of Urology, Hospital CUF Descobertas, Lisbon, Portugal
e-mail: pbargao@gmail.com

B. Graça, MD • M.F. Coelho, MD • F. Ferrito, MD
F.C. Gomes, MD
Department of Urology, Hospital Prof. Doutor Fernando Fonseca, EPE, Amadora, Portugal

J.R. Dias, MD
Department of Urology, Hospital CUF Descobertas, Lisbon, Portugal

H.R.H. Patel, MRCS, PhD, FRCS(Urol), FRCS(Eng)
Department of Urology, University Hospital North Norway, Tromsø, Norway

H.R.H. Patel et al. (eds.), *Pelvic Cancer Surgery: Modern Breakthroughs and Future Advances*,
DOI 10.1007/978-1-4471-4258-4_11, © Springer-Verlag London 2015

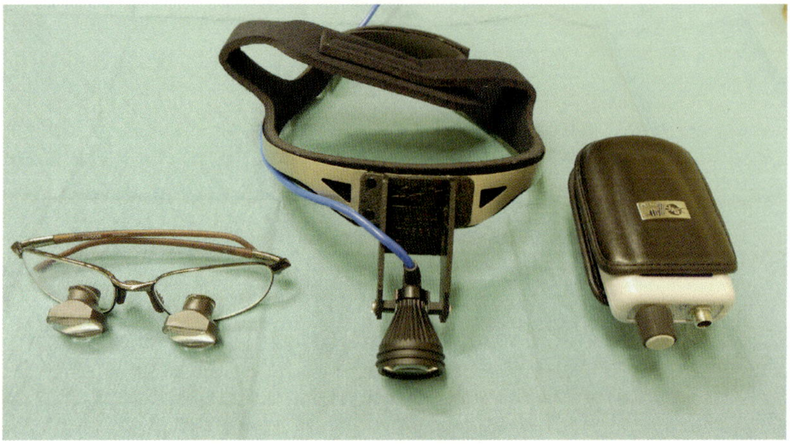

Fig. 11.1 2.5× power-loupes and fiberoptic coaxial headlight and battery

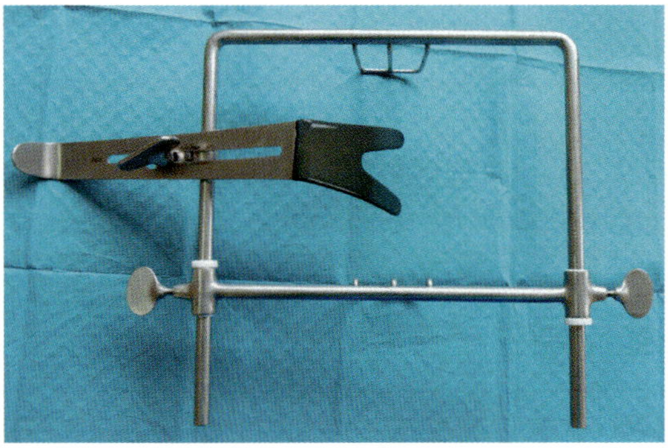

Fig. 11.2 Designed self-retractor

11.4 Incision, Exposure and Lymphadenectomy

A 16-Charrière (Ch) Foley catheter is inserted into the bladder and the balloon inflated with 10–15 cc of water. An 8–10 cm vertical midline incision made from 2 cm above the symphysis to approximately below the umbilicus provides very good exposition. The access to the Retzius space is done by opening the anterior fascia down to the pubis, splitting the rectus muscles in the midline, lifting the semilunar line and freeing the peritoneum from the internal inguinal rings and the external iliac vessels. Prostate cancer patients who are at high and intermediate risk for lymph node involvement should be submitted to extensive resection of the internal iliac lymph nodes [5–8]. Lymphadenectomy is made preferentially before the radical prostatectomy. The limits of dissection are: laterally, the upper limit of the external iliac vein and artery; caudally, the femoral canal; proximally, the bifurcation of the common iliac artery; medially, the lateral wall of the bladder; and inferiorly, the floor of the obturador fossa and the internal iliac vessels [9, 10]. It is done with the table in side-position (30°) and the aid of a Leriche spatula. Lymphatic and small vessels are ligated with small clips.

11.5 Retractor Placement

The self-retractor is placed with the Richardson type blade to fix the bladder underneath it. The assistant helps with a scissor in an upside down position.

11.6 Incision in Endopelvic Fascia

After lymph node dissection, all fatty tissue covering the endopelvic fascia and surrounding superficial Santorini's complex is removed. The outer layer of the endopelvic fascia is incised medial to the tendinous arc extending posteriorly with gentle lateral separation of the levator muscle with scissors and the aid of a peanut. It is essential to open, very well and posteriorly, this plan for freeing completely both sides of the prostate, facilitating the later approach to lateral pedicles. The endopelvic fascia is then incised

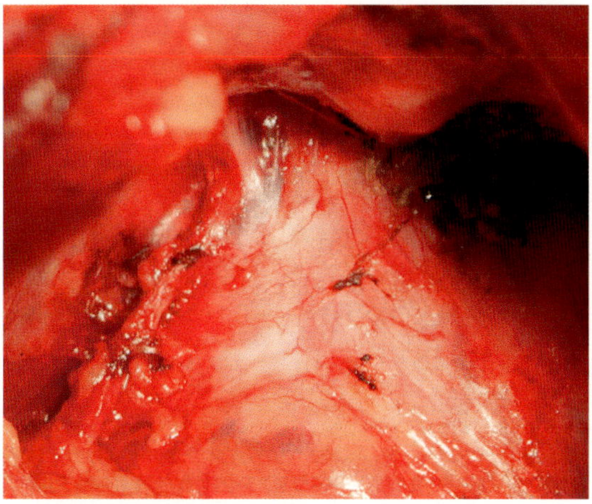

Fig. 11.3 Puboprostatic ligament

anteriorly up to the puboprostatic ligaments. This is done in both sides.

11.7 Division of Puboprostatic Ligaments

The superficial dorsal venous complex is situated between these ligaments anteriorly and the deep dorsal venous complex posteriorly. Pushing the anterior surface of the prostate backwards allows the exposition of these ligaments, facilitating its dissection and section with scissors. A right-angled forceps passing behind them can be used. Care must be taken not to hit veins that are most of the time just behind (Fig. 11.3). This maneuver allows the release of the prostate from the pubic symphysis.

11.8 Bunching and Division of the Dorsal Venous Complex

Opening laterally the second layer of the endopelvic fascia and the periprostatic fascia, from the apex to the bladder neck, will allow the preservation of the neurovascular bundles (NVB). These are rolled and separated laterally with the help of a peanut. This facilitates the bunching, with a Babcock clamp, of the dorsal venous complex that includes the ventral portions of the endopelvic and periprostatic fascia (Fig. 11.4).

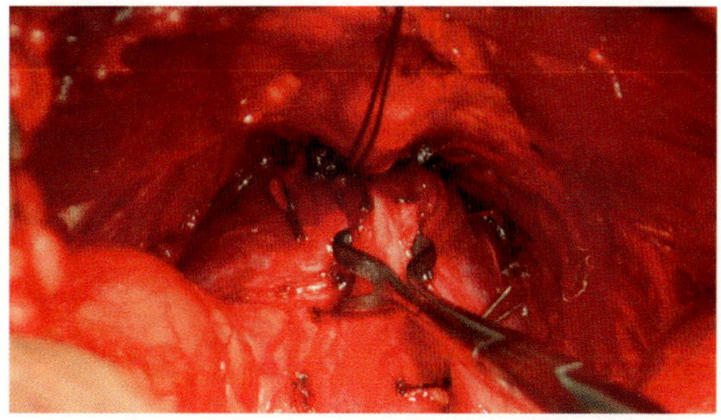

Fig. 11.4 Bunching of the dorsal venous complex with separation of the NVB from the lateral surface of the prostate

Its ligation is made with one 1-polyglactine absorbable suture over the prostate apex and another near the bladder neck. The transection of the Santorini's plexus just above the prostato-urethral junction is done with scalpel or scissors.

11.9 Apical Prostatic Dissection

The prostatic apex is approached by careful dissection along the ventral surface of the prostate towards the membranous urethra. Perfect view of this step can be achieved by gently pulling the prostate and the intraprostatic urethra upwards with a Gil-Vernet retractor. The advantage of open surgery is enabling the use of the index finger to better isolate the apex thus avoiding positive surgical margins at this difficult step. Urethra is dissected laterally by opening scissors longitudinally, achieving a maximal urethral length and an integral preservation of striated sphincter [11]. If necessary, bleeding from the Santorini's plexus is controlled by an eight figure horizontal 0-polyglactine absorbable suture, encircling the plexus.

11.10 Release of Neurovascular Bundles Starting Backwards at the Urethroprostatic Angle

At this time it is possible to continue the NVB preservation backwards by clipping the perforating vessels and pushing them down. The prostatic apex is now completely released, enabling a full view of the membranous urethra (Fig. 11.5).

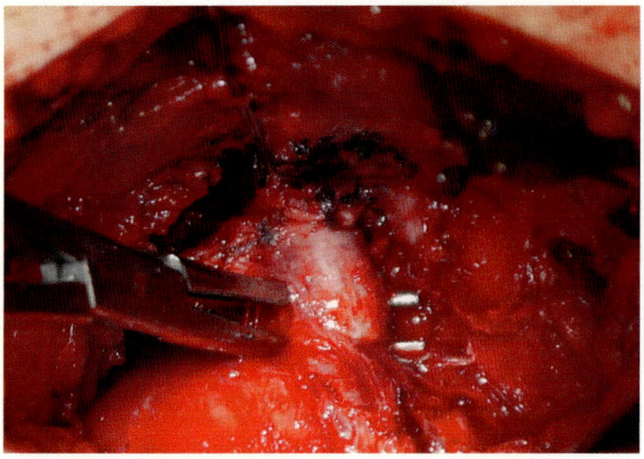

Fig. 11.5 Apical prostatic dissection

11.11 Division of Anterior Urethra and Setting the Urethral Sutures

With the 16-Ch Foley catheter still in place it is possible to transect the anterior and lateral surfaces of the urethra with the scalpel. The catheter is pulled cut and its stub hold by the assistant with a straight Kelly forceps but without making significant traction on the prostate. With the aid of an in-and-out movement of a Mercier catheter, four 2–0 double semicircular (5/8) needle polyglactin sutures are placed. This is done without cutting the posterior surface of the urethra, thereby preventing its retraction down to the pelvic floor. This step allows the visualization of all the stub length and the passage of the sutures merely in the urethra, not picking the levator ani muscle. Posterior and anterior sutures are placed in an inside-out movement, at 5 and 7 o'clock position, medial to the NVB and at 2 and 11, respectively. It is taken approximately 10 mm of the urethra length. The sutures are individually attached to the surgical drapes with mosquito forceps for later vesicourethral anastomosis. These four sutures are sufficient for a good anastomosis.

11.12 Division of the Posterior Urethra and Rectourethralis Muscle

The division of the posterior urethra is made with the scalpel at the level of the distal verumontanum after passing underneath it a right-angled forceps

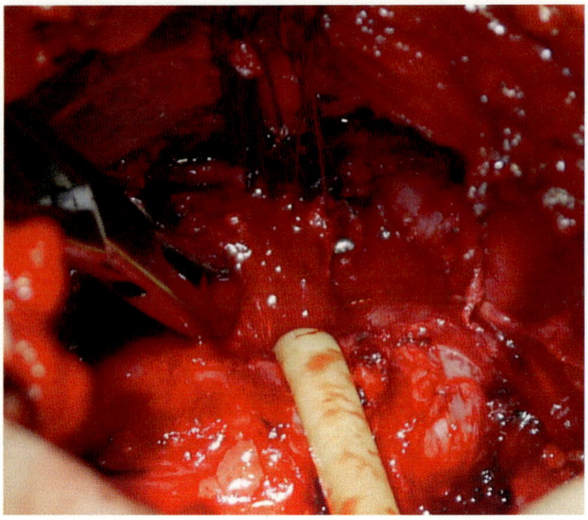

Fig. 11.6 Division of the posterior urethra and rectourethralis muscle

(Fig. 11.6). Once the urethra is sectioned, the rectourethralis muscle becomes evident. It is variable in strength and thickness. Sometimes muscle fibers are sparse and index finger easily recognizes the right plane between the prostate and the rectum. Sometimes it is a real muscular plate that needs to be incised and dissected with scissors.

11.13 Posterior Release and Ligation of Lateral Prostatic Pedicles

The index finger can easily reach up the seminal vesicles. In non-nerve sparing procedure, the NVB are completely resected and ligations with 2-0 polyglactin sutures are made close to the rectum. In the NVB preservation, small clips are used on the very little complexes of perforating vessels and nerve fibers close to the prostate. Electrocautery is never used. These maneuvers are done by ambidextrous technique with index fingertips positioned posterolaterally for constant haptic feedback [12]. Dissection continues up to the lateral surface of the seminal vesicles. In selected patients with smaller unilateral and non-apical cT3a prostate cancer, a contralateral nerve-sparing dissection can be done. Most of the authors, such as Sokoloff and Brendler [13], consider that cT3b tumors and palpable lesion at the apex are absolute contraindications for the nerve-sparing technique.

11.14 Dissection of the Seminal Vesicles and Vas Deferens

The Denonvillier's fascia is horizontally sharply incised at the posterior surface of the transition between prostate and the insertion of seminal vesicles and vas deferens, allowing the access to these structures. The vas deferens are dissected, isolated, clipped and cut. The seminal vesicles undergo the same dissection, down to the tip where vessels are clipped, without causing any trauma by squeezing, pulling or tearing to the adjacent plexus running along their dorsolateral aspect. Patients at very low risk of seminal vesicle invasion can be identified with high accuracy with an equally nomogram [14]. Zlotta et al. concluded that "complete resection of seminal vesicle may not be oncologically necessary in all patients when PSA levels are below 10 ng/ml." Their data showed that patients with biopsy Gleason scores <7 and less than 50 % of biopsies with prostate cancer involvement, have a low probability of SV invasion [15]. Other studies showed that patients submitted to seminal vesicle sparing technique can have a beneficial impact on erectile [16] and urinary function [17]. In these cases, we do the preservation, transecting them and leaving its tips intact. Prostate at this time is completely mobilized posteriorly and laterally up to the bladder neck.

11.15 Bladder Neck Preservation

According to current data, bladder-neck preservation has no negative impact on positive surgical margins (PSM) rates and these are rare at bladder-neck [18–22]. Higher stage tumors are associated with significantly higher PSM rates [20, 23]. When performed by experienced surgeons PSM rates are comparable [18]. Nevertheless long-term results on oncological outcome are pending [18]. We perform bladder neck-sparing surgery in almost all cases of low- and intermediate-risk cancer groups, if it is anatomical possible. This step starts with an anterior approach of the vesico-prostatic plan. The division is made with sharp dissection with scissors and continues with blunt dissection made with the scissors closed. Circular fibers of the bladder neck are very well seen and preserved [18, 19]. Lateral adherences between prostate and bladder base are dissected and ligated or clipped until the bladder neck is entirely circled (Fig. 11.7).

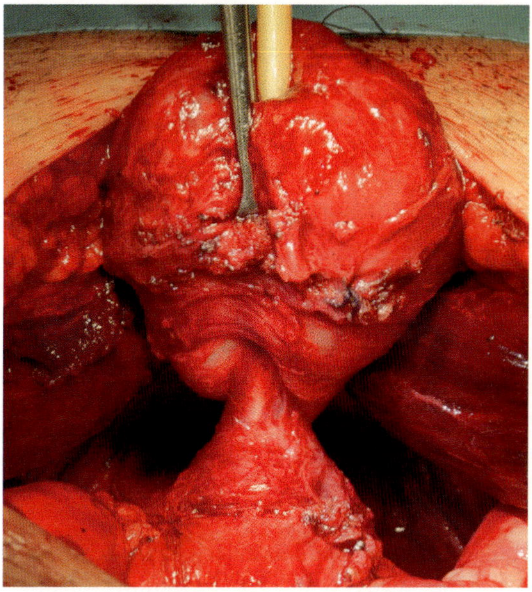

Fig. 11.7 Bladder neck preservation

11.16 Posterior Musculofascial Reconstruction and Vesicourethral Anastomosis

In 2001 Rocco et al. described a technique for restoration of the posterior aspect of the rhabdosphincter. They showed that this modification to the standard Walsh procedure, shortened time to continence after RRP [24, 25]. Since then, many surgeons have applied this technique—either as it was described or with some modification to open, laparoscopic and robotic assisted RP. A recent systematic review of the literature done by Rocco et al. [26] showed that it improves early return of continence within the first 30 days after radical prostatectomy while continence rates after 90 days were not affected. We also achieved good results so we systematically perform it before doing the anastomosis. It consists in a reconstruction, with a 2–0 polyglactin suture, of the rhabdosphincter and the proximal cutting edge of the Denonvilliers's fascia. This fixation is then done to the posterior wall of the bladder about 2 cm dorsocephalad to the bladder neck.

The quality of the vesicourethral anastomosis will directly influence urinary leakage, stricture formation and continence [27]. Before making the anastomosis between the bladder neck and the urethral stub, hemostasis is checked. If necessary, small clips are placed or 3–0 polyglactin selective sutures made. The bed of the seminal vesicles is approximated with an eight figure 2–0 polyglactin suture to avoid bleeding and development of hematomas. Like Studer et al. [28] suggests, we no more do the eversion of the bladder mucosa, advocated by Walsh for many years, for preventing bladder neck contractures.

Posterior sutures are passed inside-out throw the bladder neck grasping 10 mm of tissue. A 20-Ch two ways silicon catheter is inserted and the balloon not inflated in order to avoid inadvertent damage during the passage of the anterior sutures. These are passed in the same way as the posterior ones. The bladder is taken down near the urethral stub with the aid of a swab. Sutures are adjusted and straightened for a perfect sliding knot, starting with the posterior ones. Only now the catheter's balloon is inflated with 10–15 ml of water. Gentle traction on the catheter is made and bladder rinsed to ensure any leakage. Diuretics can be given to dilute any residual hematuria.

11.17 Drain Placement and Wound Closure

A closed suction drain (Redivac™) is inserted through a separate small skin incision, lateral to the rectus muscle, taking care not to injure the inferior epigastric vessels. It is attached to the skin with a 1 silk stitch. Wound is closed with a running 1 polyglactin suture and staples.

11.18 Perioperative and Postoperative Care

Advances in the perioperative and postoperative care of patients undergoing RRP continues to increase due to the improvements of the technique. Most patients discharge on postoperative day 2. Drains are removed before discharge when drainage is inferior to 50 cc/24 h. Catheter remains in place for 15 days and antibiotics are given for a 5–7 days period and on the day for catheter removal.

11.19 Summary

RRP still remains the gold standard surgery for prostate cancer which other techniques are compared to. Developments in the technique over the last 20 years and the permanent progress in certain steps, allowed the overlapping results of minimally invasive techniques, including intraoperative blood loss and postoperative recovery. The possibility of surgery with spinal anesthesia without limit forced position and use of tactile are some of the advantages of RRP.

Key Points

- Loupes and fiberoptic headlight
- Excellent exposition of operative field
- Control of dorsal vein complex without the need for transfusion
- Meticulous apical dissection
- Complete sphincter preservation and maximal urethral length
- Urethral transection near the verumontanum
- Neurovascular bundle release at prostate apex before urethral transection
- Bladder neck preservation without reconstruction
- Posterior musculofascial reconstruction
- Four vesicourethral sutures for optimal anastomosis

References

1. Millin T. Retropubic prostatectomy a new extravesical technique: report on 20 cases. Lancet. 1945;2(6380): 693–6.
2. Myers RP. Improving the exposure of the prostate in radical retropubic prostatectomy: longitudinal bunching of the deep venous plexus. J Urol. 1989;142:1282.
3. Walsh PC. Anatomic radical prostatectomy: evolution of the surgical technique. J Urol. 1998;160:2418.
4. Schostak M, Matischak K, Müller M, et al. New perioperative management reduces bleeding in radical retropubic prostatectomy. BJU Int. 2005;96(3):316–9.
5. Briganti A, Chun FK, Salonia A, et al. Validation of a nomogram predicting the probability of lymph node invasion based on the extent of pelvic lymphadenectomy in patients with clinically localized prostate cancer. BJU Int. 2006;98(4):788–93.
6. Heidenreich A, Varga Z, Von Knobloch R. Extended pelvic lymphadenectomy in patients undergoing radical prostatectomy: high incidence of lymph node metastasis. J Urol. 2002;167:1681–6.
7. Djavan B, Kazzazi A, Dulabon L, et al. Indications and trends in pelvic lymph node dissection for prostate cancer. Eur Urol. 2011;10(Supp):e38–43.
8. Heidenreich A, Bastian P, Bellmunt J et al. Guidelines on prostate cancer. EAU 2012;49–50.
9. Bader P, Burhard FC, Markwalder R, Studer UE. Is a limited lymph node dissection an adequate staging procedure for prostate cancer? J Urol. 2002;168:514–8.
10. Heidenreich A, Ohlmann CH, Polyakov S. Anatomical extent of pelvic lymphadenectomy in patients undergoing radical prostatectomy. Eur Urol. 2007;52:29–37.
11. Shlomm T, Heinzer H, Steuber T, et al. Full functional-length urethral sphincter preservation during radical prostatectomy. Eur Urol. 2011;60:320–9.
12. Hubanks J, Umbreit E, Karnes R, et al. Open radical retropubic prostatectomy using high anterior release of the levator fascia and constant haptic feedback in bilateral neurovascular bundle preservation plus early postoperative phosphodiesterase type 5 inhibition: a contemporary series. Eur Urol. 2012;61:878–84.
13. Sokoloff M, Brendler C. Indication and contraindication for nerve-sparing radical prostatectomy. Urol Clin N Am. 2001;28(3):535–43.
14. Gallina A, Chun FK, Briganti A, et al. Development and split-sample validation of a nomogram predicting the probability of seminal vesicle invasion at radical prostatectomy. Eur Urol. 2007;52(1):98–105.
15. Zlotta AR, Roumeguère T, Ravery V, et al. Is seminal vesicle ablation mandatory for all patients undergoing radical prostatectomy? A multivariate analysis on 1283 patients. Eur Urol. 2004;46(1):42–9.
16. Sanda MG, Dunn R, Wei J. Seminal vesicle sparing technique is associated with improved sexual HRQOL outcome after radical prostatectomy. J Urol. 2002;167:151 (A606).
17. John H, Hauri D. Seminal vesicle-sparing radical prostatectomy: a novel concept to restore early urinary continence. Urology. 2000;55:820–4. Crossref.
18. Nyarangi-Dix J, Radtke J, Hadaschik B et al. Impact of complete bladder-neck preservation on urinary continence, quality of life and surgical margins after radical prostatectomy: a randomized controlled single-blind trial. J Urol 2012. pii:S0022–5347(12)04972–5
19. Brunocilla E, Pultrone C, Pernetti R, et al. Preservation of the smooth muscular internal (vesical) sphincter and of the proximal urethra during retropubic radical prostatectomy: description of the technique. Int J Urol. 2012;19(8):783–5.
20. Poon M, Ruckle H, Bamshad BR, et al. Radical retropubic prostatectomy: bladder neck preservation versus reconstruction. J Urol. 2000;163(1):194–8.
21. Razi A, Yahyazadeh SR, Sedighi Gilani MA, et al. Bladder neck preservation during radical retropubic prostatectomy and postoperative urinary continence. Urol J. 2009;6(1):23–6.
22. Patel VR, Coelho RF, Rocco B, et al. Positive surgical margins after robotic assisted radical prostatectomy: a multi-institutional study. J Urol. 2011;186(2):511–6.
23. Terakawa T, Miyake H, Tanaka K, et al. Surgical margin status of open versus laparoscopic radical prostatectomy specimens. Int J Urol. 2008;15(8):704–7.
24. Rocco F, Carmignani L, Acquati P, et al. Early continence recovery after open radical prostatectomy with restoration of the posterior aspect of the rhabdosphincter. Eur Urol. 2007;52:376–83.
25. Rocco F, Carmignani L, Acquati P, et al. Restoration of posterior aspect of rhabdosphincter shorten continence time after radical retropubic prostatectomy. J Urol. 2006;175:2201–6.
26. Rocco B, Cozzi G, Spinelli M, et al. Posterior musculofascial reconstruction after radical prostatectomy: a systematic review of the literature. Eur Urol. 2012;62:779–90.
27. Wang R, Wood Jr DP, Hollenbeck BK, et al. Risk factors and quality of life for post-prostatectomy vesicourethral anastomotic stenosis. Urology. 2012;79(2):449–57.
28. Kessler T, Burkhard F, Studer U. Nerve-sparing open radical retropubic prostatectomy. Eur Urol. 2007;51:90–7.

Laparoscopic Radical Prostatectomy

12

Panagiotis S. Kallidonis, Evangelos N. Liatsikos, Peter Tenke, Minh Do Hoang, Alan S. McNeill, Stavros Kontogiannis, Ioannis Georgiopoulos, Anja Dietel, and Jens-Uwe Stolzenburg

12.1 Introduction

Laparoscopic radical prostatectomy (LRP) was first performed by Schuessler et al., in 1992 with disappointing results in terms of operative time [1]. Guillonneau et al. further developed the technique and successfully performed LRP with acceptable operative time [2]. Currently, the procedure represents a standard of care for localized and locally advanced prostate cancer in numerous institutions worldwide. The technique of LRP was initially based on the open technique and practically replicated its surgical steps. In addition, similar to open radical prostatectomy (ORP) trifecta outcomes (cancer control, urinary continence and potency) were achieved by LRP with the additional advantage of reduced blood loss, post-operative pain and probably superior cosmesis [3, 4]. The extraperitoneal approach of LRP was introduced in 1997 by Raboy et al. and currently is well represented by the Endoscopic Extraperitoneal Radical Prostatectomy (EERPE) [5, 6]. Over the course of time, both approaches to laparoscopic radical prostatectomy (LRP and EERPE) have evolved. Several modifications including neurovascular bundle preservation, bladder neck sparing and posterior fascial reconstruction techniques have been incorporated to the procedures. We herein present the technique and outcome of LRP in terms of oncological, functional efficacy and surgical efficacy.

P.S. Kallidonis, MD, PhD(Urol), MSc(Clin Pharma) (✉)
E.S. Liatsikos, MD, PhD • S. Kontogiannis, MD.
I. Georgiopoulos, MD
Department of Urology, University of Patras,
Patras, Greece
e-mail: pkallidonis@yahoo.com

P. Tenke, MD, PhD
Department of Urology, Jahn Ferenc South Pest
Hospital, Budapest, Hungary

M.D. Hoang, MD, PhD • A. Dietel, MD, PhD
J.-U. Stolzenburg, PhD, FRCS (Ed), FRCS (Eng)
Department of Urology, University of Leipzig,
Leipzig, Germany

A.S. McNeill, BM BS, FRCS(Eng, Ed), FRCS(Urol)
Department of Urology, Western General Hospital,
Edinburgh, UK

12.2 Technique and Evolution

The comparison among the transperitoneal and extraperitoneal approaches to laparoscopic radical prostatectomy has been a field of intensive clinical research and a number of studies have been published. This comparison showed that the extraperitoneal approach has advantages in terms of bowel related morbidity [7–9]. Nevertheless, the approach is associated with a higher rate of lymphocele and does not allow the performance of extended lymphadenectomy over the bifurcation of the common iliac artery [10]. As a result, the selection of the approach depends on the indications, experience and preference of the surgical team.

The introduction of nerve-sparing technique, where oncologically appropriate, significantly

H.R.H. Patel et al. (eds.), *Pelvic Cancer Surgery: Modern Breakthroughs and Future Advances*,
DOI 10.1007/978-1-4471-4258-4_12, © Springer-Verlag London 2015

improved the outcomes of LRP and EERPE with a faster recovery of continence and significantly improved post-operative erectile function [11–13]. An additional refinement of the neurovascular bundle (NVB) preservation technique based on recent anatomical evidence is the intrafascial nerve-sparing dissection which allows the additional preservation of peri-prostatic fascias and the nerve fibers included in the fascias resulting in improved potency outcome (Fig. 12.1a, b) [13, 14]. Several modifications such as puboprostatic ligament preservation have also been proposed with investigators reporting variable outcome regarding the contribution of these techniques to faster continence recovery [15]. Bladder neck sparing and posterior fascial reconstruction have also been reported to have a beneficial impact on postoperative continence [16–19].

The surgical steps of the procedure are almost identical, with minor modifications amongst the investigators with exception of the extraperitoneal or transperitoneal access [6–8, 21]. The patient is in Trendelenburg position and five trocars are usually placed (three 5 mm, two 12 mm). A 12 mm trocar is inserted in the umbilicus for the insertion of the optics. Another 12 mm trocar is positioned approximately two fingers-breadths medial to the left anterior superior iliac spine. A 5 mm trocar is inserted two fingers-breadths medial to the left of the midline, two-thirds of the way between the pubis and the umbilicus. Another 5 mm trocar is positioned in the right pararectal line cranially and one more is inserted medial to the right anterior superior iliac spine. Balloon dissection under direct visualization and insufflation of the preperitoneal space for the creation of the operative field follows in the case of the extraperitoneal approach.

In the transperitoneal approach, dissection of the lower peritoneum takes place without any balloon dilation and access to the prostate is achieved. Minor differences in the sequence of the steps of the procedure have been described by various investigators [20, 21]. The Intrafascial nerve-sparing EERPE is presented as a technical example [14].

An incision is made bilaterally in the periprostatic fascia at the reflection of the puboprostatic ligaments over the prostate and the plane between the prostate and fascias is developed. The latter plane allows the gradual detachment of the prostate from the fasciae surrounding the organ. Dissection of the bladder neck is then performed with careful mobilization of the branches of the NVBs while incising the dorsal bladder neck. The dissection is then continued dorsally and the seminal vesicles are mobilized with sharp and blunt dissection. The Denonviller's fascia is detached from the prostate by blunt dissection strictly in the midline with the direction of the dissection towards the apex of the prostate. Blunt

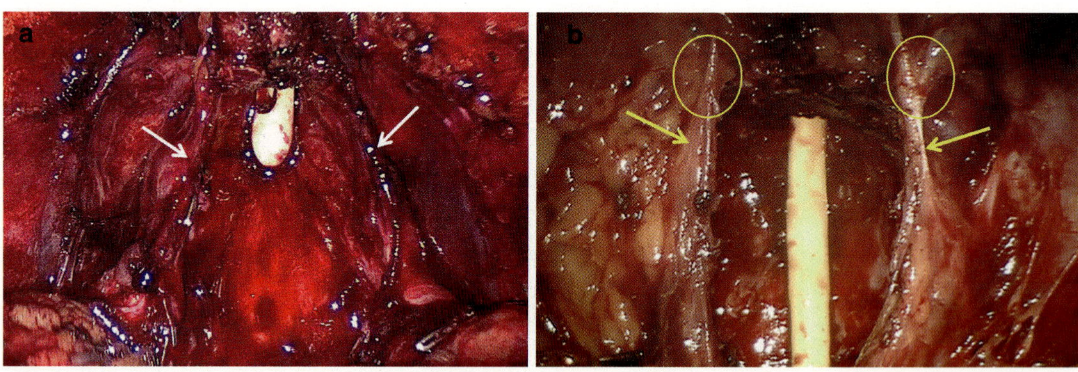

Fig. 12.1 (**a**) Bilateral interfascial nerve-sparing technique has been performed. The prostate has been removed and the neurovascular bundles have not been excised (*white arrows*). The lateral endopelvic fascia is incised bilaterally. The next step of the procedure is the performance of the vesicourethral anastomosis. (**b**) Bilateral intrafascial nerve preservation of the neurovascular bundles has been performed (*yellow arrows*). During the intrafascial approach the lateral endopelvic fascia is not incised. The puboprostatic ligaments have been preserved (*yellow circles*). The puboprostatic ligaments represent a landmark for the intrafascial approach as the dissection of the periprostatic fascias is initiated over the prostate at the reflection of the puboprostatic ligaments

dissection takes place for the detachment of the prostatic pedicles from the surrounding fascias while clipping and careful cutting of the prostatic pedicles is performed. Ligation of the Santorini's plexus by Vicryl 2-0 suture follows. The prostate is transected sharply from the external sphincter and the urethra. The vesicourethral anastomosis is performed with usually by nine interrupted sutures and the specimen is extracted for the accomplishment of the procedure.

Regarding nerve-sparing technique, energy-free dissection is utilized in order to preserve as much nerve fibers of the NVBs as possible. Although, the extent of anatomic dissection remains under investigation, intrafascial dissection is associated with improved post-operative potency in comparison to the interfascial approach [13, 14, 22].

12.3 Functional Results

Continence

Postoperative continence rates were high since the introduction of LRP [23]. In fact, the first reports on the outcome of the technique included data from large series of patients and showed continence rates between 75 and 80 % over a 6-months follow-up period [24, 25]. Large prospective studies have reported continence rates even greater than 93 % [26, 27]. Olsson et al. studied a large population by the use of validated questionnaires for a period of 12 months. At 6 months, none of the patients used more than one pad daily while 56.8 % of the patients reported no leakage at all [28]. The EPIC questionnaire was used by Link et al. for the assessment of postoperative continence and observed that 93.4 % of the patients were continent at 12 months follow-up [29]. Rassweiler et al. have reported continence rates of 33 % for their series at discharge from the hospital and 97 % after 12 months. The steep learning curve of the procedure seems to be an obstacle for centers that are not specialized in laparoscopy [30]. Other investigators confirmed the positive results with continence rates up to 97 % and follow-up periods up to 2 years [4, 31].

EERPE has offered comparable results to those of LRP [6, 13, 32]. A study by Stolzenburg et al. including 2,400 patients showed that 71.7 % of the patients were continent at 3 months after surgery and 94.7 % were continent at 12 months [6]. The intrafascial EERPE demonstrated even more promising results with a continence rate of 72.7 % at 3 months postoperatively, 85.3 % at 6 months, and 94.3 % at 12 months [13]. Similar experience with the extraperitoneal approach was presented by Rozet et al. [33]. The authors reported continence in 84 % of the patients and only 7 % of them using one-pad daily during the first year of follow-up.

Conflicting data are currently available regarding possible factors that influence postoperative continence. Several refinements of the LRP and EERPE have been proposed in an attempt to accelerate the postoperative recovery of continence.

Milhoua et al. suggested that large prostate size could be associated with a delay in recovery of post-operative continence [34]. In addition, factors related to the prostate cancer have not been recognized to predict post-operative continence [35]. Previous surgery of the prostate does not seem to significantly influence the postoperative continence. Menard et al. and Stolzenburg et al. reported high continence rates in patients that had previously undergone Transurethral Resection of the Prostate (TURP) and the results are based on long follow-up periods up to 2 years [36, 37]. Nevertheless, careful dissection of the urethra from the prostate and insertion of ureteral stents for the visualization of the ureteral orifices intraoperatively are advised during the performance of LRP/EERPE in the above patient population.

Careful bladder neck preservation has been proven to provide additional benefit in early postoperative continence without any influence on positive surgical margin (PSM) rates in several comparative studies [18, 19, 38]. Thus, the bladder neck stump after the dissection of the prostate from the bladder should remain as narrow as possible in order to allow faster recovery of continence. NVB preservation may be associated with faster recovery of continence [13, 39]. Posterior musculofascial reconstruction has also been proposed to have an impact in the faster recovery of postoperative continence. In fact, a recent systematic review reported an improvement of continence rates in the first 30 days after surgery, PSMs are similar to the patients without reconstruction and complication rates remain controversial [17]. Excellent long-term results on continence have been reported by several investigators. It should be noted that a significant improvement in continence rates is not expected beyond the first 12 months [40, 41].

Erectile Function and Potency

The quality of life of patients that have undergone radical prostatectomy is significantly influenced by the preservation of erectile function and potency (erections sufficient for intercourse). The recovery of potency and the time in which it occurs after LRP is related to the age and preoperative potency of the patient. The performance of nerve-sparing technique is a predominant factor for the recovery of potency [29]. In addition, the preservation of accessory pundendal artery has also got a favorable impact on the recovery of potency and should be considered in patients that have the latter anatomical structure [42, 43].

The first experience with the preservation of the prostatic NVBs demonstrated improved potency rates in comparison to conventional technique. Although potency after non-nerve-sparing LRP was observed in 41 % of the cases, unilateral and bilateral nerve-sparing resulted in potency rates of 44 and 53 %, respectively [44]. Moreover, Roumeguere et al. showed that more spontaneous erections were present in patients who underwent LRP in comparison to those of the open approach [45].

Patients younger than 60 years of age have been reported to have potency rates ranging between 61 and 78.6 % over a 2-year follow up period [26, 32]. In the extraperitoneal approach, overall potency rates of 44 and 72 % were reported for unilateral and bilateral NVB preservation in a 12-month follow-up period. Higher rates of potency were observed in younger patients (below 55 years of age) with the respective figures to be 50 and 84.9 % [6].

The intrafascial approach is based on recent anatomical data that document the presence of a wide nerve fiber distribution in the fascias surrounding the prostate. Thus, a more extensive preservation of the NVBs and the surrounding prostatic fascias has been proposed with the introduction of the intrafascial nerve-sparing approach [13]. A significant benefit in postoperative continence has been documented in 200 patients undergoing intrafascial EERPE in comparison to those undergoing interfascial (conventional NVB preservation) [22]. Potency rates in patients who underwent bilateral intrafascial nerve-sparing technique were 93.5 % (for patients <55 years old), 83.3 % (for patients 55–65 years old), and 60 % (for patients >65 years old) at 12 months. The respective potency figures for the bilateral interfascial group were 77.1, 50, and 40 %. The overall potency rates are also favorable for the intrafascial approach: 82.8 % versus 64.8 % for the interfascial group. Other investigators reported rates up to 97 % in patients treated by intrafascial nerve-sparing after 1-year [46]. Nevertheless, the above results were not confirmed by other investigators [47]. It is important to note that the oncological outcome does not seem to be compromised by the intrafascial dissection [13, 47]. The use of athermal, energy-free technique during a nerve-sparing LRP/EERPE has been suggested by several investigators since the use of ultrasonic scissors or bipolar coagulation at the site of NVBs has a documented disadvantage in postoperative potency (Fig. 12.2a, b) [48]. The preservation of seminal vesicles has been also proposed by Shah et al. to have a favorable impact to potency. Nevertheless, additional studies are necessary for the extraction of solid results regarding this technique [49]. Long-term results on potency showed a slight but not significant improvement of potency at 24 months [40].

12.4 Oncological Results

The main criterion used to assess the oncological efficacy of radical prostatectomy is the presence or absence of PSMs. Additional factors of interest are the level of post-operative PSA and more spe-

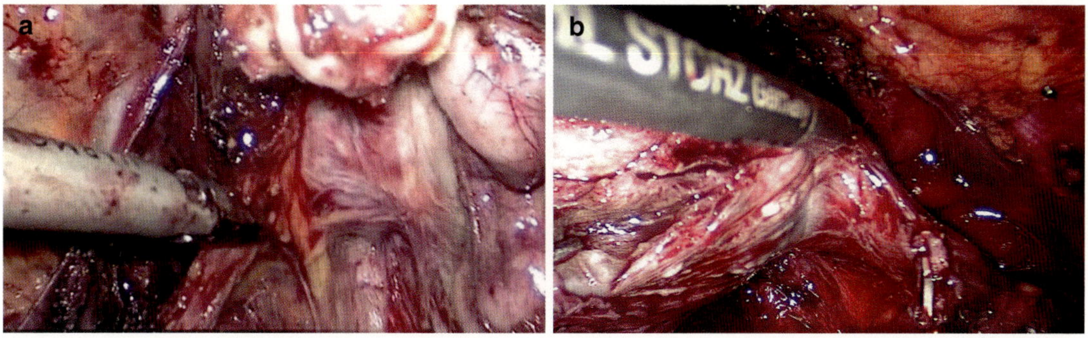

Fig. 12.2 (**a**) The use of thermal energy during the dissection of the neurovascular bundles has been proven to result in injury to the nerve fibers and significantly comprise the outcome of the nerve-sparing technique. The image shows the dissection of the neurovascular bundle with the use of ultrasonic scissors during the performance of non nerve-sparing approach. (**b**) The neurovascular bundle is meticulously dissected with the consecutive use of clips and blunt dissection. No energy instruments are used in the vicinity of the neurovascular bundles

cifically, PSA recurrence (described in literature as PSA >0.2 ng/mL and confirmed by a second measurement), the clinical progression and the progression-free survival [4, 50]. Prostate size does not represent a parameter for patient selection to undergo LRP. Nevertheless, prostate sizes smaller than 30 g are related to a higher rate of PSMs [51, 52]. Techniques of nerve reconstruction, such as sural nerve grafting, have been associated with increasing risk of PSMs [53]. Moreover, previous training of the surgeon in open or laparoscopic techniques does not have an impact to the oncological outcome [54].

The learning curve seems to have an impact to the PSM rate according to a recent meta-analysis which showed inferior PSM rates in LRP in comparison to RALP cases performed by surgeons in their learning curve [55]. Other investigators concluded that a surgeon early in the learning curve of LRP probably does not result in increased rate of PSMs [56]. The oncological results of LRP are similar to those of ORP and the PSMs are detected in the same sites in both approaches [4, 56]. Short-term oncological results reported by Salomon et al. showed PSM and 3-year progression free survival rates to be 20.6 and 86.2 % in pT2 cases, respectively. The rates were similar among LRP and ORP [57]. Similar results were also documented by Roumeguere et al. [45]. A comparison of transperitoneal and extraperitoneal approach did not demonstrate any significant difference in PSM rates among the approaches [8, 9].

In a prospective study including 1,000 patients Guilloneau et al. reported progression free survival at 3 years post-operatively. They observed 80 and 94 % progression free survival rates (overall rate 90.5 %) in patients with and without PSMs, respectively. Factors influencing the PSM rates were Gleason Score, clinical stage (TNM), pathological stage and preoperative PSA level [50]. Rozet et al. reported an overall PSM rate of 17.7 % as well as 14.6 and 25.6 % in pT2 and in pT3 cases, respectively [33].

Five-year progression free survival rate of 78.8 % was reported by Goeman et al. in a series of patients who underwent extraperitoneal LRP. PSM rates were 17.9 % for pT2, 44.8 % for pT3 and 71.4 % for pT4a tumors [32]. In a large population of patients Stolzenburg et al. [6] observed overall PSM rate of 16.4 %. The PSM rate for patients in pT2 stage was 8 and 35.6 % in pT3 stage. The long-term results on PSM and biochemical recurrence rates showed that the laparoscopic approach does not compromise the oncological outcome [40, 41, 58].

12.5 Complications

Complication rates for LRP and EERPE range between 2 and 17 % [59, 60]. The Table 12.1 summarizes most frequent complications and management. Vascular complications, including vessel injury, bleeding and the formation of hematomas represent the most common perioperative compli-

Table 12.1 Incidence and management of frequent complications of LRP and EERPE [59–63]

Complication	Rates (%)	Management	Tips
Injury of inferior epigastric vessels	0–6	Bipolar coagulation Clipping Suturing of the bleeding vessel on the abdominal wall	Careful inspection of all the trocar sites for active bleeding before and after the removal
External iliac vein injury		Endoscopic repair with 4–0 prolene Conversion to open laparotomy	Insufflation pressure can tamponade venous bleeding and makes endoscopic repair possible
Santorini plexus injury		Increase of gas insufflation to 20 mmHg and bipolar coagulation Retraction of the catheter to tamponade bleeding	Can be avoided by careful ligation of the plexus and careful inspection-coagulation after apical dissection
Bowel injury	0.47	Endoscopic repair with two-layer suturing Parenteral feeding for a minimum of 3 days Non-residual enteral feeding for a minimum of 6 days	Symptoms are presented within 2 weeks after surgery Careful inspection of trocars during insertion Careful apical dissection
Lymphocele	3–14	Percutaneous drainage Sclerotherapy Laparoscopic fenestration	A combination of bipolar coagulation, harmonic scalpel dissection and clipping in order to prevent lymphorrhea
Ureteral and bladder injury	0.1–0.2	Endoscopic repair	Infuse 200 mL saline into the bladder to confirm watertight status Infuse indigo carmine and furosemide for inspection of the ureter Preoperative insertion of double-J stents in patients with previous TURP is crucial
Port-related hernia	0.2	Open repair	Possible at the 12 mm trocar insertion sites and during specimen removal
Anastomotic leakage	0.7–7	Extra sutures at the anastomosis Revision of anastomosis if leakage is persistent	Prolonged catheterization is necessary
Urinary retention	2–3.1	Foley catheterization for 2–3 days	

cations of LRP/EERPE (89.4 % of all complications) and an incidence up to 6 % of all cases has been reported [59–63]. Hemorrhage from the inferior epigastric vessels (during trocar insertion), the Santorini's plexus, or the external iliac vein are common intra-operative complications [59–63]. Hematomas are also common post-operatively and arise from the NVBs or epigastric vessels. Rectal and intestinal injuries are reported with an incidence of 9 % of the cases and tend to be severe and life-threatening if they are not recognized intraoperatively [59–63].

Ureteric injuries, anastomotic leakage or acute urinary retention can also occur. In cases of anastomotic leakage, if placing a mono-J catheter is not enough, the anastomosis can be strengthened with more interrupted sutures or revised with an endoscopic neo-anastomosis, if not controlled properly. However, careful checking whether the anastomosis is functional and watertight intraoperatively is of crucial importance. In some cases, early removal of the catheter can lead to acute urinary retention due to anastomotic stricture. In these cases, a further period of catheterization generally resolves the issue [61].

Pelvic lymphadenectomy is related to the formation of lymphoceles, especially in the case of the extraperitoneal approach. Laparoscopic fenestration of the peritoneum intraoperatively prevents lymphocele formation during EERPE [10]. The incidence of this complication is approximately 4 % [59–63]. Rare complications such as gas embolism, obturator nerve injury, deep venous thrombosis, and prolonged ileus have been also reported [59–63].

Comparison of LRP to Alternative Approaches

Recent meta-analysis has shown that LRP has similar results in terms of potency, complications, blood loss and operative time in comparison to Robot-assisted Laparoscopic Radical Prostatectomy (RALP). Only three studies have demonstrated an earlier return to continence in the case of RALP [64]. A meta-analysis revealed that continence and erectile function were similar among LRP, ORP and RALP. PSMs were similar for LRP but higher for ORP when these procedures were compared to the results of RALP [65]. Another recent meta-analysis on the PSM status and complications reported a significantly higher PSM rate with LRP in pT2 patients in comparison to RALP. Nevertheless, the authors stated that these results should be carefully interpreted due to the inhomogenicity of the included studies. Complication rates were similar among the approaches with favorable outcome in blood loss and hospitalization time for LRP and RALP in comparison to ORP [55]. Biochemical recurrence free rates have been reported to be similar among approaches in a recent review of the literature [66].

The cost-effectiveness of LRP over ORP has been proven and the evidence show that the higher cost of equipment and instruments is balanced by the shorter hospital stay, fewer transfusions and less analgesic requirement [67]. When all approaches were compared in terms of cost, RALP was the most expensive with LRP following and ORP to be associated with the lower costs. Although the cost of disposable instruments for LRP were calculated to be higher than ORP at least in the US health system, the overall cost for hospitalization was lower for LRP. RALP had significant costs for equipment and maintenance which made the procedure far more expensive especially with a case-load of patients up to 126 per year [68].

Conclusion

LRP has stood the test of time and represents a standard of care for the surgical treatment of prostate cancer. The constant evolution of techniques, the introduction of newer equipment, and the accumulation of experience of many institutions worldwide have provided functional, oncological and surgical outcomes comparable to the available alternative surgical approaches. In addition, further improvements in long-term results are regularly being reported in literature and document the efficacy of the method over the years. The combination of comparable results, cost-effectiveness and minimally invasive approach make LRP more appealing and affordable than ORP or RALP in numerous surgical centers worldwide.

Key Points

- Laparoscopic radical prostatectomy is an established standard of surgical management of prostate cancer.
- The extraperitoneal approach is associated with lower intra-abdominal complications.
- Transperitoneal approach has lower lymphocele formation rate.
- Nerve-sparing technique accelerates the recovery of continence.
- Intrafascial nerve-sparing is associated with the highest potency rates.
- Continence rates are up to 97 % of the cases at 12 months.
- Bladder neck preservation and posterior musculofascial reconstruction result in faster recovery of continence

- The oncological outcome is similar to the alternative approaches for radical prostatetomy. Long-term results are available.
- The complication rates are to the alternative approaches for radical prostatetomy.
- The cost-effectiveness of the technique has been proven.

References

1. Schuessler WW, Kavoussi LR, Clayman RV, Vancaille T. Laparoscopic radical prostatectomy: initial case report. J Urol. 1992;147:246A, Abstract no. 130.
2. Guillonneau B, Cathelineau X, Barret E, Rozet F, Vallancien G. Laparoscopic radical prostatectomy: technical and early oncological assessment of 40 operations. Eur Urol. 1999;36(1):14–20.
3. Coelho R. Retropubic, laparoscopic and robot assisted radical prostatectomy: a critical review of outcomes reported by high-volume centers. J Endour. 2010;24(12):2003–15.
4. Rassweiler J, et al. Laparoscopic radical prostatectomy: functional and oncological outcomes. Curr Opin Urol. 2004;14(2):75–82.
5. Raboy A, Ferzli G, Albert P. Initial experience with extraperitoneal endoscopic radical retropubic prostatectomy. Urology. 1997;50:849–53.
6. Stolzenburg JU, Kallidonis P, Minh D, Dietel A, Häfner T, Dimitriou D, Al-Aown A, Kyriazis I, Liatsikos EN. Endoscopic extraperitoneal radical prostatectomy: evolution of the technique and experience with 2400 cases. J Endour. 2009;23(9): 1467–72.
7. Stolzenburg JU, Truss MC, Bekos A, Do M, Rabenalt R, Stief CG, Hoznek A, Abbou CC, Neuhaus J, Dorschner W. Does the extraperitoneal laparoscopic approach improve the outcome of radical prostatectomy? Curr Urol Rep. 2004;5(2):115–22.
8. Ruiz L, et al. Comparison of early oncologic results of laparoscopic radical prostatectomy by extraperitoneal versus transperitoneal approach. Eur Urol. 2004;46(1):50–4; discussion 54–6.
9. Erdogru T, et al. Comparison of transperitoneal and extraperitoneal laparoscopic radical prostatectomy using match-pair analysis. Eur Urol. 2004;46(3):312–9; discussion 320.
10. Stolzenburg JU, Wasserscheid J, Rabenalt R, Do M, Schwalenberg T, McNeill A, Constantinides C, Kallidonis P, Ganzer R, Liatsikos E. Reduction in incidence of lymphocele following extraperitoneal radical prostatectomy and pelvic lymph node dissection by bilateral peritoneal fenestration. World J Urol. 2008;26:581–6.
11. Su LM, Link RE, Bhayani SB, Sullivan W, Pavlovich CP. Nerve-sparing laparoscopic radical prostatectomy: replicating the open surgical technique. Urology. 2004;64(1):123–7.
12. Stolzenburg JU, Truss MC, Do M, Rabenalt R, Pfeiffer H, Dunzinger M, Aedtner B, Stief CG, Jonas U, Dorschner W. Evolution of endoscopic extraperitoneal radical prostatectomy (EERPE)—technical improvements and development of a nerve-sparing, potency-preserving approach. World J Urol. 2003;21(3):147–52.
13. Stolzenburg JU, et al. Intrafascial nerve-sparing endoscopic extraperitoneal radical prostatectomy. Eur Urol. 2008;53(5):931–40.
14. Cusumano S, et al. Feasibility, technique, and principles of tension- and energy-free laparoscopic radical prostatectomy with lateral intrafascial dissection of the neurovascular bundles with the use of a high-definition optical device. J Endourol. 2008; 22(9):1981–7.
15. Stolzenburg JU, Liatsikos EN, Rabenalt R, Do M, et al. Nerve sparing endoscopic extraperitoneal radical prostatectomy- Effect of puboprostatic ligament preservation on early continence and positive surgical margins. Eur Urol. 2006;49:103–12.
16. Rocco B, Gregori A, Stener S, Santoro L, Bozzola A, Galli S, Knez R, Scieri F, Scaburri A, Gaboardi F. Posterior reconstruction of the rhabdosphincter allows a rapid recovery of continence after transperitoneal videolaparoscopic radical prostatectomy. Eur Urol. 2007;51(4):996–1003.
17. Rocco B, Cozzi G, Spinelli MG, Coelho RF, Patel VR, Tewari A, Wiklund P, Graefen M, Mottrie A, Gaboardi F, Gill IS, Montorsi F, Artibani W, Rocco F. Posterior musculofascial reconstruction after radical prostatectomy: a systematic review of the literature. Eur Urol. 2012;62(5):779–90.
18. Goeman L, Salomon L, Hoznek A, De La Taille A, Vordos D, Yiou R, Abbou CC. Radical laparoscopic prostatectomy: should we do bladder neck preservation or a reconstruction? Curr Urol Rep. 2006;7(2):93–5.
19. Stolzenburg JU, Kallidonis P, Hicks J, Do M, Dietel A, et al. Effect of bladder neck preservation during endoscopic extraperitoneal radical prostatectomy on urinary continence. Urol Int. 2010;85(2):135–8.
20. Rassweiler J, Schulze M, Teber D, Marrero R, Seemann O, Rumpelt J, Frede T. Laparoscopic radical prostatectomy with the Heilbronn technique: oncological results in the first 500 patients. J Urol. 2005;173(3):761–4.
21. Gill IS, Zippe CD. Laparoscopic radical prostatectomy: technique. Urol Clin North Am. 2001;28(2):423–36.
22. Stolzenburg JU, Kallidonis P, Do M, Dietel A, et al. A comparison of outcomes for interfascial and intrafascial nerve-sparing radical prostatectomy. Urology. 2010;76(3):743–8.
23. Guillonneau B, et al. Laparoscopic radical prostatectomy: assessment after 240 procedures. Urol Clin North Am. 2001;28(1):189–202.

24. Guillonneau B, et al. Laparoscopic radical prostatectomy: assessment after 550 procedures. Crit Rev Oncol Hematol. 2002;43(2):123–33.
25. Abbou CC, et al. Laparoscopic radical prostatectomy: preliminary results. Urology. 2000;55(5):630–4.
26. Mariano MB, et al. Laparoscopic radical prostatectomy: 10 years experience. Int Braz J Urol. 2009;35(5):565–71; discussion 571–2.
27. Murphy DG, et al. Operative details and oncological and functional outcome of robotic-assisted laparoscopic radical prostatectomy: 400 cases with a minimum of 12 months follow-up. Eur Urol. 2009;55(6):1358–66.
28. Olsson LE, et al. Prospective patient-reported continence after laparoscopic radical prostatectomy. Urology. 2001;58(4):570–2.
29. Link RE, et al. Health related quality of life before and after laparoscopic radical prostatectomy. J Urol. 2005;173(1):175–9; discussion 179.
30. Rassweiler J, et al. Laparoscopic radical prostatectomy with the Heilbronn technique: an analysis of the first 180 cases. J Urol. 2001;166(6):2101–8.
31. Salomon L, et al. Urinary continence and erectile function: a prospective evaluation of functional results after radical laparoscopic prostatectomy. Eur Urol. 2002;42(4):338–43.
32. Goeman L, et al. Long-term functional and oncological results after retroperitoneal laparoscopic prostatectomy according to a prospective evaluation of 550 patients. World J Urol. 2006;24(3):281–8.
33. Rozet F, et al. Extraperitoneal laparoscopic radical prostatectomy: a prospective evaluation of 600 cases. J Urol. 2005;174(3):908–11.
34. Milhoua PM, et al. Issue of prostate gland size, laparoscopic radical prostatectomy, and continence revisited. Urology. 2008;71(3):417–20.
35. Novara G, et al. Evaluating urinary continence and preoperative predictors of urinary continence after robot assisted laparoscopic radical prostatectomy. J Urol. 2010;184(3):1028–33.
36. Menard J, et al. Laparoscopic radical prostatectomy after transurethral resection of the prostate: surgical and functional outcomes. Urology. 2008;72(3):593–7.
37. Do M, Haefner T, Liatsikos E, Kallidonis P, Hicks J, Dietel A, Horn LC, Rabenalt R, Stolzenburg JU. Endoscopic extraperitoneal radical prostatectomy after previous transurethral resection of prostate: oncologic and functional outcomes of 100 cases. Urology. 2010;75(6):1348–52.
38. Katz R, Salomon L, Hoznek A, de la Taille A, Antiphon P, Abbou CC. Positive surgical margins in laparoscopic radical prostatectomy: the impact of apical dissection, bladder neck remodeling and nerve preservation. J Urol. 2003;169(6):2049–52.
39. Takenaka A, Soga H, Sakai I, Nakano Y, Miyake H, Tanaka K, Fujisawa M. Influence of nerve-sparing procedure on early recovery of urinary continence after laparoscopic radical prostatectomy. J Endourol. 2009;23(7):1115–9.
40. Verze P, Scuzzarella S, Martina GR, Giummelli P, Cantoni F, Mirone V. Long-term oncological and functional results of extraperitoneal laparoscopic radical prostatectomy: one surgical team's experience on 1,600 consecutive cases. World J Urol. 2013; 31(3):529–34.
41. Busch J, Stephan C, Herold A, Erber B, Kempkensteffen C, Hinz S, Lein M, Weikert S, Miller K, Magheli A. Long-term oncological and continence outcomes after laparoscopic radical prostatectomy: a single-centre experience. BJU Int. 2012;110(11 Pt C):E985–90.
42. Matin SF. Recognition and preservation of accessory pudendal arteries during laparoscopic radical prostatectomy. Urology. 2006;67(5):1012–5.
43. Secin FP, et al. Positive surgical margins and accessory pudendal artery preservation during laparoscopic radical prostatectomy. Eur Urol. 2005;48(5):786–92; discussion 793.
44. Anastasiadis AG, et al. Radical retropubic versus laparoscopic prostatectomy: a prospective comparison of functional outcome. Urology. 2003;62(2):292–7.
45. Roumeguere T, et al. Radical prostatectomy: a prospective comparison of oncological and functional results between open and laparoscopic approaches. World J Urol. 2003;20(6):360–6.
46. Greco F, et al. Laparoscopic vs open retropubic intrafascial nerve-sparing radical prostatectomy: surgical and functional outcomes in 300 patients. BJU Int. 2010;106(4):543–7.
47. Neill MG, et al. Does intrafascial dissection during nerve-sparing laparoscopic radical prostatectomy compromise cancer control? BJU Int. 2009;104(11): 1730–3.
48. Levinson AW, Su LM. Laparoscopic radical prostatectomy: current techniques. Curr Opin Urol. 2007;17(2):98–103.
49. Shah SJ, Goyal V, Sachar R, Nath AK, Jain N, Kapadia K. Seminal vesicle sparing laparoscopic radical prostatectomy using a low-energy source: better continence and potency. Indian J Urol. 2009;25(2): 199–202.
50. Guillonneau B, et al. Laparoscopic radical prostatectomy: oncological evaluation after 1,000 cases a Montsouris Institute. J Urol. 2003;169(4):1261–6.
51. Frota R, et al. The effect of prostate weight on the outcomes of laparoscopic radical prostatectomy. BJU Int. 2008;101(5):589–93.
52. Chang CM, et al. The impact of prostate size in laparoscopic radical prostatectomy. Eur Urol. 2005;48(2):285–90.
53. Zorn KC, et al. Long-term functional and oncological outcomes of patients undergoing sural nerve interposition grafting during robot-assisted laparoscopic radical prostatectomy. J Endourol. 2008;22(5): 1005–12.
54. Frede T, et al. Laparoscopic radical prostatectomy—impact of training and supervision. Minim Invasive Ther Allied Technol. 2005;14(2):104–8.

55. Tewari A, Sooriakumaran P, Bloch DA, Seshadri-Kreaden U, Hebert AE, Wiklund P. Positive surgical margin and perioperative complication rates of primary surgical treatments for prostate cancer: a systematic review and meta-analysis comparing retropubic, laparoscopic, and robotic prostatectomy. Eur Urol. 2012;62(1):1–15.
56. Martorana G, et al. Laparoscopic radical prostatectomy: oncological evaluation in the early phase of the learning curve comparing to retropubic approach. Arch Ital Urol Androl. 2004;76(1):1–5.
57. Salomon L, et al. Outcome and complications of radical prostatectomy in patients with PSA <10 ng/ml: comparison between the retropubic, perineal and laparoscopic approach. Prostate Cancer Prostatic Dis. 2002;5(4):285–90.
58. Hruza M, Bermejo JL, Flinspach B, Schulze M, Teber D, Rumpelt HJ, Rassweiler JJ. Long-term oncological outcomes after laparoscopic radical prostatectomy. BJU Int. 2013;111(2):271–80.
59. Liatsikos E, et al. Prevention and management of perioperative complications in laparoscopic and endoscopic radical prostatectomy. World J Urol. 2008;26(6):571–80.
60. Stolzenburg JU, et al. Complications of endoscopic extraperitoneal radical prostatectomy (EERPE): prevention and management. World J Urol. 2006; 24(6):668–75.
61. Guillonneau B, et al. Perioperative complications of laparoscopic radical prostatectomy: the Montsouris 3-year experience. J Urol. 2002;167(1):51–6.
62. Tozawa K, et al. Evaluation of operative complications related to laparoscopic radical prostatectomy. Int J Urol. 2008;15(3):222–5.
63. Rabbani F, et al. Comprehensive standardized report of complications of retropubic and laparoscopic radical prostatectomy. Eur Urol. 2010;57(3):371–86.
64. Moran PS, O'Neill M, Teljeur C, Flattery M, Murphy LA, Smyth G, Ryan M. Robot-assisted radical prostatectomy compared with open and laparoscopic approaches: a systematic review and meta-analysis. Int J Urol. 2013;20(3):312–21.
65. Ficcara V, Novara G, Artibani W, Cestari A, et al. Retropubic, laparoscopic and robot-assisted radical prostatectomy: a systematic review and cumulative analysis of comparative studies. Eur Urol. 2009;55:1037–63.
66. Lim SK, Kim KH, Shin TY, Rha KH. Current status of robot-assisted laparoscopic radical prostatectomy: how does it compare with other surgical approaches? Int J Urol. 2013;20(3):271–84.
67. Al-Shaiji TF, Kanaroglou N, Thom A, Prowse C, Comondore V, Orovan W, Piercey K, Whelan P, Winter L, Matsumoto ED. A cost-analysis comparison of laparoscopic radical prostatectomy versus open radical prostatectomy: the McMaster Institute of Urology experience. Can Urol Assoc J. 2010; 4(4):237–41.
68. Bolenz C, Gupta A, Hotze T, Ho R, Cadeddu JA, Roehrborn CG, Lotan Y. Cost comparison of robotic, laparoscopic, and open radical prostatectomy for prostate cancer. Eur Urol. 2010;57(3):453–8.

Extraperitoneal Robot-Assisted Radical Prostatectomy

13

Vineet Agrawal and Jean V. Joseph

13.1 Introduction

For organ confined prostate cancer, radical prostatectomy remains the gold standard form of surgical management [1]. When performed using the open approach, this procedure is generally carried out extraperitoneally, by accessing the space of Retzius, preserving the integrity of the peritoneal cavity. With widespread adoption of robot assisted radical prostatectomy [2, 3], however, fewer surgeons have adopted the extraperitoneal approach compared to the transperitoneal route to gain access and to perform the procedure.

This chapter will focus mainly on our stepwise technique of extraperitoneal robot assisted radical prostatectomy based on experience in over 2,000 cases. The transperitoneal approach to robot assisted radical prostatectomy has been described elsewhere in this book.

V. Agrawal, MD, FRCS Ed(Urol), FEBU
Department of Urology, University of Rochester Medical Center, Rochester, NY, USA

J.V. Joseph, MD, MDA, MBA (✉)
Section of Laparoscopic and Robotic Surgery, University of Rochester Medical Center, Rochester, NY, USA
e-mail: jean_joseph@urmc.rochester.edu

13.2 Step-Wise Description

Patient Positioning

Proper patient positioning facilitates the procedure while avoiding potential position-related injuries. The patient should be secured to the operating table to avoid sliding when placed in the Trendelenburg position. The table should be properly padded to avoid pressure sores particularly with lengthy procedures. We use a vacuum bean bag (Hug-U-Vac™, Allen Medical Systems, Acton, MA) (Fig. 13.1), which wraps along the patient sides and shoulders keeping him in a fixed position throughout the procedure. Chest straps can be used but should not be too tight to allow adequate chest expansion with ventilation. The arms are placed alongside the body in egg-crate protective foam to lessen the risk of brachial plexus injuries. We use a split leg table which allows access to the perineum, keeping the legs straight avoiding calf compression. Pneumatic compression stockings are used with the legs secured using tape. Leg abduction should be kept to a minimum to avoid dislocation. Patients with a history of hip fractures should be positioned before induction of anesthesia to ascertain the limit of hip mobility. Once the robot is docked, or positioned between the patient's legs, the legs should be brought as close to the midline as possible to allow a more anatomical position if further abduction is not

H.R.H. Patel et al. (eds.), *Pelvic Cancer Surgery: Modern Breakthroughs and Future Advances*,
DOI 10.1007/978-1-4471-4258-4_13, © Springer-Verlag London 2015

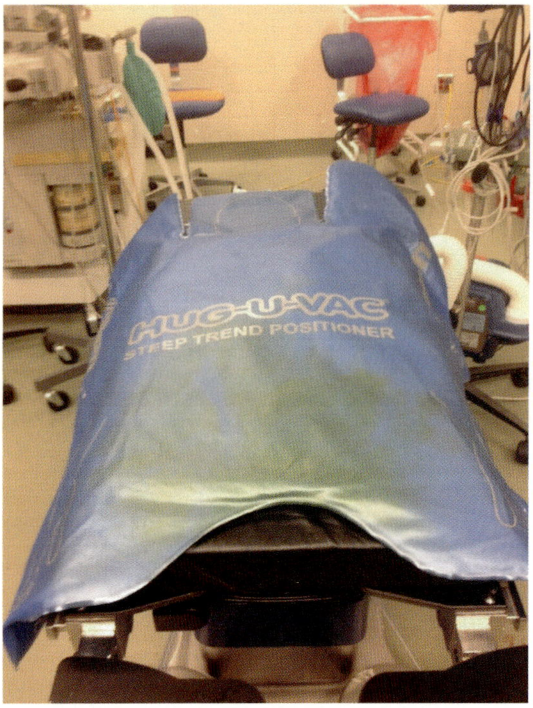

Fig. 13.1 Vacuum bean bag (Hug-U-VacTM, Allen Medical Systems, Acton, MA) to secure patient to the operating table

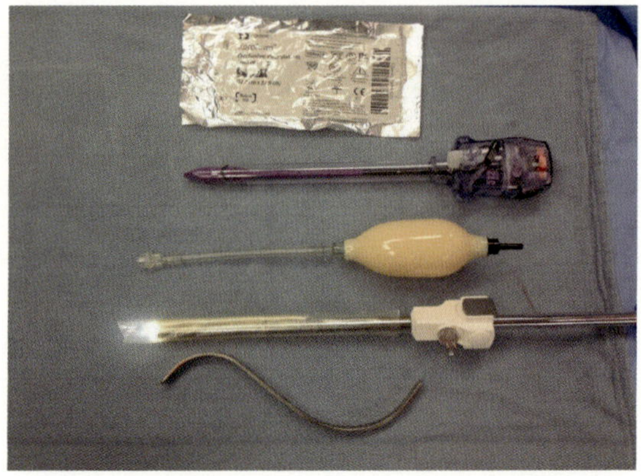

Fig. 13.2 Instruments used during creation of the extraperitoneal space. From *top* to *bottom*: Xeroform gauze, long smooth trocar with no ridges (12 mm 512 XD, Ethicon Endo-Surgery, Cincinnati, Ohio), balloon pumping mechanism, OMS-XB2 Extraview™ balloon dilator with the 0° laparoscope placed inside the uninflated balloon, "S" retractor

necessary. The legs should be brought together at the end of the procedure prior to reversal from anesthesia.

Compared to the exaggerated Trendelenburg position often used with the transperitonal approach (in order to move the bowels out of the operative field), the extraperitoneal approach allows for a much lesser degree of tilt (about 10–15°).

Access

The main difference between the extraperitoneal and transperitoneal route to performing a robot assisted radical prostatectomy is the access. This consists of creation of the extraperitoneal space and the placement of trocars. Except for minor modifications, all the subsequent steps are similar. With experience, the creation of the extraperitoneal space and trocar placement can be achieved in less than 15 min in the majority of the patients.

Creating the Extraperitoneal Space

Our favored approach is an open Hasson "cut-down" technique. The approach is obtained consistently in a controlled manner with clear visualization of anatomical landmarks. Alternatively, the Visiport optical trocar or the blunt Ethicon Excel optical trocar can be used, as has been described by others [4].

The instruments required to create the potential extraperitoneal space include a OMS-XB2 (Oval) Extraview™ balloon dilator trocar (Autosuture, Norwalk, CT) or a spacemaker ™ trocar, a 0° laparoscope, 2 S-shaped retractors and a 15 cm long smooth trocar (12 mm 512 XD, Ethicon Endo-Surgery, Cincinnati, Ohio) (Fig. 13.2). We prefer to use a separate scope for this step. The robotic camera and scope system are difficult to maneuver due to their weight.

After a 3 cm left peri-umbilical skin incision, the subcutaneous tissue is bluntly dissected to expose the anterior rectus sheath. A 1 cm incision is made in the latter and an S-shaped retractor is used to sweep the underlying belly of the rectus muscles laterally, to bring the posterior rectus sheath into view. Once the latter is visualized, the balloon dilator is inserted in the space of Retzius, with the scope placed inside the uninflated balloon. The tip of the balloon should be angled

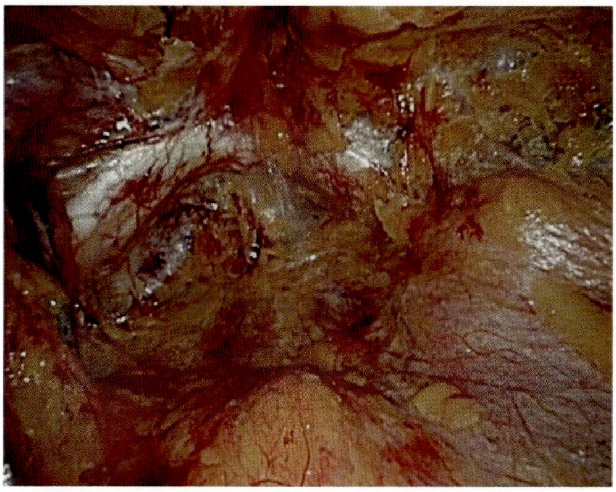

Fig. 13.3 View of the pubic symphysis and extraperitoneal space at the end of balloon dilatation

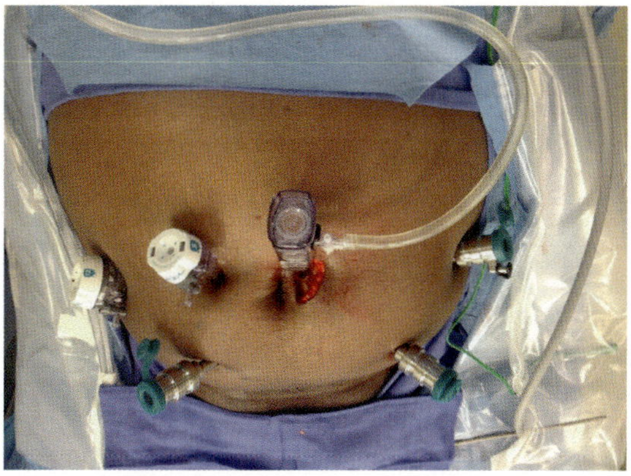

Fig. 13.4 Six trocar "W" configuration. View from the head end. Fourth robotic arm trocar on the left side

upward and toward the midline, to avoid inadvertent injury to the posterior rectus sheath, or access to the peritoneal cavity. There should normally be some resistance from the linea alba until the balloon dilator is passed below the semi-circular line of Douglas. With the start of balloon inflation, the space of Retzius and the retropubic fat are dissected bringing the pubic symphysis into view (Fig. 13.3). The other important landmarks are the inferior epigastric vessels (one artery, two veins) laterally which are visualized on both sides. The external iliac vessels with their attached epigastric tributaries should not be overstretched. Bleeding if present will be noted at this stage with insufflation of the extraperitoneal space. A torn vessel from a branch of the epigastric vessels can be seen at this stage, and can be controlled with a clip. Overdilatation should be avoided as subsequent deflation leads to bleeding. The balloon dilator is removed after deflation and a 15 cm long trocar with the 0° scope is introduced in the space thus created. The key to our approach is the use of this smooth trocar with no ridges. It is useful in the creation of the extra space required for trocar placement cephalad and laterally. This 10/12 mm trocar is wide enough to accommodate the robotic scope. CO_2 insufflation of the extraperitoneal space is carried out through the same trocar up to a pressure of 15 mmHg. Under direct vision, the space is further enlarged by retracting the scope into the trocar and using the beveled tip of the trocar (insinuated under the inferior epigastric vessels) to bluntly sweep the peritoneum posterolaterally on either side. It is important to stay between the abdominal wall muscle anteriorly and transversalis fascia posteriorly to avoid creating an inadvertent peritoneotomy which should be suspected if there is billowing. Care should also be taken not to dissect through the overlying muscle fibers. We routinely place a Xeroform gauze around the trocar to prevent CO_2 leakage at the camera trocar site. We also use a purse string suture in the fascia to narrow the opening around the trocar and to secure the latter in place. The movements necessary to develop the extraperitoneal space laterally widen the fascial opening, causing leakage of air around the trocar. To lessen air leakage, a balloon tip trocar can be used for this. We prefer the application of the gauze, which quickly seals the opening, obviating the need for trocar exchange.

Trocar Insertion

Robot-assisted procedures call for particular consideration in trocar placement in order to avoid robotic arms collision. A distance of 10 cm between all robotic working arm trocars is important.

Our practice has evolved from a 5-trocar technique to a 6-trocar arrangement in a "W" configuration (Fig. 13.4) during a 4-arm daVinci extraperitoneal robotic prostatectomy. In total, three 8 mm daVinci metal robotic trocars and two disposable assistant trocars (one 12 mm, 150 cm long Excel 512 XD trocar, and one 5 mm trocar)

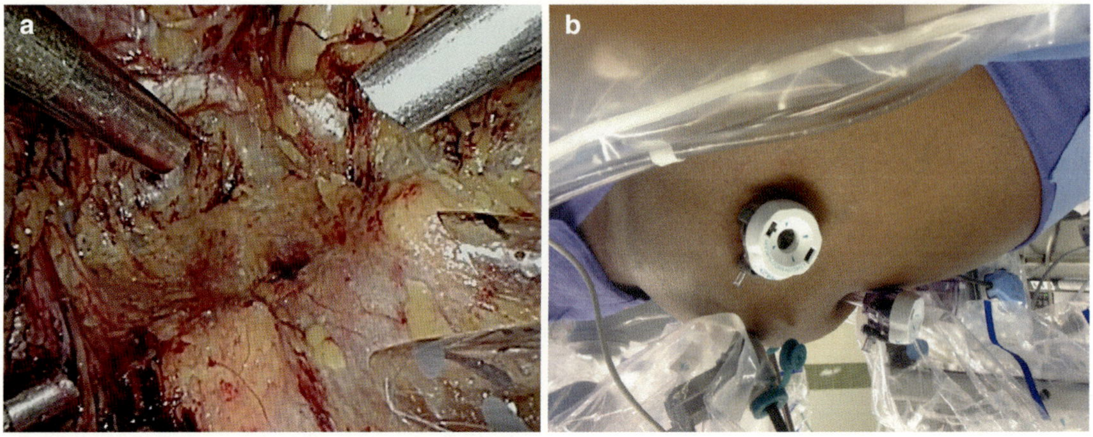

Fig. 13.5 (**a**) View through the laparoscope of the trocars at the end of their placement. A working robotic trocar with the fourth arm robot trocar on the left side of the patient, and the right working robotic trocar with the two assistant trocars (12 and 5 mm) on the right side of the patient. (**b**) View from the right side following docking of the robot. Minimal Trendenlenburg position is employed. Selective insufflation of the lower abdomen can be appreciated

are used in addition to the 12 mm infra-umbilical camera trocar. The 12 mm assistant trocar is used for passage of clips/ sutures while the 5 mm assistant trocar is used for suction/irrigation.

Once an adequate space is created, and the peritoneum pushed cephalad and laterally, the 12 mm right assistant trocar is introduced 5 cm medial to the anterior superior iliac spine along a line joining this anatomical landmark to the umbilicus. The assistant trocars can be placed on either side, based on the surgical team's preference.

The trocar for the fourth robotic arm is placed opposite to the assistant's (5 cm cephalad and medial to the anterior superior iliac spine) and guided toward the pubic symphysis under direct vision. We use a hypodermic needle to guide the site of insertion of the two remaining robotic working trocars on either side. They are generally placed 10 cm caudal and lateral to the umbilicus on either side, forming a triangle with the latter. Using the needle as a guide to identify the path of the trocars minimizes the risk of inadvertent injury to the epigastric vessels. The trocars for the robotic working arms are placed lateral to the respective epigastric vessels, at a more perpendicular angle to the abdominal wall to avoid robotic arms collision. Trocar tunneling should be avoided, as it will restrict motion of the trocars. For the remaining 5 mm assistant trocar which is placed 5 cm lateral to the umbilicus on the right side, the dissection is performed in a more medial and cephalad direction. The robot is docked once all the trocars are in place (Fig. 13.5).

We start the procedure with a Maryland bipolar grasper in the left hand, monopolar scissors in the right hand, and Prograsp forceps in the fourth arm. The only other robotic instruments needed are two needle holders used during dorsal vein ligation and completion of vesicourethral anastomosis to be described later. Instruments used by the assistant include suction/irrigation, blunt tip graspers, clip applier and specimen entrapment bag. A 0° scope is used throughout the procedure.

Division of Endopelvic Fascia and Ligation of the Dorsal Venous Complex

The first step following docking of the robot is to incise the endopelvic fascia. One of the advantages of the extraperitoneal approach is evident in this step. The bladder take-down step is eliminated. The endopelvic fascia is often visualized through the balloon dilator as the space is created.

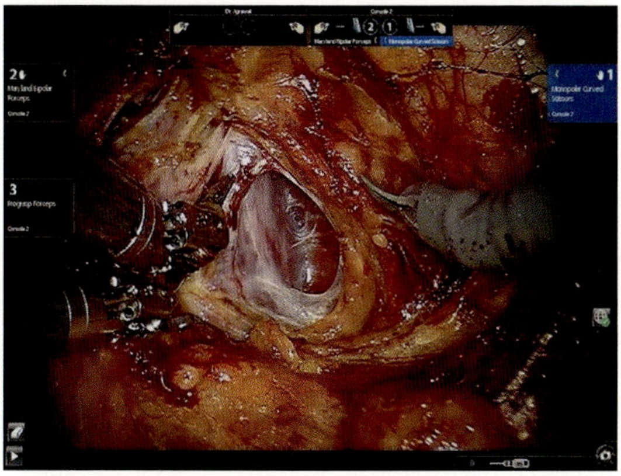

Fig. 13.6 Incision of the endopelvic fascia

If the fascia is not visualized, the loose fatty tissue in the space of Retzius is easily swept off the fascia with all vessels cauterized to ensure hemostasis. Beginning the dissection on the right side and using the left arm to retract the prostate medially, the best plane to enter the endopelvic fascia is identified which is usually a window along the mid portion of the prostate. Allowing air to get behind the fascia helps further delineate the anatomy (Fig. 13.6). This is a generally an avascular plane and can be opened using scissors without cautery. The incision extends from the base of the prostate up to the puboprostatic ligaments. The proper plane of the dissection is where the prostate surface and the pelvic floor muscles are visualized. Once in this plane, the prostatic attachments can be separated by a gentle sweeping motion, pushing the muscles laterally. Dissection toward the puboprostatic ligaments should be performed away from the dorsal venous complex to prevent its inadvertent injury. A combination of delicate sharp as well as blunt dissection is used to free the muscular attachments at the apex of the prostate. We prefer to transect the puboprostatic ligaments as this thins out the dorsal venous complex allowing better coaptation or cinching down of the suture used for its control. Further dissection of the apex of the prostate allows the exposure of the notch between the dorsal venous complex and the urethra where the suture used for venous ligation is placed. We use a barbed V-lock suture on a SH needle to place a figure of eight suture to control the DVC. The needle is held at the junction of its proximal one third at a 30° angle. Guiding it in the correct direction from right to left, parallel to the dorsal venous complex is very important. The tip of the needle is directed toward the previously exposed notch and twisting the needle using the endowrist rather than sliding the needle across the DVC is preferred. The needle should be retrieved following its curve to avoid tearing of dorsal venous complex veins. The suture can be tied, or anchored to the symphysis following dorsal vein ligation. If the needle is placed too posterior, this may lead to capture of the Foley catheter. One should suspect this if the knot does not hold when the vein is being tied. The needle holders should be directed in an anterior-posterior direction during knot tying. Caudal or lateral movement of the needle holders may lead to bleeding due to rubbing of the pubic bones.

Bladder Neck Dissection

In order to expose the plane between the bladder and the prostate, the fourth arm is used to retract the bladder in a postero-cephalad direction. For the novice, where to commence the bladder neck dissection can be challenging. Identifying the waist where the perivesical fat attenuates over the prostate and grasping the tissue with bipolar forceps, taking care not to include the prostate, is a useful starting point. We prefer starting this dissection lateral to the bladder neck where the longitudinal bladder fibers can be easily seen. We use a "burn and push" technique rather than overuse of the cautery to develop the plane between the bladder and the prostate as the latter can lead to creation of multiple planes. The funnel of the bladder neck should be followed to maintain a proper plane. It is very useful to establish this plane laterally and then follow it towards the midline from either side. Following dissection of the anterior bladder neck and confirmation of the correct plane of dissection, a greater appreciation of the planar anatomy between the bladder neck and the prostate can be made on either side. We prefer to transect the bladder neck sharply in the midline. We believe that avoidance of cautery during this step minimizes the risk of bladder neck contracture. The posterior bladder neck fibers are swept off the prostate using a combination of sharp and blunt dissection. Care is taken to carry the dissection in a postero-cephalad direction to follow the normal contour of the prostate which extends cephalad (Fig. 13.7). Identification of the plane between the posterior bladder neck and prostate laterally, and following it medially, minimizes the risk of "button hole" in the posterior bladder neck which may risk injury to the ureteral orifices. Proper traction is important during the bladder neck dissection and the fourth arm is adjusted progressively to help with this.

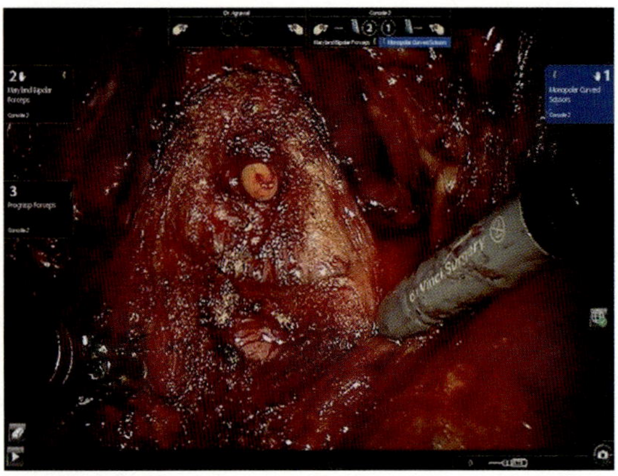

Fig. 13.7 Bladder neck dissection. View following transection of the bladder neck, with catheter in the prostatic urethra. Following the correct plane is important

Seminal Vesicles Dissection

This is a relatively easier step once one enters the right plane behind the bladder. With the bladder neck retracted cephalad, the longitudinal muscle fibers crossing posterior to the bladder are transected in the midline to allow visualization of the ampulla of both vasa and the attached seminal vesicles (Fig. 13.8a). The vas is dissected with the aid of the bipolar forceps, grasped and a clip is applied enbloc encompassing the artery to the vas which runs between the vas and the adjoining seminal vesicle (Fig. 13.8b). It is useful to stay as anterior as possible, avoiding the roots of the vessels, to avoid injury to the neurovascular bundles coursing posteriorly in nerve sparing cases. Clips are preferred at this stage to avoid thermal energy. Next, the seminal vesicles are dissected laterally with individual clipping of vessels. The vas and its respective seminal vesicles are retracted anteriorly. As there are no attachments to the seminal vesicles posteriorly, the bipolar forceps can be used to push Denonvillier's fascia away from the seminal vesicles leading to their complete visualization. We find that the fourth arm is useful in retracting both the vasa and the attached seminal vesicles anteriorly. This helps expose and stretch

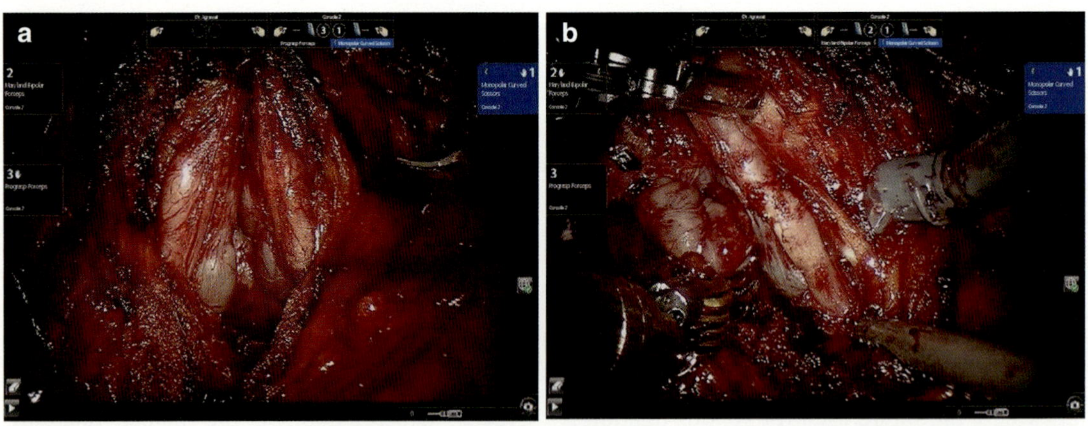

Fig. 13.8 (**a**) Vas and seminal vesicles visualized at the beginning of their dissection. (**b**) Artery to the right vas being dissected in preparation for its enbloc clipping with its vas

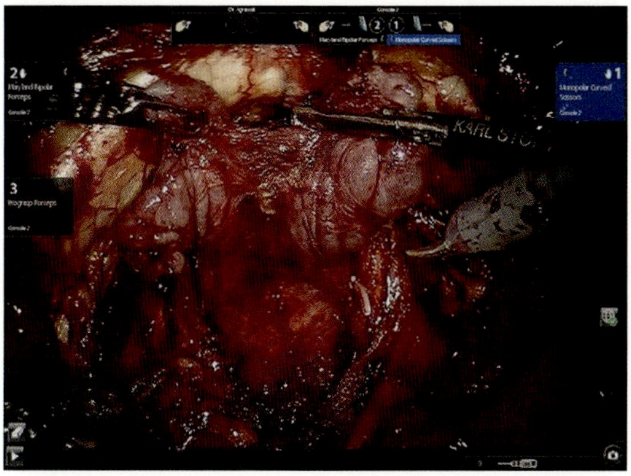

Fig. 13.9 Posterior prostate dissection. Both the vas and their respective seminal vesicles have been lifted anteriorly to expose the Denonvillier's fascia

Denonvilliers fascia, in preparation for the posterior prostate dissection.

Posterior Prostate Dissection

Denonvillier's fascia is incised transversely exposing the yellow peri-rectal fat (Fig. 13.9). The rectum is dissected bluntly off the prostate caudally to the level of the prostatic apex. The plane between Denonvillier's fascia and the prostatic fascia is developed bluntly using bipolar forceps spread open and pushing posteriorly away from the prostate.

Neurovascular Bundle Dissection

Our preference is for a combined antegrade and retrograde dissection for the nerve-sparing. The fourth arm is used to retract the prostate anteriorly and to the opposite side of the neurovascular bundle being dissected. This helps to visualize the course of the neurovascular bundles along the lateral aspect of the prostate. The characteristics of the cancer, and intraoperative digital rectal exam dictate the extent of the nerve sparing. The pedicle is dissected sequentially using clips to control vessels entering the base of the prostate (Fig. 13.10). Medial retraction of the base of the prostate facilitates visualization of the interfascial plane between the endopelvic and periprostatic fascia which is sharply divided. Gentle sweeping motion with the scissors opened helps further establish the plane along the lateral surface of the prostate. Once the intended level of nerve sparing on the lateral surface of the prostate is identified, the tissues at the base of the prostate are further dissected exposing the posterior surface of the prostate. Once the neurovascular bundle is released at the prostatic base, there is a clear distinction between the surface of the prostate and the neurovascular bundle. Further clipping of any remaining attachment between the neurovascular bundle and the prostatic base is often needed in order to release the remaining bundle along its course. Following release of the neurovascular bundle from the prostate base, the prostate is retracted upward, the interfascial plane is followed caudally, pushing the neurovascular bundle off the prostate. We do not recommend an intrafascial dissection due to a high risk of positive margins in patients with extracapsular invasion, and the risk of capsulotomy which can compromise cancer control.

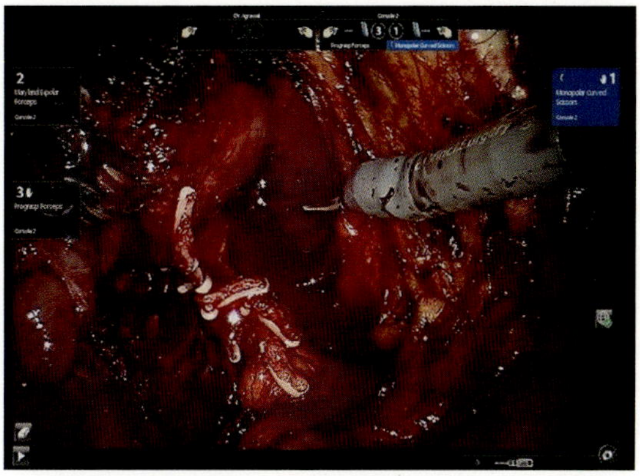

Fig. 13.10 Right neurovascular bundle preservation with clips (athermal technique)

Dissection of Prostatic Apex and Urethra

The fourth arm is used to retract the prostate in a postero-cephalad direction. Once the assistant passes the catheter through the prostate, the previously ligated dorsal vein complex is sharply transected down to the level of the longitudinal

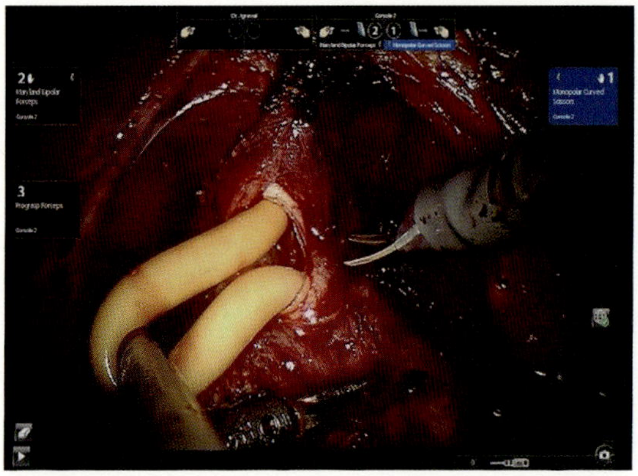

Fig. 13.11 Transection of the posterior urethra at the apex

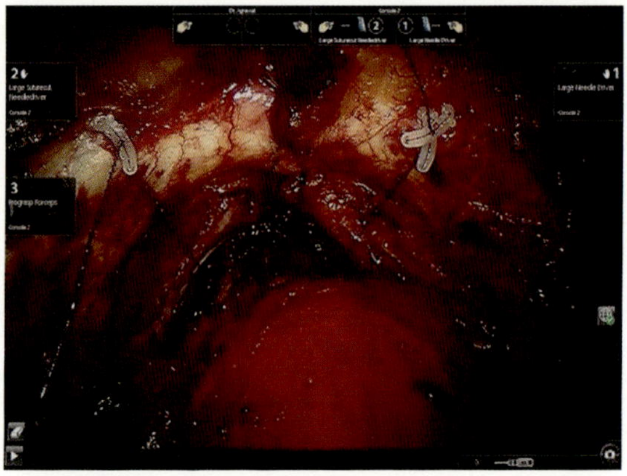

Fig. 13.12 Anterior suspension of posterior reconstruction sutures, suspending the bladder neck

urethral fibers. Occasionally the dorsal vein suture may fall due to posterior retraction. It can be sewn without difficulty. To facilitate this and to limit bleeding, intra-abdominal pressure can be raised temporarily up to 20 mmHg. The fourth arm can be used to lift the prostate anteriorly, compressing the dorsal vein, while the surgeon gets the suture ready to oversew the venous complex. The preservation of the dorsal vein suture should never be at the expense of transecting the prostatic apex, risking a positive apical margin. If the neurovascular bundles have been spared, they should be inspected and further dissected away from the apex to avoid injury. The neurovascular bundles can be tethered to the prostatic apex and injured at that level. The prostate is then retracted cephalad to put the urethra on stretch. After confirmation that the Foley catheter is in place, the anterior surface of the urethra is sharply transected leaving a clear margin on the prostate. Once the Foley catheter is visualized, it is picked up and retracted cephalad by the assistant. This tents up the posterior surface of the urethra and allows sharper dissection of the prostate (Fig. 13.11). The posterior prostate often extends more caudally than the anterior aspect, therefore, this transection should be carried out with great care, being mindful of possible prostatic apical tissue extending caudally. Once the prostate is free, it is inspected and placed in a 10 mm Endocatch specimen retrieval bag (Covidien, Mansfield, MA) and pulled out of the pelvis away from the operative field until it is extracted at the end of the procedure. Rectal wall integrity is ensured at this point.

Posterior Reconstruction

Two interrupted 9-in., 3-0 barbed polyglactin V-lock sutures on an RB-1 needle are used for posterior reconstruction. This approximates the posterior rhabdosphincter with Denonvillier's fascia incorporating the longitudinal fibers posterior to the bladder which were previously covering the seminal vesicles. This posterior reconstruction helps bring the bladder neck close to the urethra in preparation for the anastomosis. More recently, we have been suspending the posterior reconstruction sutures to the pubic symphysis, stabilized using hem-o-lok clips (the suspension is carried out after completion of the vesicourethral anastomosis). This maneuver keeps the urethro-sphincteric complex anteriorly in its intrapelvic location (Fig. 13.12).

Vesico-Urethral Anastomosis

The anastomosis is carried out in a continuous manner using two separate 2-0 polyglactin sutures on a RB-1 needle cut to 9 in. One suture is used to first complete the posterior layer, while another is used for the anterior aspect of the anastomosis. The posterior layer of the anastomosis is carried out in a clockwise direction (5–11'o clock position) while the anterior layer is completed in the opposite direction. The anterior layer starts at the 4'o clock position and moves in an anticlockwise direction until it meets the other suture. The two sutures are tied separately, providing two distinct suture lines, avoiding reliance on a single knot. A 20 Fr Foley catheter is passed into the bladder under vision before cinching and tying the anterior suture. Sutures should be pulled perpendicular to the urethra to avoid tearing of the longitudinally oriented urethral fibers. Application of perineal pressure by the assistant, and decreasing the pneumoperitoneum to 8–10 mmHg, are useful steps to allow the bladder neck and urethra to come into proximity and allow mucosa to mucosa apposition. The bladder is irrigated to verify the watertightness of the anastomosis.

Specimen Delivery and Completion of the Procedure

On completion of the anastomosis, the robot is disconnected. A 19 Fr closed suction Blake drain is placed under vision in the retropubic space. It is introduced via the 12 mm trocar which is then withdrawn. The trocars for the left and right robotic arms close to the epigastric vessels are removed under vision to ensure there is no bleeding from these vessels or their tributaries. The fascial opening at the peri-umbilical camera trocar site is widened just enough to extract the specimen. It is then closed with several interrupted figure-of-eight 0 polyglactin sutures. Occasionally, a small opening is required in the posterior rectus sheath and peritoneum to release intraperitoneal trapped air if present. This opening is closed with a single 0 polygalactin suture. The remaining fascial openings do not have to be closed, given their extraperitoneal location. Local anesthetic is used to infiltrate the skin openings, which are closed with interrupted subcuticular 3-0 Monocryl sutures.

13.3 Post-operative Course

The patient is admitted to the post anesthesia care unit, and later transferred to the 23-h stay unit. Clear liquid diet followed by regular diet is allowed as tolerated. Patients are ambulated within 4 h of surgery. Ketorolac and opiates are used for pain management. The former is administered every 6 h while the latter is used on demand, using a PCA (patient controlled analgesia) administration device. Two doses of intravenous antibiotics and subcutaneous heparin are administered 8 h apart. The drain is removed when the output is minimal post ambulation during an 8-h period. We do not routinely draw labs unless indicated. Most of our patients are discharged within 23 h. The Foley catheter is removed after 7–10 days in the office. Cystograms are not routinely performed unless there is bleeding or suspicion of leakage at the anastomotic site. Patients are instructed in pelvic floor or Kegel exercises which they commence the day after removal of the catheter. Penile rehabilitation is also initiated using Tadalafil in preoperatively potent patients without contraindications, who had a nerve sparing procedure.

13.4 Advantages and Disadvantages of the Extraperitoneal Approach

The main reasons for the perceived disadvantages of the extraperitoneal approach include unfamiliarity with access and instruments, difficulty in spacing the trocars especially with the use of the fourth arm, relatively limited working space, and an increased risk of lymphocele formation following pelvic lymph node dissection. In addition, if an extended pelvic lymphadenectomy is indicated, the alternative transperitoneal approach may afford a better exposure of the cephalad limits of the template of dissection. Tension on the anastomosis is often cited as a potential disadvantage of the extraperitoneal approach, given the urachal attachments are unaltered. As with open retropubic prostatectomy which is generally performed extraperitoneally, there is no meaningful tension on the anastomosis once completed. The initial sutures are indeed under some tension, which is quickly redistributed, or relieved with the placement of additional sutures. Approximating the posterior urethra to the posterior bladder neck is helpful in eliminating possible tension, facilitating the anastomosis. We routinely decrease the pressure in the working space to 8 or 10 mmHg to ease reapproximation of the cephalad-displaced bladder to the urethra. The application of perineal pressure is also helpful at this stage, lessening the risk of urethral tearing. The perceived disadvantages of the extraperitoneal approach can be easily eliminated with experience.

There are several advantages of the extraperitoneal route. These include the need for less steep Trendelenburg positioning. This is helpful in patients with poor pulmonary reserve. Diaphragmatic expansion is less compromised, allowing proper ventilation, diminishing possible associated complications. The limited Trendelenburg also lessens the risk of position-related neuropraxia, which is more likely when the patient's body weight is shifted to the shoulders, with possible brachial plexus compression. The extraperitoneal route avoids all potential intraperitoneal adhesions making this the route of choice for patients with prior extensive and/or multiple bowel surgeries as the risk of injury to the intra-abdominal organs during adhesiolysis is avoided. This approach gives rapid access to the target organ. The bladder takedown step is eliminated. The peritoneum acts as a natural barrier obviating the need for bowel retraction from the operative surgical field as can be seen with the transperitoneal approach. This potentially lessens the incidence of paralytic ileus, as bowel handling is avoided and hence relatively faster recovery [5]. In addition, this route allows containment of bleeding or urine leak in the confined extraperitoneal space, should any of these occur.

Conclusion

Since the first publication on the use of the extraperitoneal approach to robot assisted radical prostatectomy [6], there have been further reports of surgical technique and functional and oncological outcome from high volume centers using the extraperitoneal approach for robot assisted prostatectomy [7–10]. These have demonstrated equivalence in functional outcome between the two approaches.

A recent meta-analysis (one randomized controlled trial and five case-control studies) comparing the perioperative outcome between the extraperitoneal (n = 530) and the transperitoneal route (n = 537) showed that while there were no differences in estimated blood loss, hospital stay or margin positivity, the operative time and complications were more favorable with the extraperitoneal approach [11]. A recent study looked at recovery following the extraperitoneal approach comparing it to the transperitoneal approach found that using the validated CARE (Convalescence and Recovery evaluation) questionnaire, patients undergoing the EP approach showed improved recovery [5].

At our medical center, we routinely use both the extraperitoneal and transperitoneal approaches. The approach is individualized based on patient factors. With experience, more challenging cases such as an obese patient [12] and large prostates with enlarged median lobes can be carried out safely with the extraperitoneal approach. It can be a very advantageous approach in certain patients. We have performed robot assisted radical prostatectomy via the extraperitoneal route in patients with a pelvic kidneys [13], or following kidney transplant [14]. In the latter, compared to the transperitoneal approach, the risk of damaging the ureter of the transplanted kidney is certainly reduced. With a history of multiple previous accesses to the abdominal cavity, including peritoneal dialysis, complex adhesions that are likely to be encountered in such patients can be avoided.

The majority of patients are candidates for the extraperitoneal approach. In our view, the only contraindication to this route is in a patient who has had the extraperitoneal space created during a previous procedure such as in mesh herniorraphy, especially where bilateral meshes are placed. This renders the space obliterated and re-creation of the space inevitably leads to multiple peritoneotomies.

While it is true that the transperitoneal approach is felt to be easier by most surgeons, overall the extraperitoneal approach is less invasive. Ultimately, the choice of approach depends upon patient factors and surgeon training. Training in carrying out the extraperitoneal route to performing a robot assisted radical prostatectomy adds to the surgical armamentarium of any surgeon carrying out this procedure.

Key Points

- Proper patient positioning is critical as it facilitates the procedure while avoiding potential position-related injuries.
- The main difference between the two approaches is the access i.e., creating the pneumoperitoneum and the trocar placement. Except for minor modification, all the subsequent steps are similar.
- Robotic-assisted procedures call for particular consideration in trocar placement in order to avoid robotic arms collision. A distance of 10 mms cms between all robotic working arm trocars is important.
- One of the advantages of the extraperitoneal approach is evident at the beginning of the intraoperative procedure as the "bladder take down" step is eliminated.
- Following the correct plane during bladder neck dissection is paramount.
- Anterior suspension of the posterior reconstruction stitch may help in earlier return of urinary continence
- Two separate sutures are used for vesicourethral anastomosis to avoid relying on a single knot.
- One contraindication to this route is a patient who has had the extraperitoneal space created during a previous procedure such as in mesh herniorraphy, especially where bilateral meshes have been placed. This renders the space obliterated and re-creation of the space inevitably leads to multiple peritoneotomies.
- The advantages of the extraperitoneal route include the need for less steep Trendelenburg positioning (which is useful in a patient with poor pulmonary reserve) thereby lessening the risk of position-related neuropraxia, avoidance of intraperitoneal adhesions making this the route of choice for patients with prior extensive and/or multiple bowel surgeries as the risk of injury to the intra-abdominal organs during adhesionolysis is avoided, rapid access to the target organ, peritoneum acting as a natural barrier obviating the need for bowel retraction from the operative surgical field, less pain, and a lesser incidence of paralytic ileus as bowel handling is avoided and hence relatively faster recovery.
- Fewer surgeons use the extraperitoneal approach to performing a robot assisted radical prostatectomy compared to the transperitoneal approach. However, there are certain benefits associated with the extraperitoneal approach. Training in carrying out the extraperitoneal route to performing a robot assisted radical prostatectomy adds to the surgical armamentarium of any surgeon carrying out this procedure.

References

1. Bill-Axelson A, Holmberg L, Garmo H, Rider JR, Taari K, Busch C, Nordling S, Häggman M, Andersson SO, Spångberg A, Andrén O, Palmgren J, Steineck G, Adami HO, Johansson JE. Radical prostatectomy or watchful waiting in early prostate cancer. N Engl J Med. 2014;370(10):932–42.
2. Mirheydar HS, Parsons JK. Diffusion of robotics into clinical practice in the United States: process, patient safety, learning curves, and the public health. World J Urol. 2013;31(3):455–61.

3. Yuh BE, Hussain A, Chandrasekhar R, Bienko M, Piacente P, Wilding G, Menon M, Peabody J, Guru KA. Comparative analysis of global practice patterns in urologic robot-assisted surgery. J Endourol. 2010;24(10):1637–44.
4. Hajdinjak T, Oakley NE. Use of optical dilating trocar for initial access during extraperitoneal laparoscopic radical prostatectomy. J Endourol. 2007;21(9):1089–92.
5. Jacobs BL, Montgomery JS, Dunn RL, Weizer AZ, Miller DC, Wood DP, Wolf Jr JS, Zhang Y, Wei JT, Hollenbeck BKA. Comparison of extraperitoneal and intraperitoneal approaches for robotic prostatectomy. Surg Innov. 2012;19(3):268–74.
6. Gettman MT, Hoznek A, Salomon L, Katz R, Borkowski T, Antiphon P, Lobontiu A, Abbou CC. Laparoscopic radical prostatectomy: description of the extraperitoneal approach using the da Vinci robotic system. J Urol. 2003;170(2 Pt 1):416–9.
7. Joseph JV, Rosenbaum R, Madeb R, et al. Robotic extraperitoneal radical prostatectomy: an alternative approach. J Urol. 2006;175:945–51.
8. Chung JS, Kim WT, Ham WS, et al. Comparison of oncological results, functional outcomes, and complications for transperitoneal versus extraperitoneal robot-assisted radical prostatectomy: a single surgeon's experience. J Endourol. 2011;25(5):787–92.
9. Horstmann M, Vollmer C, Schwab C, Kurz M, Padevit C, Horton K, John H. Single-centre evaluation of the extraperitoneal and transperitoneal approach in robotic-assisted radical prostatectomy. Scand J Urol Nephrol. 2012;46(2):117–23.
10. Ploussard G, Salomon L, Parier B, Abbou CC, de la Taille A. Extraperitoneal robot-assisted laparoscopic radical prostatectomy: a single-center experience beyond the learning curve. World J Urol. 2013;31(3):447–53.
11. Joo Yong L, Jong Chan K, Kyu Hyun K, Richilda Red D, Kwang Hyun K, Hye Young L, Jae Seung C, Kang Su C, Won Sik H, Young Deuk C. Comparison of perioperative outcomes and complications of transperitoneal versus extraperitoneal robot-assisted radical prostatectomy: a meta-analysis. J Urol. 2013;189(4):e352.
12. Boczko J, Madeb R, Golijanin D, Erturk E, Mathe M, Patel HR, Joseph JV. Robot-assisted radical prostatectomy in obese patients. Can J Urol. 2006;13(4):3169–73.
13. Boczko J, Joseph JV. Robot-assisted extraperitoneal radical prostatectomy in a patient with a pelvic kidney. Urology. 2006;68(5):1122.e3–4.
14. Ghazi A, Erturk E, Joseph JV. Modifications to facilitate extraperitoneal robot-assisted radical prostatectomy post kidney transplant. JSLS. 2012;16(2):314–9.

Diagnostic and Endoscopic Management of Bladder Tumors

14

Eleanor R. Ray and Anup Patel

14.1 Introduction

Bladder cancer management is underpinned by endoscopic diagnosis and therapy by transurethral resection (TURBT), particularly for non-muscle invasive bladder cancer (NMIBC).

The first working Nitze/Leiter cystoscope, appeared in 1878. The Stern-McCarthy resectoscope, which closely resembles today's instruments, had evolved by the late 1920s. The Harold Hopkins rod lens system and Karl Storz fiber optics of the 1950s–1960s respectively, followed by video-endoscopy, truly revolutionized endourology. Digital and high definition images have now made bladder tumor endo-visualization outstanding.

Despite remarkable urothelial images, accurate diagnosis of bladder cancer, particularly the detection of primary carcinoma-in-situ (CIS), is difficult, as flat tumors often devoid of surface urothelium can be hard to characterize. Residual tumors are common after standard TURBT in 27–65 % of patients undergoing routine second resection [1, 2]. In a much cited meta-analysis of 2,410 patients in 63 centers, after TURBT of multifocal tumors, the 3 months 'recurrence' rate ranged from 7.4 to 45.8 %. This significant variability was attributed to surgeon skill and the technique used [3] and relate to quality assurance in Urology.

Over the last 20 years, endourology for bladder cancer has seen rapid advancements. Much of the new technology and concepts are still exciting work in progress. In this chapter we evaluate the current position with options for different energy sources and techniques, which seek to improve upon the traditional TURBT operation, and review adjuncts which could improve tumor detection, possibly allowing better future characterization of benign and malignant urothelial lesions in situ.

14.2 Diagnosis and Initial Tumor Management

Painless visible hematuria is the classic presenting feature of bladder cancer. A high index of suspicion should be maintained for patients with asymptomatic non-visible hematuria, unexplained storage lower urinary tract symptoms, or painful bladder syndromes [4, 5].

Imaging

Most patients are diagnosed with bladder cancer at flexible cystoscopy, but the majority will also

E.R. Ray, MBBCh, BSc, MS, FRCS(Urol)
Department of Urology, University College Hospital London, London, UK

A. Patel, BSc(Hons), MBBS, MS, FRCS(Urol) (✉)
Department of Urology, Royal London Hospital at Barts Health NHS Trust, London, UK
e-mail: AnupPatel666@gmail.com

H.R.H. Patel et al. (eds.), *Pelvic Cancer Surgery: Modern Breakthroughs and Future Advances*,
DOI 10.1007/978-1-4471-4258-4_14, © Springer-Verlag London 2015

have had some initial investigative imaging. Virtual cystoscopy has recently explored the potential for a "scan" to replace invasive endoscopy. The first reported CTVC was in 1996 by Vining [6]. In a small study of 25 patients with bladder cancer undergoing CTVC, all 38 lesions detected were cystoscopically confirmed, 17 were <1 cm (including one measuring 2×3 mm), 7 were sessile, 5 were wall thickenings, and 35/38 (88 %) were confirmed malignant [7]. In other studies sensitivity for bladder cancer ranged 94–100 %, specificity 40–71 %, with 97 % PPV and 55 % NPV [8–10]. Since then, technical refinements such as air insufflation of the bladder with a urethral catheter, supine and prone scanning, 3-dimensional reconstruction, and analysis by software with interactive intraluminal navigation and a surface-rendering algorithm, have increased the sensitivity for bladder lesions. A meta-analysis including 3,084 patients comparing CT, MRI, and US virtual cystoscopy, found that CT virtual cystoscopy (CTVC) proved to be superior. At 95 % CI, sensitivity and specificity respectively for bladder tumor were: CT 93.9 and 98 %; MRI 90.8 and 94.5 %; and US 77.9 and 96.2 % [11].

CTVC has the advantages of being able to serially investigate patients with ongoing hematuria, those where bladder access is difficult, and those with inaccessible bladder diverticula. However, it cannot detect CIS, has not yet been assessed or validated in randomized trials, and involves a considerable ionizing radiation dose. Although it may be combined with a CT urogram for the primary investigation of hematuria, radiation based imaging will never replace a simple flexible cystoscopy for bladder cancer endosurveillance over many years. Therefore, the best virtual cystoscopy cannot yet replace cystoscopy.

Urine Cytology and Other Urine Markers

The standard and still most widely used noninvasive test for bladder cancer is voided urine cytology. A fresh cytological evaluation has a sensitivity and specificity of >90 % to detect high grade urothelial cancer, and is useful to detect CIS [12, 13]. Correct urine cytology analysis requires significant operator expertise, is costly, and has poor sensitivity for low-grade urothelial cancer.

Other urine based tests exploiting molecular markers—either laboratory analysis (e.g. UroVysion, Microsatellite analysis, gene microarray, ImmunoCyt, BTA TRAK), or point-of-care tests (NMP22, BTA Stat), have been developed in an attempt to improve upon cytology. In a systematic review of 71 studies reporting the performance of biomarkers and cytology in detecting bladder cancer, with 95 % CI, overall sensitivity was highest for ImmunoCyt, an immunocytological test which measures two antigens found in the urine of patients with bladder cancer [84 % (77–91 %)] and lowest for cytology [44 % (38–51 %)], whereas specificity was highest for cytology [96 % (94–98 %)] and lowest for ImmunoCyt [75 % (68–83 %)] [14]. Fluorescence in-situ-hybridization (FISH) had the highest median sensitivity (95 %) for detecting high-risk bladder cancer, and both FISH and ImmunoCyt had median sensitivities of 100 % for CIS.

NMP22 BladderChek is the most widely used point-of-care test with a higher sensitivity overall for bladder cancer than urine cytology. In a meta-analysis of five studies involving 2,426 participants, the median sensitivity for bladder cancer was 65 % (50–85 %) [14]. However, the low specificity 81 % (40–87 %) limits its routine clinical use.

Current evidence suggests that no urine biomarker can replace urine cytology for the detection of high grade bladder cancer, and no urine test, alone or in combination, can yet replace cystoscopy which is still standard of care for the diagnosis and surveillance up of bladder cancer.

Cystoscopy and TURBT

The cornerstone of bladder cancer management is the initial cystoscopy, bladder mapping, TURBT, and examination under anesthesia. The aims of the operation are to obtain tissue for a histological diagnosis and accurate cancer staging

Table 14.1 American Joint Committee on Cancer TNM staging for bladder cancer, IUCC 2002 [86]

Primary tumor (T)
Tx: Primary tumor cannot be assessed
T0: No evidence of primary tumor
Ta: Noninvasive papillary carcinoma
Tis: Carcinoma in situ (i.e., flat tumor)
T1: Tumor invades subepithelial connective tissue (lamina propria)
T2: Tumor invades muscle
pT2a: Tumor invades superficial muscle (inner half)
pT2b: Tumor invades deep muscle (outer half)
T3: Tumor invades perivesical tissue
pT3a: Microscopically
pT3b: Macroscopically (extravesical mass)
T4: Tumor invades any of the following: prostate, uterus, vagina, pelvic wall, or abdominal wall
T4a: Tumor invades the prostate, uterus, vagina
T4b: Tumor invades the pelvic wall, abdominal wall
Regional lymph nodes (N)
Nx: Regional lymph nodes cannot be assessed
N0: No regional lymph node metastasis
N1: Metastasis in a single lymph node, =2 cm in greatest dimension
N2: Metastasis in a single lymph node, >2 cm but =5 cm in greatest dimension; or multiple lymph nodes, =5 cm in greatest dimension
N3: Metastasis in a lymph node, >5 cm in greatest dimension
Distant metastasis (M)
Mx: Distant metastasis cannot be assessed
M0: No distant metastasis
M1: Distant metastasis

Table 14.2 1973 WHO histological tumor grading [87]

Urothelial papilloma
Grade 1 (G1)—well differentiated
Increase in number of urothelial cell layers, some loss of normal cellular orientation. No invasion
Grade 2 (G2)–moderately differentiated
Increased mitotic activity and loss of cellular polarity
Nuclei more abnormal and show variable staining
Grade 3 (G3)—poorly differentiated
Cells very poorly differentiated with loss of cellular cohesion. Invasion often seen

Table 14.3 The 2004 WHO/ISUP consensus classification [88]

Normal
Normal—may include cases formerly "mild dysplasia"
Hyperplasia
Flat
Papillary
Flat lesions with atypia
Reactive (inflammatory)
Atypia of unknown significance
Dysplasia (low grade intraurothelial neoplasia)
Carcinoma in situ (high grade intraurothelial neoplasia)
Papillary neoplasms
Papilloma
Inverted papilloma
Papillary neoplasm of low malignant potential (PUNLMP)
Papillary carcinoma, low grade
Papillary carcinoma, high grade
Invasive neoplasms
Lamina propria invasion
Muscularis propria (detrusor) invasion

(Tables 14.1, 14.2, and 14.3). It is critical to differentiate NMIBC from muscle invasive bladder cancer (MIBC), and it is essential to adequately sample the muscularis propria. At second resection when there is no muscle in the original specimen, 49 % of patients were upstaged compared with 14 % when muscle was present [2, 15]. A diagnosis of concomitant CIS should be sought, as its presence can significantly change prognosis and management. The EAU guidelines recommend separate resection of the tumor base and resection margins to achieve these endpoints [16].

Accurate histological diagnosis and staging ensures appropriate treatment, and in NMIBC, complete tumor clearance reduces 'recurrence' and improves the effectiveness of adjuvant intravesical therapies [17]. A 'radical' TURBT is not recommended as monotherapy for MIBC, but 'maximal' TURBT forms part of contemporary multimodal bladder preservation therapy for MIBC. A complete TURBT has been demonstrated to increase the rate of complete response to chemoradiotherapy (from 63 to 74 %) and reduce the need for salvage radical cystectomy (from 50 to 29 %) [18, 19].

The overall incidence of TURBT complications was 5.1 % of 2,821 patients in one study

[20], but rises with increasing tumor size and multifocality. Bladder perforation is one of the most devastating complications. Open surgery for bladder perforation was required in 15 of 4,144 (0.36 %) patients in one retrospective cohort series, two of whom died of the iatrogenic injury [21]. Although carrying out traditional monopolar (MP) TURBT under full muscle paralysis, not overfilling the bladder, and use of short bursts of diathermy, can reduce the incidence of obturator nerve stimulation which can lead to bladder perforation, this can be avoided by the use of alternative energy sources.

14.3 Evolving TURBT

Bipolar TURBT (BP-TURBT)

Monopolar (MP-) TURBT has been the gold standard operation for bladder cancer. BP-TURBT is inherently safer, by reducing the chance of obturator nerve stimulation and by better hemostasis. Using a similar resectoscope and loop, plasmakinetic BP-TURBT uses transferable skills giving a short learning curve.

MP-TURBT and BP-TURBT have been compared in randomized [22–24] and non-randomized studies [25]. Those receiving BP-TURBT had no/lower risk of bladder perforation and a day shorter catheterization and hospitalization times. One group found that bladder perforation with BP-TURBT, was more likely with higher power, and abolished it by reducing the energy setting from 160 W cut /80 W coagulation to 50/40 W [26]. BP-TURBT may have advantages beyond less morbidity. In one randomized study less residual tumor was found in the bipolar group (9.3 % vs. 20.8 %) [24]. One could speculate that improved hemostasis and less char allows better tumor visibility, allowing more thorough resection. No difference in the quality of bladder tumor chips submitted for histological evaluation was found when MP-TURBT and BP-TURBT specimens were compared blindly [27].

Bipolar plasmavaporization of bladder tumors with the button 'mushroom' electrode instead of a resecting loop, is an ablative technique which may be useful for managing the bulk of large volume tumors or small recurrences [24, 28]. Biopsies of the tumor and tumor base are required as no tissue specimen is obtained using this technique.

The En-bloc Resection

Another possible recurrence mechanism is that traditional piecemeal TURBT may scatter tumor cells into the bladder lumen from where they could implant into the freshly cut and other urothelial surfaces [29]. Adjuvant single shot chemotherapy, as recommended for all patients by the EAU guidelines [16], was conceptualized to prevent cell implantation, thus overcoming this TURBT shortcoming [30]. En-bloc bladder tumor resection with a margin of normal tissue refines the surgical technique itself, for a more oncologically sound operation and may reduce NMIBC recurrence while providing a better a surgical specimen [31].

The EAU guidelines recommend that tumors <1 cm should be resected en-bloc [16]. A literature review reveals diverse techniques of en-bloc resection, but also that larger tumors can safely be managed thus.

En-bloc resection was described in 1997 using a bespoke arched resection electrode [32]. Other groups have used a knife electrode, a J-shaped needle, or more recently, the Holmium laser [33–36]. One group carried out en-bloc resection of tumors measuring 0.5–4.5 cm using the Collins knife in 41/46 (89 %) consecutive patients. The five tumors that could not be resected en-bloc were at the bladder neck [37]. Another group reported en-bloc polypectomy using a 7Fr monopolar lasso-like snare electrode passed through a cystoscope for tumors <5 cm. A margin of en-bloc normal bladder wall cannot be excised with the tumor by this method, and some tumors required bisection in order to be removed, but it was suggested that the majority of specimens could be withdrawn with the cystoscope or within a mesh net, reducing tumor cell scatter [38]. Fritsche combined a water jet dissector and needle knife (HybridKnife). The water jet at 30 atm elevated the tumor on the superficial layer of the muscularis propria on a bleb of saline thus facilitating en-bloc resection. The users found it easy to learn, with no additional morbidity [39].

Perhaps the most interesting technique is bladder tumor excision using an end firing laser fiber. It is a precise surgical tool, which negates obturator nerve stimulation risk. Both Holmium and Thulium lasers have been used for bladder cancer. Several small studies found Holmium laser bladder tumor resection (HoLBRT) to be technically safe and histologically uncompromised [33, 40–42]. A large non-randomized comparison of 101 HoLBRT and 111 MP-TURBT in primary tumors found operative time to be longer, but fewer complications, and shorter catheterization and hospitalization by 1 day, in the HoLBRT group [43]. En-bloc resection was possible in 84.9 % of 152 tumors, except for anterior wall tumors. Although the study was not designed to detect a difference in recurrence rates, after mean follow up of 34 months, during which all patients received adjuvant intravesical chemotherapy, no difference in recurrence was seen.

In a small six patient study, all histological specimens obtained after Thulium laser bladder tumor resection included deep muscle layer sampling, and there was no residual tumor at re-resection 6 weeks later [44].

Lasers are probably the best surgical tools for en-bloc bladder tumor resection. The current literature describes HoLBRT as a safe technique but efficacy evaluation in large prospective randomized trials is lacking.

14.4 Adjuncts to TURBT: Improving Tumor Detection

Significant evidence exists to prove that after an apparently visually complete resection, residual tumor frequently remains. A second, or re-resection, for patients with high-risk bladder cancer manages some of this residual disease, and in patients with low-risk disease, residual cancer may be detected as 'recurrence' at the first 3 month check cystoscopy. The more contemporary approach however, is to try to improve the first operation.

Photodynamic Diagnosis (PDD)

In the 1970s Kelly and Snell used PDD successfully to detect bladder tumors in cystectomy specimens using intravenous hematoporphyrin derivative and ultraviolet (UV) wavelength 390–420 nm light [45]. This technique utilized the heme biosynthetic pathway (Fig. 14.1). Kriegmair and colleagues, carried out a series of groundbreaking clinical studies using an intravesical photosensitizer 5-aminolevulinic acid (5ALA) in the 1990s [46–49]. This was the beginning of the modern era of clinically feasible PDD for bladder cancer.

The third generation, regulatory approved, photosensitizer is hexylaminolevulinate (HAL). HAL causes tumors to fluorescence red contrasting against blue normal urothelium (Fig. 14.2).

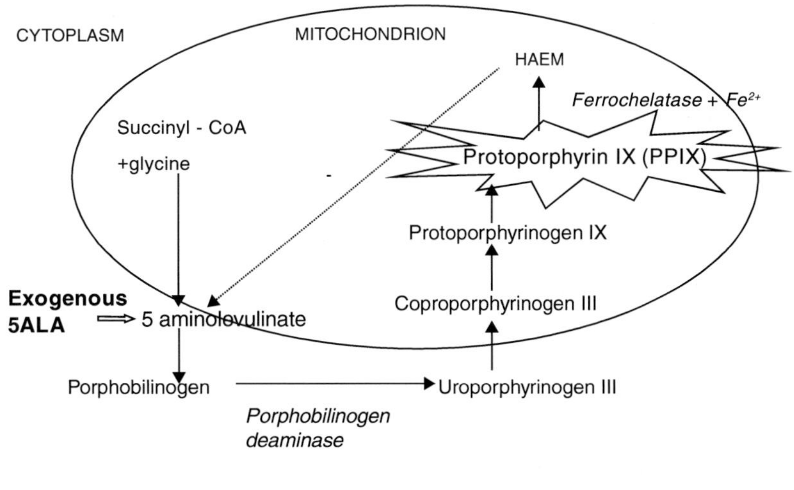

Fig. 14.1 Heme biosynthetic pathway. When the negative feedback mechanism of heme on 5ALA is overcome by exogenous 5ALA the fluorescent molecule protoporphyrin IX (PPIX) accumulates selectively in tumor cells

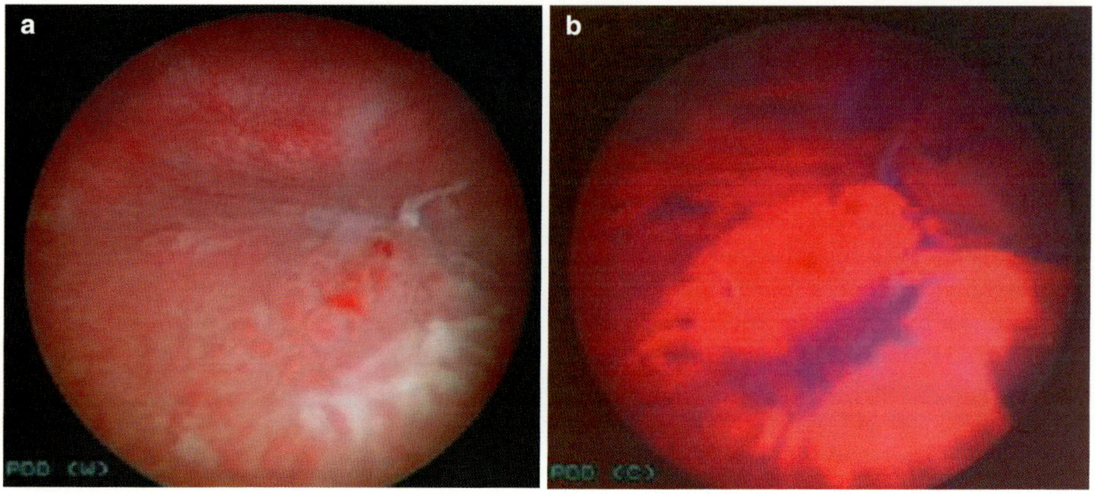

Fig. 14.2 Photodynamic diagnosis with hexylaminolevulinate. (**a**) *White* light cystoscopy, (**b**) PDD assisted cystoscopy gives a clearer indication of the extent of the tumor: histology low grade G2pTa + carcinoma in situ

In addition to a safe, effective photosensitizer administered intravesically, PDD also requires a UV light source, narrow fluid light cables, a cystoscope modified with filters, and a CCD camera which allows the switch between white and blue light.

A systematic review of the literature including 27 studies and 2,949 patients confirmed that PDD using either 5ALA or HAL had higher sensitivity for tumor than white light cystoscopy (WLC) (92 % vs. 71 %), but lower specificity (57 % vs. 72 %) at both patient and biopsy levels [14]. This difference was most pronounced for high-risk tumors where at the biopsy level, median sensitivity was 99 % vs. 67 %. Most importantly, improved tumor detection translated into reduced residual tumor and recurrence at 2 years. PDD assisted MP-TURBT resulted in statistically significantly fewer residual tumors [RR 0.37 (95 % CI, 0.20–0.69)]; and a small but statistically significant improvement in recurrence free survival (RFS) [RR 1.37 (95 % CI, 1.18–1.59)].

An unpublished meta-analysis of eight HAL-PDD studies including 2,231 patients found similar results. HAL-PDD detected 13.2 % more pTa tumors, 39.8 % more CIS lesions, and 24.6 % more CIS patients. Patients with new bladder cancer and recurrence benefitted. Recurrence at 12 months was lower in the PDD group at 34.5 % compared with 45.4 % in the WLC group [50]. Denzinger reported 80 % RFS at 8 years after PDD for patients with T1 high grade NMIBC compared with 52 % after WLC [51] suggesting a durable effect on recurrence. For progression, although PDD assisted TURBT slightly favored WLC, patient numbers were small, confidence intervals were wide, and the differences were not statistically significant [14, 52, 53].

Despite these convincing meta-analyses, recent studies have challenged the efficacy of PDD. Schumacher found high recurrence rates with no statistically significant difference at 1 year after WLC or 5ALA-PDD (53.1 % vs 50.4 %) [53].

Additionally, two trials using HAL and a routine single dose of intravesical chemotherapy for all patients found conflicting outcomes. A UK randomized trial of patients newly presenting with bladder cancer failed to show a statistically significant difference in 1 year recurrence after WLC or HAL-PDD (20 % vs. 15 %) [54]. However, in the trial by Karaolides, large differences in recurrence were seen at 18 months after WLC and HAL-PDD (49.4 % vs. 17.5 %) [55].

The improved detection of CIS is one of the undisputed attributes of PDD. Sensitivity ranges 92–97 % for HAL-PDD compared with 58–68 % for WLC [52, 56–58]. PDD should be considered for all patients with high grade cancer cells in the urine and an apparent absence of visible tumor in the bladder at WLC.

PDD undoubtedly improves tumor detection at the level of the urothelium: at the resection margin, satellite lesions, multifocal tumor, and CIS. What is still not categorically clear is whether PDD-assisted resection results in reduced long term recurrence. The results of good quality randomized trials, with and without adjunctive routine instillation chemotherapy and early re-resection, have demonstrated conflicting evidence. Although easy to learn, PDD requires a significant economical investment, while its clinical effectiveness is still to be completely realized.

Narrow Band Imaging

Digital imaging allows the incorporation of other technologies such as Narrow Band Imaging (NBI). White light is filtered to produce 415 nm blue and 540 nm green wavelengths which are absorbed by hemoglobin. On the NBI image blood vessels, which are more numerous in tumors, appear black, increasing the contrast between tumor and normal urothelium (Fig. 14.3). Bryan et al. first published results on the use of NBI in flexible cystoscopic assessment of recurrent NMIBC in 2008 and found it to be a technique which was easily adopted by new users [59, 60]. NBI, like PDD, can assist endoscopic tumor detection by achieving adequate resection margins.

A systematic review and meta-analysis of NBI assisted WLC in 1,040 patients demonstrated that NBI detected an additional 17 % bladder cancer patients with an additional 24 % tumor detection [61, 62], and an additional 28 % CIS

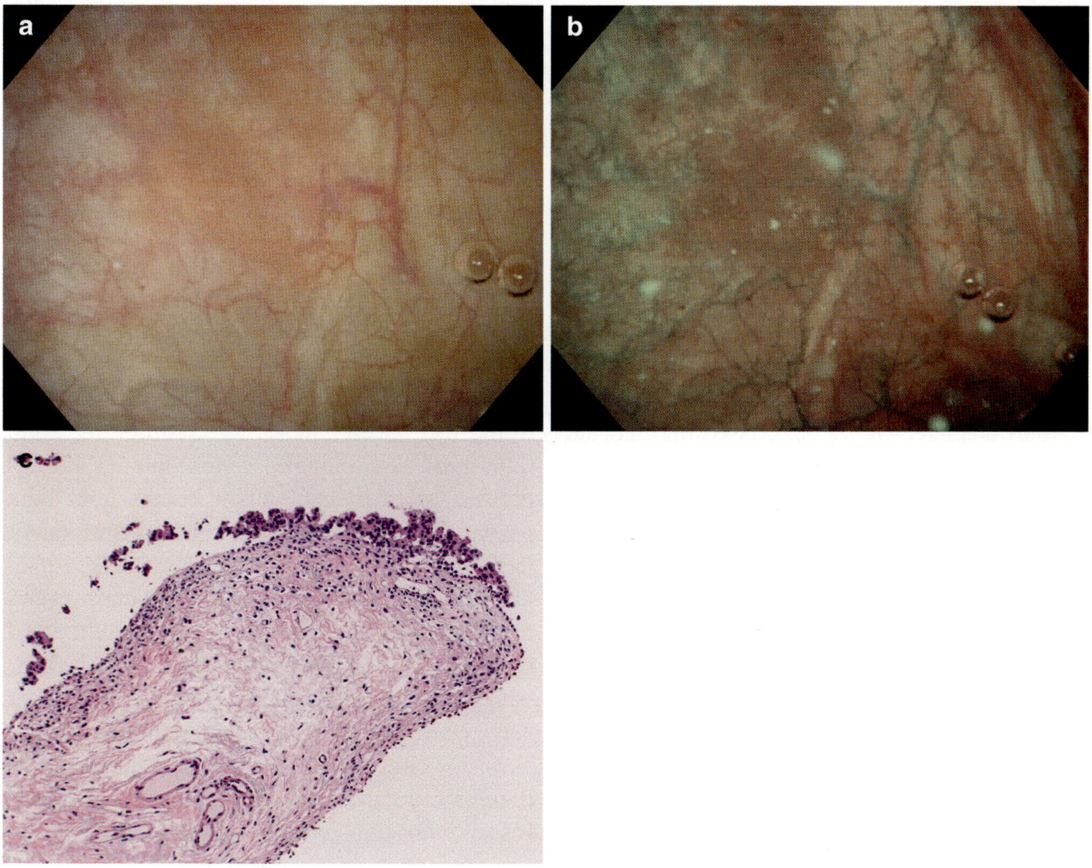

Fig. 14.3 Narrow Band Imaging (NBI) of area of bladder Carcinoma in situ (**a**) White light Cystoscopy, (**b**) NBI, (**c**) histology of targeted biopsy (Courtesy of Prof. Seiji Naito, Dept. Urology, Kyushu University, Fukuoka, Japan)

detection. Two prospective randomized studies have assessed the effect of NBI on bladder tumor recurrence [23, 63]. Geavlete found that residual tumor was significantly lower in the groups assessed with NBI (6.3 % vs. 17.5 %), which translated into significantly lower recurrence at 1 year (7.9 % vs. 17.8 %) [23]. Naselli found that after NBI, recurrence was significantly lower than in the WLC group at 3 months (3.9 % vs. 16.7 %) and at 1 year (32.9 % vs. 51.4 %) [63]. NBI was also found useful for the assessment patients with positive urine cytology for cancer, but no visible WLC disease (5/12 [42 %] had bladder cancer detected by NBI) [64].

These results are comparable to PDD, but NBI is potentially more cost-efficient as it requires only cystoscopes with NBI capability, in contrast to PDD, which involves preparation, time, and consumables.

14.5 Adjuncts to TURBT: Real Time Assessment of Bladder Lesions

Optical Coherence Tomography (OCT)

The use of OCT (Niris System: Imalux) was first reported in the human bladder in 1997 [65]. It uses near infrared light interferometry to visualize tissue microstructure in cross section. A 2.7 mm diameter OCT fiber passed through the cystoscope allows visualization of a small field of view with 2–3 mm penetration depth down to the muscularis propria. OCT offers the possibility of real time bladder lesion assessment detected by WLC, PDD, or NBI. In one small study, it was possible to differentiate between normal bladder, chronic inflammation, squamous metaplasia, severe dysplasia, and urothelial carcinoma [66]. It may also be valuable in the assessment of the extent of tumor depth, complimenting PDD and NBI, which assess the tumor lateral extent, for more complete resection.

In studies comparing OCT and histopathology, the sensitivity for cancer was 100 %; for detection of invasion of the lamina propria 90–100 %; and for detection of muscle invasive cancer 100 %, with a specificity of only 65–89 % [67–70].

Schmidbauer found that by combining PDD and OCT the specificity of PDD alone was increased from 78.6 to 97.9 % [71]. High magnification cystoscopy is a newer technique of NBI which can be used to look for neoangiogenesis and vascular patterns characteristic of a neoplasm, on suspect lesions [72]. OCT is not in common clinical use yet.

Raman Spectroscopy

This is a technique in which the Raman effect of light is used to assess the molecular composition of a bladder lesion. Like OCT it also has the potential for real-time assessment of bladder lesions. However, although it has shown some success in the assessment of cancer cell grade in urine [73], and the differentiation of cancerous from benign bladder biopsies with 84 % accuracy [74], only ex-vivo studies exist. In vivo endoscopic use has been unsuccessful due to poor specificity, but newly developed confocal Raman probes show some promise ex-vivo [75].

Confocal Laser Endomicroscopy

This new endoscopic technique has been adapted from the gastroenterology setting to rigid (2.6 mm) and flexible cystoscopic (1.4 mm) probes, which transmit a low energy laser light source to a urothelium after administration of intravenous or intravesical fluorescein (as urothelium lacks autofluorescence). The larger probes give a real time microscopic cellular architectural view akin to high power light microscopy (LM) with a 60–100 μm depth and a 240 μm field of view, while the smaller probes are more akin to a "low-power LM view" with 600 μm field of view. Presently, it can be used to evaluate urothelium, vessels, muscle and fat, but cannot evaluate nuclear detail or be combined with HAL, is subjective, requires a 15–20 min evaluation time, and lacks multicenter studies [76].

Bladder Surveillance

Flexible cystoscopic surveillance has largely replaced rigid cystoscopy. New diagnostic techniques and concepts are also influencing surveillance and management of recurrence.

PDD and NBI

PDD is feasible via flexible cystoscopy, but the expense, preparation and need to repeat PDD at the time of general anesthetic have prevented its widespread adoption in routine surveillance programs [77–79]. Conversely, NBI does not require any special preparation and therefore is ideally suited to the outpatient setting. Herr demonstrated that by introducing regular NBI into the surveillance program for a 3 year period, the median recurrence free interval could be extended in patients with a recent history of tumor recurrence from 13 to 29 months [80].

Holmium Laser Tumor Ablation

Holmium laser fulguration at 10 W via the same flexible cystoscope is ideally suited for small low-risk tumors in high anesthetic risk patients. Flexible cystoscopy PDD may be attractive if Holmium laser ablation were immediately available when tumor was detected [81]. Soler-Martinez reported on the feasibility of laser tumor ablation, although patients had intravenous sedation in addition to topical urethral 2 % lidocaine [82]. All but one patient preferred it to TURBT, and visual analog pain scales were low. Jönler found that Holmium laser ablation of recurrent tumors was feasible and acceptable by patients under local anesthetic alone [83].

Active Surveillance

Active surveillance is the cystoscopic surveillance of a bladder cancer without intervention. Such an approach may be attractive for patients with recurrent low risk cancer and significant comorbidity. In a prospective cohort matched study of 64 patients with low risk tumors, 6.5 % progressed in stage (none to MIBC), and 17.2 % progressed in grade [84] over a median surveillance period of 10.3 months. Such an approach is not advocated in any guidelines, as more safety determinations are required.

Surveillance After Bladder Preservation Therapy for MIBC

Evidence of tumor at first check cystoscopy after bladder preservation treatment indicates need for salvage cystectomy for fit patients. However, the best surveillance schedule for patients having a complete response to radical chemoradiotherapy is not clear. Recommendations from a recent systematic review advocated a general anesthetic check cystoscopy at 3 months and at 15–36 months, when recurrence was most likely. Otherwise flexible cystoscopy surveillance should continue for at least 10 years [85].

Key Points

- Cystoscopy and TURBT are at the foundation of bladder cancer diagnosis and management of NMIBC
- Virtual cystoscopy cannot yet replace diagnostic or surveillance cystoscopy
- No urine based molecular marker can replace cystoscopy or voided urine cytology
- The gold standard monopolar TURBT is flawed
- Bipolar TURBT is safer and is easy to adopt
- En-bloc laser tumor resection is safer and has the potential to reduce tumor recurrence
- PDD and NBI both improve tumor detection and may improve long term tumor recurrence
- PDD or NBI is recommended to investigate patients with malignant urine cytology, with no endoscopic white light evidence of disease

- Techniques like OCT, Raman spectroscopy, and confocal laser endomicroscopy, may in the future allow in vivo assessment of abnormal urothelial lesions
- Novel surveillance strategies for NMIBC including NBI and PDD assisted flexible cystoscopy, local anesthetic laser ablation, and active surveillance are intriguing developments

References

1. Schips L, Augustin H, Zigeuner R, Trummer H, Pummer K, Hubmer G. Is second transurethral resection justified in patients with newly diagnosed superficial bladder cancer? Eur Urol. 2000;37(Suppl.2):111.
2. Schwaibold HE, Sivalingam S, May F, Hartung R. The value of a second transurethral resection for T1 bladder cancer. BJU Int. 2006;97(6):1199–201.
3. Brausi M, Collette L, Kurth K, van der Meijden AP, Oosterlinck W, Witjes JA, et al. Variability in the recurrence rate at first follow-up cystoscopy after TUR in stage Ta T1 transitional cell carcinoma of the bladder: a combined analysis of seven EORTC studies. Eur Urol. 2002;41(5):523–31.
4. Elias K, Svatek RS, Gupta S, Ho R, Lotan Y. High-risk patients with hematuria are not evaluated according to guideline recommendations. Cancer. 2010;116(12):2954–9.
5. Khadra MH, Pickard RS, Charlton M, Powell PH, Neal DE. A prospective analysis of 1,930 patients with hematuria to evaluate current diagnostic practice. J Urol. 2000;163(2):524–7.
6. Vining DJ, Zagoria RJ, Liu K, Stelts D. CT cystoscopy: an innovation in bladder imaging. AJR Am J Roentgenol. 1996;166(2):409–10.
7. Karabacak OR, Cakmakci E, Ozturk U, Demirel F, Dilli A, Hekimoglu B, et al. Virtual cystoscopy: the evaluation of bladder lesions with computed tomographic virtual cystoscopy. Can Urol Assoc J. 2011;5(1):34–7.
8. Singh I, Mehrotra G, Jaura MS, Agarwal V, Tandon A, Joshi M. Virtual cystoscopy (pneumo-cystoscopy)-its utility in the prospective evaluation of bladder tumor. Indian J Urol. 2012;28(2):164–8.
9. Amin MF, Abd El Hamid AM. The diagnostic accuracy of multidetector computed tomography with multiplanar reformatted imaging and virtual cystoscopy in the early detection and evaluation of bladder carcinoma: comparison with conventional cystoscopy. Abdom Imaging. 2013;38(1):184–92.
10. Kuehhas FE, Weibl P, Tosev G, Schatzl G, Heinz-Peer G. Multidetector computed tomography virtual cystoscopy: an effective diagnostic tool in patients with hematuria. Urology. 2012;79(2):270–6.
11. Qu X, Huang X, Wu L, Huang G, Ping X, Yan W. Comparison of virtual cystoscopy and ultrasonography for bladder cancer detection: a meta-analysis. Eur J Radiol. 2011;80(2):188–97.
12. Habuchi T, Marberger M, Droller MJ, Hemstreet III GP, Grossman HB, Schalken JA, et al. Prognostic markers for bladder cancer: international consensus panel on bladder tumor markers. Urology. 2005;66(6 Suppl 1):64–74.
13. Lokeshwar VB, Habuchi T, Grossman HB, Murphy WM, Hautmann SH, Hemstreet III GP, et al. Bladder tumor markers beyond cytology: international consensus panel on bladder tumor markers. Urology. 2005;66(6 Suppl 1):35–63.
14. Mowatt G, Zhu S, Kilonzo M, Boachie C, Fraser C, Griffiths TR, et al. Systematic review of the clinical effectiveness and cost-effectiveness of photodynamic diagnosis and urine biomarkers (FISH, ImmunoCyt, NMP22) and cytology for the detection and follow-up of bladder cancer. Health Technol Assess. 2010;14(4):1–331. iv.
15. Herr HW. The value of a second transurethral resection in evaluating patients with bladder tumors. J Urol. 1999;162(1):74–6.
16. Babjuk M, Oosterlinck W, Sylvester R, Kaasinen E, Bohle A, Palou-Redorta J, et al. EAU guidelines on non-muscle-invasive urothelial carcinoma of the bladder, the 2011 update. Eur Urol. 2011;59(6):997–1008.
17. Herr HW. Restaging transurethral resection of high risk superficial bladder cancer improves the initial response to bacillus Calmette-Guerin therapy. J Urol. 2005;174(6):2134–7.
18. Coen JJ, Zietman AL, Kaufman DS, et al. Trimodality therapy in the management of muscle-invasive bladder cancer: a selective organ-sparing approach. In: Lerner SP, Schoenberg MP, Sternberg CN, editors. Textbook of bladder cancer. Oxford: Taylor & Francis; 2006. p. 569–77.
19. Mak RH, Zietman AL, Heney NM, Kaufman DS, Shipley WU. Bladder preservation: optimizing radiotherapy and integrated treatment strategies. BJU Int. 2008;102(9 Pt B):1345–53.
20. Collado A, Chechile GE, Salvador J, Vicente J. Early complications of endoscopic treatment for superficial bladder tumors. J Urol. 2000;164(5):1529–32.
21. Golan S, Baniel J, Lask D, Livne PM, Yossepowitch O. Transurethral resection of bladder tumour complicated by perforation requiring open surgical repair—clinical characteristics and oncological outcomes. BJU Int. 2011;107(7):1065–8.
22. Del RA, Pace G, Masciovecchio S, Saldutto P, Galatioto GP, Vicentini C. Plasmakinetic bipolar versus monopolar transurethral resection of non-muscle invasive bladder cancer: A single center randomized controlled trial. Int J Urol. 2013;20(4):399–403.
23. Geavlete B, Multescu R, Georgescu D, Stanescu F, Jecu M, Geavlete P. Narrow band imaging cystoscopy and bipolar plasma vaporization for large nonmuscle-

invasive bladder tumors—results of a prospective, randomized comparison to the standard approach. Urology. 2012;79(4):846–51.

24. Geavlete B, Multescu R, Georgescu D, Jecu M, Dragutescu M, Geavlete P. Innovative technique in nonmuscle invasive bladder cancer-bipolar plasma vaporization. Urology. 2011;77(4):849–54.
25. Xishuang S, Deyong Y, Xiangyu C, Tao J, Quanlin L, Hongwei G, et al. Comparing the safety and efficiency of conventional monopolar, plasmakinetic, and holmium laser transurethral resection of primary non-muscle invasive bladder cancer. J Endourol. 2010;24(1):69–73.
26. Gupta NP, Saini AK, Dogra PN, Seth A, Kumar R. Bipolar energy for transurethral resection of bladder tumours at low-power settings: initial experience. BJU Int. 2011;108(4):553–6.
27. Wang DS, Bird VG, Leonard VY, Plumb SJ, Konety B, Williams RD, et al. Use of bipolar energy for transurethral resection of bladder tumors: pathologic considerations. J Endourol. 2004;18(6):578–82.
28. Canter DJ, Ogan K, Master VA. Initial North American experience with the use of the Olympus button electrode for vaporization of bladder tumors. Can J Urol. 2012;19(2):6211–6.
29. Albarran J, Imbert L. Les Tumeurs du Rein. Paris: Masson et Cie; 2006. p. 452–9.
30. Tolley DA, Parmar MK, Grigor KM, Lallemand G, Benyon LL, Fellows J, et al. The effect of intravesical mitomycin C on recurrence of newly diagnosed superficial bladder cancer: a further report with 7 years of follow up. J Urol. 1996;155(4):1233–8.
31. Ray ER, O'Brien TS. Should urologists be spending more time on the golf course? BJU Int. 2007;100(4):728–9.
32. Kawada T, Ebihara K, Suzuki T, Imai K, Yamanaka H. A new technique for transurethral resection of bladder tumors: rotational tumor resection using a new arched electrode. J Urol. 1997;157(6):2225–6.
33. Das A, Gilling P, Fraundorfer M. Holmium laser resection of bladder tumors (HoLRBT). Tech Urol. 1998;4(1):12–4.
34. Lodde M, Lusuardi L, Palermo S, Signorello D, Maier K, Hohenfellner R, et al. En bloc transurethral resection of bladder tumors: use and limits. Urology. 2003;62(6):1089–91.
35. Saito S. Transurethral en bloc resection of bladder tumors. J Urol. 2001;166(6):2148–50.
36. Ukai R, Kawashita E, Ikeda H. A new technique for transurethral resection of superficial bladder tumor in 1 piece. J Urol. 2000;163(3):878–9.
37. Naselli A, Introini C, Germinale F, Spina B, Puppo P. En bloc transurethral resection of bladder lesions: a trick to retrieve specimens up to 4.5 cm. BJU Int. 2012;109(6):960–3.
38. Maurice MJ, Vricella GJ, MacLennan G, Buehner P, Ponsky LE. Endoscopic snare resection of bladder tumors: evaluation of an alternative technique for bladder tumor resection. J Endourol. 2012;26(6):614–7.
39. Fritsche HM, Otto W, Eder F, Hofstadter F, Denzinger S, Chaussy CG, et al. Water-jet-aided transurethral dissection of urothelial carcinoma: a prospective clinical study. J Endourol. 2011;25(10):1599–603.
40. Hossain MZ, Khan SA, Salam MA, Hossain S, Islam R. Holmium YAG laser treatment of superficial bladder carcinoma. Mymensingh Med J. 2005; 14(1):13–5.
41. Muraro GB, Grifoni R, Spazzafumo L. Endoscopic therapy of superficial bladder cancer in high-risk patients: holmium laser versus transurethral resection. Surg Technol Int. 2005;14:222–6.
42. Zhong C, Guo S, Tang Y, Xia S. Clinical observation on 2 micron laser for non-muscle-invasive bladder tumor treatment: single-center experience. World J Urol. 2010;28(2):157–61.
43. Zhu Y, Jiang X, Zhang J, Chen W, Shi B, Xu Z. Safety and efficacy of holmium laser resection for primary nonmuscle-invasive bladder cancer versus transurethral electroresection: single-center experience. Urology. 2008;72(3):608–12.
44. Wolters M, Kramer MW, Becker JU, Christgen M, Nagele U, Imkamp F, et al. Tm:YAG laser en bloc mucosectomy for accurate staging of primary bladder cancer: early experience. World J Urol. 2011;29(4):429–32.
45. Kelly JF, Snell ME. Hematoporphyrin derivative: a possible aid in the diagnosis and therapy of carcinoma of the bladder. J Urol. 1976;115(2):150–1.
46. Kriegmair M, Baumgartner R, Hofstetter A: Intravesikale Instillation von Delta-Aminol~tvulins~mre (ALA)–Eine neue Methode zur photodynamischen Diagnostik und Therapie. Lasermedizin. 1992;8:83.
47. Kriegmair M, Baumgartner R, Knuechel R, Steinbach P, Ehsan A, Lumper W, et al. Fluorescence photodetection of neoplastic urothelial lesions following intravesical instillation of 5-aminolevulinic acid. Urology. 1994;44(6):836–41.
48. Kriegmair M, Baumgartner R, Knuchel R, Stepp H, Hofstadter F, Hofstetter A. Detection of early bladder cancer by 5-aminolevulinic acid induced porphyrin fluorescence. J Urol. 1996;155(1):105–9.
49. Kriegmair M, Zaak D, Stepp H, Stepp H, Baumgartner R, Knuechel R, et al. Transurethral resection and surveillance of bladder cancer supported by 5-aminolevulinic acid-induced fluorescence endoscopy. Eur Urol. 1999;36(5):386–92.
50. Burger M, Grossman HB, Droller MJ, Schmidbauer J, Hermann GG, Dragoescu O, et al. Photodynamic diagnosis of non-muscle invasive bladder cancer with hexaminolevulinate cystoscopy: a meta-analysis based on raw data. 1–11–2012. Ref Type: unpublished work.
51. Denzinger S, Burger M, Walter B, Knuechel R, Roessler W, Wieland WF, et al. Clinically relevant reduction in risk of recurrence of superficial bladder cancer using 5-aminolevulinic acid-induced fluorescence diagnosis: 8-year results of prospective randomized study. Urology. 2007;69(4):675–9.
52. Geavlete B, Multescu R, Georgescu D, Jecu M, Stanescu F, Geavlete P. Treatment changes and long-term recurrence rates after hexaminolevulinate

(HAL) fluorescence cystoscopy: does it really make a difference in patients with non-muscle-invasive bladder cancer (NMIBC)? BJU Int. 2012;109(4):549–56.
53. Schumacher MC, Holmang S, Davidsson T, Friedrich B, Pedersen J, Wiklund NP. Transurethral resection of non-muscle-invasive bladder transitional cell cancers with or without 5-aminolevulinic Acid under visible and fluorescent light: results of a prospective, randomised, multicentre study. Eur Urol. 2010;57(2):293–9.
54. Ray ER, Chatterton K, Wilby D, Khan MS, Thomas K, O'Brien TS. A prospective randomised trial of Hexylaminolevulinate (HAL) assisted transurethral resection (TURBT) plus single shot intravesical Mitomycin C (MMC) versus white light TURBT plus single shot MMC in newly presenting bladder cancer. BJU Int. 2011;108(S1):8. Ref Type: Abstract.
55. Karaolides T, Skolarikos A, Bourdoumis A, Konandreas A, Mygdalis V, Thanos A, et al. Hexaminolevulinate-induced fluorescence versus white light during transurethral resection of noninvasive bladder tumor: does it reduce recurrences? Urology. 2012;80(2):354–9.
56. Fradet Y, Grossman HB, Gomella L, Lerner S, Cookson M, Albala D, et al. A comparison of hexaminolevulinate fluorescence cystoscopy and white light cystoscopy for the detection of carcinoma in situ in patients with bladder cancer: a phase III, multicenter study. J Urol. 2007;178(1):68–73.
57. Jocham D, Witjes F, Wagner S, Zeylemaker B, van Moorselaar J, Grimm MO, et al. Improved detection and treatment of bladder cancer using hexaminolevulinate imaging: a prospective, phase III multicenter study. J Urol. 2005;174(3):862–6.
58. Schmidbauer J, Witjes F, Schmeller N, Donat R, Susani M, Marberger M. Improved detection of urothelial carcinoma in situ with hexaminolevulinate fluorescence cystoscopy. J Urol. 2004;171(1):135–8.
59. Bryan RT, Shah ZH, Collins SI, Wallace DM. Narrow-band imaging flexible cystoscopy: a new user's experience. J Endourol. 2010;24(8):1339–43.
60. Bryan RT, Billingham LJ, Wallace DM. Narrow-band imaging flexible cystoscopy in the detection of recurrent urothelial cancer of the bladder. BJU Int. 2008;101(6):702–5.
61. Li K, Lin T, Fan X, Duan Y, Huang J. Diagnosis of narrow-band imaging in non-muscle-invasive bladder cancer: a systematic review and meta-analysis. Int J Urol. 2013;20(6):602–9.
62. Zheng C, Lv Y, Zhong Q, Wang R, Jiang Q. Narrow band imaging diagnosis of bladder cancer: systematic review and meta-analysis. BJU Int. Dec 2012;110(11 Pt B):E680-7.
63. Naselli A, Introini C, Timossi L, Spina B, Fontana V, Pezzi R, et al. A randomized prospective trial to assess the impact of transurethral resection in narrow band imaging modality on non-muscle-invasive bladder cancer recurrence. Eur Urol. 2012;61(5):908–13.
64. Zhu YP, Shen YJ, Ye DW, Wang CF, Yao XD, Zhang SL, et al. Narrow-band imaging flexible cystoscopy in the detection of clinically unconfirmed positive urine cytology. Urol Int. 2012;88(1):84–7.
65. Sergeev A, Gelikonov V, Gelikonov G, Feldchtein F, Kuranov R, Gladkova N, et al. In vivo endoscopic OCT imaging of precancer and cancer states of human mucosa. Opt Express. 1997;1(13):432–40.
66. Zagaynova EV, Streltsova OS, Gladkova ND, Snopova LB, Gelikonov GV, Feldchtein FI, et al. In vivo optical coherence tomography feasibility for bladder disease. J Urol. 2002;167(3):1492–6.
67. Karl A, Stepp H, Willmann E, Buchner A, Hocaoglu Y, Stief C, et al. Optical coherence tomography for bladder cancer—ready as a surrogate for optical biopsy? Results of a prospective mono-centre study. Eur J Med Res. 2010;15(3):131–4.
68. Manyak MJ, Gladkova ND, Makari JH, Schwartz AM, Zagaynova EV, Zolfaghari L, et al. Evaluation of superficial bladder transitional-cell carcinoma by optical coherence tomography. J Endourol. 2005;19(5):570–4.
69. Goh AC, Tresser NJ, Shen SS, Lerner SP. Optical coherence tomography as an adjunct to white light cystoscopy for intravesical real-time imaging and staging of bladder cancer. Urology. 2008;72(1):133–7.
70. Ren H, Waltzer WC, Bhalla R, Liu J, Yuan Z, Lee CS, et al. Diagnosis of bladder cancer with microelectromechanical systems-based cystoscopic optical coherence tomography. Urology. 2009;74(6):1351–7.
71. Schmidbauer J, Remzi M, Klatte T, Waldert M, Mauermann J, Susani M, et al. Fluorescence cystoscopy with high-resolution optical coherence tomography imaging as an adjunct reduces false-positive findings in the diagnosis of urothelial carcinoma of the bladder. Eur Urol. 2009;56(6):914–9.
72. Jichlinski P, Lovisa B. High magnification cystoscopy in the primary diagnosis of bladder tumors. Curr Opin Urol. 2011;21(5):398–402.
73. Shapiro A, Gofrit ON, Pizov G, Cohen JK, Maier J. Raman molecular imaging: a novel spectroscopic technique for diagnosis of bladder cancer in urine specimens. Eur Urol. 2011;59(1):106–12.
74. Crow P, Molckovsky A, Stone N, Uff J, Wilson B, WongKeeSong LM. Assessment of fiberoptic near-infrared raman spectroscopy for diagnosis of bladder and prostate cancer. Urology. 2005;65(6):1126–30.
75. Barman I, Dingari NC, Singh GP, Kumar R, Lang S, Nabi G. Selective sampling using confocal Raman spectroscopy provides enhanced specificity for urinary bladder cancer diagnosis. Anal Bioanal Chem. 2012;404(10):3091–9.
76. Sonn GA, Jones SN, Tarin TV, Du CB, Mach KE, Jensen KC, et al. Optical biopsy of human bladder neoplasia with in vivo confocal laser endomicroscopy. J Urol. 2009;182(4):1299–305.
77. Loidl W, Schmidbauer J, Susani M, Marberger M. Flexible cystoscopy assisted by hexaminolevulinate induced fluorescence: a new approach for bladder cancer detection and surveillance? Eur Urol. 2005;47(3):323–6.

78. Witjes JA, Moonen PM, van der Heijden AG. Comparison of hexaminolevulinate based flexible and rigid fluorescence cystoscopy with rigid white light cystoscopy in bladder cancer: results of a prospective Phase II study. Eur Urol. 2005;47(3):319–22.
79. Hermann GG, Mogensen K, Toft BG, Glenthøj A, Pedersen HM. Outpatient diagnostic of bladder tumours in flexible cystoscopes: evaluation of fluorescence-guided flexible cystoscopy and bladder biopsies. Scand J Urol Nephrol. 2011;46(1):31–6.
80. Herr HW, Donat SM. Reduced bladder tumour recurrence rate associated with narrow-band imaging surveillance cystoscopy. BJU Int. 2011;107(3):396–8.
81. Thomas K, O'Brien T. Blue-sky thinking about blue-light cystoscopy. BJU Int. 2009;104(7):887–9.
82. Soler-Martinez J, Vozmediano-Chicharro R, Morales-Jimenez P, Hernandez-Alcaraz D, Vivas-Vargas E, Santos Garcia-Vaquero I, et al. Holmium laser treatment for low grade, low stage, noninvasive bladder cancer with local anesthesia and early instillation of mitomycin C. J Urol. 2007;178(6):2337–9.
83. Jonler M, Lund L, Bisballe S. Holmium: YAG laser vaporization of recurrent papillary tumours of the bladder under local anaesthesia. BJU Int. 2004;94(3):322–5.
84. Hernandez V, Alvarez M, la PE D, Amaruch N, Martin MD, De la Morena JM, et al. Safety of active surveillance program for recurrent nonmuscle-invasive bladder carcinoma. Urology. 2009;73(6):1306–10.
85. Sapre N, Anderson P, Foroudi F. Management of local recurrences in the irradiated bladder: a systematic review. BJU Int. 2012;110 Suppl 4:51–7.
86. Sobin LH, Wittekind C. TNM classification of malignant tumours. 6th ed. Chichester/West Sussex: Wiley; 2002.
87. Mostofi FK, Sobin LH, Torloni H. International histological classification of tumours. Geneva: World Health Organisation; 1973.
88. Epstein JI, Amin MB, Reuter VR, Mostofi FK. The World Health Organization/international society of urological pathology consensus classification of urothelial (transitional cell) neoplasms of the urinary bladder. Bladder Consensus Conference Committee. Am J Surg Pathol. 1998;22(12):1435–48.

15 Bladder Preservation Approaches

Mathew Oommen, Janet Colli, and Raju Thomas

15.1 Introduction

The management of muscle invasive bladder cancer is challenging because of the daunting task of discussing the appropriate therapeutic options and prognosis for the patient. The gold standard for muscle invasive bladder cancer is open radical cystectomy, extended pelvic lymph node dissection with appropriate choice for urinary diversion based on a multitude of factors. In certain subsets, patients who are either poor surgical candidates or strongly wish to preserve their bladders, despite the risk of disease progression must consider other less invasive treatment modalities. This chapter will attempt to discuss current therapies available for patients that are not candidates for a standard radical cystectomy. As with open radical cystectomy, laparoscopic and robot assisted radical cystectomy have slowly gained acceptance as viable options for the treatment of bladder cancer. However, even in the most experienced hands, there is a significant risk of perioperative and postoperative complications. A multi-institutional study by Smith and colleagues suggested a 30 % complication rate [1]. In addition to the removal of the bladder, the extended pelvic lymph node dissection has its own set of complications. Radical cystectomy series have confirmed that the two most common sites of lymph node involvement are the obturator/hypogastric and external iliac lymph node chains [2]. A smaller percentage will also drain into the sacral or common iliac lymph nodes. Therefore, a standard template for pelvic lymph node dissection for radical cystectomy should include the common iliac, internal iliac, external iliac, and obturator packets on both sides [3]. In conjunction with the radical cystectomy, a thorough pelvic lymph node dissection incorporates longer operative time and major complications which can be immediately noted at the time of surgery or may be delayed in presentation. The immediate complications associated with a lymph node dissection include major vascular injury, as well as damage and/or transection of nerves running in close proximity to the lymphatic packets.

Post operative complications of extended lymph node dissections include symptomatic lymphocele formation and the increased risk of thromboembolic events [4].

These factors must be considered in patients who may not tolerate a radical cystectomy with a pelvic lymph node dissection. A study by Chamie and colleagues [5] suggested that there is no significant overall survival benefit in older patients when comparing a radical cystectomy versus a bladder sparing approach. Of note, there is a group of patients that regardless of age will adamantly refuse to entertain any procedure that involves the removal of the bladder, even if a neobladder is offered to maintain anatomic

M. Oommen, MD • J. Colli, MD
R. Thomas, MD, FACS, MHA (✉)
Department of Urology, Tulane University School of Medicine, New Orleans, LA, USA
e-mail: rthomas@tulane.edu

H.R.H. Patel et al. (eds.), *Pelvic Cancer Surgery: Modern Breakthroughs and Future Advances*,
DOI 10.1007/978-1-4471-4258-4_15, © Springer-Verlag London 2015

continuity. These patients are few, but difficult to treat knowing the progressive nature of invasive bladder cancer.

15.2 Imaging

One of the most difficult aspects of a bladder preservation approach for radical transurethral resection of bladder tumor or partial cystectomy is the inability to accurately evaluate tumor margins at time of surgery. Recently, many new technologies have been evaluated or are in the process of being evaluated for real time diagnostic accuracy. Macroscopic imaging techniques that appear to aid in the detection of bladder malignancies during cystoscopy include both narrow band imaging (NBI) and photodynamic diagnosis (PDD) with the use of photosensitive protoporphyrin analogs such as 5-aminolevulinic acid (5-ALA) or hexaminolevulinate 9 (HAL) [6]. NBI uses a light source that filters standard white light into wavelengths of 415 and 540 nm. This causes a more stark contrast between benign mucosa and capillaries that absorb hemoglobin. A popular aspect of NBI is that there is no need for intravesical instillation of any contrast agents. PDD uses a combination of blue light with a wavelength of 375–440 nm and intravesical photosensitizing agents. The two most promising agents currently are 5-ALA and HAL. PDD requires the placement of the intravesical agent at least an hour prior to cystoscopy. Both NBI and PDD have false positive rates of at least 34 % [7]. Microscopic real time imaging has also gained traction with the use of confocal laser endomicroscopy and optical coherence tomography. Both of these modalities are still under investigation and need other modalities to help identify lesions of interest on a larger scale.

15.3 Therapeutic Options

When deciding between bladder sparing approaches for the treatment of bladder cancer, there are a few options and combinations available at this time. Current treatment modalities include:

- Surgical (radical TURBT, open partial cystectomy, laparoscopic partial cystectomy with or without robotic assistance)
- Radiation therapy
- Chemotherapy
- Combination of all these modalities

Surgical options for bladder preservation include radical transurethral resection of bladder tumor (TURBT) and partial cystectomy by correlating with imaging modalities.

15.4 Radical TURBT

When performing a radical TURBT, certain technical aspects of the procedure must be considered. Monopolar transurethral resection of bladder tumors has been around since the 1940s and is still the most commonly used technology around the world. However, we suggest using bipolar cautery when available. This method allows for the use of normal saline as the irrigation solution, which eliminates the need for intravesical instillation of sterile water. Monopolar TURBT, which uses sterile water, increases the risk of fluid absorption and hyponatremia, especially when there is a prolonged operative course or known risk of bladder perforation. Special considerations based on the tumor location must be considered. For lesions located in the lateral aspects of the bladder, the transmitted energy may stimulate an obturator reflex. A sudden movement during resection may result in bladder perforation. There should be an appropriate communication between the surgeon and the anesthesia team prior to the procedure. The patient should be on muscle relaxants before any lateral wall resection is attempted. When resecting around or over the ureteral orifices, remember to have the generator power setting on cut, not the coagulation setting, as the coagulation function may be more likely to cause scarring and possible long-term upper urinary tract damage. Fluid management during the entire case is paramount during a transurethral case, especially if monopolar cautery is used (Fig. 15.1). After performing a radical TURBT, it is important to not only biopsy the resection bed, separately but also, the peripheral margins

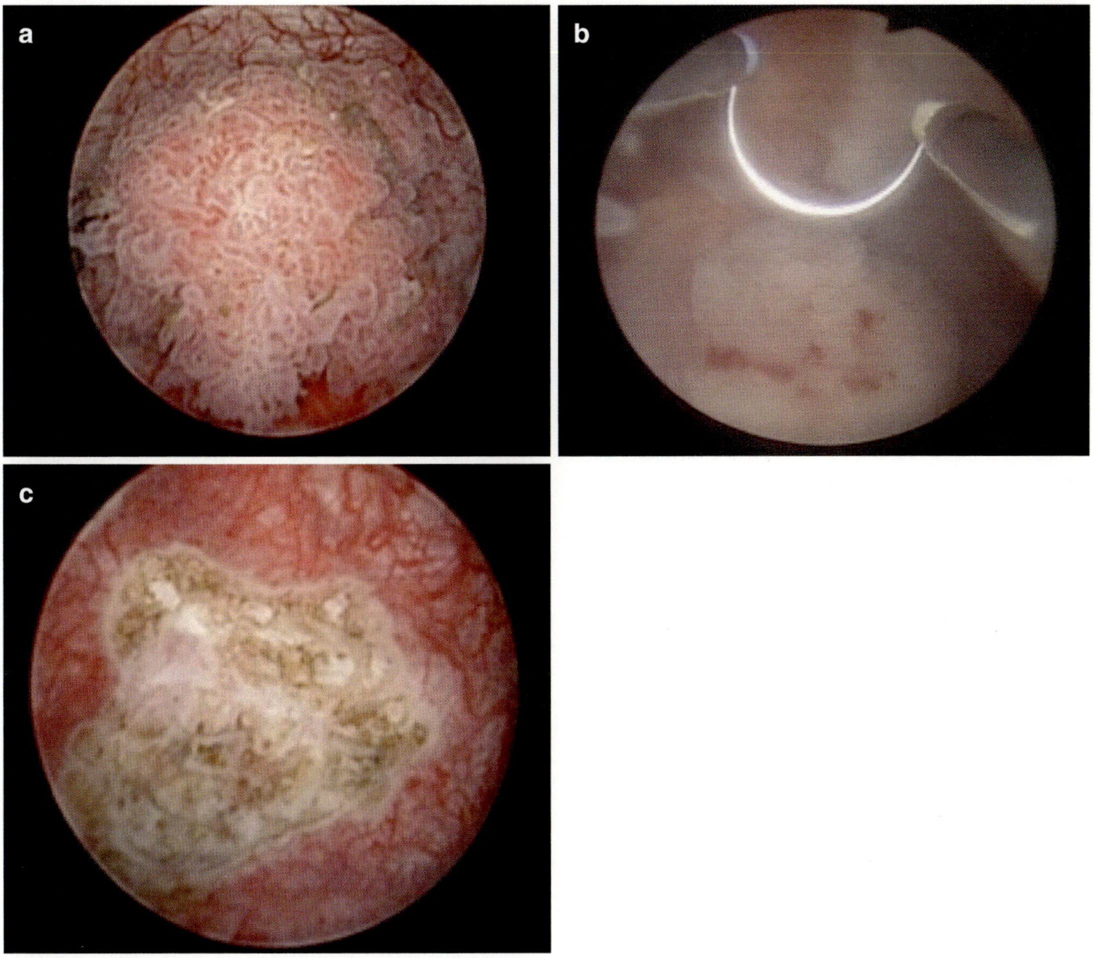

Fig. 15.1 (**a**) Bladder lesion. (**b**) Bipolar resectoscope. (**c**) Post transurethral resection image

of the resection site. We recommend sending these specimens in separate containers for more accurate staging. Negative biopsies appear to correlate with better long-term survival outcomes in patients undergoing a radical TURBT as the sole form of therapy [8]. In case of doubts about negative radical TURBT margins, a repeat procedure is recommended in 6–12 weeks.

15.5 Partial Cystectomy

Partial cystectomy provides a feasible approach in a select group of bladder cancer patients who meet certain qualifying criteria. Though it does maintain a conventional voiding mechanism and erectile function, not all patients are appropriate candidates. Patients with urachal carcinoma, solitary tumor located in a bladder diverticulum, dome, or posterolateral aspect of the bladder are optimal candidates assuming there is no evidence of carcinoma in situ (CIS) elsewhere in the bladder at time of random bladder biopsies. Transurethral prostatic biopsies are recommended to complete the staging process. There should be enough space to allow for wide excision without need for ureteral reimplantation. Partial cystectomy allows for a full thickness resection of the diseased bladder, with adequate negative margins, as well as a concomitant pelvic lymph node dissection. Kassouf and colleagues reported that only 5 out of 37 patients who underwent partial cystectomy subsequently required a radical cystectomy. Of these five patients, only one patient died of bladder cancer with a median of 37 months of follow-up from the time of delayed cystectomy [9]. Patients undergoing partial cystectomy must understand that they must be compliant for lifelong cystoscopic evaluation if they choose this treatment option. The gold standard for performing partial cystectomy is the open surgical approach. However, recent advances in minimally invasive surgery may allow for a laparoscopic or robotic resection of a portion of the bladder.

15.6 Technique for Open Partial Cystectomy

The patient is placed in supine position with slight Trendelenburg and the abdomen and genitalia are prepped and draped giving access to the genitalia for sterile Foley catheter placement, which should be placed within the sterile surgical field. A regional or general anesthetic approach may be used for the procedure. All visible bladder tumors should always be resected prior to consideration for partial cystectomy. This is to minimize any risk of tumor spillage. The bladder may be accessed via a transperitoneal or extraperitoneal approach. If the lesion or diverticulum is posterior, a transperitoneal approach is suggested. Sometimes, if there is a possibility for difficult identification of the tumor site at time of resection, cystoscopic marking with either fulguration or dye should be considered at the time of surgery. A low vertical midline incision is used to enter the peritoneal cavity. Of note, a Maylard incision may be considered if the patient has strong reservations against a midline incision. Once the peritoneal cavity is entered, a pelvic lymph node dissection can be performed in the standard fashion. To aid in the dissection of the bladder, it may help to fill the bladder slightly with sterile water and clamp the Foley catheter. Overly distending the bladder may make it more susceptible to perforation at time of dissection.

It is important to quickly identify anatomic landmarks that help in the further mobilization of the bladder and facilitate partial cystectomy. The medial umbilical ligament can be followed to the superior vesical artery. The artery can then be ligated on the side of the bladder lesion. This will help further mobilize the bladder. The vas deferens on that side may be identified and mobilized or transected as needed. It is recommended that the perivesical fat directly over the suspected tumor area remain attached to the bladder. If the lesion is on the posterior wall, the peritoneum overlying the posterior bladder may be incised. This will allow the rectum to be mobilized off the bladder, if needed giving access to the posterior wall. All adjacent bowel contents should be packed away so as to avoid any contamination from spillage. Once the bowel is packed away from the field surrounding the bladder, the bladder is evaluated and the tumor location is verified. This can be accomplished via manual palpation or with concomitant cystoscopy. If cystoscopy is needed, the Foley catheter should be removed in a manner to avoid tumor spillage.

Once the site of the tumor has been verified, 2–0 delayed absorbable sutures are placed to help elevate the bladder at time of cystotomy and partial cystectomy. The Foley catheter has been unclamped and the bladder has been completely drained at this point. The bladder is incised and the tumor is removed with an approximate 2 cm margin is excised. Special care should be paid to the location of the ureteral orifices. Frozen biopsies at the margin sites are suggested if there are any questions at the time of resection. A standard two-layer closure with a 2–0 delayed absorbable suture is recommended. The bladder may be filled with 150–200 cc of sterile water to confirm a watertight closure. Once the stay sutures have been removed, and the Foley catheter is draining appropriately, an abdominal drain is placed in a dependent location of the pelvis. The drain should stay in for at least 5–7 days and output should be monitored prior to its removal at an outpatient setting. Since the closed suction drain is intraperitoneal and there is concern regarding the amount of fluid present in the drain, a creatinine level of the drain fluid should be obtained. The Foley catheter should stay in place for at least 1 week. A cystogram is performed prior to removal of the catheter to check for any contrast extravasation.

15.7 Robot Assisted Partial Cystectomy

The technique for robot assisted partial cystectomy shares a similar trocar set up with techniques for robot assisted radical cystectomy [10] (Fig. 15.2). Once general anesthesia is adequate, a Foley catheter and orogastric tube is placed. The patient is placed in a modified low lithotomy position and the operating table is placed in steep Trendelenburg position. Special care is given to adequately pad and secure the patient to avoid any movement of the patient while the robot is docked. This will prevent pressure related complications. The abdomen is shaved, prepped, and draped in the standard fashion. Access and insufflation techniques are per surgeon preference. At our institution, unless there is a significant history of multiple abdominal surgeries and risk of bowel adhesions, the Veress needle is placed in a supraumbilical incision and a 12 mm blunt dilating trocar is placed through the same incision.

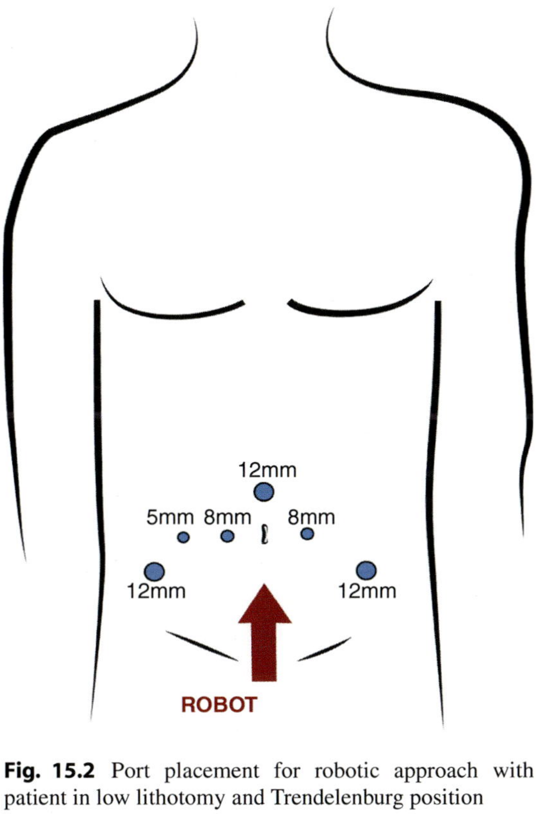

Fig. 15.2 Port placement for robotic approach with patient in low lithotomy and Trendelenburg position

If there is any worry about midline adhesions, an off site entry is performed. The off set teaching laparoscope is used to perform lysis of adhesions when multiple ports are not feasible secondary to multiple intestinal adhesions to aid in proper dissection.

The da Vinci Surgical Robotic System Si type (Intuitive Surgical Inc., Sunnyvale, CA) is utilized with all four arms being docked. Assistant 12 and 5 mm trocars are placed in addition to the camera port and three robotic working ports. The camera port is usually placed about 3–5 cm above the umbilicus. If the partial cystectomy is for urachal pathology, the camera is placed slightly higher. Once the robot is docked, the dissection is performed with the help of a bedside assistant. Our standard technique is to identify the bilateral medial umbilical ligaments and start the dissection at the level of the urachus and continue down just lateral to the medial umbilical ligament thereby completely dissecting and developing the space of Retzius. This helps to drop the bladder completely for ease of mobilization. As much perivesical fat must be left adherent to the bladder as possible. If the tumor or diverticulum is easily visualized then a 2 cm margin is used to excise the tumor (Fig. 15.3a). Special care should be taken to avoid any urine or tumor spillage. The use of traction sutures and ensuring that the Foley catheter is draining properly will help avoid spillage of tumor. One may also place a small lap pad around the incision site. We find that placing a Keith needle with a traction suture just over the pubic symphysis and into the detrusor helps to elevate the bladder without the need for an additional 5 mm trocar. If the tumor location is not easily visualized, flexible cystoscopy by the bedside surgeon can help to localize the lesion. In certain cases, a cystotomy is performed away from the presumed location of the tumor and the tumor identified with gross inspection. Once the tumor or margins of the diverticulum are identified, careful dissection with a wide surgical margin is performed. The specimen is immediately placed in a laparoscopic retrieval sac. The subsequent defect is closed with a 2.0-delayed absorbable suture using a standard two-layer closure (Fig. 15.3b). We recommend filling the bladder

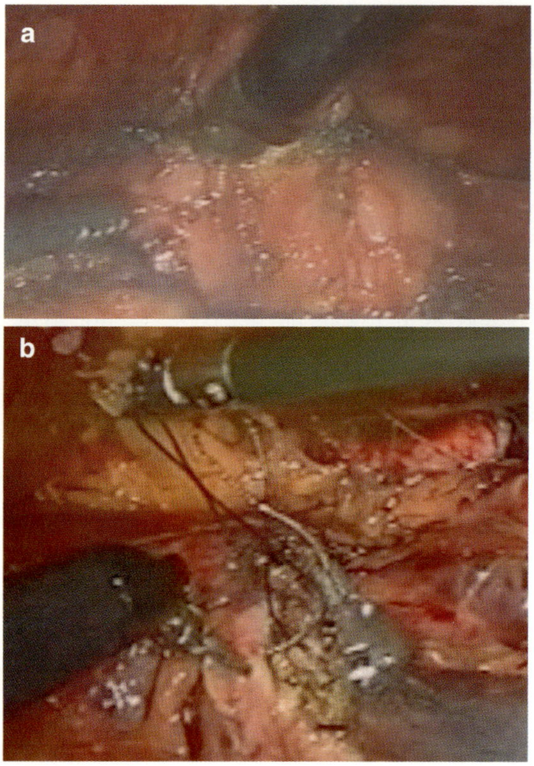

Fig. 15.3 (**a**) Resection of bladder lesion with wide margin. (**b**) Two layer closure with 3–0 delayed absorbable suture

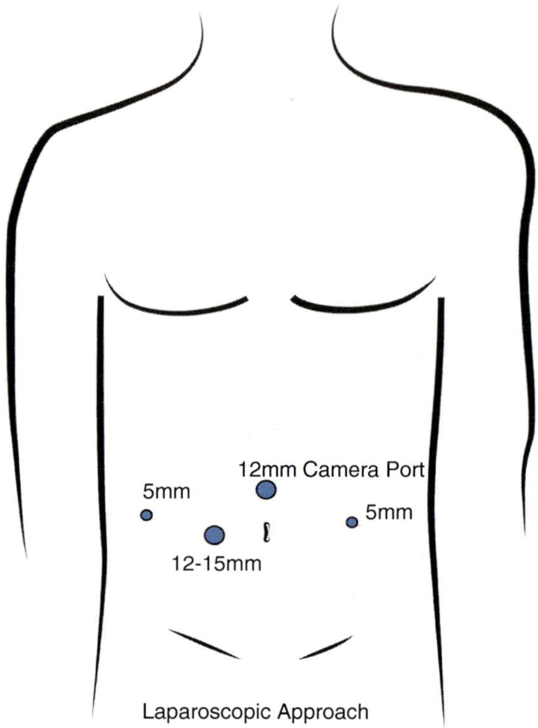

Fig. 15.4 Port placement for laparoscopic approach

with roughly 150–200 cc of fluid to evaluate for any leak. Once the anastomosis is deemed water tight, an intra-abdominal drain is left in place through one of the 8 mm robotic ports. The specimen is extracted via a small infraumbilical vertical midline or Pfannenstiel incision, depending on prior scars or patient preference. The drain is usually left in place for approximately 5–7 days and the Foley catheter is left in place 10–14 days. Prior to removing of the Foley catheter, a cystogram is performed to ensure no extravasation of contrast.

15.8 Laparoscopic Partial Cystectomy

Once treatment options have been discussed and a minimally invasive bladder sparing approach is desired, a laparoscopic partial cystectomy is a feasible option. This may be an appropriate option, especially in centers lacking access to robotic technology. Factors such as patient body habitus, prior abdominal surgeries, ability to tolerate pneumoperitoneum, and surgeon's laparoscopic experience must all be considered to maximize patient safety and achieve a favorable oncological outcome. A pure laparoscopic approach is highly dependent on surgeon experience. The bladder reconstruction requires significant intracorporeal suturing expertise. As discussed for the open technique, flexible cystoscopy is suggested to help with localization of the tumor. This can be performed at the beginning of the procedure or at the time of resection. The patient is placed in low lithotomy position with a small bump placed to slightly elevate the ipsilateral hemipelvis. We suggest a four-port arrangement (Fig. 15.4) using a 12 mm camera port with an additional 12–15 mm port and two 5 mm ports placed in a fan pattern. The 12 mm trocar is helpful for the passage of needles and the use of any larger cutting/coagulation devices. A Keith needle may be passed trancutaneously for placement of any traction sutures. This prevents the need for any additional trocars but still allows for adequate positioning of the bladder prior to the resection. The dissection and suturing technique is similar to what is mentioned for the robotic technique. One additional caveat is the placement of a 5 mm port just superior to the pubic symphysis if an additional retractor is needed.

15.9 Trimodal Therapy

In select patients with early tumor stage, small tumor size, radical TURBT with negative biopsies, absence of hydronephrosis, and no evidence of carcinoma in situ, studies suggest a multi-disciplinary approach may hold promise. Many centers have looked at combining a radical TURBT with a mixture of chemotherapy and radiation therapy followed by cystoscopy with additional consolidation radiotherapy if there is no evidence of recurrence. Five year overall survival ranged from 48 to 62 % [11]. This approach does pose certain challenges such as getting all the various services on board and deciding who will have primary responsibility for the long term care of the patient. However, as more patients live longer with more complex comorbidities, this type of combined therapy may be become a more acceptable treatment option.

Key Points

- Radical cystectomy does not always give a survival advantage in older patients with bladder cancer
- Radical TURBT, in the appropriate patient, can be curative
- Negative biopsies at time of TURBT correlate with better long term survival
- Transperitoneal approach allows for better visualization of the posterior bladder at time of open partial cystectomy
- Ligation of the superior vesicle artery on the ipsilateral side may help with mobilization
- Fulguration or submucosal dye injection via cystoscopy may help identify the lesion at time of partial cystectomy
- Partial cystectomy should not be considered in tumors located on the trigone and adjacent to the ureteral orifices
- Trimodal therapy using radical TURBT, radiotherapy, and chemotherapy may yield comparable long term outcomes in select patients
- All patients undergoing bladder sparing approaches must be counseled strongly about the importance of lifelong follow up with cystoscopy, cytology, and imaging
- Patients should be made aware of all available treatment options at time of diagnosis

References

1. Smith AB, Raynor M, Amling CL, Busby JE, Castle E, Davis R, et al. Multi-institutional analysis of robotic radical cystectomy for bladder cancer: perioperative outcomes and complications in 227 patients. J Laparoendosc Adv Surg Tech. 2012;22(1):17–21.
2. Stein JP, Skinner DG. The role of lymphadenectomy in high-grade invasive bladder cancer. Urol Clin N Am. 2005;32(2):187–97.
3. Gakis G, Efstathiou J, Lerner SP, Cookson MS, Keegan KA, Guru KA, et al. ICUD-EAU International Consultation on Bladder Cancer 2012: radical cystectomy and bladder preservation for muscle-invasive urothelial carcinoma of the bladder. Eur Urol Eur Assoc Urol. 2012;6:1–13.
4. Raboy A, Adler H, Albert P. Extraperitoneal endoscopic pelvic lymph node dissection: a review of 125 patients. J Urol. 1997;158(6):2202–4.
5. Chamie K, Hu B, deVere White RW, Ellison LM. Cystectomy in the elderly: does the survival benefit in younger patients translate to the octogenarians? BJU Int. 2008;102(3):284–90.
6. Liu JJ, Droller MJ, Liao JC. New optical imaging technologies for bladder cancer: considerations and perspectives. J Urol. 2012;188(2):36–8. Elsevier Inc.
7. Ray ER, Chatterton K, Khan MS, Chandra A, Thomas K, Dasgupta P, O'Brien TS. Hexylaminolaevulinate fluorescence cystoscopy in patients previously treated with intravesical bacille Calmette-Guérin. BJU Int. 2010;105(6):789–94.
8. Olsona E, Iborra I, Ricos JV, Monros JL, Casanova J, Calabuig C. Feasibility of transurethral resection

for muscle infiltrating carcinoma of the bladder: long-term follow-up of a prospective study. J Urol. 1998;159:95–8.
9. Kassouf W, Swanson D, Kamat AM, Leibovici D, Siefker-Radtke A, Munsell MF, et al. Partial cystectomy for muscle invasive urothelial carcinoma of the bladder: a contemporary review of the M. D. Anderson Cancer Center experience. J Urol. 2006;175(6):2058–62.
10. Allaparthi S, Ramanathan R, Balaji KC. Robotic partial cystectomy for bladder cancer: a single-institutional pilot study. J Endourol. 2010;24(2): 223–7.
11. Khosravi-Shahi P, Cabezón-Gutiérrez L. Selective organ preservation in muscle-invasive bladder cancer: review of the literature. Surg Oncol. 2012;21(1): e17–22. Elsevier Ltd.

Radical Cystectomy: Robotic, Laparoscopic, Open and Partial

16

James E. Ferguson, Raj S. Pruthi, and Michael E. Woods

16.1 Bladder Cancer Epidemiology

Bladder cancer is a common disease with over 70,000 new cases and almost 15,000 deaths in the US in 2011 [1]. Untreated, muscle invasive bladder cancer is a lethal disease with a 2-year mortality rate approaching 85 % [2]. In addition to its morbidity and mortality, bladder cancer is the most expensive cancer to diagnose, treat, and survey, with a per-patient lifetime cost of $96,500 [3, 4]. In the United States and other developed countries, urothelial carcinoma (UC) represents 90 % of bladder cancers, with squamous cell carcinoma and adenocarcinoma comprising the majority of the remaining histologies. The predominant risk factors for developing UC of the bladder are age and environmental exposures, especially to tobacco smoke and aromatic amines from dyes and industrial chemicals. In addition, males are three to four times more likely to develop bladder cancer than females, presumably due to higher rates of carcinogenic exposures.

The prognosis and treatment for UC of the bladder is largely determined by the level of cellular de-differentiation (grade), and the depth of invasion (stage). According to the World Health Organization 2004 guidelines, bladder cancer grade is dichotomized to either low- or high-grade. Staging is based on the American Joint Committee on Cancer TNM staging system, which can be divided into two main groups: non-muscle invasive (Ta, T1, Tis, which are all superficial to the muscularis propria), and muscle invasive (T2–T4). Non-muscle invasive bladder cancers (NMIBC) generally carry a favorable prognosis and are amenable to transurethral resection (TURBT) and instillation of intravesical therapies. Conversely, muscle invasive bladder cancer is by definition high-grade, carries a poorer prognosis, and is usually treated with radical cystectomy and urinary diversion, with or without systemic chemotherapy.

Of all incident cases of bladder cancer, 70 % are non-muscle invasive, of which roughly two-thirds are low grade [5, 6]. The low-grade tumors commonly recur after treatment (48–71 %), however they rarely progress to muscle invasive disease (2–12 %). On the other hand, high-grade non-muscle invasive carcinomas have a high rate of both recurrence (55 %) and stage progression (27–61 %) within 3 years after treatment [7].

For muscle invasive bladder cancer and high-grade NMIBC that is recurrent or persistent despite TURBT and intravesical therapies, the standard of care is radical cystectomy combined with bilateral pelvic lymphadenectomy and urinary diversion. In addition, perioperative systemic chemotherapy in the setting of muscle invasive disease has been shown to provide a

J.E. Ferguson, MD • M.E. Woods, MD
R.S. Pruthi, MD (✉)
Division of Urology, Department of Surgery, University of North Carolina, Chapel Hill, NC, USA
e-mail: raj_pruthi@med.unc.edu; rpruthi@med.unc.edu

H.R.H. Patel et al. (eds.), *Pelvic Cancer Surgery: Modern Breakthroughs and Future Advances*,
DOI 10.1007/978-1-4471-4258-4_16,

survival benefit, with patients with extravesical disease (≥pT3) receiving the most benefit [8].

16.2 Open Radical Cystectomy Outcomes, Past and Present

Open radical cystectomy (ORC) is the gold standard treatment for muscle invasive bladder cancer. In 2001, Stein et al. published a landmark paper describing the outcomes of over 1,000 radical cystectomy patients between 1971 and 1997 [9]. The overall recurrence-free survival at 5 and 10 years was 68 and 66 %, respectively. Twenty-four percent of patients had lymph node involvement and their recurrence free survival at 5 years was significantly lower (35 %) than patients with node-negative disease (78 %). The median time to recurrence was 12 months, of which approximately 75 % were distant (non-pelvic) metastases. There was a 2.5 % mortality rate within 30 days, and a 90-day overall complication rate of 28 %. These findings were corroborated in another large study of 507 ORC patients in which the 5-year recurrence-free and overall survival was 62 and 59 %, respectively, with a mean follow-up of 45 months. This cohort of patients had a mean age of 66, 57 % were > pT2, and 24 % were lymph node positive. Similar to Stein et al. extravesical disease and lymph node positivity were associated with poorer prognosis, and the majority of cancer-related deaths occurred in the first 2 years [10].

In 2004, Herr et al. analyzed the outcomes of the Bladder Cancer Collaborative Group in an attempt to better define surgical benchmarks for radical cystectomy. Studying outcomes from 1,091 radical cystectomies by 16 experienced surgeons from four institutions between 2000 and 2002, they concluded that pathologic goals for surgeons performing radical cystectomies should include a positive margin rate lower than 10 % and a lymph node yield of greater than ten [11]. These findings were corroborated by a prospective study which showed improved overall survival in patients with negative margins and > ten lymph nodes dissected, independent of other factors [12]. It should be noted however, that ten dissected lymph nodes represents a minimum rather than a goal, as there is linear relationship between lymph node positivity and overall number of lymph nodes removed [13].

Despite improvements in surgical technique and post-operative care pathways, radical cystectomy remains a morbid surgical procedure. In 2008, Lowrance et al. reported a minor and major complication rate of 38 and 7 %, respectively, with a 30-day mortality rate of 1.7 % [14]. In a large prospective study of over 1,000 patients between 1995 and 2005, Shabsigh et al. found the perioperative complication rates to be much higher (64 % within 90 days, with 13 % being high-grade) when using a strict complication reporting system. These complications were dominated by gastrointestinal events (29 %), infections (25 %), and wound-related complications (15 %). The 90-day mortality rate was found to be 2.7 %, 65 % of which was due to cardiopulmonary events [15].

16.3 Robotic-Assisted Radical Cystectomy

In an attempt to decrease perioperative morbidity, minimally invasive surgery has been applied to radical cystectomy. Due to a combination of the familiarity of urologists with the Da Vinci robotic system (Intuitive Surgical, Sunnyvale CA), as well as the technical challenges of pelvic surgery with a pure laparoscopic approach, robot-assisted radical cystectomy (RARC) has emerged as the most widely utilized minimally invasive approach in the United States [16]. Since the first reported case series in 2003, there has been a significant increase in the use of the robotic technique for bladder cancer surgery [17]. In theory, the robotic approach should provide superior visualization, decrease blood loss, and improve patient convalescence due to decreased incision length, retractor injury, and bowel manipulation leading to shorter length of stay. However with these theoretical advantages come the potential disadvantages of increased operative time and cost, as well as concerns over pathologic compromise secondary to loss of tactile feedback and thoroughness of pelvic lymph node dissection. A growing number of single and multi-institution case series described below have supported the continued utilization of RARC.

16.4 Perioperative Outcomes of RARC

With regards to perioperative outcomes, small prospective studies (including two randomized trials) have shown non-inferiority or superiority of RARC compared to ORC in terms of mortality, blood loss, transfusion requirement, hospital stay, narcotic use, and time to resumption of diet. In a randomized prospective trial of ORC vs RARC enrolling 40 patients, Nix et al. found that RARC patients experienced less estimated blood loss, quicker return of bowel function, and lower use of inpatient narcotics compared to the ORC patients [18]. Ng et al. showed in a prospective, non-randomized cohort study of 187 consecutive patients that the 30-day overall Clavien complication rate was higher in the open group compared with the robotic group (ORC 59 % vs RARC 41 %, p=0.04), as well as the rate of major complications at 90 days (30 % vs 10 %, p=0.007) [19]. In addition, post-operative length of stay has been found to be significantly shorter in RARC patients by several authors on retrospective analysis [19–21] (Table 16.1). A recent meta-analysis of the head-to-head comparisons of RARC vs ORC has reinforced the above findings [31]. However, these advantages come at the expense of longer operative time in the robotic approach, which has been demonstrated by multiple studies [32, 33]. Whether these perioperative improvements result in more rapid patient convalescence after hospital discharge is an area of active investigation.

16.5 Pathologic Outcomes

While long-term survival data continue to mature, pathologic outcomes such as lymph node yield and surgical margin status have been evaluated as surrogate markers of surgical quality during RARC. Critics of the robotic approach have focused on the ability to perform an adequate pelvic lymph node dissection, and have expressed concerns that the robotic approach results in poorer lymph node dissection [34]. In a multi-institutional international RARC database from 15 institutions, 527 patients underwent robotic lymphadenectomy and 83 % of them had a lymph node count of greater than ten [28]. Using this same series, positive surgical margins occurred in 6.8 % of patients [29]. Importantly, 36 % of this cohort harbored extravesical (≥pT3) disease, a number comparable to prior open series. Smith et al. reported in another multi-institution RARC case series of 227 patients an average lymph node yield of 18 and a positive surgical margin rate of 2 % [35]. Abaza et al. demonstrated that performing an extended lymph node dissection robotically resulted in equivalent lymph node yield compared with open surgery in a non-randomized comparison [36]. In a prospective cohort study, Richards et al. compared 70 consecutive patients (35 ORC vs 35 RARC) with equal rates of extravesical (40 %) and lymph node positive disease (29 %) and found a lower positive margin rate in RARC (3 %) compared to ORC (9 %) and equivalent lymph node yield [37]. Finally, two randomized prospective trials comparing ORC and RARC examined several perioperative outcomes including lymph node yield, and found RARC to be non-inferior to ORC. In the study by Nix et al. lymph node yield was not different between groups, and no positive surgical margins were identified in either group [18]. Parekh and colleagues recently published results of a RCT with 20 patients in each arm and found the average lymph node yield to be 23 in the ORC group and 11 in the RARC group (p=0.135), and positive margin rate to be identical at 5 % in each group. These findings were despite a higher rate of extravesical disease in the RARC group (50 % vs 35 %) [38]. Using these surrogate surgical outcomes, oncologic efficacy of RARC appears comparable to ORC. However, these data must still be interpreted with caution as retrospective studies are inherently susceptible to selection bias, and the randomized prospective studies have been small. These head-to-head studies are summarized in Table 16.2.

Table 16.1 Outcomes of ORC and RARC case series

ORC series	n	Years	% male	Age	Peri-op death %	PSM %	LNY	%≤pT2	%≥pT3	+LN%	% neoadjuvant chemo	Follow up (months)	Complication rate	LOS (day)	% IC	5-year RFS
Stein et al. (2001) [9]	1,054	1971–1997	80	66	2.5 %	NR	NR	51	49	24 %	5 %	120	28 % (30 days)	NR	25	68 %
Madersbacher et al. (2003) [10]	507	1985–2000	80	66	2	NR	NR	48	52	24 %	0	45	NR	NR	41 %	62
Hautmann et al. (2006) [22]	788	1986–2003	83	63	5 (90 day)	NR	NR	67 %	33 %	18 %	0	31	NR	NR	25	68
Manoharan et al. (2009) [23]	432	1992–2007	80	69	2	5	10	61	39	21	13	38	33	NR	56	64
RARC series																
Kauffman et al. (2011) [24]	85	2006–2008	79	73	NR	6	19	63	36	16	20	18	41	5.5	71	71 (2 years)
Pruthi et al. (2010) [25]	100	2006–2009	73	65	0	0	19	67	33	20	5	21	36	4.9	61	85 (2 years)
Martin et al. (2010) [26]	59	2005–2009	NR	NR	0	NR	NR	48	52	34	17	25	NR	NR	81	72 (3 years)
Kahn et al. (2011) [27]	50	2004–2008	88	66	0	2	17	72	28	NR	12	NR	34	10	90	NR
IRCC [28, 29]	527	2003–2009	79	69	NR	7	18	65	35	20	NR	NR	NR	NR	NR	NR
Hayn et al. (2011) [30]	164	2005–2010	79	68	1	8.5	22	50	50	29	8	8	64	NR	93	NR

ORC open radical cystectomy, *RARC* robot-assisted radical cystectomy, *PSM* positive surgical margin, *LNY* lymph node yield, *LOS* length of stay, *IC* ileal conduit, *RFS* recurrence free survival, *IRCC* International Robotic Cystectomy Consortium, *NR* not reported

Table 16.2 Outcomes of head-to-head studies comparing RARC to ORC

	Study design	# of patients	Complication %	PSM %	LNY (count)	LOS (days)	2-years RFS
Richards et al. (2010) [37]	R	35/35	60 v 66	3 v 9	15 v 16	7 v 8	NR
Nepple et al. (2012) [33]	R	36/29	NR	14 v 14	14 v 17	7.9 v 9.6	67 % v 58 %
Ng et al. (2010) [19]	P	83/104	41 v 59	7 v 9	15.7 v 17.9	5.5 v 8	NR
Styn et al. (2012) [32]	P	50/100	66 v 62	16 v 11	15.2 v 14.3	9.5 v 10.2	NR
Abaza et al. (2012) [36]	P	35/120	NR	6 v 7	36.9 v 37.5	NR	NR
Nix et al. (2010) [18]	RCT	21/20	33 v 50	0	18.5 v 18.3	5.1 v 6	NR
Parakeh et al. (2012) [38]	RCT	20/20	25 v 25	5 v 5	11 v 23	6 v 6	NR

Reported as counts or percentages for RARC v ORC
ORC open radical cystectomy, *RARC* robot assisted radical cystectomy, *OR* odds ratio, *PSM* positive surgical margin rate, *LNY* lymph node yield, *LOS* length of stay, *P* prospective, *R* retrospective, *RCT* randomized controlled trial, *NR* not reported

16.6 Survival Outcomes

While perioperative and pathologic outcomes are certainly important, oncologic outcomes as defined by recurrence-free survival (RFS) and overall survival (OS) are paramount. While the current survival outcomes of most RARC series are less than 3 years, no survival differences have been identified when compared with ORC series [25, 39, 40]. Martin et al. reported oncologic outcomes in a RARC cohort of 59 patients with a mean follow-up of 25 months [26]. Overall survival rates at 12 and 36 months were 82 and 69 %, respectively, and disease-specific survival rates were 82 and 72 %. This compares favorably to contemporary open radical cystectomy series [9]. Even in patients with node-positive disease, a high risk group where differences in surgical technique should be seen in intermediate survival outcomes, Mmeje et al. found no difference in RFS compared with previous open cohorts [41]. They reported that lymph-node positive patients treated with RARC had a 3-year recurrence-free survival of 43 % and the local recurrence rate was 6 %, demonstrating excellent local disease control with robotic surgery. Again, however, the above data should be interpreted with caution as they are retrospective and non-randomized.

Several prospective randomized trials comparing robotic to open radical cystectomy are currently underway. First, a 15-site multi-institution study with 2-year recurrence-free survival as its primary endpoint is currently accruing in the United States (NCI study #NCT01157676). The accrual target of this study is 160 patients in each arm. Secondary endpoints include peri-operative outcomes (EBL, blood transfusion, operative time, length of stay, analgesic requirement), pathologic outcomes (lymph node yield and positive surgical margins), 90-day complications, post-operative convalescence, and quality of life measures. It should be completed within 5 years. Next, a single institution study at Memorial Sloan Kettering Cancer center is currently underway with 90-day complications as a primary end point and a number of secondary endpoints including EBL, operative time, positive surgical margins, lymph node yield, and 2-year cancer recurrence with an accrual goal of 210 patients (NCI study # NCT01076387). Finally, a single-institution European study termed CORAL comparing open, laparoscopic, and robotic cystectomy has been mentioned in abstract form, but the full details are not yet known [42].

16.7 Partial Cystectomy: Open, Laparoscopic, and Robotic

In addition to radical cystectomy, minimally-invasive surgery has also been utilized to perform partial cystectomy; an operation with relatively rare indications including symptomatic bladder diverticula, bladder endometriosis, and urachal adenocarcinoma. The use of partial cystectomy for urothelial carcinoma is considered only in rare circumstances.

Traditionally, open partial cystectomy (OPC) for urachal carcinoma has been performed along with bilateral pelvic lymph node dissection (PLND). In the most complete series of OPC for urachal adenocarcinoma, out of 50 patients, Herr et al. found a 5-year recurrence free survival rate of 90 % in patients with localized disease [43]. Positive surgical margins, peritoneal involvement, and positive lymph nodes conferred poor prognosis. In their series, 18 % of patients had positive surgical margins, the median lymph node yield was 14 (with 16 % lymph node positivity), and 18 % of patients suffered a local recurrence (most of which who harbored a positive surgical margin). No peri-operative data such as complications, OR time, length of stay, or EBL were reported.

Laparoscopic partial cystectomy (LPC) with PLND is a technically challenging procedure, and our knowledge of the procedure is based on a few small case series. Mariano et al. performed LPC with PLND on six patients with urothelial carcinoma of the bladder with mean operative time of 200 min, mean EBL of 200 cc, mean hospital length of stay of 4 days (range 2–6), with no reported complications. There were no recurrences with a mean follow-up of 30 months. Lymph node yield and positive margin status were not reported [44]. Wadhwa et al. reported their findings with three patients with urachal adenocarcinoma who underwent LPC and PLND. The average OR time was 180 min, the lymph node yield ranged from 8 to 11, and no recurrences were found at a mean follow up of 6 months [45]. Finally, Colombo et al. described the findings of six patients (three with urachal adenocarcinoma, three with urothelial carcinoma) treated with LPC without PLND. Mean operative time was 110 min, EBL was 70 cc, LOS was 2.5 days, and no positive surgical margins were found. No recurrences were seen after a mean follow up of 28.5 months [46].

Similar to LPC, the literature pertaining to robotic partial cystectomy (RPC) is sparse, which prevents robust conclusions. Allaparthi et al. reported three cases (two of urothelial CA of bladder, one of urachal adenocarcinoma) treated with RPC without PLND. Average operative time was 165 min, EBL was 20 cc, and mean hospital length of stay was 3 days (range 2–5). There was one readmission for bowel obstruction and no recurrences with follow-up ranging from 3 to 10 months [47]. Kim et al. showed similar results for a cohort of four patients treated with RPC without PLND [48]. Due to the rarity of the operation, no head-to-head comparisons of RPC or LPC to OPC have been performed to evaluate patient convalescence, peri-operative outcomes, and oncologic effectiveness.

16.8 Future Directions in Bladder Cancer Surgery

While we await randomized prospective data on the relative effectiveness of RARC, further innovations are beginning to be reported. Radical cystectomy using laparoendoscopic single site surgery (LESS) has been reported in small series of patients [49, 50]. While outcomes are favorable with operative times around 5 h, average EBL of 217 cc, negative margins with adequate lymph node yield, and a short length of stay (6 days), patient numbers were small (eight patients), and the authors concluded that the procedure was feasible, but technically challenging with a steep learning curve. In order to avoid the post-operative pain associated with the peri-umbilical midline incision necessary for extracorporeal urinary diversion, intracorporeal techniques have been developed (Fig. 16.1) [51–54]. However, the

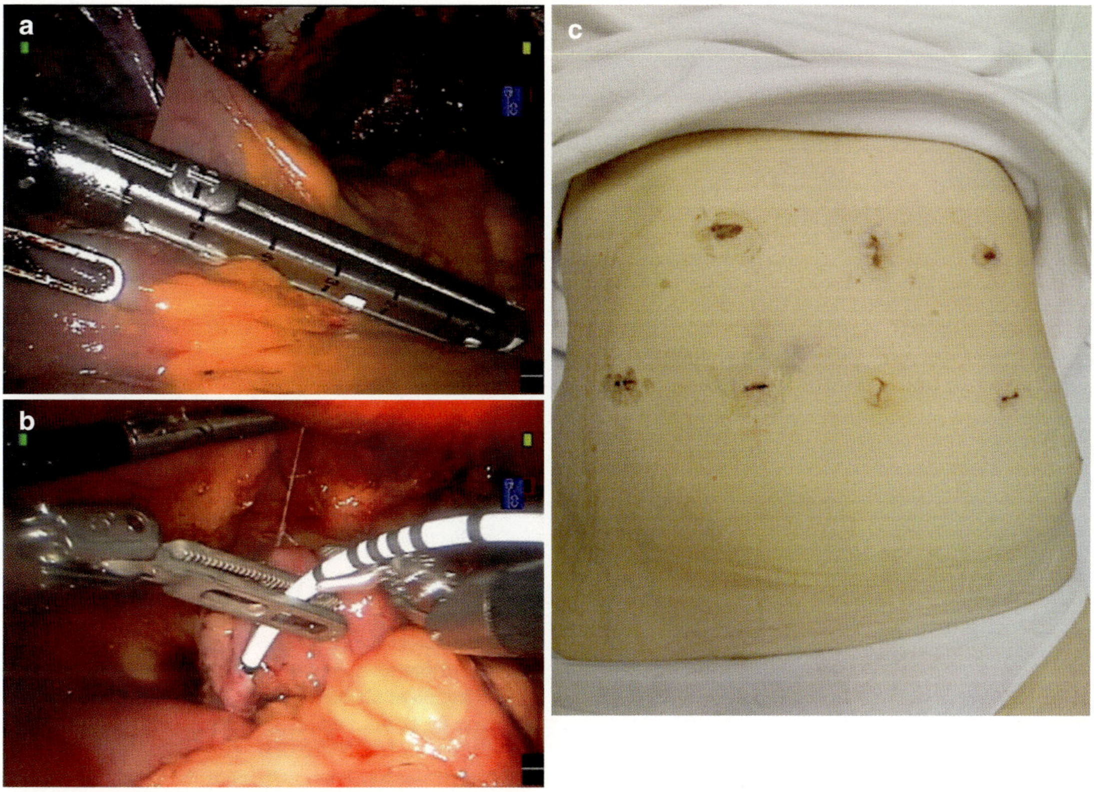

Fig. 16.1 (**a**) An endovascular stapler is used to divide the bowel and mesentery during intracorporeal diversion. (**b**) Ureteral stent placement performed by the robotic surgeon. (**c**) Post-operative image of female patient who underwent robotic radical anterior pelvic exenteration, bilateral pelvic lymphadenectomy, and intracorporeal orthotopic ileal neobladder. Of note, the specimen was placed in an impermeable sac and withdrawn through a small incision in the posterior vaginal wall

overall surgical time, while decreased from initial laparoscopic reports, is still substantially increased compared to an extracorporeal diversion, which has so far prevented widespread adoption of these techniques. Finally, while not specific to robotic bladder cancer surgery, efforts to avoid the use of bowel in urinary conduit formation and its attendant high rates of post-operative complications have led to a current trial using bioengineered tubularized synthetic conduits coated with urothelium derived from stem cells (NCT#01087697) [55]. The possibility of non-bowel conduits with intracorporeal anastomoses raises the exciting possibility of maximizing the benefits of laparoscopic/robotic surgery for the management of bladder cancer in the future.

16.9 Summary

While ORC remains the gold standard treatment for muscle-invasive bladder cancer, preliminary data using surrogate outcomes suggests that RARC may be at least non-inferior to ORC. Studies to date have been mostly retrospective, and are susceptible to selection bias. Large ongoing randomized clinical trials will answer the important question of whether RARC is truly equivalent to ORC in oncologic terms, and whether the added financial costs and operative times are recouped in improved patient convalescence.

Key Points

- Open radical cystectomy (ORC) is the gold standard treatment for muscle invasive bladder cancer.
- Robot-assisted radical cystectomy (RARC) is an evolving procedure in urology and is currently being compared to the gold standard of ORC.
- Several prospective, randomized controlled trials comparing RARC with ORC using recurrence free survival as the primary endpoint are currently underway.
- Current conclusions on the comparability of RARC and ORC are based on prospective series using intermediate-term survival and surrogate oncologic end points as well as retrospective data comparing well-matched cohorts.
- Peri-operative outcomes such as blood loss, narcotic requirement, complications, hospital length of stay, and complication rates appear equivalent or improved for RARC.
- Pathologic outcomes such as lymph node yield and positive margin status are similar between the approaches.
- Medium-term (3-year) progression free- and overall survival appears similar between RARC and ORC series.
- Robotic partial cystectomy is feasible and provides another minimally invasive option for this procedure.
- Intracorporeal urinary diversion performed robotically is technically challenging, but current efforts are underway to minimize the surgical time devoted to this approach.
- Laparoendoscopic single site surgery has been successfully applied to radical cystectomy.

References

1. Jemal A, Siegel R, Ward E, Hao Y, Xu J, Thun MJ. Cancer statistics, 2009. CA Cancer J Clin. 2009;59(4):225–49.
2. Prout GR, Marshall VF. The prognosis with untreated bladder tumors. Cancer. 1956;9(3):551–8.
3. Racioppi M, Palermo G, D'Addessi A, Pinto F, Sacco E, D'Agostino D, et al. Hot topics in urological health economics. A mini review. Arch Ital Urol Androl. 2012;84(2):47–52.
4. Donat SM. Evaluation and follow-up strategies for superficial bladder cancer. Urol Clin N Am. 2003;30(4):765–76.
5. Holmang S, Andius P, Hedelin H, Wester K, Busch C, Johansson SL. Stage progression in Ta papillary urothelial tumors: relationship to grade, immunohistochemical expression of tumor markers, mitotic frequency and DNA ploidy. J Urol. 2001;165(4):1124–8; discussion 1128–30.
6. Samaratunga H, Makarov DV, Epstein JI. Comparison of WHO/ISUP and WHO classification of noninvasive papillary urothelial neoplasms for risk of progression. Urology. 2002;60(2):315–9.
7. Montironi R, Lopez-Beltran A. The 2004 WHO classification of bladder tumors: a summary and commentary. Int J Surg Pathol. 2005;13(2):143–53.
8. Grossman HB, Natale RB, Tangen CM, Speights VO, Vogelzang NJ, Trump DL, et al. Neoadjuvant chemotherapy plus cystectomy compared with cystectomy alone for locally advanced bladder cancer. N Engl J Med. 2003;349(9):859–66.
9. Stein JP, Lieskovsky G, Cote R, Groshen S, Feng AC, Boyd S, et al. Radical cystectomy in the treatment of invasive bladder cancer: long-term results in 1,054 patients. J Clin Oncol. 2001;19(3):666–75.
10. Madersbacher S, Hochreiter W, Burkhard F, Thalmann GN, Danuser H, Markwalder R, et al. Radical cystectomy for bladder cancer today—a homogeneous series without neoadjuvant therapy. J Clin Oncol. 2003;21(4):690–6.
11. Herr H, Lee C, Chang S, Lerner S. Standardization of radical cystectomy and pelvic lymph node dissection for bladder cancer: a collaborative group report. J Urol. 2004;171(5):1823–8; discussion 1827–8.
12. Herr HW, Faulkner JR, Grossman HB, Natale RB, deVere White R, Sarosdy MF, et al. Surgical factors influence bladder cancer outcomes: a cooperative group report. J Clin Oncol. 2004;22(14):2781–9.
13. Capitanio U, Suardi N, Shariat SF, Lotan Y, Palapattu GS, Bastian PJ, et al. Assessing the minimum number of lymph nodes needed at radical cystectomy in patients with bladder cancer. BJU Int. 2009;103(10):1359–62.
14. Lowrance WT, Rumohr JA, Chang SS, Clark PE, Smith Jr JA, Cookson MS. Contemporary open radical cystectomy: analysis of perioperative outcomes. J Urol. 2008;179(4):1313–8; discussion 8.

15. Shabsigh A, Korets R, Vora KC, Brooks CM, Cronin AM, Savage C, et al. Defining early morbidity of radical cystectomy for patients with bladder cancer using a standardized reporting methodology. Eur Urol. 2009;55(1):164–74.
16. Challacombe BJ, Rose K, Dasgupta P. Laparoscopic radical and partial cystectomy. J Minim Access Surg. 2005;1(4):188–95.
17. Menon M, Hemal AK, Tewari A, Shrivastava A, Shoma AM, El-Tabey NA, et al. Nerve-sparing robot-assisted radical cystoprostatectomy and urinary diversion. BJU Int. 2003;92(3):232–6.
18. Nix J, Smith A, Kurpad R, Nielsen ME, Wallen EM, Pruthi RS. Prospective randomized controlled trial of robotic versus open radical cystectomy for bladder cancer: perioperative and pathologic results. Eur Urol. 2010;57(2):196–201.
19. Ng CK, Kauffman EC, Lee MM, Otto BJ, Portnoff A, Ehrlich JR, et al. A comparison of postoperative complications in open versus robotic cystectomy. Eur Urol. 2010;57(2):274–81.
20. Martin AD, Nunez RN, Castle EP. Robot-assisted radical cystectomy versus open radical cystectomy: a complete cost analysis. Urology. 2011;77(3):621–5.
21. Pruthi RS, Wallen EM. Robotic assisted laparoscopic radical cystoprostatectomy: operative and pathological outcomes. J Urol. 2007;178(3 Pt 1):814–8.
22. Hautmann RE, Gschwend JE, de Petriconi RC, Kron M, Volkmer BG. Cystectomy for transitional cell carcinoma of the bladder: results of a surgery only series in the neobladder era. J Urol. 2006;176(2):486–92; discussion 491–2.
23. Manoharan M, Ayyathurai R, Soloway MS. Radical cystectomy for urothelial carcinoma of the bladder: an analysis of perioperative and survival outcome. BJU Int. 2009;104(9):1227–32.
24. Kauffman EC, Ng CK, Lee MM, Otto BJ, Wang GJ, Scherr DS. Early oncological outcomes for bladder urothelial carcinoma patients treated with robotic-assisted radical cystectomy. BJU Int. 2011;107(4):628–35.
25. Pruthi RS, Nielsen ME, Nix J, Smith A, Schultz H, Wallen EM. Robotic radical cystectomy for bladder cancer: surgical and pathological outcomes in 100 consecutive cases. J Urol. 2010;183(2):510–4.
26. Martin AD, Nunez RN, Pacelli A, Woods ME, Davis R, Thomas R, et al. Robot-assisted radical cystectomy: intermediate survival results at a mean follow-up of 25 months. BJU Int. 2010;105(12):1706–9.
27. Khan MS, Elhage O, Challacombe B, Rimington P, Murphy D, Dasgupta P. Analysis of early complications of robotic-assisted radical cystectomy using a standardized reporting system. Urology. 2011; 77(2):357–62.
28. Hellenthal NJ, Hussain A, Andrews PE, Carpentier P, Castle E, Dasgupta P, et al. Lymphadenectomy at the time of robot-assisted radical cystectomy: results from the international robotic cystectomy consortium. BJU Int. 2010;107(4):642–6.
29. Hellenthal NJ, Hussain A, Andrews PE, Carpentier P, Castle E, Dasgupta P, et al. Surgical margin status after robot assisted radical cystectomy: results from the International Robotic Cystectomy Consortium. J Urol. 2010;184(1):87–91.
30. Hayn MH, Hellenthal NJ, Seixas-Mikelus SA, Mansour AM, Stegemann A, Hussain A, et al. Is patient outcome compromised during the initial experience with robot-assisted radical cystectomy? Results of 164 consecutive cases. BJU Int. 2011;108(6):882–7.
31. Li K, Lin T, Fan X, Xu K, Bi L, Duan Y, et al. Systematic review and meta-analysis of comparative studies reporting early outcomes after robot-assisted radical cystectomy versus open radical cystectomy. Cancer Treat Rev. 2013;39(6):551–60.
32. Styn NR, Montgomery JS, Wood DP, Hafez KS, Lee CT, Tallman C, et al. Matched comparison of robotic-assisted and open radical cystectomy. Urology. 2012;79(6):1303–8.
33. Nepple KG, Strope SA, Grubb 3rd RL, Kibel AS. Early oncologic outcomes of robotic vs. open radical cystectomy for urothelial cancer. Urol Oncol. 2013;31(6):894–8.
34. Studer UE, Collette L. Robot-assisted cystectomy: does it meet expectations? Eur Urol. 2010; 58(2):203–4.
35. Smith AB, Raynor M, Amling CL, Busby JE, Castle E, Davis R, et al. Multi-institutional analysis of robotic radical cystectomy for bladder cancer: perioperative outcomes and complications in 227 patients. J Laparoendosc Adv Surg Tech A. 2012;22(1):17–21.
36. Abaza R, Dangle PP, Gong MC, Bahnson RR, Pohar KS. Quality of lymphadenectomy is equivalent with robotic and open cystectomy using an extended template. J Urol. 2012;187(4):1200–4.
37. Richards KA, Hemal AK, Kader AK, Pettus JA. Robot assisted laparoscopic pelvic lymphadenectomy at the time of radical cystectomy rivals that of open surgery: single institution report. Urology. 2010;76(6):1400–4.
38. Parekh DJ, Messer J, Fitzgerald J, Ercole B, Svatek R. Perioperative outcomes and oncologic efficacy from a pilot prospective randomized clinical trial of open versus robotic assisted radical cystectomy. J Urol. 2012;24.
39. Kauffman EC, Ng CK, Lee MM, Otto BJ, Wang GJ, Scherr DS. Early oncological outcomes for bladder urothelial carcinoma patients treated with robotic-assisted radical cystectomy. BJU Int. 2010;107(4):628–35.
40. Murphy DG, Challacombe BJ, Costello AJ. Outcomes after robot-assisted laparoscopic radical prostatectomy. Asian J Androl. 2009;11(1):94–9.
41. Mmeje CO, Nunez-Nateras R, Nielsen ME, Pruthi RS, Smith A, Wallen EM, et al. Oncologic outcomes for lymph node-positive urothelial carcinoma patients treated with robot assisted radical cystectomy: With mean follow-up of 3.5 years. Urol Oncol. 2013;31(8):1621–7.
42. Choudhury SM, Mahesan NM, Elhage O, Khan MS, Dasgupta P. Oncological outcomes of robot-assisted radical cystectomy. BJU Int. 2011;108(11):1679–80.

43. Herr HW, Bochner BH, Sharp D, Dalbagni G, Reuter VE. Urachal carcinoma: contemporary surgical outcomes. J Urol. 2007;178(1):74–8; discussion 78.
44. Mariano MB, Tefilli MV. Laparoscopic partial cystectomy in bladder cancer—initial experience. Int Braz J Urol. 2004;30(3):192–8.
45. Wadhwa P, Kolla SB, Hemal AK. Laparoscopic en bloc partial cystectomy with bilateral pelvic lymphadenectomy for urachal adenocarcinoma. Urology. 2006;67(4):837–43.
46. Colombo Jr JR, Desai M, Canes D, Frota R, Haber GP, Moinzadeh A, et al. Laparoscopic partial cystectomy for urachal and bladder cancer. Clinics (Sao Paulo). 2008;63(6):731–4.
47. Allaparthi S, Ramanathan R, Balaji KC. Robotic partial cystectomy for bladder cancer: a single-institutional pilot study. J Endourol. 2010;24(2):223–7.
48. Kim DK, Lee JW, Park SY, Kim YT, Park HY, Lee TY. Initial experience with robotic-assisted laparoscopic partial cystectomy in urachal diseases. Korean J Urol. 2010;51(5):318–22.
49. Kaouk JH, Goel RK, White MA, White WM, Autorino R, Haber GP, et al. Laparoendoscopic single-site radical cystectomy and pelvic lymph node dissection: initial experience and 2-year follow-up. Urology. 2010;76(4):857–61.
50. Ma LL, Bi H, Hou XF, Huang Y, Wang GL, Zhao L, et al. Laparoendoscopic single-site radical cystectomy and urinary diversion: initial experience in China using a homemade single-port device. J Endourol. 2012;26(4):355–9.
51. Canda AE, Atmaca AF, Altinova S, Akbulut Z, Balbay MD. Robot-assisted nerve-sparing radical cystectomy with bilateral extended pelvic lymph node dissection (PLND) and intracorporeal urinary diversion for bladder cancer: initial experience in 27 cases. BJU Int. 2012;110(3):434–44.
52. Goh AC, Gill IS, Lee DJ, de Castro Abreu AL, Fairey AS, Leslie S, et al. Robotic intracorporeal orthotopic ileal neobladder: replicating open surgical principles. Eur Urol. 2012;62(5):891–901.
53. Haber GP, Campbell SC, Colombo Jr JR, Fergany AF, Aron M, Kaouk J, et al. Perioperative outcomes with laparoscopic radical cystectomy: "pure laparoscopic" and "open-assisted laparoscopic" approaches. Urology. 2007;70(5):910–5.
54. Pruthi RS, Nix J, McRackan D, Hickerson A, Nielsen ME, Raynor M, et al. Robotic-assisted laparoscopic intracorporeal urinary diversion. Eur Urol. 2011;57(6):1013–21.
55. Atala A. Tissue engineering of human bladder. Br Med Bull. 2011;97:81–104.

17 Orthotopic Bladder Substitution

Scott M. Cheney and Erik P. Castle

17.1 Introduction

Orthotopic bladder substitution is an important tool in the armamentarium of the urologist for urinary diversion after cystectomy. Techniques for orthotopic neobladders were described in the early 1900s, however the procedure did not gain traction with urologists until the late 1970s and 1980s when studies were published on the feasibility of this type of diversion in men [1]. Various techniques have been introduced since the initial work by Camey and LeDuc, such as the Hautmann "W" neobladder [2], the Studer Pouch [3] and the T-pouch [4]. Initially, the neobladder was only considered in male patients because the risk of incontinence in the female was felt to be too high. In the 1990s, however, studies demonstrated acceptable continence outcomes in women with neobladders [5]. Although orthotopic urinary diversion is a more time-consuming procedure for the urologist and demands vigorous maintenance by the patient, it is a rewarding procedure and has similar short and long term complications with simpler forms of diversion [6].

The ileal conduit with a Bricker uretero-ileal anastomosis remains the most commonly used form of diversion [7]. Drawbacks to the ileal conduit include the risk of retrograde reflux of urine, uretero-ileal anastomotic stricture, renal deterioration, pyelonephritis, stomal stenosis, and peristomal hernia. Use of an orthotopic neobladder avoids many of these drawbacks and more closely resembles native voiding function, and when an appropriate patient is selected for this diversion, acceptable long-term outcomes are observed [8].

This chapter focuses on the general principles, proper patient selection, operative techniques, complications, and outcomes of orthotopic urinary diversions.

17.2 General Principles

A neobladder should resemble the function of the native bladder as closely as possible. This includes formation of a compliant reservoir with adequate capacity (400–500 mL) and maintenance of continence. Orthotopic diversions do not retain the ability to contract in a coordinated manner, therefore patients void with the assistance of gravity and valsalva maneuvers coupled with relaxation of the rhabdosphincter. Most patients with neobladders do not require self-intermittent catheterization (SIC), but this may be needed in a minority of patients who do not empty (approximately 12 % in women and 9.5 % in men) [9, 10].

Another important concept in orthotopic diversion is detubularization of the bowel segment and formation of a spherical diversion. The Law of Laplace states that the tension in the wall of a

S.M. Cheney, MD • E.P. Castle, MD (✉)
Department of Urology, Mayo Clinic,
Phoenix, AZ, USA
e-mail: castle.erik@mayo.edu

H.R.H. Patel et al. (eds.), *Pelvic Cancer Surgery: Modern Breakthroughs and Future Advances*,
DOI 10.1007/978-1-4471-4258-4_17, © Springer-Verlag London 2015

Table 17.1 Formulas for calculating the wall tension of a vessel using the Law of Laplace

Sphere	T=PR/2
Cylinder	T=PR

T wall tension (resistance to internal vessel pressure), *P* internal pressure, *R* radius

Table 17.2 Indications for orthotopic neobladder

Renal funtion: eGFR >35–40 mL/min
Liver function: low risk of hyperammonemia
Absence of severe urethral stricture disease
Absence of Inflammatory Bowel Disease (IBD) or short-gut syndrome
Adequate manual dexterity/mental function
Absence of UC in prostatic urethra (men) or bladder neck (women)
Impaired rhabdosphincter

container (T) is proportional to the pressure (P) of the container's contents and its radius (R) [11]. When comparing wall tension in a sphere (neobladder) versus a cylinder (tubularized bowel), the law dictates that the wall tension of the sphere is one half that of the cylinder given the same pressure and radius (see Table 17.1) [11].

Camey and LeDuc illustrated this concept in comparing their initial orthotopic diversions. Their first neobladder used tubularized bowel and demonstrated high intraluminal pressures [1]. This problem was remedied with use of detubularized bowel in their later diversions [12].

17.3 Patient Selection

The most common indication for orthotopic urinary diversion is radical cystectomy for muscle invasive urothelial carcinoma (UC). The characteristics of the cancer are critical to choosing the correct diversion, and sound oncological judgment should never be compromised to obtain a better functional outcome. In men, the highest risk for urethral recurrence of UC is in patients who have involvement of the prostatic urethra [13]. While some have advocated pre-cystectomy biopsies of the distal prostatic urethra, it is generally felt that the most accurate information about prostatic involvement comes from intra-operative frozen section. This information is critical to the decision to proceed with neobladder or convert to an ileal conduit. Tumor multifocality, and orthotopic diversion (versus conduit) are also associated with urethral recurrence, but to a much lesser degree than prostatic urethral involvement [13]. Interestingly, carcinoma in situ (CIS) and pathologic stage at radical cystectomy are not predictive of urethral recurrence.

In women, studies have shown that the bladder neck is not necessary to obtain acceptable continence rates after neobladder formation (90 % daytime and 57 % nighttime continence) [14]. Sparing the external urethral sphincter along with creation of a capacious neobladder provides for excellent continence. In terms of cancer control, women with UC or atypia at the bladder neck at the time of cystectomy should be strongly advised against orthotopic diversion [15]. Likewise, UC invasion of the vagina or cervix portends an unacceptably high risk for urethral recurrence and these patients should not receive a neobladder.

Renal and hepatic function are important factors to consider when performing orthotopic neobladder. Use of ileum in the urinary tract carries the risk for hyperchloremic, hypokalemic metabolic acidosis. Urinary solutes, such as urea, potassium, ammonium, and bicarbonate, are absorbed in higher quantities than would be absorbed in an ileal conduit because of the greater surface area. Patients with a creatinine level less than 1.7 mg/dL and an eGFR greater than 35–40 mL/min are considered acceptable candidates for neobladder [16]. Liver function must also be adequate to prevent hyperammonemia with the increased resorption of solute that occurs with a neobladder (See Table 17.2).

Treatment of other pelvic malignancies, such as prostate and cervical cancer, with pelvic radiation is a common risk factor for bladder cancer [17]. The prevalence of prior radiation in patients undergoing radical cystectomy in large series is approximately 8 % [18]. This predicts a higher long-term incontinence rate and higher perioperative complication rate; however, a neobladder can be safe and effective in a very appropriately selected patient with a history of pelvic radiation [19].

Other factors are also important to the choice of urinary diversion. In general, the overall health status of the patient should be evaluated by the physician to determine if the patient will be able to adequately care for the neobladder. Age is not an absolute contra-indication to neobladder formation but older patients who are debilitated and have multiple medical co-morbidities are often not as dexterous or well suited to maintain a neobladder, especially if SIC is required. An ileal conduit is easier to sustain and eliminates the risk of needing SIC. Urethral stricture disease is not an absolute contraindication for neobladder; however, if the degree of stricture is severe, orthotopic diversion should not be used. Prior prostate or urethral surgery may also add a level of complexity to the urethral dissection and anastomosis, but this does not preclude neobladder formation. Extra care must be taken during the dissection around the urethra in order to maintain the rhabdosphincter. Body mass index (BMI) is another consideration for the type of diversion to be performed. Obese patients may have a fat, short mesentery and when coupled with a thick abdominal wall, an ileal conduit can be difficult to construct. A neobladder in these patients often alleviates these problems and avoids post-operative issues with ischemia to the distal conduit segment. Before neobladder formation in these patients; however, the surgeon must also ensure that part of the bowel segment reaches the pelvis for urethral anastomosis (See Table 17.2).

17.4 Surgical Preparation

Surgical preparation depends on the type of bowel to be used. Use of a bowel prep for ileal diversions has not demonstrated any short or long-term benefit [20]. For neobladders involving colon, a clear liquid diet and full bowel prep the day before surgery are recommended along with an enema 1–2 h before surgery. Colonoscopy is also warranted to rule out malignancy prior to use of this bowel segment.

Deep vein thrombosis (DVT) prophylaxis is used prior to incision for radical cystectomy and a broad spectrum antibiotic covering skin and enteric flora is also recommended.

17.5 Bowel Segment

Urologists have a variety of options available for orthotopic diversions and each segment has advantages and disadvantages. Surgeon preference is the most important consideration, but this must be adapted to each patient specifically in order to obtain the best outcome possible.

Ileum is the most common segment used in neobladders because it the most compliant and affords the lowest filling pressure [21]. It is easily mobilized into the pelvis and most urologists are familiar with the properties of this bowel. The main disadvantage to use of ileum is the risk of vitamin B-12 deficiency. This is avoided by leaving the distal-most segment of ileum intact. Ileum may also be unacceptable for use because of inflammatory bowel disease (IBD). As described earlier, the metabolic abnormality associated with this bowel segment is hyperchloremic hypokalemic metabolic acidosis. Chronically, this can lead to bone demineralization as bone serves as a buffer to chronic acidosis in these patients. Periodic bone mineral density analysis is recommended and bony complications associated with this bowel segment can often be prevented with potassium citrate.

Colon is the second most frequently used bowel segment in orthotopic diversions. Colon is generally less distensible and results in higher pressures than neobladders using ileum alone. Like ileal neobladders, hyperchloremic hypokalemic metabolic acidosis can occur with use of colon and this is also treated with potassium citrate.

Stomach and jejunum are rarely used in orthotopic diversion because of the associated metabolic complications and because of the difficulty mobilizing these segments down into the pelvis for urethral anastomosis. Use of stomach can cause hypochloremic hypokalemic metabolic alkalosis and can result in hematuria dysuria syndrome. Use of jejunum causes hypochloremic hyperkalemic hyponatremic metabolic acidosis and results in severe dehydration.

17.6 Techniques for Orthotopic Diversion

Numerous techniques are used by urologists to fold bowel segments into a reservoir for orthotopic diversion and most of these have acceptable long-term outcomes. The most important consideration for the surgeon is the use of a familiar technique that can be perfected and replicated with each diversion. Generally, the bowel is detubularized to prevent high pressure contractions and non-absorbable suture is avoided to prevent a nidus for stone formation.

Ureteral stents are placed before final closure of the neobladder. The stents are either brought out percutaneously, through the urethra, or left in the bladder and removed cystoscopically later. A suprapubic tube is optional and may be left to maximize drainage during the healing process. An intraperitoneal drain is also left in place to drain any leakage and prevent abscess formation.

We describe some of the most commonly used techniques using ileum for creating a neobladder; however, it should be recognized that there are many other options and variations to the techniques that are described herein.

Hautmann "W" Ileal Neobladder

Hautmann first described his technique for neobladder formation in 1988 [2]. Seventy centimeters (cm) of terminal ileum is harvested and folded into a "W" with an equal length for each limb of the W. The bowel is detubularized along the anti-mesenteric border and the inner-most aspect of each limb is sutured together. A buttonhole incision on the distal aspect of one of the limbs is created and the urethral anastomosis completed. The ureters are anastomosed to the neobladder in an end-to-side fashion, and the outside edges of the W are closed to each other in a

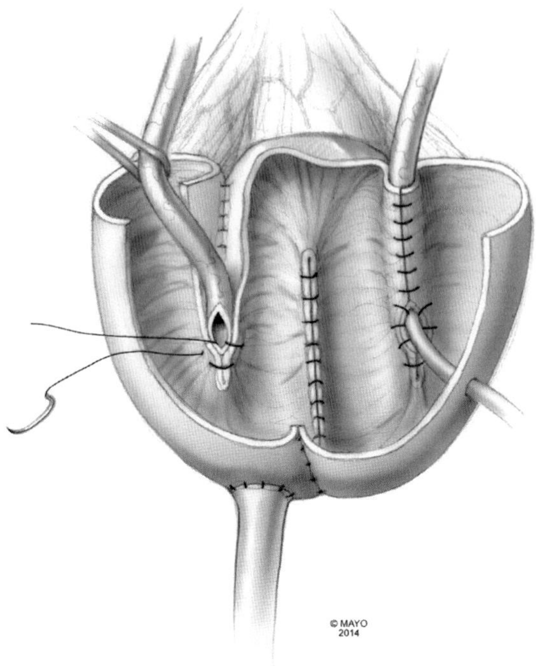

Fig. 17.1 Hautmann neobladder: a Hautmann neobladder utilizes 70 cm of terminal ileum folded into a W configuration (By permission of Mayo Foundation for Medical Education and Research. All rights reserved)

side-to-side fashion (See Fig. 17.1). The advantages to this technique are the large capacity which decreases nocturnal incontinence, and the ability to leave the ends of the W long if the ureters are short. The main disadvantage also stems from the large size of this diversion. As the neobladder matures and expands with time, patients can experience an increase in absorption of urinary solutes and also have a higher risk of retention.

A variation of this technique, called the serous-lined extra-mural tunnel, was first described by Abol-Enein in dogs and eventually tested in humans [22]. Forty centimeters of terminal ileum are used instead of 70 cm. A trough is made for the ureters between the first and second limbs, as well as the third and fourth limbs of the W. The ureters are then laid into the troughs, spatulated, and anastomosed to the mucosa at the inside corners of the W. The bowel mucosa is then closed over the top of the ureter in each trough, and the neobladder is closed in side-to-side fashion, similarly to Hautmann's technique. The serous troughs serve as an anti-refluxing mechanism, but also increase the risk of distal ureteral obstruction. A very long ureteral length is necessary for this diversion, so this is not possible unless the distal ureters are free of UC (Fig. 17.1).

Studer Ileal Neobladder

This neobladder is the most commonly performed orthotopic diversion because it is simple to construct and gives the urologist a great deal of flexibility with the uretero-ileal and urethral anastomoses. A 50–60 cm segment of terminal ileum is isolated, detubularized, and folded into a "U" configuration, leaving the proximal 10–15 cm segment (chimney) tubularized and isoperistaltic for ureteral anastomosis. The bottom half of the U is folded vertically and prior to closure, the urethral anastomosis is performed. The ureters are anastomosed to the chimney with the Bricker or Wallace technique (See Fig. 17.2).

This simple, elegant diversion avoids the use of staples, accommodates short ureters, has a low rate of anastomotic stricture, and provides for excellent continence rates [23].

T-Pouch Ileal Neobladder

The T-pouch was described by Stein and Skinner [4] and is similar to the anti-refluxing anastomotic technique of the serous lined tunnel. Forty-four centimeters of terminal ileum are harvested and the proximal 8–10 cm are left tubularized and isoperistaltic for uretero-ileal anastomosis. The distal portion of the bowel segment is detubularized and folded into a U configuration. A trough in the upper aspect of the U is created for the distal part of the tubularized segment to lie. The mucosa of the bowel segments is sutured together and the bowel is then closed over this segment. The distal half of the U is then folded vertically and closed after stent placement and urethral anastomosis (See Fig. 17.3). This technique preserves an anti-refluxing mechanism and avoids the increased risk of ureteral stricture that was historically seen with the Koch pouch.

Uretero-Neobladder Anastomosis

There has been considerable debate in the literature regarding use of anti-refluxing ureteral anastomosis for urinary diversion. Long term renal deterioration is observed with refluxing anastomoses in a significant proportion of patients, and was more common in patients receiving ileal conduit (36 %) versus Studer Neobladder (21 %) [24]. Patients with neobladders usually void by valsalva maneuvers which can create reflux of urine. Not only does this cause a "waterhammer" effect on the kidney, but it also causes reflux of bacteria into the upper tracts, increasing the risk for pyelonephritis and scarring. This is a critical problem in children, but also effects adults with urinary diversions. Approximately 30 % of patients with a neobladder have asymptomatic bacteriuria and 58 % will have a urinary tract infection (UTI) by 5 years after diversion [25]. The surgeon must weigh the benefit of prevention of bacterial reflux with the increased risk of stenosis with an anti-refluxing anastomosis.

17.7 Urethral Dissection and Anastomosis

In both men and women, extreme care should be taken during dissection near the membranous urethra and its surrounding attachments. Large suture bites through the pelvic floor muscles and rhabdosphincter should be avoided. In men, a nerve sparing approach is felt to help maintain continence. In women, the anterior vaginal wall should be spared if oncologically feasible to preserve sexual function. When a strip of vagina must be taken with the bladder, an omental flap between the vagina and neobladder should be employed to prevent formation of a fistula [26]. The apex of the vagina should then be suspended to the uterosacral ligaments if possible.

Sub Figures are Overlapped, Please Check

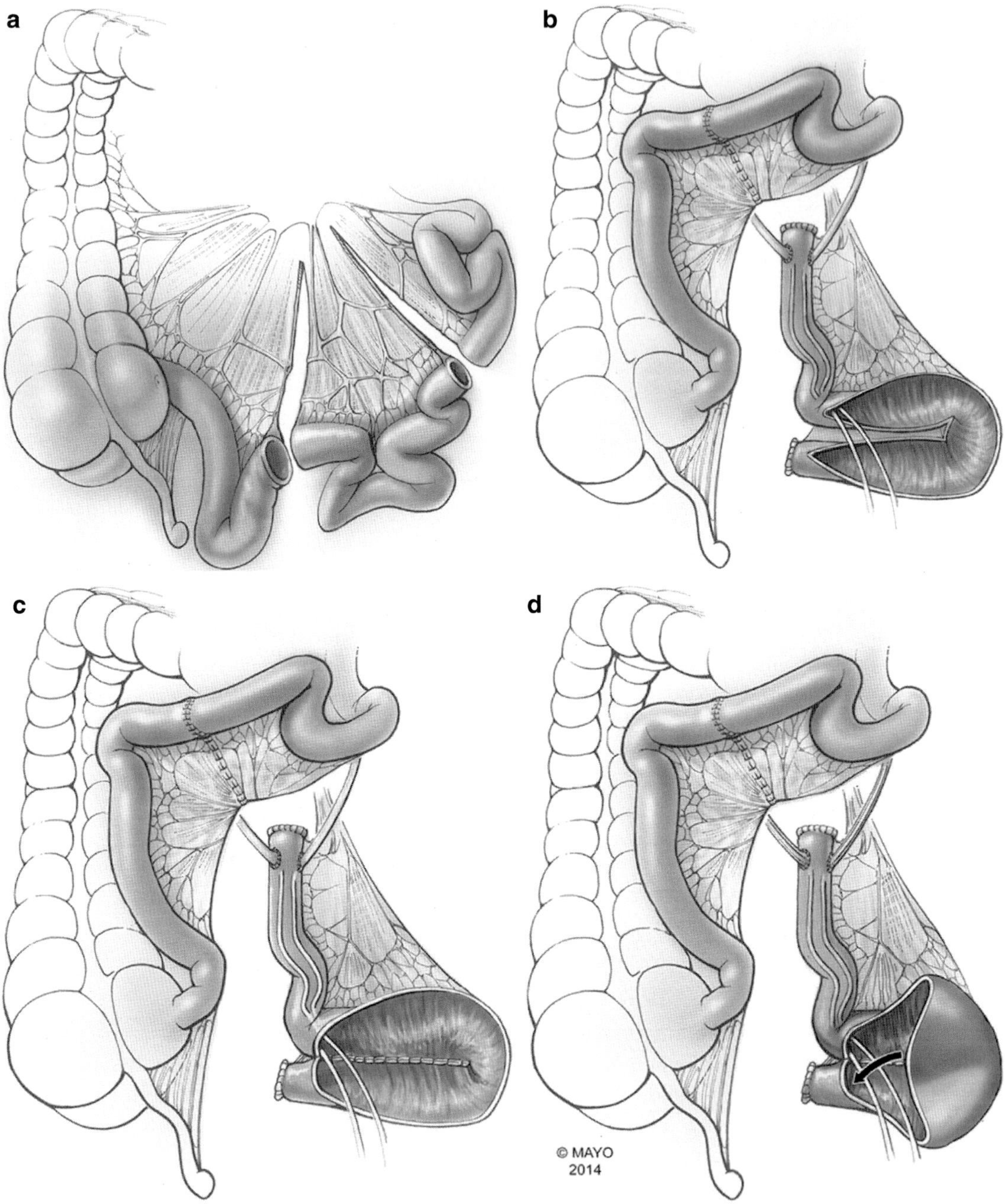

Fig. 17.2 Studer neobladder: the Studer neobladder is formed with a tubularized "chimney" to prevent retrograde reflux of urine. The distal bowel segment is folded into a U configuration and folded on itself to resemble a sphere. **a**) Isolate and harvest 50–60 cm; **b**) ureters anastomosed to the 10 to 15 cm chimmney; **c**) U-shape created from detubularized ileum; **d**) the pouch is folded on itself to create a sphere; and **e**) final closure of the Studer pouch with stents externalized (By permission of Mayo Foundation for Medical Education and Research. All rights reserved)

e

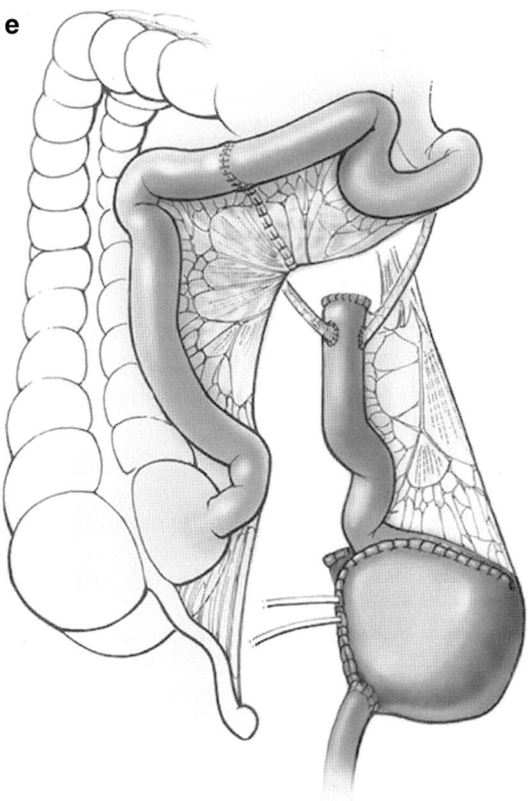

Fig. 17.2 (continued)

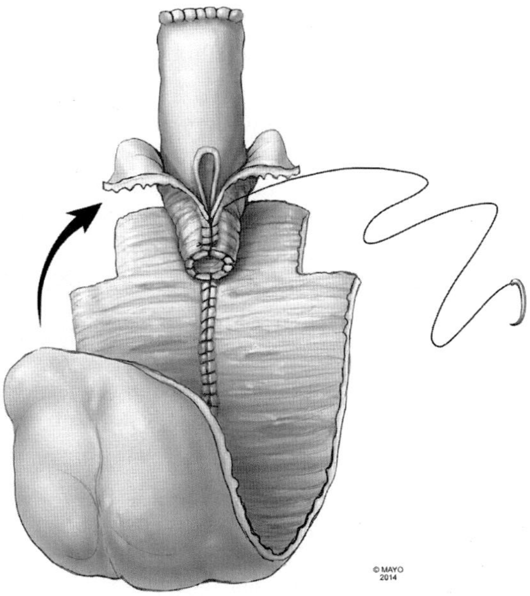

Fig. 17.3 T pouch neobladder: the T pouch neobladder utilizes a separate proximal bowel segment to create a non-refluxing serous-lined tunnel. The distal bowel segment is folded into a U configuration (By permission of Mayo Foundation for Medical Education and Research. All rights reserved)

17.8 Complications and Outcomes

It is imperative to accurately counsel patients who are considering a neobladder so they can anticipate the rigorous upkeep and understand the benefits and pitfalls of the operation.

Complications with cystectomy and urinary diversion are commonplace. It is important to note that the complication rate with orthotopic diversion is not significantly different to that of ileal conduit formation. Gastrointestinal problems and urine leak are among the most common early complications. Urine leak should be treated initially with diversion using nephrostomy tubes followed by exploration and repair if the leak does not heal spontaneously. Long-term complications include small bowel obstruction (SBO), ureteral/urethral anastomotic stricture, incontinence, and pouch perforation.

Maintenance of continence is the most important quality of life issue for patients with neobladders. There is generally an early period of poor continence/recovery that gradually improves over 6–12 months as the neobladder stretches and the rhabdosphincter is trained [14]. Night-time incontinence is generally more commonplace (20–50 %) than daytime incontinence (7 %). Risk factors for incontinence are increasing age, use of colon, and lack of a nerve sparing approach [27]. If incontinence is significantly bothersome, procedures such as placement of an artificial urinary sphincter (AUS), sling, or bulking agent can alleviate this issue.

Urinary retention is also a significant issue for some patients with neobladders, occurring in 2–6 % in large series [27, 28]. There are many etiologies for retention, including a capacious reservoir, stricture disease, mucus plugging, poor voiding technique, and vaginal prolapse. This is usually more common in females due to angulation between the neobladder and urethra. SIC is usually curative of this problem and prevents UTIs due to urinary stasis. Detailed patient instruction following catheter removal is imperative to proper emptying, although some patients need long-term SIC despite adequate technique.

17.9 Robot-Assisted Intracorporeal Neobladder

Robotic technology has allowed urologists to adapt minimally invasive techniques to many different operations, including radical prostatectomy, partial nephrectomy, sacrocolpopexy, and radical cystectomy. Historically, robotic surgeons would generally extend a mid-line port or make an infraumbilical incision to perform the urinary diversion. Several surgeons recently described successful intracorporeal diversion, including ileal conduit and orthotopic neobladder [29–32]. This is a challenging procedure but has been described as successful with similar early complication rates and favorable outcomes when compared to the open alternative [32].

17.10 Summary

Orthotopic urinary diversion is a safe, well-established surgical option for patients undergoing cystectomy. A properly selected patient can expect voiding function that more closely resembles normal voiding and has the potential to avoid chronic renal deterioration seen with other types of urinary diversions. With diligent follow-up care and maintenance, most patients will have excellent long-term urinary function.

References

1. Camey M, Le Duc A. L'enterocystoplastie avec cystoprostatectomie totale pour cancer de la vessie. Ann d'Urol. 1979;13:114–23.
2. Hautmann RE, Egghart G, Frohneberg D, Miller K. The ileal neobladder. J Urol. 1988;139:39–42.
3. Studer UE, Ackermann D, Casanova GA, Zingg EJ. Three years' experience with an ileal low pressure bladder substitute. Br J Urol. 1989;63:43–52.
4. Stein JP, Lieskovsky G, Ginsberg DA, Bochner BH, Skinner DG. The T pouch: an orthotopic ileal neobladder incorporating a serosal lined ileal antireflux technique. J Urol. 1998;159:1836–42.
5. Borirakchanyavat S, Aboseif SR, Carroll PR, Tanagho EA, Lue TF. Continence mechanism of the isolated female urethra: an anatomical study of the intrapelvic somatic nerves. J Urol. 1997;158:822–6.
6. Parekh DJ, Gilbert WB, Kock MO, Smith Jr JA. Continent urinary reconstruction versus ileal conduit: a contemporary single-institution comparison of perioperative morbidity and mortality. Urology. 2000;55:852–5.
7. Gore JL, Saigal CS, Hanley JM, Schonlau M, Litwin MS. Variations in reconstruction after radical cystectomy. Cancer. 2006;107:729–37.
8. Hautmann RE, de Petriconi RC, Volkmer BG. 25 years of experience with 1000 neobladders: long-term complications. J Urol. 2011;185:2207–12.
9. Nagele U, Kuczyk M, Anastasiadis G, Sievert KD, Seibold J, Stenzl A. Radical cystectomy and orthotopic bladder replacement in females. Eur Urol. 2006;50:249–57.
10. Ahmadi H, Skinner EC, Simma-Chiang C, Miranda G, Cai J, Penson DF, Daneshmand S. Urinary functional outcome following radical cystoprostatectomy and ileal neobladder reconstruction in male patients. J Urol. 2013;189(5):1782–8.
11. Basford JR. The Law of Laplace and its relevance to contemporary medicine and rehabilitation. Arch Phys Med Rehabil. 2002;83(8):1165–70.
12. Camey M. Detubularized U-shaped cystoplasty (Camey 2). Curr Surg Technol Urol. 1990;3:1–6.
13. Boorjan SA, Kim SP, Weight CJ, Cheville JC, Thapa P, Frank I. Risk factors and outcomes of urethral recurrence following radical cystectomy. Eur Urol. 2011;60(6):1266–72.
14. Granberg CF, Boorjan SA, Crispen PL, Tollefson MK, Farmer SA, Frank I, Blute ML. Functional and oncological outcomes after orthotopic neobladder reconstruction in women. BJUI. 2008;102(11):1551–5.
15. Wu SD, Simma-Chang V, Stein JP. Pathology guidelines for orthotopic urinary diversion in women with bladder cancer: a review of the literature. Rev Urol. 2006;8(2):54–60.
16. Hautmann RE. Urinary diversion: ileal conduit to neobladder. J Urol. 2003;169:834–42.
17. Shirodkar SP, Kishore TA, Soloway MS. The risk and prophylactic management of bladder cancer after various forms of radiotherapy. Curr Opin Urol. 2009;19(5):500–3.
18. Stein JP, Lieskovsky G, Cote R, Groshen S, Feng AC, Boyd S, Skinner E, Bochner B, Thangathurai D, Mikhail M, Raghavan D, Skinner DG. Radical cystectomy in the treatment of invasive bladder cancer: long-term results in 1,054 patients. J Clin Oncol. 2001;19:666–75.
19. Kim HL, Steinberg GD. Complications of cystectomy in patients with a history of pelvic radiation. Urology. 2001;58:557–60.

20. Tabibi A, Simforoosh N, Basiri A, Ezzatnejad M, Abdi H, Farrokhi F. Bowel preparation versus no preparation before ileal urinary diversion. Urology. 2007;70(4):654–8.
21. Santucci RA, Park CH, Mayo ME, Lange PH. Continence and urodynamic parameters of continent urinary reservoirs: comparison of gastric, ileal, ileocolic, right colon, and sigmoid segments. Urology. 1999;54(2):252–7.
22. Abol-Enein H, Ghoneim MA. Optimization of uretero-intestinal anastomosis in urinary diversion: an experimental study in dogs. III. A new antireflux technique for uretero-ileal anastomosis: a serous-lined extramural tunnel. Urol Res. 1993;21(2):135–9.
23. Studer UE, Burckard FC, Schumacher M, Kessler TM, Thoeny H, Fleischmann A, Thalmann GN. Twenty years experience with an ileal orthotopic low pressure bladder substitute—lessons to be learned. J Urol. 2006;176:161–6.
24. Jin XD, Roethlisberger S, Burkhard FC, Birkhaueser F, Thoeny HC, Studer UE. Long-term renal function after urinary diversion by ileal conduit or orthotopic ileal bladder substitution. Eur Urol. 2012;61(3):491–7.
25. Wood Jr DP, Bianco Jr FJ, Pontes JE, Heath MA, DaJusta D. Incidence and significance of positive urine cultures in patients with an orthotopic neobladder. J Urol. 2003;169:2196–9.
26. Tunuguntla HS, Manoharan M, Gousse AE. Management of neobladder-vaginal fistula and stress incontinence following radical cystectomy in women: a review. World J Urol. 2005;3(4):231–5.
27. Hautmann RE, DePetriconi R, Gottfried HW, Kleinschmidt K, Mattes R, Paiss T. The ileal neobladder: complications and functional results in 363 patients after 11 years of followup. J Urol. 1999;161:422–7.
28. Abol-Enein H, Ghoneim MA. Functional results of orthotopic ileal neobladder with serous-lined extramural ureteral reimplantation: experience with 450 patients. J Urol. 2001;165:1427–32.
29. Johnson D, Castle E, Pruthi R, Woods ME. Robotic intracorporeal urinary diversion: ileal conduit. J Endourol. 2012;26(12):1566–9.
30. Pruthi RS, Nix J, McRackan D, Hickerson A, Nielsen ME, Raynor M, Wallen EM. Robot-assisted laparoscopic intracorporeal urinary diversion. Eur Urol. 2010;57:1013–21.
31. Tyritzis SI, Hosseini A, Jonsson M, Adding C, Nilsson A, Wiklund NP. Robot-assisted intracorporeal formation of the ileal neobladder. J Endourol. 2012;26(12):1–6.
32. Goh AC, Gill IS, Lee DJ, de Castro Abreu AL, Fairey AS, Leslie S, Berger AK, Daneshmand S, Sotelo R, Gill KS, Xie HW, Chu LY, Aron M, Desai MM. Robotic intracorporeal ileal neobladder: replicating open surgical principles. Eur Urol. 2012;62:891–901.

Techniques of Urinary Diversion

18

Richard E. Hautmann

18.1 Introduction

Radical cystectomy and urinary diversion have been assessed the highest relative value in terms of difficulty of the surgery for any procedure in urology. They are also the most difficult laparoscopic or robotic procedures and more so if the diversion is performed totally intracorporeally. The risk of cystectomy and urinary diversion is based not only on the technical challenges of the procedure but also on the nature of the patient's need. The incidence of bladder cancer increases continually with advancing age; thus, the responsibility of providing optimal surgical treatment for elderly and possibly frail patients is common among urologists. Improvement in patient rehabilitation is noteworthy through continent cutaneous diversions and neobladders and better enterostomal therapy support. In this context, there must remain continued emphasis on refining the surgical technique of radical cystectomy and urinary diversion to provide utmost safety for the patient [1, 2]. Unfortunately, not a single randomized controlled study within the field of urinary diversion exists. A recent International Consultation on Urological Diseases (ICUD) has looked at published evidence and produced recommendations. They form the basis of this chapter [1, 2]. This expert opinion is based on almost 16,000 diversions and radical cystectomies. This ICUD committee represents a well-balanced combination of pioneering institutions of any type of diversion, high volume centers and surgeons, as well as data from low volume institutions, plus a leading pediatric urology institution and the Swedish registry for bladder cancer, which reports any case from Sweden, including treatment, that has been observed in the respective period (Table 18.1).

Some conclusions from Table 18.1 are:

- Only 3/11 institutions have experience with any type of diversion
- Anal diversions play no role in the US, but are of value in pediatric patients and in the third world.
- Continent cutaneous diversions play a secondary role; even former pioneering institutions use it with decreasing frequency.
- Conduit (42.2 %) and neobladder (38 %) are the standard diversions at large centers.
- Truly population-based data from the USA and from the Swedish Bladder Cancer Registry (S. Jahnson, Linköping, Sweden) show a neobladder rate in the range of 15 %; with increasing hospital volume the neobladder/continent diversion rate approaches 75 %, addressing the impact of hospital volume on the use of continent reconstruction.

Table 18.1 includes data of seven pioneering institutions of UD. Their average annual RC caseload is 80 (range: 27–100). The Swedish

R.E. Hautmann, MD, MD hon
Department of Urology, University of Ulm, Neu-Ulm, Germany
e-mail: richard.hautmann@uni-ulm.de

H.R.H. Patel et al. (eds.), *Pelvic Cancer Surgery: Modern Breakthroughs and Future Advances*, DOI 10.1007/978-1-4471-4258-4_18, © Springer-Verlag London 2015

Registry includes all RCs performed annually. With a minimum of seven RC centers required for Sweden, the annual caseload would be 30. A minimum annual caseload of 25 RCs done by not more than two surgeons is the basis of a high-volume surgeon. An additional 15–20 cases performed by the next generation of high-volume surgeons under the supervision of the actual high-volume surgeons defines 40–45 RCs per year as a high-volume center [1].

18.2 General Aspects of Urinary Diversion

Urinary Diversion and Real Function

Urinary diversion into bowel segments is not inherently damaging to the kidneys. In general, renal function after diversion into continent detubularized reservoirs compares favorably with ileal conduit diversion. However, the literature is insufficient to recommend one form of diversion over another. There remains a long-term risk of renal deterioration, which is often asymptomatic, and thus close follow-up is necessary for all patients who have undergone urinary diversion in order to identify correctable causes early.

Those with renal pathology prior to surgery seem to be at greatest risk of postoperative renal deterioration. Serum creatinine is an imprecise measure of renal function. Isotopic GFR measurement will detect renal function deterioration most accurately and at an early stage. The latter, however, is not available to all patients. In these situations, follow-up with serum creatinine and ultrasound should be followed by diuresis renography if upper tract dilation is seen. Early intervention for physical obstruction often results in a sustained improvement in renal function [2].

Secondary Tumors After Urinary Diversion

Patients who have undergone conduit diversion, continent cutaneous diversion, or orthotopic bladder substitution do not seem to be at increased risk of secondary malignancy. By comparison, the risk is slightly higher after cystoplasty, albeit not increased enough to support endoscopic surveillance. However, the present knowledge regarding gastric cystoplasty is insufficient, and hence patients should be followed after such surgery. Furthermore, yearly colonoscopy is recommended in cases involving ureterosigmoidostomy, beginning 10 years after the procedure [2].

Complications

Radical cystectomy and urinary diversion are two steps of one operation. However, the literature notoriously reports on complications of radical cystectomy, ignoring that the vast majority of complications are diversion-related [3]. Surgical morbidity following urinary diversion is significant and, when strict reporting guidelines are incorporated, higher than previously published (20–57 %). Accurate reporting of postoperative complications after radical cystectomy is essential for counseling patients, combined modality treatment planning, clinical trial design, and assessment of surgical success [3].

Urinary Diversion After Pelvic Irradiation

Tumor recurrence in patients who had received definitive radiation therapy may be followed by salvage radical cystectomy. Historically, these patients have been considered to have a risk of significant postoperative morbidity and unsatisfactory functional results. Complications have been attributed to radiation damage to the ureter and bowel, resulting in increased rates of anastomotic problems, upper urinary tract obstruction, and infection. Therefore, most centers use supravesical urinary diversion with a transverse colonic segment or cutaneous ureterostomy.

During pelvic radiotherapy for cancer, the cecal pole as well as parts of the ascending colon, appendix and ileum are exposed to considerable doses of radiation. Since these segments of bowel are used for reservoir and afferent segment

Table 18.1 Numbers and types of urinary diversions (%) performed by the authors

	#RC	Period	Neo-bladder	Cont. cut	Conduit	UC TUUC	Anal	Unknown no diversion	Others
Ann Arbor	643	95–04	45.1	1.4	53.5	–	–	–	–
	962	00–09	40.0	2.0	58.0	–	–	0.9	–
Bern	611	85–99	51.5	1.5	42.5	1.6	2.5	–	0.4
	708	00–10	51.0	8.0	39.0	1.5	0.5	–	0.1
Kassel	765	94–10	30.2	6.8	60.5	0.7	2.0	0.1	–
Los Angeles	1,359	71–01	51.6	25.8	22.3	–	–	–	0.3
	1,012	00–10	74.2	5.3	20.2	–	–	0.3	–
Lund	119	00–04	28.6	31.1	40.3	–	–	–	–
	134	04–09	6.0	30.6	63.4	–	–	–	–
Mainz	335	68–80	–	–	55.0	–	45	–	–
	593	81–90	2.0	33	41.0	–	15	–	9
	982	91–00	6.0	39	41.0	–	12	–	2
	1,023	01–10	15.0	24	53.0	–	4	–	4
Mansoura	3,157	80–04	39.1	3.5	34.4	–	23.1	–	–
Norwich	246	02–09	10.6	–	89.4	–	–	–	–
Swedish/Registry	158	1997	19.0	19	55.0	–	–	7	–
	221	2003	17.0	12	70.0	–	–	1	–
	208	2006	9.0	6	80.0	–	–	5	–
	229	2008	15.0	4	81.0	–	–	–	–
Ulm	1,613	86–09	66.0	0.4	22.0	10.0	1.3	0.2	–
Vanderbilt	789	00–07	35.5	0.4	63.5	–	0.1	–	0.5
Total	15,867		38.0	10.4	42.2	1.2	7.5	0.1	0.8

construction, it is plausible that the high complication rate that was observed was secondary to radiation damage of the intestinal segments.

Since radiation damage is historically known to increase with time, these aspects are especially important when evaluating complications of surgical procedures in irradiated patients, Proper patient selection for salvage surgery has also contributed to the improvements in long-term outcome. Selection of appropriate surgical candidates for salvage therapy depends on several factors: recurrent prostate or bladder cancer versus gastrointestinal or gynecologic cancer, extent of recurrent disease, and existence of fistula formation. It is believed that patients with more advanced local disease, refractory voiding symptoms related to a fibrosed non-functional bladder, or severe symptoms related to other complications associated with the prior irradiation will be better served with cystectomy and lower urinary tract reconstruction. Based on the published long-term experience, salvage surgery (cystoprostatectomy, anterior exenteration) with orthotopic lower urinary tract reconstruction is a safe, effective procedure that can provide a potential curative intervention and a functional lower urinary tract for properly selected patients in whom previous definitive radiation therapy has failed, with results only marginally worse as compared to nun-irradiated patients, at least in high volume centers [2].

18.3 Continent Diversion

Orthotopic Bladder Substitution in Men

The extent of pelvic disease has little bearing on the appropriateness of a neobladder. If pelvic recurrence does develop, it does not usually have a significant impact on the function of a neobladder and patients who have positive pelvic nodes can achieve good functional results.

The risk of urethral recurrence after a neobladder is generally 5–10 % and it usually occurs in the first 3 years when it does happen. A high risk is a contraindication to a neobladder, but prediction of risk is not simple. Reported risk factors for urethral recurrence include multifocal disease, carcinoma in situ, prior intravesical chemotherapy, ureteric disease, and urothelial cancer in the distal prostatic urethra. Nevertheless, an intraoperative frozen section of the resection margin is considered sufficient by many centers. Biopsies done before cystectomy also enable discussion of the result with the patient, who then has greater certainly that orthotopic bladder substitution will be possible at the time of cystectomy [1].

Age and Motivation

Although there is no age cut-off for a neobladder, in practice many patients over the age of 70 years will opt for a simpler conduit urinary diversion as the postoperative course is less arduous and urinary incontinence is less likely. The motivation of the patient is probably the most important factor when considering their suitability for a neobladder, although it is difficult to assess this objectively. Patients must be prepared to commit to the long-term follow-up program necessary.

Sphincter Function

Urinary continence after orthotopic bladder substitution depends, amongst other factors, on adequate urethral sphincter function. Caution should be exercised before offering orthotopic bladder substitution in patients with significant urethral strictures.

Surgical Technique

If tumor characteristics permit, then nerve sparing should be attempted. This can be bilateral if disease is not muscle-invasive, or unilateral if there is lateralized muscle-invasive disease. In men, the nerves are at particular risk dorsolateral to the seminal vesicles, in the vesicoprostatic angle, and in the region of the prostatic apex (Fig. 18.1).

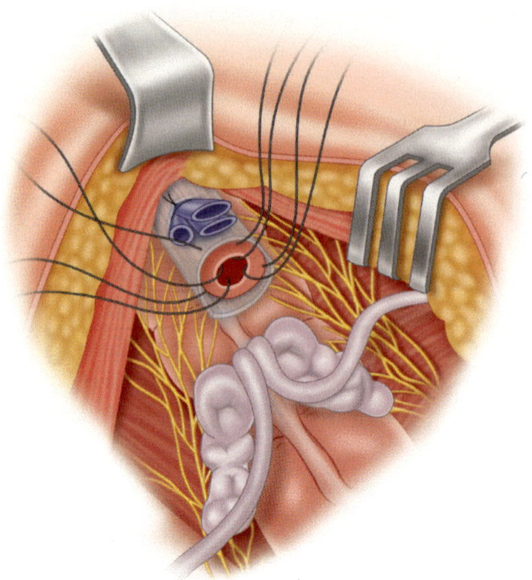

Fig. 18.1 Final situation after nerve- and seminal vesicle sparing radical cystectomy: The procedure starts as a standard nerve-sparing radical prostatectomy (RP). After transection of the urethra with Denonvillier's fascia still intact, vasa deferentia and seminal vesicles are transected at the base of the prostate, and the trigone is undermined to the space of Douglas. The cystectomy is completed in ascending or preferably descending fashion (Reprinted from Hautmann et al. [6]. With permission from Elsevier)

Reservoir Configuration

A neobladder must be a low-pressure reservoir of adequate capacity and must empty to completion. If this is so, the upper urinary tracts will be preserved, and metabolic disturbance will be minimal. Many surgical techniques have been reported but some key factors are alike. Detubularization and a spherical shape ensure that an orthotopic bladder substitute has low pressure and maximum volume for the length of bowel used (Fig. 18.2). Popular techniques include an ileal afferent limb orthotopic bladder substitute using 55 cm of distal ileum, preserving the 25 cm of terminal ileum, and the W-shaped classical ileal neobladder.

A simple end-to-side freely refluxing anastomosis into an afferent limb of a low pressure orthotopic reconstruction (Fig. 18.3) is sufficient.

Minimally-Invasive Surgery

There is increasing interest in laparoscopic and robotic cystectomy, with either intracorporeal or

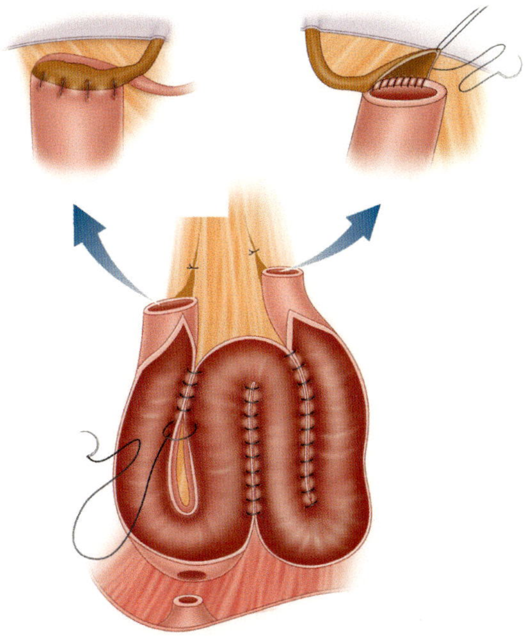

Fig. 18.2 W-shaped reconfiguration of the intestinal segment after detubularization and asymmetric incision of the ileal wall at the site of the anastomosis to the urethra, forming a U-shaped flap. Refluxing ileo-ureteral anastomosis using chimneys of a 3–5 cm afferent limb on each side

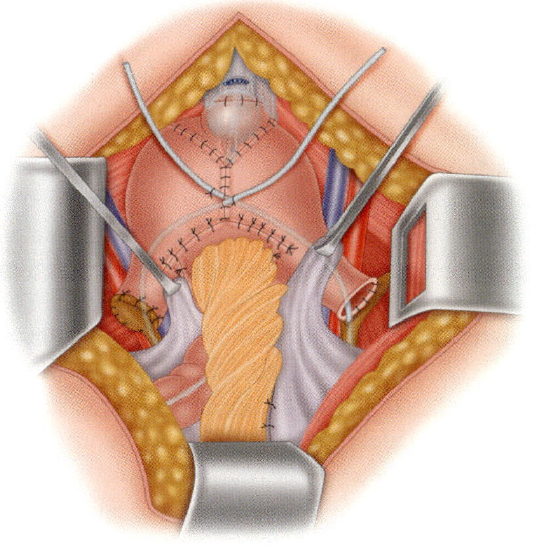

Fig. 18.3 Completely extraperitoneal localization of neobladder as well as ileo-urethral and ileo-ureteral anastomoses

management and regular long-term follow-up of patients with an orthotopic bladder substitute. The key issues are achieving a capacity of 400–500 mL, residual free voiding of sterile urine, and the treatment of any outlet obstruction [1].

Orthotopic Diversion in Females

A number of the contraindications to continent diversion are identical for men and women. These include the basic requirements of adequate renal function, available healthy bowel, and a functional urethral sphincter. Pre existing incontinence is a relative contraindication for women considering a neobladder. A woman with stress urinary incontinence may be willing to continue to wear pads rather than deal with a stoma, or may be considered for a sling or Burch procedure at the time of diversion with planned self catheterization. Age alone is not a criterion for offering continent diversion. Women over age 75 are at higher risk of incontinence but some of them will have excellent neobladder function [1].

Complications

Most of the early and late complications of women undergoing radical cystectomy and neobladder are identical to those of men and are managed in a similar fashion. Two complications are different in female patients:

- Pouch-vaginal Fistula
- Urinary Retention

Urinary retention is clearly more common in women than men undergoing orthotopic diversion. Such retention may occur early, but often appears after a year or more of good neobladder function and emptying. In the Ulm series of 116 women, the rate of retention increased steadily over time to approximately 50 % by 5 years. The etiology has been debated, but most authors believe it is due to a mechanical kink in the urethra-pouch anastomosis as the full pouch falls posteriorly during Valsalva maneuver. This can often be documented on a lateral straining cystogram. However, not all patients with retention have this finding. Other suggested etiologies include autonomic denervation of the urethral stump or disordered reinnervation resulting in inability to relax the sphincter [2].

Treatment of retention is intermittent catheterization. Transurethral resection of an urethral fold and open reduction of the pouch size with anterior fixation to the abdominal wall have also been described. It is clear that every woman undergoing neobladder reconstruction should be advised that intermittent catheterization may be required for adequate emptying and must be willing and able to learn how to perform this. Many women who are dry but require self-catheterization seem quite happy with the diversion in spite of this [2].

It is reasonable to advise against neobladder reconstruction for a woman with invasive bladder neck involvement or suspected invasion of the vaginal wall or cervix. However, such patients may be considered for neobladder diversion if intraoperative frozen section of the urethral margin is negative. It appears that overall 60–70 % of women undergoing cystectomy might be reasonable candidates for continent diversion [2].

Continent Cutaneous Urinary Diversion

The modern era of continent urinary diversion began 30 years ago with the introduction of continent cutaneous diversion, which at that time was represented by the Kock pouch. Since then, numerous techniques for this type of diversion have been described, but some of these appeared only once in the literature, indicating that they were associated with technical problems, high complication rates, and suboptimal functional results. Today, only a handful of methods are in use, and, in general, they are the second choice after orthotopic bladder substitution for patients undergoing radical cystectomy.

Indications

In patients with bladder cancer undergoing radical cystectomy, the main indication for continent cutaneous diversion is when urethral removal is deemed necessary due to a high risk of recurrence of urothelial carcinoma. The risk can be estimated based on the pathology report from the preoperative transurethral resection biopsies of the prostate. Such biopsies should be taken from the bladder neck to the verumontanum on both sides before cystectomy. Relying on frozen sections of the urethra obtained during surgery may be dangerous because of the risk of a false negative report from the pathologist. Urothelial cell carcinoma locates in the urethra or involving prostatic ducts or stroma is the main indication for urethrectomy.

In female patients, biopsies should also be obtained from the bladder neck, and, if positive urethrectomy should be performed. Furthermore, it is necessary to exercise caution if there is a tumor close to the bladder neck, as well as in cases involving widespread CIS. Optimal knowledge regarding the urothelial pathology of the lower urinary tract is of importance when informing and discussing with the patient preoperatively.

Some patients may prefer continent diversion to orthotopic reconstruction because of the risk of urine leakage after the latter procedure.

The Outlet

- Intussuscepted ileal nipple valve
- Mainz pouch I
- Appendix
- Tapered/stapled ileal outlet
- Indiana pouch
- Lundiana pouch
- Serous-lined extramural valve/T-pouch

Continent cutaneous diversion has a place as an option for reconstruction of the urinary tract in patients who undergo cystectomy. The main indications seem to be in patients in whom urethrectomy has to be performed and in those in whom the prospect of possible urine leakage after orthotopic neobladder is repugnant. Multiple techniques have been described. However, many of them are too complicated to gain widespread acceptance. Simplicity characterizes the appendiceal outlet and the outlet of the different modifications of the Indiana pouch, and excellent functional results can be obtained. However, complications from the pouch and the outlet are not infrequent and lifelong surveillance of these patients is necessary [1, 2].

18.4 Incontinent Diversion

Conduit Urinary Diversion

Urinary conduit using ileum is the most commonly performed conduit procedure. Studies comparing ileal or colonic urinary conduit diversion have documented fairly similar long- and short-term complication rates. It is likely that ileum is used more commonly because it is the technically simplest conduit to perform. Acknowledging this, there are still settings where it is preferable that colon, as opposed to ileum, be used. Specifically, in the setting of patients with short bowel syndrome or in patients who have had prior irradiation of the ileum or distal ureters, a colonic conduit should be considered. Another setting where a sigmoid colon conduit should be considered is in the patient who is undergoing en bloc resection of the colon or rectum, as this may eliminate the need for an additional bowel anastomosis [1, 2].

Nevertheless, ileal conduit diversion remains the most commonly used method for reconstructing the urinary tract in conjunction with radical cystectomy. It is probably technically easier than continent reconstruction. However, the complications, early as well as late, are legion. It is difficult to draw definitive comparisons with other diversion techniques as surgical techniques have improved markedly over the last 25 years, and few series report comparable long-term outcomes (>20 years) in patients with neobladders.

Ureterosigmoidostomy

Regarding this type of diversion, there is no really new information. This corresponds to conduit diversion.

Although the mortality and initial morbidity following ureterosimoidostomy have been significantly reduced, some inherent chronic complications remain problematic.

18.5 Palliative Urinary Diversion

The issue of palliation and urinary diversion centers around two issues: (1) management of elderly/geriatric patients with muscle-invasive bladder cancer in whom radical cystectomy/urinary diversion is associated with a considerable morbidity and mortality, and (2) patients with tumor-induced upper urinary tract dilatation and renal insufficiency in a palliative setting.

Cutaneous Ureterostomy

This is the most popular form of alternative non-bowel type of diversion in elderly patients or in a palliative setting. Operative time is short, and renal function is not a selection factor. Construction of a single stoma in the lateral or midline position is generally feasible and ensures easy care with minimal patient discomfort (Table 18.2).

Defunctionalization of the Contralateral Renal Unit

If only one kidney is diverted and urine continues to flow downstream, it may be necessary to defunctionalize the latter. These patients are usually poor candidates for nephrectomy. In a previously obstructed kidney, ligation of the ureter usually causes significant pain and spontaneous ureteral recanalization. In these cases, renal arterial embolization should be considered [2].

Percutaneous Nephrostomy

Drainage of an obstructed upper urinary tract caused by a locally advanced or metastatic urothelial cancer leads to an ethical dilemma—is such drainage going to facilitate treatment with chemotherapy or radiotherapy, or is it perpetuating and allowing other problems to develop? Only patients with specific cancers (e.g., prostate

Table 18.2 Advantages and disadvantages of conduit and UC/TUUC UD

	UC/TUUC	Conduit
Advantages	Safe and easy	Safe and reliable
	Fast	Gold standard of UD
	Short LOS	Most frequently used UD
	Low perioperative complication rate	Low stomal stenosis rate
	Easy access to upper tract	No metabolic complications
	QoL acceptable	QoL high
Disadvantages	Stomal stenosis rate high	Complications are legend
		Complications increase linear to time
	Lifelong need mono/double J	Abdominal procedure
	Difficult with short ureters	Risk of intestinal leakage
		Risk of parastomal hernia
	UTI	UTI
	Skin reaction	Longer LOS
		More difficult access to upper tract

UD urinary diversion, *UC* cutaneous ureterostomy, *TUUC* trans-uretero-ureterostomy, *LOS* length of stay, *QoL* quality of life

cancer) that progress slowly by nature may substantially benefit from the procedure. Bilateral nephrostomies are generally poorly tolerated and usually only the renal unit with the better function should be diverted by nephrostomy. Subcutaneous pyelovesical diversion ensures a better quality of life than classical percutaneous nephrostomy in cancer patients at the palliative stage [2].

These data suggest that in patients with a limited life expectancy permanent stents might be an option.

The decision regarding bladder sparing or radical cystectomy in the elderly/geriatric patient with invasive bladder cancer should be based on tumor stage and comorbidity best quantified by a validated score, such as the Charlson score. Chronological age is of limited relevance. Cutaneous ureterostomy is the most popular non-bowel urinary diversion in this setting, providing adequate quality of life. The issue of decompression of an obstructed urinary tract in a patient with advancing pelvic malignancy (particularly bladder cancer) remains a difficult clinical situation. The indication for drainage should only be made when the views and wishes of the patient and caregivers are taken into account. The prognosis remains very poor.

18.6 Current Status of the Urinary Bladder in Regenerative Medicine

There are possible advantages offered by regenerative medicine over currently available treatment. A tissue-engineered bladder augment or neobladder lined by autologous urothelium (rather than intestinal epithelium) could be predicted to overcome most of the complications associated with conventional enterocystoplasty. The risks and complications associated with intestinal resection in poor-risk patients undergoing cystectomy for bladder cancer might also be obviated by the availability of a tissue-engineered urinary conduit.

The ideal material for bladder augmentation or substitution would, therefore, combine the compliance conferred by smooth muscle with a urinary barrier, as provided by the urothelium.

An ideal tissue engineered urinary bladder would mimic the range of functions fulfilled by the normal healthy bladder. Adequate compliance is critical to the low pressure storage of urine and protection of the upper urinary tract. As normal bladder function is dependent on a complex interplay between neuronal circuits, detrusor muscle and sphincteric complex, the creation of a functioning neobladder may in fact represent one of the most challenging tasks for tissue engineering. However, as an interim approach, it seems reasonable to assume that clean intermittent catheterization can be relied upon to substitute for the voiding component of bladder function.

The long term durability of tissues arising from implanted cell-scaffold constructs will need to be addressed in future studies, especially in pediatric patients in whom the regenerated tissue would be retained over their remaining life-time [4].

The mechanisms of urothelial tissue regeneration in vivo are still poorly understood and, although the presence of slow-cycling cells in rat urothelium has been described a distinct resident human urothelial stem cells populations has not yet been identified. Isolated human urothelial cells show a highly proliferative phenotype, but enter a senescent state after a finite number of cell divisions in vitro. It will be clinically relevant to assess whether ex vitro urothelium shows a long term regenerative capacity in vivo [4]. The potential to acquire full voiding function by a reconstructed urinary bladder is questionable. Although smooth muscle cell contraction has been reported from cultured smooth muscle cells and different studies have indicated the formation of neuronal structures, a voluntarily-controlled voiding function seems unlikely, particularly where the graft exceeds a critical size.

18.7 Alloplastic Bladder Substitution

Although artificial substitution of the bladder would be desirable due to the physical, psychological, technical, and economic benefits, an alloplastic material with compatible properties to the human body has yet to be discovered. So, the answer to the question "are we making progress?" must be unequivocal "no" or "not sufficient." Indeed, the repeated failure of this therapeutic approach has been one of the factors prompting researchers to explore tissue engineering and other alternatives to conventional enterocystoplasty. Inter-professional collaboration, recent advances in technology, and innovations in tissue engineering may help in developing suitable alloplastic prosthesis. Therefore both urologists, as well as engineers and the industry need to give this matter a serious attention [5].

18.8 Summary

At high volume hospitals, orthotopic reconstruction has become the procedure of choice for urinary diversion. In these patients, the construction of a neobladder allows the elimination of a stoma and preservation of body image without compromising the cancer control. However, the patient must be committed to the labor-intensive rehabilitation process. He or she must also have adequate manual dexterity to perform self-catheterization should it become necessary. When involvement of the lower urinary tract by tumor excludes the use of a neobladder, a continent cutaneous reservoir may still offer some advantages over an ileal conduit. For patients who are not candidates for either type of continent diversion, the ileal loop remains a time-honored option.

Key Points

- Radical cystectomy and urinary diversion have been assessed the highest relative value of difficulty of the surgery of any procedure in urology, resulting in a low acceptance of neobladder reconstruction as seen from population-based data.
- The perioperative and long-term complication rate is significant, even in the most experienced hands, and higher than previously published.
- The morbidity of the procedure is up to 75 % diversion-related.
- This type of surgery should only be performed at high volume hospitals.
- If it is done with the intent to cure high volume surgeons prefer orthotopic reconstruction whenever possible (80 %).

- CCUD is second choice after orthotopic reconstruction and used in cases when the reservoir cannot be anastomosed to the urethra.
- Anal diversions are used in rare circumstances.
- Conduit UD remains the gold standard, against whom the others have to be measured.
- Incontinent diversion including UC, TUCC are done for palliation.
- UD into bowel segments is not interherently damaging to the kidneys as compared to anal UD.
- Conduit, CCUD and orthotopic reconstruction are not at increased risk of secondary malignancy.
- Meticulous follow up after any type of UD is mandatory.

References

1. Hautmann RE, Volkmer BG, Abol-Enein H, Davidsson T, Gudjonsson S, Hautmann S, et al. ICUD-EAU Internationl Consultation on Bladder Cancer 2012: urinary diversion. Eur Urol 2013;63:67–80.
2. Hautmann RE, Volkmer BG, Abol-Enein H, Davidsson T, Gudjonsson S, Hautmann SH, et al. Urinary diversion. In: Soloway M, Khoury S, editors. Bladder cancer. 2nd ed. Vienna: International Consultation on Bladder Cancer – ICUD-EAU; 2012. 2012. Distributor: EDITIONS 21, 5 Boulevard Flandrin – 75016 Paris – France (2012).
3. Hautmann RE, de Petriconi RC, Volkmer BG. Lessons learned from 1,000 neobladders: the 90-day complication rate. J Urol. 2010;184:990–4.
4. Wezel F, Southgate J, Thomas DFM. Regenerative medicine in urology. BJU Int. 2011;108:1046–65.
5. Cosentino M, Breda A, Palou J, Caffaratti J, Villavicencio H. Alloplastic bladder substitution: are we making progress? J Tissue Eng Regen Med. 2012;1(5):343–9.
6. Hautmann RE, Hautmann O, Volkmer BG, Hautmann S. Nerve-sparing radical cystectomy: a new technique. Eur Urol Suppl. 2010;9:428–12.

Single Port Surgery in the Pelvis: Current and Future Feasibility

19

Dinesh Samarasekera, Riccardo Autorino, and Abhay Rane

19.1 Introduction

Laparoendoscopic single site surgery (LESS) has been conceived with the aim of minimizing the morbidity associated with laparoscopic surgery [1]. A broad spectrum of urologic procedures has been shown to be feasible with LESS, including radical nephrectomy and prostatectomy [2, 3].

A number of studies comparing standard urologic laparoscopy to urologic LESS have been reported [4–8]. Overall, these studies suggest that LESS is not inferior to laparoscopic surgery with regards to perioperative outcomes, with a trend towards improved cosmesis and less post-operative pain.

However, it has been recognized that LESS is significantly more challenging, especially when complex reconstruction or intracorporeal suturing is required. The need to cross instruments at the abdominal wall to facilitate dissection results in a significant mental challenge, due to the resulting reverse handedness. Other challenges include instrument collision, lack of triangulation, and in-line vision. A number of strategies were developed to overcome these difficulties, including curved and articulating instruments, flexible endoscopes, and needlescopic accessory ports/instruments [9].

Despite these advances, conventional LESS remains challenging and it requires extensive surgeon experience in laparoscopy and stringent patient selection to achieve successful outcomes [10].

Robotic-assisted laparoscopic surgery offers several advantages when compared to standard laparoscopic surgery, including better visualization, ergonomics, dexterity, and precision. For these same reasons, it was postulated that the application of robotics could facilitate LESS by overcome some of the aforementioned constraints. Kaouk et al. [11] reported the first experience with robotic LESS (R-LESS) in 2008 and immediately noted that intracorporeal suturing and dissection were easier, as compared with standard LESS.

Since then there have been numerous reports and refinements in technique from the same group, for a number different of urologic procedures [12–14]. However, despite the advantages provided by the current da Vinci® robotic platform, R-LESS is not free of challenges. Although solutions are currently under development [15, 16], we are in the infancy of R-LESS.

D. Samarasekera, MD, FRCSC
Glickman Urologic and Kidney Institute, Cleveland Clinic, Cleveland, OH, USA

R. Autorino, MD, PhD, FEBU
Urology Institute, University Hospitals Case Western Reserve University, Cleveland, OH, USA

A. Rane, MS, FRCS (Urol) (✉)
Department of Urology, East Surrey Hospital, Redhill, UK
e-mail: a.rane@btinternet.com

H.R.H. Patel et al. (eds.), *Pelvic Cancer Surgery: Modern Breakthroughs and Future Advances*, DOI 10.1007/978-1-4471-4258-4_19, © Springer-Verlag London 2015

Both conventional LESS and R-LESS have been successfully employed for pelvic malignancies in general surgery, gynecology, and urology [17–19]. This chapter will highlight current applications and challenges as well as future perspectives of LESS in pelvic urologic surgery.

19.2 Patient Selection and Current Indications in Pelvic Surgery

Theoretically, all patients who are eligible for laparoscopic surgery should be eligible for LESS [20]. However, patient selection for LESS in reported series has been more rigorous as compared to standard laparoscopy, despite that fact that the procedures were done by experienced laparoscopic surgeons.

Kaouk et al. [10] performed a multi-institutional review of 1,076 cases (only 3 % were pelvic surgery). Mean age was 52.1 ± 16.9 years, BMI was 25 ± 4.2 kg/m^2, and ASA was 1.7 ± 0.7. Patients tended to be younger, non-obese, and of low surgical risk.

However, as more surgeons gain experience, it is logical to expect that more challenging cases will be attempted, as this was seen with pure laparoscopy. Furthermore, wide adaptation of the robotic platform to LESS, will further aid this progression.

Regarding, more specifically, pelvic surgery, a variety of indications for LESS has been investigated thus far (Table 19.1).

Table 19.1 Pelvic LESS procedures

Indication	LESS procedure
Prostate adenocarcinoma	Radical prostatectomy
TCC bladder	Radical cystoprostatectomy
BPH	Simple prostatectomy (STEP)
Reconstruction	Bladder diverticulectomy
	Ureteral reimplantation
	Vesico-vaginal fistula repair
	Sacrocolpopexy

19.3 LESS Prostate Surgery

Simple Prostatectomy

The open simple prostatectomy remains the gold standard in surgical therapy for prostates larger than 80 g [21]. However, there is still the potential for significant morbidity associated with this procedure, including significant hemorrhage. A number of centers have recently reported their experience with single-port transvesical enucleation of the prostate (STEP) as a minimally invasive alternative. For this procedure ports are placed through the bladder, and the prostate adenoma is enucleated. Desai et al. [22] described their experience with 34 cases in 2010. The mean prostate volume estimated by transrectal ultrasonography was 102.5 mL and the mean baseline prostate-specific antigen level was 6.7 ng/mL. A TriPort (Advanced Surgical Concepts, Wicklow, Ireland) multichannel port was placed into the bladder under direct cystoscopic vision, and pneumovesium of 15 mmHg was achieved. The adenoma was then enucleated with electrocautery or ultrasonic shears, by creating a circumferential mucosal incision at the bladder neck. A stay suture (2-0 polyglactin on CT-X needle) was placed through the intravesical adenoma and brought out percutaneously using a Carter-Thomason device, to facilitate retraction. In patients with a small intravesical component (19/34 of patients), enucleation of the distal apical adenoma was done with finger dissection by disconnecting the valve of the TriPort. Mean OR time was 116 min and EBL was 360 mL. There were two conversions to the open procedure. Major complications included one death, which was due to hemorrhage/coagulopathy in a Jehovah's Witness who refused transfusion. One patient experienced a rectal injury. At 8 months follow-up mean American Urologic Association symptom score was 3, maximum urinary flow rate was 44 ml/s, and post-void residual was 30 mL. No patients developed incontinence. Wang et al. [23] performed the STEP procedure in nine patients with a mean prostate size of 83.8 ± 19.9 mL. Using a similar technique, a TriPort was placed in a preperitoneal fashion into the bladder. Mean OR time was 160.9±30.4 min, and EBL was 418.8±282.76 mL. One case was converted to open prostatectomy because of difficulties with TriPort insertion. At 12 months post procedure, the mean Qmax was 22.7±4.62 mL/s, PVR was 36.1±40.02 mL, and IPSS was 4.1±1.36. Fareed et al. [24] reported their experience with STEP, using the DaVinci surgical robot. Nine patients underwent R-STEP with a GelPort (Applied Medical, Santa Margarita, CA) as the access platform (Fig. 19.1). Robotic instruments consisted of a 5-mm Schertel grasper and harmonic scalpel. Mean gland size was 146.4 mL (83–304 mL) based on trans-rectal ultrasound. Mean OR time was 3.8 h (2.75–4.75), and EBL was 584.4 mL (150–1,200). One patient required conversion to an open prostatectomy, and was excluded from the analysis. Two patients required cystoscopy, fulguration, and clot evacuation post-operatively for clot retention. Additionally one patient developed a DVT which required anti-coagulation, and one patient suffered a peri-operative myocardial infarction, requiring admission to the ICU. At 1 month follow up mean IPSS was 4.83 (2–15), Q_{max} was 20.1 mL/s (6–36), and PVR was 75.75 m; (0–360). The authors concluded that while R-LESS is technically feasible and effective in treating bladder outlet obstruction, they found a high rate of complications in their study (Table 19.2).

Radical Prostatectomy

Kaouk et al. first reported a series of conventional LESS radical prostatectomy [3]. Four patients (mean age 63 years, mean BMI 29 kg/m2; mean PSA 5.50 ng/dl; no prior history of pelvic surgery) were selected to have the procedure. All were clinical stage T1c, with a Gleason score 3+3 in two, and 3+4 in two patients. An open Hassan technique was used to insert a Uni-X™ single access (Pnavel Systems) multichannel port through a 1.8 cm umbilical incision into the peritoneal cavity. Then, a 5 mm Endoeye scope (Olympus) with a flexible tip and articulating graspers (Novare Surgical Systems, Cupertino, CA, USA) were used (Fig. 19.2a). The surgeons reported that these instruments were helpful in providing effective retraction during dissection, but difficulty was noted with applying adequate anterior traction on the seminal vesicles and vas deferens while at the same time retracting the bladder cephalad to gain exposure to the rectum.

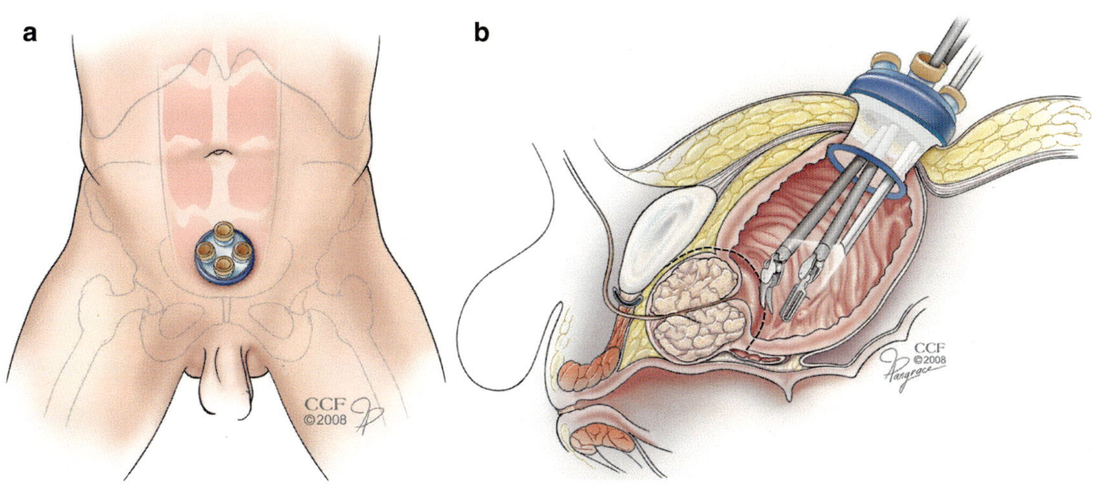

Fig. 19.1 Illustration of R-STEP. (**a**) Gel-port located in the suprapubic area; (**b**) 12mm robotic scopeand two 5mm robotic instruments introduced thorugh the Gel-port inserted in tranvesically through the bladder dome. The 30° lens are angled upwords in order to minimize instrument clashing

Table 19.2 LESS transvesical prostate enucleation series

Ref.	# of pts.	Procedure	Prostate volume (mL)	Port	OR time (min)	EBL (mL)	Conversions/extra ports	Complications	IPSS/Qmax (mL/s)
Desai et al. [22]	34	STEP	102.5	TriPort	116	360	2 (to open surgery)	1 death (perioperative hemorrhage) 1 rectal injury 5 perioperative hemorrhage 1 UTI	3/44 of (8 months)
Wang et al. [23]	9	STEP	83.8	TriPort	160.9	418.8	1 (to open surgery)	1 UTI 1 urethral stricture	4.1/22.7 of (12 months)
Fareed et al. [24]	9	R-STEP	146.4	GelPort	228	584.4	1 (to open surgery)	1 MI 1 DVT 2 perioperative hemorrhage	4.83/20.1 of (1 month)
Lee et al. [25]	7	STEP	100.8	Home made	191.86	600	None	1 transfusion	11.43/17.14 of (3 months)

For this reason apical dissection of the prostate was done first, prior to releasing the vas deferens and seminal vesicles completely. A lymph node dissection was performed in one patient only. Although the 5 mm LigaSure (Valley Lab) was used to take the pedicles, the neurovascular bundles were released with cold scissors. The urethro-vesical anastomosis was completed with interrupted 2-0 Vicryl sutures on SH needles (Fig. 19.2b). The knots were tied externally and advanced into the pelvis with a knot pusher. At the end of the procedure the prostate was delivered by extending the umbilical incision up to 2–3 cm. There were no urine leaks when the anastomosis was tested intraoperatively by filling the bladder with saline. Additionally there were no conversions to either standard laparoscopy, or open prostatectomy. Mean OR time was 4.75 h, and EBL was 287 mL. On follow-up, three patients were continent (using 0 or 1 pad for security). Follow up was too short to determine potency outcomes. One patient developed a recto-urethral fistula, which was treated with a mucosal advancement flap. Two patients had a positive margin but their PSA remained undetectable on short-term follow up. The authors concluded that while LESS radical prostatectomy was technically feasible, there was considerable difficulty with intracorporeal suturing and knot tying. They postulated that application of the robotic platform might overcome the challenges with conventional LESS.

Caceres et al. reported the largest LESS prostatectomy series of 31 patients using the KeyPort multi-channel single site umbilical system (Richard Wolf GmbH, Knittlingen, Germany), in conjunction with a new DuoRotate system (Richard Wolf) [26]. The system incorporates bent instruments with double rotation, and allows for precise movement at the tips of the instruments after alignment of the arms. The majority of patients had intermediate risk disease (45.8 %) according to D'Amico stratification [27]. An additional 3.5 mm port placed in the right iliac fossa was used by the assistant for suction/retraction, and was also used by the primary surgeon during the urethrovesical anastomosis to facilitate suturing. They also used "marionette" sutures

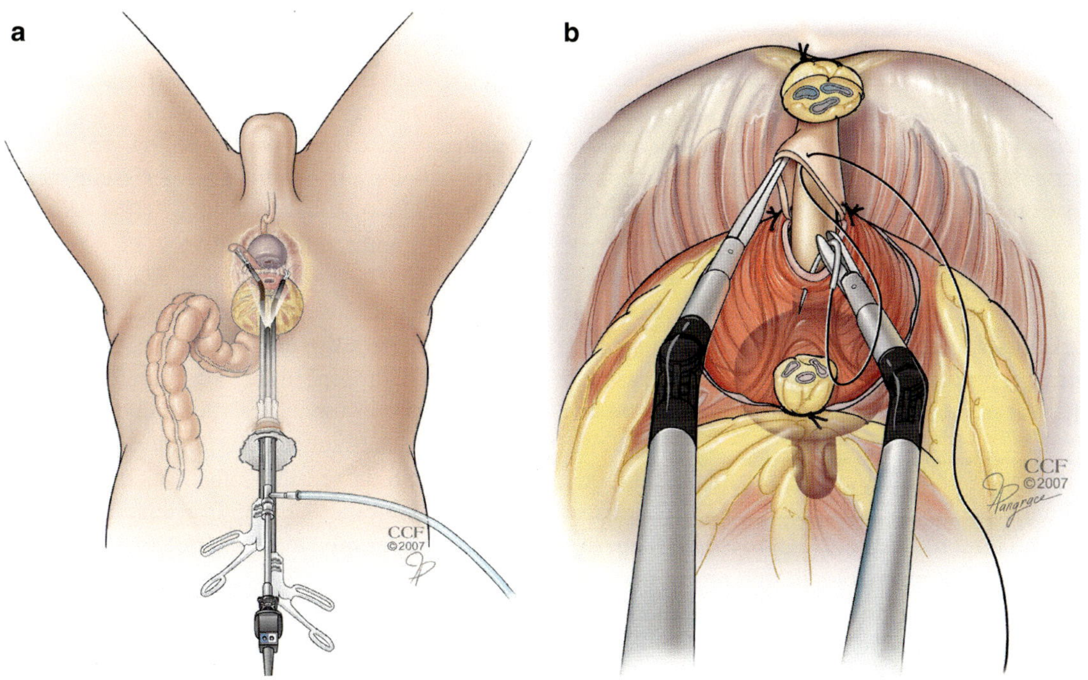

Fig. 19.2 Illustration of LESS radical prostatectomy. (**a**) Set-up with multichannel port and in-line instruments and scope (**b**) detail of urethro-vesical anastomosis using articulating instruments

to retract the bladder cephalad during dissection of the prostate. The anastomosis was completed with a running barbed polyglyconate suture V-LOC 90 2–0 (Covidien). There were no conversions to standard laparoscopy, or intraoperative complications. Mean OR time was 207 min (120–390) and EBL was 258 mL (200–500). Nerve sparing was performed in ten patients (32.3 %) and a lymph node dissection was done in eight (25.8 %). At 20 weeks post procedure, 33 % were fully continent. With regards to potency, 3/10 of patients who had an athermal nerve sparing procedure had a SHIM score of >21 at 20 weeks. Five patients had a focal positive margin. Two patients experience major complications. One patient had a rectal injury and presented 2 days post-op with peritonitis. He underwent a diverting colostomy. Another patient developed respiratory acidosis due to a prolonged OR time (390 min) and required admission to the intensive care unit post-operatively.

Zhu et al. [28] performed a LESS RP using an extraperitoneal approach in six patients. Mean age was 74.7 years (74–76) and BMI was 23.8 kg/m2 (19.5–32.2). Mean PSA was 8.49 ng/mL (1.53–19.4) and prostate volume was 45.5 ml (27.2–63.3). Three patients were cT2a and the remaining three were cT3a. On TRUS biopsy, two patients had Gleason 6 disease, and four patients had Gleason 7 (3+4=1 patient, 4+3=3 patients) Standard laparoscopic instruments were used in conjunction with a QuadPort (Olympus, Tokyo, Japan) and a 0° Olympus EndoEYE 5 mm flexible tip videolaparoscope. The extra-peritoneal space was developed using a balloon device. Nerve-sparing was not performed in this series of patients, and the harmonic scalpel was used to control the prostate pedicles. Mean OR time was 252.5 min (190–305) and EBL was 300 mL (100–500). There were no intraoperative complications or conversions to standard laparoscopy/open surgery. Long-term oncologic outcomes were not presented, but there were no positive margins, and all patients had an undetectable PSA at 1 month. Additionally all six patients were completely continent (0 pads/day) at 12 months post-operatively. Again, like previous studies, the authors reported that LESS RP is feasible, but found intracorporeal suturing during the urethrovesical anastomosis challenging.

A number of groups have reported their experience with R-LESS radical prostatectomy [29, 30], the largest including 20 patients by White et al. [14]. They used a single-site approach, with a SILS port and two 8 mm standard robotic trocars (or one 8 mm and one 5 mm trocar) placed through separate fascial incisions (Fig. 19.3). Standard 8 mm EndoWrist (Intuitive Surgical) monopolar shears and a 5 mm EndoWrist Schertel grasper were used during dissection. The majority of patients were D'Amico low risk (45 %). Mean age was 60.4 years, and mean BMI was 25.4 kg/m^2. Because the fourth arm was not used, retraction was accomplished by assistant suction or marionette sutures. Mean OR time was 187.6 min, and EBL was 128.8 mL. There was one conversion to standard robotic prostatectomy because of a large median lobe and need for more effective retraction. Also, two cases required an additional 8 mm port placed outside of the umbilical incision due to issues with triangulation and leakage of gas from the SILS port. There were four positive margins, but no patients experienced biochemical recurrence at 1 year follow up. The authors also reported a trend towards improved urinary continence, with five patients completely pad free over the follow up period. Three patients underwent an interfascial nerve sparing technique, and one had SHIM score of >21 at 3 months post-operatively. Five patients had a leak at the urethrovesical anastomosis on cystogram done 1 week post surgery, and required an additional week of catheterization. One patient experienced urosepsis and was admitted to the ICU 45 days postoperatively, but recovered with intravenous antibiotics. The authors concluded that R-LESS is feasible, and less challenging than conventional LESS. Instrument clashing was virtually eliminated by staggering the robotic trocars, and marionette sutures allowed for effective retraction despite inability to use the fourth arm. Assistant-driven retraction with the suction was also important, and facilitated by placing a 15–30° downward bend, in the distal one third of the instrument (Table 19.3).

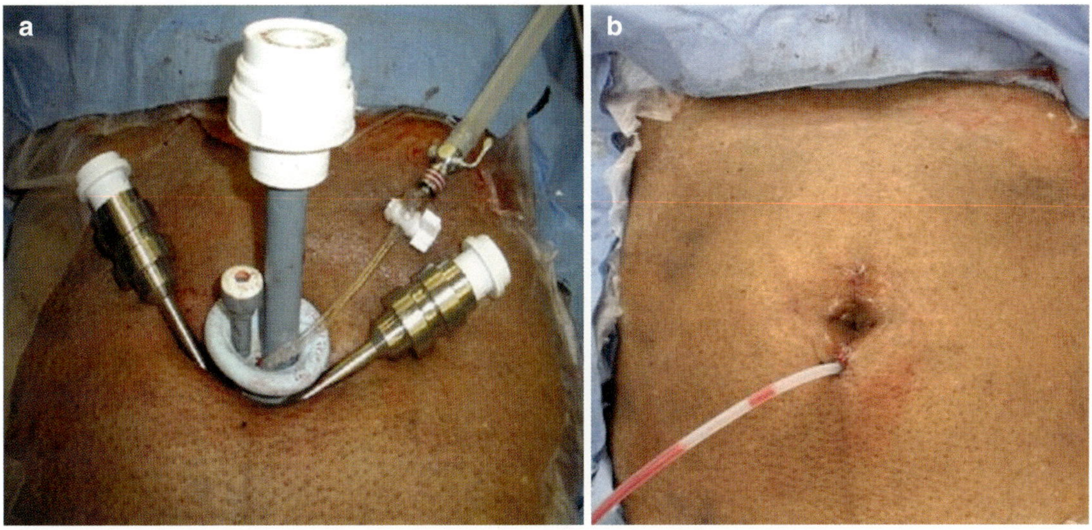

Fig. 19.3 Port configuration for R-LESS radical prostatectomy: (**a**) SILS port (Covidien) and two 8 mm standard robotic trocars (or one 8 m and one 5 mm trocar) placed through separate fascial incisions; (**b**) final aspect of umbilical incision (Photos courtesy of Dr. Jihad Kaouk, Cleveland Clinic)

19.4 LESS Bladder Surgery

Radical Cystectomy

There is considerably less experience with LESS radical cystectomy, with only a few cases reported in the literature. Kaouk et al. [32] reported their experience with conventional LESS radical cystectomy in three patients (two male, one female; mean age 73 years, mean BMI 28 kg/m^2). Access was gained in a similar fashion to their reported LESS radical prostatectomy series, using the UniX multichannel port (Pnavel Systems). A steerable, 5-mm laparoscope (Olympus Surgical) was used with flexible 5 mm instruments. Bladder pedicles were taken with either the 5 mm Harmonic Scalpel (Ethicon Endo-Surgery), 5-mm Ligasure (Valleylab) or Hem-o-Lok clips (Weck Closure Systems). A full lymph node dissection was carried out up to the bifurcation of the aorta. For diversion, all patients had an ileal conduit, which was constructed extracorporeally by extending the peri-umbilical incision. Mean OR time was 315 min, and mean EBL was 217 mL. There were no intraoperative complications, or conversions to standard laparoscopy or the open technique. All surgical margins were negative, and patients were free of recurrent or metastatic disease at 2-year follow up.

More recently, Ma et al. [33] reported the Chinese experience with LESS radical cystectomy in five male patients using a homemade port constructed using an inverted polycarbonate cone device, and a surgical glove. Standard laparoscopic instruments were used for dissection. Mean age was 62.2 years, and BMI was 23.64 kg/m^2. All patients underwent a standard lymph node dissection. Two patients had a cutaneous ureterostomy as their diversion, and the remaining three had an ileal conduit. Mean OR time for the extirpative portion of the procedure was 208.2 min, and mean EBL was 270 mL. Average length of stay in hospital was 19.5 days, and 4/5 of patients developed an ileus post-operatively (mean duration 9.75 days). One patient developed a small bowel obstruction that resolved spontaneously. One patient suffered a peri-operative MI related to a blood transfusion, and expired. The surviving patients remained disease free on latest follow-up (mean follow up 143 (110–173) days).

Lin et al. [34] performed a LESS radical cystectomy, lymph node dissection, and orthotopic ileal neobladder in 12 patients with muscle

Table 19.3 LESS radical prostatectomy series

Ref.	# of pts.	Procedure	Port	OR time (min)	EBL (mL)	Conversions/ extra ports	Complications	Margins	Potency	Continence	PSA (ng/dL)
Kaouk et al. [3]	4	LESS RRP	Uni-X	285	287	None	1 rectourethral fistula	2 positive	F/U not sufficient	3 patients dry (0–1 pads/ day)	<0.03
Caceres et al. [26]	31	LESS RRP	KeyPort	207	258	None (all cases had 2.5 mm port in RIF)	1 rectal injury 1 resp. acidosis 1 transfusion 1 UTI	5 positive	3/10 of patients had SHIM>21 (20 weeks)	33 % continent at 12 weeks	F/U not sufficient
Zhu et al. [28]	6	LESS RRP (extraperitoneal)	QuadPort	252.5	300	None	None reported	All negative	Non-NS procedure	All continent at 12 months (0 pads)	<0.03 (1 month)
Wen et al. [31]	6	LESS RRP	QuadPort/ Home Made	265	230	None	None reported	All negative	3/6 of patients had erections (3 months)	4 pts. (0 pads) 2 pts. (1 pad) at 6 months	<0.03 (3 months)
White et al. [14]	20	R-LESS RRP	SILS port	187.6	128.8	1 (standard robotic prostatectomy) 2 required extra 8 mm port	1 ileus 1 transfusion 1 PE 1 urosepsis	4 positive	3 pts underwent NS → 1 had SHIM>21 at 3 months	5 pts. (0 pads) at 12 months	<0.03 (5.9 months)

RRP radical retropubic prostatectomy, *RIF* right iliac fossa, *PE* pulmonary embolus, *NS* nerve-sparing invasive bladder cancer. A homemade port which consisted of a surgical glove was also used for access. The ileal neo-bladder was constructed extracorporeally and was subsequently sutured to the urethral stump laparoscopically. The procedures were actually considered "hybrid-LESS," as a separate sub-umbilical port was placed for the laparoscope. Nevertheless, all procedures were completed successfully without need for conversion. Median OR time was 383 min, and EBL was 150 mL. All surgical margins were negative, and at a mean follow-up of 16.1 months, all patients were free of recurrent or metastatic disease. Three patients received adjuvant chemotherapy for positive lymph nodes, or pT3a disease. Furthermore patients had good functional outcomes with regards to their neo-bladder. At 12 months mean pouch capacity, PVR, and maximal flow rate were 369 mL (230–640 mL), 42 mL (0–180 mL), and 12.1 mL/s (7.1–28 mL/s), respectively. No patients experienced urinary retention or stricture disease. The authors reported that the extra sub-umbilical incision for the laparoscope facilitated lymph-node dissection and suturing of the neo-bladder to the urethral stump, without compromising the cosmetic results. They found that the initial incision often had to be extended anyways, to extract the specimen (Table 19.4).

Bladder Diverticulectomy

Bladder diverticula are essentially a herniation of urothelium through the detrusor muscle of the bladder wall. They are classified as either congenital or acquired, and acquired diverticula are typically seen in the setting of bladder outlet obstruction. Indications for bladder diverticulectomy include chronic urinary tract infection, stones within the diverticlum, malignancy, or upper tract deterioration secondary to reflux/obstruction. Both transurethral-endoscopic, and open surgical approaches have been utilized. However typically the endoscopic approach is reserved for poor surgical candidates, and open surgery remains the gold standard. In an effort to reduce the morbidity of an open diverticulectomy, minimally invasive approaches have been developed, including LESS. Stolzenberg et al. [35] used a TriPort and a combination of bent and conventional laparoscopic instruments to perform trans-peritoneal diverticulectomies in four patients. Prior to resection a stent was placed in the ureter on the side of the diverticulum, and an 18F foley was advanced into the diverticulum under fluoroscopic guidance. The balloon was then inflated, to guide dissection. Following resection of the diverticulum the bladder was closed by absorbable interrupted sutures. Saline was then instilled into the bladder via the foley catheter, to check for any leakage. Median OR time was 130 min (101–154 min) and blood loss was minimal. There were no complications and pain scores were minimal on post-operative day three. Follow-up cystogram was done in each patient after catheter removal, and there were no leaks. Roslan et al. [36] described their technique of transvesical LESS diverticulectomy in three male patients. After a 1.5 cm incision was made 2 cm above the pubic symphisis, a TriPort+ was inserted using an unbladed introducer into the bladder under cystoscopic guidance. Pneumovesicum was then created and the diverticular sac was dissected transvesically using 5-mm laparoscopic instruments. To facilitate resection, an extragrasper was placed transurethrally into the bladder. The bladder wall defect was then closed with an absorbable 3–0 running suture (The V-Loc 90 Absorbable Wound Closure Device, Covidien, Norwalk, CT), and a foley catheter was left in place. After removal of the TriPort, only the skin incision was sutured closed. Routine cystography was not performed prior to catheter removal. Mean OR time was 128 min, and there were no complications. Both of these studies illustrate the fact that LESS bladder diverticulectomy is feasible and safe, and may be approached in a transvesical or transperitoneal fashion.

Ureteroneocystotomy

Both extra-vesical and transvesical ureteral reimplantation have been attempted using the

Table 19.4 LESS radical cystectomy and lymph node dissection series

Ref.	# of pts.	Procedure	Port	Diversion	OR time	EBL	Conversions/ extra ports	Complications	Oncologic outcomes
Kaouk et al. [32]	3	LESS radical cystectomy+LND	UniX	Ileal conduit (extracorporeal)	315	217	None	None reported	All margins negative; no recurrence/mets at 2 years
Ma et al. [33]	5	LESS radical cystectomy+LND	Home made	Cutaneous ureterostomy (2) Ileal conduit (3) (extracorporeal)	208.2 (extirpative portion)	270	None	1 death (peri-op MI) 1 transfusion	All margins negative; no recurrence/mets (mean F/U 143 days)
Lin et al. [34]	12	LESS radical cystectomy+LND	Home made	Orthotopic ileal neobladder (extracorporeal)	383	150	All pts had extra sub-umbilical port for laparoscope	1 bowel obstruction Delirium (1 pt.) Prolonged lymphatic drainage (2 pts.)	All margins negative; no recurrence/mets (mean F/U 16.1 months)

LND lymph node dissection

LESS approach. Desai et al. [37] reported on their first 100 LESS cases, two of which were ureteral reimplantation. Operative times were 210 and 140 min, with an EBL of 100 and 250 mL, respectively. Two additional needle-scopic ports were used to facilitate triangulation and retraction during suturing. Roslan et al. [38] used their experience with transvesical LESS, and performed a ureteral reimplantation in a 39 years old female with vesicoureteric reflux. Like their transvesical diverticulectomy series, they used a TriPort with was placed directly in to the bladder. The procedure took 250 min to complete, and blood loss was reported as minimal. The ureter was dissected and the 5 cm terminal portion was transected. A 4 cm submucosal tunnel was then created, and the ureter was brought through this tunnel near the fundus of the bladder. Diuretic renography and an ultrasound at 6 months post-op revealed resolution of her hydronephrosis, and no evidence of persistent reflux or obstruction.

Vesicovaginal Fistula Repair

The most common cause of a vesicovaginal fistula (VVF) in the industrialized world is inadvertent bladder injury at the time of pelvic gynecologic or urologic surgery. This occurs most commonly during a hysterectomy, when an unrecognized cystotomy is made near the vaginal cuff. Both the abdominal and transvaginal routes of repair have been extensively used, with the transvaginal approach being less morbid [39]. However fistulas that are high in the vaginal cuff can be difficult to repair by this route. Abdel-Karim et al. first reported their experience with conventional laparoscopic VVF repair in 2010 [40], and subsequently LESS VVF repair [41]. Five patients underwent transperitoneal LESS VVF repair, with omental interposition. An extra 5 mm port was used to facilitate intracorporeal suturing and triangulation. There were no complications, or conversions to standard laparoscopy or open surgery. Mean follow up was 8 ± 3.2 months, and all patients were continent with no recurrence of their fistulae.

19.5 LESS Reconstructive Surgery

Sacralcolpopexy

Sacralcolpopexy is an effective technique for repair of a pelvic-organ prolapse (POP) in young patients who desire to continue with sexual intercourse, as vaginal shortening is minimal. Open, pure laparoscopic [42], and robotic approaches [43] have been described. White et al. [44] compared a cohort of 30 patients with POP who underwent sacralcolpopexy. Ten patients underwent conventional laparoscopic repair, ten had a robotic repair, and ten had a LESS repair. There were no differences amongst the three groups with regards to OR time, EBL, visual analog pain scores at discharge, or duration of hospitalization. At 6 months follow-up 27 patients underwent repeated POP-Q scoring which revealed excellent apical support and no recurrence of their prolapse. Tome et al. [45] described their LESS approach in one patient with a stage IV (POP-Q) vaginal vault prolapse. They used a homemade multichannel port (Alexis wound retractor and surgical glove) and clips, rather than knots for securing the mesh. At 3 months post surgery, the patient was a stage 0, and experienced no complications. LESS sacralcolpopexy appears technically feasible with excellent results, however it seems an extra-port is helpful to facilitate intracorporeal suturing during repair.

19.6 Summary

Laparoendoscopic single-site surgery continues to evolve, with improvements in technique and instrumentation. Issues with triangulation, clashing, and visualization have been addressed with articulating instruments and endoscopes, and application specific access platforms. Additionally considerable laparoscopic expertise is required before attempting LESS. The technique has been applied to a number of different pelvic oncology procedures, spanning the fields of Gynecology, Urology, and General Surgery.

Comparative analysis between standard laparoscopy and LESS exist, which reveal while

LESS is not inferior with regards to most perioperative outcomes, it is much more technically demanding. However, the main benefit of LESS seems to be the potential for better cosmetic outcomes as it represents a step towards truly "scarless" surgery.

The application of robotics to LESS (R-LESS) has addressed many of the limitations seen with the conventional technique. The endowrist™ technology allows for superior dissection, triangulation, and intra-corporeal suturing. However R-LESS is still in its infancy, as the current iteration of the DaVinci robotic platform has not been designed for LESS. As a result of the bulky extracorporeal profile, instrument clashing and limited space at the bedside remain important issues. Solutions such as the DaVinci Single-site™ platform (Fig. 19.4) have been designed to address these challenges, however their full clinical potential has not yet been reached as further testing is required.

The ideal robotic platform for R-LESS would be low profile, task specific, and would allow for deployment through a single incision. Additionally the instruments would be articulating, and there would be effective triangulation and retraction. Further advancements in the field of robotic surgery are necessary before truly scarless LESS becomes widely adapted.

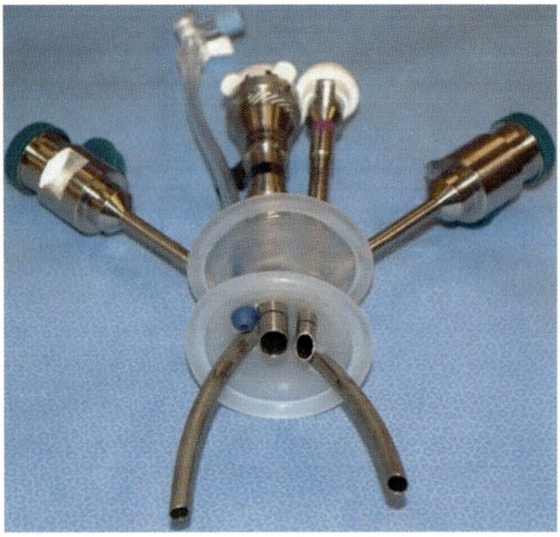

Fig. 19.4 DaVinci single-site surgery access platform

Key Points

- LESS is equivalent to conventional laparoscopic surgery with regards to perioperative outcomes with a trend towards improved cosmesis and less post-operative pain
- Radical prostatectomy, radical cystectomy, are the most common pelvic surgeries that LESS has been used for
- LESS is significantly more challenging, especially when complex reconstruction or intracorporeal suturing is required
- Experience with laparoscopic surgery and a training program is suggested before a surgeon undertakes LESS
- Instrument clashing and difficulties achieving triangulation can make LESS challenging
- The DaVinci robotic platform has been applied to conventional LESS to address some of the difficulties
- Bulky external design, lack of space for the assistant at the bedside, and clashing of the robotic arms are challenges facing R-LESS
- Devices such as the DaVinci single site platform have been designed to address some of the limitations of R-LESS
- The future of R-LESS is task specific surgical robots with a low external profile, ability to be deployed through a single incision, and with robust articulating instruments that restore intracorporeal triangulation

References

1. Autorino R, Stein RJ, Lima E, et al. Current status and future perspectives in laparoendoscopic single-site and natural orifice transluminal endoscopic urological surgery. Int J Urol. 2010;17:410–31.
2. Rané A, Rao P, Rao P. Single-port-access nephrectomy and other laparoscopic urologic procedures using a novel laparoscopic port (R-port). Urology. 2008;72(2):260–3.

3. Kaouk JH, Goel RK, Haber GP, et al. Single port laparoscopic radical prostatectomy. Urology. 2008;72:1190–3.
4. Raman JD, Bagrodia A, Cadeddu JA. Single-incision, umbilical laparoscopic versus conventional laparoscopic nephrectomy: a comparison of perioperative outcomes and short-term measures of convalescence. Eur Urol. 2009;55:1198–206.
5. Tracy CR, Raman JD, Bagrodia A, et al. Perioperative outcomes in patients undergoing conventional laparoscopic versus laparoendoscopic single-site pyeloplasty. Urology. 2009;74:1029–34.
6. Raybourn 3rd JH, Rane A, Sundaram CP. Laparoendoscopic single site surgery for nephrectomy as a feasible alternative to traditional laparoscopy. Urology. 2010;75:100–3.
7. Jeong BC, Park YH, Han DH, et al. Laparoendoscopic single-site and conventional laparoscopic adrenalectomy: a matched case control study. J Endourol. 2009;23:1957–60.
8. Canes D, Berger A, Aron M, et al. Laparo-endoscopic single site (LESS) versus standard laparoscopic left donor nephrectomy: matched-pair comparison. Eur Urol. 2010;57:95–101.
9. Autorino R, Cadeddu JA, Desai MM, et al. Laparoendoscopic single site and natural orifice transluminal endoscopic surgery in urology: a critical analysis of the literature. Eur Urol. 2011;59:26–45.
10. Kaouk JH, Autorino R, Kim FJ, et al. Laparoendoscopic single-site surgery in urology: worldwide multi-institutional analysis of 1076 cases. Eur Urol. 2011;60:998–1005.
11. Kaouk JH, Goel RK, Haber GP, et al. Robotic single-port transumbilical surgery in humans: initial report. BJU Int. 2008;103:366–9.
12. Stein RJ, White WM, Goel RK, et al. Robotic laparoendoscopic single-site surgery using GelPort as the access platform. Eur Urol. 2010;57:132–7.
13. White MA, Autorino R, Spana G, et al. Robotic laparoendoscopic single-site radical nephrectomy: surgical technique and comparative outcomes. Eur Urol. 2011;59:815–22.
14. White MA, Haber G-P, Autorino R, et al. Robotic laparoendoscopic single-site radical prostatectomy: technique and early outcomes. Eur Urol. 2010;58:544–50.
15. Joseph RA, Goh AC, Cuevas SP, et al. Chopstick surgery: a novel technique improves surgeon performance and eliminates arm collision in robotic single-incision laparoscopic surgery. Surg Endosc. 2010;24:1331–5.
16. Haber GP, White MA, Autorino R, et al. Novel robotic da Vinci instruments for laparoendoscopic single-site surgery. Urology. 2010;76:1279–8.
17. Rodríguez RM, Pavón JM, de la Portilla F, Sillero EP, Dussort JM, Padillo J. Robotic-assisted total mesorectal excision with the aid of a single-port device. Surg Innov. 2013;20(4):NP3–5. doi: 10.1177/1553350611434643.
18. Fader AN, Escobar PF. Laparoendoscopic single-site surgery (LESS) in gynecologic oncology: technique and initial report. Gynecol Oncol. 2009;114:157–61.
19. Nam EJ, Kim SW, Lee M, et al. Robotic single-port transumbilical total hysterectomy: a pilot study. J Gynecol Oncol. 2011;22:120–6.
20. De Sio M, Quattrone C, Damiano R, et al. Patient selection for LESS urological surgery. Arch Esp Urol. 2012;65(3):280–4.
21. Ou R, You M, Tang P, et al. A randomized trial of transvesical prostatectomy versus transurethral resection of the prostate for prostate greater than 80 mL. Urology. 2010;76:958.
22. Desai MM, Fareed K, Berger AK, et al. Single-port transvesical enucleation of the prostate: a clinical report of 34 cases. BJU Int. 2010;105(9):1296–300.
23. Wang L, Liu B, Yang Q, et al. Preperitoneal single-port transvesical enucleation of the prostate (STEP) for large-volume BPH: one-year follow-up of Qmax, IPSS, and QoL. Urology. 2012;80(2):323–8.
24. Fareed K, Zaytoun OM, Autorino R, et al. Robotic single port suprapubic transvesical enucleation of the prostate (R-STEP): initial experience. BJU Int. 2012;110(5):732–7.
25. Lee JY, Han JH, Moon HS, et al. Single-port transvesical enucleation of the prostate for benign prostatic hyperplasia with severe intravesical prostatic protrusion. World J Urol. 2012;30(4):511–7.
26. Caceres F, Cabrera PM, Garcia-Tello A, et al. Safety study of umbilical single-port laparoscopic radical prostatetomy with a new DuoRotate System. Eur Urol. 2012;62:1143–9.
27. D'Amico AV, Whittington R, Malkowicz SB, et al. Predicting prostate specific antigen outcome preoperatively in the prostate specific antigen era. J Urol. 2001;166(6):2185–8.
28. Zhu G, Zhang YQ, Grange P, et al. Laparoendoscopic single-site radical prostatectomy: technique and initial outcomes. Chin Med J (Engl). 2012;125(21):3815–20.
29. Barret E, Sanchez-Salas R, Cathelineau X, et al. Re: initial complete laparoendoscopic single-site surgery robotic assisted radical prostatectomy (LESS-RARP). Int Braz J Urol. 2009;35:92–3.
30. Leewansangtong S, Vorrakitkatorn P, Amornvesukit T, et al. Laparo-endoscopic single site (LESS) robotic radical prostatectomy in an Asian man with prostate cancer: an initial case report. J Med Assoc Thai. 2010;93:383–7.
31. Wen XQ, Huang WT, Situ J, et al. Single-port laparoscopic radical prostatectomy: initial experience and technical points to reduce its difficulties. Chin Med J (Engl). 2011;124(23):4092–5.
32. Kaouk JH, Goel RK, White MA, et al. Laparoendoscopic single site radical cystectomy and pelvic lymph node dissection: initial experience and 2-year follow-up. Urology. 2010;76:857–61.

33. Ma L, Bi H, Hou X, et al. Laparoendoscopic single-site radical cystectomy and urinary diversion: initial experience in China using a homemade single-port device. J Endourol. 2012;26:355–9.
34. Lin T, Huang J, Han J, et al. Hybrid laparoscopic endoscopic single-site surgery for radical cystoprostatectomy and orthotopic ileal neobladder: an initial experience of 12 cases. J Endourol. 2011;25:57–63.
35. Stolzenburg JU, Do M, Kallidonis P, et al. Laparoendoscopic single-site bladder diverticulectomy: technique and initial experience. J Endourol. 2011;25(1):85–90.
36. Roslan M, Markuszewski MM, Kłącz J, et al. Laparoendoscopic single-port transvesical diverticulectomy: preliminary clinical experience. J Endourol. 2012;26(8):975–9.
37. Desai MM, Berger AK, Brandina R, et al. Laparoendoscopic single-site surgery: initial hundred patients. Urology. 2009;74:805.
38. Roslan M, Markuszewski MM, Kłącz J, et al. Laparoendoscopic single-site transvesical ureteroneocystostomy for vesicoureteral reflux in an adult: a one-year follow-up. Urology. 2012;80(3):719–23.
39. Eilber KS, Kavaler E, Rodriguez LV, et al. Ten-year experience with transvaginal vesicovaginal fistula repair using tissue interposition. J Urol. 2003; 169(3):1033–6.
40. Abdel-Karim AM, Mousa A, Hasouna M, Elsalmy S. Laparoscopic transperitoneal extravesical repair of vesicovaginal fistula. Int Urogynecol J. 2011;22(6): 693–97. doi:10.1007/s00192-010-1334-7.
41. Abdel-Karim AM, Moussa A, Elsalmy S. Laparoendoscopic single-site surgery extravesical repair of vesicovaginal fistula: early experience. Urology. 2011;78(3):567–71.
42. Sundaram CP, Venkatesh R, et al. Laparoscopic sacrocolpopexy for the correction of vaginal vault prolapse. J Endourol. 2004;18(7):620–3.
43. Daneshgari F, Paraiso MF, et al. Robotic and laparoscopic female pelvic floor reconstruction. BJU Int. 2006;98(Suppl.1):62–8.
44. White WM, Goel RK, Swartz MA, et al. Single-port laparoscopic abdominal sacral colpopexy: initial experience and comparative outcomes. Urology. 2009;74(5):1008–12.
45. Tome AL, Tobias-Machado M, Correa WF. Laparoendoscopic single-site (LESS) sacrocolpopexy: feasibility and efficacy of knotless procedure performed with conventional instruments. Int Urogynecol J. 2011;22(7):885–7.

20 Radical Perineal Prostatectomy

Lance J. Coetzee and Gregory B. Boustead

20.1 Introduction

Radical perineal prostatectomy was first described by Young in 1905 for the management of clinically localized prostate cancer. Young described the "supra sphincteric approach" later modified in 1939 by Belt describing the "sub sphincteric approach." Both procedures, based on wide excision of the prostate usually resulted in erectile impotence [1, 2]. The radical perineal prostatectomy technique was the treatment of choice for clinically localized prostate cancer until the mid 1970s when Walsh and associates described technical modifications to the retro-pubic approach with an anatomical description of the dorsal venous complex (DVC) and neurovascular bundles (NVB) responsible for maintaining erectile function. This approach was familiar to many urologists used to operating in the retro-pubic space. In this pre-PSA era, when nearly 60 % of prostate cancers diagnosed were T3 tumors, access to the pelvic lymph nodes through the retropubic approach was an additional advantage of the retropubic approach. In 1988 Weldon et al. described the nerve sparing radical perineal prostatectomy with potency preservation similar to the retro-pubic nerve sparing procedure [3]. Further modifications by one of the authors (Coetzee) with the use of pediatric instruments excluding any mechanical retractors, has eliminated traction on the NVB and improved potency rates to 70–80 % in men who were potent pre-operatively, particularly those under the age of 65 year.

In the pre-PSA era, nearly 60 % of patients were diagnosed with stage C (T3) prostatic carcinoma, but since 1989 the introduction of PSA testing has resulted in stage migration towards T1C prostate cancer and nearly 75 % of patients' diagnosed today have non-palpable disease. Nomograms have assisted in determining the potential risk of lymph node involvement [4–6], leading to renewed interest in radical perineal prostatectomy, which could provide equivalent cancer control with a reduced morbidity. Despite the introduction of the laparoscopic and robotic approaches, cancer control rates have remained very similar to open approaches [7–9].

In the last 5 years there has been renewed interest in the importance of pelvic lymphadenectomy as well as limited versus extended pelvic lymphadenectomy and the impact of this on not only staging, but also on possible survival [10, 11]. The impact on survival versus improved staging is as yet uncertain with a long-term follow up. In most contemporary series, a statistical risk analysis using nomograms can determine the risk of possible lymphatic spread [12, 13]. Pelvic

L.J. Coetzee, MD
Consultant Urological Surgeon, Pretoria Urology Hospital, 1162 Pretorius Street, Pretoria, South Africa

G.B. Boustead (✉)
Consultant Urological Surgeon & Clinical Director, Herts & South Bedsfordshire Urological Cancer Centre, Lister Hospital, Stevenage, UK
e-mail: mrboustead@btconnect.com

H.R.H. Patel et al. (eds.), *Pelvic Cancer Surgery: Modern Breakthroughs and Future Advances*,
DOI 10.1007/978-1-4471-4258-4_20, © Springer-Verlag London 2015

lymphadenectomy is not performed if the risk falls below 5–7 %. In fact a decisional analysis would suggest that pelvic lymph node dissection is unnecessary in the subset of patients where the risk of nodal involvement is less than 18 % [14].

20.2 Indications and Limitations of the Perineal Approach

The classic indications include any pT1–2, Nx-0, M0 prostate cancer. Radical perineal prostatectomy is the favored approach in the following circumstances:

- Previous abdominal sepsis, adhesions or multiple laparotomies
- Problematic mesh inguinal and incisional hernia repairs, both open and laparoscopic
- Previous anterior resection or abdomino-perineal excision of rectum (APER)
- Renal transplant patients [15]
- Previous retro-pubic surgery
- Pelvic vascular surgery

Advantages to the radical perineal prostatectomy include reduced blood loss, excellent access to the apex of the prostate with maximal preservation of the sub-sphincteric urethral length with resultant early regaining of urinary incontinence. In experienced hands clear visualization of the NVB responsible for potency preservation, early mobilization and regaining of bowel function due to extra-peritoneal surgery conducted entirely beneath the pelvic floor.

A limitation of the perineal operation has been the inability to access pelvic lymph nodes through the same incision as with the retro-pubic approach. We favor a 5 cm supra-pubic mini-laparotomy, giving access to the pelvic lymph nodes up to the internal iliac arteries in all but the most obese of patients [16]. Saito and colleagues demonstrated the feasibility of sampling the pelvic lymph nodes via the perineal incision, while a combined laparoscopic lymphadenectomy has been described.

Contra-indications to perineal prostatectomy would include:

- Severe ankylosis of the hips
- Unstable total hip replacements
- Prior history of rectal operations, recto-cutaneous fistula or perirectal abscess
- Massive prostates size (relative in experienced hands)
- Morbid obesity if ventilation pressures are too high (relative- see below)

Boczko and Melman reported their series in 100 patients with a BMI of greater than 30 kg/m^2. They reported no major difficulties performing RPP with no need for blood transfusion [17].

20.3 Patient Selection and Pre-operative Preparation

Pre-operative Counseling and Planning Nerve Sparing Versus Wide Excision

Radical prostatectomy has become a procedure judged by not only the cancer cure rates, but also the ability to preserve the functional outcomes of potency and urinary continence, especially in the younger potent patients. Planning nerve sparing radical prostatectomy has improved in T1C or suspected T3a disease with pre-op staging MRI scans, and is particularly useful in patients with high volume or intermediate to high risk Gleason grade or even a patient in the intermediate d'Amico risk category group. The pre-operative MRI scans also allows the surgeon to counsel the patient about the possibility nerve sparing versus wide excision. It is important to emphasize that the primary goal of the surgery should be curative and that the nerve sparing option although desirable, is not the number one priority. The surgeon's discretion to the type of nerve sparing or not should be accepted by the patient and preferably the partner as well in the pre-operative counseling session.

Pre-hospital Preparation

Patients undergo pre-operative assessment 7–10 days prior to surgery with FBC, U&E, urinalysis and blood group and save without cross matching and MRSA screening. Given that most men considering radical prostate surgery are ASA risk I-II, specific anesthetic review is rarely required. We have stopped any autologous blood donation, as this is not cost effective. Patients receive a single dose of Coloprep bowel preparation 12 h before their surgery.

Immediate Pre-operative Preparation in the Operating Room

In the operating room, the patient is given a spinal or caudal injection of Marcaine with opiates for immediate and post-operative pain control for the first 12–24 h. The patients are positioned in the extended dorsal lithotomy position attempting to get the perineum parallel to the floor (Fig. 20.1) so that the perineal incision allows the prostate to be approached through the base of the triangular pelvic entrance between the ischial tuberosities. If this is not done, the surgeon tends to operate through the narrower sub-pubic arch of the apex of the triangular entrance to the pelvis that restricts the view. This is especially important in patients with larger prostates above 50 g. Rarely the anesthetist may encounter raised ventilation pressures in large patients, which can usually be overcome by minor patient repositioning.

20.4 Surgical Technique

An inverted horseshoe incision is made with clearance of the anal verge by roughly 2 cm all round. A curved Lowsley retractor is passed down the urethra into the bladder. The incision is roughly square shaped with rounding of the edges. This gives a broad based flap and has been found to have less of an incidence of midline wound break down due to ischemia with retraction of the skin margins.

Following the development of the ischio-rectal fossa the central tendon is identified and a finger passed beneath the central muscle/tendon anterior to the rectal wall and the central tendon divided allowing the rectum to drop away, opening the approach to the prostate. Following the division of the central tendon, the space either side of the central tendon is developed exposing the anterior rectal wall and the recto-urethralis muscle which is placed on stretch by double gloving and placing the index finger of the left hand (right handed surgeon) through the anus and retracting directly posteriorly towards the floor. The central tendon is then cut back with sharp dissection (this is usually an avascular structure and provided it is thinned out and only the tendon is cut). Within two to three centimeters back the midline space opens up and the prostate can usually be visualized in the depths of the incision. The two lateral wings of remaining muscle either side of the central tendon are divided a short way back, but not as far as the central tendon. These muscular structures are continuous with the layer in which the neuro-vascular bundle is housed and it is felt that by not cutting them back against the prostate that the neuro-vascular bundle is afforded some protection (see Fig. 20.2).

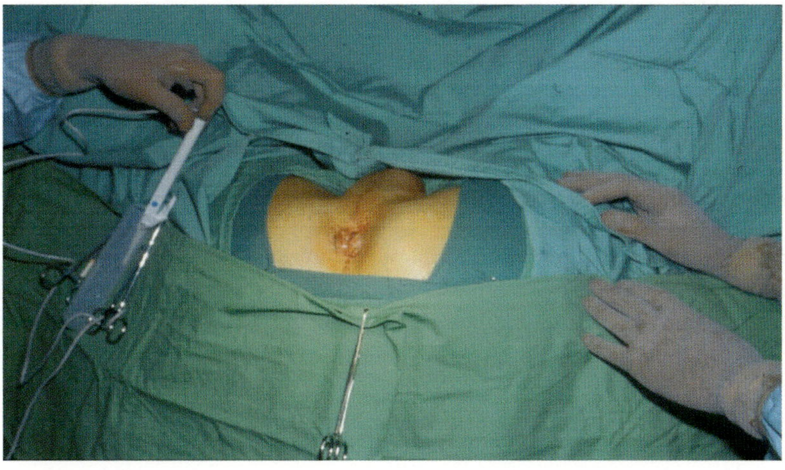

Fig. 20.1 Patient draped and positioned with the perineum parallel to the floor

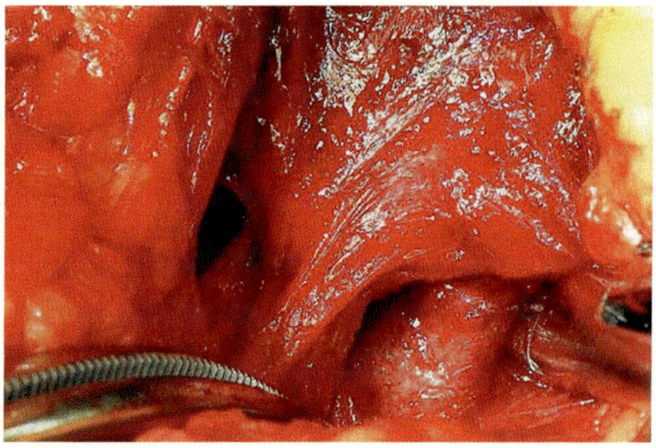

Fig. 20.2 Exposure of the urethra under the neuro-vascular bundles

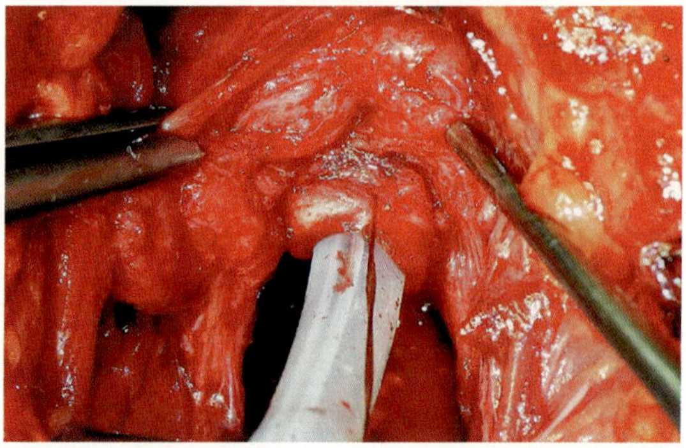

Fig. 20.3 Divided urethra with a Foley catheter in place (tagged with suture) between the neuro-vascular bundles. The limited space available working between the neuro-vascular fascia is visible

The down side of this is that the visualization of the prostate is slightly more limited. It has been our policy over the last 8 years not to use any instrumentation for retraction as this places the nerve bundles on stretch and although it may improve the visualisation of the prostate for the surgeon, it is usually not necessary with the instruments we use. I find it very useful to use two small stainless steel pediatric spatula (1 and 1.5 cm wide) which can be bent and hooked in behind the neuro-vascular bundles to gently retract these off the prostate while the connections with the prostate are divided with or without small liga-clips on visible blood vessels. The urethral prostatic junction is then cleaned and the length of urethra below the sphincter exposed. A right angle Mieke or Lahey clamp passed behind the urethra between the urethra and the dorsal vena complex, gently opened to separate the dorsal complex off the urethra and the urethra is then divided against the Lowsley retractor. The retractor is withdrawn and a holding suture placed through the urethra before it is totally divided (Fig. 20.3). A long Ellis clamp placed in the urethral opening into the prostate allows the prostate to be manipulated and the dorsal venous complex to be gently shifted back towards the bladder neck. The alternative is the placement of straight Lowsley retractor into the bladder which then can be used to manipulate the prostate and also to clearly delineate the vesico-prostatic junction. This is recommended in the early learning phase of one's surgical experience. Hereafter the plane is developed between the prostate and the bladder by cutting down at 90° with a right-angled scissors opening the bladder neck area and visualizing the internal surface of the bladder. This automatically creates two lateral pedicles between the bladder and the prostate, which can then be clipped and sharply divided or cut with a Harmonic scalpel. The tissue lateral to the seminal vesicles represents the vascular pedicles which are clipped and divided. The prostate is lifted and approached from the posterior aspect with division of Denonvilliers and the anterior rectal fascia covering the posterior aspect of the prostate. This fascia and with it the rectum can then be gently swept off the vesicles, allowing the rectum to drop away out of harm's way. The seminal vesicles can either be dissected out completely or truncated, clipped and divided. We seldom remove more than two-thirds of the vesicles as we believe if there is infiltration beyond this point, the surgery becomes a non-curative procedure and the risk of disturbing the vesical nerve plexus at the apex of the vesicle does not justify the wide dissection posterior to the bladder. We perform a circumferential bladder neck frozen section biopsy to establish a clear bladder neck margins particularly in patients with suspected T4 cancer infiltrating the bladder neck. We routinely use a posterior racket handle reconstruction, and don't believe preservation of the bladder neck plays a major role in the regaining of urinary incontinence. Sutures are placed after visualizing the ureters and progressed from the 6 o' clock position towards 12 o' clock. After two to three stitches have been placed, a running 4-O monocryl suture everts the mucosal lining from 12 to 4 o'clock and 12 to 8 o'clock. An 18 French Biocath urethral catheter is then passed and the anastomotic sutures in the urethra placed at 1, 11, 5, 7, 3 and 9 o'clock positions. The 3 o'clock and 9 o'clock sutures are placed at a later stage once the racket handle has been completed and the urethral opening closed to the required caliber from posterior. The urethral-vesical anastomosis is then carried out under direct vision (this is one of the big advantages of the perineal approach) and once completed can be inspected and additional sutures placed to stabilize the anastomosis. The rectal wall is the checked for any possible injuries. The wound is irrigated and checked for any residual bleeding from the lateral pedicles. The wound is closed in layers with zero absorbable glycolic acid fat sutures with an 8 mm pencil drain in the right lower corner of the wound, caprosyn sutures in the vertical arms of the suture and a 4-O V-lock suture sub-cuticularly along the apex of the wound. The legs are then lowered and the patient, after leaving the operating room, is returned to the post-surgical ward and depending on the facilities, either to a general surgical ward or to a high care ward [2, 18, 19].

Lymphadenectomy

In the high risk patients, Gleason 7 or higher, PSA above 15 and clinical T3 cancers, or patients with suspected seminal vesicle infiltration, a pre-radical prostatectomy mini laparotomy is done through a 5 cm suprapubic incision and frozen sections is done on the lymph nodes. Although it is very rare that in a patient who otherwise qualifies for a radical prostatectomy due to clinical organ confined disease and acceptable risk profile, would be disqualified due to bulky nodal disease and this is done mainly as a staging procedure. It is done under the same anesthetic and adds roughly 30 min to the surgery.

20.5 Post-operative Management

Patients can usually start eating and drinking immediately as there is no abdominal wound in the majority of cases (even with a small extra-peritoneal mini-lap incision). The risk of deep vein thrombosis is extremely low because the legs are at a higher level than the heart during the time of the entire procedure, the patient is still covered with prophylactic anti-coagulation with low molecular weigh heparins and elasticated stockings for the first few days of the hospital stay and in high-risk patients the first 14 days following their surgery.

The patients are mobilized and resume normal diet on day 1 and encouraged to walk actively. Emphasis is placed on wound care and keeping the wound dry especially the apical part of the incision in the midline raphae which can, because of its poor blood supply, sometimes show slight delayed healing. Since using the sub-cuticular V-lock suture over the last 2–3 years, we have seen very few problems in this area. An oral stool softener (not a laxative) is given daily until the first bowel movement. The patients are usually discharged on the second or third post-operative day once they have had their first bowel movement. It is important allow the patient access to the surgeon/nurse practitioner if he has any concerns about wound infection, pain control, bowel activity etc. The Foley-catheter is usually removed between 10 and 14 days depending on the size of the patient, the ease of the surgery and the general confidence level of the surgeon following the procedure with regards to the vesico-urethral anastomosis. We now seldom do a retrograde urethrogram/cystogram prior to removing a catheter, unless concerned in very obese patients for example, about the integrity of the anastomosis.

20.6 Complications and Their Management

Overall the peri-operative variables show the safety of the perineal approach (Table 20.1) The risk of peri-operative of complications is

Table 20.1 Peri-operative variables after 1,764 consecutive

Variable	Result (mean and range)
Age	Mean 61 years (42–78)
PSA	Mean 8 ng/ml (0.2–37)
Operative time	141 min (93–185)
Prostate weight	38 g (15–142)
Catheterization	14 days (9–29)
Hospital stay	3.2 days (2–20)

Table 20.2 Complications in our series of 1,764 consecutive radical perineal prostatectomies

Complication	Incidence (%)
Wound infection	4.0
UTI/orchitis within 30 days surgery	4.1
Bladder neck stenosis	1.6
Urine leak	1
Lower limb neurapraxia	0.001
Pulmonary embolism	0.1
Sub-vesical hematoma	0.3
Ileus	0.001
Urinary fistula	0.001

low as summarized in our series of over 1,700 cases (Table 20.2). The incidence of rectal injury in our combined series of 1,786 patients over a 17 year period is 0.003 %. Two of these patients had a loop colostomy for 6 weeks. The others were repaired primarily during the operation and recovered uneventfully. This is well below the quoted incidence of 1 % and significantly below the 4 % incidence reported by Bishoff et al. [20]. Rectal injuries not recognized at the time of surgery usually require a loop diverting colostomy for 6–8 weeks. Important is to confirm closure of the fistula prior to the closing of the colostomy. Those injuries recognized intra-operatively are closed in two layers using absorbable sutures. Anal stretch and a period of bowel rest with antibiotic cover followed by a low residue diet for a week allows the majority of these injuries to heal without incident.

Late development of a fecal fistula is rare and this can be repaired by the same trans perineal approach with freeing up of the tissue well back from the fistula and closing this with a 4-O monocryl suturing at least two layers. Hereafter tissue inter-position either with the patient's own tissue or a collagen patch is recommended. To date we have repaired a number of post laparoscopic recto-vesical fistulae (possibly unrecognized due to abdominal insufflation) but only two following radical perineal prostatectomy (0.001 %).

At the time of catheter removal patients are warned about minor stress incontinence that can take 2–4 weeks for regaining of urine control and the patient is issued with protective pads. More than 50 % of the patients in our series have been dry within 24 h to the extent that they do not require any external protection, 25 % are dry within 2 weeks and the remainder usually within the first 4–6 weeks. In patients who do have delayed return of urine control, any external collecting device such as condom catheter or penile clamp is strongly discouraged especially in the early healing phase up to 6 months. Following this peri-urethral bulking, the male advance sling, and AMS 800 sphincter are options in patients with significant leakage, which in our series was less than 1 %.

In the odd patient who has difficulty to pass urine or develops urine retention, the catheter is usually re-inserted for a further week. Late episodes of poor urine flow or retention, although extremely uncommon, are usually managed with a careful dilatation of what is usually an anastomotic stricture. Given the careful eversion of the bladder mucosa during the surgery and the mucosa to mucosa anastomosis, this is seldom seen however.

Neurapraxia due to the exaggerated lithotomy position has been described. This is seldom seen provided the surgical time is limited to less than 2 h. Isolated nerve injuries may occur due to patient positioning but are preventable with use of generous gel foam padding. Rhabdomyolysis has been described but is extremely rare and tends to be associated with very long periods of surgery above 4 h. As the average time for our surgery was between 110 and 140 min, we did not in our series see a single case of rhabdomyolysis and myoglobinuria [21].

20.7 Outcomes After Radical Perineal Prostatectomy

Cancer Control

Few large contemporary series of radical perineal prostatectomy (RPP) have published oncological outcomes, since the landmark publication from Duke University in 1999 [9]. We evaluated cancer control in 1,320 men after RPP over a 13 year period. Mean follow up was 61 ± 40 months (Range 12–157). At the time of the analysis 1,270 patients were alive and remain under surveillance, 22 patients have died, (9 prostate cancer; 13 other causes). Twenty-eight patients are lost to follow up. Median pre-operative PSA of 7.2 ng/ml; the pathological staging were T2a 9 %; T2b 66 %; T3 25 %. Positive surgical margin rate was 16 % for pT2 and 43 % for pT3. Kaplan-Meier estimates of actuarial PSA survival as a function of surgical margin status (months) are shown in Fig. 20.4 below. Overall survival at 5 years was 94 % (93.0–95.5) and at 10 years was 94 % (93.0–95.5).

RPP therefore offers excellent cancer control and overall survival at 10 years. As shown in other large RP series, pT3 disease, PSA >10, and positive surgical margins are significant risk factors for PSA recurrence [22].

Continence

In our series we defined using no external protection urinary continence. To date the risk of significant stress incontinence in over 1,764 patients is 2 %. Some risk factors for delayed urine control are the following:

- Large apical tumors,
- Morbidly obese patients,
- Patients with previous trans-urethral resection of their prostate;
- Poorly controlled diabetic patients

To date three artificial sphincters and five male slings have been placed in our series.

Potency

In our series we defined potency as being able to achieve penetrative intercourse with/or without added PDE5 inhibitors. Overall potency rates were 70 % in patients under 65 years of age, rising to 84 % in men under 55 years with no other co-morbidities, with organ confined disease and no sign of a capsular encroachment or penetration. In our early experience using external retraction in the same population group, potency rates were lower at of 53 %.

Our patients are started on Tadalafil 5 mg per day or Vardenafil daily for the first 3–6 months,

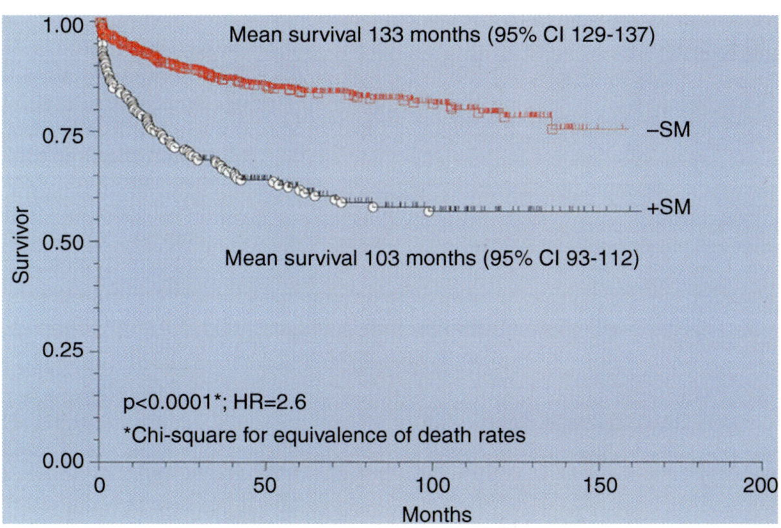

Fig. 20.4 Kaplan-Meier actuarial risk of PSA failure stratified by surgical margin status

followed by intracavernous injection therapy if there is no response to PDE5 inhibitors. Harris et al. reported that after 12 months 50 % of patients who underwent unilateral nerve sparing radical perineal prostatectomy and 70 % of patients who underwent bilateral nerve sparing radical perineal prostatectomy were able to achieve an erection adequate for intercourse with or without the use of PDF 5 inhibitors [23].

20.8 Summary

Radical perineal prostatectomy remains as relevant today as when it was first described more than a century ago. Despite the increasing popularity of laparoscopic and robotic surgery, not every patient qualifies for these approaches, and these patients should not be denied the option of surgical treatment based on contraindications to a single surgical approach. In these patients the perineal approach is an excellent alternative, offering ease of access, good visualization, low blood loss, ability to preserve the neuro-vascular bundles and potency, early post operative mobilization and short hospital stay, particularly to patients with low and intermediate risk disease, providing cure rates comparable with any other approach while keeping salvage options open should they be required at a later stage. This procedure is also especially relevant in developing countries, where access to first world technology and intensive care facilities in the post-op period may be limited which these patients seldom require due to the low morbidity of the surgery.

Key Points

- Avoids dorsal vein complex, minimizing blood loss and <1 % transfusion rate
- Minimal analgesic requirement
- Early mobilization and short hospital stay
- No thromboembolic problems
- Position discourages venous bleeding and encourages organ perfusion
- Low complication rates
- Excellent urinary continence
- Potency preservation with modified, minimal retraction technique
- Equivalent cancer control to other approaches
- Extremely cost effective

References

1. Young HH. VIII. Conservative perineal prostatectomy: the results of two years' experience and report of seventy-five cases. Ann Surg. 1905;41(4):549–57.
2. Belt E, Turner RD. A study of 229 consecutive cases of total perineal prostatectomy for cancer of the prostate. J Urol. 1957;77(1):62–77. Epub 1957/01/01.
3. Weldon VE, Tavel FR. Potency-sparing radical perineal prostatectomy: anatomy, surgical technique and initial results. J Urol. 1988;140(3):559–62. Epub 1988/09/01.
4. Blute ML, Bergstralh EJ, Partin AW, Walsh PC, Kattan MW, Scardino PT, et al. Validation of Partin tables for predicting pathological stage of clinically localized prostate cancer. J Urol. 2000;164(5):1591–5. Epub 2000/10/12.
5. Pound CR, Walsh PC, Epstein JI, Chan DW, Partin AW. Radical prostatectomy as treatment for prostate-specific antigen-detected stage T1c prostate cancer. World J Urol. 1997;15(6):373–7. Epub 1997/01/01.
6. Bluestein DL, Bostwick DG, Bergstralh EJ, Oesterling JE. Eliminating the need for bilateral pelvic lymphadenectomy in select patients with prostate cancer. J Urol. 1994;151(5):1315–20. Epub 1994/05/01.
7. Guillonneau B, Vallancien G. Laparoscopic radical prostatectomy: the Montsouris technique. J Urol. 2000;163(6):1643–9. Epub 2000/05/08.
8. Weldon VE, Tavel FR, Neuwirth H. Continence, potency and morbidity after radical perineal prostatectomy. J Urol. 1997;158(4):1470–5. Epub 1997/09/25.
9. Iselin CE, Robertson JE, Paulson DF. Radical perineal prostatectomy: oncological outcome during a 20-year period. J Urol. 1999;161(1):163–8. Epub 1999/02/26.
10. Heidenreich A, Varga Z, Von Knobloch R. Extended pelvic lymphadenectomy in patients undergoing radical prostatectomy: high incidence of lymph node metastasis. J Urol. 2002;167(4):1681–6. Epub 2002/03/26.
11. Bader P, Burkhard FC, Markwalder R, Studer UE. Is a limited lymph node dissection an adequate staging procedure for prostate cancer? J Urol. 2002;168(2):514–8; discussion 518. Epub 2002/07/20.
12. Briganti A, Larcher A, Abdollah F, Capitanio U, Gallina A, Suardi N, et al. Updated nomogram predicting lymph node invasion in patients with prostate cancer undergoing extended pelvic lymph node dissection: the essential importance of percentage of

positive cores. Eur Urol. 2012;61(3):480–7. Epub 2011/11/15.
13. Kattan MW. Re: updated nomogram to predict pathologic stage of prostate cancer given prostate-specific antigen level, clinical stage, and biopsy Gleason score (Partin tables) based on cases from 2000 to 2005. Eur Urol. 2007;52(5):1528. Epub 2007/11/07.
14. Meng MV, Carroll PR. Is it necessary to do staging pelvic lymph node dissection for T1c prostate cancer? Curr Urol Rep. 2001;2(3):237–41. Epub 2002/06/27.
15. Yiou R, Salomon L, Colombel M, Patard JJ, Chopin D, Abbou CC. Perineal approach to radical prostatectomy in kidney transplant recipients with localized prostate cancer. Urology. 1999;53(4):822–4. Epub 1999/04/10.
16. Parra RO, Boullier JA, Rauscher JA, Cummings JM. The value of laparoscopic lymphadenectomy in conjunction with radical perineal or retropubic prostatectomy. J Urol. 1994;151(6):1599–602. Epub 1994/06/01.
17. Boczko J, Melman A. Radical perineal prostatectomy in obese patients. Urology. 2003;62(3):467–9. Epub 2003/08/30.
18. Weldon VE. Technique of modern radical perineal prostatectomy. Urology. 2002;60(4):689–94. Epub 2002/10/19.
19. Hudson PB. Symposium on the prostate. Perineal prostatectomy. Urol Clin North Am. 1975;2(1):69–83. Epub 1975/02/01.
20. Bishoff JT, Motley G, Optenberg SA, Stein CR, Moon KA, Browning SM, et al. Incidence of fecal and urinary incontinence following radical perineal and retropubic prostatectomy in a national population. J Urol. 1998;160(2):454–8. Epub 1998/07/29.
21. Price DT, Vieweg J, Roland F, Coetzee L, Spalding T, Iselin C, et al. Transient lower extremity neurapraxia associated with radical perineal prostatectomy: a complication of the exaggerated lithotomy position. J Urol. 1998;160(4):1376–8. Epub 1998/09/29.
22. Boustead GBC, Coetzee LJE. MP-16.10: cancer control following radical perineal prostatectomy. Urology. 2009;74(4):S122.
23. Harris MJ. The anatomic radical perineal prostatectomy: an outcomes-based evolution. Eur Urol. 2007;52(1):81–8. Epub 2006/11/07.

Management of Pelvic Retroperitoneal Tumors

21

Steven M. Lucas

21.1 Management of Pelvic Retroperitoneal Tumors

Retroperitoneal tumors of the pelvis are commonly encountered in urology. This is due to the reflection of the peritoneum, which reflects over the dome of the bladder, leaving the majority of the bladder, prostate, seminal vesicles, and ureters in the retroperitoneum. While some cancers are commonly encountered such as prostate cancer and bladder cancer, others are infrequently encountered, such as tumors of the seminal vesicles. Often pelvic tumors encountered in the retroperitoneum require not only extirpation, but also pelvic lymphadenectomy, reconstruction, and multimodal treatments. Through improvements in laparoscopic and robotic techniques, many of these tumors are now treated in a minimally invasive manner. In this chapter, the different types of retroperitoneal urologic tumors are reviewed with emphasis on the controversies of lymphadenectomy, multimodal therapy, and minimally invasive therapy.

S.M. Lucas, MD
Department of Urology, Wayne State University
School of Medicine, Detroit, MI, USA
e-mail: smlucas@med.wayne.edu

21.2 Prostate Cancer

Prostate cancer is the most commonly encountered pelvic retroperitoneal tumor in urology. While it is discussed in other chapters, there are some aspects of treatment that bear debate. The indication for pelvic lymphadenectomy and its extent is one topic. Another is the comparative efficacy of minimally invasive prostatectomy and open prostatectomy.

Due to stage migration of prostate cancer in recent years, the rate of lymph node metastases has significantly declined. This is mirrored in the declining use of PLND in the U.S.A. at the time of radical prostatectomy with a median of 4LN removed during open surgery and three during minimally invasive prostatectomy [1, 2]. Recent guidelines from the AUA and EUA reserve PLND for high risk and intermediate and high risk patients respectively [3]. The NCCN guidelines in 2011 changed the recommendation for PLND if the nomogram risk is at least 2 %, down from 7 % [3]. None of these specify to what extent the lymphadenectomy should be performed. Comparisons of standard lymphadenectomy (SLND includes external iliac and obturator nodes, Fig. 21.1) and extended lymphadenectomy (ELND includes SLND plus internal iliac nodes and common iliac nodes up to the level of the ureter, Fig. 21.1) demonstrate increased node positivity with ELND [3–5]. However, it is not clear whether biochemical recurrence is altered [3]. In an analysis of 52 patients (1,469 lymph

H.R.H. Patel et al. (eds.), *Pelvic Cancer Surgery: Modern Breakthroughs and Future Advances*,
DOI 10.1007/978-1-4471-4258-4_21, © Springer-Verlag London 2015

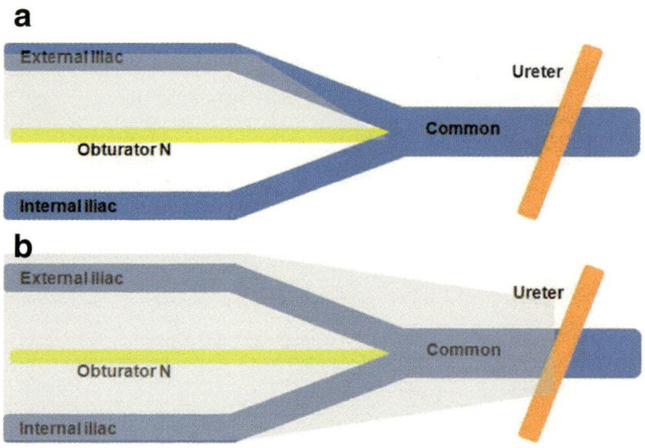

Fig. 21.1 (**a**) Standard lymph node dissection for prostate cancer includes the lymph nodes adjacent to the external iliac vein and the obturator fossa, extending from the node of Cloquet to the confluence of the external and internal iliac veins. (**b**) Extended lymph node dissection includes the standard template and the nodes adjacent to the internal iliac vein and common iliac vessels up to the ureter

nodes) undergoing ELND, positive lymph nodes were found in the standard template in 71 % of lymph nodes removed, 16 % along the internal iliac vein, and 13 % by the common iliac vein (32) [4]. Among lymph node positive patients, 63 % had positive nodes outside the standard template [4]. Comparing ELND (54 patients), SLND (231), and no lymphadenectomy (207), Liss et al. found positive lymph nodes in 24.1 % ELND versus 3.4 % SLND [3]. In high risk patients, positive lymph nodes were found in 29.3 % ELND versus 12.3 % SLND. There was no difference in overall complications and clinically significant lymphoceles occurred in 0 ELND and 3.4 % SLND [3]. However, there was no difference in biochemical recurrence noted. Similarly, Yuh et al. compared 202 ELND with a historical cohort of 204 SLND, performed in the 2 years prior to starting ELND [5]. Median lymph node yield and lymph node positivity was significantly higher for ELND, 21.5 versus 7 and 10 % versus 4 % respectively. Symptomatic lymphoceles occurred in 2.5 % ELND and 2.9 % SLND. Thrombotic complications occurred in 1 % ELND and 2.9 % SLND [5]. Though higher diagnostic yield was achieved with ELND with little change in complications in these series, one barrier to this may be the learning curve required. In a review of 500 cases, plateus for OR time, lymphadenectomy-specific complications, and lymph node count occurred after 130, 40, and 150 cases [6]. However, plateus are influenced by case selection and may not be a measure of competence, making the learning curve unrealistically steep.

Since the emergence of robotic prostatectomy (RARP), its oncologic efficacy relative to open prostatectomy (RRP) has been debated. In a recent meta-analysis of robotic prostatectomy, 13 series that compared RARP (3,917) to RRP (4,241) demonstrated no difference in positive surgical margins (847 and 820 cases for each, HR = 1.2, p = 0.19) [7]. There was also no difference in biochemical recurrence between RARP and RRP (HR = 0.9, p = 0.53). Positive margins were also similar for laparoscopic prostatectomies. In a separate meta-analysis, urinary incontinence was slightly less for RARP (7.5 %) than RRP (11.9 %) at 12 months (HR = 1.53, CI95 % = 1.04–2.53) [8]. Finally, the same authors performed a meta-analysis evaluating potency rates following RARP and RRP, demonstrating a slight advantage at 12 months with RARP (OR: 2.84, CI95 %: 1.46–5.43) [9]. Though slight advantages were seen for functional outcomes, true comparison of technique was limited in these meta-analyses, given wide variation in patients, outcome definitions and reporting.

21.3 Bladder Cancer

Though bladder cancer is discussed in other chapters, several crucial aspects regarding its management are still debated. The therapeutic effect of lymphadenectomy and the extent is one such topic. Another is the comparison between open and laparoscopic or robotic cystectomy. Finally, the benefit and timing of perioperative chemotherapy is debated.

In patients undergoing radical cystectomy, 25–30 % were found to have positive lymph nodes [10–12]. Along with grade and stage at transurethral resection, the presence of lymphovascular invasion and preoperative hydronephrosis predicted lymph node metastasis [13–15]. Many

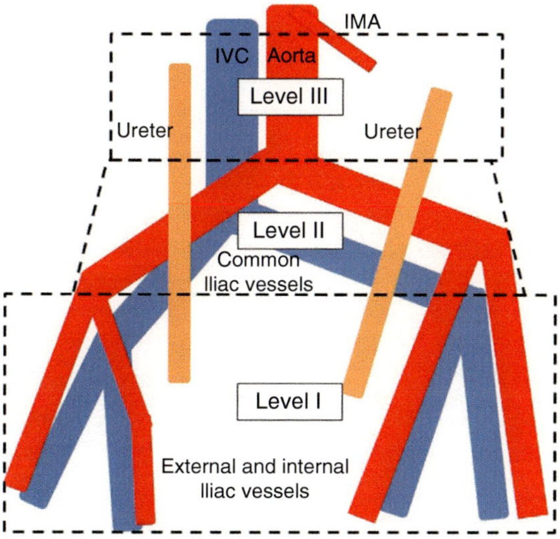

Fig. 21.2 Three levels of template dissection relevant to bladder cancer. *Level 1*: external iliac nodes, internal iliac nodes, obturator, and deep obturator nodes. *Level 2*: Common iliac, presacral and presciatic nodes. *Level 3*: Para-aortic, interaortocaval, and paracaval lymph nodes below the inferior mesenteric artery

series have attempted to delineate a minimum number of nodes as measure of extent, ranging from 10 to 16 [16]. However, one large series showed increasing survival benefit with increasing node counts [17]. Additionally, lymph node counts are affected by patient anatomy, and specimen collection, processing, and interpretation [18]. Lymph node extent was better defined by template, which can be divided into three levels (Fig. 21.2). Rates of node positive ranged from 21 to 31 % for level I, 9 to 19 % for level II, and 7 to 13 % for level III [19–21]. Additionally, the necessary extent for lymph node dissection was affected by the rate of skip metastases observed which range from 2 to 8 % of cases with positive nodes in level II [12, 20, 22], and 0–6 % for level III [20, 21], though many series have found the latter to be rare. While an extended lymphadenectomy versus a limited dissection (approximating level 1) has shown improved survival [11, 23], a recent comparison of superextended up to the inferior mesenteric artery (level III) showed no benefit over lymphadenectomy up to the proximal common iliac arteries (level II) [24]. The survival benefit of extended lymphadenectomy is also clouded by stage migration.

Systemic chemotherapy has also been shown to improve survival in patients undergoing radical cystectomy. In the neoadjuvant setting, a randomized trial comparing 153 treated with MVAC versus 154 without chemotherapy showed a median survival benefit of 77 months vs 46 months ($p=0.05$) [25]. In terms of cancer specific survival, there were 54 deaths due to bladder cancer in the neoadjuvant group and 77 in the group treated with surgery alone, $HR=1.66$ (CI95 %: 1.22–2.45). Similarly, a meta-analysis of 11 trials comparing platinum based neoadjuvant chemotherapy with surgery alone demonstrated a benefit in overall survival (HR: 0.86, CI95 %: 0.77–0.95) [26]. In the adjuvant setting, Svatek et al. retrospectively reviewed 3,947 patients from 11 different institutions, finding improved survival with adjuvant chemotherapy (HR: 0.83, CI95 %: 0.72–0.97 %) [27]. Direct comparison of neoadjuvant chemotherapy versus adjuvant chemotherapy is inadequate in the current literature. However, Eldefrawy et al. demonstrated that patients who received neoadjuvant chemotherapy were more likely to complete the planned cycles of chemotherapy (83.5 %) than those receiving adjuvant chemotherapy (35.5 %) [28]. The reason for this may be due to the difficult recovery that is required following radical cystectomy with urinary diversion.

Through increased robotic experience, many institutions have performed minimally invasive radical cystectomies with lymph node dissection. Several series demonstrated similar oncologic efficacy and complications between robotic and open cystectomy with less blood loss at the expense of typically longer operative times (Table 21.1) [29–34]. Lymph node yield and the proportion of cases with positive lymph nodes were similar for both modalities. Type of urinary diversion did not vary, though it is not clear what proportion were performed by an intracorporeal method.

21.4 Distal Ureteral Cancer

Upper tract urothelial-cell carcinoma accounts for 5 % of urothelial carcinomas [35]. Nearly 70 % of ureteral tumors occur in the distal ureter, which is

Table 21.1 Comparison of the outcomes of robotic and open cystectomy

	N	EBL(ml)/ transfuse %	OR time	Complications %	LOS d	Positive margin %	LN
Nix et al. [29]	RC- 21	258[a]	4.2[a]	33	5.1	0	18 (12–30)
	OC- 20	575	3.5	50	6.0	0	18 (8–30)
Parekh et al. [30]	RC- 20	400[a]/0	300[a] (245–366)	20 (Cl >1)	6	5	11 (9–21.5)
	OC- 20	800/2	285 (240–321)	20 (Cl >1)	6	5	23 (15–28)
Styn et al. [31]	RC- 50	350[a]/4[a]	459	28.1 (Cl >2)	9.5	2	14.3 ± 9.1
	OC-100	475/24	349	21.3 (Cl >2)	10.2	2	15.2 ± 9.5
Knox et al. [32]	RC-58	276[a]	7.8[a] ± 1.5	43		7	
	OC-84	1,522	6.6 ± 1.25	65		8	
Gondo et al. [33]	RC-11	656[a]/0[a]		54		9.1	20.6[a]
	OC-15	1,788/40		75		20	14.1
Nepple et al. [34]	RC-36	675[a]/39[a]	410		7.9	6	17 (12–20)
	OC-29	1,497/83	345		9.6	7	14 (10–20)

[a]Denotes a statistically significant difference between the two treatment modalities in that particular series

Table 21.2 Comparison of the oncologic outcomes of nephroureterectomy and distal ureterectomy for distal ureteral tumors

Series	Number of patients	Median follow-up (months)	Cancer-specific survival (%)	P
Dalpiaz et al. [40]	RNU: 42	51.5	5 years: 78	0.92
	DU: 49		5 years: 77	
Simonato et al. [41]	DU: 73	87	5 years: 94.1	
Colin et al. [43]	RNU: 416	26	5 years: 86.3	0.99
	DU: 52		5 years: 87.9	
Jeldres et al. [42]	RNU: 1,222	30	5 years: 82.2	>0.05
	DU: 569		5 years: 86.6	
Lehmann et al. [44]	RNU: 91	96	10 year pTa/1: 87	0.271
	DU: 51		10 year pT2-4: 36	
Giannarini et al. [45]	RNU: 24	58	5 years: 66	0.896
	DU: 19		5 years: 64	

found in the pelvis [35]. Radical nephroureterectomy is the gold standard treatment for high grade and invasive tumors of the upper tract. In a recent multi-institutional review of 1,363 patients, cancer-specific survival following nephroureterectomy was 78.3 ± 1.3 and 72.9 ± 1.4 % at 3 and 5 years respectively [36]. Imaging with CT urogram is the modality of choice for diagnosing distal ureteral tumors [37]. Cytology can be helpful as positive cytology has been associated with muscle-invasive and higher stage tumors [38]. Ureteroscopy is a useful diagnostic adjunct, when the diagnosis is uncertain, and it can determine tumor grade in 90 % of cases [39].

While nephroureterectomy is the gold standard therapy for invasive upper tract tumors, distal ureterectomy may have a similar outcome to nephroureterectomy in managing invasive or high grade tumors in the distal ureter. Initially performed for cases in which renal preservation was imperative (i.e., solitary kidney), distal ureterectomy is increasingly offered electively to reduce the development of chronic kidney disease, thereby avoiding associated cardiovascular morbidity and maximizing adjuvant chemotherapy options. Recently, several series demonstrated similar oncologic efficacy of segmental ureterectomy versus nephroureterectomy for distal ureteral tumors (Table 21.2) [40–45]. Follow-up of these patients demonstrated that recurrence in the ipsilateral upper tract was low. For example, Dalpiaz et al. noted two patients with such recurrence at 63 and 45 months after surgery, both were alive after nephroureterectomy [40]. When planning a distal ureterectomy, diagnostic ureteroscopy was avoided in several of the series for fear of seeding the proximal upper urinary tract. Additionally, performance of lymphadenectomy during nephroureterectomy or distal ureterectomy was done sparingly in many of the series [40, 41, 43]. Although lymphadenectomy is beneficial in bladder urothelial carcinoma, a similar benefit for upper tract urothelial cancer has not been definitively shown [46]. Furthermore, the precise boundaries for lymphadenectomy for upper tract TCC is not clearly defined. In the multi-institutional review, Margulis et al. found that lymphadenectomy was performed in 48 % of cases [36].

Although theoretical, the benefit of platinum-based chemotherapy was assumed due to the success of this regimen in bladder cancer, but there is considerably less data for its support for the treatment of upper tract TCC. In one study of neoadjuvant chemotherapy (which compared 43 patients receiving neoadjuvant chemotherapy with 107 historical controls), Margulis et al. demonstrated a reduction in stage pT2 or higher disease (46.5 % versus 65.4 %) and pT3 or higher disease (27.9 % versus 47.7 %) at the time of surgery in patients treated with neoadjuvant chemotherapy [47]. In two separate multi-institutional studies, adjuvant chemotherapy had minimal impact on cancer-specific survival [48, 49].

Minimally invasive distal ureterectomy with reconstruction for distal ureteral cancer was reported in some series [50–54]. Schimpf et al. reported 11 patients, of which 5 were for ureteral cancer, with median operative time of 189 min [50]. One intraoperative complication, an iliac vein injury, was repaired intraoperatively. Three patients underwent psoas hitch and two underwent boari flap. There were two recurrences noted, both in the ipsilateral pelvis treated with nephroureterectomy. All patients were free of disease at follow-up. Glinianski et al. reported nine patients undergoing distal ureterectomy of which six had a psoas hitch, with a mean operative time was 252 min [51]. There were no intraoperative complications, and all margins were negative. One patient each had pT1,2, and 3 disease, and five patients had high grade urothelial carcinoma. During follow-up five patients had superficial bladder cancer, and one patient had superficial recurrence in the renal pelvis. In general patients undergoing distal ureterectomy by minimally invasive means tended to be of lower grade and stage. Robotic port placement was achieved with the camera cephalad to the umbilicus, with three trocars and one assistant port placed laterally in a configuration similar to robotic prostatectomy [50, 53].

21.5 Seminal Vesicle Tumors

Tumors of the seminal vesicle most often occur due to spread from other tumors. Primary cancers of the seminal vesicle are very rare, with 51 reported in a review in 2002 [55]. The most common histology of these tumors is adenocarcinoma. Diagnosis is supported by increased levels of CA-125 [55]. Primary seminal vesicle adenocarcinomas do not produce PSA or CEA [56]. Useful imaging studies include pelvis CT [57] and pelvic MRI [58], which has the advantage of improved soft tissue resolution to help delineate the extent of the tumor. Method of histologic diagnosis varied, but 30 % were diagnosed by transrectal biopsy, 25 % by transurethral resection, and 45 % at the time of open surgery [55].

While prognosis was historically poor, recent reports demonstrated prolonged recurrence-free survival over 3 years, likely due to earlier diagnosis [55]. Primary treatment involved surgical resection. Early reports recommended excision of the prostate and seminal vesicles, due to frequent involvement of the ejaculatory ducts [59]. In tumors without evidence of invasion into the prostate, vesiculectomy may be performed [55]. Conversely, patients with more advanced tumors may benefit from cystoprostatectomy with urinary diversion. Surgery with negative margins offered the best chance of cure as it is not clear whether radiation or chemotherapy improved outcomes [56, 60]. Androgen deprivation therapy was reported to have efficacy in some series [61,

62]. Other histologies of primary seminal vesicle tumors include sarcoma, germ cell tumors, and squamous carcinomas [63, 64].

Conclusion

Urologic retroperitoneal tumors span a wide variety of tumor types. However, treatment of many of these tumors not only involves removal of the offending organ, but also involve regional lymphadenectomy. The efficacy and extent of such lymphadenectomy is still debated. With improvements in minimally invasive tools and techniques, minimally invasive treatments have been increasingly applied to what was once a difficult tumor location to reach. Further monitoring of the safety and efficacy of these treatment are warranted, and they should be applied in the appropriately selected cases.

Key Points

- Retroperitoneal urologic pelvic tumors arise in the prostate, bladder, ureters and seminal vesicles.
- Extended pelvic lymph node dissection increases the diagnosis of lymph node metastasis in high risk prostate cancer patients.
- Robotic prostatectomy demonstrates similar oncologic efficacy to open prostatectomy in terms of surgical margins and biochemical recurrence. Further research is need to validate the slight advantage in functional outcomes with robotic prostatectomy.
- Lymphadenectomy at the time of cystectomy is best measured by template and not count. While extended lymphadenectomy should be performed, whether this should be extended to the inferior mesenteric artery is debatable.
- Neoadjuvant and adjuvant chemotherapy have been shown to improve survival in patients with bladder cancer.
- Robotic cystectomy has been successful in early series.
- Distal ureterectomy has similar efficacy to nephroureterectomy for appropriately selected distal ureteral tumors.
- The role of chemotherapy and lymphadenectomy needs to be more clearly defined in the treatment of distal ureteral tumors.
- Distal ureterectomy, including complex reconstruction can be done in a minimally invasive fashion.
- Tumors of the seminal vesicle are rare, and surgery is the key component of treatment.

References

1. Hu JC, Prasad SM, Gu X, et al. Determinants of performing radical prostatectomy pelvic lymph node dissection and the number of lymph nodes removed in elderly men. Urology. 2011;77:402–6.
2. Feifer AH, Elkin EB, Lowrance WT, et al. Temporal trends and predictors of pelvic lymph node dissection in open or minimally invasive radical prostatectomy. Cancer. 2011;117:3933–42.
3. Liss MA, Palazzi K, Stroup SP, Jabaji R, Raheem OA, Kane CJ. Outcomes and complications of pelvic lymph node dissection during robotic-assisted radical prostatectomy. World J Urol. 2013;31:481–8.
4. Heck MM, Retz M, Bandur M, et al. Topography of lymph node metastases in prostate cancer patients undergoing radical prostatectomy and extended lymphadenectomy: results of a combined molecular and histopathologic mapping study. Eur Urol. 2014;66(2):222–9.
5. Yuh BE, Ruel NH, Mejia R, Novara G, Wilson TG. Standardized comparison of robot-assisted limited and extended pelvic lymphadenectomy for prostate cancer. BJU Int. 2013;112:81–8.
6. Eden CG, Zacharakis E, Bott S. The learning curve for laparoscopic extended pelvic lymphadenectomy for intermediate- and high-risk prostate cancer: implications for compliance with existing guidelines. BJU Int. 2013;112:346–54.
7. Novara G, Ficarra V, Mocellin S, et al. Systematic review and meta-analysis of studies reporting oncologic outcome after robot-assisted radical prostatectomy. Eur Urol. 2012;62:382–404.
8. Ficarra V, Novara G, Rosen RC, et al. Systematic review and meta-analysis of studies reporting urinary continence recovery after robot-assisted radical prostatectomy. Eur Urol. 2012;62:405–17.
9. Ficarra V, Novara G, Ahlering TE, et al. Systematic review and meta-analysis of studies reporting potency

rates after robot-assisted radical prostatectomy. Eur Urol. 2012;62:418–30.
10. Stein JP, Lieskovsky G, Cote R, et al. Radical cystectomy in the treatment of invasive bladder cancer: long-term results in 1,054 patients. J Clin Oncol. 2001;19:666–75.
11. Dhar NB, Klein EA, Reuther AM, Thalmann GN, Madersbacher S, Studer UE. Outcome after radical cystectomy with limited or extended pelvic lymph node dissection. J Urol. 2008;179:873–8; discussion 178.
12. Steven K, Poulsen AL. Radical cystectomy and extended pelvic lymphadenectomy: survival of patients with lymph node metastasis above the bifurcation of the common iliac vessels treated with surgery only. J Urol. 2007;178:1218–23; discussion 1223–4.
13. Resnick MJ, Bergey M, Magerfleisch L, Tomaszewski JE, Malkowicz SB, Guzzo TJ. Longitudinal evaluation of the concordance and prognostic value of lymphovascular invasion in transurethral resection and radical cystectomy specimens. BJU Int. 2011;107:46–52.
14. Stimson CJ, Cookson MS, Barocas DA, et al. Preoperative hydronephrosis predicts extravesical and node positive disease in patients undergoing cystectomy for bladder cancer. J Urol. 2010;183:1732–7.
15. Karakiewicz PI, Shariat SF, Palapattu GS, et al. Precystectomy nomogram for prediction of advanced bladder cancer stage. Eur Urol. 2006;50:1254–60; discussion 1261–2.
16. Morgan TM, Kaffenberger SD, Cookson MS. Surgical and chemotherapeutic management of regional lymph nodes in bladder cancer. J Urol. 2012;188:1081–8.
17. Koppie TM, Vickers AJ, Vora K, Dalbagni G, Bochner BH. Standardization of pelvic lymphadenectomy performed at radical cystectomy: can we establish a minimum number of lymph nodes that should be removed? Cancer. 2006;107:2368–74.
18. Parkash V, Bifulco C, Feinn R, Concato J, Jain D. To count and how to count, that is the question: interobserver and intraobserver variability among pathologists in lymph node counting. Am J Clin Pathol. 2010;134:42–9.
19. Leissner J, Ghoneim MA, Abol-Enein H, et al. Extended radical lymphadenectomy in patients with urothelial bladder cancer: results of a prospective multicenter study. J Urol. 2004;171:139–44.
20. Miocinovic R, Gong MC, Ghoneim IA, Fergany AF, Hansel DE, Stephenson AJ. Presacral and retroperitoneal lymph node involvement in urothelial bladder cancer: results of a prospective mapping study. J Urol. 2011;186:1269–73.
21. Dorin RP, Daneshmand S, Eisenberg MS, et al. Lymph node dissection technique is more important than lymph node count in identifying nodal metastases in radical cystectomy patients: a comparative mapping study. Eur Urol. 2011;60:946–52.
22. Vazina A, Dugi D, Shariat SF, Evans J, Link R, Lerner SP. Stage specific lymph node metastasis mapping in radical cystectomy specimens. J Urol. 2004;171:1830–4.
23. Abol-Enein H, Tilki D, Mosbah A, et al. Does the extent of lymphadenectomy in radical cystectomy for bladder cancer influence disease-free survival? A prospective single-center study. Eur Urol. 2011;60:572–7.
24. Zehnder P, Studer UE, Skinner EC, et al. Super extended versus extended pelvic lymph node dissection in patients undergoing radical cystectomy for bladder cancer: a comparative study. J Urol. 2011;186:1261–8.
25. Grossman HB, Natale RB, Tangen CM, et al. Neoadjuvant chemotherapy plus cystectomy compared with cystectomy alone for locally advanced bladder cancer. N Engl J Med. 2003;349:859–66.
26. Advanced Bladder Cancer (ABC) Meta-analysis Collaboration. Neoadjuvant chemotherapy in invasive bladder cancer: update of a systematic review and meta-analysis of individual patient data. Eur Urol. 2005;48:202–5; discussion 205–6.
27. Svatek RS, Shariat SF, Lasky RE, et al. The effectiveness of off-protocol adjuvant chemotherapy for patients with urothelial carcinoma of the urinary bladder. Clin Cancer Res. 2010;16:4461–7.
28. Eldefrawy A, Soloway MS, Katkoori D, Singal R, Pan D, Manoharan M. Neoadjuvant and adjuvant chemotherapy for muscle-invasive bladder cancer: the likelihood of initiation and completion. Indian J Urol. 2012;28:424–6.
29. Nix J, Smith A, Kurpad R, Nielsen ME, Wallen EM, Pruthi RS. Prospective randomized controlled trial of robotic versus open radical cystectomy for bladder cancer: perioperative and pathologic results. Eur Urol. 2010;57:196–201.
30. Parekh DJ, Messer J, Fitzgerald J, Ercole B, Svatek R. Perioperative outcomes and oncologic efficacy from a pilot prospective randomized clinical trial of open versus robotic assisted radical cystectomy. J Urol. 2013;189:474–9.
31. Styn NR, Montgomery JS, Wood DP, et al. Matched comparison of robotic-assisted and open radical cystectomy. Urology. 2012;79:1303–8.
32. Knox ML, El-Galley R, Busby JE. Robotic versus open radical cystectomy: identification of patients who benefit from the robotic approach. J Endourol. 2013;27:40–4.
33. Gondo T, Yoshioka K, Nakagami Y, et al. Robotic versus open radical cystectomy: prospective comparison of perioperative and pathologic outcomes in Japan. Jpn J Clin Oncol. 2012;42:625–31.
34. Nepple KG, Strope SA, Grubb 3rd RL, Kibel AS. Early oncologic outcomes of robotic vs. open radical cystectomy for urothelial cancer. Urol Oncol. 2011;31:894–8.
35. Munoz JJ, Ellison LM. Upper tract urothelial neoplasms: incidence and survival during the last 2 decades. J Urol. 2000;164:1523–5.
36. Margulis V, Shariat SF, Matin SF, et al. Outcomes of radical nephroureterectomy: a series from the upper tract urothelial carcinoma collaboration. Cancer. 2009;115:1224–33.
37. Dillman JR, Caoili EM, Cohan RH, Ellis JH, Francis IR, Schipper MJ. Detection of upper tract urothelial

neoplasms: sensitivity of axial, coronal reformatted, and curved-planar reformatted image-types utilizing 16-row multi-detector CT urography. Abdom Imaging. 2008;33:707–16.
38. Brien JC, Shariat SF, Herman MP, et al. Preoperative hydronephrosis, ureteroscopic biopsy grade and urinary cytology can improve prediction of advanced upper tract urothelial carcinoma. J Urol. 2010; 184:69–73.
39. Tavora F, Fajardo DA, Lee TK, et al. Small endoscopic biopsies of the ureter and renal pelvis: pathologic pitfalls. Am J Surg Pathol. 2009;33:1540–6.
40. Dalpiaz O, Ehrlich G, Quehenberger F, Pummer K, Zigeuner R. Distal ureterectomy is a safe surgical option in patients with urothelial carcinoma of the distal ureter. Urol Oncol. 2014;32(1):34.e1–8.
41. Simonato A, Varca V, Gregori A, et al. Elective segmental ureterectomy for transitional cell carcinoma of the ureter: long-term follow-up in a series of 73 patients. BJU Int. 2012;110:E744–9.
42. Jeldres C, Lughezzani G, Sun M, et al. Segmental ureterectomy can safely be performed in patients with transitional cell carcinoma of the ureter. J Urol. 2010;183:1324–9.
43. Colin P, Ouzzane A, Pignot G, et al. Comparison of oncological outcomes after segmental ureterectomy or radical nephroureterectomy in urothelial carcinomas of the upper urinary tract: results from a large French multicentre study. BJU Int. 2012;110:1134–41.
44. Lehmann J, Suttmann H, Kovac I, et al. Transitional cell carcinoma of the ureter: prognostic factors influencing progression and survival. Eur Urol. 2007;51:1281–8.
45. Giannarini G, Schumacher MC, Thalmann GN, Bitton A, Fleischmann A, Studer UE. Elective management of transitional cell carcinoma of the distal ureter: can kidney-sparing surgery be advised? BJU Int. 2007;100:264–8.
46. Roupret M, Zigeuner R, Palou J, et al. European guidelines for the diagnosis and management of upper urinary tract urothelial cell carcinomas: 2011 update. Eur Urol. 2011;59:584–94.
47. Matin SF, Margulis V, Kamat A, et al. Incidence of downstaging and complete remission after neoadjuvant chemotherapy for high-risk upper tract transitional cell carcinoma. Cancer. 2010;116:3127–34.
48. Hellenthal NJ, Shariat SF, Margulis V, et al. Adjuvant chemotherapy for high risk upper tract urothelial carcinoma: results from the upper tract urothelial carcinoma collaboration. J Urol. 2009;182:900–6.
49. Audenet F, Yates DR, Cussenot O, Roupret M. The role of chemotherapy in the treatment of urothelial cell carcinoma of the upper urinary tract (UUT-UCC). Urol Oncol. 2013;31(4):407–13.
50. Schimpf MO, Wagner JR. Robot-assisted laparoscopic distal ureteral surgery. JSLS. 2009;13:44–9.
51. Glinianski M, Guru KA, Zimmerman G, Mohler J, Kim HL. Robot-assisted ureterectomy and ureteral reconstruction for urothelial carcinoma. J Endourol. 2009;23:97–100.
52. Allaparthi S, Ramanathan R, Balaji KC. Robotic distal ureterectomy with boari flap reconstruction for distal ureteral urothelial cancers: a single institutional pilot experience. J Laparoendosc Adv Surg Tech A. 2010;20:165–71.
53. Roupret M, Harmon JD, Sanderson KM, et al. Laparoscopic distal ureterectomy and anastomosis for management of low-risk upper urinary tract transitional cell carcinoma: preliminary results. BJU Int. 2007;99:623–7.
54. Gerber E, Dinlenc CZ, Wagner JR. Laparoscopic distal ureterectomy for low grade transitional cell carcinoma. J Urol. 2003;169:2295.
55. Thiel R, Effert P. Primary adenocarcinoma of the seminal vesicles. J Urol. 2002;168:1891–6.
56. Ohmori T, Okada K, Tabei R, et al. CA125-producing adenocarcinoma of the seminal vesicle. Pathol Int. 1994;44:333–7.
57. Sussman SK, Dunnick NR, Silverman PM, Cohan RH. Carcinoma of the seminal vesicle: CT appearance. J Comput Assist Tomogr. 1986;10:519–20.
58. Navallas M, Vargas HA, Akin O, et al. Primary seminal vesicle adenocarcinoma. Clin Imaging. 2011;35:480–2.
59. Smith Jr BA, Webb EA, Price WE. Carcinoma of the seminal vesicle. J Urol. 1967;97:743–50.
60. Oxley JD, Brett MT, Gillatt DA, Burton P. Seminal vesicle carcinoma. Histopathology. 1999;34:562–3.
61. Benson Jr RC, Clark WR, Farrow GM. Carcinoma of the seminal vesicle. J Urol. 1984;132:483–5.
62. Gohji K, Kamidono S, Okada S. Primary adenocarcinoma of the seminal vesicle. Br J Urol. 1993;72:514–5.
63. Wang J, Yue X, Zhao R, Cheng B, Wazir R, Wang K. Primary squamous cell carcinoma of seminal vesicle: an extremely rare case report with literature review. Int Urol Nephrol. 2013;45:135–8.
64. Yao XD, Hong YP, Ye DW, Wang CF. Primary yolk sac tumor of seminal vesicle: a case report and literature review. World J Surg Oncol. 2012;10:189.

Management of Erectile Dysfunction After Radical Prostatectomy

22

John P. Mulhall, Craig F. Donatucci, Kelly A. Chiles, and Hartwig Büttner

22.1 Introduction

Men undergoing radical prostatectomy (RP) require management of the sexual dysfunction sequelae that accompanies this surgery. Erectile dysfunction (ED) is the most common sexual dysfunction following RP, and has a prevalence of anywhere from 20 to 90 % [1]. It is important for prostatectomists to appreciate, however, that ED is not the only sexual dysfunction encountered by patients and their partners. The "burden of cure" which men face after radical prostatectomy encompasses many facets of sexual satisfaction and intimacy (Table 22.1).

The significant discrepancy in the quoted ED prevalence after RP stems from multiple causes. ED is defined as the consistent inability to obtain or maintain an erection sufficient for sexual activity for at least 3 months duration. This definition is liberally applied throughout the published literature, and there is often no distinction between men who have spontaneous return of erections after RP and men who continue to require erectogenic agents for the duration of their lives. Men who require these aids are still recorded as having "return of erectile function" for the purposes of publication, despite this being significantly different from their baseline function. In many instances, there is no formal assessment of erectile function through the use of validated instruments such as the International Index of Erectile Function (IIEF questionnaire). Merely asking patients "have your erections returned" is an inadequate means of determining erectile function, yet unfortunately this is a common method for determining published outcomes. In addition, the formal evaluation of the effect of RP on erectile function is confounded by the definition of "nerve sparing" being subjectively assessed by the prostatectomist given the lack of any objective way to determine the nerve-sparing status. Retrospective studies often do not include the entire population of men who underwent RP, and the introduction of this selection bias clearly impacts results. Furthermore, duration of follow-up is limited, and there is limited data on ED prevalence beyond several years after surgery. This is important to appreciate because although we know that there is an immediate decline in function after RP that often improves over time, very little is understood regarding the role RP

J.P. Mulhall, MD, FECSM
Male Sexual and Reproductive Medicine Program, Memorial Sloan Kettering Cancer Center, New York, NY, USA

C.F. Donatucci, MD
Department of Men's Health, Eli Lilly & Company, Indianapolis, IN, USA

K.A. Chiles, MD, MSc
Male Reproductive Medicine and Microsurgery, Department of Urology, Weill Cornell Medical College, New York, NY, USA

H. Büttner, MD, FECSM (✉)
Medical Department, Men's Health ACE (Australia, Canada, Europe), Lilly Deutschland GmbH, Bad Homburg v.d.H., Germany
e-mail: buettnerh@lilly.com

H.R.H. Patel et al. (eds.), *Pelvic Cancer Surgery: Modern Breakthroughs and Future Advances*,
DOI 10.1007/978-1-4471-4258-4_22, © Springer-Verlag London 2015

Table 22.1 Prevalence of sexual dysfunctions after RP

Dysfunction	Prevalence (%)
Erectile dysfunction	20–90
Climacturia	14–28
Arousal incontinence	93
Orgasmic dysfunction (anorgasmia, delayed orgasm, dysorgasmia, decreased orgasm intensity)	18–46
Reduced penile size	68–71
Peyronie's disease	16

plays in the patient's long-term erectile function as they undergo the natural process of aging or cope with the ramifications of additional co-morbidities such as diabetes or hypertension.

Optimal evaluation of erectile function would include a prospective baseline pre-RP assessment as well as repeated post-RP evaluations over time. EF should be evaluated in a way that incorporates all aspects of sexual dysfunction into the surgeon's queries and utilizes objective, validated instruments. Because of the obvious limitations within the published literature, prostatectomists should be encouraged to maintain their own prospective databases in order to be able to accurately inform their patients regarding what their specific functional outcomes truly are.

22.2 Pathophysiology of Erectile Dysfunction After Radical Prostatectomy

Erectile Dysfunction after radical prostatectomy differs from ED due to other causes. Post prostatectomy ED is associated with a life changing diagnosis (cancer); the onset of post prostatectomy ED can be immediate and post prostatectomy ED is relatively refractory to simple therapy (ED response rates to phosphodiesterase type 5 inhibitor (PDE5i) therapy are the lowest of all etiological categories) at least in the first 12 months after surgery. The introduction of nerve-sparing radical prostatectomy reduced direct surgical injury and interruption of the neurovascular bundle, yet even careful low trauma surgical maneuvers can lead to neuropraxia [2]. The cavernous nerve is located on the postero-lateral aspect of the seminal vesicle and the prostate, ascends to the 1 o'clock position and 11 o'clock position along the membranous urethra under the pubic bone and penetrates the hilum of the penis to enervate the corpora cavernosa [3]. Quinlan et al. reported the first series documenting the potential impact of nerve sparing; of 503 patients who were potent preoperatively, 342 (68 %) remained potent at 18 months, though these were self-reports gathered in the era before validated patient reported outcome instruments were introduced [4]. While it has been reported that the advent of robotic surgical techniques appears to have diminished the ED seen after prostatectomy, this has not yet definitively translated into better functional erectile outcomes [5]. Traction, thermal injury and ischemia due to associated vascular injury still accompany all operative techniques (open, conventional laparoscopic and robot-assisted laparoscopic prostatectomy).

The pathophysiology leading to ED after radical prostatectomy has been well documented by Hatzimouratidis et al. and there is significant animal data in the literature to support this mechanism [6]. Neuropraxia is, to a degree, an expected outcome of prostatectomy while complete neural destruction may occur when nerve-sparing is not clinically indicated or possible. The reduction or complete loss of erectile function after radical prostatectomy is a consequence of the cumulative or even synergistic response to multiple injuries of the erectile mechanism.

The response to neural injury or loss is immediate and is initiated at the genetic level. Neuromodulatory treatment strategies resulting in improved erectile function currently suffer from a lack of knowledge of the complex genetic changes that orchestrate the molecular systems involved in recovery. Initial investigation of the neuro-reparative processes at the gene level was performed by User et al. using nascent gene expression technology [7]. Penile tissue from Sprague Dawley (SD) rats was harvested 48 h after bilateral cavernous nerve injury. Of a possible 8,000 genes analyzed in the array, 126 were found to be significantly altered; 79 were up regulated and 47 genes down regulated. The dominant class of genes activated did not appear to be directly involved in erectile function. Recognizing that erectile recovery was primarily dependent on neuro-regenerative properties, Calenda et al. turned away from the penis, which is the target tissue of enervation, to the injured peripheral nerve itself as the focus of examination [8]. These investigators used the major pelvic ganglion as the target for gene expression analysis in a SD rat model; two time points were examined representing acute (48 h) and chronic (14 days) after bilateral cavernous nerve injury. A significant number (265) of neuro-reparative and neuro-protective genes were uniquely up-regulated acutely, 54 genes uniquely up-regulated at chronic time point, and 60 additional genes were up-regulated at both time points. In addition to genes involved in inflammation and immune responses, genes involved in tissue differentiation, neural growth, and proliferation were significantly involved in the response to injury. Further research based on this novel approach may lead to tailored neuro-modulatory therapy with the hope of significant recovery of pre-surgical erectile function.

With surgical neural injury and loss, cessation of daily and nocturnal erections occurs, leading to significant cavernosal hypoxia with attendant microstructural consequences. Schwartz et al. reported on two groups of post prostatectomy patients who underwent pre-operative penile biopsy, the first group received sildenafil 50 mg every other night for 6 months and the second 100 mg of sildenafil every other night [9]. While a minority of patients returned for a second penile biopsy, there was a difference in percentage of smooth muscle content between the groups; patients receiving 100 mg of sildenafil demonstrated an increase in the percentage of smooth muscle. Despite limitations, this manuscript contributed in part to the concept of chronic PDE5i therapy as a possible penile rehabilitation.

Several authors have utilized a model of radical prostatectomy induced ED in SD rats demonstrating that cavernous nerve injury leads to generation of multiple cytokines (Transforming Growth Factor β[beta], Endothelin1) and significant apoptosis of penile erectile tissue [10, 11], followed by fibrosis [12], depending in part on the severity of the injury. Using the same model of RP induced ED, Leungwattanakij et al. documented increases in hypoxia-inducible factor-1a-(HIF-1a), TGFβ[beta] and collagen I and III (all markers of fibrosis), in penile tissue [13]. Gross morphometric changes in the penis occur subsequent to cavernous nerve injury in this rat model. Penile fibrosis and loss of smooth muscle lead to failure of the veno-occlusive mechanism and the development of erectile dysfunction.

The correlation between the degree of neurovascular injury and the severity of morphometric change and subsequent development of ED was confirmed in a later study by Özden et al. [14]. These investigators used a rat model of ED and compared bilateral cavernous nerve injury (BCN) to unilateral cavernous nerve injury (UCN) and sham operated animals; a subset of animals in each group were given sildenafil after injury. The BCN animals had the largest decrease in penile weight and smooth muscle apoptosis, while UCN animals demonstrated less severe loss of penile weight and apoptosis.

Radical prostatectomy may injure more than just the cavernous nerve. Accessory pudendal arteries (APA's) are vessels that arise in a supra-diaphragmatic location. Such arteries often course close to the prostate and travel beneath the pubic bone. In some patients, these arteries represent a major source of arterial inflow to the corpora cavernosa. It is estimated that APA's occur in 30 % of men based on laparoscopic or robotic prostatectomy studies. Neurovascular injury subsequent to radical prostatectomy was documented by Aboseif et al. who evaluated 20 patients with intracavernosal injection (ICI) of prostaglandin E1 (PGE1) with subsequent duplex Doppler ultrasound evaluation of the cavernosal arteries [15]. At 1 year post surgery 8/20 (40 %) had reduced erectile hardness in response to the ICI PGE1 with accompanying decreased in arterial blood flow.

Several morphometric reports document the effects of neurovascular injury with subsequent fibrosis and apoptosis after radical prostatectomy. Penile measurements were made from the symphysis pubis to the mid glans in the stretched penis in 31 men before and 3 months after radical prostatectomy; nearly half of the men experienced a loss of penile length ±1 cm, and an additional 23 % had loss between 0 and 1 cm [16]. A larger series of 124 men undergoing reported by Savoie et al. confirmed that morphometric penile changes were measurable men 3 months after radical prostatectomy [17].

22.3 Rehabilitation and Preservation of Erectile Function After Prostatectomy

Rehabilitation or optimal preservation of natural EF after radical prostatectomy represents the ultimate goal for patients and a challenge for the practicing urologist.

Neuropraxia leads to an impairment of erectile responsiveness to sexual stimuli as well as a reduction of nocturnal and morning erections and is associated with a persistent hypoxia of penile corpora cavernosa, evident immediately following prostatectomy.

Montorsi et al. [18] first suggested the concept of penile rehabilitation, based on the preservation of EF through the improvement of tissue-oxygenation to prevent from endothelial dysfunction and cavernosal smooth-muscle fibrosis.

However, to date no strategy investigated provides the definite answer, and a clear goal for these patients is also to improve EF early after surgery and to retain the best response to PDE5i if they require assistance.

The concept of penile rehabilitation with PDE5i is supported by several well-designed preclinical studies [19]. Promotion of EF-recovery, improvement of the smooth-muscle-to-collagen ratio, reduction of cavernosal apoptotic index, preservation of endothelial function, and neuroprotection during nerve damage have been proven in animal models [19].

In clinical practice, rehabilitative concepts using different PDE5i and schedules for administration are widely adopted based on their potential antifibrotic and neuroprotective properties, but its use is so far not fully supported by high evidence data. While chronic administration of short-acting PDE5i such as sildenafil-citrate or vardenafil HCL has been shown to increase the rate of EF recovery as compared to placebo [20, 21], no study has demonstrated higher efficacy on penile rehabilitation with PDE5i with its chronic use as compared to the respective on-demand administration schedules.

One of the main criticisms of these studies lies in the type of PDE5i used. Both sildenafil-citrate and vardenafil-HCL are characterized by a relatively short half-life, which may prevent them from reaching coverage over a full dosing-interval with a single daily administration. In contrast, the longer half-life of tadalafil confers to this drug the optimal pharmacokinetic profile for its use in the rehabilitative setting with a once-daily administration [22]. However, Montorsi et al. could not demonstrate higher efficacy on unassisted EF with once-daily tadalafil (5 mg) as compared to on-demand administration of 20 mg in a multicenter, randomized, double-blind trial (REACTT) [23]. Chronic use of once-daily tadalafil 5 mg given for 9 months was not superior to tadalafil 20 mg given on demand or to placebo in EF recovery rates at the end of a 6-weeks wash-out (primary endpoint of the trial). Further criticisms of the design of REACTT and all other published evidence are the improper patient selection (men at low risk of postoperative ED) and the relatively short duration of the study-period, as the ultimate rehabilitation analyses should ideally performed at 18–24 months post NSRP [24, 25].

Therefore, none of the currently available PDE5i showed higher efficacy on rehabilitation of unassisted EF within a time-period of approximately 1 year post surgery when administered once-daily as compared to on demand dosing following RP in well-designed, prospective, randomized trials.

However, in the REACTT-Trial, treatment with tadalafil 5 mg once daily provided significant benefit on recovery of assisted EF, as indicated by a significant improvement of achieving penile tumescence (Sexual Encounter Profile Question 1, SEP1) both at the end of the 9-month randomized double-blind, double-dummy treatment phase as well as at the end of the open-label phase at month 13.5 versus placebo, whereas on-demand treatment with tadalafil 20 mg was not significantly superior to placebo at month 13.5. Improvements of successful intercourse (SEP3) were statistically significant versus placebo only for tadalafil once daily and exceeded the minimal clinically important difference (MCID) after double-blind treatment. Results of this trial indicate that active treatment early after NSRP improves responsiveness to PDE5i also in the further course of post-surgery follow-up, as shown by significantly improved SEP3 yes-responses (55.3 %, post-hoc ANCOVA) after re-challenge with tadalafil once-daily during the 3-month open-label treatment, with (absolute) 17.5 % less per-patient yes-responses to SEP3 after OLT in those patients with no active treatment during DBT.

REACTT is the first randomized controlled trial providing evidence that chronic inhibition of PDE5 with tadalafil once daily significantly protects from penile length loss post RP. Similar results confirming chronic PDE5-inhibition protects penile length following prostatectomy have recently been published by Berookhim and colleagues from Memorial Sloan Kettering Cancer Center [26].

22.4 Treating Erectile Dysfunction in Radical Prostatectomy Patient

PDE5 Inhibitors

Multiple treatment modalities are available for men after RP, and a rudimentary understanding of the various options are important for anyone counseling patients (Table 22.2). Even more salient is the concept that EF recovery is a long-term process, and the degree of recovery at 2 years is often significantly better than what patients experienced 6 months after surgery [27].

First-line therapy for ED after RP is the use of a phosphodiesterase type 5 inhibitor. There is no evidence that any one member of this family of drugs is more efficacious than another, and it is reasonable to consider the patient's/couple's sexual dynamics and financial constraints when choosing which drug to prescribe [28]. Although 85 % of men will not respond to PDE5i at 6 months, over time up to 70 % of men will achieve penetration hardness erections after RP with PDE5i use [29, 30]. The degree of success is directly related to the degree of nerve sparing, and men with bilateral nerve sparing surgery clearly have better outcomes with PDE5i [31].

Intracavernosal Injections

Intracavernosal injections are a highly effective although initially anxiety-provoking treatment for ED. Multiple medications and combinations are available, however, a combination of alprostadil, phentolamine, and papaverine (also known as trimix) is the most common formulation utilized by sexual medicine practitioners in the USA. Appropriate counseling for patients will alleviate the vast majority of anxiety, and it is routine practice for patients to undergo in-office training using two teaching visits to ensure proper injection technique and dose titration. Although the response rate is lower after RP and there is a higher drop-out rate in this population, it has been established that a significant cause of ICI attrition is secondary to patients converting to being PDE5i responders or having return of their natural erectile function [32].

Vacuum Erection Device

The vacuum erection device (VED) uses negative pressure to pull venous blood into the erectile bodies and superficial veins; a constriction band needs to be applied to the base of the penis in order to maintain the erection. VED can be used in combination with another erectogenic aid with improvement in patient satisfaction with the quality of their erection. In conjunction with PDE5i, VEDs increased the number of patients with penetration rigid erections to over 90 % compared to 57 % on PDE5i alone [33]. Another utility of the VED may be preventing penile

Table 22.2 Comparison of ED treatments after RP

Treatment	Success rates (%)	Pros	Cons
PDE5i	80	Oral therapy Have glans tumescence with erection	Side effects include headache, GERD, chromotopsia, muscle aches Cannot be used in men taking nitrates Could be cost prohibitive
ICI	>50	Initially anxiety provoking Erection occurs within 15 min without stimulation Inexpensive	Can only use up to three times a week Risk of priapism (less than 3 %) No glans tumescence
IUA	40	Glans tumescence occurs with erection	Painful urethritis is common (at least 20 %) Inconsistent erections (50 % of time does not work in men who initially responded) Most expensive drug treatment
VED	75	Can be effective even after IPP removal with severe penile fibrosis Inexpensive	Cosmetically questionable with engorged superficial veins and cold, blue penis Constriction band may be uncomfortable Not recommended in men on blood thinners or with decreased penile sensation (risk of pressure injuries)
IPP	>90	Highly effective Immediate erection upon activation	Most invasive Risk of infection and malfunction No glans tumescence

PDE5i phosphodiesterase type 5 inhibitors, *GERD* gastroesophageal reflux disease, *ICI* intracorporeal injections, *IUA* intraurethral alprostadil; *VED* vacuum erection device, *IPP* inflatable penile prosthesis

volume loss after RP, although the seminal objective studies remain to be performed [34, 35].

Intraurethral Alprostadil Suppository

Intraurethral alprostadil (IUA) involves insertion of a small pellet into the first inch of the urethra. Patients must be standing to encourage absorption of the medication across the urethra, through the corpus spongiosum, and into the corpora cavernosum. Unfortunately for the 40 % of men post-RP who do respond to this medication, IUA is inconsistent, as it fails to result in erection in up to 50 % of administrations [36].

Penile Implant Surgery

Inflatable penile prosthesis (IPP) surgery warrants special attention not only because of its impressive patient satisfaction rates, but because the surgery itself is more complicated in men who have undergone RP. A three-piece IPP consists of two cylinders placed within the corpora cavernosum, a pump placed with the scrotum, and a reservoir. Traditionally, the reservoir has been placed retroperitoneally in the space of Retzius, however, this space can often be obliterated in men who are post-RP. Ectopic reservoir placement refers to placement within the abdominal wall between the rectus abdominis and the transversalis fascia. In men with pre-existing ED who would require an IPP even before undergoing RP, it is possible to undergo simultaneous IPP and RP [37]. In these instances, however, some surgeons place only the reservoir during RP and leave the cylinder/pump placement till some months after the RP. For patients who have a pre-existing IPP who are to undergo a RP, it is recommended that they be prescribed antibiotics to help reduce the risk of infection that exposure to urine might cause. Inflating the implant during the RP may assist the operative dissection by deflating the reservoir.

Key Points

- Erectile Dysfunction is only one of many potentially debilitating sexual sequelae after RP.
- ED and sexual sequelae outcomes within the literature are often embellished because of limited reporting of negative outcomes, patient selection bias in published reports, and a lack of objective determination of erectile function
- The "burden of cure" which men and their partners face after radical prostatectomy encompasses many facets of sexual satisfaction and intimacy
- Neurovascular injury subsequent to prostatectomy leads to impaired erectile function, hypoxia and ultimately in fibrosis and reduction of smooth-muscle content in the corpora cavernosa
- To date, no concept of drug-assisted rehabilitation has shown to improve patients' natural erectile function within approximately 1 year following surgery
- ED treatment includes not only the use of PDE5i, but also an awareness of the use of ICI, VED, IUA, and IPP and an understanding of which men who may most benefit from each specific treatment modality
- Daily tadalafil has been shown in a randomized, placebo controlled trial to reduce penile length loss after RP
- IPP placement is associated with unique considerations if it is placed pre-RP, during RP, or post-RP and close consultation with a sexual medicine expert will improve patient satisfaction rates

References

1. Tal R, Alphs HH, Krebs P, Nelson CJ, Mulhall JP. Erectile function recovery rate after radical prostatectomy: a meta-analysis. J Sex Med. 2009;6:2538–46.
2. Walsh PC, Donker PJ. Impotence following radical prostatectomy: insight into etiology and prevention. J Urol. 1982;128:492–97.
3. Breza J, Aboseif SE, Orvis BR, Lue TF, Tanago EA. Detailed anatomy of penile neurovascular structures: surgical significance. J Urol. 1989;141:437–43.
4. Quinlan DM, Epstein JL, Carter BS, Walsh PC. Sexual function following radical prostatectomy: influence of preservation of neurovascular bundles. J Urol. 1991;145:998–1002.
5. Ficarra V, Novara G, Ahlering TE, Costello A, Eastham JA, Graefen M, Guazzoni G, Menon M, Mottrie A, Patel VR, Van der Poel H, Rosen RC, Tewari AK, Wilson TG, Zattoni F, Montorsi F. Systematic review and meta-analysis of studies reporting potency rates after robot-assisted radical prostatectomy. Eur Urol. 2012;62:418–30.
6. Hatzimouratidis K, Burnett AL, Hatzichristou D, McCullough AR, Montorsi F, Mullhall JP. Phosphodiesterase type 5 inhibitors in postprostatectomy erectile dysfunction: a critical analysis of the basic science rationale and clinical application. Eur Urol. 2009;55:334–47.
7. User HM, Zelner DJ, McKenna KE, McVary KT. J Urol. 2003;170:298–301.
8. Calenda G, Strong TD, Pavlovich CP, Schaeffer EM, Burnett AL, Yu W, Davies KP, Bivalacqua TJ. Whole genome microarray of the major pelvic ganglion after cavernous nerve injury: new insights. BJU Int. 2012;109:1552–64.
9. Schwartz EJ, Wong P, Graydon RJ. Sildenafil protects intracorporal smooth muscle after radical retropubic prostatectomy. J Urol. 2004;171:771–74.
10. Klein LT, Miller MI, Buttyan R, Raffo AJ, et al. Apoptosis in the rat penis after denervation. J Urol. 1997;158:626–30.
11. User HM, Hairston JH, Zelner DJ, McKenna KE, et al. Penile weight and cell subtype specific changes in a post-radical prostatectomy model of erectile dysfunction. J Urol. 2003;169:1175–9.
12. Iacono F, Gianella R, Somma P, Manno G, et al. Histologic alterations in cavernous tissue after radical prostatectomy. J Urol. 2005;173:1673–6.
13. Leungwattanakij S, Bivalacqua TJ, Usta MF, Yang DY, et al. Cavernous neurotomy causes hypoxia and fibrosisin rat corpus cavernosum. J Androl. 2003;24:239–45.
14. Özden E, Öztürk B, Kosan M, Tezel GG, et al. Effect of sildenafil citrate on penile weight and physiology of cavernous smooth muscle in a post-radical prostatectomy model of erectile dysfunction in rats. Urology. 2011;77:761.e1–761.e7
15. Aboseif S, Shinohara K, Breza J, Benard F, et al. Role of penile vascular injury in erectile dysfunction after radical prostatectomy. Br J Urol. 1994;73:75–82.
16. Munding MD, Wessells HB, Dalkin BL. Pilot study of changes in stretched penile length 3 months after radical prostatectomy. Urology. 2001;58:567–9.

17. Savoie M, Kim SS, Soloway M. A prospective study measuring penile length in men treated by radical prostatectomy for prostate cancer. J Urol. 2003;169: 162–4.
18. Montorsi F, Guazzoni G, Strambi LF, Da Pozzo LF, et al. Recovery of spontaneous erectile function after nerve-sparing radical reteropubic prostatectomy with and without early intracavernous injections of alprostadil: results of a prospective randomized trial. J Urol. 1997;158:1408–10.
19. Mulhall JP, Bivalacqua TJ, Becher EF. Standard operating procedure for the preservation of erectile function outcomes after radical prostatectomy. J Sex Med. 2013;10:195–203.
20. Padma-Nathan H, McCullough AR, Levine LA, Lipshultz LI, et al. Randomized, double-blind, placebo-controlled study of postoperative nightly sildenafil citrate for the prevention of erectile dysfunction after bilateral nerve-sparing radical prostatectomy. Int J Impot Res. 2008;20:479–86.
21. Montorsi F, Brock G, Lee J, Shapiro J, et al. Effect of nightly versus on-demand vardenafil on recovery of erectile function in men following bilateral nerve-sparing radical prostatectomy. Eur Urol. 2008;54: 924–31.
22. Wrishko R, Sorsaburo S, Wong D, Strawbridge A, et al. Safety, efficacy and pharmacokinetic overview of low-dose daily administration of tadalafil. J Sex Med. 2009;6:2039–48.
23. Montorsi F, Brock G, Stolzenburg JU, Mulhall J, et al. Effects of tadalafil treatment on erectile function recovery following bilateral nerve-sparing radical prostatectomy: a randomised placebo-controlled study (REACTT). Eur Urol. 2014;65:587–96.
24. Castiglione F, Nini A, Briganti A. Penile rehabilitation with phosphodiesterase type 5 inhibitors after nerve-sparing radical prostatectomy: are we targeting the right patients? Eur Urol. 2014;65:663–4.
25. Kilminster S, Müller S, Menon M, Joseph JV, et al. Predicting erectile function outcome in men after radical prostatectomy for prostate cancer. BJU Int. 2011;110:422–6.
26. Berookhim BM, Nelson CJ, Kunzel B, Mulhall JP, et al. A Prospective analysis of penile length changes following radical prostatectomy. BJU Int. 2013. doi:10.1111/bju.12443 BJU Int. 2014;113:E131–6.
27. Rabbani F, Schiff J, Piecuch M, et al. Time course of recovery of erectile function after radical retropubic prostatectomy: does anyone recover after 2 years? J Sex Med. 2010;7:3984–90.
28. Smith 2nd WB, McCaslin IR, Gokce A, Mandava SH, et al. PDE5 inhibitors: considerations for preference and long-term adherence. Int J Clin Pract. 2013;67: 768–80.
29. Katz D, Bennett NE, Stasi J, Eastham JA, et al. Chronology of erectile function in patients with early functional erections following radical prostatectomy. J Sex Med. 2010;7:803–9.
30. Raina R, Lakin MM, Agarwal A, Sharma A, et al. Long-term effect of sildenafil citrate on erectile dysfunction after radical prostatectomy: 3-year follow-up. Urology. 2003;62:110–5.
31. Montorsi F, McCullough A. Efficacy of sildenafil citrate in men with erectile dysfunction following radical prostatectomy: a systematic review of clinical data. J Sex Med. 2005;2:658–67.
32. Coombs PG, Heck M, Guhring P, Narus J, et al. A review of outcomes of an intracavernosal injection therapy programme. BJU Int. 2012;110:1787–91.
33. Baniel J, Israilov S, Segenreich E, Livne PM. Comparative evaluation of treatments for erectile dysfunction in patients with prostate cancer after radical retropubic prostatectomy. BJU Int. 2001;88:58–62.
34. Zippe C, Nandipati K, Agarwal A, Raina R. Sexual dysfunction after pelvic surgery. Int J Impot Res. 2006;18:1–18.
35. Köhler TS, Pedro R, Hendlin K, Utz W, et al. A pilot study on the early use of the vacuum erection device after radical retropubic prostatectomy. BJU Int. 2007;100:858–62.
36. Costabile RA, Spevak M, Fishman IJ, Govier FE, et al. Efficacy and safety of transurethral alprostadil in patients with erectile dysfunction following radical prostatectomy. J Urol. 1998;160:1325–8.
37. Ramsawh HJ, Morgentaler A, Covino N, Barlow DH, et al. Quality of life following simultaneous placement of penile prosthesis with radical prostatectomy. J Urol. 2005;174:1395–8.

Management of Incontinence After Pelvic Malignancy

23

Patrick McKenzie and Gopal Badlani

23.1 Introduction

After successful management of Pelvic malignancies, one of the main quality of life issues is urinary incontinence. The etiology of this is as varied as the management. A correct diagnosis of the cause goes a long way to manage the patient presenting with incontinence. Although there are common pathways, differences in male and female anatomy as well as difference in physiology requires us to look at the two in separate algorithms. The etiology of incontinence can be attributed to neural interruption resulting in bladder dysfunction or the failure of the outlet, i.e. sphincteric dysfunction.

23.2 Urinary Incontinence Following Pelvic Surgery or Radiation in a Male

Voiding dysfunction in men undergoing surgery or radiation for pelvic malignancy is a common occurrence. Urologic surgeries for malignancies such as the bladder or prostate are the most common causes of voiding dysfunction; however abdominoperineal resection can cause incontinence as well. In patients with neobladder creation post cystectomy, nocturnal enuresis is a common issue and it occurs in 6–25 % of patients depending on the type of neobladder [1–3]. Daytime continence rates are much higher. This is presumed to be due to decrease in the outlet resistance from relaxation of the voluntary component of the external sphincter as well as the higher volume of urine at night. Incontinence after abdominoperineal resection can be due to overflow from detrusor failure in the immediate post-operative period while delayed presentation can be due to loss of compliance or bladder denervation.

Quality of life 2 years after treatment for prostate cancer shows wide variability. Radical prostatectomy had the largest negative impact on urinary incontinence while differences between external radiation and brachytherapy were relatively small [4]. Of note, patients undergoing brachytherapy had a moderate increase in urinary irritation compared either the external beam radiation therapy or prostatectomy groups. Urinary symptoms, as quantified by IPSS, have been shown to exacerbate acutely over the 1–3 months post treatment with brachytherapy with return to pretreatment baseline levels over the following 9–18 months [5]. When comparing open radical retropubic prostatectomy (ORRP) to robot assisted laparoscopic radical prostatectomy (RALRP) quality-of-life outcomes are not statistically significant. Patients undergoing salvage treatments for failed

P. McKenzie, MD
Department of Urology, Wake Forest University, Winston-Salem, NC, USA

G. Badlani, MD (✉)
Department of Urology, Wake Forest University Baptist Medical Center, Winston-Salem, NC, USA
e-mail: gbadlani@wakehealth.edu

H.R.H. Patel et al. (eds.), *Pelvic Cancer Surgery: Modern Breakthroughs and Future Advances*,
DOI 10.1007/978-1-4471-4258-4_23, © Springer-Verlag London 2015

cancer control, however, had dissatisfaction and regret rates which were higher than patients undergoing RALRP [6]. Multiple studies have quoted a 56–89 % 1 year urinary continence rates in patients undergoing prostatectomy [7, 8]. In these studies the majority of patients reached continence at 7–8 months and patients that were incontinent at 18 months rarely regained continence. In the majority of these patients mean urinary function and incontinence did not recover to preoperative baseline after prostatectomy; however, this did not add distress because mean urinary bother returned to pre-prostatectomy levels.

Urinary incontinence post treatment for cancer of the prostate is most commonly due to the sphincteric dysfunction, associated detrussor overactivity secondary to a stricture, or poor compliance post radiation (Table 23.1). Desautel et al. found that sphincteric incontinence was the most common cause of urine leakage following retropubic prostatectomy (RRP), followed by detrusor instability/poor compliance, detrusor hypoactivity, and stricture formation [9]. In patients undergoing RRP, this group also found urethral scarring and anastomotic stricture, as demonstrated on flexible cystoscopy and fluoroscopic cystourethrography, occurred in 67 % of patients, which, in 38 % of the patients, was confounded by detrusor instability.

The risk of urethral stricture after prostate cancer therapy ranges from 1.1 to 8.4 % depending on cancer treatment type [10]. This risk was highest after radical prostatectomy or brachytherapy plus external beam radiotherapy and in those with advanced age or obesity. Multiple series have quoted between a 0.7 and 29 % bladder neck contracture rates for RRP [11–13]. It is believed that the etiology of bladder neck contractures are related to urine leakage, periurethral hematoma, lack of mucosa to mucosa anastomosis, devascularization of the bladder neck or urethral segment, and prolonged catheterization. In a large series Geary et al. found a 0.5–9 % bladder neck contracture rate which often occurred several years after RRP [14]. They found technical factors that increased the risk of anastomotic stricture included excessive blood loss intraoperatively and urinary extravasation, while a previous history of TURP or EBRT also increased the risk of stricture. The contracture rate is considerable better for patients undergoing robotic prostatectomy, with an average of less than 1 % contracture rate [15–17]. Patients undergoing radiation therapy for prostate cancer have a 2.2–35 % urinary stricture rate as well as an increased risk of urinary retention [18, 19].

Table 23.1 Causes of incontinence after pelvic surgery for malignancy or radiation in a male

Bladder causes
1. Over activity of the bladder from obstruction secondary to: (a) RT (radiotherapy), (b) Seeds (brachytherapy), (c) Urethral stricture after radical prostatectomy (RRP)
2. Loss of compliance secondary to: (a) Denervation post APR (abdomino-perineal resection), (b) Post RT for pelvic cancers (prostate, bladder, rectum)
3. Overflow: (a) Denervation (post APR, post radical prostatectomy), (b) Neobladder
4. Outlet/sphincteric incontinence: (a) Post radical prostatectomy (b) Post cysto-prostatectomy (c) TURP post RT/brachytherapy/cryotherapy)

23.3 Urinary Incontinence Following Pelvic Surgery or Radiation in a Female

Female voiding dysfunction following pelvic radiation or pelvic surgery can be related to a variety of issues including bladder dysfunction and bladder outlet disorders (Table 23.2). Bladder overactivity in this group can be related to neurologic injury, decreased compliance, bladder outlet obstruction, inflammation, irritation, or pain. During radical hysterectomy or abdominal perineal resection, posterior dissection along the bladder can lead to denervation of the bladder or urethra leading to urinary retention and/or intrinsic sphincter deficiency. Women that undergo abdominoperineal resection and/or radiation for rectal cancer have an increased incidence of

Table 23.2 Causes of incontinence after pelvic surgery for malignancy or radiation in a female

Bladder	
	Retention/overflow: post radical hysterectomy, APR (denervation)
	Loss of compliance: post RT for carcinoma of cervix, ovarian or rectal malignancy
	Fistula formation: post-surgical, post RT, vesico vaginal, ureterovaginal
Outlet	
	Post neo bladder, post RT resulting in ISD

urinary incontinence and detrusor overactivity [20]. Decreased outlet resistance in this group results from damage to the innervation of structural elements of the smooth and/or striated sphincter or damage that impairs the support of the bladder outlet in the female. A special consideration is outlet obstruction following neobladder creation which is reported to occur in 1.2–2.5 % of women undergoing neobladder creation [21, 22]. In patients with neobladder creation urinary leakage due to overflow incontinence and urethral stricture are common. A decrease in bladder compliance can also lead to lower urinary tract symptoms in women following pelvic surgery or radiation [23]. The decrease in compliance can either be related to neurologic injury at the time of surgery or delayed neurologic injury following pelvic radiation. Radiation can also cause remodeling of the detrusor muscle [24] and this damage long-term leads to a decrease in compliance and bladder function [25, 26].

A unique situation following radiation or surgery for pelvic malignancy in female patients is fistula formation. The most common cause of vesicovaginal fistula (VVF) formation is surgical injury during gynecologic, urologic, or other pelvic surgery [27, 28]. The incidence of fistula after hysterectomy is estimated to be 0.1–0.2 % [29]. Cervical, vaginal, and endometrial carcinoma are the most common causes of malignant VVF which account for 3–5 % of VVF [30]. Pelvic radiation is also a cause of urinary fistula and usually occurs several years after radiation treatment [31]. There have been numerous studies which have estimated the VVF rate after pelvic radiation to be between 0.6 and 2.0 % [32–34]. Another complication of pelvic surgery and radiation is ureterovaginal fistula formation. The most common cause for ureterovaginal fistulae is surgical injury to the distal ureter which includes ureteral laceration or transection, avulsion, crush injury, suture ligation, and/or ureteral ischemia due to compromise of the vascular supply or electrocautery injury. The incidence of ureteral injury during pelvic surgery has been estimated to be between 0.5 and 2.5 % [35].

23.4 Patient Workup

A careful history is pertinent in diagnosing the likely physiologic mechanism for voiding dysfunction and devising a treatment plan. The physician should document predisposing factors for voiding dysfunction which may have been present prior to the pelvic surgery or pelvic radiation including: (1) Neurologic symptoms or spinal issues or surgeries, (2) Metabolic issues including diabetes mellitus control, (3) Benign prostatic hyperplasia, (4) Detrusor overactivity, and (5) Stress urinary incontinence. It has been documented that patients with prior BPH and detrusor overactivity will have their symptoms worsen with pelvic radiation. It is therefore, important to document these pre-existing conditions when evaluating a patient with new onset voiding complaints following pelvic radiation or surgery. The onset of symptoms can also shed light on the likely etiology. For example, immediate onset of urinary issues following discontinuation of the Foley catheter may be related detrusor overactivity versus urinary tract infection versus bladder neck or urethral irritation. Urinary fistula, however, presents days to months to years after the treatment whereas issues with compliance or strictures usually present several months to years after the initial surgery or pelvic radiation. Acute exacerbation of mild leaking usually point to urinary tract infection versus gradual onset of mild leaking which can represent overflow incontinence.

Further history should focus on the progression of symptoms over time. Issues with compliance and detrusor overactivity usually worsen over time while sphincteric incontinence usually gets better over time up until 18 months post procedure. The time of day that the urinary dysfunction occurs is also important in determining likely etiology. Urinary leakage that occurs during the day especially with change in position is more likely to be sphincteric incontinence due to gravity. Detrusor overactivity will often present as episodic urinary leakage or urge. Urinary leakage that occurs at night can also be related to detrusor overactivity, but overflow incontinence, storage issues such as compliance and issues with bladder augments capacity or neobladder capacity must also be considered. Patients with continuous daytime and nighttime leakage may be due to overflow incontinence versus urinary fistula. In all of these scenarios it is important to consider the associated voiding pattern. Are these patients having frequency with small volumes to suggest overflow or sphincteric incontinence or frequency with large volumes to suggest overactive bladder? Does the patient have associated urgency, a weak stream, hesitancy, straining or pushing to urinate? Is gross hematuria present and is it initial, continuous, or terminal hematuria to help delineate between stricture, radiation cystitis, or sloughing post radiation? All of these associated urinary complaints are key in steering any further workup and the treatment plan. It is also helpful to illicit any previous workup or treatments the patient underwent for their symptoms and the timing of assessments and treatments.

Following an appropriate detailed history the clinician should focus on a detailed neurologic, abdominal, and genitourinary exam when evaluating patients with voiding complaints following pelvic radiation or surgery. Assess for abdominal fullness or discomfort related to a full bladder or the presence of a colostomy or non-healing wound. It is important to assess overall strength and sensation when trying to rule out systemic disease where voiding dysfunction is the initial complaint and the timing of pelvic surgery or radiation is a coincidence. The physician should also assess perigenital sensation, rectal tone, ability to contract the pelvic floor, and bulbarcavernosal reflex as part of the routine workup if the rectum is present. In women vaginal support should be assessed especially in patients who have had an anterior exenteration, hysterectomy, or a neobladder creation. Urethral obstruction due to anterior overcorrection is more likely in the neobladder population. Concomitant radiation therapy can also increase the risk of induration or irritation of the labia, urethra, or vagina in this population, and it has been shown to increase the risk or fistula formation. It is, therefore, important to document these findings during your initial evaluation.

During the initial evaluation the patients should have a UA to look for hematuria and to rule out UTI as the cause of the voiding complaints, and a post void residual (PVR) to rule out retention. If UTI is present treat accordingly and see the patient back to ensure the voiding symptoms have resolved. If retention is found the patient should be taught clean intermittent catheterization (CIC) if the patient is able to do so, and if not, a Foley catheter should be placed. If the catheter cannot be passed in a male and retention is present these patients should undergo flexible cystoscopy followed by wire passage, stricture dilation, and catheter placement. If UTI and urinary retention has been ruled out, the patient should be instructed to complete a voiding diary prior to their follow-up appointment to further assess the severity and chronology of their voiding dysfunction. The majority of patients with these complex presentations should undergo a pressure flow study or videourodynamics (VUDS) to further assess the etiology and severity of their voiding dysfunction. During VUDS it is important to document initial flow and PVR along with filling compliance, Valsalva leak point pressure (VLPP), and detrusor leak point pressure (DLPP). These parameters will assist in delineating stricture, detrusor overactivity, detrusor underactivity, denervation, and poor compliance as cause for the patients voiding dysfunction as well as assess the risk for upper tract deterioration. If sphincteric incontinence is suspected and cannot be demonstrated with catheter in place, the urethral catheter should be removed and leaking assessed using rectal pressure as VLPP.

23.5 Treatment Options

After proper identification of the cause of the voiding complaint, it is important to counsel patients on the various treatment options. Detrusor overactivity in both male and female patients can be managed by first treating the underlying cause, i.e. obstruction, followed by anticholinergics in patients with refractory detrusor overactivity. Botox can also be offered in this population, but the patient must be counseled on the 5–10 % risk of retention and the need to do CIC following Botox administration. Patients who are unwilling to accept CIC should not be offered intravesical Botox as a treatment for their detrusor overactivity.

In patients with urinary retention following pelvic surgery or radiation, the etiology of their retention is important in determining the appropriate treatment. Patients with retention due to prostatic obstruction can be offered CIC versus TURP. Post radiation, however, sphincteric incontinence after TURP is more likely [36]. Individuals with urinary retention with normal bladder compliance can be managed with indwelling Foley catheter versus CIC versus suprapubic tube placement depending on patient preference and dexterity. In patient with poor bladder compliance, however, it is important to add anticholinergics or Botox to the treatment algorithm in order to promote dryness in between catheterization and decrease urinary leakage with the catheter in place. In patients with retention due to stricture the least aggressive treatment would be to dilate and leave an indwelling catheter for 3–5 days. Patients receiving this treatment must be warned that this is only a temporizing measure and that the stricture is very likely to recur without further treatment or daily catheterizations. Another treatment option for male patients with urethral stricture is direct vision internal urethrotomy (DVIU). This can be accomplished with either an endoscopic cold knife or laser and this treatment has good short and mid-term results. The best results are obtained by DVIU followed by daily catheterizations to maintain urethral patency. It is also important that patients undergoing this treatment be counseled that their incontinence may worsen due to damage to the sphincter, especially if the patient had prior radiation. In male patients with sphinteric incontinence following radical prostatectomy, the pad weight should determine the appropriate treatment, i.e. in patients with pad counts of less than two a male sling can be offered, whereas in patients with higher pad counts, an artificial urinary sphincter should be considered.

Special situations that lead to voiding dysfunction following pelvic surgery or radiation include urinary fistula formation, incontinent and continent diversion. After the initial diagnosis of a urinary fistula immediate management or control of the urinary leakage is important. Urine management with indwelling catheters, pads, or nephrostomy tubes early on is important in the management of urinary fistula since it will decrease the incidence of skin breakdown and related complications. A small number of urinary fistulas will close with conservative management, however the majority of fistulas, especially fistulas related to radiation, will require surgical intervention. Often times, repair and reconstruction of urinary fistulae are complex and these repairs should be approached on a case by case basis. The majority of these complex repairs will require extensive experience as well as innovative and improvisational techniques including a variety of tissue or muscle flaps. After definitive repair, recurrence of the fistula may be due to a variety of patient factors including malignancy, nutritional issues, tissue ischemia, or a host of surgical issues, including persistent distal urinary obstruction, technical issues with the surgery, or inadequate postoperative urinary drainage. In patients with radiation related fistulas it is important to close the fistula with a muscle flap to provide adequate vascular supply to the area to promote healing and to prevent fistula recurrence.

In male patients with recurrent urethral stricture or dystrophic calcifications, in the setting of incontinence and/or upper tract deterioration, continent versus incontinent urinary diversion must be considered. This is especially true in patients with recurrent stricture or calcifications following EBRT or brachytherapy that have previously been managed with aggressive endoscopic resection. The type of urinary diversion should be based on a host of patient factors including body habitus, comorbidities, previous surgeries, upper tract status, and patient compliance. Female patients with decreased bladder compliance with concomitant upper tract changes following either pelvic surgery or radiation should also be counseled on urinary diversion in order to improve quality of life and prevent further upper tract deterioration.

23.6 Summary

Voiding dysfunction and urinary incontinence following pelvic malignancy surgery or radiation is often complex and requires a detailed history, workup and management strategy. Patients should be counseled on treatment options as well as the complications associated with each treatment. Improved Quality of life should be the goal in these patients, however, patient expectations should be realistic. Practitioners should be cautious with patient expectations since lower urinary tract symptoms are unlikely to fully resolve following treatment. Detrusor overactivity without obstruction can be managed with anticholinergics or Botox. Urinary retention without obstruction can be managed with CIC with or without anticholinergics or Botox. Urethral obstruction in men can be managed with DVIU versus resection depending on the etiology, but the physician should counsel the patient on post procedure incontinence from intrinsic sphincter deficiency. Most common treatment for male incontinence post prostatectomy remains a male sling and an artificial urinary sphincter. These treatments have the ability to restore the quality of life in a majority of patients. Previous radiation therapy leads to a variety of upper and lower urinary tract issues and it offers unique challenges in management. In patients with high grade outlet obstruction refractory to endoscopic management or poor bladder compliance with upper tract deterioration, urinary diversion should be considered as a management strategy.

Urinary Incontinence Post Pelvic Malignancy: Key Points

- Rule out retention
- Rule out outlet obstruction
- Rule out Bladder over activity
- Assess bladder compliance
- Functional bladder capacity
- VLPP, DLPP
- Patient's mental ability to learn CIC or use of devices
- Hand dexterity to be able to do CIC or use the artificial urinary sphincter
- Expectations of "normal" versus control.
- Fistula with complex repair.

References

1. Hautmann RE. Urinary diversion: ileal conduit to neobladder. J Urol. 2003;169(3):834–42. doi:10.1097/01.ju.0000029010.97686.eb. PubMed PMID: 12576795.
2. Stein JP, Dunn MD, Quek ML, Miranda G, Skinner DG. The orthotopic T pouch ileal neobladder: experience with 209 patients. J Urol. 2004;172(2):584–7. doi:10.1097/01.ju.0000131651.77048.73. PubMed PMID: 15247737.
3. Studer UE, Danuser H, Hochreiter W, Springer JP, Turner WH, Zingg EJ. Summary of 10 years' experience with an ileal low-pressure bladder substitute combined with an afferent tubular isoperistaltic segment. World J Urol. 1996;14(1):29–39. PubMed PMID: 8646238.
4. Guedea F, Ferrer M, Pera J, Aguilo F, Boladeras A, Suarez JF, et al. Quality of life two years after radical prostatectomy, prostate brachytherapy or external beam radiotherapy for clinically localised prostate cancer: the Catalan Institute of Oncology/Bellvitge Hospital experience. Clin Transl Oncol. 2009;11(7):470–8. PubMed PMID: 19574206.
5. Williams SG, Millar JL, Duchesne GM, Dally MJ, Royce PL, Snow RM. Factors predicting for urinary morbidity following 125iodine transperineal prostate brachytherapy. Radiother Oncol. 2004;73(1):33–8. doi:10.1016/j.radonc.2004.07.026. PubMed PMID: 15465143.
6. Lepor H. Status of radical prostatectomy in 2009: is there medical evidence to justify the robotic approach? Rev Urol. 2009;11(2):61–70. PubMed PMID: 19680527; PubMed Central PMCID: PMC2725307.
7. Novara G, Ficarra V, D'Elia C, Secco S, Cioffi A, Cavalleri S, et al. Evaluating urinary continence and

preoperative predictors of urinary continence after robot assisted laparoscopic radical prostatectomy. J Urol. 2010;184(3):1028–33. doi:10.1016/j.jur0.2010.04.069. PubMed PMID: 20643426.

8. Litwin MS, Lubeck DP, Spitalny GM, Henning JM, Carroll PR. Mental health in men treated for early stage prostate carcinoma: a posttreatment, longitudinal quality of life analysis from the Cancer of the Prostate Strategic Urologic Research Endeavor. Cancer. 2002;95(1):54–60. doi:10.1002/cncr.10651. PubMed PMID: 12115317.
9. Desautel MG, Kapoor R, Badlani GH. Sphincteric incontinence: the primary cause of post-prostatectomy incontinence in patients with prostate cancer. NeurourolUrodyn. 1997;16(3):153–60. PubMed PMID: 9136137.
10. Elliott SP, Meng MV, Elkin EP, McAninch JW, Duchane J, Carroll PR, et al. Incidence of urethral stricture after primary treatment for prostate cancer: data from CaPSURE. J Urol. 2007;178(2):529–34; discussion 34. doi:10.1016/j.jur0.2007.03.126. PubMed PMID: 17570425.
11. Igel TC, Barrett DM, Segura JW, Benson Jr RC, Rife CC. Perioperative and postoperative complications from bilateral pelvic lymphadenectomy and radical retropubic prostatectomy. J Urol. 1987;137(6):1189–91. PubMed PMID: 3586152.
12. Foote J, Yun S, Leach GE. Postprostatectomy incontinence. Pathophysiology, evaluation, and management. Urol Clin North Am. 1991;18(2):229–41.
13. Rudy DC, Woodside JR, Crawford ED. Urodynamic evaluation of incontinence in patients undergoing modified Campbell radical retropubic prostatectomy: a prospective study. J Urol. 1984;132(4):708–12. PubMed PMID: 6471217.
14. Geary ES, Dendinger TE, Freiha FS, Stamey TA. Incontinence and vesical neck strictures following radical retropubic prostatectomy. Urology. 1995;45(6):1000–6. PubMed PMID: 7771001.
15. Cathelineau X, Rozet F, Vallancien G. Robotic radical prostatectomy: the European experience. Urol Clin North Am. 2004;31(4):693–9, viii. doi:10.1016/j.uc1.2004.06.001. PubMed PMID: 15474596.
16. Menon M, Shrivastava A, Bhandari M, Satyanarayana R, Siva S, Agarwal PK. Vattikuti Institute prostatectomy: technical modifications in 2009. Eur Urol. 2009;56(1):89–96. doi:10.1016/j.eurur0.2009.04.032. PubMed PMID: 19403236.
17. Patel VR, Palmer KJ, Coughlin G, Samavedi S. Robot-assisted laparoscopic radical prostatectomy: perioperative outcomes of 1500 cases. J Endourol/Endourol Soc. 2008;22(10):2299–305. doi:10.1089/end.2008.9711. PubMed PMID: 18837657.
18. Crook J, McLean M, Catton C, Yeung I, Tsihlias J, Pintilie M. Factors influencing risk of acute urinary retention after TRUS-guided permanent prostate seed implantation. Int J Radiat Oncol Biol Phys. 2002;52(2):453–60. PubMed PMID: 11872292.
19. Bucci J, Morris WJ, Keyes M, Spadinger I, Sidhu S, Moravan V. Predictive factors of urinary retention following prostate brachytherapy. Int J Radiat Oncol Biol Phys. 2002;53(1):91–8. PubMed PMID: 12007946.
20. Tekkis PP, Cornish JA, Remzi FH, Tilney HS, Strong SA, Church JM, et al. Measuring sexual and urinary outcomes in women after rectal cancer excision. Dis Colon Rectum. 2009;52(1):46–54. doi:10.1007/DCR.0b013e318197551e. PubMed PMID: 19273955.
21. Nam JK, Kim TN, Park SW, Lee SD, Chung MK. The Studer orthotopic neobladder: long-term (more than 10 years) functional outcomes, urodynamic features, and complications. Yonsei Med J. 2013;54(3):690–5. doi:10.3349/ymj.2013.54.3.690. PubMed PMID: 23549816; PubMed Central PMCID: PMC3635617.
22. Hautmann RE, de Petriconi RC, Volkmer BG. 25 years of experience with 1,000 neobladders: long-term complications. J Urol. 2011;185(6):2207–12. doi:10.1016/j.jur0.2011.02.006. PubMed PMID: 21497841.
23. Gondi V, Bentzen SM, Sklenar KL, Dunn EF, Petereit DG, Tannehill SP, et al. Severe late toxicities following concomitant chemoradiotherapy compared to radiotherapy alone in cervical cancer: an inter-era analysis. Int J Radiat Oncol Biol Phys. 2012;84(4):973–82. doi:10.1016/j.ijrobp.2012.01.064. PubMed PMID: 22898381.
24. Kraft M, Oussoren Y, Stewart FA, Dorr W, Schultz-Hector S. Radiation-induced changes in transforming growth factor beta and collagen expression in the murine bladder wall and its correlation with bladder function. Radiat Res. 1996;146(6):619–27. PubMed PMID: 8955711.
25. Hamada K, Kihana T, Kataoka M, Yoshioka S, Nishio S, Matsuura S, et al. Urinary disturbance after therapy for cervical cancer: urodynamic evaluation and beta2-agonist medication. Int Urogynecol J Pelvic Floor Dysfunct. 1999;10(6):365–70. PubMed PMID: 10614971.
26. Pisarska M, Sajdak S. Lower urinary tract function after postoperative radiotherapy in the treatment of cervical cancer. Eur J Gynaecol Oncol. 2003;24(6):490–4. PubMed PMID: 14658587.
27. Tancer ML. Observations on prevention and management of vesicovaginal fistula after total hysterectomy. Surg Gynecol Obstet. 1992;175(6):501–6. PubMed PMID: 1448730.
28. Symmonds RE. Incontinence: vesical and urethral fistulas. Clin Obstet Gynecol. 1984;27(2):499–514. PubMed PMID: 6744702.
29. Harris WJ. Early complications of abdominal and vaginal hysterectomy. Obstet Gynecol Surv. 1995;50(11):795–805. PubMed PMID: 8545085.
30. Gerber GS, Schoenberg HW. Female urinary tract fistulas. J Urol. 1993;149(2):229–36. PubMed PMID: 8426392.
31. Zoubek J, McGuire EJ, Noll F, DeLancey JO. The late occurrence of urinary tract damage in patients successfully treated by radiotherapy for cervical carcinoma. J Urol. 1989;141(6):1347–9. PubMed PMID: 2724431.

32. Perez CA, Grigsby PW, Lockett MA, Chao KS, Williamson J. Radiation therapy morbidity in carcinoma of the uterine cervix: dosimetric and clinical correlation. Int J Radiat Oncol Biol Phys. 1999;44(4):855–66. PubMed PMID: 10386643.
33. Emmert C, Kohler U. Management of genital fistulas in patients with cervical cancer. Arch Gynecol Obstet. 1996;259(1):19–24. PubMed PMID: 8933925.
34. Alert J, Jimenez J, Beldarrain L, Montalvo J, Roca C. Complications from irradiation of carcinoma of the uterine cervix. Acta Radiol Oncol. 1980;19(1):13–5. PubMed PMID: 6246724.
35. Gilmour DT, Dwyer PL, Carey MP. Lower urinary tract injury during gynecologic surgery and its detection by intraoperative cystoscopy. Obstet Gynecol. 1999;94(5 Pt 2):883–9. PubMed PMID: 10546778.
36. Kollmeier MA, Stock RG, Cesaretti J, Stone NN. Urinary morbidity and incontinence following transurethral resection of the prostate after brachytherapy. J Urol. 2005;173(3):808–12. doi:10.1097/01.ju.0000152698.20487.0e. PubMed PMID: 15711274.

Part III

Gynecologic

24 Imaging of Gynecological Cancers

Ayshea Hameeduddin and Nandita M. deSouza

24.1 Introduction

Imaging plays a crucial role in staging pelvic cancer. The assessment of disease presence, location and extent profoundly affects the decision for surgery, its timing in relation to neoadjuvant therapies and in planning the optimal surgical procedure. Information required of imaging is to accurately identify the presence of tumor, and describe its volume, margins and spread beyond the organ of origin. In the pelvis, where several soft tissues lie in close proximity, contrast between them is of primary importance. Early imaging techniques relied on attenuation of X-ray irradiation thus generating contrast based on differences in tissue density. Over the last 25 years, techniques such as magnetic resonance imaging and positron emission tomography have revolutionized the type of imaging information available for describing disease prior to surgery as well as in evaluating the post-surgical pelvis.

Demands on the quality and the nature of the imaging information required also change with advances in therapeutic options. Surgical procedures that limit the extent of resection (for instance to offer fertility-sparing options) necessitate very accurate delineation of small cervical lesions and their relation to the internal os. At the other end of the spectrum, exenterative procedures, which are being more widely performed, require the complete extent of the tumor to be delineated, including depiction of adjacent fat planes and involvement of pelvic side-walls and neurovascular structures. In ovarian cancer, identification of the extent of peritoneal disease affects resectability and the timing of surgery in relation to chemotherapy. Increasingly, therefore, new imaging techniques are employed that enable not only the morphological delineation of the tumor but also aid recognition of tumor deposits by identifying abnormal areas of tissue function such as vascularity, increased cellular density resulting from proliferative activity of tumors, glucose metabolism and membrane turnover. By combining morphological and functional imaging characteristics, there is now overwhelming evidence that tumor staging and follow-up in gynecological malignancies is improved.

A. Hameeduddin, MBBS, BA, MSc (✉)
Department of Imaging,
Bart's Cancer Centre,
St. Bartholomew's Hospital, London, UK
e-mail: ayshea.hameeduddin@bartshealth.nhs.uk

N.M. deSouza, MR, FRCP, FRCR
CRUK/EPSRC Cancer Imaging Centre,
Institute of Cancer Research, Royal Marsden Hospital,
Downs Road, Sutton, Surrey SM2 5PT, UK

H.R.H. Patel et al. (eds.), *Pelvic Cancer Surgery: Modern Breakthroughs and Future Advances*,
DOI 10.1007/978-1-4471-4258-4_24, © Springer-Verlag London 2015

24.2 Advances in Imaging Techniques for Gynecological Cancers

Ultrasound

Transabdominal and transvaginal ultrasound (TVS) are widely utilized in the assessment of endometrial thickness, characterization of adnexal masses and detection of recurrence. Ultrasound is a validated technique as part of the Risk of Malignancy Index (RMI) for ovarian cancer, which is a useful pre-operative tool [1]. Implementation of three-dimensional (3D) TVS has improved the morphological assessment of adnexal masses by allowing detection of small papillary excrescences and focal mural irregularities which are associated with malignancy [2]. Advances in transvaginal color Doppler sonography (TV-CDS) have allowed the assessment of tumor neovascularity, which is increased in malignancy. When combined with morphological features, this functional data has increased the accuracy of determining benign from malignant adnexal masses [3]. Further refinements such as dynamic contrast-enhanced TVS using microbubbles allow detection of microvascular tumor networks. Microbubble ultrasound has been shown to have higher sensitivity and specificity than conventional TVS for detecting stage 1 ovarian carcinoma [3].

Computerized Tomography

Computerized Tomography (CT) has a crucially important role in the pre-operative staging of gynecological malignancy, particularly in detecting metastases. Modern multi-detector computed tomography (MDCT) using 64 slice or 256 slice scanners, allows the rapid acquisition of volumetric data-sets of the chest, abdomen and pelvis in less than 10 s with vast improvements in spatial and temporal resolution. Multi-planar reconstruction in axial, coronal and sagittal dimensions facilitates more accurate assessment of disease status. Intravenous [4] and oral [5] contrast to opacify bowel loops provides high accuracy of detection of peritoneal deposits.

Magnetic Resonance Imaging

Conventional magnetic resonance imaging (MRI) is established in the detection, staging and evaluation of response to treatment of gynecological cancers. Contrast enhanced images allow the differentiation of neoplastic from normal tissue. Dynamic contrast enhanced MRI (DCE-MRI) involves the acquisition of images before, during and after contrast administration; temporal resolution depends on the selected coverage but typically the uterus can be sampled every 20–30 s with a 3 mm spatial resolution whilst retaining signal to noise ratio for images to be of sufficient diagnostic quality. The difference in degree and rate of enhancement between tumor and surrounding stroma can vary, so that multiple images acquired over several minutes provides optimal visualization of the tumor. In endometrial cancer the tumor enhances more slowly than normal myometrium with the greatest difference at 50–120 s post contrast. In cervical cancer, DCE-MRI helps distinguish recurrent disease from radiation fibrosis [6]. There is an emerging body of evidence to support the use of DCE-MRI for characterizing indeterminate adnexal lesions using semi-quantitative analysis and threshold criteria applied to the rate of contrast wash-in within the mass. An increase in specificity compared with conventional MRI in correctly characterizing benign and malignant masses has been shown using this method [7].

Diffusion-weighted (DW) MRI is a functional imaging technique that quantifies the thermally driven, random movement of water protons within tissue, which are hampered by membrane boundaries. It thus generates tissue contrast based on intrinsic features that reflect tissue cellularity and integrity of cell membrane boundaries; diffusion restriction characterizes tumors where cell density is higher and membrane boundaries more numerous relative to normal tissue. DW-MRI is useful in identifying malignant disease, detecting peritoneal and serosal implants, recurrent disease and when patients are unable to tolerate intravenous extrinsic contrast agents. Early studies suggest further utility in predicting cancer grade and treatment outcomes [8]. With further refinements in the analysis methodologies of these functional MRI techniques there is now expanding clinical application for their use as predictive and prognostic biomarkers [9].

The type of receiver coil used in MRI and the placement in relation to the suspected disease profoundly affects the signal to noise ratio of the images, and thus their diagnostic quality. In particular, techniques such as DW-MRI, which are inherently low in signal to noise ratio, benefit from optimal receiver coil arrangements. In gynecological cancer, a notable development has been an endovaginal coil to image early stage cervical cancer; this has significantly improved delineation of early stage 1 tumors, allowing selection of patients for fertility-sparing procedures such as tracheletomy.

Positron Emission Tomography/ Computerized Tomography

Combined PET and CT scanners allow integrated functional and anatomical image acquisition. ^{18}F-FDG is a radioactive glucose analog that is taken up by cells which have a high glucose turnover including cancerous tissue. The analog is phosphorylated and therefore trapped within the cell; positron emission detected from the ^{18}F radioisotope label reflects increased cellular metabolic activity. PET/CT is used in lymph node detection, recurrent disease, evaluation of metastases and in complex cases which pose a diagnostic dilemma. New radiopharmaceuticals which target tumor angiogenesis (radiolabeled Vascular Endothelial Growth Factor), tissue hypoxia (^{64}Cu, ^{18}F misonidazole), cell membrane constituents (^{11}C-acetate, ^{11}C-methionine) and receptor studies ^{18}F-fluoro-17β[beta]-estradiol (FES) are currently used in the research setting [10–12]. The production of hardware that combines PET and MRI is challenging; such systems are limited in number at selected institutions and their clinical utility is under evaluation.

24.3 Imaging the Primary Site (T-Staging)

Cervical Cancer

The mainstay of management of organ-confined (stage 1) cervical cancer is surgical, whereas extension into the parametrial tissues or adjacent vagina usually indicates a preference for primary chemoradiotherapy. Accurate T-staging with imaging is of critical importance in determining optimal management. Moreover, the opportunity for fertility-sparing procedures such as trachelectomy or even just a repeat extended therapeutic cone biopsy is of increasing demand in a population where child-bearing is increasingly postponed. T2-W MRI provides the best image contrast for T-staging cervical cancer and is superior to CT both in detecting disease (sensitivity 75 vs 51 %, $p<0.005$) and staging accuracy (77 vs 69 %, $p<0.025$, [13]. Multiplanar acquisitions are possible and three planes orthogonal to the cervix are preferred to assess anterior/posterior and cranio-caudal extension (sagittal plane) and lateral extension into parametria (coronal and axial planes) [14]. It is also possible to acquire data in 3-D and reconstruct images in the desired planes, although acquisition times are longer and therefore prone to motion artifact.

Tumor volumetry is an important feature of imaging assessment; it has been shown that the size of the tumor is an important prognostic indicator [15]. Tumor volume is also related to the likelihood of lymph node involvement [16]. Volumes obtained from MRI images correlate well with those derived from histomorphometric methods, but less well with clinical stage [17]. Derivations of volume are often done using dimension measurements in three planes and assuming an ovoid shape, however, tumor margins are often irregular and more accurate estimates may be obtained by outlining tumor on every slice and multiplying by slice thickness. In small tumors, where volumetry may well affect the type of surgical management, this approach is preferred. In larger lesions, accurate estimations of volume are a useful prognostic indicator [15].

Although the use of contrast enhancement for detecting tumor within the cervix or describing its extent has been explored, evidence indicates that it is not warranted as the contrast between the intermediate signal-intensity tumor and the low signal-intensity cervical stroma on T2-W imaging is diagnostically adequate with contrast-enhancement providing no additional benefit. The use of dynamic-contrast enhanced studies is largely limited to defining the vascular fraction of tumor in order to deliver adaptive radiotherapy [18] or to identify a hypoxic fraction and relate it to treatment outcome [19].

The use of an endovaginal receiver coil allows a fourfold increase in signal detection from the cervix [20] and thus an equivalent improvement in spatial resolution that improves detection of Stage 1 cervical lesions [21, 22]. T2-W images of sub-millimeter resolution enable delineation of 5 mm lesions with 100 % accuracy [23]. However, as patients are often referred following cone-biopsy, the addition of DW-MRI to the T2-W MRI is required to improve the sensitivity of the technique (56–89 % with little loss in specificity in tumors with a median longitudinal diameter of 1.1 cm) [24] (Fig. 24.1). This type of image is of particular advantage when assessing patients for fertility-sparing surgical options where delineation of small lesions and their extension into the endocervical canal is required. Exophytic lesions with little endocervical extension are best demarcated on sagittal and coronal images and the length of uninvolved endocervical canal can be determined [24]. The technique also requires the reporting radiologist to perform a vaginal examination which has the added advantage of being able to combine clinical and radiological information.

Parametrial extension can be assessed on both CT and MRI, although image contrast is better on the latter. Both result in false-positives from interpreting inflammatory soft tissue strands as invasive tumor; comparison with hysterectomy specimens showed an accuracy of 87% for MRI, 80% for CT and 82.5 % for examination under anesthesia [25]. Images transverse to the cervix are preferred [26]. There is no advantage in using fat-suppression [27], neither does contrast-enhancement provide additional benefits (accuracy of parametrial extension 83 % on T2-W images compared with 72 % for gradient–enhanced, T1-W fat suppressed images, [28]. More recently, diffusion-weighted imaging, which is proving of major benefit in diagnosis of soft-tissue tumors, has been successfully employed to improve detection of small cervical tumors: combining the information from the apparent diffusion coefficient maps derived from DW-MRI sequences with the standard T2-W data improves sensitivity and specificity from 56 and 75 % respectively to 89 and 67 % respectively [24].

Endometrial Cancer

As the primary management of endometrial cancer is surgical, T-staging of the tumor is done at histopathology. However, accurate T-staging on pre-operative imaging serves to guide the need for nodal dissection and the use of adjuvant therapies.

T2-W MRI is the preferred modality for T-staging the tumor; CT lacks contrast between tumor and myometrium. On T2-W imaging the abnormal uterus has a well-defined zonal anatomy in post-menarche, pre-menopausal women with a high signal intensity endometrial stripe, a low signal-intensity inner myometrium (junctional zone) and an intermediate signal intensity outer myometrium. In these cases, definition of an intermediate signal intensity endometrial tumor against the low signal intensity junctional zone can be relatively clear, making the assessment of myometrial invasion fairly straightforward. However, endometrial cancer primarily affects the post-menopausal age group where the zonal anatomy of the uterus disappears and the junctional zone increases in signal intensity. In these cases, outlining the extent of invasion of tumor into the myometrium lacks contrast on T2-W imaging and the use of gadolinium to highlight a poorly vascular tumor against a much more avidly enhancing myometrium is often used. However, contrast-enhanced images need to be acquired dynamically with a temporal resolution of <30 s in order to be sufficiently

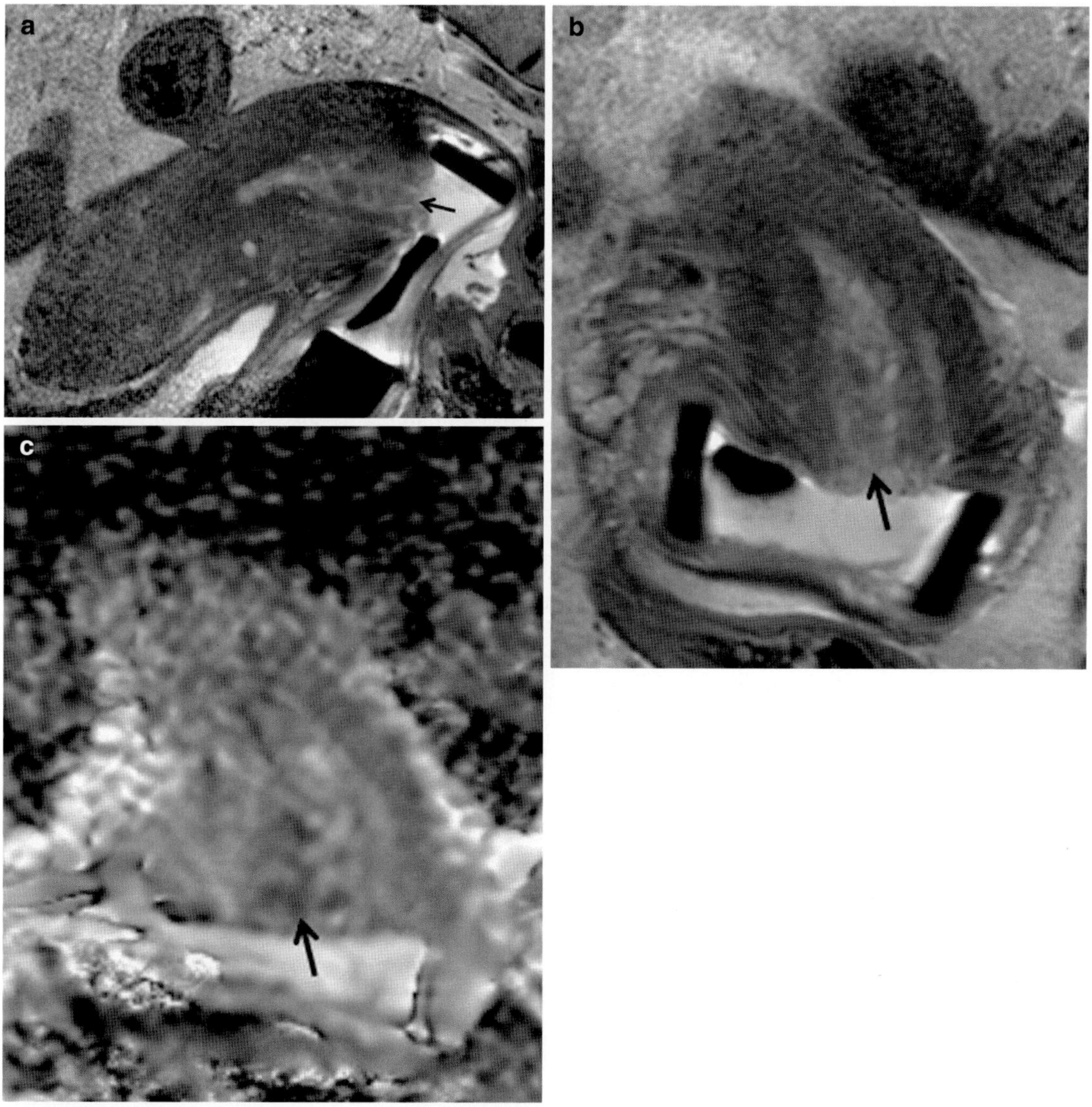

Fig. 24.1 T2-weighted fast spin-echo transverse (**a**) and coronal (**b**) MR images and corresponding coronal ADC map (**c**) obtained using an endovaginal coil in a woman with stage Ib1 tumor. An area of diffuse abnormal intermediate signal intensity (*arrows*) is seen on T2-weighted images (**a**, **b**), which corresponds with area of restricted diffusion in (**c**) (*arrow*), lending greater confidence to diagnosis of invasive cervical carcinoma

accurate, as after 3 min, enhancement of the tumor itself and washout of contrast from the myometrium mean that these structures become isointense with each other and contrast between them is lost. The need for high temporal resolution images acquired dynamically results in a compromise on spatial resolution, with pixel sizes of 3–5 mm and leads to a loss of sensitivity for T-staging. In postmenopausal women, the accuracy in estimating myometrial invasion with T2-W images, contrast-enhanced T1-W images, and DCE-MRI was 66.7, 77.8, and 92.6 %, respectively [29]. In a more recent study of 45 women, Nasi et al. showed that gadolinium enhancement with better temporal resolution had a global sensitivity and specificity of 90.6 and 93.3 %, respectively, with a mean Negative Predictive Value of 96,3 % and a mean Positive Predictive Value of 88 % compared to the FSE T2-W sequence (global sensitivity and specificity of 80.6 and 87.6 %, respectively, mean Negative Predictive Value 92.6 %, mean Positive Predictive Value 86 %) giving contrast-enhanced sequences a higher staging accuracy (95 % vs. 78 %) [30]. DCE-MRI images in combination with T2-W sequences give more accurate assessment of myometrial invasion [31] (Fig. 24.2). Deep myometrial invasion (>50 %) is associated with a 40 % risk of nodal metastases so that MRI has an important role in distinguishing superficial from deep myometrial invasion. More recently, DW-MRI has been shown in preliminary studies to have superior diagnostic accuracy in the assessment of myometrial invasion and significantly higher staging accuracy compared with DCE-MRI [32]. In a retrospective study of 48 patients, Beddy et al. showed diagnostic accuracy, sensitivity, and specificity, respectively, of 90, 84, and 100 % for DWI vs 71, 61, and 88 % for DCE-MRI. DW-MRI has also been successfully employed in differentiating benign from malignant endometrial lesions: derived apparent diffusion coefficient values have been shown to be significantly lower in malignant disease ($0.84 \pm 0.19 \times 10^{-3}$ mm^2/s vs. $1.58 \pm 0.36 \times 10^{-3}$ mm^2/s, [$P < 0.01$]) [33–35].

A minimum of two planes is required to delineate the tumor against the inner myometrium. The sagittal plane which visualizes the longitudinal axis of the endometrial cavity and a plane truly transaxial to the uterine body to image the uterus in cross-section are preferred. Spatial resolution is optimized to achieve an in-plane pixel size of 0.5 mm with a 3–4 mm slice thickness; this can be accomplished while maintaining a sufficient signal to noise ratio within the capability of most 1.5 and 3 T scanners with an external pelvic array coil. Smaller pixels merely result in an increase in image noise and a reduction in diagnostic accuracy.

Lesions within the endometrial cavity are often hemorrhagic, particularly if there has been a recent biopsy or curettage. This is a common diagnostic pitfall and can lead to an overestimation of disease burden or extent. It is therefore imperative to acquire T1-W images where

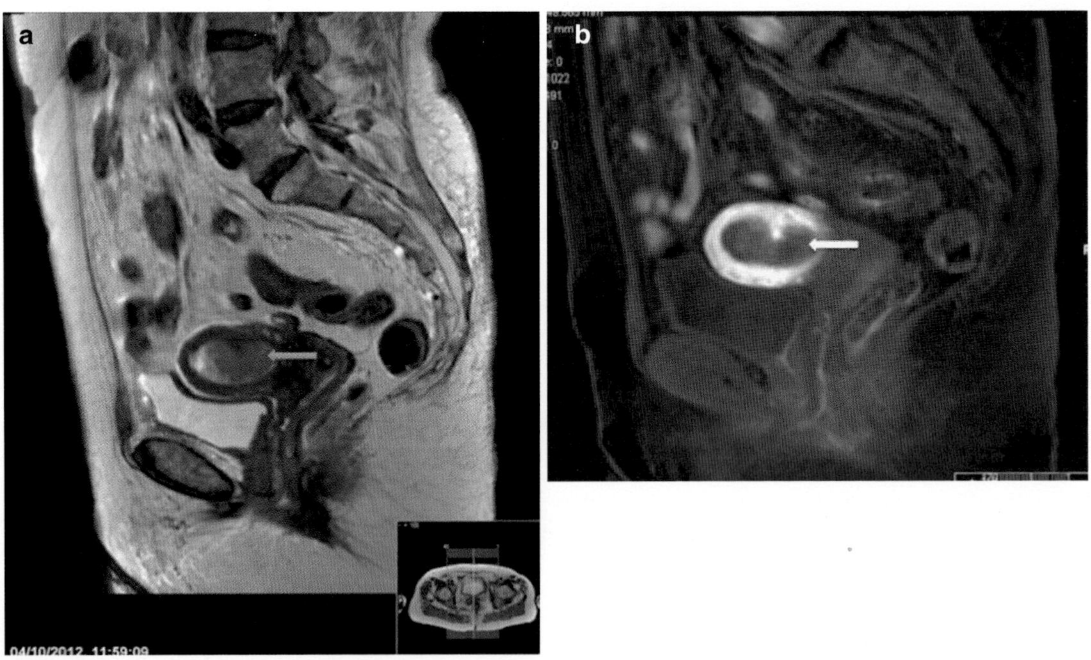

Fig. 24.2 T2-weighted sagittal image (**a**) and DCE image (**b**) in a woman with stage 1a endometrial carcinoma. An intermediate T2 signal intensity mass is distending the endometrial cavity (**a**, *blue arrow*). The myometrium enhances avidly on the DCE image and the tumor enhances less avidly (**b**, *white arrow*), therefore invasion of the myometrium is more easily visualized, in this case there is minimal invasion

sub-acute hemorrhage is easily recognized as high signal-intensity within the endometrial cavity. The irregular margins, nodularity and nodular nature of the tumor mass have also been used to differentiate endometrial stromal sarcoma from endometrial cancer [36] although in an organ where tissue sampling is relatively simple, the need for this histological differentiation on imaging is unlikely to have major clinical impact.

Ovarian Cancer

Ovarian cancer is usually recognized late because of lack of symptoms. By the time women present with abdominal distension and discomfort peritoneal dissemination is widespread with ascites. Previous studies have investigated ultrasound for screening, but these have not proved cost-effective [37]. In >3,500 women at high risk of ovarian or fallopian tube cancer screened at 37 UK centers, annual transvaginal ultrasound and serum CA125 screening had positive and negative predictive values of 25.5 % (95 % CI, 14.3–40.0) and 99.9 % (95 % CI, 99.8–100) respectively at the incident screen [38]. The longer term follow up from this study is ongoing and due to report in 2015.

Ovarian cancer is recognized by complex partly solid, partly cystic masses within one or both ovaries as disease is frequently bilateral. The solid components are in the form of nodules, septations or papilliform fronds and when recognized in these patterns are characteristic of epithelial ovarian cancer. Rarer histological subtypes (cystadenocarcinomas, endometroid adenocarcinoma and clear cell variants) may also be recognized by classical appearances of the solid components of the masses on T2-W imaging [39]. For example, granulose cell tumors are predominantly solid intermediate signal-intensity homogenous masses with small, often punctuate cystic/necrotic components. Conventional and contrast-enhanced MR imaging also are useful to evaluate morphologic features, including lesion complexity, signal intensity, and enhancement of solid areas. At dynamic contrast-enhanced MR imaging with semiquantitative analysis, early enhancement characteristics may help differentiate some complex benign and malignant lesions. Diffusion-weighted imaging has a limited but useful role in evaluating adnexal masses: Those with a hypointense solid area on both diffusion-weighted (b = 1,000 s/mm^2) and T2-weighted images are likely benign, whereas those that are hyperintense on diffusion-weighted images (b = 1,000 s/mm^2) with intermediate signal intensity on T2-weighted images are likely malignant [40].

The extent of peritoneal disease is still best 'evaluated' on CT because it enables coverage from the dome of the diaphragms to the pelvic floor within a few seconds. The associated ascites provides a low density background against which the nodules and plaques of peritoneal disease are outlined. The use of contrast agents both in CT and MRI has been explored, but their use does not provide advantages over unenhanced images [41]. Ovarian lesions generally are poorly enhancing and are not highlighted within a mesentery where normal vascular enhancement is prominent or against normally enhancing bowel wall. DCE-CT and MRI techniques lack the coverage of the whole abdomen and pelvis with sufficient spatial and temporal resolution [6]. Their utility is therefore confined to characterizing single lesions that require better delineation [42] (Fig. 24.3).

Newer techniques such as DW-MRI are revolutionizing the imaging assessment of ovarian cancer, as not only is image contrast improved but they are also quantitative [43, 44]. On heavily DW images (high b-value) tumor appears bright against a dark background and is therefore easily recognized (Fig. 24.4). However, normal bowel wall also shows diffusion restriction and appears bright so that it is difficult to separate serosal deposits from normal bowel. Use of threshold values of the apparent diffusion coefficient is advocated to enable this differentiation. In future use of such thresholds and automated segmentation of lesions will enable estimations of the volume of burden of solid disease which can then be measured in longitudinal studies on chemotherapy. It should also be possible to use such information for assessing the optimal timing for

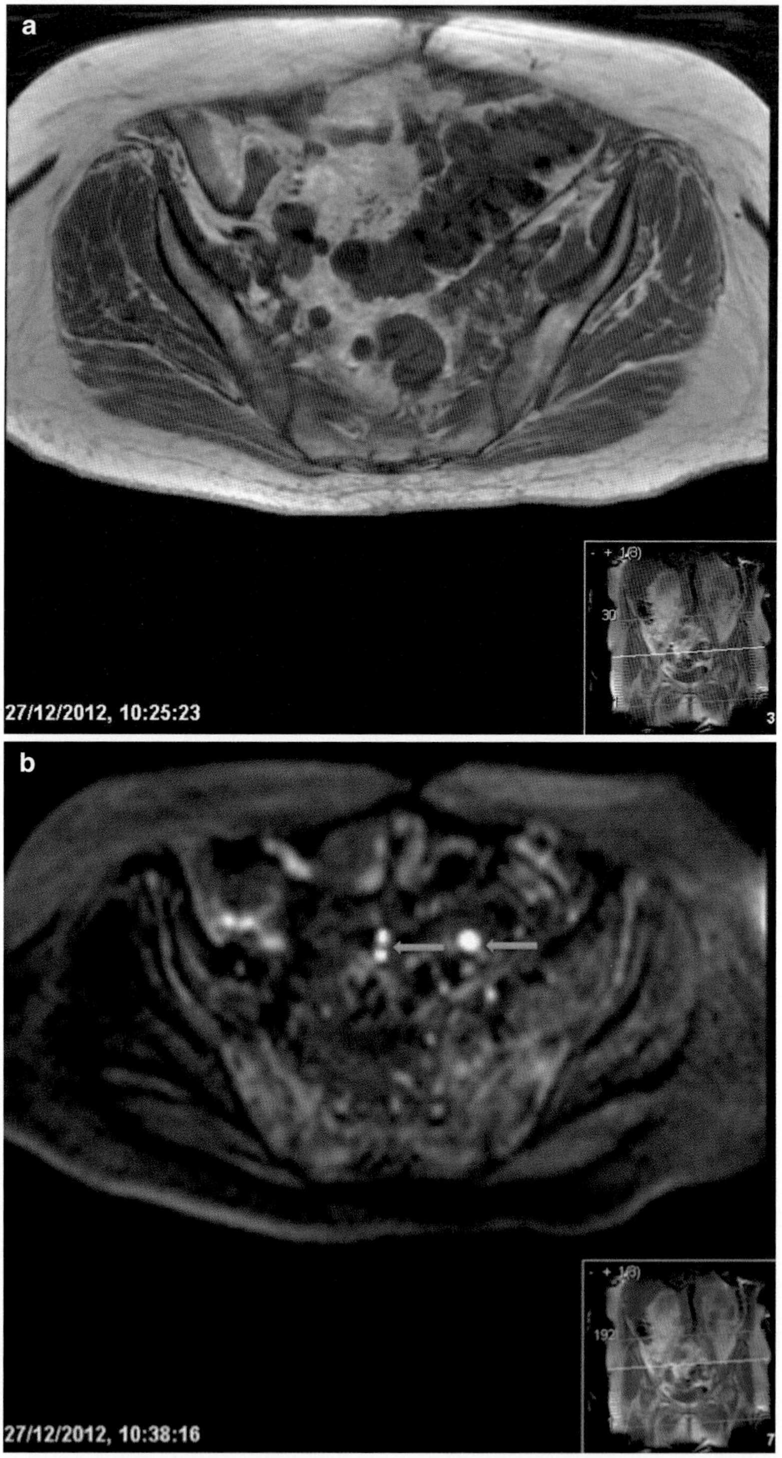

Fig. 24.3 T1-weighted axial image of the pelvis (**a**) and corresponding b1200 DW-MRI image (**b**) and sagittal T2-weighted image (**c**) in a woman with ovarian carcinoma. Diverticular disease is present in the sigmoid colon and the signal intensity of peritoneal and serosal deposits is similar to bowel making assessment of deposits difficult on T1-weighted images (**a**). DW-MRI increases the conspicuity of disease, image (**b**) demonstrates three areas of bright signal (*blue arrows*), the larger lesion is a serosal deposit and the two smaller lesions correlate with small peritoneal deposits seen on image (**c**) (*white arrow*)

Fig. 24.3 (continued)

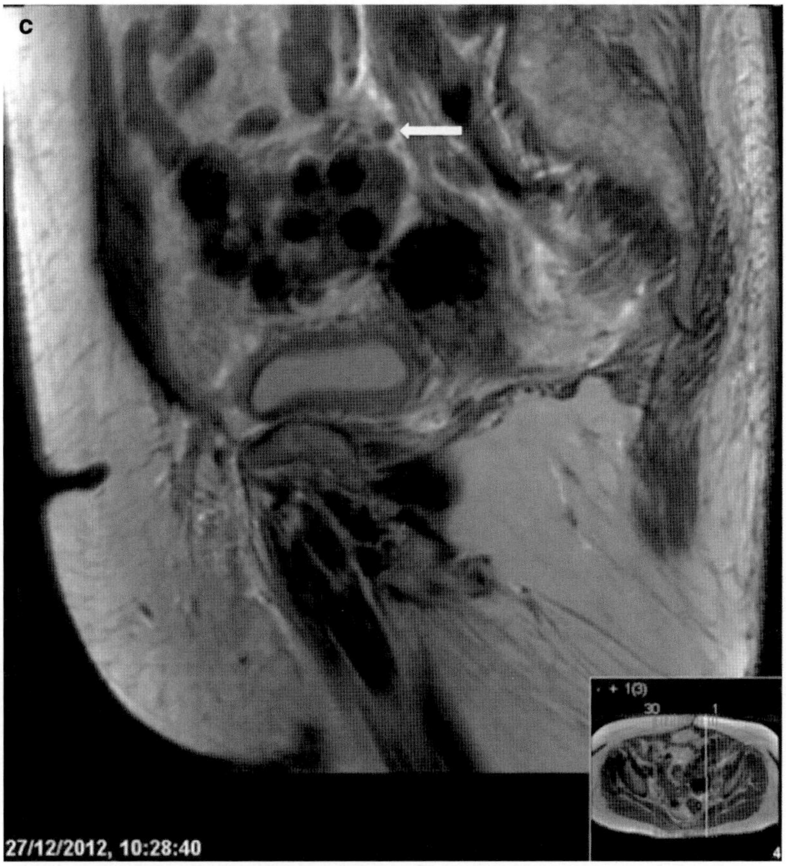

debulking disease within a course of chemotherapy, thus individualizing and optimizing the surgical management in these patients.

24.4 Imaging Nodal Stations (N-Staging)

Cervical Carcinoma

Lymph node status is the single most important prognostic factor in cervical cancer [10]. The 5-year survival rate without nodal metastases is estimated at 85 %, this reduces to 71 % with the presence of pelvic lymph nodes [45]. Lymphatic spread occurs first to the local paracervical and parametrial nodes, obturator nodes are frequent sites of disease and spread to iliac chains, para-aortic and retroperitoneal nodes although largely contiguous may not be necessarily so. Pre-operative imaging assessment aims to identify nodal disease which would require combined chemotherapy and radiation therapy rather than surgery (Fig. 24.5). Morphological features which suggest involved lymph nodes include round shape, irregular outline and size greater than 10 mm—however using this size cut-off on CT and MRI yields a low sensitivity [46]. If a parametrial lymph node is greater than 5 mm this is regarded as suspicious. Yang et al. showed that central nodal necrosis has a 100 % positive predictive value for metastases in squamous cell carcinoma of the cervix [47]. Signal intensity similar to the primary tumor also suggests nodal involvement. DWI-MRI has shown potential in detecting metastatic nodes; although some studies show significantly lower ADC values in diseased nodes compared to benign nodes [8] there is significant overlap in values which reduces specificity.

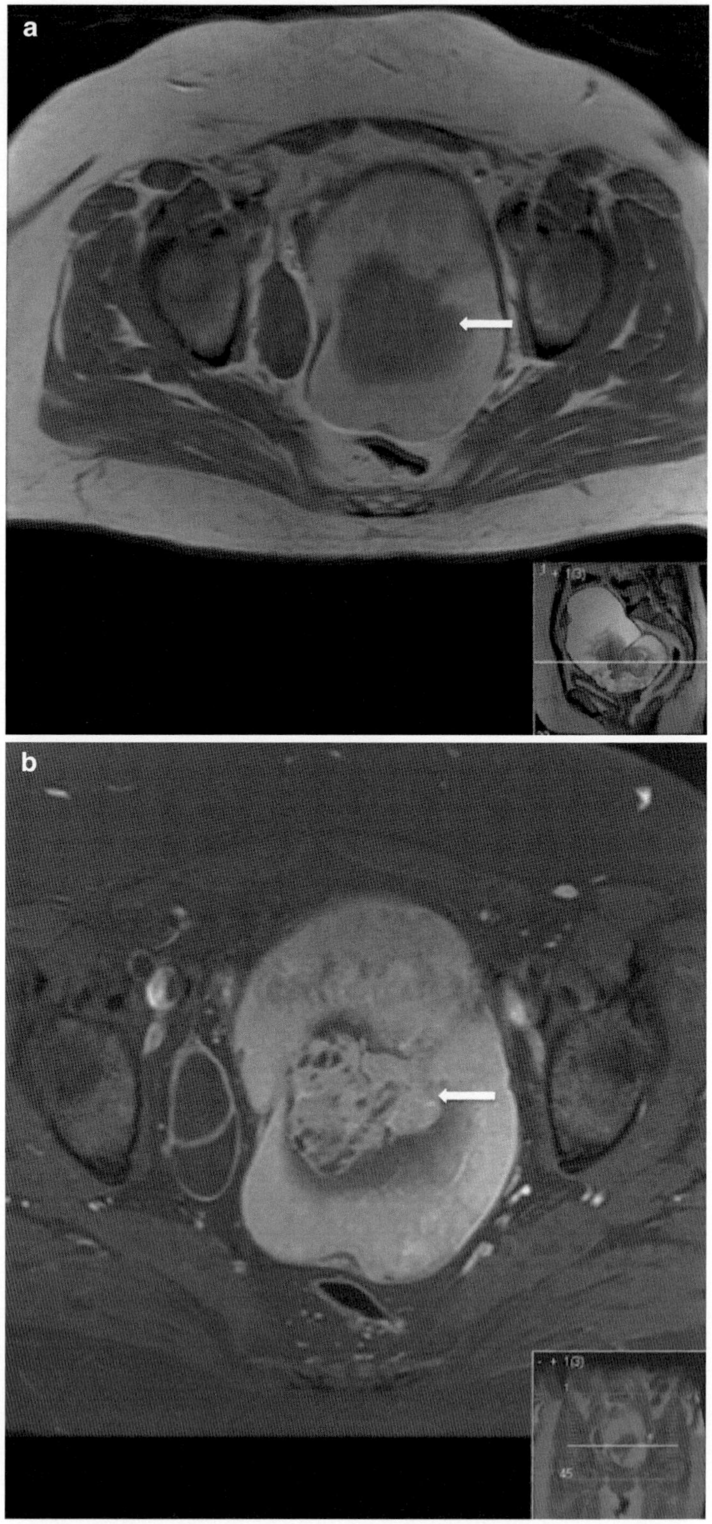

Fig. 24.4 T2-weighted axial image through the pelvis (**a**) with corresponding contrast enhanced image (**b**), b1200 DW-MRI (**c**) and corresponding ADC map (**d**) in a woman with a mucinous adenocarcinoma of the left ovary. The left adnexal mass has a high T2 signal intensity cystic component and an intermediate T2-signal intensity central solid component (**a**, *arrow*). The solid component enhances heterogeneously (**b**, *arrow*). On the high b-value DW image the solid area returns bright signal (**c**, *arrow*) with corresponding dark signal on the ADC map (**d**, *arrow*)

Fig. 24.4 (continued)

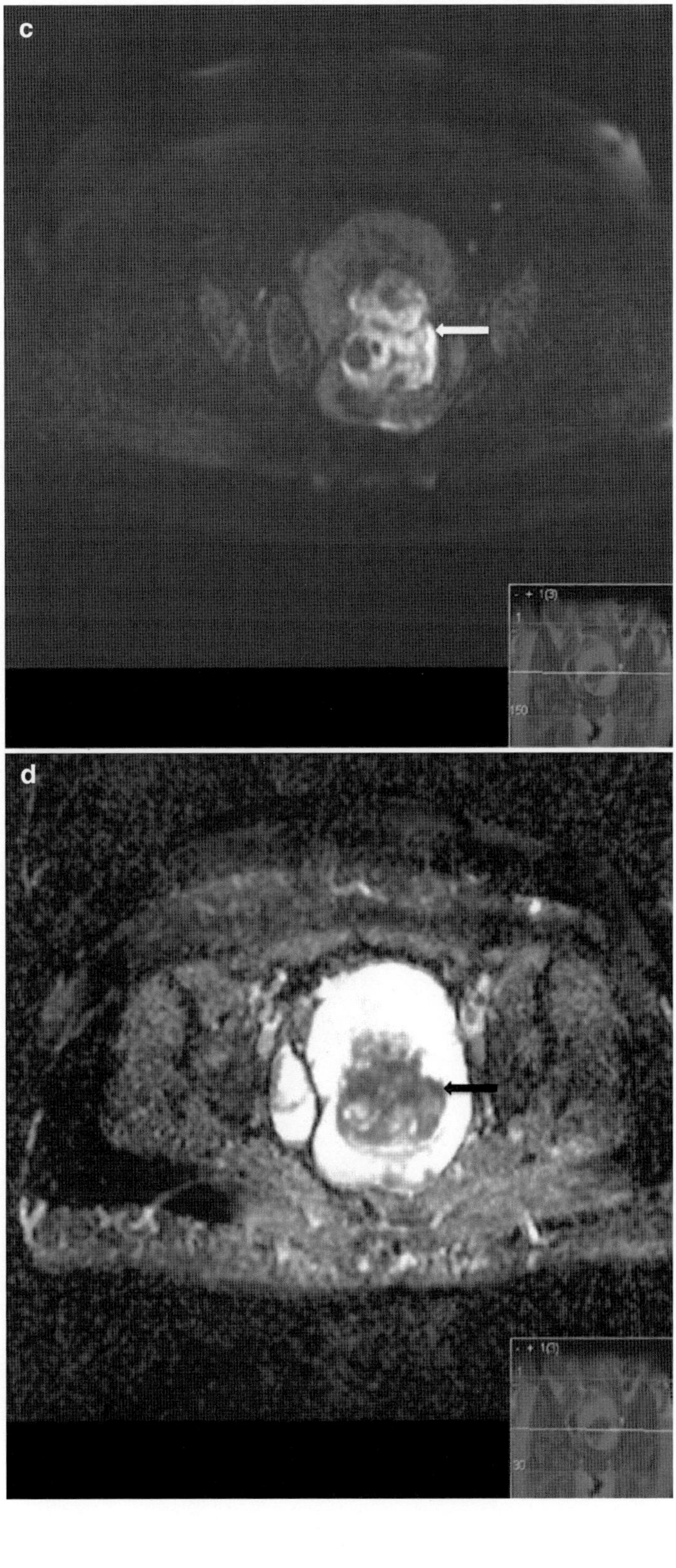

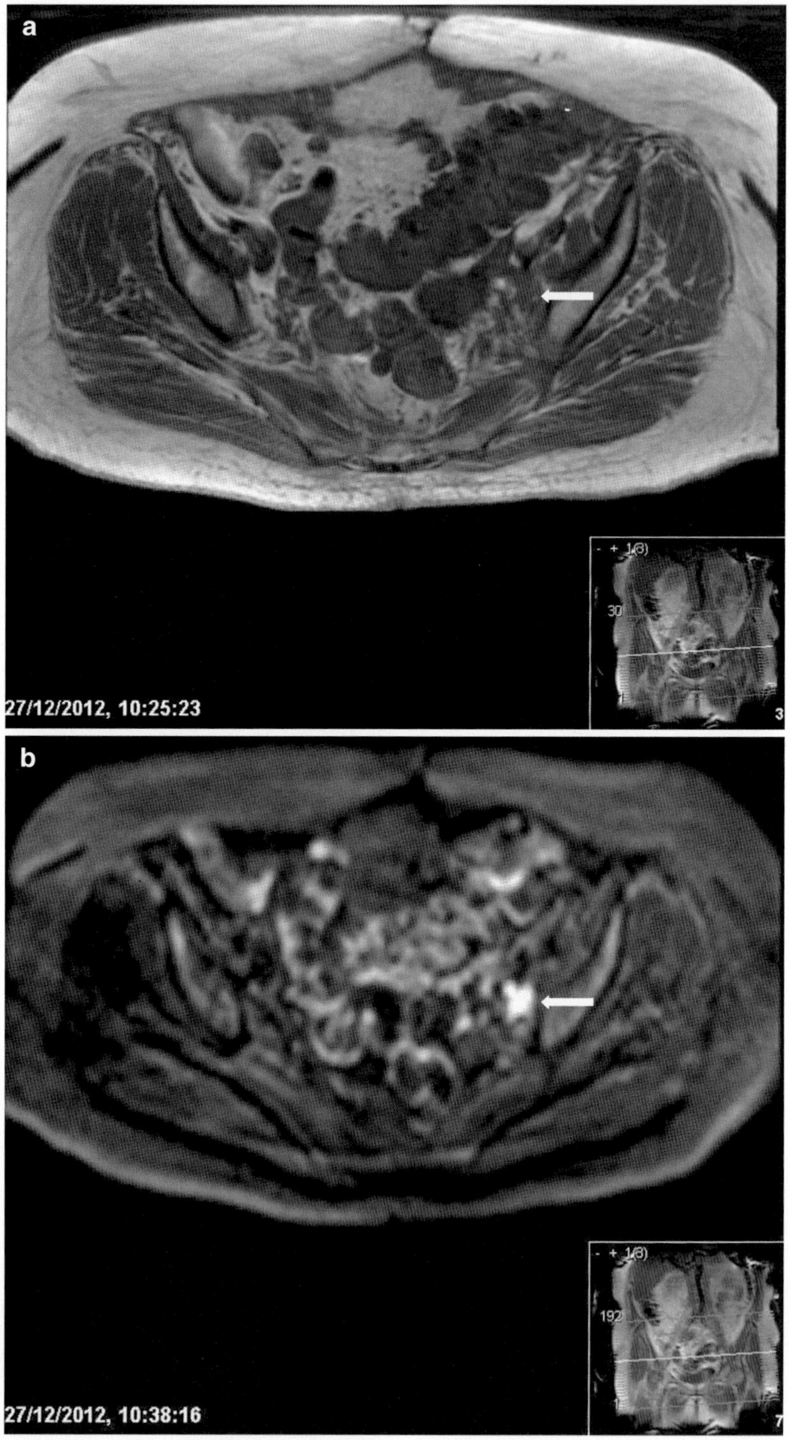

Fig. 24.5 T1-weighted axial image through the pelvis (**a**) and corresponding high b-1200 value DW-MRI image (**b**) and ADC map (**c**) in a patient with stage IIb cervical carcinoma. The 9 mm left external iliac node is of similar intensity to the bowel and vessels (**a** *arrow*), however the lymph node demonstrates restricted diffusion appearing very bright on the DW image (**b**) and dark on the ADC map (**c**) highlighting the value of functional MRI

Fig. 24.5 (continued)

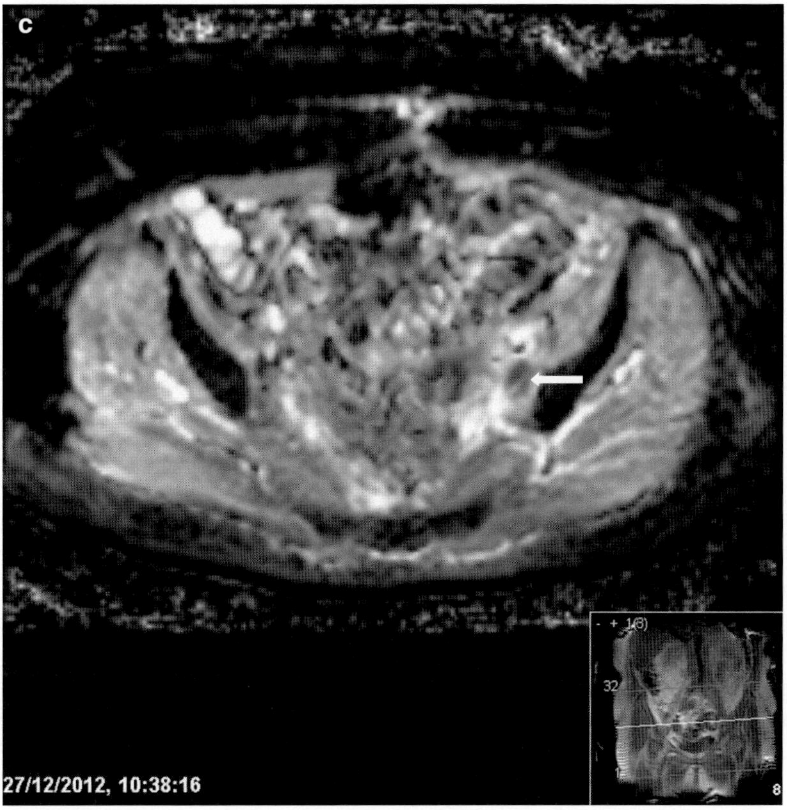

^{18}F-FDG PET/CT has been shown to be superior to MRI in detecting pelvic and para-aortic nodal disease in later stages of disease (FIGO II and greater), with sensitivities between 60 and 100 % and specificities between 55 and 95 % compared with MRI sensitivities of 71 % with no loss in specificity [47, 48]. Early work has shown that combining information from PET and MRI has higher accuracy compared to ^{18}F-FDG PET/CT in nodal detection [49], but remains to be corroborated in larger studies.

Endometrial Carcinoma

Lymphadenectomy is part of the surgico-pathological staging of endometrial cancer but is not performed in all centers. In low FIGO stage disease (<1B) lymphadenectomy may not be performed so that pre-operative imaging is particularly important in optimal surgical planning. The depth of myometrial and cervical stromal invasion are key prognostic factors of nodal metastases; pelvic nodes >8 mm in short axis are generally considered enlarged and likely to be metastatic. The middle and lower uterus drain to regional lymph nodes in the parametrium, paracervical and obturator nodes (stage IIIC disease), whilst the upper uterus drains to common iliac and para-aortic chains. The presence of enlarged para-aortic lymph nodes is associated with the highest impact on prognosis and indicates stage IIIC2 disease [50].

As with cervical carcinoma ^{18}F-FDG-PET/CT is useful in the detection of nodal metastases in endometrial cancer. A recent meta-analysis has shown that the overall pooled estimates for sensitivity and specificity of ^{18}F-FDG-PET or PET/CT scans in the detection of pelvic and/or para-aortic metastasis were 63.0 % (95 % CI, 48.7–75.7 %) and 94.7 % (95 % CI, 90.4–97.4 %), respectively with an overall diagnostic accuracy of 89.5 % [51]. MRI lymphography using iron-oxide nanoparticles showed promising results in preliminary studies

[46], but awaits larger scale multicenter trials when the contrast agent becomes available.

Ovarian Carcinoma

Primary lymph node drainage from the ovaries is to the para-aortic lymph nodes, secondary drainage occurs through the broad ligament to obturator, internal and external iliac lymph nodes and through the round ligament to inguinal lymph nodes. The presence of regional lymph nodes stages the disease as FIGO IIIC and is associated with a 5-year survival of 34 % [10]. Supra-renal para-aortic lymph nodes may result in a patient being unsuitable for primary surgical resection underlining the importance of imaging in pre-operative assessment. In the evaluation of nodal disease, ^{18}F-FDG-PET/CT is the most accurate imaging technique available, as it is capable of identifying metastatic deposits in nodes deemed unenlarged by size criteria on morphological imaging. Yoshida et al. demonstrated malignant involvement in normal sized lymph nodes in ovarian cancer and showed that ^{18}F-FDG-PET/CT improved staging accuracy from 53 to 87 % when compared with CT alone [52].

24.5 Imaging Metastatic Spread (M-Staging)

Nearly 80 % of patients with endometrial cancer present with stage 1 disease; hematogenous spread to other organs and bones is rare at presentation. The lungs are the commonest site involved [53] and sometimes peritoneal deposits are seen. Similarly, distant spread of cervical cancer to the lungs, liver and bones can occur but is rare at presentation. In contrast, the majority of patients with ovarian cancer often present with advanced disease due to the general non-specific nature of associated symptoms. Peritoneal metastases outside the pelvis including subcapsular liver deposits and/or regional lymph node metastases are common at presentation. Stage IV disease is recognized when metastatic deposits are identified beyond the peritoneal cavity or within liver parenchyma. Surgical staging is the gold-standard but increasingly where treatment is with primary chemotherapy followed by interval debulking surgery, a "staging CT" is common place with a quoted accuracy of 70–90 % [54].

CT allows detection of peritoneal disease, ascites, nodal, visceral and bone disease which aids surgical planning. Detection of peritoneal deposits depends on a number of factors, size (over 1 cm), presence of ascites, and administration of oral and intravenous contrast. Calcified deposits are easier to detect on CT. In the absence of disseminated disease, primary debulking surgery is recommended. If disease is widespread, the likelihood of suboptimal surgical debulking is high and primary chemotherapy is given. In these cases, image-guided biopsy may be necessary to provide a definitive histological diagnosis. CT features which suggest a high risk of suboptimal cytoreduction, such as extensive subhepatic disease, also may be used to select patients for laparoscopic evaluation prior to laparotomy.

Additional roles for CT are in diagnosing primary peritoneal carcinoma which cannot be distinguished from ovarian cancer pathologically as well as in identifying ovarian metastases from a gastrointestinal, breast or pancreatic primary tumor.

Newer techniques such as DW-MRI are now being increasingly investigated in whole body protocols for identifying metastases, but data acquisition techniques are still variable across scanners and, unless rigorously conducted, the examinations can be prone to significant image artifact. DWI-MRI has proven useful in detection of small peritoneal, serosal and subcapsular liver deposits which are seen as bright signal intensity areas on high b-values. DWI-MRI is also useful in detecting low volume peritoneal disease and identifying lesions in difficult anatomical locations for example the right sub-diaphragmatic space, although correlation with conventional imaging is necessary [43].

24.6 Imaging Response and Recurrence

Disease response on DW-MRI is recognized as an increase in ADC because of an increase in apoptosis and necrosis within the tumor mass increasing extracellular space and allowing more free water diffusion within the tissue. A sound basis for applying thresholds of response and non-response depends on establishing a robust measurement and understanding the limitations, particularly in a multicenter setting where equipment variations affect the reproducibility of the technique [55]. In ovarian cancer, although 18F-FDG PET/CT is still the norm for follow-up and for detecting recurrence (Fig. 24.6), DW-MRI of the pelvis and abdomen is being increasingly recognized [56]. It is currently under evaluation in a multicenter clinical trial, and may replace CT in assessing response and relapse in this disease not only because of its high sensitivity, but also because of its provision of quantifiable data. Its reproducibility is of importance in this disease

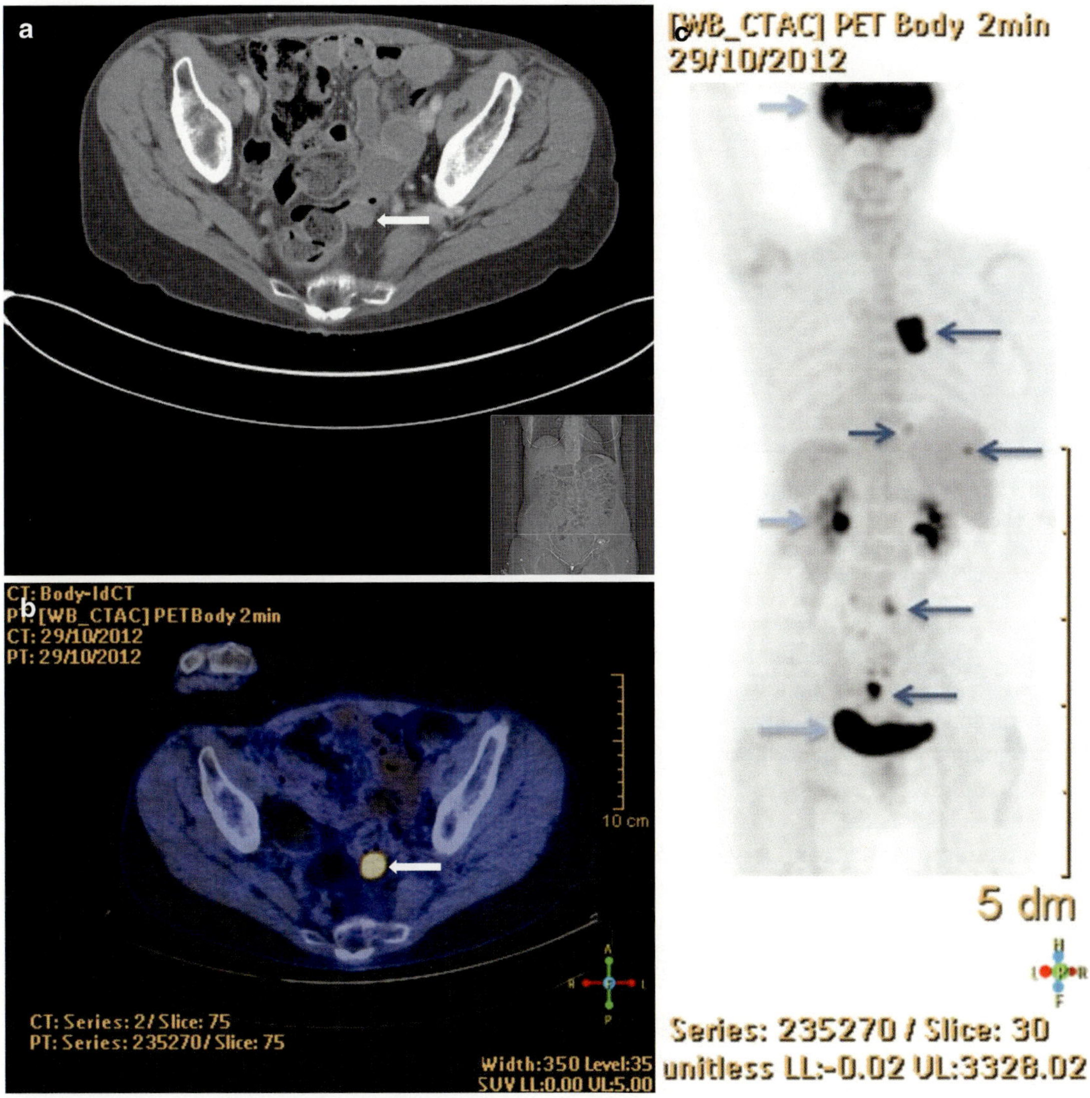

Fig. 24.6 Axial contrast enhanced CT image through the pelvis (**a**) corresponding fused PET/CT image (**b**) and whole-body coronal MIP 18F-FDG-PET image (**c**) in a woman with recurrent ovarian cancer. There is a pelvic peritoneal deposit posterior to a small bowel loop (**a**, *arrow*) which has similar appearances to bowel and could easily be overlooked on CT, however there is intense tracer uptake on the fused PET/CT (**b**, *arrow*) consistent with a metastatic deposit. Image (**c**) demonstrates the extent of widespread metastatic disease (*dark blue arrows*) including a metastatic right hilar lymph node mass, sub-centimeter supra-diaphragmatic node, intra-parenchymal liver deposit, iliac chain lymph nodes and the pelvic deposit (from *top* to *bottom*). Pale *blue arrows* demonstrate normal uptake in the brain and excretion within the kidneys and bladder

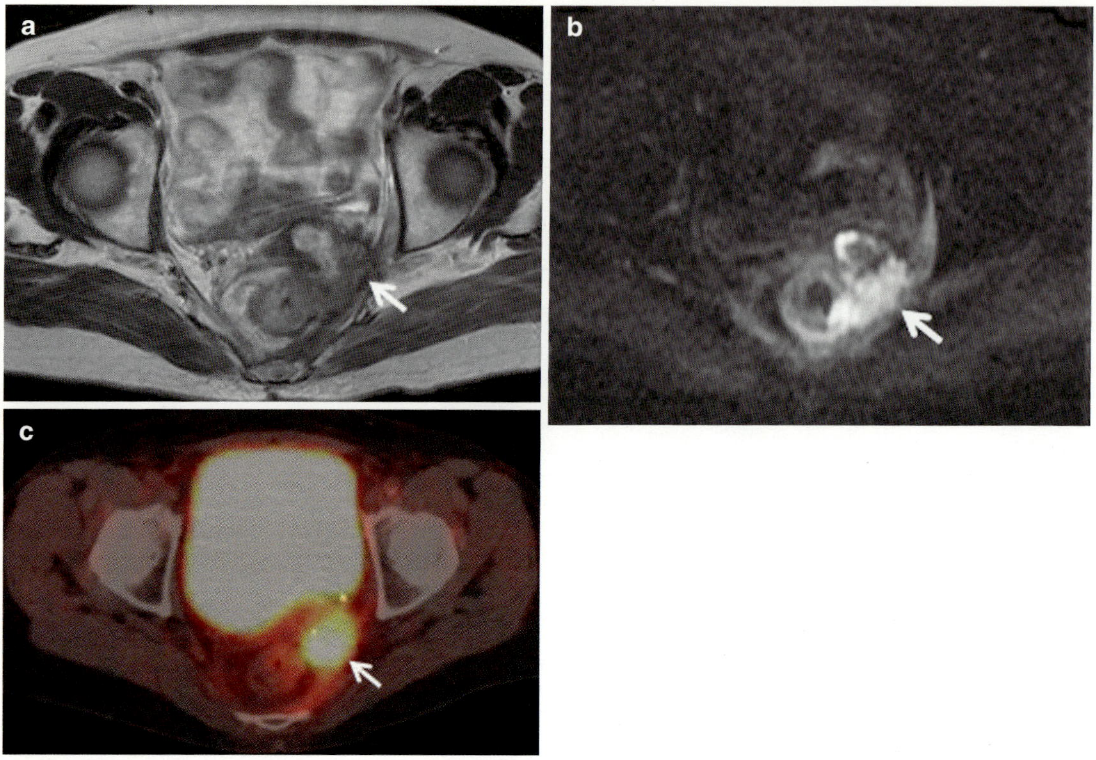

Fig. 24.7 T2-W fast spin-echo transverse image through the middle of the true pelvis (**a**) and corresponding diffusion-weighted MRI b = 900 mm^2/s images (**b**) show a recurrent endometrial tumor (**a**, *arrow*) as a mass of restricted diffusion in (**b**) (*arrow*) involving the left pelvic side-wall. An 18F-FDG PET scan at the same level (**c**) shows a marked increase in glucose metabolism in the pelvic side-wall mass (*arrow*)

where intensive longitudinal follow-up is required to recognize a pattern of relapse and remission and implement appropriate chemotherapeutic regimens as patients develop treatment related toxicities or become resistant to selected chemotherapeutic agents.

In imaging recurrence in cervical and endometrial cancer, morphological methods such as helical CT and T2-W MRI are still the norm, but increasingly DCE techniques, DW-MRI (Fig. 24.7) and ^{18}F-FDG PET/CT are being routinely used. Most research efforts have, however, focussed on the early prediction of recurrence. In cervical cancer, a study by Mayr et al. showed that the tenth centile value of the signal-intensity on contrast enhanced images [1] and the 3D tumor volume 2–2.5 weeks into therapy could independently predict disease recurrence (hazard ratio [HR], 2.6; 95 % confidence interval [95 % CI], 1.0–6.5 [P = .04] and HR, 1.9; 95 % CI, 1.1–3.5 [P = .03], respectively) and death (HR, 1.9; 95 % CI, 1.0–3.5 [P = .03] and HR, 1.9; 95 % CI, 1.2–2.9 [P = .01], respectively), and were superior to clinical prognostic factors [57]. Similarly, in a study of 80 patients, the mean ADC of primary cervical cancer was shown to be an independent predictive factor for disease recurrence [58], however, tumor volume was not interrogated in this analysis. Failure of metabolic response after treatment is another predictive factor for recurrence: in a series of 238 patients with cervical cancer, 38 % subsequently recurred; all of these had failed to show a metabolic response (24 % local, 76 % distant) on post treatment 18F-FDG PET done within 8–16 weeks of completion of chemoradiotherapy [59]. Kang et al. [60] developed a web-based nomogram for predicting recurrence in cervical cancer based on data from 434 patients in four institutions. They showed that four parameters were significantly associated with distant recurrence: pelvic and para-aortic nodal positivity on ^{18}F-FDG-PET, non-squamous cell histology, and pre-treatment serum squamous cell carcinoma antigen levels.

In endometrial cancer, records from eight institutions that provided data on 282 patients with recurrence showed that recurrent sites were, vaginal vault 12.4 %, central pelvis 18.0 %, pelvic side-wall 4.9 % lymph-node 13.8 %, distant metastases 45.3 % and both distant relapse and local relapse 5.3 % [61]. This indicates that a whole body technique such as CT or ^{18}F-FDG PET/CT is indicated in the follow-up of patients with endometrial cancer. The sensitivity, specificity, positive and negative predictive values, and accuracy of ^{18}F-FDG PET/CT for detecting recurrence have been shown to be 88.9, 93.6, 94.1, 88, and 91 %, respectively [62]. Eventually whole body DW-MRI may replace these, but requires the technique to be refined to reduce significant artifact and be available cost-effectively to providers within a time-frame tolerable to patients (current methods require a 45 min scan time).

24.7 Summary

Radiological assessment of gynecological malignancies currently is not incorporated into the FIGO staging systems however non-invasive anatomical and functional imaging modalities are routinely utilized and essential in the diagnosis, detection, staging of disease and in shaping the patients treatment pathway. Advances in technology have led to more powerful equipment including high field strength MRI scanners, development of endocervical coils, hybrid PET/CT and multidetector CT scanners. In parallel, new imaging techniques enabled by these hardware advances, in particular DCE-MRI, DW-MRI and PET/CT have furthered the capability to detect small sites of active disease. These techniques are being more widely used in the assessment of treatment response, distinguishing residual sites of disease from post-treatment changes and in identifying early recurrence.

Future directions include the clinical utilization of PET/MRI scanners which capitalize on the exquisite soft tissue resolution of MRI and the functional potential of new PET probes. However, it remains to be seen whether PET/MRI can improve diagnostic accuracy above the established described techniques and whether it will be incorporated into primary assessment of tumors. As imaging techniques continue to evolve they will enable us to interrogate tumor biology and the effects of sophisticated treatment modalities. New radiotracers that inform on biological mechanisms and metabolic pathways may prove useful biomarkers of tumor response to targeted drugs in an era of personalized medicine.

References

1. Bharwani N, Reznek RH, Rockall AG. Ovarian cancer management: the role of imaging and diagnostic challenges. Eur J Radiol. 2011;78(1):41–51.
2. Fleischer AC, Milam MR, Crispens MA, Shappell HW. Sonographic depiction of intratumoral vascularity with 2- and 3-dimensional color Doppler techniques. J Ultrasound Med. 2005;24(4):533–7.
3. Fleischer AC, Lyshchik A, Hirari M, Moore RD, Abramson RG, Fishman DA. Early detection of ovarian cancer with conventional and contrast-enhanced transvaginal sonography: recent advances and potential improvements. J Oncol. 2012;2012:302858.
4. Satoh Y, Ichikawa T, Motosugi U, Kimura K, Sou H, Sano K, Araki T. Diagnosis of peritoneal dissemination: comparison of 18F-FDG PET/CT, diffusion-weighted MRI, and contrast-enhanced MDCT. AJR Am J Roentgenol. 2011;196(2):447–53 [Comparative Study].
5. Otero HJ, Yap JT, Patak MA, Erturk SM, Israel DA, Johnston CJ, Sakellis C, Rybicki FJ, Van den Abbeele AD, Ros PR. Evaluation of low-density neutral oral contrast material in PET/CT for tumor imaging: results of a randomized clinical trial. AJR Am J Roentgenol. 2009;193(2):326–32 [Randomized Controlled TrialResearch Support, Non-U.S. Gov't].
6. Sala E, Rockall A, Rangarajan D, Kubik-Huch RA. The role of dynamic contrast-enhanced and diffusion weighted magnetic resonance imaging in the female pelvis. Eur J Radiol. 2010;76(3):367–85.
7. Bernardin L, Dilks P, Liyanage S, Miquel ME, Sahdev A, Rockall A. Effectiveness of semi-quantitative multiphase dynamic contrast-enhanced MRI as a predictor of malignancy in complex adnexal masses: radiological and pathological correlation. Eur Radiol. 2012;22(4):880–90.
8. Punwani S. Diffusion weighted imaging of female pelvic cancers: concepts and clinical applications. Eur J Radiol. 2011;78(1):21–9.

9. Punwani S. Contrast enhanced MR imaging of female pelvic cancers: established methods and emerging applications. Eur J Radiol. 2011;78(1):2–11.
10. Lai G, Rockall AG. Lymph node imaging in gynecologic malignancy. Semin Ultrasound CT MR. 2010;31(5):363–76.
11. Lewis JS, Laforest R, Dehdashti F, Grigsby PW, Welch MJ, Siegel BA. An imaging comparison of 64Cu-ATSM and 60Cu-ATSM in cancer of the uterine cervix. J Nucl Med. 2008;49(7):1177–82.
12. Torizuka T, Kanno T, Futatsubashi M, Okada H, Yoshikawa E, Nakamura F, Takekuma M, Maeda M, Ouchi Y. Imaging of gynecologic tumors: comparison of (11)C-choline PET with (18)F-FDG PET. J Nucl Med. 2003;44(7):1051–6.
13. Ozsarlak O, Tjalma W, Schepens E, Corthouts B, Op de Beeck B, Van Marck E, Parizel PM, De Schepper AM. The correlation of preoperative CT, MR imaging, and clinical staging (FIGO) with histopathology findings in primary cervical carcinoma. Eur Radiol. 2003;13(10):2338–45.
14. Sala E, Wakely S, Senior E, Lomas D. MRI of malignant neoplasms of the uterine corpus and cervix. AJR Am J Roentgenol. 2007;188(6):1577–87 [Review].
15. Soutter WP, Hanoch J, D'Arcy T, Dina R, McIndoe GA, DeSouza NM. Pretreatment tumour volume measurement on high-resolution magnetic resonance imaging as a predictor of survival in cervical cancer. BJOG. 2004;111(7):741–7 [Evaluation Studies].
16. Burghardt E, Baltzer J, Tulusan AH, Haas J. Results of surgical treatment of 1028 cervical cancers studied with volumetry. Cancer. 1992;70(3):648–55.
17. Burghardt E, Hofmann HM, Ebner F, Haas J, Tamussino K, Justich E. Magnetic resonance imaging in cervical cancer: a basis for objective classification. Gynecol Oncol. 1989;33(1):61–7 [Comparative Study].
18. Dimopoulos JC, Petrow P, Tanderup K, Petric P, Berger D, Kirisits C, Pedersen EM, van Limbergen E, Haie-Meder C, Potter R. Recommendations from Gynaecological (GYN) GEC-ESTRO Working Group (IV): basic principles and parameters for MR imaging within the frame of image based adaptive cervix cancer brachytherapy. Radiother Oncol. 2012;103(1):113–22 [Research Support, Non-U.S. Gov't].
19. Mayr NA, Huang Z, Wang JZ, Lo SS, Fan JM, Grecula JC, Sammet S, Sammet CL, Jia G, Zhang J, Knopp MV, Yuh WT. Characterizing tumor heterogeneity with functional imaging and quantifying high-risk tumor volume for early prediction of treatment outcome: cervical cancer as a model. Int J Radiat Oncol Biol Phys. 2012;83(3):972–9 [Research Support, N.I.H., Extramural].
20. Gilderdale DJ, de Souza NM, Coutts GA, Chui MK, Larkman DJ, Williams AD, Young IR. Design and use of internal receiver coils for magnetic resonance imaging. Br J Radiol. 1999;72(864):1141–51 [Research Support, Non-U.S. Gov'tReview].
21. de Souza NM, Dina R, McIndoe GA, Soutter WP. Cervical cancer: value of an endovaginal coil magnetic resonance imaging technique in detecting small volume disease and assessing parametrial extension. Gynecol Oncol. 2006;102(1):80–5.
22. de Souza NM, Whittle M, Williams AD, Sohail M, Krausz T, Gilderdale DJ, McIndoe GA, Soutter WP. Magnetic resonance imaging of the primary site in stage I cervical carcinoma: a comparison of endovaginal coil with external phased array coil techniques at 0.5T. J Magn Reson Imaging. 2000;12(6):1020–6 [Comparative Study].
23. Charles-Edwards E, Morgan V, Attygalle AD, Giles SL, Ind TE, Davis M, Shepherd J, McWhinney N, de Souza NM. Endovaginal magnetic resonance imaging of stage 1A/1B cervical cancer with A T2- and diffusion-weighted magnetic resonance technique: effect of lesion size and previous cone biopsy on tumor detectability. Gynecol Oncol. 2011;120(3):368–73.
24. Charles-Edwards EM, Messiou C, Morgan VA, De Silva SS, McWhinney NA, Katesmark M, Attygalle AD, De Souza NM. Diffusion-weighted imaging in cervical cancer with an endovaginal technique: potential value for improving tumor detection in stage Ia and Ib1 disease. Radiology. 2008;249(2):541–50 [Research Support, Non-U.S. Gov't].
25. Kim SH, Choi BI, Han JK, Kim HD, Lee HP, Kang SB, Lee JY, Han MC. Preoperative staging of uterine cervical carcinoma: comparison of CT and MRI in 99 patients. J Comput Assist Tomogr. 1993;17(4):633–40.
26. de Souza NM, McIndoe GA, Soutter WP, Krausz T, Chui KM, Hughes C, Mason WP. Value of magnetic resonance imaging with an endovaginal receiver coil in the pre-operative assessment of Stage I and IIa cervical neoplasia. Br J Obstet Gynaecol. 1998;105(5):500–7.
27. Lam WW, So NM, Yang WT, Metreweli C. Detection of parametrial invasion in cervical carcinoma: role of short tau inversion recovery sequence. Clin Radiol. 2000;55(9):702–7.
28. Sironi S, Bellomi M, Villa G, Rossi S, Del Maschio A. Clinical stage I carcinoma of the uterine cervix value of preoperative magnetic resonance imaging in assessing parametrial invasion. Tumori. 2002;88(4):291–5.
29. Joja I, Asakawa M, Asakawa T, Nakagawa T, Kanazawa S, Kuroda M, Togami I, Hiraki Y, Akamatsu N, Kudo T. Endometrial carcinoma: dynamic MRI with turbo-FLASH technique. J Comput Assist Tomogr. 1996;20(6):878–87 [Comparative Study].
30. Nasi F, Fiocchi F, Pecchi A, Rivasi F, Torricelli P. MRI evaluation of myometrial invasion by endometrial carcinoma. Comparison between fast-spin-echo T2w and coronal-FMPSPGR Gadolinium-Dota-enhanced sequences. Radiol Med. 2005;110(3):199–210 [Comparative Study Evaluation Studies].
31. Frei KA, Kinkel K, Bonel HM, Lu Y, Zaloudek C, Hricak H. Prediction of deep myometrial invasion in patients with endometrial cancer: clinical utility of

contrast-enhanced MR imaging-a meta-analysis and Bayesian analysis. Radiology. 2000;216(2):444–9.
32. Beddy P, Moyle P, Kataoka M, Yamamoto AK, Joubert I, Lomas D, Crawford R, Sala E. Evaluation of depth of myometrial invasion and overall staging in endometrial cancer: comparison of diffusion-weighted and dynamic contrast-enhanced MR imaging. Radiology. 2012;262(2):530–7 [Comparative Study].
33. Takeuchi M, Matsuzaki K, Nishitani H. Diffusion-weighted magnetic resonance imaging of endometrial cancer: differentiation from benign endometrial lesions and preoperative assessment of myometrial invasion. Acta Radiol. 2009;50(8):947–53.
34. Tamai K, Koyama T, Saga T, Morisawa N, Fujimoto K, Mikami Y, Togashi K. The utility of diffusion-weighted MR imaging for differentiating uterine sarcomas from benign leiomyomas. Eur Radiol. 2008;18(4):723–30.
35. McVeigh PZ, Syed AM, Milosevic M, Fyles A, Haider MA. Diffusion-weighted MRI in cervical cancer. Eur Radiol. 2008;18(5):1058–64.
36. Ueda M, Otsuka M, Hatakenaka M, Sakai S, Ono M, Yoshimitsu K, Honda H, Torii Y. MR imaging findings of uterine endometrial stromal sarcoma: differentiation from endometrial carcinoma. Eur Radiol. 2001;11(1):28–33.
37. De Priest PD, DeSimone CP. Ultrasound screening for the early detection of ovarian cancer. J Clin Oncol. 2003;21(10 Suppl):194s–9 [Review].
38. Rosenthal AN, Fraser L, Manchanda R, Badman P, Philpott S, Mozersky J, Hadwin R, Cafferty FH, Benjamin E, Singh N, Evans DG, Eccles DM, Skates SJ, Mackay J, Menon U, Jacobs IJ. Results of annual screening in phase I of the United kingdom familial ovarian cancer screening study highlight the need for strict adherence to screening schedule. J Clin Oncol. 2013;31(1):49–57.
39. Saini A, Dina R, McIndoe GA, Soutter WP, Gishen P, de Souza NM. Characterization of adnexal masses with MRI. AJR Am J Roentgenol. 2005;184(3):1004–9.
40. Mohaghegh P, Rockall AG. Imaging strategy for early ovarian cancer: characterization of adnexal masses with conventional and advanced imaging techniques. Radiographics. 2012;32(6):1751–73.
41. Sala E, De Souza N, Lee SI, Atri M, Hricak H. Ovarian cancer: the role of functional imaging as an end point in clinical trials. Int J Gynecol Cancer. 2010;20(6):971–8 [Review].
42. Tamada T, Sone T, Tanimoto D, Higashi H, Miyoshi H, Egashira N, Yamamoto A, Imai S. MRI appearance of primary giant ovarian leiomyoma in a hysterectomised woman. Br J Radiol. 2006;79(946):e126–8 [Case Reports Review].
43. Kyriazi S, Collins DJ, Morgan VA, Giles SL, de Souza NM. Diffusion-weighted imaging of peritoneal disease for noninvasive staging of advanced ovarian cancer. Radiographics. 2010;30(5):1269–85.
44. Kyriazi S, Kaye SB, de Souza NM. Imaging ovarian cancer and peritoneal metastases—current and emerging techniques. Nat Rev Clin Oncol. 2010;7(7):381–93 [Review].
45. Tsai CS, Lai CH, Wang CC, Chang JT, Chang TC, Tseng CJ, Hong JH. The prognostic factors for patients with early cervical cancer treated by radical hysterectomy and postoperative radiotherapy. Gynecol Oncol. 1999;75(3):328–33.
46. Rockall AG, Sohaib SA, Harisinghani MG, Babar SA, Singh N, Jeyarajah AR, Oram DH, Jacobs IJ, Shepherd JH, Reznek RH. Diagnostic performance of nanoparticle-enhanced magnetic resonance imaging in the diagnosis of lymph node metastases in patients with endometrial and cervical cancer. J Clin Oncol. 2005;23(12):2813–21.
47. Yang WT, Lam WW, Yu MY, Cheung TH, Metreweli C. Comparison of dynamic helical CT and dynamic MR imaging in the evaluation of pelvic lymph nodes in cervical carcinoma. AJR Am J Roentgenol. 2000;175(3):759–66.
48. Choi HJ, Roh JW, Seo SS, Lee S, Kim JY, Kim SK, Kang KW, Lee JS, Jeong JY, Park SY. Comparison of the accuracy of magnetic resonance imaging and positron emission tomography/computed tomography in the presurgical detection of lymph node metastases in patients with uterine cervical carcinoma: a prospective study. Cancer. 2006;106(4):914–22.
49. Kim SK, Choi HJ, Park SY, Lee HY, Seo SS, Yoo CW, Jung DC, Kang S, Cho KS. Additional value of MR/PET fusion compared with PET/CT in the detection of lymph node metastases in cervical cancer patients. Eur J Cancer. 2009;45(12):2103–9.
50. Todo Y, Kato H, Kaneuchi M, Watari H, Takeda M, Sakuragi N. Survival effect of para-aortic lymphadenectomy in endometrial cancer (SEPAL study): a retrospective cohort analysis. Lancet. 2010;375(9721):1165–72.
51. Chang MC, Chen JH, Liang JA, Yang KT, Cheng KY, Kao CH. 18F-FDG PET or PET/CT for detection of metastatic lymph nodes in patients with endometrial cancer: a systematic review and meta-analysis. Eur J Radiol. 2012;81(11):3511–7 [Research Support, Non-U.S. Gov't].
52. Yoshida Y, Kurokawa T, Kawahara K, Tsuchida T, Okazawa H, Fujibayashi Y, Yonekura Y, Kotsuji F. Incremental benefits of FDG positron emission tomography over CT alone for the preoperative staging of ovarian cancer. AJR Am J Roentgenol. 2004;182(1):227–33.
53. Patel S, Liyanage SH, Sahdev A, Rockall AG, Reznek RH. Imaging of endometrial and cervical cancer. Insights Imaging. 2010;1(5–6):309–28.
54. Sohaib SA, Reznek RH. MR imaging in ovarian cancer. Cancer Imaging. 2007;7(Spec No A):S119–29.
55. Tofts PS, Collins DJ. Multicentre imaging measurements for oncology and in the brain. Br J Radiol. 2011;84(Spec No 2):S213–26 [Research Support, Non-U.S. Gov't Review].

56. Kyriazi S, Collins DJ, Messiou C, Pennert K, Davidson RL, Giles SL, Kaye SB, Desouza NM. Metastatic ovarian and primary peritoneal cancer: assessing chemotherapy response with diffusion-weighted MR imaging—value of histogram analysis of apparent diffusion coefficients. Radiology. 2011;261(1):182–92.
57. Mayr NA, Yuh WT, Jajoura D, Wang JZ, Lo SS, Montebello JF, Porter K, Zhang D, McMeekin DS, Buatti JM. Ultra-early predictive assay for treatment failure using functional magnetic resonance imaging and clinical prognostic parameters in cervical cancer. Cancer. 2010;116(4):903–12 [Comparative Study Research Support, N.I.H., Extramural Validation Studies].
58. Nakamura K, Joja I, Nagasaka T, Fukushima C, Kusumoto T, Seki N, Hongo A, Kodama J, Hiramatsu Y. The mean apparent diffusion coefficient value (ADCmean) on primary cervical cancer is a predictive marker for disease recurrence. Gynecol Oncol. 2012;127(3):478–83.
59. Schwarz JK, Siegel BA, Dehdashti F, Grigsby PW. Metabolic response on post-therapy FDG-PET predicts patterns of failure after radiotherapy for cervical cancer. Int J Radiat Oncol Biol Phys. 2012;83(1):185–90.
60. Kang S, Nam BH, Park JY, Seo SS, Ryu SY, Kim JW, Kim SC, Park SY, Nam JH. Risk assessment tool for distant recurrence after platinum-based concurrent chemoradiation in patients with locally advanced cervical cancer: a Korean gynecologic oncology group study. J Clin Oncol. 2012;30(19):2369–74.
61. Carrara L, Gadducci A, Landoni F, Maggino T, Scambia G, Galletto L, Lissoni AA, Fuso L, Zola P, Sartori E. Could different follow-up modalities play a role in the diagnosis of asymptomatic endometrial cancer relapses?: an Italian multicentric retrospective analysis. Int J Gynecol Cancer. 2012;22(6):1013–9 [Comparative Study Multicenter Study].
62. Sharma P, Kumar R, Singh H, Jeph S, Sharma DN, Bal C, Malhotra A. Carcinoma endometrium: role of 18-FDG PET/CT for detection of suspected recurrence. Clin Nucl Med. 2012;37(7):649–55.

Pathology of Gynecologic Cancers 25

C. Blake Gilks

25.1 Ovarian, Tubal and Peritoneal Neoplasms

Introduction

The ovary can give rise to an extraordinary range of tumor types, reflecting the complex function and structure of this relatively small organ [1]. Ovarian neoplasms are classified based on the cell of origin, with profound differences between different tumor types with respect to behavior and response to therapy. For example, malignant germ cell tumors are treated differently than high-grade serous carcinomas (a tumor in the surface epithelial-stromal category and the most common malignant ovarian tumor), and have a much better prognosis [2]. Accurate classification of ovarian tumors based on histopathological assessment is therefore critically important in planning treatment. Tumors within the surface epithelial-stromal category can also arise from the fallopian tube or peritoneum [3], and in cases of advanced stage carcinomas, where there is involvement of ovaries, tubes and peritoneum, it may be difficult or impossible to determine the primary site with certainty.

C.B. Gilks, MD, FRCPC
Department of Pathology and Laboratory Medicine, Vancouver General Hospital, Vancouver, BC, Canada
e-mail: blake.gilks@vch.ca

Surface Epithelial-Stromal Carcinomas

Carcinomas of surface epithelial-stromal type account for more than 90 % of ovarian malignancies. There have been recent advances in our understanding of ovarian carcinomas, and it is now appreciated that the five main subtypes (accounting for more than 98 % of cases) are different diseases, with differences in genetic risk factors, precursor lesions, molecular events during oncogenesis, patterns of spread, and response to standard chemotherapy (summarized in Table 25.1) [4]. These subtypes are, in descending order of frequency: high-grade serous (70 %), clear cell (10 %), endometrioid (10 %), mucinous (3 %), and low-grade serous (2 %) (percentages are based on data from British Columbia, Canada, and Washington DC USA) [5]. For patients with advanced stage (stage III or IV) disease at presentation, more than 90 % are high-grade serous carcinomas; in contrast, most stage I carcinomas are non-serous types. Gross Findings: Most ovarian carcinomas are advanced stage high-grade serous carcinomas. The ovarian involvement in these cases is typically bilateral and consists of 10–20 cm solid and cystic masses with areas of hemorrhage and necrosis, and obvious ovarian surface involvement by soft friable exophytic tumor deposits. Most clear cell, endometrioid and mucinous carcinomas are smooth surfaced, and the mucinous carcinomas are noteworthy for attaining huge sizes in some patients. Microscopic Findings: High-grade

H.R.H. Patel et al. (eds.), *Pelvic Cancer Surgery: Modern Breakthroughs and Future Advances*,
DOI 10.1007/978-1-4471-4258-4_25, © Springer-Verlag London 2015

Table 25.1 Characteristics of ovarian carcinoma subtypes

	HGSC	CCC	EC	MC	LGSC
Genetic risk factors	BRCA1/2	Lynch syndrome	Lynch syndrome	None known	None known
Precursor lesions	Serous tubal intraepithelial carcinoma	Endometriosis	Endometriosis	Not known	Serous borderline tumor
Molecular abnormalities	P53, BRCA1, BRCA2, HR defects[a]	PI3K, ARID1A, MMR[b]	PTEN, beta-catenin, ARID1A, MMR[b]	KRAS, HER2	BRAF, KRAS, NRAS
Stage at presentation	III	I	I	I	I–III
Response to platinum chemotherapy	Chemosensitive	Chemoresistant	Chemosensitive	Chemoresistant	Chemoresistant

[a]*HR defects* homologous recombination defects
[b]*MMR* loss of expression of DNA mismatch repair enzyme(s)

serous carcinomas show a variety of architectural patterns, including papillary, solid, glandular, and transitional-like architecture, but all consist of cells with high-grade nuclear features and very high mitotic rates. Foci of identical cells in the fallopian tube mucosa are referred to as serous tubal intraepithelial carcinoma (STIC) and are regarded as the precursor lesion of most high-grade serous carcinomas that in the past were designated as being primary ovarian, tubal or peritoneal high-grade serous carcinomas [3]. Clear cell carcinomas can also show solid, papillary and glandular architectural patterns, but the cells have clear or eosinophilic cytoplasm, high-grade nuclear features, and a lower mitotic rate than is seen in high-grade serous carcinomas. Endometrioid carcinomas are morphologically indistinguishable from the more common endometrioid carcinomas of the endometrium, are usually glandular and low grade, and frequently have areas of squamous differentiation. Mucinous carcinomas are recognized by their glandular architecture and intracellular mucin. Low-grade serous carcinomas are distinguished from high-grade serous carcinomas by the presence of less than threefold variability in nuclear size [6]. Low-grade serous carcinomas contain numerous psammoma bodies (laminated calco-spherules produced by the tumor cells) in most cases. These five subtypes can be reproducibly diagnosed based on routine histopathological assessment [7] and representative photomicrographs of these five ovarian carcinoma subtypes are shown in Fig. 25.1.

Borderline Tumors

These epithelial neoplasms are characterized by atypia but, unlike the carcinomas, they lack invasion. The same cell types seen in ovarian carcinomas can be encountered as borderline tumors, but serous and mucinous types account for the large majority of borderline tumors. Borderline serous tumors (also referred to as serous tumors of low-malignant potential, or atypical proliferative serous tumors) are characterized by extra-ovarian implants in 20–40 % of cases [8]. If these implants show invasion, the behavior is identical to that of low-grade serous carcinoma. If there is no evidence of invasion in either the ovarian tumor(s) or extra-ovarian implants, a more indolent course can be anticipated, so careful histopathological examination for evidence of invasion is critical in accurate prognostication in these cases. Grossly, serous borderline tumors lack the hemorrhage and necrosis seen in high-grade serous carcinomas, and the papillary structures, whether projecting into cyst cavities or from the ovarian surface, have delicate uniform appearance. Mucinous borderline tumors are invariably stage Ia at presentation, and recurrences are rare. Borderline endometrioid and clear cell tumors are rare, and all reported cases to date have behaved in a benign fashion.

Sex Cord-Stromal Tumors

Adult-type granulosa cell tumors are the most common malignant tumor in this category. Other malignant sex cord-stromal tumors (Sertoli-Leydig cell tumor, fibrosarcoma, sex cord tumor with annular tubules) are very rare. Adult-type granulosa cell tumors, macroscopically, are typically smooth surfaced and confined to the ovary at presentation; on sectioning blood-filled cysts are common. Microscopically they consist of uniform cells with scant cytoplasm, resembling normal granulosa cells. A somatic activating point mutation in the FOXL2 gene is pathognomonic for adult-type granulosa cell tumors [9].

Germ Cell Tumors

More than 98 % of ovarian germ cell tumors are benign cystic teratomas. Malignant germ cell tumors fall into two general categories. The primitive germ cell tumors occur in young women (peak incidence in second and third decades), and can show a variety of histological patterns that are indistinguishable from their more common counterparts in the testis. These are all rare, and include dysgerminoma, yolk sac tumor (endodermal sinus tumor), choriocarcinoma, embryonal carcinoma, and mixed tumors [1]. The second category is malignancies arising in a benign cystic teratoma. These are a result of malignant transformation of one of the components of the teratoma, the peak incidence is in the sixth decade, and squamous cell carcinomas account for more than 90 % of such cases, with occasional cases of intestinal-type adenocarcinoma, thyroid carcinoma, melanoma or other malignancies encountered.

Other Tumors

Metastasis account for most other ovarian tumors, and consideration of any clinical history of prior malignancy is important in cases of unusual ovarian tumors [10]. Ovarian metastases may be the presenting finding, but more commonly are identified at the same time as the primary tumor, or thereafter. An extraordinarily wide range of tumor types, apart from those described previously, may be also be encountered as primary ovarian neoplasms, including tumor types more commonly encountered at other sites, such as lymphoma and melanoma, and rare ovarian tumors of uncertain histogenesis, such as small cell carcinoma of hypercalcemic type.

25.2 Uterine Corpus

Introduction

Cancers of the uterine corpus are predominantly derived from endometrial glandular epithelial cells (endometrial adenocarcinoma), with small number of cases derived from either endometrial stromal cells (endometrial stromal sarcomas) or smooth muscle cells (leiomyosarcomas). In the past, carcinosarcomas, high-grade biphasic tumors of endometrium showing both epithelial and stromal differentiation, were classified with the sarcomas, but based on molecular evidence they are best considered to be endometrial carcinomas with metaplastic (sarcomatous) growth [11].

Carcinomas

Endometrial carcinomas arise through two different pathways, and these are referred to as Type 1 and Type 2 carcinomas [12]. The Type 1 carcinomas account for approximately 90 % of cases and are associated with estrogen excess (obesity, infertility, estrogen producing tumors such as granulosa cell tumor, exogenous hormonal therapy) and the precursor lesion is atypical hyperplasia of the endometrium. Most Type 1 tumors are low-grade (grade 1 or 2) endometrioid carcinomas. Type 2 carcinomas arise in an estrogen independent fashion and the patients tend to be older and not obese, the precursor lesion is endometrial intraepithelial carcinoma, and the prototypical Type 2 tumor is serous carcinoma of the endometrium. It is now clear that these Type 1 and Type 2 designations, which were derived based on consideration of epidemiological data, refer to loose clinicopathological clusters and do not correspond to specific histopathological tumor types. As can be seen from Fig. 25.2, some serous carcinomas arise from low-grade endometrioid carcinomas, in patients with increased estrogenic stimulation of the endometrium, as a result of acquired mutations during tumor progression, while some arise de novo, from endometrial intraepithelial carcinoma, in a background of atrophic endometrium [13]. Gross Findings: Endometrial carcinomas present as exophytic masses projecting into the endometrial cavity. When large, they may prolapse through the cervical os. The tumor is typically friable and soft, and there may be extensive necrosis. Myometrial invasion, cervical involvement, serosal implants or extrauterine spread may be seen, and are more common in high-grade endometrial carcinomas. Microscopic Findings: Endometrial carcinomas, like other ovarian carcinomas, are subclassified based on cell type. Endometrioid, serous, and clear cell subtypes, and carcinosarcomas together account for almost all cases of endometrial carcinoma. Endometrioid carcinomas are composed of glandular epithelial cells resembling normal endometrial epithelium, but with significant nuclear atypia and increased mitotic activity. Squamous differentiation and mucinous metaplasia are common. Endometrioid carcinomas are graded based on the percent solid non-squamous growth as grade 1 (<5 % solid), grade 2 (6–50 % solid), or grade 3 (>50 % solid) [14]. Grade 1 and 2 tumors are considered low grade, account for most endometrioid carcinomas, and a majority are stage Ia at presentation. All serous carcinomas, clear cell carcinomas, and carcinosarcomas of the endometrium are considered high-grade [1]. Serous and clear cell carcinomas resemble their counterparts in the ovary, and most commonly show papillary or solid architecture, although glandular architecture is also commonly encountered. The tumor cell nuclei show high-grade features and there is a brisk mitotic rate. Carcinosarcomas have both a high-grade carcinoma and high-grade sarcoma component; the sarcoma can be homologous (i.e. composed of cell types normally found in the uterus, such as smooth muscle or endometrial stromal cells) or heterologous (e.g. malignant cartilage, skeletal muscle, adipose tissue etc.).

Sarcomas

Within the category of uterine sarcoma, there are (1) leiomyosarcomas, of smooth muscle origin, (2) endometrial stromal sarcomas, of endometrial stromal cell origin, and (3) high-grade undifferentiated sarcomas, which probably are a mixed group of cases, including poorly differentiated leiomyosarcomas and endometrial stromal sarcomas, in which morphological features of smooth muscle or endometrial stromal cell origin, respectively, have been lost, and poorly differentiated carcinosarcomas in which the carcinomatous component has been overgrown. Leiomyosarcomas show complex genetic abnormalities, and once cases of benign mimics of leiomyosarcoma are excluded (e.g. mitotically active leiomyoma, leiomyoma with bizarre nuclei, etc.) are aggressive neoplasms [15]. They consist of fascicles or bundles of spindle cells with markedly atypical nuclei and eosinophilic cytoplasm, that stain positively for markers of smooth muscle differentiation, such as desmin and h-caldesmon. There is no one feature that allows distinction between leiomyomas and leiomyosarcomas, apart from metastasis, and a combination of infiltrative margin, mitotic activity, cytological atypia, and coagulative tumor cell necrosis are used in the diagnosis of leiomyosarcoma [16]. Rare tumors have morphological features intermediate between leiomyoma and leiomyosarcoma, and a designation of "smooth muscle tumor of uncertain malignant potential" (STUMP) can be used for those cases. Endometrial stromal sarcomas, unlike leiomyosarcomas, are characterized genetically by recurrent translocations. In low-grade endometrial stromal sarcomas the chromosomal translocation t7:17, bringing together the JAZF1 and SUZ12 genes, is the most common genetic abnormality in low-grade endometrial stromal sarcoma

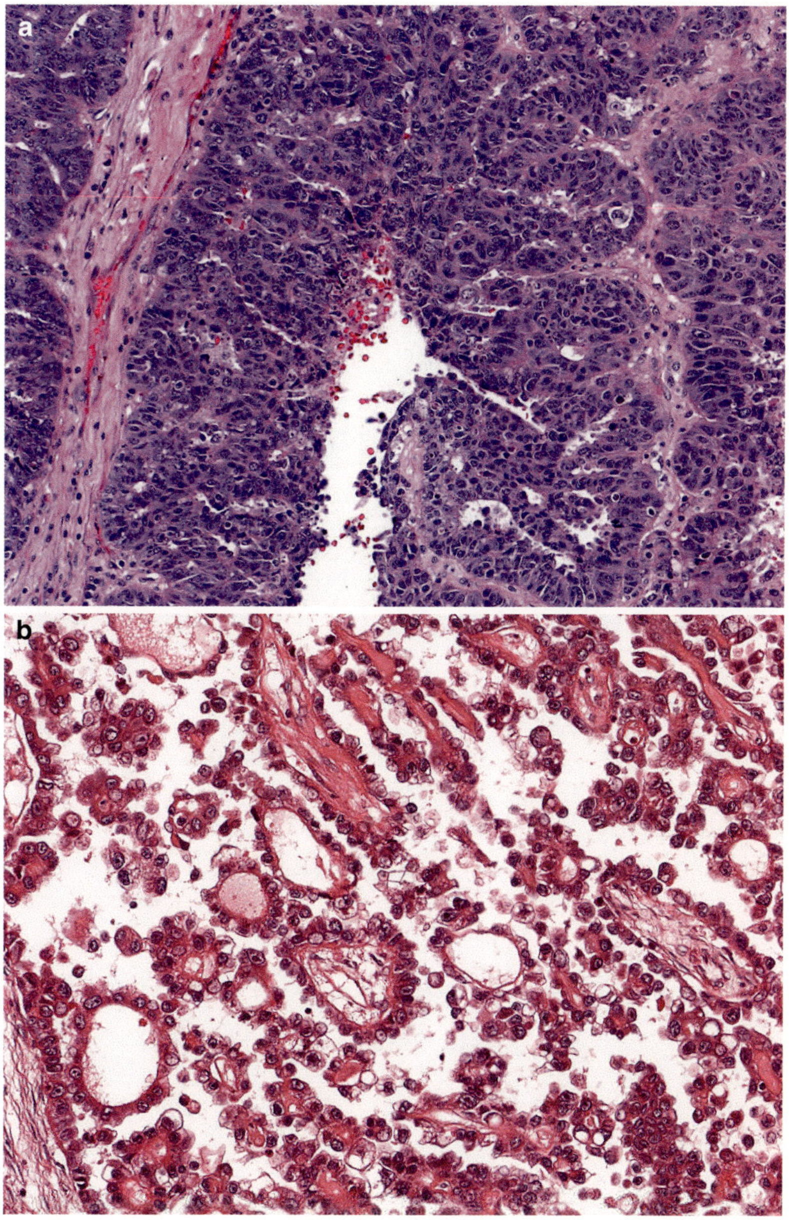

Fig. 25.1 The five subtypes of ovarian surface epithelial-stromal carcinoma. (**a**) High-grade serous carcinoma, showing stratification and tufting of markedly atypical cells. (**b**) Clear cell carcinoma, with prominent papillary architecture and cells with clear cytoplasm, (**c**) Endometrioid carcinoma, showing both glandular architecture and low-grade cytological features. (**d**) Mucinous carcinoma, with occasional tumor cells showing intracytoplasmic mucin vacuoles (goblet cells). (**e**) Low-grade serous carcinoma, with uniform cells, showing less than threefold variation in nuclear size, and a low mitotic rate

Fig. 25.1 (continued)

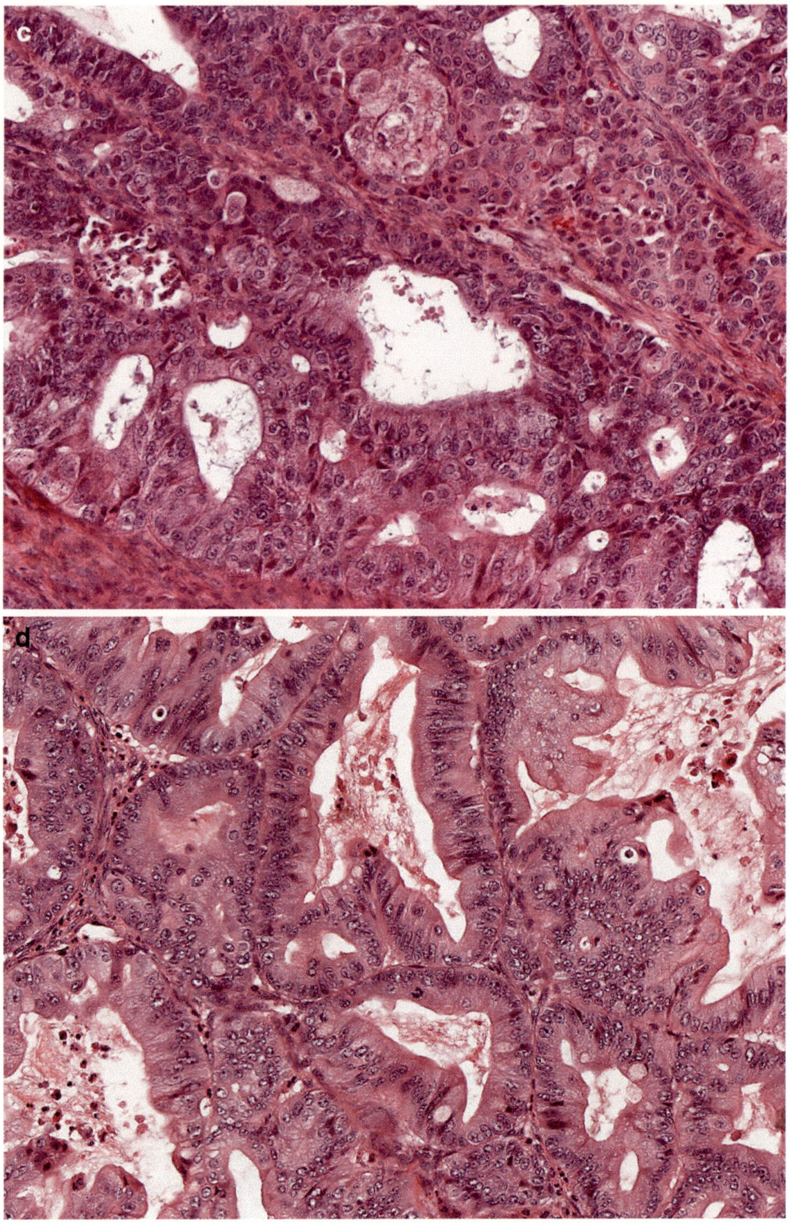

Fig. 25.1 (continued)

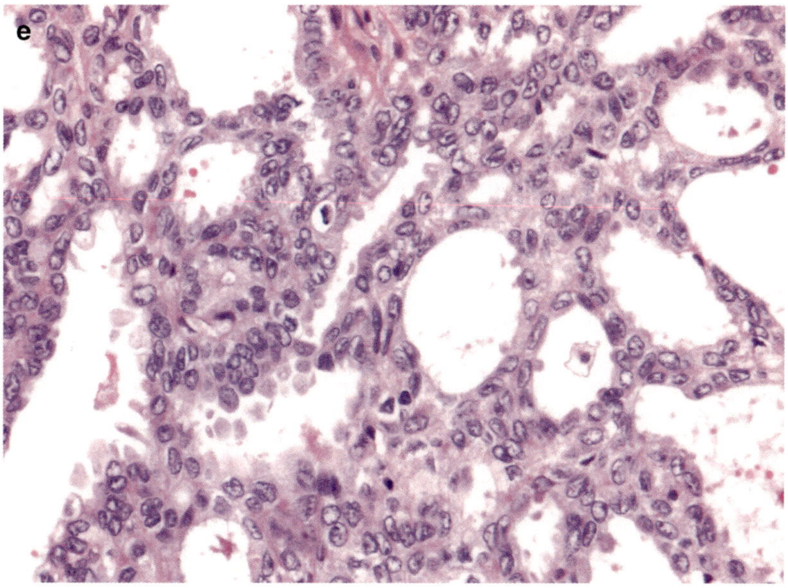

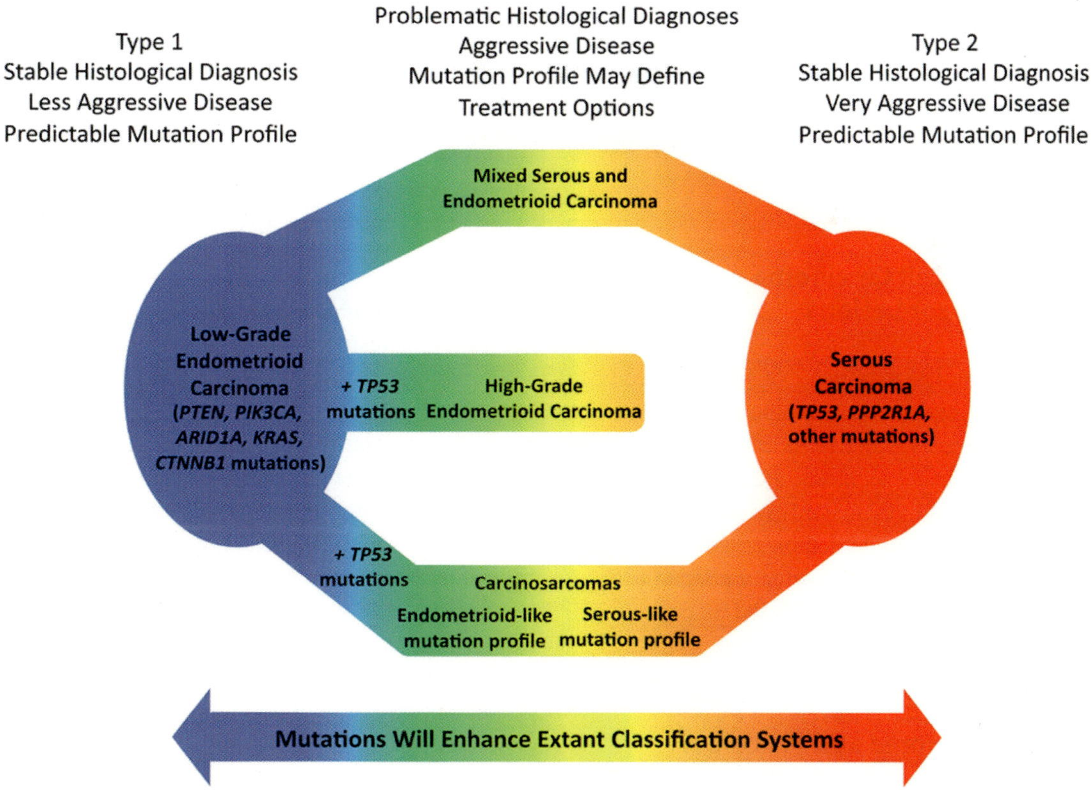

Fig. 25.2 While most endometrial carcinomas can be fit into either the Type 1 or Type 2 category (shown on the *left* and *right*, respectively), a significant number of cases fall somewhere in the middle, and based on clinical, pathological and/or genetic features are intermediate between typical Type 1 and Type 2 endometrial carcinomas (From McConechy et al. [13])

[17], while high-grade stromal sarcomas are characterized by t10:17 translocations [18]. Endometrial stromal sarcomas are characterized by cells with scant cytoplasm, and prominent small blood vessels, resembling the spiral arterioles of the normal endometrium. Mitotic figures are present, being more common in the high-grade endometrial stromal sarcomas. The high-grade undifferentiated sarcomas consist of pleomorphic cells which often show differentiation along heterologous lineages, such as cartilage or skeletal muscle. Mitotic rates are high, and abnormal mitotic figures common.

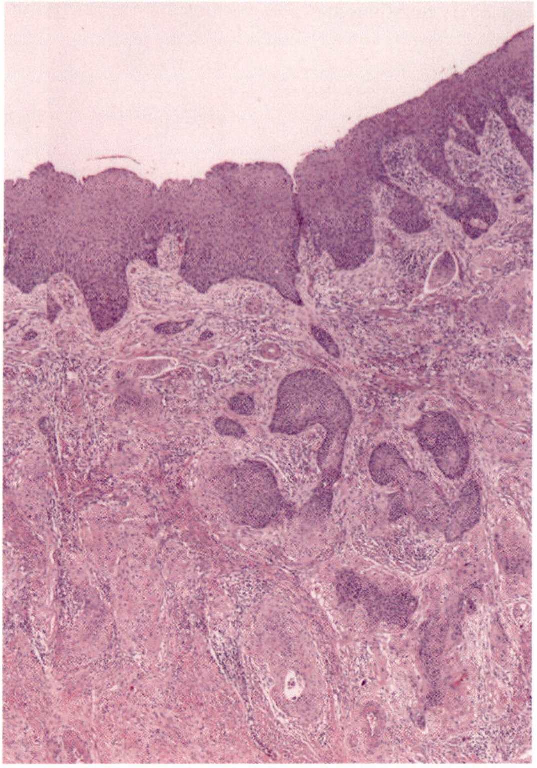

Fig. 25.3 Squamous cell carcinoma of the cervix with stromal invasion, seen as irregularly shaped nests of cells in the stroma, beneath the overlying high-grade squamous epithelial lesion (HSIL)

25.3 Uterine Cervix

Introduction

Almost all cervical malignancies are carcinomas, and are etiologically linked to human papilloma virus (HPV) infection [1]. These carcinomas preferentially occur in the region of the squamocolumnar junction, and can be squamous cell carcinomas, adenocarcinomas, or an admixture of squamous cell and adenocarcinoma.

Squamous Cell Carcinoma and Precursor Lesions

The precursor lesion of invasive squamous cell carcinoma is high-grade squamous intraepithelial lesion (HSIL), also referred to, in the cervix, as cervical intraepithelial neoplasia, grade 2 or 3 (CIN2 or CIN3) [19]. In the vast majority of such lesions high-risk HPV types can be demonstrated. The earliest sign of invasion is seen as irregular small nests of cells or individual cells beneath the basement membrane, with a desmoplastic host response (Fig. 25.3).

Adenocarcinoma and Precursor Lesions

The precursor lesion of invasive adenocarcinoma of the cervix is adenocarcinoma in situ (AIS). AIS frequently co-exists with HSIL. Cervical cytology screening is less sensitive in detection of glandular lesions of the cervix, compared to HSIL. Early invasive lesions arising in AIS are difficult to recognize reproducibly, as the stromal reaction common in early invasive squamous cell carcinoma and the pattern of invasion as individual cells and small irregular nests of cells is less common in adenocarcinoma, compared to squamous cell carcinoma. Unlike the situation in ovarian and endometrial carcinoma, where adenocarcinomas can be meaningfully subclassified based on tumor cell type, there is little agreement on subclassification of cervical adenocarcinomas based on cell type. Rare cases of cervical adenocarcinoma are not related to HPV, including the so-called "adenoma malignum" or gastric-like variant, which can occur in association with Peutz-Jehger syndrome, or sporadically, unrelated to the syndrome [20].

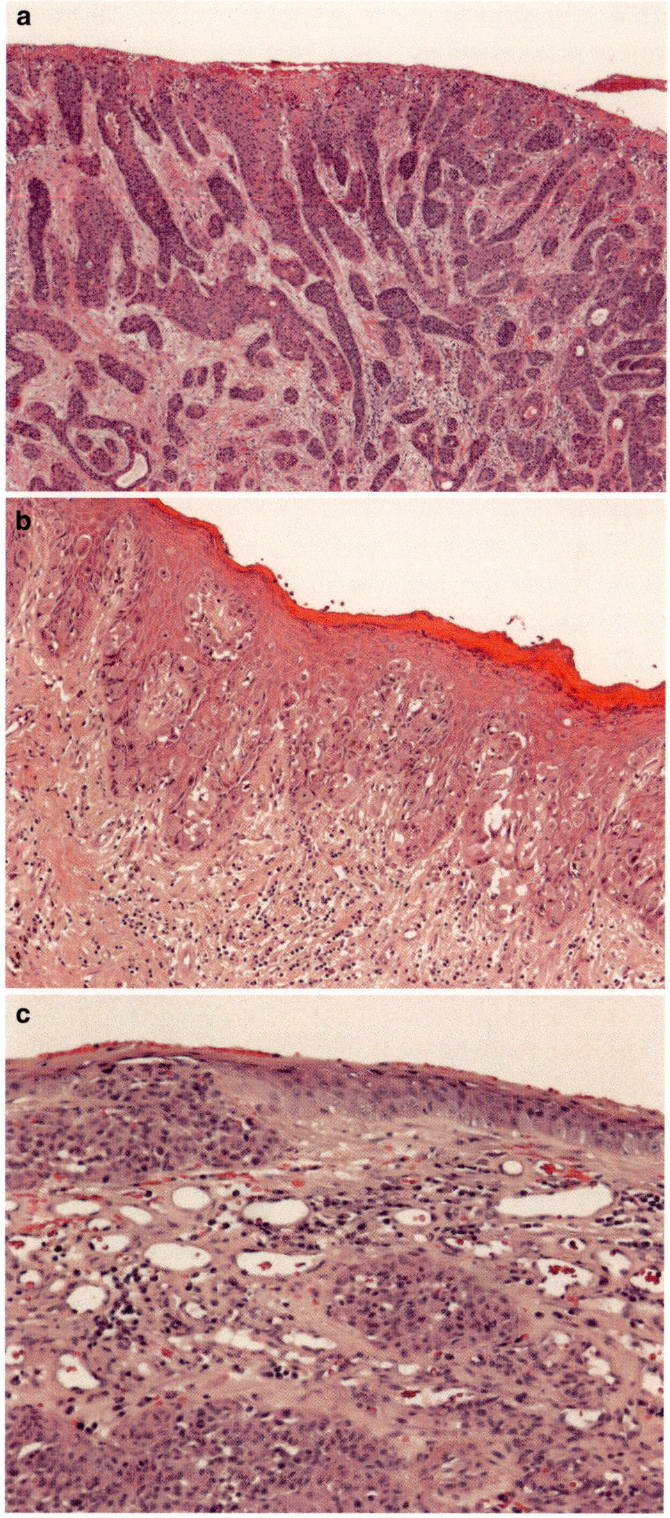

Fig. 25.4 (**a**) Invasive vulvar squamous cell carcinoma, with overlying vulvar intraepithelial neoplasia. (**b**) Paget's disease of the vulva, with large vacuolated neoplastic cells interspersed between the benign squamous epithelial cells. There is no invasion of the underlying stroma. (**c**) Invasive vulvar melanoma: the tumor cells are amelanotic, and there is a single nest of cells at the epidermal-dermal junction, representing the in situ component of this tumor

25.4 Vagina

A large majority of vaginal cancers are HPV-associated squamous cell carcinomas. The precursor lesion is high-grade squamous intraepithelial lesion (HSIL), which in the vagina can also be referred to as vaginal intraepithelial neoplasia, grade 2 or 3 (VaIN 2 or VaIN 3) [19]. The morphological features are identical to those seen in the more common squamous cell carcinomas of cervix and vulva.

25.5 Vulva

Introduction

Vulvar cancers are predominantly squamous cell carcinomas, with significant but lesser numbers of cases of Paget's disease (primary vulvar adenocarcinoma) and malignant melanoma (Fig. 25.4). The distinction between these entities, based on biopsy, may require the use of immunostains, because of sometimes overlapping morphological features.

Squamous Cell Carcinoma

Of the squamous cell carcinomas, there are roughly equal numbers of HPV associated and non-HPV associated cases (Table 25.2), although there is considerable geographic variability in this ratio [21]. The precursor of HPV associated squamous cell carcinoma is high-grade squamous intraepithelial lesion (HSIL), referred to in the vulva as high-grade vulvar intraepithelial neoplasia (high-grade VIN), or vulvar intraepithelial neoplasia grade 2 or 3 (VIN 2 or VIN 3) [19]. The morphological features are identical to HSIL appearing elsewhere in the female genital tract, except that surface keratinization is more common. Non-HPV associated squamous cell carcinoma is frequently seen in association with lichen sclerosis, an inflammatory condition associated with immune-mediated damage and increased turnover of the vulvar epithelium. The precursor lesion of non-HPV associated squamous cell carcinoma of the vulva can be very deceptively bland, so called differentiated vulvar intraepithelial neoplasia, or dVIN [22]. Although the features of VIN associated with non-HPV squamous cell carcinoma can be very cytologically bland, there also may be significant atypia present. Unlike the HPV-associated HSIL lesions, p53 mutations are common in dVIN. Invasive squamous cell carcinoma of HPV and non-HPV associated types are morphologically similar, although the non-HPV associated carcinomas are more likely to be lower grade and keratinizing. At the time of writing, although there are differences between HPV associated and non-HPV associated squamous cell carcinoma of vulva, summarized in Table 25.2, treatment does not differ, and HPV testing is not routinely performed.

Table 25.2 HPV versus non-HPV associated vulvar squamous cell carcinoma

	HPV	Non-HPV
Age	Fourth to sixth decade	Sixth to ninth decade
Etiology	Oncogenic viral infection	Chronic inflammation (lichen sclerosis)
Precursor	HSIL (VIN)[a], usual type	dVIN[b]
Biomarker expression	p16 overexpression	Abnormal p53 expression
Outcome[c]	Favorable	Less favorable (more likely to have nodal mets, recur locally)

[a]*HSIL (VIN)* high-grade squamous intraepithelial lesion (vulvar intraepithelial neoplasia)
[b]*dVIN* differentiated vulvar intraepithelial neoplasia
[c]Differences in outcomes for the HPV and non-HPV vulvar squamous cell cancers are speculative at present, and definitive studies are needed

Paget's Disease

Paget's disease is a primary vulvar adenocarcinoma, and in most instances is in situ at the time of diagnosis and remains in situ thereafter. It is characterized by large cells with abundant cytoplasm present in the epidermis, including appendages. These neoplastic cells, referred to as Paget cells, are concentrated in the basal layer of the epidermis, but also appear within the more superficial layers of the epidermal squamous epithelium (so-called Pagetoid spread). These cells can be difficult or impossible to distinguish from malignant squamous cells or melanoma cells on routine stains; immunostaining is routinely used for diagnosis and the cells of Paget's disease strongly express cytokeratin 7, unlike squamous cells or melanoma cells [23]. There is often a prominent host inflammatory reaction to Paget's disease and this can make assessment of invasion difficult. When there is invasion, which appears as single cells and small, irregularly shaped nests of cells infiltrating dermal stroma, unless it is only a few cells/nests, there is significant risk of nodal metastasis. Paget's disease, which is a primary vulvar adenocarcinoma, must be distinguished from the much less common secondary involvement of the vulva by adenocarcinoma, most commonly arising from the anorectal mucosa or endocervix, or transitional cell carcinoma of bladder or urethra. This secondary vulvar involvement has been referred to as Paget's disease in the past, which has led to significant confusion.

Melanoma

Malignant melanoma of the vulva is morphologically and molecularly similar to melanoma arising at other non-sun exposed sites. Occasional cases of in situ melanoma, with cytologically malignant melanocytes confined to the basal layer of the epidermis, are encountered, but most vulvar melanomas are deeply invasive at the time of presentation. Melanoma cells may be pigmented or non-pigmented (amelanotic), and the pigment may be seen macroscopically or only present focally, and therefore only visible microscopically. It is the non-pigmented or amelanotic melanomas that are the most challenging to diagnose. Melanomas are notable for their wide range of growth patterns, from spindle cells, mimicking sarcoma, to epithelioid cells, mimicking squamous cell carcinoma. The presence of a in situ component at the epidermal/dermal junction can be an aid to diagnosis, but it is usual, in amelanotic cases, to resort to immunostaining for melanoma specific markers (S-100, Melan-A, HMB-45, microphthalmia transcription factor) to confirm a diagnosis of melanoma. As is the case with other mucosal melanomas, BRAF mutations are rare in vulvar melanoma, so that BRAF inhibitors are rarely a therapeutic option [24].

References

1. Tavassoli FA, Deville P. World health organization classification of tumours: pathology and genetics of tumours of the breast and female genital tract. Lyon: IARC Press; 2003.
2. Low JJ, Ilancheran A, Ng JS. Malignant ovarian germ-cell tumours. Best Pract Res Clin Obstet Gynaecol. 2012;26(3):247–55.
3. Crum CP, Drapkin R, Kindelberger D, Medeiros F, Miron A, Lee Y. Lessons from BRCA: the tubal fimbria emerges as an origin for pelvic serous cancer. Clin Med Res. 2007;5(1):35–44.
4. Conklin CMJ, Gilks CB. Differential diagnosis and clinical relevance of ovarian carcinoma subtypes. Expert Rev Obstet Gynecol. 2012;8(1):1–16.
5. Köbel M, Kalloger SE, Huntsman DG, et al. Differences in tumor type in low-stage versus high-stage ovarian carcinomas. Int J Gynecol Pathol. 2010;29(3):203–11.
6. Malpica A, Deavers MT, Lu K, et al. Grading ovarian serous carcinoma using a two-tier system. Am J Surg Pathol. 2004;28(4):496–504.
7. Köbel M, Kalloger SE, Baker PM, et al. Diagnosis of ovarian carcinoma cell type is highly reproducible: a transcanadian study. Am J Surg Pathol. 2010;34:984–93.
8. Longacre TA, McKenney JK, Tazelaar HD, Kempson RL, Hendrickson MR. Ovarian serous tumors of low malignant potential (borderline tumors): outcome based study of 276 patients with long-term (>or =5year) follow-up. Am J Surg Pathol. 2005;29:707–23.
9. Shah SP, Köbel M, Senz J, et al. Mutation of FOXL2 in granulosa-cell tumors of the ovary. N Engl J Med. 2009;360(26):2719–29.
10. Yemelyanova AV, Vang R, Judson K, Wu LS, Ronnett BM. Distinction of primary and metastatic mucinous tumors involving the ovary: analysis of size and laterality data by primary site with reevaluation of an algorithm for tumor classification. Am J Surg Pathol. 2008;32(1):128–38.
11. McCluggage WG. Uterine carcinosarcomas (malignant mixed Mullerian tumors) are metaplastic carcinomas. Int J Gynecol Cancer. 2002;12(6):687–90.
12. Bohkman JV. Two pathogenetic types of endometrial carcinoma. Gynecol Oncol. 1983;15(1):10–7.

13. McConechy MK, Ding J, Cheang MCU, et al. Use of mutation profiles to refine the classification of endometrial carcinomas. J Pathol. 2012;228(1):20–30.
14. Zaino RJ, Kurman RJ, Diana KL, Morrow CP. The utility of the revised International Federation of Gynecology and Obstetrics histologic grading of endometrial adenocarcinoma using a defined nuclear grading system a Gynecologic Oncology Group study. Cancer. 1995;75(1):81–6.
15. D'Angelo E, Spagnoli LG, Prat J. Comparative clinicopathologic and immunohistochemical analysis of uterine sarcomas diagnosed using the World Health Organization classification system. Hum Pathol. 2009;40(11):1571–85.
16. Bell SW, Kempson RL, Hendrickson MR. Problematic smooth muscle neoplasms: a clinicopathologic study of 213 cases. Am J Surg Pathol. 1994;18(6):535–58.
17. Chiang S, Ali R, Melnyk N, et al. Frequency of known gene rearrangements in endometrial stromal tumors. Am J Surg Pathol. 2011;35:1364–72.
18. Lee C-H, Mario-Enriquez A, Ou W, et al. The clinicopathologic features of YWHAE-FAM22 endometrial stromal sarcomas: a histologically high-grade and clinically aggressive tumor. Am J Surg Pathol. 2012;36(9):641–53.
19. Darragh TM, Colgan TJ, Cox JT, et al. The lower anogenital squamous terminology standardization project for HPV-associated lesions: background and consensus recommendations from the College of American Pathologists and the American Society for Colposcopy and Cervical Pathology. Int J Gynecol Pathol. 2013;32(1):76–115.
20. Kusanagi Y, Kojima A, Mikami Y, et al. Absence of high-risk human papillomavirus (HPV) detection in endocervical adenocarcinoma with gastric morphology and phenotype. Am J Pathol. 2010;177(5):2169–75.
21. van der Avoort IA, Shirango H, Hoevenaars BM, et al. Vulvar squamous cell carcinoma is a multifactorial disease following two separate and independent pathways. Int J Gynecol Pathol. 2006;25(1):22–9.
22. Kokka F, Singh N, Faruqi A, Gibbon K, Rosenthal AN. Is differentiated vulval intraepithelial neoplasia the precursor lesion of human papilloma virus-negative vulval squamous cell carcinoma? Int J Gynecol Cancer. 2011;21(7):1297–305.
23. Crawford D, Nimmo M, Clement PB, et al. Prognostic factors in Paget's disease of the vulva: a study of 21 cases. Int J Gynecol Pathol. 1999;18(4):351–9.
24. Edwards RH, Ward MR, Wu H, et al. Absence of BRAF mutations in UV-protected mucosal melanomas. J Med Genet. 2004;41(4):270–2.

Screening for Gynaecological Cancers

26

Aleksandra Gentry-Maharaj, Jatinderpal Kalsi, and Usha Menon

26.1 Introduction

Screening is the identification of unrecognized disease in an apparently asymptomatic population using tests, examinations or other procedures leading to earlier diagnosis compared to clinical presentation of the disease [1]. In cancer screening, the main goal is to reduce mortality from the disease, either by preventing the cancer (in those where a premalignant condition exists) or diagnosing it earlier (when treatment is more effective).

Cancer specific criteria exist that outline which cancers could benefit most from screening and build on the WHO criteria for all diseases [2, 3]. Screening needs to achieve high sensitivity (percentage of patients with cancer correctly identified as a result of a positive test), specificity (percentage of the population without cancer correctly identified as a result of a negative test), positive predictive value (PPV, percentage of patients with a positive test that have the cancer, true positives) and negative predictive value (NPV, percentage of patients with a negative test that do not have the cancer, true negatives) if it is to be effective when applied to the population at large. The primary considerations in a national screening program are outlined in Table 26.1 [3].

A. Gentry-Maharaj, PhD • J. Kalsi, PhD
U. Menon, MBBS, MD(Res), FRCOG (✉)
Department of Women's Cancer,
Gynaecological Cancer Research Centre,
University College London,
Institute for Women's Health, London, UK
e-mail: u.menon@ucl.ac.uk

Gynecological Cancers

Worldwide cervical, ovarian and uterine/endometrial cancers accounted for an estimated 17 % of all new cancer cases in women and 14.6 % of all female cancer deaths in 2008 [4]. These rates are expected to rise due to aging of the world's population, the obesity epidemic and the unhealthy lifestyle choices [5]. It is estimated that if these current trends persist, an increase in incidence and mortality rates from gynecologic cancers of 66 % and 62 % respectively would be observed by 2030 [4]. Screening, as an approach to reduce incidence and mortality from gynaecological cancer is being discussed in this chapter.

Cervical Cancer

Cervical cancer is the third most common cancer in women and the fourth leading cause of death in women with 529,800 new cases and an estimated 275,000 deaths reported worldwide in 2008 [4, 5]. The majority of new cases (453,300) and deaths (242,000) occur in the developing nations. The highest incidence and mortality are

H.R.H. Patel et al. (eds.), *Pelvic Cancer Surgery: Modern Breakthroughs and Future Advances*,
DOI 10.1007/978-1-4471-4258-4_26,

Table 26.1 Key issues to consider in a national screening program

1	Effectiveness	There is sufficient scientific evidence that the screening program is effective
2	Need	Program is set up as there is a recognized need for screening
3	Clear objectives	There are clear objectives of screening set up at the outset
4	Defined target population	General population—usually age criteria used High risk—currently based on family history or specific gene mutations
5	Screening	Screening tests Screening strategy Frequency of testing
6	Infrastructure	Staff Equipment Facilities IT systems
7	Quality assurance	Setting of standards, monitoring, training of personnel
8	Program evaluation	Should be specified from the start
9	Compliance with screening	Monitoring and recall systems
10	Informed choice	Detailed information leaflets, websites, helpline
11	Equity and access to screening	For the whole target population

in Africa, South-Central Asia and South America whilst the lowest are in North America, New Zealand/Australia. These differences in part reflect access to well-organized screening programs which when properly implemented have been associated with significant reductions (50–90 %) in mortality [6]. The challenge now is to implement programs in low/middle income countries [7].

Cervical cancer is a sexually transmitted disease which is caused by Human Papilloma Virus (HPV). Typically the disease develops over two to three decades, with well-defined pre-malignant lesions termed cervical intraepithelial neoplasia (CIN). Depending on the degree of severity of neoplastic change observed histologically, these are graded CIN1 (low), CIN 2 (moderate) and CIN 3 (severe). The majority of lesions resolve and only a small proportion progress to cancer.

Current efforts are focused on identifying those lesions which are most likely to progress to cancer. Approximately 40 HPV genotypes have been identified as having the ability to infect the genital tract in humans [8, 9]. Fifteen of these 40 genotypes have been classed as high risk for cervical cancer [10]. The most prevalent types of HPV are HPV16 and HPV18 and account for 71 % of all cervical cancer cases [11], whilst HPV16, HPV18 and HPV45 are jointly responsible for 94 % of adenocarcinomas. A key factor in cancer development is persistence of infection with oncogenic HPV types. Other risk factors include early age of sexual activity, co-infection with other STD related microorganisms, long term use of contraceptives, multiparity, multiple partners and smoking [12].

26.2 Screening Tests

Cervical Cytology

Papanicoloau test (Pap-smear) based on exfoliative cytology is the primary test in many countries [12, 13]. It has a wide range of specificity (14–97 %) and sensitivity (11–99 %) [14]. Due to issues related to sampling and interpretation errors, liquid based cytology (LBC) was introduced in the mid-1990s to 2000s [15]. LBC was recommended as the primary test in the NHS cervical screening program in England and Wales [16] with a changeover to this technology in 2008 [12]. Whether LBC is a better test than Pap-smear remains to be determined, as recent meta-analysis demonstrated similar performance of both screening tests for histologically confirmed CIN 2 or worse [17].

Visual Inspection Tests

Cytology-based screening is expensive and resource intensive and needs a well-organized infrastructure for repeat testing and for these reasons is not feasible in low resource setting. Alternative screening strategies have been developed [18, 19]. These mainly rely on visual inspection of the cervix, either after application of 3–5 % acetic acid (VIA), visual inspection with a magnifying glass (VIAM) or visual inspection after Lugol's iodine (VILI). Although a subjective test, VIA still has similar sensitivity and specificity of 14–95 % and 14–98 % respectively as Pap-smear [19]. Single round of VIA, followed by immediate colposcopy and treatment in a cluster randomized controlled trial (RCT) in India resulted in significant reduction (35 %) in mortality at 7 years [20].

Table 26.2 Sensitivity and specificity of screening tests for detection of high grade CIN or cervical cancer

Screening test	Sensitivity (%)	Specificity (%)
Pap-smear [14]	11–99[a]	14–97[a]
Liquid based cytology [17]	57.1[a,b]	97[a, b]
HR HPV DNA testing using hybrid capture [29]	98	86.8
HR HPV DNA testing using careHPV [28]	90	84.2
VIA [19]	14–95[a]	14–98[a]
VILI [30]	68.1	90.8

Meta-analysis results used where available
HR HPV high risk HPV, *VIA* visual inspection with acetic acid, *VILI* visual inspection after Lugol's iodine
[a]Meta-analysis
[b]Pooled estimates

HPV Testing

As virtually all cervical cancer cases (99.7 %) are due to HPV, the attention has focused on detection of viral DNA [21]. Several assays for HPV have been developed; either DNA hybridization or PCR based assays which determine the presence of high risk genotypes. HPV testing is incorporated in the screening strategies in a number of countries, including the UK [12, 13, 22]. These assays have mainly been used to triage women who have equivocal smears or for checking samples for proof of cure.

To further refine identification of lesions most likely to progress, more recent assays focus on detecting the HPV viral oncoproteins E6 and E7, which are closely associated with the process of malignant transformation in cervical cancer. Compared to cytology, HPV tests are more reproducible, stable over a range of ages, have a higher NPV and better sensitivity but specificity is lower [23–26]. Combination with cytology yields higher sensitivities [27].

The performance of various screening tests is outlined in Table 26.2 [14, 17, 19, 28–30].

HPV as a Primary Test in Cervical Cancer Screening

As HPV testing has a high NPV, it may allow extension of the screening interval in cervical cancer. Recent data suggests that this can be as much as up to 6 years [31]. For these reasons, HPV has been suggested as a primary test in cervical cancer screening. A pilot of HPV testing with reflex cytology has recently been announced in the UK [32]. To avoid unnecessary repeat testing and treatment in younger women where lesions are often due to transient infections, it has been suggested that HPV testing should begin at 29 years of age (POBASCAM trial) [33] or even later (NTCC trial) [34].

In low resource settings, a single screening episode using primary HPV screening [35] can achieve a significant reduction in advanced cancers and 50 % mortality reduction at 7 years. Superior performance of HPV compared to VIA in detecting CIN2–3 lesions has also been reported [36].

As existing HPV DNA assays are expensive and results are only available after several hours, alternative HPV tests are being developed for LMIC settings where a 'screen and treat' approach is considered as the best strategy. A low cost assay, careHPV (Quiagen) is in late development for use in rural or remote communities. This assay has demonstrated higher sensitivity (90 %) for identifying moderate or severe cervical disease (CIN 2+) compared to either VIA (41 %) or LBC (85 %). The test requires no electricity or running water and results are available in 2.5 hours [28].

HPV testing, in addition, lends itself to self-sampling allowing access to cervical cancer screening to a greater number of women. Self-collected samples perform well in assays and the performance of the test is comparable to those collected by healthcare professionals [37, 38].

Impact of Vaccination on Cervical Screening

Cervical cancer is currently the only cancer for which vaccination is advocated by the WHO [39]. Currently there are two HPV vaccines against HPV16 and HPV18, Gardasil (Merck, USA) and Cervarix (GSK, UK), which are highly effective in preventing high grade abnormalities [40] and in modeling studies have been suggested to confer protection up to 20 years [41]. HPV vaccination programs target adolescent girls, mainly aged 12–17 years, with reduction in CIN3+ incidence in young women <18 years already reported. Screening should still continue in those that have not been vaccinated.

26.3 Ovarian and Fallopian Tube Cancer

Ovarian cancer accounts for 4 % of cancers diagnosed in women, with women having a 1.3 % [42] life time risk of developing ovarian cancer [43]. Worldwide, over 225,000 new cases are diagnosed and 140,000 deaths occur each year [43]. Ovarian cancer is the most fatal of all gynaecological cancers. Incidence rates are highest in the USA and Northern Europe and lowest in Africa and Asia. Majority of cases (90 %) occur in women over the age of 50 with the remaining 10 % occurring in younger women who have familial predisposition to the disease. Around 80–85 % of cancers are epithelial in origin. Serous epithelial ovarian cancer (EOC) is the most common histological subtype which usually presents at advanced stages and has the poorest outcomes [44]. Five year survival rates decrease sharply from 90 % in women diagnosed with early stage disease to 30–40 % in those with advanced disease [45], thus implying that earlier detection by screening may have an impact on mortality.

Although currently there are no national screening programs for ovarian cancer anywhere in the world, major efforts have been made into investigating whether screening can impact on mortality from the disease, both in the ***general population*** (age >50) and those at ***high risk*** (age >35 and a family history of ovarian and/or breast cancer). The latter women have a lifetime risk of developing ovarian cancer of approximately >10 % [46] with those with germline mutations in the BRCA1 gene (40–50 %) and BRCA2 mutations (11–26 %) having much higher risk [47]. In women with Lynch syndrome, the lifetime risk of developing ovarian cancer is about 8–12 % [48].

26.4 Screening Strategies

The screening strategies investigated over the past three decades have used the serum tumour marker CA125 and ultrasound.

Primary Ultrasound Screening with Repeat Ultrasound as a Second Line Test

Transvaginal ultrasound scanning (TVS) to assess ovarian size and morphology is used to screen for ovarian cancer [49, 50] as it gives a superior view of the pelvic organs and is acceptable to the women [51]. However in postmenopausal women, ovaries can be difficult to visualize although this can be overcome through quality assurance and monitoring [52]. In parallel with the models developed to distinguish benign from malignant adnexal masses in patients presenting with symptoms [53], algorithms have been developed in asymptomatic women undergoing screening [54, 55]. Both are based on the fact that certain ovarian features (papillary projections, complex ovarian cysts with wall abnormalities or solid areas) are strongly associated with the presence of malignancy compared to others (septal thickness, unilocular ovarian cysts <10 cm in diameter and inclusions cysts) [56–58]. Women with complex ovarian cysts at primary screening have repeat scans in 6 weeks to decrease false positive rates as many lesions can resolve spontaneously.

So far, two large studies/trials have investigated the performance of ultrasound-based strategy in ovarian cancer screening.

The University of Kentucky Ovarian Cancer Screening Trial is a single-arm single center ultrasound screening study involving 25,327 women who underwent annual screening between 1987 and 2005. The study has reported encouraging sensitivity/specificity with 9.3 operations carried out per case detected. A stage shift was observed with 82 % of the primary ovarian cancers being early stage (I/II) [54]. Recently, the study reported increased survival in those that were screened [59]. However, as this was not an RCT, it is very likely that a healthy volunteer affect and other biases contributed to the apparent impact of screening [60].

The performance of a TVS-only strategy has been investigated in an RCT. In the ultrasound arm of the general population trial, the UK Collaborative Trial of Ovarian Cancer Screening (UKCTOCS), where 202,638 post-menopausal women aged 50–74 years were randomized to either control or annual screening with ultrasound or a multimodal strategy in a 2:1:1 fashion [55, 61] (www.ukctocs.org.uk). In addition to the effect of ovarian cancer on mortality, the trial is also investigating the acceptability, compliance, costs, and performance characteristics of the two screening strategies, ultrasound and CA125-based, and the physical and psychological morbidity of screening. The results of the prevalence screen suggests inferior performance of ultrasound screening alone (19 surgeries per case of primary ovarian/FT cancer) compared to the multimodal strategy (3 surgeries per case detected) [55]. Mortality results are expected in 2015.

Primary CA125 Screening with Ultrasound as a Second Line Test

The discovery that CA125 was raised 5 years in advance of ovarian cancer [62] led to it being investigated as a screening test. 2.9 % of healthy postmenopausal women have elevated CA125 levels, limiting its use as a stand-alone test [63]. This has been overcome by using TVS as a second-line test in a multimodal screening strategy [64, 65] with TVS interpretation based on ovarian morphology [66, 67]. The interpretation of CA125 has been further improved by incorporating age, menopausal status and the rate of change of CA125 values over time into a statistical algorithm (Risk of Ovarian Cancer, ROC) [68–70]. In a RCT of 13,582 postmenopausal women, aged over 50, the ROC algorithm demonstrated high specificity (99.8 %) and PPV (19 %) for primary invasive EOC [70].

The only ovarian cancer screening trial in the general population to use the ROC algorithm is UKCTOCS [55, 61]. In the multimodal arm, CA125 is interpreted using the ROC algorithm to triage the women into low, intermediate and elevated risk. Those at intermediate risk have a repeat CA125 in 12 weeks, whereas those with elevated risk are referred for a transvaginal scan and repeat CA125 in 6 weeks. On the prevalence screen, this strategy had very encouraging sensitivity (89 %) [55] which was maintained at the incidence screens [71].

In the women at high risk (due to a family history of ovarian/breast cancer or mutations in genes such as BRCA1/2) annual screening is not regarded as effective [72, 73]. As most of the cancers detected in this group of women are high grade serous EOCs which progress rapidly, a shorter screening interval has been suggested. A screening strategy incorporating CA125 interpreted using the ROC algorithm and annual TVS has been investigated in the UK Familial Ovarian Cancer Screening Study (UKFOCSS), which is a prospective screening study involving 5,732 women [74]. The only results available from this trial are those from Phase I where 3,563 women at high risk underwent annual screening with CA125 using a cut-off and TVS. Although sensitivity for detection of incident OC/FT was encouraging (81.3 % if occult cancers were classified as false negatives and 87.5 % classified as true positives), only 4 (30.8 %) of 13 incident screen-detected OC/FTCs were detected at stage I/II. Advanced stage OC (>IIIC) was more likely detected in those diagnosed over a year from the last screen compared to those diagnosed within a year of screening (85.7 % v 26.1 %; P=0.009). UKFOCSS Phase I results further confirm that annual screening does not lead to detection of early-stage disease [74]. Results of the performance of four-monthly screening with ROC are expected in 2015 from UKFOCSS Phase II and the US trials, the GOG-199 study and the US Cancer Genetics Network trial [75]. Current recommendation remains that women at high risk should undergo genetic counseling with a view to risk reducing surgery once they have completed their family.

To further improve performance characteristics, a number of marker panels alone or in combination with CA125 have been evaluated with little success. The exception is Human Epididymis protein 4 (HE4) which is elevated in EOC but not in benign gynecologic conditions [76]. HE4 as an additional screening marker to CA125 is currently being investigated in the Novel Markers Trial [77].

Primary Screening with Both TVS and CA125

TVS and CA125 have been has been used together in primary screening in order to increase sensitivity. The downside is an increase in false positive screens. Two large trials undertaken over the last three decades have evaluated this strategy.

The Japanese Shizuoka Cohort Study of Ovarian Cancer Screening [78] was an RCT of 82,487 low-risk postmenopausal women who were screened using an annual ultrasound and CA125 using a cut-off. Encouraging sensitivity of 77.1 % and specificity of 99.9 % were reported [78]. The women in the screened arm were more likely to be detected at early stage (63 %) compared to the control arm (38 %). The mortality impact has however not been reported.

The US Prostate, Lung, Colorectal and Ovarian (PLCO) Cancer Screening Trial enrolled 78,237 women aged 55–74 years, with 34,202 women randomized to ovarian cancer screening. Women were screened using a combination of serum CA125 (using a 35 kU/L cut-off), and transvaginal ultrasound for 3 years followed by CA125 alone for a further 2 years. During four annual screens in 34,261 postmenopausal women, 89 invasive ovarian/ peritoneal cancers were detected, of which 60 were screen detected. Overall, 19.5 surgeries were performed per screen-detected cancer [79]. No mortality benefit was found at a median follow up of 12.4 years [80]. Furthermore, in those who had surgery and were not found to have cancer, the complication rate was 15 % [80]. The results need to be interpreted with caution, as 40.6 % of the women were diagnosed after screening ended. Furthermore, CA125 was interpreted using an absolute cut-off (rather than a time series algorithm), and management of screen positives was at the discretion of the treating clinician (rather than via a well-defined protocol) [81].

The details of the four large ovarian cancer screening trials in the general population are outlined in Table 26.3 [54, 55, 59, 78–80].

Following the review of the PLCO mortality data, the US Preventive Services Task Force (USPSTF) has reaffirmed their previous recommendation that ovarian cancer screening is not advocated [82]. However, they state that the impact of a time series algorithm-based strategy on mortality from UKCTOCS is eagerly awaited.

Other Early Detection Strategies

Symptoms for ovarian cancer are non-specific until the disease is in advanced stages. Most commonly reported symptoms experienced by the women 3–6 months prior to diagnosis are abdominal (77 %), gastrointestinal (70 %), pain (58 %), constitutional (50 %), urinary (34 %),

Table 26.3 Outline of the key findings of the four major ovarian cancer screening trials

Ovarian cancer screening trials in the general population					
	University of Kentucky study [54, 59]	Japanese Shizuoka cohort study of ovarian cancer screening [78]	Prostate Lung Colorectal Ovarian Cancer screening trial (PLCO) [79, 80]	UK Collaborative Trial of Ovarian Cancer Screening (UKCTOCS) [55]	
Study/RCT	Single arm prospective study	RCT	RCT	RCT	RCT
Cohort	25,327	41,688	34,261	50,078	48,230
1st line test	TVS	TVS + CA125 (>35 kU/L)	TVS + CA125 (>35 kU/L)	CA125 interpreted using the Risk of Ovarian Cancer (ROC) algorithm	TVS
2nd line test	TVS	TVS + CA125	TVS + CA125	TVS	TVS
Sensitivity	81 % for primary OC/FT cancer; 76.3 % for primary invasive OC/FT cancer	77.1 % for primary OC/FT cancer	69.5 % for primary OC/FT/PP cancer; 68.2 % for primary invasive OC/FT/PP cancer when compared to the other trials	89.4 % for primary OC/FT cancer; 89.5 % for invasive disease	84.9 % for primary OC/FT cancer; 75 % for invasive disease
Stage (I/II)	82 %	63 %	28 %	47 %	50 %
Proportion of participants who underwent screen positive surgery	1.4 %	0.7 %	3.4 %	0.2 %	1.7 %
Mortality/survival	Longer 5-year survival: 74.8 % for women in the screened arm compared to 53.7 % in unscreened women (from the same institution treated by the same surgical and chemotherapeutic protocols) (P<0.001)	Stage shift: 63 % of women in the screened group detected with Stage I compared to 38 % of the control women	No mortality benefit: No difference in OC deaths between the two arms (118 in the screened arm, 100 in the control arm)	Mortality data awaited in 2015	
Current status	Completed	Completed	Completed	Follow up	

and pelvic (26 %) with gynecologic symptoms being the least common [83]. The frequency and severity of symptoms are higher in women with ovarian cancer than in those with other conditions and appear not to be related to stage of the cancer [84, 85]. Goff et al. have developed a symptom index [86] that may help in identifying women with ovarian cancer but there is concern about whether it has adequate performance characteristics (sensitivity of 64 %, specificity of 88 %) as a stand-alone screen. On using the symptom index to select women to undergo CA125 and HE4 testing, the specificity improved to 98.5 % at a decrease in sensitivity to 58 % [87]. More recently, the data form the DoVE pilot project, where women who presented with symptoms underwent screening with serum CA125 and TVS, suggested that this approach can pick up more cancers than that reported from screening studies [88]. However, we feel that only large trials using this approach will be able to answer confirm these preliminary findings.

Increasingly, there are efforts to institute national ovarian cancer symptom awareness campaigns in women and primary care physicians [89–92].

Future Developments

Recent progress which has immediate implication for ovarian cancer screening is the increasing evidence that ovarian cancer is a heterogeneous disease with well-defined genetic and phenotypic subtypes. Some authors group the latter into Type I (low-grade serous, low-grade endometrioid, clear cell, mucinous and transitional/Brenner) carcinomas which are slow growing and have good prognosis and more aggressive Type II (high grade serous, high grade endometrioid, undifferentiated tumours and carcinosarcomas) [93]. In the future, the focus of screening is likely to be invasive EOC with different strategies for detecting Type I (TVS based) versus Type II (marker time profile based) cancers. Unlike cervical cancer, the view over the past few decades has been that a pre-malignant lesion for ovarian cancer does not exist and therefore all efforts were focused on detecting early-stage disease [94, 95]. However, most researchers now accept that the origins of a majority of ovarian cancers may not be in the ovary but elsewhere in the Mullerian tract [96]. Crum et al. have identified premalignant serous tubal intraepithelial cancer (STIC) lesions in the distal fallopian tube and suggested a model of 'fimbrial-ovarian' serous neoplasia, with a proportion of serous ovarian cancers starting as STIC lesions and spreading to the ovary [97]. This development raises the possibility of primary prevention. Work is already underway to identify these lesions in vitro [98].

26.5 Endometrial Cancer

Similar to ovarian cancer, cancer of the uterus is more common in the industrialized nations [99]. In the UK, 7,835 women were diagnosed with uterine cancers in 2009 and 1,937 died of the disease [99]. Since the early 1990s, the incidence of endometrial cancer in the UK has increased by 40 % [100]. In view of the rising obesity, decrease in fertility and aging population, it is likely that these rates of endometrial cancer will rise further, making it a significant public health concern [101].

Screening for Endometrial Cancer

As most (95 %) of the women who develop endometrial cancer present with abnormal vaginal bleeding and are diagnosed with early stage disease, screening is not currently recommended. However, the presence of a precursor lesion, atypical endometrial hyperplasia (AEH), raises the possibility of primary prevention as in cervical cancer. Screening is currently only recommended in women with Lynch Syndrome (LS) or Hereditary Nonpolyposis Colorectal Cancer (HPNCC) [102, 103] whose risk of endometrial cancer by age 70 ranges from 54 % in MLH1 mutation carriers, 21 % in MSH2 to 16 % in MSH6 [104]. Women with LS also have an 8–10 % lifetime risk of ovarian cancer. Although the efficacy of such endometrial screening remains unproven, women are offered screening with annual TVS and endometrial biopsy from the age of 35 [105–107]. There is lack of consensus on an appropriate cut-off value for endometrial thickness (ET) on TVS screening in asymptomatic premenopausal women, and interval cancers are known to occur [108, 109]. The superior performance of annual outpatient hysteroscopy and endometrial sampling over TVS was reported in a prospective observational cohort study of 41 LS women attending a tertiary high-risk familial gynecological cancer clinic [110] with four cases of endometrial cancer/AEH detected using this approach compared to two by TVS. It confirms the guidance on the need for endometrial sampling in these women.

There has been limited enthusiasm to explore screening for endometrial cancer in the general population in view of its good prognosis. However, when diagnosed at late stage, the survival rates are very similar to those of ovarian cancer where major efforts have been made in the last few decades to detect the disease early through screening [55, 80]. In 2001, Fleischer et al. reported detecting one case of endometrial cancer and four cases of AEH on TVS screening of 1,926 asymptomatic postmenopausal women from the general population [111]. More recent data from 37,038 women in the ultrasound arm of UKCTOCS demonstrated that in the general population, ET cut-off of 5 and 10 mm had a sensitivity of 80.5 and 54.1 %, at a specificity 85.7 and 97.2 %, respectively. A 5 mm cut-off would result in 56, whereas 10 mm in 17 diagnostic interventions per case detected [112]. A logistic regression model incorporating epidemiological data (oral contraceptive pill use, age at menarche, number of pregnancies, weight, age, and history of cancer), was able to stratify women according to risk of endometrial cancer. The quarter at most risk included 40 % of endometrial cancers or AEH cases [112]. Work is underway to improve this risk stratification strategy by adding hormonal factors/novel biomarkers so that screening can be offered only to those at highest risk.

In general population screening, endometrial sampling is limited to those with increased ET. It can be performed using either Pipelle endometrial biopsy or hysteroscopy. The former, though well-established and easily performed as an outpatient procedure, has a 10 % procedure failure rate and inadequate tissue yield [113] especially in post-menopausal women. Furthermore, cancers have been reported to be missed on Pipelle alone. Outpatient hysteroscopy is increasingly the gold-standard and is tolerated as well as endometrial sampling [114]. Hysteroscopy has an advantage over TVS and Pipelle as it can detect pathology missed by both tests [115, 116]. Although accepted as the gold standard, it still has an 8–11 % failure rate [117, 118].

26.6 Summary

Cervical cancer screening will continue to be the gold standard for cancer screening. Primary HPV testing with cytology triage is the most likely future strategy over the next 5 years with molecular tests focusing on HPV16, 18 and 45 genotypes and markers of malignant transformation. In low resource settings, organized screening programs using cheap reliable tests and population education are likely to be widely implemented. Future efforts need to focus on maximal coverage, quality assurance of the screening programs and provision of appropriate treatment facilities. This together with the increasing global pool of vaccinated women is likely to impact on disease incidence and mortality.

Currently ovarian cancer screening is not recommended. The results of the large prospective ovarian cancer screening trials, UKFOCSS in high-risk women and UKCTOCS in low-risk women, will determine whether this will change in the near future. It is envisaged that novel insights into ovarian cancer biology and heterogeneity coupled with biomarker discovery using pre diagnostic samples from the large trials and individualized interpretation based on marker profile with time will result in effective novel screening strategies.

The rise in endometrial cancer is alarming. There is already a call for action by the UN in tackling the negative impact of unhealthy lifestyles on the incidences of cancers. The current strategies for endometrial screening have high sensitivity but poor specificity. The research focus will be on building risk prediction models that can identify women from the general population at highest risk of developing the disease.

Key Points

Cervical cancer

- Organized screening programs can reduce incidence and mortality from cervical cancer as the disease has a long premalignant phase with easily identifiable and treatable lesions
- Even a single round of screening yields mortality benefit, supporting use of 'screen and treat' strategies in LMIC
- HPV testing, especially with development of low cost alternatives for use in LMIC, is likely to increasingly be the primary test for cervical cancer screening
- Primary prevention through vaccination programs have been initiated in pre-adolescent girls aged 12–17 in over 100 countries

Ovarian cancer

- Ovarian cancer screening continues not to be recommended with screening in the PLCO trial not showing any mortality benefit
- The largest RCT, UKCTOCS, utilizing a novel risk based interpretation of CA125 profile will report in 2015
- Recent developments in understanding the disease heterogeneity and natural history are likely to influence the development of novel screening approaches aimed at detection of premalignant lesions and low volume disease

Endometrial cancer

- The incidence of endometrial cancer is rising due to rise in obesity, decreasing parity and aging population
- Screening using endometrial sampling is recommended for women at high risk (Lynch Syndrome)
- Screening is not currently recommended in the general population as women are usually symptomatic and diagnosed in early stages
- Screening using TVS in the general population is sensitive but has high false positive rates and better strategies for risk stratification are required

References

1. Morrison A. Screening in chronic disease. New York: Oxford University Press; 1992.
2. Wilson JM, Jungner YG. Principles and practice of mass screening for disease. Bol Oficina Sanit Panam. 1968;65(4):281–393.
3. WHO. Revisiting Wilson and Jungner in the genomic age: a review of screening criteria over the past 40 years. 2013 [cited 2013 20/01/2013]; Available from: http://www.who.int/bulletin/volumes/86/4/07–050112/en/.
4. GLOBOCAN. GLOBOCAN 2008—estimated cancer incidence, mortality, prevalence and disability-adjusted life years (DALYs) worldwide in 2008. 2008 [cited 2012 24/12/2012]; Available from: http://globocan.iarc.fr/.
5. Jemal A, Bray F, Center MM, Ferlay J, Ward E, Forman D. Global cancer statistics. CA Cancer J Clin. 2011;61(2):69–90.
6. Castle PE. Gynecological cancer: more evidence supporting human papillomavirus testing. Nat Rev Clin Oncol. 2012;9(3):131–2.
7. ACCP. Recent evidence on cervical cancer screening in low-resource settings. 2011 [cited 2013 20/01/2013]; Available from: http://www.alliance-cxca.org/files/ACCP_cxca_screening_2011.pdf.
8. Bernard HU, Burk RD, Chen Z, van Doorslaer K, Hausen H, de Villiers EM. Classification of papillomaviruses (PVs) based on 189 PV types and proposal of taxonomic amendments. Virology. 2010;401(1):70–9.
9. Schiffman M, Herrero R, Desalle R, Hildesheim A, Wacholder S, Rodriguez AC, Bratti MC, Sherman ME, Morales J, Guillen D, Alfaro M, Hutchinson M, Wright TC, Solomon D, Chen Z, Schussler J, Castle PE, Burk RD. The carcinogenicity of human papillomavirus types reflects viral evolution. Virology. 2005;337(1):76–84.
10. Munoz N, Bosch FX, de Sanjose S, Herrero R, Castellsague X, Shah KV, Snijders PJ, Meijer CJ. Epidemiologic classification of human papillomavirus types associated with cervical cancer. N Engl J Med. 2003;348(6):518–27.
11. de Sanjose S, Quint WG, Alemany L, Geraets DT, Klaustermeier JE, Lloveras B, Tous S, Felix A, Bravo LE, Shin HR, Vallejos CS, de Ruiz PA, Lima MA, Guimera N, Clavero O, Alejo M, Llombart-Bosch

A, Cheng-Yang C, Tatti SA, Kasamatsu E, Iljazovic E, Odida M, Prado R, Seoud M, Grce M, Usubutun A, Jain A, Suarez GA, Lombardi LE, Banjo A, Menendez C, Domingo EJ, Velasco J, Nessa A, Chichareon SC, Qiao YL, Lerma E, Garland SM, Sasagawa T, Ferrera A, Hammouda D, Mariani L, Pelayo A, Steiner I, Oliva E, Meijer CJ, Al-Jassar WF, Cruz E, Wright TC, Puras A, Llave CL, Tzardi M, Agorastos T, Garcia-Barriola V, Clavel C, Ordi J, Andujar M, Castellsague X, Sanchez GI, Nowakowski AM, Bornstein J, Munoz N, Bosch FX. Human papillomavirus genotype attribution in invasive cervical cancer: a retrospective cross-sectional worldwide study. Lancet Oncol. 2010;11(11):1048–56.

12. NHSCSP. NHS Cervical Screening Programme—Audit of invasive cervical cancer. 2011 [cited 2012 24/12/2012]: Available from: http://www.cancerscreening.nhs.uk/cervical/publications/nhscsp-audit-invasive-cervical-cancer-201107.pdf.
13. Moyer VA. Screening for cervical cancer: U.S. Preventive Services Task Force recommendation statement. Ann Intern Med. 2012;156(12):880–91. W312.
14. Fahey MT, Irwig L, Macaskill P. Meta-analysis of Pap test accuracy. Am J Epidemiol. 1995;141(7):680–9.
15. Albrow R, Kitchener H, Gupta N, Desai M. Cervical screening in England: the past, present, and future. Cancer Cytopathol. 2012;120(2):87–96.
16. NICE. National Institute for Health and Clinical Excellence—Guidance on the use of liquid-based cytology for cervical screening. 2003 [cited 2012 24/12/2012]; Available from: http://publications.nice.org.uk/guidance-on-the-use-of-liquid-based-cytology-for-cervical-screening-ta69.
17. Arbyn M, Bergeron C, Klinkhamer P, Martin-Hirsch P, Siebers AG, Bulten J. Liquid compared with conventional cervical cytology: a systematic review and meta-analysis. Obstet Gynecol. 2008;111(1):167–77.
18. Cronje HS. Screening for cervical cancer in the developing world. Best Pract Res Clin Obstet Gynaecol. 2005;19(4):517–29.
19. Sankaranarayanan R, Nessa A, Esmy PO, Dangou JM. Visual inspection methods for cervical cancer prevention. Best Pract Res Clin Obstet Gynaecol. 2012;26(2):221–32.
20. Sankaranarayanan R, Esmy PO, Rajkumar R, Muwonge R, Swaminathan R, Shanthakumari S, Fayette JM, Cherian J. Effect of visual screening on cervical cancer incidence and mortality in Tamil Nadu, India: a cluster-randomised trial. Lancet. 2007;370(9585):398–406.
21. Walboomers JM, Jacobs MV, Manos MM, Bosch FX, Kummer JA, Shah KV, Snijders PJ, Peto J, Meijer CJ, Munoz N. Human papillomavirus is a necessary cause of invasive cervical cancer worldwide. J Pathol. 1999;189(1):12–9.
22. Saslow D, Solomon D, Lawson HW, Killackey M, Kulasingam SL, Cain J, Garcia FA, Moriarty AT, Waxman AG, Wilbur DC, Wentzensen N, Downs Jr LS, Spitzer M, Moscicki AB, Franco EL, Stoler MH, Schiffman M, Castle PE, Myers ER. American Cancer Society, American Society for Colposcopy and Cervical Pathology, and American Society for Clinical Pathology screening guidelines for the prevention and early detection of cervical cancer. CA Cancer J Clin. 2012;62(3):147–72.
23. Cuzick J, Clavel C, Petry KU, Meijer CJ, Hoyer H, Ratnam S, Szarewski A, Birembaut P, Kulasingam S, Sasieni P, Iftner T. Overview of the European and North American studies on HPV testing in primary cervical cancer screening. Int J Cancer. 2006;119(5):1095–101.
24. Mayrand MH, Duarte-Franco E, Rodrigues I, Walter SD, Hanley J, Ferenczy A, Ratnam S, Coutlee F, Franco EL. Human papillomavirus DNA versus papanicolaou screening tests for cervical cancer. N Engl J Med. 2007;357(16):1579–88.
25. Zhao FH, Lin MJ, Chen F, Hu SY, Zhang R, Belinson JL, Sellors JW, Franceschi S, Qiao YL, Castle PE. Performance of high-risk human papillomavirus DNA testing as a primary screen for cervical cancer: a pooled analysis of individual patient data from 17 population-based studies from China. Lancet Oncol. 2010;11(12):1160–71.
26. Arbyn M, Sasieni P, Meijer CJ, Clavel C, Koliopoulos G, Dillner J. Chapter 9: clinical applications of HPV testing: a summary of meta-analyses. Vaccine. 2006;24 Suppl 3:S3/78–89.
27. Koliopoulos G, Arbyn M, Martin-Hirsch P, Kyrgiou M, Prendiville W, Paraskevaidis E. Diagnostic accuracy of human papillomavirus testing in primary cervical screening: a systematic review and meta-analysis of non-randomized studies. Gynecol Oncol. 2007;104(1):232–46.
28. Qiao YL, Sellors JW, Eder PS, Bao YP, Lim JM, Zhao FH, Weigl B, Zhang WH, Peck RB, Li L, Chen F, Pan QJ, Lorincz AT. A new HPV-DNA test for cervical-cancer screening in developing regions: a cross-sectional study of clinical accuracy in rural China. Lancet Oncol. 2008;9(10):929–36.
29. Cuzick J, Bergeron C, von Knebel Doeberitz M, Gravitt P, Jeronimo J, JLMM C, Lorincz AT, Sankaranarayanan R, JFS P, Szarewski A. New technologies and procedures for cervical cancer screening. Vaccine. 2012;30 Suppl 5:F107–16.
30. Murillo R, Luna J, Gamboa O, Osorio E, Bonilla J, Cendales R. Cervical cancer screening with naked-eye visual inspection in Colombia. Int J Gynaecol Obstet. 2010;109(3):230–4.
31. Kitchener HC, Gilham C, Sargent A, Bailey A, Albrow R, Roberts C, Desai M, Mather J, Turner A, Moss S, Peto J. A comparison of HPV DNA testing and liquid based cytology over three rounds of primary cervical screening: extended follow up in the ARTISTIC trial. Eur J Cancer. 2011;47(6):864–71.
32. Wise J. Pilot study will assess whether HPV test should replace smears to screen for cervical cancer. BMJ. 2012;344:e3744.

33. Rijkaart DC, Berkhof J, Rozendaal L, van Kemenade FJ, Bulkmans NW, Heideman DA, Kenter GG, Cuzick J, Snijders PJ, Meijer CJ. Human papillomavirus testing for the detection of high-grade cervical intraepithelial neoplasia and cancer: final results of the POBASCAM randomised controlled trial. Lancet Oncol. 2012;13(1):78–88.
34. Ronco G, Giorgi-Rossi P, Carozzi F, Confortini M, Dalla Palma P, Del Mistro A, Ghiringhello B, Girlando S, Gillio-Tos A, De Marco L, Naldoni C, Pierotti P, Rizzolo R, Schincaglia P, Zorzi M, Zappa M, Segnan N, Cuzick J. Efficacy of human papillomavirus testing for the detection of invasive cervical cancers and cervical intraepithelial neoplasia: a randomised controlled trial. Lancet Oncol. 2010;11(3):249–57.
35. Sankaranarayanan R, Nene BM, Shastri SS, Jayant K, Muwonge R, Budukh AM, Hingmire S, Malvi SG, Thorat R, Kothari A, Chinoy R, Kelkar R, Kane S, Desai S, Keskar VR, Rajeshwarkar R, Panse N, Dinshaw KA. HPV screening for cervical cancer in rural India. N Engl J Med. 2009;360(14):1385–94.
36. Denny LA, Wright Jr TC. Human papillomavirus testing and screening. Best Pract Res Clin Obstet Gynaecol. 2005;19(4):501–15.
37. Nobbenhuis MA, Helmerhorst TJ, van den Brule AJ, Rozendaal L, Jaspars LH, Voorhorst FJ, Verheijen RH, Meijer CJ. Primary screening for high risk HPV by home obtained cervicovaginal lavage is an alternative screening tool for unscreened women. J Clin Pathol. 2002;55(6):435–9.
38. Petignat P, Faltin DL, Bruchim I, Tramer MR, Franco EL, Coutlee F. Are self-collected samples comparable to physician-collected cervical specimens for human papillomavirus DNA testing? A systematic review and meta-analysis. Gynecol Oncol. 2007;105(2):530–5.
39. WHO. World Health Organization: human papillomavirus vaccines. WHO position paper. Wkly Epidemiol Rec. 2009;84:118–31.
40. Tay SK. Cervical cancer in the human papillomavirus vaccination era. Curr Opin Obstet Gynecol. 2012;24(1):3–7.
41. David MP, Van Herck K, Hardt K, Tibaldi F, Dubin G, Descamps D, Van Damme P. Long-term persistence of anti-HPV-16 and -18 antibodies induced by vaccination with the AS04-adjuvanted cervical cancer vaccine: modeling of sustained antibody responses. Gynecol Oncol. 2009;115(3 Suppl):S1–6.
42. National Cancer Institute. Surveillance, Epidemiology, and End Results (SEER) Program - Stat Fact Sheets: Ovary Cancer. 2011; Available from: http://seer.cancer.gov/statfacts/html/ovary.html.
43. CRUK. Ovarian cancer incidence statistics. 2008 [cited 2012 25/12/2012]; Available from: http://www.cancerresearchuk.org/cancer-info/cancerstats/types/ovary/incidence/.
44. Seidman JD, Horkayne-Szakaly I, Haiba M, Boice CR, Kurman RJ, Ronnett BM. The histologic type and stage distribution of ovarian carcinomas of surface epithelial origin. Int J Gynecol Pathol. 2004;23(1):41–4.
45. CRUK. Ovarian cancer survival statistics. 2010 [cited 2012 25/12/2012]; Available from: http://www.cancerresearchuk.org/cancer-info/cancerstats/types/ovary/survival/ovarian-cancer-survival-statistics#By4.
46. Rosenthal A, Jacobs I. Familial ovarian cancer screening. Best Pract Res Clin Obstet Gynaecol. 2006;20(2):321–38.
47. Chen S, Parmigiani G. Meta-analysis of BRCA1 and BRCA2 penetrance. J Clin Oncol. 2007;25(11):1329–33.
48. Dunlop MG, Farrington SM, Carothers AD, Wyllie AH, Sharp L, Burn J, Liu B, Kinzler KW, Vogelstein B. Cancer risk associated with germline DNA mismatch repair gene mutations. Hum Mol Genet. 1997;6(1):105–10.
49. Campbell S, Goessens L, Goswamy R, Whitehead M. Real-time ultrasonography for determination of ovarian morphology and volume. A possible early screening test for ovarian cancer? Lancet. 1982;1(8269):425–6.
50. DePriest PD, Gallion HH, Pavlik EJ, Kryscio RJ, van Nagell Jr JR. Transvaginal sonography as a screening method for the detection of early ovarian cancer. Gynecol Oncol. 1997;65(3):408–14.
51. Gentry-Maharaj A, Sharma A, Burnell M, Ryan A, Amso NN, Seif MW, Turner G, Brunell C, Fletcher G, Rangar R, Fallowfield L, Campbell S, Jacobs I, Menon U. Acceptance of transvaginal sonography by postmenopausal women participating in the United Kingdom Collaborative Trial of Ovarian Cancer Screening. Ultrasound Obstet Gynecol. 2013;41(1):73–9.
52. Sharma ABM, Gentry-Maharaj A, Campbell S, Amso NN, Seif MW, Fletcher G, Brunel C, Turner G, Rangar R, Ryan A, Jacobs I, Menon U. Quality Assurance and its impact on ovarian visualisation rates in the Multicentre United Kingdom Collaborative Trial of Ovarian Cancer Screening (UKCTOCS) Forthcoming April 2015.
53. Timmerman D, Ameye L, Fischerova D, Epstein E, Melis GB, Guerriero S, Van Holsbeke C, Savelli L, Fruscio R, Lissoni AA, Testa AC, Veldman J, Vergote I, Van Huffel S, Bourne T, Valentin L. Simple ultrasound rules to distinguish between benign and malignant adnexal masses before surgery: prospective validation by IOTA group. BMJ. 2010;341:c6839.
54. van Nagell JR, DePriest PD, Ueland FR, DeSimone CP, Cooper AL, McDonald JM, Pavlik EJ, Kryscio RJ. Ovarian cancer screening with annual transvaginal sonography: findings of 25,000 women screened. Cancer. 2007;109(9):1887–96.
55. Menon U, Gentry-Maharaj A, Hallett R, Ryan A, Burnell M, Sharma A, Lewis S, Davies S, Philpott S, Lopes A, Godfrey K, Oram D, Herod J, Williamson K, Seif MW, Scott I, Mould T, Woolas R, Murdoch J, Dobbs S, Amso NN, Leeson S, Cruickshank D, McGuire A, Campbell S, Fallowfield L, Singh N, Dawnay A, Skates SJ, Parmar M, Jacobs I. Sensitivity and specificity of multimodal and ultrasound screening for ovarian cancer, and stage distribution of

detected cancers: results of the prevalence screen of the UK Collaborative Trial of Ovarian Cancer Screening (UKCTOCS). Lancet Oncol. 2009;10(4):327–40.
56. Sharma A, Gentry-Maharaj A, Burnell M, Fourkala EO, Campbell S, Amso N, Seif MW, Ryan A, Parmar M, Jacobs I, Menon U. Assessing the malignant potential of ovarian inclusion cysts in postmenopausal women within the UK Collaborative Trial of Ovarian Cancer Screening (UKCTOCS): a prospective cohort study. BJOG. 2012;119(2):207–19.
57. Sharma A, Apostolidou S, Burnell M, Campbell S, Habib M, Gentry-Maharaj A, Amso N, Seif MW, Fletcher G, Singh N, Benjamin E, Brunell C, Turner G, Rangar R, Godfrey K, Oram D, Herod J, Williamson K, Jenkins H, Mould T, Woolas R, Murdoch J, Dobbs S, Leeson S, Cruickshank D, Fourkala EO, Ryan A, Parmar M, Jacobs I, Menon U. Risk of epithelial ovarian cancer in asymptomatic women with ultrasound-detected ovarian masses: a prospective cohort study within the UK collaborative trial of ovarian cancer screening (UKCTOCS). Ultrasound Obstet Gynecol. 2012;40(3):338–44.
58. Modesitt SC, Pavlik EJ, Ueland FR, DePriest PD, Kryscio RJ, van Nagell Jr JR. Risk of malignancy in unilocular ovarian cystic tumors less than 10 centimeters in diameter. Obstet Gynecol. 2003;102(3):594–9.
59. van Nagell JR, Miller RW, DeSimone CP, Ueland FR, Podzielinski I, Goodrich ST, Elder JW, Huang B, Kryscio RJ, Pavlik EJ. Long-term survival of women with epithelial ovarian cancer detected by ultrasonographic screening. Obstet Gynecol. 2011;118(6):1212–21.
60. Jacobs I, Menon U. Can ovarian cancer screening save lives? The question remains unanswered. Obstet Gynecol. 2011;118(6):1209–11.
61. Menon U, Gentry-Maharaj A, Ryan A, Sharma A, Burnell M, Hallett R, Lewis S, Lopez A, Godfrey K, Oram D, Herod J, Williamson K, Seif M, Scott I, Mould T, Woolas R, Murdoch J, Dobbs S, Amso N, Leeson S, Cruickshank D, McGuire A, Campbell S, Fallowfield L, Skates S, Parmar M, Jacobs I. Recruitment to multicentre trials—lessons from UKCTOCS: descriptive study. BMJ. 2008;337:a2079.
62. Zurawski Jr VR, Orjaseter H, Andersen A, Jellum E. Elevated serum CA 125 levels prior to diagnosis of ovarian neoplasia: relevance for early detection of ovarian cancer. Int J Cancer. 1988;42(5):677–80.
63. Bonfrer JM, Korse CM, Verstraeten RA, van Kamp GJ, Hart GA, Kenemans P. Clinical evaluation of the Byk LIA-mat CA125 II assay: discussion of a reference value. Clin Chem. 1997;43(3):491–7.
64. Jacobs IJ, Skates SJ, MacDonald N, Menon U, Rosenthal AN, Davies AP, Woolas R, Jeyarajah AR, Sibley K, Lowe DG, Oram DH. Screening for ovarian cancer: a pilot randomised controlled trial. Lancet. 1999;353(9160):1207–10.
65. Jacobs I, Davies AP, Bridges J, Stabile I, Fay T, Lower A, Grudzinskas JG, Oram D. Prevalence screening for ovarian cancer in postmenopausal women by CA 125 measurement and ultrasonography. BMJ. 1993;306(6884):1030–4.
66. Menon U, Talaat A, Jeyarajah AR, Rosenthal AN, MacDonald ND, Skates SJ, Sibley K, Oram DH, Jacobs IJ. Ultrasound assessment of ovarian cancer risk in postmenopausal women with CA125 elevation. Br J Cancer. 1999;80(10):1644–7.
67. Menon U, Talaat A, Rosenthal AN, Macdonald ND, Jeyerajah AR, Skates SJ, Sibley K, Oram DH, Jacobs IJ. Performance of ultrasound as a second line test to serum CA125 in ovarian cancer screening. BJOG. 2000;107(2):165–9.
68. Skates SJ, Xu FJ, Yu YH, Sjovall K, Einhorn N, Chang Y, Bast Jr RC, Knapp RC. Toward an optimal algorithm for ovarian cancer screening with longitudinal tumor markers. Cancer. 1995;76(10 Suppl):2004–10.
69. Skates SJ, Menon U, MacDonald N, Rosenthal AN, Oram DH, Knapp RC, Jacobs IJ. Calculation of the risk of ovarian cancer from serial CA-125 values for preclinical detection in postmenopausal women. J Clin Oncol. 2003;21(10 Suppl):206s–10.
70. Menon U, Skates SJ, Lewis S, Rosenthal AN, Rufford B, Sibley K, Macdonald N, Dawnay A, Jeyarajah A, Bast Jr RC, Oram D, Jacobs IJ. Prospective study using the risk of ovarian cancer algorithm to screen for ovarian cancer. J Clin Oncol. 2005;23(31):7919–26.
71. Jacobs IRA, Skates S, Habib M, Apostolidou S, Singh N, Benjamin E, Gentry-Maharaj A, Burnell M, Kalsi J, Dawnay A, Sharma A, Gunu R, Godfrey K, Oram D. Herod J, Williamson K, Seif MW, Jenkins H, Mould T, Woolas R, Murdoch J, Dobbs S, Amso N, Leeson S, Cruickshank D, Fallowfield L, Campbell S, Parmar M, Menon U, for the UKCTOCS Group, editors. Performance characteristics of multimodal screening with serum CA125 in the United Kingdom Collaborative Trial of Ovarian Cancer Screening (UKCTOCS). Paper presented at the National Cancer Research Institute (NCRI) conference, 5th Nov 2012, Liverpool.
72. Stirling D, Evans DG, Pichert G, Shenton A, Kirk EN, Rimmer S, Steel CM, Lawson S, Busby-Earle RM, Walker J, Lalloo FI, Eccles DM, Lucassen AM, Porteous ME. Screening for familial ovarian cancer: failure of current protocols to detect ovarian cancer at an early stage according to the international federation of gynecology and obstetrics system. J Clin Oncol. 2005;23(24):5588–96.
73. Hermsen BB, Olivier RI, Verheijen RH, van Beurden M, de Hullu JA, Massuger LF, Burger CW, Brekelmans CT, Mourits MJ, de Bock GH, Gaarenstroom KN, van Boven HH, Mooij TM, Rookus MA. No efficacy of annual gynaecological screening in BRCA1/2 mutation carriers; an observational follow-up study. Br J Cancer. 2007;96(9): 1335–42.
74. Rosenthal AN, Fraser L, Manchanda R, Badman P, Philpott S, Mozersky J, et al. Results of annual screening in phase I of the United Kingdom familial ovarian cancer screening study highlight the need for

strict adherence to screening schedule. J Clin Oncol 2013;31(1):49–57.
75. Skates SJ, Mai P, Horick NK, Piedmonte M, Drescher CW, Isaacs C, Armstrong DK, Buys SS, Rodriguez GC, Horowitz IR, Berchuck A, Daly MB, Domchek S, Cohn DE, Van Le L, Schorge JO, Newland W, Davidson SA, Barnes M, Brewster W, Azodi M, Nerenstone S, Kauff ND, Fabian CJ, Sluss PM, Nayfield SG, Kasten CH, Finkelstein DM, Greene MH, Lu K. Large prospective study of ovarian cancer screening in high-risk women: CA125 cut-point defined by menopausal status. Cancer Prev Res (Phila). 2011;4(9):1401–8.
76. Montagnana M, Lippi G, Ruzzenente O, Bresciani V, Danese E, Scevarolli S, Salvagno GL, Giudici S, Franchi M, Guidi GC. The utility of serum human epididymis protein 4 (HE4) in patients with a pelvic mass. J Clin Lab Anal. 2009;23(5):331–5.
77. A trial using novel markers to predict malignancy in elevated-risk women. 2010 [25/12/2012]; Available from: http://clinicaltrials.gov/ct2/show/NCT01121640.
78. Kobayashi H, Yamada Y, Sado T, Sakata M, Yoshida S, Kawaguchi R, Kanayama S, Shigetomi H, Haruta S, Tsuji Y, Ueda S, Kitanaka T. A randomized study of screening for ovarian cancer: a multicenter study in Japan. Int J Gynecol Cancer. 2008; 18(3):414–20.
79. Partridge E, Kreimer AR, Greenlee RT, Williams C, Xu JL, Church TR, Kessel B, Johnson CC, Weissfeld JL, Isaacs C, Andriole GL, Ogden S, Ragard LR, Buys SS. Results from four rounds of ovarian cancer screening in a randomized trial. Obstet Gynecol. 2009;113(4):775–82.
80. Buys SS, Partridge E, Black A, Johnson CC, Lamerato L, Isaacs C, Reding DJ, Greenlee RT, Yokochi LA, Kessel B, Crawford ED, Church TR, Andriole GL, Weissfeld JL, Fouad MN, Chia D, O'Brien B, Ragard LR, Clapp JD, Rathmell JM, Riley TL, Hartge P, Pinsky PF, Zhu CS, Izmirlian G, Kramer BS, Miller AB, Xu JL, Prorok PC, Gohagan JK, Berg CD. Effect of screening on ovarian cancer mortality: the Prostate, Lung, Colorectal and Ovarian (PLCO) Cancer Screening Randomized Controlled Trial. JAMA. 2011;305(22):2295–303.
81. Menon U, Gentry-Maharaj A, Jacobs I. Ovarian cancer screening and mortality. JAMA. 2011;306(14):1544; author reply -5.
82. Moyer VA, Force USPST. Screening for ovarian cancer: U.S. Preventive Services Task Force reaffirmation recommendation statement. Ann Intern Med. 2012;157(12):900–4.
83. Goff BA, Mandel L, Muntz HG, Melancon CH. Ovarian carcinoma diagnosis. Cancer. 2000;89(10):2068–75.
84. Olson SH, Mignone L, Nakraseive C, Caputo TA, Barakat RR, Harlap S. Symptoms of ovarian cancer. Obstet Gynecol. 2001;98(2):212–7.
85. Goff BA, Mandel LS, Melancon CH, Muntz HG. Frequency of symptoms of ovarian cancer in women presenting to primary care clinics. JAMA. 2004;291(22):2705–12.
86. Goff BA, Mandel LS, Drescher CW, Urban N, Gough S, Schurman KM, Patras J, Mahony BS, Andersen MR. Development of an ovarian cancer symptom index: possibilities for earlier detection. Cancer. 2007;109(2):221–7.
87. Andersen MR, Goff BA, Lowe KA, Scholler N, Bergan L, Drescher CW, Paley P, Urban N. Use of a symptom index, CA125, and HE4 to predict ovarian cancer. Gynecol Oncol. 2010;116(3):378–83.
88. Gilbert L, Basso O, Sampalis J, Karp I, Martins C, Feng J, Piedimonte S, Quintal L, Ramanakumar AV, Takefman J, Grigorie MS, Artho G, Krishnamurthy S. Assessment of symptomatic women for early diagnosis of ovarian cancer: results from the prospective DOvE pilot project. Lancet Oncol. 2012;13(3):285–91.
89. DoH. Department of Health—Key messages for ovarian cancer for members of the public. 2008 [cited 2012 25/12/2012]; Available from: http://www.ovarian.org.uk/media/8815/ovarian_cancer_kms_final.pdf.
90. DoH. Department of Health—Key messages for ovarian cancer for health professionals. 2009; Available from: http://www.dh.gov.uk/en/Publicationsandstatistics/Publications/PublicationsPolicyAndGuidance/DH_110534.
91. TGCF. The Gynecologic Cancer Foundation—First National Consensus on Ovarian Cancer Symptoms—Symptoms Education Imperative for Earlier Diagnosis. 2007 [cited 2012 25/12/2012]; Available from: http://www.wcn.org/downloads/GCF_Press_Release_June2007.pdf.
92. NICE. Ovarian cancer: the recognition and initial management of ovarian cancer. 2011 [16/01/2013]; Available from: http://www.nice.org.uk/nicemedia/live/13464/54194/54194.pdf.
93. Kurman RJ, Shih IM. The origin and pathogenesis of epithelial ovarian cancer: a proposed unifying theory. Am J Surg Pathol. 2010;34(3):433–43.
94. Menon U, Jacobs I. Screening for ovarian cancer. Best Pract Res Clin Obstet Gynaecol. 2002;16(4):469–82.
95. Gentry-Maharaj A, Menon U. Screening for ovarian cancer in the general population. Best Pract Res Clin Obstet Gynaecol. 2012;26(2):243–56.
96. Dubeau L. The cell of origin of ovarian epithelial tumours. Lancet Oncol. 2008;9(12):1191–7.
97. Crum CP, Drapkin R, Miron A, Ince TA, Muto M, Kindelberger DW, Lee Y. The distal fallopian tube: a new model for pelvic serous carcinogenesis. Curr Opin Obstet Gynecol. 2007;19(1):3–9.
98. Williams RM, Flesken-Nikitin A, Ellenson LH, Connolly DC, Hamilton TC, Nikitin AY, Zipfel WR. Strategies for high-resolution imaging of epithelial ovarian cancer by laparoscopic nonlinear microscopy. Transl Oncol. 2010;3(3):181–94.
99. CRUK. Uterine cancer statistics. 2009 [cited 2012 25/12/2012]; Available from: http://www.cancerresearchuk.org/cancer-info/cancerstats/types/uterus/?script=true.

100. CRUK. Uterine (womb) cancer incidence statistics. 2009 [cited 2012 25/12/2012]; Available from: http://www.cancerresearchuk.org/cancer-info/cancerstats/types/uterus/incidence/.
101. Bray F, Dos Santos Silva I, Moller H, Weiderpass E. Endometrial cancer incidence trends in Europe: underlying determinants and prospects for prevention. Cancer Epidemiol Biomarkers Prev. 2005; 14(5):1132–42.
102. Lynch HT, Krush AJ. The cancer family syndrome and cancer control. Surg Gynecol Obstet. 1971;132(2):247–50.
103. Lynch HT, Smyrk T. Hereditary nonpolyposis colorectal cancer (Lynch syndrome). An updated review. Cancer. 1996;78(6):1149–67.
104. Bonadona V, Bonaiti B, Olschwang S, Grandjouan S, Huiart L, Longy M, Guimbaud R, Buecher B, Bignon YJ, Caron O, Colas C, Nogues C, Lejeune-Dumoulin S, Olivier-Faivre L, Polycarpe-Osaer F, Nguyen TD, Desseigne F, Saurin JC, Berthet P, Leroux D, Duffour J, Manouvrier S, Frebourg T, Sobol H, Lasset C, Bonaiti-Pellie C. Cancer risks associated with germline mutations in MLH1, MSH2, and MSH6 genes in Lynch syndrome. JAMA. 2011;305(22):2304–10.
105. Smith RA, Cokkinides V, Brawley OW, Smith RA, Cokkinides V, Brawley OW. Cancer screening in the United States, 2009: a review of current American Cancer Society guidelines and issues in cancer screening. CA Cancer J Clin. 2009; 59(1):27–41.
106. Lindor NM, Petersen GM, Hadley DW, Kinney AY, Miesfeldt S, Lu KH, Lynch P, Burke W, Press N. Recommendations for the care of individuals with an inherited predisposition to Lynch syndrome: a systematic review. JAMA. 2006;296(12):1507–17.
107. Hendriks YM, de Jong AE, Morreau H, Tops CM, Vasen HF, Wijnen JT, Breuning MH, Brocker-Vriends AH. Diagnostic approach and management of Lynch syndrome (hereditary nonpolyposis colorectal carcinoma): a guide for clinicians. CA Cancer J Clin. 2006;56(4):213–25.
108. Dove-Edwin I, Boks D, Goff S, Kenter GG, Carpenter R, Vasen HF, Thomas HJ. The outcome of endometrial carcinoma surveillance by ultrasound scan in women at risk of hereditary nonpolyposis colorectal carcinoma and familial colorectal carcinoma. Cancer. 2002;94(6):1708–12.
109. Rijcken FE, Mourits MJ, Kleibeuker JH, Hollema H, van der Zee AG. Gynecologic screening in hereditary nonpolyposis colorectal cancer. Gynecol Oncol. 2003;91(1):74–80.
110. Manchanda R, Saridogan E, Abdelraheim A, Johnson M, Rosenthal AN, Benjamin E, Brunell C, Side L, Gessler S, Jacobs I, Menon U. Annual outpatient hysteroscopy and endometrial sampling (OHES) in HNPCC/Lynch syndrome (LS). Arch Gynecol Obstet. 2012;286(6):1555–62.
111. Fleischer AC, Wheeler JE, Lindsay I, Hendrix SL, Grabill S, Kravitz B, MacDonald B. An assessment of the value of ultrasonographic screening for endometrial disease in postmenopausal women without symptoms. Am J Obstet Gynecol. 2001;184(2):70–5.
112. Jacobs I, Gentry-Maharaj A, Burnell M, Manchanda R, Singh N, Sharma A, Ryan A, Seif MW, Amso NN, Turner G, Brunell C, Fletcher G, Rangar R, Ford K, Godfrey K, Lopes A, Oram D, Herod J, Williamson K, Scott I, Jenkins H, Mould T, Woolas R, Murdoch J, Dobbs S, Leeson S, Cruickshank D, Skates SJ, Fallowfield L, Parmar M, Campbell S, Menon U. Sensitivity of transvaginal ultrasound screening for endometrial cancer in postmenopausal women: a case-control study within the UKCTOCS cohort. Lancet Oncol. 2011;12(1):38–48.
113. Dijkhuizen FP, Mol BW, Brolmann HA, Heintz AP. The accuracy of endometrial sampling in the diagnosis of patients with endometrial carcinoma and hyperplasia: a meta-analysis. Cancer. 2000; 89(8):1765–72.
114. Elmasry K, Davies AJ, Evans DG, Seif MN, Reynolds K. Strategies for endometrial screening in the Lynch syndrome population: a patient acceptability study. Fam Cancer. 2009;8(4):431–9.
115. Pasqualotto EB, Margossian H, Price LL, Bradley LD. Accuracy of preoperative diagnostic tools and outcome of hysteroscopic management of menstrual dysfunction. J Am Assoc Gynecol Laparosc. 2000;7(2):201–9.
116. Tahir MM, Bigrigg MA, Browning JJ, Brookes ST, Smith PA. A randomised controlled trial comparing transvaginal ultrasound, outpatient hysteroscopy and endometrial biopsy with inpatient hysteroscopy and curettage. Br J Obstet Gynaecol. 1999;106(12):1259–64.
117. Lecuru F, Le Frere Belda MA, Bats AS, Tulpin L, Metzger U, Olschwang S, Laurent-Puig P. Performance of office hysteroscopy and endometrial biopsy for detecting endometrial disease in women at risk of human non-polyposis colon cancer: a prospective study. Int J Gynecol Cancer. 2008;18(6):1326–31.
118. Lecuru F, Metzger U, Scarabin C, Le Frere Belda MA, Olschwang S, Laurent Puig P. Hysteroscopic findings in women at risk of HNPCC. Results of a prospective observational study. Fam Cancer. 2007;6(3):295–9.

Inherited Gene Mutations in Gynecological Oncology

27

Adam N. Rosenthal and Lucy E. Side

27.1 Introduction

Up to 10 % of ovarian and endometrial cancers are associated with an inherited genetic predisposition to cancer. A rare cervical cancer (adenoma malignum or minimal deviation adenocarcinoma) is associated with an inherited gene mutation. In this chapter, we describe these heritable mutations, their gynecological cancer risks and current management recommendations.

Identifying familial predisposition to malignancy offers opportunities for cancer prevention in individuals and their relatives. Reproductive options including pre-implantation genetic diagnosis can enable gene-carriers to have unaffected children [1]. More recently, targeted cancer therapies have been developed, utilizing defective DNA repair mechanisms in some inherited cancers [2]. Consequently, failure to identify inherited malignancies can limit treatment and reproductive options.

The germline mutations known to increase the risk of gynecological malignancy occur in tumor suppressor genes (TSG) (Table 27.1). Importantly, these are inherited in an autosomal dominant way and can be passed to offspring paternally as well as maternally. They show incomplete penetrance i.e. not all mutation-carriers develop cancer. Generally inactivation of both maternally and paternally derived alleles of a TSG is required for cancer development. This is Knudsen's 'two hit hypothesis.' In the case of germline mutations, where all an individual's cells carry a mutated allele, acquired mutation, deletion or hypermethylation of the remaining allele inactivates the gene, and renders the cell vulnerable to cancer development. This mechanism explains the earlier age of onset of inherited cancers.

A.N. Rosenthal, PhD, MRCOG (✉)
Department of Women's Health,
University College London Hospitals NHS
Foundation Trust & Department of Women's Cancer,
UCL EGA Institute for Women's Health, London, UK
e-mail: adam.rosenthal@ucl.ac.uk

L.E. Side, MD, MB, BCh
Department of Women's Cancer, UCL EGA Institute
for Women's Health & North East Thames Regional
Genetics Service, Great Ormond Street Hospital,
London, UK

27.2 Determining Risk

It is good practice to take a family history of cancer when a patient is seen for the first time; criteria are shown in Table 27.2. If this suggests an inherited predisposition, then referral to Clinical Genetics services should be offered. This ensures access to (1) accurate risk-assessment, (2) explanation of genetic testing and its implications (3) enrolment in screening programs and clinical trials and (4) referral to a surgeon experienced in risk-reducing procedures. Identifying a predisposition to cancer can affect the patient's psychological and physical well-being and has implications for their blood-relatives. This requires sensitive handling.

H.R.H. Patel et al. (eds.), *Pelvic Cancer Surgery: Modern Breakthroughs and Future Advances*,
DOI 10.1007/978-1-4471-4258-4_27, © Springer-Verlag London 2015

Table 27.1 Gene mutations increasing risk of gynecological cancer and their management options

Gene mutated	Gene function	General population gene frequency	Associated non-gynecologic cancers/other conditions (male and female)	Ovarian cancer lifetime risk	Endometrial cancer lifetime risk	Other associated gynecologic cancers	Gynecologic surgical prophylaxis and efficacy	Chemo prophylaxis options for gynecologic cancers	Gynecologic surveillance and efficacy	Successful PGD reported	Comment
BRCA genes											
BRCA1	dsDNA repair/HR	1 in 800 (AJ 1 in 40)	BC (approx. 60 % by age 70 year for female, lower for male), prostate risk 3-fold, pancreatic risk 2-fold	39–65 %	2 % with tamoxifen use	None	RRSO offers complete protection against tubal and OC risk. Residual (~4 %) risk of PPC remains	COCP may protect against OC but needs to be offset against further increased risk of BC and is not recommended solely for risk-reduction pre-RRSO	6-monthly TVS and CA125a. Evidence of good sensitivity but majority of cancers detected are high stage	Yes	1. Risk of occult cancer detection as a result of RRSO 2. BC risk-reduction if surgery performed premenopausally 3. Mucinous/non-epithelial OC not known to be BRCA-associated
BRCA2	dsDNA repair/HR	1 in 800 (AJ 1 in 40)	BC (approx. 50 % by age 70 year for female, lower for male), prostate risk 5-fold, pancreatic risk 4-fold, melanoma risk 3-fold, stomach 3-fold, gallbladder 5-fold	11–37 %	2 % with tamoxifen use	None				Yes	
Lynch syndrome (HNPCC) genes											
MLH1 *MSH2* *MSH6* *PMS2* *EPCAM*	MMR MMR MMR MMR Inactivates *MSH2*	1 in 600–2,000 (*MLH1* 50 %, *MSH2* 40 %, *MSH6* 7–10 %, *PMS2* <5 %, *EPCAM* 1 %)	CRC, EC, OC, renal pelvis/ureteric cancers, small bowel cancers, sebaceous skin tumors; possible BC and Prostate (BC and prostate risk controversial)	3–33 %	40–60 % (highest risk in *MSH6*)	None	Hysterectomy + BSO offers complete protection against EC/OC. Case reports of PPC following surgery – uncertain if risk increased	Aspirin may reduce EC risk. Levonorgestrel IUS may reduce EC risk (unproven efficacy) COCP might reduce EC/OC risk (unproven efficacy)	Consider annual TVS and CA125 ± outpatient hysteroscopy + endometrial biopsy (unproven efficacy)	Yes Yes No No	Bowel surgeons should liaise with gynecologists if patients require surgery for bowel cancer – provides opportunity for hysterectomy + BSO at same time. Prior bowel surgery is not contra-indication to attempt at laparoscopic hysterectomy + BSO

Cowden syndrome											
PTEN	Phosphatase	1 in 125,000	BC, thyroid cancer, EC, CRC, renal cancer, Lhermitte–Duclos disease (cerebellar dysplastic gangliocytoma)	General population risk	EC 10–32 %	None	Total hysterectomy and salpingectomy offers complete protection against EC. Consider ovarian preservation depending on patient age. Hysterectomy would need to be done at age 32 to prevent 95 % of EC	Consider levonorgestrel IUS until hysterectomy (unproven efficacy). Theoretically COCP might reduce risk of endometrial cancer. However might also increase risk of breast cancer. No data on efficacy	Consider annual outpatient hysteroscopy and endometrial biopsy until has hysterectomy (efficacy unknown)	No	Presents with multiple hamartomas of ectodermal, mesodermal, and endodermal origin
Peutz-Jeghers syndrome											
STK11	Protein kinase	1 in 300,000	Breast (45–50 %), colon (39 %), stomach (29 %), pancreas (11–36 %), small bowel (13 %)	18–21 % (mostly sex cord stromal tumors – usually benign)	General population risk	cervix 10 % (minimal deviation adenocarcinoma)	Not currently recommended	No data available	Annual pelvic examination and cervical smear. Consider annual transvaginal ultrasound[a]	No	1. Sensitivity of cervical smears for adenoma malignum may be less than for cervical intra-epithelial neoplasia 2. In authors' view, surgical prophylaxis for gynecological cancers should be considered on completion of child-bearing

(continued)

Table 27.1 (continued)

Gene mutated	Gene function	General population gene frequency	Associated non-gynecologic cancers/other conditions (male and female)	Ovarian cancer lifetime risk	Endometrial cancer lifetime risk	Other associated gynecologic cancers	Gynecologic surgical prophylaxis and efficacy	Chemo prophylaxis options for gynecologic cancers	Gynecologic surveillance and efficacy	Successful PGD reported	Comment
DICER1 syndrome											
DICER1	Ribonuclease	Rare – not known	Pleuropulmonary blastoma, cystic nephroma, nasal chondromesenchymal hamartoma, ocular medulloepithelioma, familial multinodular goiter	Sertoli Leydig tumors of ovary	General population risk	None	Not reported	Not reported	No guidance available	No	Very rare. No data to justify surgical prophylaxis

dsDNA double stranded DNA, *HR* homologous recombination, *MMR* mismatch repair, *LS* Lynch syndrome, *EC* endometrial cancer, *OC* ovarian cancer, *BC* breast cancer, *PPC* primary peritoneal cancer, *CRC* colorectal cancer, *TVS* transvaginal sonography, *IUS* intra-uterine system, *BSO* bilateral salpingo-oophorectomy, *RRSO* risk reducing bilateral salpingo-oophorectomy, *HNPCC* hereditary non-polyposis colorectal cancer syndrome, *COCP* combined oral contraceptive pill.

[a]Current National Comprehensive Cancer Network® (NCCN) recommendations

Table 27.2 Family history criteria suggestive of an inherited germline mutation causing gynecological cancer

Families with ovarian or ovarian and breast cancer
≥2 individuals with ovarian cancer who are FDR[a]
One ovarian cancer[b] and 1 breast cancer <50 years who are FDR[a]
One ovarian cancer[b] and 2 breast cancers <60 years who are FDR[a]
Breast cancer in proband (≤45 years) and mother with both breast and ovarian cancer[b] (in the same person)
Breast cancer in proband (≤40 years) and sister with both breast and ovarian cancer[b] (in the same person)
Families with Lynch syndrome (HNPCC)
The family contains ≥3 individuals with a HNPCC related cancer[c], who are FDR and ≥1 case is diagnosed before 50 years and the cancers affect ≥1 generation
Families with only breast cancer
≥4 breast cancers
3 breast cancers related by FDR: one ≤30 years, or all ≤40 years, or one MBC and one bilateral breast cancer
Breast cancer in proband (≤50 years) and breast cancer in mother (age of onset being ≤30 years in one and ≤50 years in the other), or bilateral breast cancer in mother (≤40 years onset), or one MBC and one bilateral breast cancer
Two MBC (one <40 years) in the family and proband is a FDR of one of them
Families with AJ ethnicity
AJ ethnicity and any one of the following:
Breast cancer (<40 years) or bilateral breast cancer (first cancer <50 years) in proband, irrespective of family history of cancer
Breast cancer in proband (<50 years) and one FDR with breast cancer (<50 years) or ovarian cancer (any age) or MBC (any age)
Breast cancer in proband (<60 years) and one FDR with breast cancer (<40 years) or ovarian cancer (any age) or MBC (any age)
One FDR with ovarian cancer (<50 years)
FDR with breast and ovarian cancer in the same woman (any age)
Two FDR with breast cancer (<40 years)
Two MBC (<60 years) in the family and proband is a FDR of one of them

FDR first degree relative, *NHPCC* hereditary non-polyposis colorectal cancer, *MBC* male breast cancer, *AJ* Ashkenazi Jewish

[a]Criteria can be modified where paternal transmission is occurring i.e. families where affected relatives are related by second degree through an unaffected intervening male relative and there is an affected sister

[b]NB Tubal and primary peritoneal cancers may be considered equivalent to ovarian cancers

[c]HNPCC related cancers—colorectal, endometrial, ovarian, small bowel, ureteric, renal pelvic

Accurate documentation of the types of cancer in a family and their age of onset is crucial. Where possible cancer registration documents, death certificates or histopathology reports should be obtained. For example, ovarian cancer is reported correctly by family members in only two-thirds of cases [3] and some histological subtypes may not be associated with a genetic cancer predisposition [4]. This information can modify the level of risk. Fabricated family histories have been reported, emphasizing the need to confirm cancer diagnoses [5]. For Lynch syndrome, initial testing is performed on archival tumor samples and these need to be requested. Clinical Genetics services have the infrastructure for obtaining cancer documentation and tumor samples. Surgeons involved in managing women at high risk should liaise closely with them. This is a rapidly evolving field and it is likely that current guidelines on who can be offered genetic testing will be broadened.

27.3 Management Options

For women whose high-risk status is confirmed, the principal management option is risk-reducing surgery (Table 27.1). The decision to undergo surgery will be influenced by a woman's age, menopausal status and fertility wishes as well as her cancer risk [6]. Women wishing to delay surgery or those who decline surgery altogether, may wish to undergo cancer screening. Currently, no form of gynecological cancer screening has been shown to reduce mortality in high-risk families [7, 8]. If screening is performed, the woman and her clinicians need to be aware of the significant limitations and the possibility of psychological distress [9] and surgery for false-positive results [7]. Lifestyle modifications may affect risk, but should not be relied on to prevent cancer in high-risk women.

27.4 Risk-Reducing Surgery

Risk-reducing surgery is surgery to prevent the occurrence of a specific type of cancer in at-risk women. The term 'risk-reducing' is preferred to 'prophylactic' as it correctly implies that not all cancers can be prevented. In the case of risk-reducing salpingo-oophorectomy (RRSO) for women at risk of *BRCA1* and *BRCA2* mutation-associated tubal and ovarian cancer, RRSO cannot prevent primary peritoneal cancer. RRSO may reduce (but not eliminate) the risk of breast cancer when performed before natural menopause.

Health-care professionals and women considering surgery should understand that risk-reducing surgery is being offered to prevent future ill-health, not to treat an established problem. As cancer penetrance is incomplete, cancer may never develop even if surgery is not performed. There are no tests which can accurately predict whether a woman will go on to develop cancer or not, even if she is high-risk. Once she has understood her risk level she needs to balance this against the risk of surgical complications. Fortunately, the majority of women considering risk-reducing surgery are young and fit.

The types of risk-reducing surgery offered depends on which cancer(s) a woman is at risk of developing (Table 27.1):

- Risk-reducing salpingo-oophorectomy (RRSO) is offered to women at significantly increased risk of ovarian cancer (OC) and fallopian tube cancer (FTC), including BRCA1 and 2 mutation-carriers
- Risk-reducing hysterectomy and bilateral salpingo-oophorectomy (RR-HBSO) is offered to women at significantly increased risk of endometrial (EC) and OC, including women with Lynch syndrome mutations.

27.5 Occult Cancers Detected as a Result of Risk-Reducing Surgery

Women undergoing risk-reducing surgery must be informed of the possibility of finding an occult cancer. This risk can be minimized by obtaining a transvaginal ultrasound and serum CA125 prior to RRSO, and in addition an endometrial biopsy prior to RR-HBSO. However, normal results cannot completely exclude an occult OC, FTC, peritoneal or other cancer (e.g. metastatic BC). All women should be counseled pre-operatively that if an occult cancer is found, further surgery and/or chemotherapy may be necessary. Confirmation of any abnormality found at surgery depends on accurate histopathology and a second procedure will usually be needed to stage an occult cancer. Converting to a full ovarian cancer staging procedure at the time of RRSO would be a major undertaking for which women would be ill-prepared. For this reason, the authors prefer to mention the possibility of a second operation if an occult cancer is found, rather than proceed to staging surgery at the time of RRSO. The occult cancer risk depends on age and gene-status. The highest risk is for BRCA gene carriers (BRCA1 > BRCA2), and the lowest in younger women of unknown mutation status [6]; women should be counseled accordingly.

The SEE-FIM histopathology protocol [10] for analysis of tubes and ovaries is mandatory to avoid missing an occult cancer or tubal intra-epithelial carcinoma (TIC), and avoid under-treatment. TIC or small invasive tubal lesions can be missed due to diathermy artifact. A surgical protocol to minimize this possibility has been described [11]. Peritoneal washings are mandatory, as they can affect staging of any occult FTC/OC, and could indicate occult PPC [12]. Furthermore, finding an occult cancer or TIC in a woman of unknown mutation status may facilitate gene-testing.

27.6 Primary Peritoneal Cancer

Women undergoing RRSO must be warned about the future risk of Primary Peritoneal Cancer (PPC). Women who develop symptoms suggestive of PPC should seek urgent referral for investigation. As the histopathological appearances of high-grade serous cancers are similar whether they originate in the ovary, tube or peritoneum, women who develop PPC may be concerned that their RRSO was inadequate. The risk of subsequent PPC is highest for BRCA mutation-carriers. This risk may be less than previously thought, as in some older studies fallopian tubes were not removed and occult cancers may not have been identified on histopathology.

27.7 Timing of Surgery

Once risk-reducing surgery is offered, the decision about when it should be performed can be complex because of the infertility and premature menopause it induces in younger women. However, delaying surgery risks development of OC/FTC/EC. Whilst premenopausal RRSO can reduce subsequent BC risk in BRCA1/2 mutation-carriers, delaying RRSO until after natural menopause does not [13].

Surgery is only appropriate once a woman's family is complete, but young women may seek advice about RRSO before this. In BRCA1 mutation-carriers, delaying RRSO beyond 40 years is associated with a rising risk of developing OC/FTC. The age of onset of OC/FTC in BRCA2 mutation-carriers is later, and the penetrance lower than in BRCA1-carriers, so surgery may be delayed until after 40 year. Efforts should be made to offer genetic testing in a family if a woman's mutation status is unknown prior to RRSO. If this is not possible then a decision about timing needs to be made depending upon the strength of her family history. Lynch and Cowden syndrome carriers may delay surgery until after 40 years, again because of the age of onset of the endometrial cancers and the lower penetrance for OC in Lynch syndrome.

The absolute annual risk of developing OC in BRCA carriers (Table 27.3) [14] helps guide timing of surgery.

The benefit of RRSO on BC risk is well-established in women undergoing surgery under 50 years [13]. This issue is not relevant if risk-reducing mastectomies (RRM) are performed, as this reduces BC risk by 90–95 %. Taking HRT until the age of natural menopause does not negate BC risk-reduction following RRSO [13]. Women should not be dissuaded from taking HRT unless they have had BC.

Table 27.3 Annual % incidence of ovarian cancer in mutation-carriers according to age

Age group (year)	BRCA1-carrier	BRCA2-carrier
20–24	0.001	0.001
25–29	0.002	0.002
30–34	0.18	0.004
35–39	0.28	0.01
40–44	0.87	0.08
45–49	1.49	0.14
50–54	0.96	0.60
55–59	1.19	0.75

Adapted from Antoniou et al. [14]

27.8 Hormonal Considerations

HRT compliance may influence timing as surgical menopause can cause significant physical and psychological symptoms. HRT is most likely to alleviate symptoms, and to reduce the detrimental effects of premature menopause on bone strength, cardiovascular health and possibly cognitive function. Nevertheless, women undergoing RRSO must be aware that there is no guarantee that all symptoms will be alleviated by HRT, nor future medical problems prevented. Whilst RRSO results in reduced all-cause mortality in BRCA1 and also possibly BRCA2 mutation-carriers [15] median follow-up in this study was only 3.65 years. This mortality benefit might reduce over time, if RRSO increases osteoporosis or cardiovascular risks.

Women dissatisfied with HRT should be encouraged to try different doses or preparations. The following points should be considered:

- Low dose preparations are not licensed for bone-protection and generally should not be used after premenopausal RRSO.
- Transdermal HRT is associated with a lower risk of thrombosis than oral HRT.
- In studies of postmenopausal HRT, progestogens were associated with an increased BC risk compared with estrogen-only HRT [16]. Consequently, women at increased risk of BC may prefer the progestogenic component via the levonorgestrel intra-uterine system (IUS). This provides lower plasma levels than oral/transdermal progestogens. The IUS does not increase general population BC-risk [17] but data from the high-risk population is lacking. This issue must be discussed prior to RRSO, which provides the ideal opportunity for safe IUS insertion.

- There are a variety of non-hormonal treatments for menopausal symptoms and bone and cardiovascular protection, but HRT remains the most effective treatment for symptoms.

Current guidelines [18] suggest giving HRT to BRCA1/2 mutation-carriers with prior BC is contraindicated even in triple-negative tumors. Referral to specialist menopause clinicians for symptomatic BC patients should be considered. Use of Low-dose HRT should be discussed with the breast oncologist if quality of life is significantly affected by symptoms despite non-hormonal treatments.

27.9 Surgical Considerations

The benefits of any surgical procedure must outweigh the risks. This is particularly important with risk-reducing surgery, which is being done to prevent future ill-health.

Answering the following questions should guide decision-making:

1. Is cancer risk high enough to justify surgery?
2. Has this risk been confirmed through medical records/genetic testing where possible?
3. Are there comorbidities or previous operations which increase surgical risk?
4. Given the above, is the woman statistically less likely to come to harm if she undergoes surgery than if she does not undergo surgery?

Questions 1 and 2 are best answered by the Clinical Genetics team, especially when risk-reducing surgery is contemplated for a woman of unknown mutation status. The surgeon should liaise with the genetics team if their risk assessments differ (e.g. because the family history has changed).

27.10 Patient-Specific Factors

Laparoscopic RRSO in a young, fit, thin patient with no prior abdominal surgery can usually be achieved successfully with minimal risk of complications, and is frequently a day-case procedure. However, patient-specific factors may increase surgical risk to a point where surgery should not be offered:

1. Significant comorbidities: pre-operative assessment by an experienced anesthetist is necessary before deciding to proceed.
2. Surgical challenge: Obesity can make clearing bowel loops from the pelvis difficult, as can abdomino-pelvic adhesions. These cannot be assumed because a patient has undergone prior surgery. An experienced laparoscopic surgeon can often safely deal with significant adhesions without laparotomy. Patients who have undergone hysterectomy with ovarian conservation can pose a challenge, because the adnexae can be densely adherent to adjacent structures and adhesions may obscure anatomy.

All women undergoing risk-reducing surgery via a planned laparoscopic approach must be consented for possibility laparotomy, both immediate (in the event of technical difficulties/intra-operative complications) or delayed (in the event of late-presenting complications). Early discharge following laparoscopic surgery will depend on adequate home support, patient understanding of how they should be recovering and when to seek medical advice. Discharge should be backed-up with written information e.g. the Royal College of Obstetricians and Gynaecologists 'Recovering well' leaflet [19].

27.11 Type of Surgical Intervention

As with all surgery, it is prudent to perform the least invasive procedure possible to achieve the desired aims (in this case, exclusion of occult malignancy and prevention of future malignancy). For women at risk of OC/FTC only, RRSO is all that is required and hysterectomy should only be performed for benign gynecological pathology which cannot be managed by non-surgical treatments (e.g. large symptomatic fibroids). Hysterectomy is associated with a greater risk of complications compared with RRSO alone. The authors do not consider avoidance of progestogens in women requiring HRT post RRSO, nor prevention of uterine malignancy in women taking tamoxifen, as valid indications for prophylactic hysterectomy. The latter risk in BRCA-carriers is estimated to be only 2 % [20], and may in reality be lower, as recently aromatase inhibitors have been used in preference to tamoxifen following RRSO.

Proven family history or germline mutations associated with Lynch Syndrome are indications for hysterectomy. Recent data on EC penetrance in Cowden syndrome [21] suggests that hysterectomy may be justifiable for this much rarer syndrome. OC risk is not increased in Cowden syndrome, and the ovaries (but not the tubes) should be conserved if the woman is undergoing premenopausal hysterectomy. This decision should take age into account, as ovarian preservation in a woman >47 years [22] is unlikely to confer any hormonal benefit. Asking about menopausal age in blood-relatives can be helpful as this is heritable [23].

Hysterectomy should wherever possible be performed via the laparoscopic route as this facilitates obtaining peritoneal washings (see section on occult cancers) and complete removal of tubes and ovaries, which can be difficult via the vaginal route. Uterine morcellation for large uteri is acceptable providing endometrial pathology is excluded pre-operatively.

The risk of endometrial cancer is not significantly increased in *BRCA1* and *BRCA2* mutation-carriers unless they have taken tamoxifen [20]. Nevertheless, dilation and curettage (D + C) at the time of surgery is recommended to rule out occult endometrial pathology. This is particularly relevant in women with endometrial hyperplasia/cancer risk from tamoxifen and obesity. D + C is a low risk procedure, and is unlikely to be associated with uterine perforation. Hysteroscopy is not generally necessary at the time of RRSO; there is no evidence it improves detection of occult neoplasia compared with D + C alone.

27.12 Thromboprophylaxis Considerations

All patients undergoing risk-reducing surgery should be considered for peri-operative thromboprophylaxis including low molecular weight heparin. A minority will have an occult cancer and some will have taken tamoxifen. Tamoxifen is associated with increased thrombosis risk and so should be stopped 6 weeks prior to surgery [24]. When laparotomy or hysterectomy is performed, restarting tamoxifen should be delayed and low molecular weight heparin prophylaxis continued for up to 28 days. It may be appropriate for women to be switched from tamoxifen to an aromatase inhibitor following RRSO. This should be discussed with their oncologist.

27.13 Lifestyle Modifications

Epidemiological protective-factors for OC include multiparity, breast-feeding, combined oral contraceptive pill (COCP) use and tubal ligation. Neither sterilization nor having children should be advocated purely to reduce OC risk but it can be helpful for women to know that these may reduce OC risk. High-risk women considering tubal ligation should be aware that resulting adhesions could render subsequent RRSO more challenging and increase the risk of complications. If she does not wish to undergo oophorectomy as a risk-reduction measure at the time of sterilization, laparoscopic salpingectomy can be offered. This would be expected to prevent tubal cancer in BRCA1/2 mutation-carriers [25].

The COCP confers an increased BC risk in the general population and in BRCA1/2 mutation-carriers. This risk returns to baseline 10 years after ceasing usage. The risk needs to be balanced against the following points: (1) the COCP is a reliable and convenient form of contraception. (2) BRCA1/2 mutation-carriers have a high lifetime BC risk and are offered breast screening from 30 year [24]. (3) Data on COCP since 1975 have not proven an increased BC risk in BRCA1/2 carriers [26], but this remains a concern. (4) The COCP offers significant reduction in OC/EC risk. Nevertheless the COCP should not be offered solely for OC prevention if a BRCA1/2 carrier is likely to undergo RRSO. Women should be informed of the advantages and disadvantages of the COCP so they can decide if they want to use it for contraception.

Other modifiable risk-factors include lack of physical activity, obesity, and smoking. Clearly, avoidance of these offers other health benefits. Data on the use of perineal talc as an OC risk-factor is conflicting, but it is easily avoided.

None of the above environmental or reproductive factors affect OC risk to the level of carrying a predisposing mutation. Consequently, lifestyle modifications cannot be considered an equivalent alternative to RRSO.

Conclusion

Inherited gene mutations define a group of women at risk of specific gynecological cancers. Identifying such women can be challenging, but affords opportunities for effective cancer prevention in women and their blood-relatives. Risk-reducing surgery requires complex decision-making. It needs to be timed appropriately for the woman's age-dependent risk level, taking into account her fertility wishes and willingness to take HRT. Surgical procedures should take into account the types of cancer from which the woman is at risk. Screening cannot currently be recommended as a safe alternative to risk-reducing surgery. Use of the oral contraceptive pill, breastfeeding and a healthy lifestyle may reduce the risk of inherited gynecological cancers, but only surgery is guaranteed to prevent them.

Key Points

- Germline mutations that predispose to gynecological cancer are inherited in an autosomal dominant pattern with incomplete penetrance.
- The gynecological cancers they cause tend to occur at earlier ages than sporadic cancers occurring in the general population.
- Obtaining accurate documentation of cancers in the family is crucial to risk-assessment
- Not all histological subtypes of gynecological cancers are inherited.
- Currently gene testing is offered to unaffected family members only after a causative mutation is found in an affected relative. As the cost of sequencing falls, testing criteria will broaden.
- If no affected relative is available for genetic testing, calculating an individual's statistical risk on the basis of their family history is sufficient for guiding management.
- To date, no form of gynecological cancer screening in any high-risk population has been shown to reduce mortality and risk-reducing surgery is the most effective preventative measure.
- Risk-reducing surgery for BRCA1/2-carriers and breast/ovarian cancer families must include salpingectomy as well as oophorectomy (Risk Reducing Salpingo-Oophorectomy—RRSO), peritoneal washings and strict pathology protocols.
- Risk-reducing surgery in Lynch syndrome should include hysterectomy as well as RRSO, but hysterectomy is not usually offered in BRCA1/2-carriers and breast/ovarian cancer families.
- HRT should be given until the age of natural menopause if risk-reducing surgery is undertaken premenopausally, except in women who have breast cancer. The benefit of premenopausal RRSO on subsequent breast cancer risk is retained even with HRT.

References

1. Sagi M, Weinberg N, Eilat A, Aizenman E, Werner M, Girsh E, Siminovsky Y, Abeliovich D, Peretz T, Simon A, Laufer N. Preimplantation genetic diagnosis for BRCA1/2–a novel clinical experience. Prenat Diagn. 2009;29:508–13.
2. Audeh MW, Carmichael J, Penson RT, Friedlander M, Powell B, Bell-McGuinn KM, Scott C, Weitzel JN,

Oaknin A, Loman N, Lu K, Schmutzler RK, Matulonis U, Wickens M, Tutt A. Oral poly(ADP-ribose) polymerase inhibitor olaparib in patients with BRCA1 or BRCA2 mutations and recurrent ovarian cancer: a proof-of-concept trial. Lancet. 2010;376:245–51.
3. Soegaard M, Jensen A, Frederiksen K, Høgdall E, Høgdall C, Blaakaer J, Kjaer SK. Accuracy of self-reported family history of cancer in a large case-control study of ovarian cancer. Cancer Causes Control. 2008;19:469–79.
4. Lakhani SR, Manek S, Penault-Llorca F, Flanagan A, Arnout L, Merrett S, McGuffog L, Steele D, Devilee P, Klijn JG, Meijers-Heijboer H, Radice P, Pilotti S, Nevanlinna H, Butzow R, Sobol H, Jacquemier J, Lyonet DS, Neuhausen SL, Weber B, Wagner T, Winqvist R, Bignon YJ, Monti F, Schmitt F, Lenoir G, Seitz S, Hamman U, Pharoah P, Lane G, Ponder B, Bishop DT, Easton DF. Pathology of ovarian cancers in BRCA1 and BRCA2 carriers. Clin Cancer Res. 2004;10:2473–81.
5. Kerr B, Foulkes WD, Cade D, Hadfield L, Hopwood P, Serruya C, Hoare E, Narod SA, Evans DG. False family history of breast cancer in the family cancer clinic. Eur J Surg Oncol. 1998;24:275–9.
6. Manchanda R, Abdelraheim A, Johnson M, Rosenthal AN, Benjamin E, Brunell C, Burnell M, Side L, Gessler S, Saridogan E, Oram D, Jacobs I, Menon U. Outcome of risk-reducing salpingo-oophorectomy in BRCA carriers and women of unknown mutation status. BJOG. 2011;118:814–24.
7. Rosenthal AN, Fraser L, Manchanda R, Badman P, Philpott S, Mozersky J, Hadwin R, Cafferty FH, Benjamin E, Singh N, Evans DG, Eccles DM, Skates SJ, Mackay J, Menon U, Jacobs IJ. Results of annual screening in the UK familial ovarian cancer screening study (UK FOCSS phase 1) highlight need for strict adherence to screening schedule. J Clin Oncol. 2013;31:49–57.
8. Manchanda R, Saridogan E, Abdelraheim A, Johnson M, Rosenthal AN, Benjamin E, Brunell C, Side L, Gessler S, Jacobs I, Menon U. Annual outpatient hysteroscopy and endometrial sampling (OHES) in HNPCC/Lynch syndrome (LS). Arch Gynecol Obstet. 2012;286:1555–62.
9. Brain KE, Lifford KJ, Fraser L, Rosenthal AN, Rogers MT, Lancastle D, Phelps C, Watson EK, Clements A, Menon U. Psychological outcomes of familial ovarian cancer screening: no evidence of long-term harm. Gynecol Oncol. 2012;127:556–63.
10. Crum CP, Drapkin R, Miron A, Ince TA, Muto M, Kindelberger DW, Lee Y. The distal fallopian tube: a new model for pelvic serous carcinogenesis. Curr Opin Obstet Gynecol. 2007;19:3–9.
11. Manchanda R, Silvanto A, Abdelraheim A, Burnell M, Johnson M, Saridogan E, Rosenthal AN, Brunell C, Aslam N, Vashisht A, Pandis G, Jacobs I, Menon U, Benjamin E. Diathermy-induced injury may affect detection of occult tubal lesions at risk-reducing salpingo-oophorectomy. Int J Gynecol Cancer. 2012;22(5):881–8.
12. Manchanda R, Drapkin R, Jacobs I, Menon U. The role of peritoneal cytology at risk-reducing salpingo-oophorectomy (RRSO) in women at increased risk of familial ovarian/tubal cancer. Gynecol Oncol. 2012;124:185–91.
13. Eisen A, Lubinski J, Klijn J, Moller P, Lynch HT, Offit K, Weber B, Rebbeck T, Neuhausen SL, Ghadirian P, Foulkes WD, Gershoni-Baruch R, Friedman E, Rennert G, Wagner T, Isaacs C, Kim-Sing C, Ainsworth P, Sun P, Narod SA. Breast cancer risk following bilateral oophorectomy in BRCA1 and BRCA2 mutation carriers: an international case-control study. J Clin Oncol. 2005;23:7491–6.
14. Antoniou A, Pharoah PD, Narod S, Risch HA, Eyfjord JE, Hopper JL, Loman N, Olsson H, Johannsson O, Borg A, Pasini B, Radice P, Manoukian S, Eccles DM, Tang N, Olah E, Anton-Culver H, Warner E, Lubinski J, Gronwald J, Gorski B, Tulinius H, Thorlacius S, Eerola H, Nevanlinna H, Syrjäkoski K, Kallioniemi OP, Thompson D, Evans C, Peto J, Lalloo F, Evans DG, Easton DF. Average risks of breast and ovarian cancer associated with BRCA1 or BRCA2 mutations detected in case series unselected for family history: a combined analysis of 22 studies. Am J Hum Genet. 2003;72:1117–30.
15. Domchek SM, Friebel TM, Singer CF, Evans DG, Lynch HT, Isaacs C, Garber JE, Neuhausen SL, Matloff E, Eeles R, Pichert G, Van't Veer L, Tung N, Weitzel JN, Couch FJ, Rubinstein WS, Ganz PA, Daly MB, Olopade OI, Tomlinson G, Schildkraut J, Blum JL, Rebbeck TR. Association of risk-reducing surgery in BRCA1 or BRCA2 mutation carriers with cancer risk and mortality. JAMA. 2010;304:967–75.
16. Beral V, Million Women Study Collaborators. Breast cancer and hormone-replacement therapy in the Million Women Study. Lancet. 2003;362:419–27.
17. Dinger J, Bardenheuer K, Minh TD. Levonorgestrel-releasing and copper intrauterine devices and the risk of breast cancer. Contraception. 2011;83:211–7.
18. Finch A, Evans DG, Narod SA. BRCA carriers, prophylactic salpingo-oophorectomy and menopause: clinical management considerations and recommendations. Womens Health. 2012;8:543–55.
19. Recovering well – information for you after a laparoscopy. https://www.rcog.org.uk/globalassets/documents/patients/patient-information-leaflets/recovering-well/laparoscopy-recovering-well.pdf.
20. Segev Y, Iqbal J, Lubinski J, Gronwald J, Lynch HT, Moller P, Ghadirian P, Rosen B, Tung N, Kim-Sing C, Foulkes WD, Neuhausen SL, Senter L, Singer CF, Karlan B, Ping S, Narod SA, Hereditary Breast Cancer Study Group. The incidence of endometrial cancer in women with BRCA1 and BRCA2 mutations: an international prospective cohort study. Gynecol Oncol. 2013;130:127–31.
21. Riegert-Johnson DL, Gleeson FC, Roberts M, Tholen K, Youngborg L, Bullock M, Boardman LA. Cancer and Lhermitte-Duclos disease are common in Cowden syndrome patients. Hereditary Cancer Clin Pract. 2010;8:6.

22. Moorman PG, Myers ER, Schildkraut JM, Iversen ES, Wang F, Warren N. Effect of hysterectomy with ovarian preservation on ovarian function. Obstet Gynecol. 2011;118:1271–9.
23. Morris DH, Jones ME, Schoemaker MJ, Ashworth A, Swerdlow AJ. Familial concordance for age at natural menopause: results from the Breakthrough Generations Study. Menopause. 2011;18:956–61.
24. Familial breast cancer: classification and care of people at risk of familial breast cancer and management of breast cancer and related risks in people with a family history of breast cancer. National Institute for Health and Care Excellence (NICE) guideline, June 2013. https://www.nice.org.uk/guidance/cg164.
25. Dubeau L. The cell of origin of ovarian epithelial tumours. Lancet Oncol. 2008;9:1191–7.
26. Iodice S, Barile M, Rotmensz N, Feroce I, Bonanni B, Radice P, Bernard L, Maisonneuve P, Gandini S. Oral contraceptive use and breast or ovarian cancer risk in BRCA1/2 carriers: a meta-analysis. Eur J Cancer. 2010;46:2275–84.

Endoscopy in Gynecologic Oncology

28

Roberto Tozzi, Giorgio Fachechi, Kumar Gubbala, Stefano Cianci, Riccardo Garruto Campanile, and Hooman Soleymani Majd

28.1 Introduction

Endoscopic procedures have become an integral part of Gynecology. Some endoscopic devices were designed specifically for/by the gynecologist, and some procedures became quickly popular in the diagnosis and treatment of female benign conditions. The application of the same techniques to patients with malignant conditions was laborious and a significant delay occurred. The first laparoscopic hysterectomy dates back to the 1980s, but it is not until the beginning of the century that a clinical trial was published on the use of laparoscopy in endometrial cancer. Nowadays the use of endoscopy in Gynecologic Oncology is very common. The same surgical techniques performed by laparotomy have been safely and successfully reproduced at laparoscopy fully respecting the principles of cancer surgery. The reduced trauma to the body, the decreased blood loss and the diminished pain induce a faster postoperative recovery and less morbidity. Such profile provides a benefit to oncologic patients often presenting with a complex medical profile and sometime in need of adjuvant treatment. The use of endoscopy in Gynecologic Oncology has been recently sanctioned and encouraged by national and international institutes. Nonetheless the access to endoscopic techniques varies based on the patients, the institutions and the type of disease.

28.2 Cervical Cancer

Introduction

The management of patients with cervical cancer is either surgery or a combination of chemo and radiotherapy. Surgery maintains an important role especially in patients with early-stage and recurrent disease. In patients with locally advanced disease or with spread to the lymph nodes, it is largely accepted that chemoradiation is the first treatment modality, with surgery confined to patients with persistent or recurrent disease. Endoscopy has a clear role in the primary surgical treatment, with the intrinsic benefits provided over a laparotomy. In addition, it

R. Tozzi, MD, PhD (✉)
Department of Gynaecologic Oncology, Oxford Cancer Centre, Oxford University Hospital, Oxford, UK

Department of Gynaecologic Oncology, Oxford University Hospitals, Oxford, Oxfordshire, UK
e-mail: roberto.tozzi@obs-gyn.ox.ac.uk

G. Fachechi, MD • K. Gubbala • S. Cianci, MD
R.G. Campanile, MD
Department of Gynaecologic Oncology, Oxford University Hospitals, Oxford, Oxfordshire, UK

H. Soleymani Majd, MD, MRCOG
Department of Gynaecologic Oncology, Churchill Hospital, Oxford University Hospitals NHS Trust, Oxford, Oxfordshire, UK

H.R.H. Patel et al. (eds.), *Pelvic Cancer Surgery: Modern Breakthroughs and Future Advances*,
DOI 10.1007/978-1-4471-4258-4_28,

may be used to facilitate and tailor the efficacy of the chemoradiation by removing large lymph nodes or detecting microscopic metastasis.

Staging and Re-staging

FIGO staging of patients with cervical cancer is based on a clinical examination, but this has a low sensitivity and specificity. Radiology can enhance staging information. Surgical staging can provide further information to detect spread to the lymph nodes status and adjacent organs. Querleu published the first series on surgical staging in 1991 on 39 patients with early-stage cervical cancer who had laparoscopic pelvic lymphadenectomy for staging purposes [1]. Since this report numerous retrospective studies were published confirming feasibility and safety of a laparoscopic approach. In 2006, Benedetti Panici et al. [2] compared the outcomes of 168 patients who had undergone an open transperitoneal, open extraperitoneal and laparoscopic pelvic lymphadenectomy in a prospective randomized trial. They did not find statistical differences in intraoperative or postoperative complications. Postoperative recovery was faster in the laparoscopic and extraperitoneal groups. Despite a lower lymph node harvest at laparoscopy, the number of nodes was considered adequate. In 2008 Lim et al. [3] published a prospective study of 83 patients with cervical cancer stage IB2-IVA who had a pre-treatment laparoscopic staging. All patients had pelvic and para-aortic lymphadenectomy. Despite a 15.2 % rate of surgery related complications, all patients completed the planned radiotherapy. In 2013 Benedetti Panici et al. [4] reported a series of 167 consecutive patients with local advanced cervical cancer who had laparoscopic staging. Minor laparoscopy complication rate was 1 %. The median overall survival was 65 months. They concluded that laparoscopic staging is a feasible and safe procedure. Marnitz et al. [5] published in 2012 the results of a prospective study. They demonstrated that in patients with early cervical cancer, laparoscopic staging with the use of frozen section of the lymph nodes successfully tailored the treatment. In this study 90 % of the patients had no need for adjuvant treatment. They concluded that surgical staging should be used as routine procedure. In 2011 Ghezzi et al. [6] analyzed the radiation-induced bowel complications following an open or laparoscopic staging for gynecological cancers. Using multiple regression analysis they found an independent protective role of minimal-access surgery. Several cases series [7, 8] have confirmed the utility of a laparoscopic re-staging in patients with incidental finding of early stage cervical cancer following a simple hysterectomy or a sub-total hysterectomy. By means of laparoscopy, lymphadenectomy and radical parametrectomy could be performed for patients with microscopic or macroscopic tumor left behind and for those at risk of parametrial invasion. In 2012 Li et al. [9] reported 28 cases of laparoscopic nerve-sparing parametrectomy, recording two intra-operative complications. After a median follow-up of 38 months, no recurrences were recorded.

Fertility-Sparing Surgery

Fertility sparing surgery can be performed for patients with cervical cancer FIGO stage Ib1 and a tumor size less than 2 cm. Laparoscopy is used to perform the lymphadenectomy prior to a radical vaginal trachelectomy, or to perform a fully laparoscopic radical trachelectomy. Radical trachelectomy removes the cervix, the inner aspect of the parametrium and the upper third of the vagina, but retains the body of the uterus. In 2010 Kim et al. [10] reported 27 cases of laparoscopic radical trachelectomy. Six patients required transfusions, but no further complications were reported. After a median follow-up of 31 months there was one recurrence with death from disease. In 2013, Ebisawa et al. [11] evaluated obstetrical outcomes of a series of 56 patients treated with laparoscopic radical trachelectomy. They reported a pregnancy rate of 52 %, with 13 live births. Preterm premature rupture of membranes was the most common complication.

Radical Hysterectomy and Nerve-Sparing Surgery

Radical hysterectomy remains the standard of treatment for patients with stage 1bi cervical cancer. Feasibility and safety of a laparoscopic approach to radical hysterectomy is now well accepted.

Park retrospectively compared the survival and surgical outcomes of 115 laparoscopic radical hysterectomy (LRH) vs 118 open radical hysterectomy (ORH) in patients with stage IB2 to IIA2 [12]. Conversion to laparotomy occurred in two patients. There were no differences in 5-years disease-free survival (78 % vs. 77 %) and 5-years overall survival (83 % in both groups). However the estimated blood loss, length of hospital stay, time to recover bowel movement and postoperative complications favored the patients in the LRH group.

In 2004 Steed et al. [13] compared perioperative morbidity and recurrence-free survival between 71 patients treated with laparoscopic-assisted radical vaginal hysterectomy and 205 patients with radical abdominal hysterectomy. They demonstrated similar clinical outcomes but less intra-operative blood loss and shorter hospital stay in the laparoscopic group. They reported more intraoperative complications however (13 % vs. 4 %).

Hertel et al. [14] reported their experience of 200 patients operated by a laparoscopic assisted radical vaginal hysterectomy. Major intra and post-operative complications rates were 6 and 8 %, respectively. Overall 5-years survival was 83 %, but in patients with stage Ib1 and no risk factors (L0V0N0), it was as high as 98 %.

In 2012 Nam et al. [15] compared in a retrospective study, 263 ORH with 263 LRH for patients with early-stage cervical cancer. No differences in overall survival or disease free survival were found. LRH group had a shorter postoperative hospital stay and a lower estimated blood loss. Although intraoperative complication rates were similar, postoperative complication rates were less in LRH group.

Pellegrino et al. [16] published in 2009 the results of a prospective study on the surgical and clinical outcomes of 107 patients who underwent a total laparoscopic hysterectomy for stage Ib1. Conversion to laparotomy occurred in six patients. Two patients had minor intraoperative complications, while five patients needed a second surgical procedure for a postoperative complication. After a median period of follow up of 30 months, they reported 11 recurrences and a survival rate of 95 %.

In 2010 Naik et al. [17] published the first randomized phase II trial comparing laparoscopic vs abdominal radical hysterectomy. Although they reported outcomes of only 13 patients, the study confirms benefits of laparoscopic approach in terms of blood loss, hospital stay and analgesic requirement.

Traditionally radical hysterectomy is associated with a 5–10 % neurogenic bladder dysfunction, namely reduced perception of fullness, impaired urge and weakened voiding capacity. These side effects are caused by injury of the pelvic splanchnic nerves and the inferior hypogastric plexus during the dissection and resection of parametrium. Since 2000, when Possover et al. [18] described the first series of nerve-sparing radical hysterectomy, papers have confirmed the efficacy of the laparoscopic technique (LNSRH) in identifying and sparing these sympathetic and parasympathetic pelvic nerves. In 2010 Liang et al. [19] compared 82 LNSRH with 81 LRH. They reported less urinary complications in LNSRH group. After a median follow up of 22.3 months no recurrences were recorded. In 2011 Park et al. [20] in a retrospective study evaluated 125 consecutive LNSRH. They reported 13 urological complications, but they concluded that LNSRH is a feasible technique.

Pelvic Exenteration

Anterior, posterior or total exenteration is performed in selected patients with recurrent cervical cancer following radical radiotherapy. Surgery is aborted due to the presence of unresectable disease in up to 45 % of patients. An explorative laparoscopy has proved useful in the assessment of these patients, minimizing the number of patients whose exenterative surgery is abandoned [21].

Other authors have reported on a laparoscopic technique to perform pelvic exenteration for patients with cervical cancer [22, 23], demonstrating feasibility and safety of the technique. However due to the small numbers of the patients included in the studies, the oncological outcome remains to be proven.

Robotic Surgery

In the last few years, the use of robotic surgery in gynecology oncology has become more common. Several studies were published comparing different techniques of radical hysterectomy, including robotic. In 2008 Magrina et al. [24] in a case control study, compared robotic radical hysterectomy (RRH) to laparoscopy and to laparotomy. They reported 27 cases of robotic surgery. There were no significant differences in intra- or postoperative complications among the three groups, but in patients with minimal invasive surgery the blood loss and hospital stay were reduced compared to laparotomy. Similar results were obtained by Maggioni et al. [25] in a case control study. In 2008 Boggess et al. [26] compared 51 robotically assisted radical hysterectomies with 49 open radical hysterectomies. There were significant differences in blood loss, operative time and number of nodes removed in favor of the robotic group. They also reported 7.8 % vs. 16.3 % postoperative complications respectively. In an interesting review [27] Kruijdemberg et al. compared 342 robotic radical hysterectomies vs. 943 laparoscopic radical hysterectomies. They reported fewer blood transfusions in the robotic group, but a higher rate of major postoperative complications (9.6 % vs. 5.5 %). In 2013 Chong et al. [28] compared 50 consecutive robotic NSRH with a cohort of 50 LNSRH. They found that blood loss and intraoperative complication rate were significantly lower in robotic surgery. Similar results are reported from other case series [29, 30].

Robotic surgery has been used in trachelectomy also. Nick et al. [31] compared 25 open vs 12 robotic radical trachelectomy, showing similar morbidities but less blood loss and hospitalization in the robotic group. Personn et al. [32] demonstrated similar results comparing robotic trachelectomy vs. vaginal trachelectomy. Initial case reports or small series have also reported the use of robotic surgery in patients with advanced and recurrent cervical cancer.

In 2010 Lambaudie et al. [33] compared robotic vs. laparoscopy vs. laparotomy in staging of locally advanced cervical cancer. Complication rate was similar, as was the recurrence rate.

Lim et al. [34] in 2009 reported the first case of robotic pelvic exenteration for a recurrent cervical cancer with an ileal loop urinary diversion. Davis et al. [35] and Lambaudie et al. [36] published in 2010 two other small series of robotic anterior pelvic exenteration. The numbers are very small but the expansion of robotic surgery will enable more surgeons to use endoscopic surgery and abandon the traditional laparotomy.

Single Port Surgery

Single port surgery (SPS) has been reported very little in the treatment of patients with cervical cancer. In 2010 Hahn and Kim [37] reported two cases of single port laparoscopic pelvic lymph nodes dissection with a modified vaginal hysterectomy in patients with stage IA2.

Conclusions

The use of endoscopic surgery in the treatment of patients with cervical cancer has been supported by a large number of studies. Although no phase III clinical trial has been published so far, the safety and efficacy of the technique is beyond doubt and the oncologic outcomes appear equivalent to open surgery. Endoscopy delivers significant benefits for patients with cervical cancer.

28.3 Ovarian Cancer

Introduction

Ovarian cancer remains the most common cause of death from a gynecological malignancy [38]. The high lethality is due to the common presentation of advanced stage disease (75 % present with

FIGO stage 3–4). Patients with early stage display a median 90 % 5 year survival rate.

Ovarian cancer can be assessed and treated by laparotomy, laparoscopy and robotic surgery. Again, laparoscopy and robotic surgery offer multiple advantages due to the smaller incisions—less need for postoperative analgesics, quicker recovery, shorter hospital stay and a lower risk of complications such as infections, blood loss, wound infection, ileus and incisional hernias. Laparoscopy has been found to reduce the risk of post-operative incisional hernia. The reported incidence of incisional hernia through the 10/12 mm laparoscopic trocar site is 3 % [39] compared to 16.9 % following a midline laparotomy for a gynecological oncology procedure [40].

Port site recurrence has been a concern. In a study by Zivanovic, the port site recurrence rate was 1.96 % following laparoscopy for ovarian, fallopian tube or primary peritoneal cancer [41].

Primary Ovarian Cancer: Early Stage

As much as 30 % of women with apparent early stage disease have microscopic metastasis [42, 43]. Full staging of presumed early stage disease provides important prognostic information. In case of patients whose disease is upstaged, there is a recommendation for adjuvant chemotherapy. When stage I disease is confirmed, no chemotherapy is required, and in young women a fertility sparing treatment can be offered. Early stage disease can be upstaged due to microscopic tumor deposits in the omentum, pelvic and/or para-aortic lymph nodes and contra-lateral ovarian involvement.

Upstaging can occur due to intra-operative mass rupture leading to contamination of the peritoneal cavity with tumor cells. Whilst only retrospective data are provided on the prognostic effect [44], mass rupture changes the stage from potential IA to IC, with the immediate implication that chemotherapy will be prescribed in patients otherwise requiring no adjuvant treatment [45, 46]. The risk of intraoperative mass rupture is also present at laparotomy but seems to be increased by a laparoscopic approach. In view of this, laparoscopy may be more suitable for restaging procedures following a primary removal of the ovary at a previous operation. There is no risk of intraoperative mass rupture since the tumor has already been removed.

A further concern with endoscopy in ovarian cancer is that spread and implantation of ovarian cancer cells may be facilitated during laparoscopy by the CO_2 under pressure. This may be the reason for port site metastases [47, 48]. A large retrospective series has identified port-site metastasis in 20 of 1,694 patients (1.18 %) with malignant intraperitoneal disease undergoing laparoscopy. Fifteen of the 20 patients with port-site metastases had a diagnosis of fallopian tube or ovarian cancer, but only 2 patients had early stage ovarian cancer [41]. In order to reduce the risks when employing laparoscopy for the management of patients with early stage ovarian cancer there should be adequate surgical expertise, meticulous technique with limited tissue manipulation and the use of an endobag for tissue extraction.

Despite these concerns, the use of laparoscopy in early stage ovarian cancer is increasing, and data supports this development. Brookbank demonstrated 94 % 5 years disease free survival and a 100 % overall survival at a median 18 months (range 3–59) follow-up [49]. The rate of conversion to laparotomy in the literature is averagely below 5 %, with a range 3.2–10 % [50].

Robotic surgery has been used in early stage ovarian cancer. A recent study matched 25 robotic cases of epithelial ovarian cancer staging with 27 laparoscopic and 119 open cases. All patients were operated on during the same period and the groups were matched by age, BMI, type, and number of procedures done. Compared with open surgery, the robotic and laparoscopic groups had a decreased hospital stay. No difference in outcomes was reported between robotic and laparoscopic surgery. Survival was also unaffected by surgical approach [51].

Advanced Stage

Laparoscopy in patients with advanced disease has limited application. It can be used to confirm a suspected diagnosis, but this is increasing performed by radiologically guided biopsy. A second application is to predict whether cytoreductive surgery is possible. However, small volume abdominal disease may be missed at laparoscopy, particularly in areas like the small bowel and the mesentery.

The use of laparoscopy in cytoreduction in patients with presumed stage 3 primary ovarian cancer has been reported [52]. Patients had CT evidence of omental metastasis and ascites. Twenty-three cases (92 %) were successfully cytoreduced without conversion to laparotomy. Median operative time was 2.3 h and median blood loss was 340 ml. All tumors were debulked to less than 2 cm and 36 % had no residual disease.

Recurrent Ovarian Cancer

A retrospective analysis by Magrina on 52 selected patients with recurrent ovarian cancer undergoing secondary cytoreduction by laparoscopy, laparotomy or robotics was performed between January 2006 and December 2010 [51]. Robotics and laparoscopy provided similar perioperative outcomes, such as reduced blood loss and shorter hospital stay as compared to laparotomy. The comment of the author was that use of robotics is preferable when all recurrent disease can be excised without redocking and need of additional trocars. In addition it was most suitable for isolated recurrences particularly in the diaphragms, liver, peri-rectal area, and in the pelvis. Laparoscopy was preferable in the presence of limited disease and when redocking would be necessary. Laparotomy seemed preferable for patients with widespread peritoneal implants, multiple sites of recurrence, and/or extensive adhesions.

Conclusion

There is evidence to support the use of endoscopic surgery in early stage ovarian cancer management without compromising survival. Its use in advanced disease is less established with far fewer reported studies. Most studies have supported the equivalence of robotic surgery and laparoscopy in many perioperative outcomes. Some studies suggest that robotic surgery may have advantages over laparoscopy in the learning curve required to perform complex gynecological oncology procedures. However, this is entirely dependent on the surgeon and the final outcomes seem to be unchanged between laparoscopy and robotic.

28.4 Endometrial Cancer

Introduction

Endometrial cancer is the third most common cancer in women accounting for 6–9 % of all cancers in female patients [53–55]. The standard treatment for patients with early-stage endometrial cancer is surgery with a total hysterectomy (TH) and bilateral salpingo-oophorectomy with or without pelvic and para-aortic lymph node resection based on risk factors [56, 57]. A midline laparotomy has been the traditional route of choice for extended surgery with lymph node removal. However, patients with endometrial cancer frequently present with co-morbidities such as obesity, diabetes and cardio-vascular disease. The morbidity associated with a laparotomy can be substantial in this group of patients, especially with regards to infection, wound dehiscence, thrombosis and embolism [58]. The most validated alternative approach for patients with early endometrial cancer is laparoscopy. Several prospective controlled studies showed that total laparoscopic (TLH) was an effective, minimally invasive, safe alternative to total abdominal hysterectomy (TAH) for benign indications [59, 60].

Through the PubMed, EMBASE, CBM and Cochrane Review databases, eight randomized trials were found assessing the effects of TLH versus TAH in women with early-stage endometrial cancer [61–68]. A total of 3,644 women were enrolled in these trials with 2,286 women randomized to laparoscopic surgery and 1,358 randomized to laparotomy. First trial published was Fram in 2002 with 61 patients with stage I endometrial cancer. Twenty-nine patients were treated with laparoscopic assisted vaginal hysterectomy (LAVH) and bilateral salpingo-oophrectomy (BSO) ± laparoscopic pelvic lymphadenectomy (LPLA), while 32 patients were treated with the traditional laparotomy and underwent total abdominal hysterectomy (TAH) and BSO ± pelvic lymphadenectomy (PLA). Despite the limited number of patients, laparoscopic surgery was associated with less blood loss and shorter hospitalization but with longer operative time.

The multicenter randomized trial conducted by Janda (LACE, 2010) enrolled 361 patients. Although the operative time was longer in the TLH group than in the TAH group (138 min vs. 109 min; $p=0.001$), similar intra-operative adverse events were documented (TAH 5.6 % vs. TLH 7.4 % $p=0.53$); postoperatively, twice as many patients in the TAH group experienced adverse events of grade 3 or higher (23.2 % vs. 11.6 % in the TLH group; $p=0.004$). Postoperative serious adverse events occurred more in the TAH group (27 of 142 [19.0 %]) than in the TLH group (16 of 190 [7.9 %]; $p=0.002$).

Primary endpoints of Malzoni et al. in 2009 were the disease-free survival and recurrence rate. With similar surgical outcomes, laparoscopic surgery did not compromise the degree of oncological radicality required with reduced convalescence and discomfort. The disease free survival and recurrence rate were similar in both groups.

Mourits et al. in 2010 designed a multi-center trial with 21 hospitals recruiting in the Netherlands. They randomized 281 patients with stage I endometrioid adenocarcinoma or complex atypical hyperplasia. The study investigated the complication rate of TLH versus TAH showing no major differences between the two groups (major complications was 14.6 %, 27 of 185 in the TLH group versus 14.9 %, 14 of 94 in the TAH group). The patients in the TLH group were associated with significantly less blood loss, reduced use of pain medication, a shorter hospital stay ($p<0.0001$), and a faster recovery.

Tozzi et al. in 2005 published an analysis of their randomized trial commenced in 1995 with 122 patients. They identified Body Mass Index (BMI), age >65 years, weight >80 kg and one out of diabetes, hypertension, cardio-respiratory failure to be predictive of complications but a multivariate analysis identified the surgical technique (laparoscopy vs. laparotomy) to be the only significant risk factor for complications.

The largest trial so far, the GOG LAP 2 reported by Walker et al., was conducted in the US including more than 2,500 patients. Feasibility and efficacy of laparoscopic technique was compared to laparotomy. They also published 6 years recurrence and survival rates demonstrating that laparoscopy was not inferior to laparotomy: recurrence rate was 11.4 % vs. 10.2 % and overall survival (89.8 %) was the same. Quality of life (QoL) was the primary endpoint for the trial designed by Zullo et al. published in 2005 with 84 patients recruited in the study. A further long term data published in 2009 confirmed that laparoscopy provided significant benefits compared to laparotomy in terms in QoL. Survival outcomes were not different.

In the last few years robotic-assisted surgery has emerged as another minimally invasive approach for the treatment of patients with endometrial cancer. The largest series from Yu et al. [69] with 2,247 patients (median age 64 years) analyzed the utilization and hospital charges associated with robotic (RS) versus laparoscopic (LS) and open surgery (OS) in endometrial cancer patients. Median hospital stay for the RS and LS group was 1.6 compared to 3.9 days for the OS group. The hospital charge for RS was $51,569 compared to $36,492 for OS ($P<0.001$), with theater's charges ($22,600 vs. $11,272) accounting for the major difference. Coronado et al. [70] in his retrospective series enrolled 347 patients. Operative time was longer in the laparoscopy group as compared to robotics and laparotomy (218.2, 189.2, and 157.4 min respectively). Similar findings were observed for the pre- and post-operative outcomes. On the other hand the length of hospital stay was longer in the laparotomy group compared to robotics and laparoscopy (8.1, 3.5 and 4.6 days respectively). The conversion rate to laparotomy was lower for robotics (2.4 % for robotics and 8.1 % for laparoscopy, $p=0.181$). Overall complications were similar for robotics and laparoscopy (21.1 %, 28.5 %, $p=0.079$). Robotic complications were significantly lower as compared to laparotomy (21.2 vs 34.9 %, p = 0.036). No differences were found with respect to disease-free or overall survival among the three groups. The global costs were similar for the three approaches (p = 0.566). This study would possibly support the use of robotic surgery against laparoscopy.

Peiretti et al. [71] in 2009 published a series of 80 patients with early endometrial cancer during the introduction of robotic surgery. They observed a substantial change in their surgical activity. Open surgical procedures decreased from 78 to 35 % confirming that age, obesity and previous surgeries did not seemed to be a contraindication to robotic surgery. These last data would support the use of robotic surgery. However there are still areas of controversy surrounding this technology including the paucity of randomized controlled trials, long-term efficacy data, and cost-effectiveness research.

The most recent addition to the surgical portfolio of options for patients with endometrial cancer is the Single Port (SP) surgery. Fagotti [72] has reported, in a multicenter retrospective series, the first 100 cases undergoing SP surgery. Patients were all diagnosed with early stage endometrial cancer. Total hysterectomy and BSO were performed in all patients, whilst 75 patients underwent to pelvic and para-aortic lymphadenectomy. Blood loss and operative time were greater when lymphadenectomy was performed. Although this technique, has proved to be effective and safe only few reports are available and more data are required.

Conclusion

The role of endoscopic surgery is well established in the treatment of patients with endometrial cancer. Data from retrospective and prospective studies, including randomized trials, have conclusively demonstrated the superiority of endoscopy over laparotomy. Survival outcome is unaffected but morbidity is reduced. Whether robotic or single port approaches are superior to traditional laparoscopy is yet to be established.

References

1. Querleu D, Leblanc E, Castelain B. Laparoscopic pelvic lymphadenectomy in the staging of early carcinoma of the cervix. Am J Obstet Gynecol. 1991; 164(2):579–81.
2. Panici BP, Plotti F, Zullo MA, Muzii L, Manci L, et al. Pelvic lymphadenectomy for cervical carcinoma: laparotomy extraperitoneal, transperitoneal or laparoscopic approach? A randomized study. Gynecol Oncol. 2006;103(3):859–64.
3. Lim MC, Bae J, Park JY, Lim S, Kang S, Seo SS, Kim JY, Rho JW, Park SY. Experiences of pretreatment laparoscopic surgical staging in patients with locally advanced cervical cancer: results of a prospective study. J Gynecol Oncol. 2008;19(2):123–8.
4. Benedetti Panici P, Perniola G, Tomao F, Fischetti M, Savone D, Di Donato V, Angioli R, Muzii L. An update of laparoscopy in cervical cancer staging: is it a useful procedure? Oncology. 2013;85(3):160–5.
5. Marnitz S, Kohler C, Affonso RJ, Schneider A, Chiantera V, Tsounoda A, Vercellino F. Validity of laparoscopic staging to avoid adjuvant chemoradiation following radical surgery in patients with early cervical cancer. Oncology. 2012;83:346–53.
6. Ghezzi F, Cromi A, Serati, Uccella S, Formenti G, Bogani G, Vanoli P. Radiation-induced bowel complications: laparoscopic versus open staging of gynecologic malignancy. Ann Surg Oncol. 2011;18:782–91.
7. Kholer C, Tozzi R, Klemm P, et al. "Schuata sine utero" technique and results of laparoscopical-vaginal parametrectomy. Gynecol Oncol. 2003;91:359–68.
8. Buda A, Pellegrino A, Vitobello D, Meroni MG, Recalcati D, Perego P. Total laparoscopic radical parametrectomy, partial colpectomy, and pelvic lymphadenectomy in patients with occult cervical cancer. Int J Gynaecol Obstet. 2009;107(1):73–6.
9. Li J, Xu H, Chen Y, Wang D, Li Y, Liang Z. Laparoscopic nerve-sparing radical parametrectomy for occult early-stage invasive cervical cancer after simple hysterectomy. Int J Gynecol Cancer. 2012;22(8): 1383–8.
10. Kim IH, Park JY, Kim DY, et al. Fertility-sparing laparoscopic radical trachelectomy for young women with early stage cervical cancer. BJOG. 2010;117(3):340–7.
11. Ebisawa K, Takano M, Fukuda M, Fujiwara K, Hada T, Ota Y, Kurotsuchi S, Kanao H, Andou M. Obstetric outcomes of patients undergoing total laparoscopic radical trachelectomy for early stage cervical cancer. Gynecol Oncol. 2013;131:83–6.
12. Park JY, Kim DY, Kim JH, Kim YM, Kim Y, Nam JH. Laparoscopic versus open radical hysterectomy in patients with stage IB2 and IIA2 cervical cancer. J Surg Oncol. 2013;108(1):63–9.
13. Steed H, Rosen B, Murphy J, Laframboise S, De Petrillo D, Covens A. A comparison of laparascopic-assisted radical vaginal hysterectomy and radical abdominal hysterectomy in the treatment of cervical cancer. Gynecol Oncol. 2004;93:588–93.

14. Hertel H, Kohler C, Michels W, Possover M, Tozzi R, Schneider A. Laparoscopic-assisted radical vaginal hysterectomy (LARVH): prospective evaluation of 200 patients with cervical cancer. Gynecol Oncol. 2003;90:505–11.
15. Nam JH, Park JY, Kim DY, Kim JH, Kim JM, Kim YT. Laparoscopic versus open radical hysterectomy in early-stage cervical cancer: long-term survival outcomes in a matched cohort study. Ann Oncol. 2012;93:903–11.
16. Pellegrino A, Vizza E, Fruscio R, Villa A, Corrado G, et al. Total laparoscopic radical hysterectomy and pelvic lymphadenectomy in patients with Ib1 stage cervical cancer: analysis of surgical and oncological outcome. Eur J Surg Oncol. 2009;35(1):98–103.
17. Naik R, Jackson K, Lopes A, Cross P, Henry J. Laparoscopic assisted radical vaginal hysterectomy versus radical abdominal hysterectomy-a randomised phase II trial: perioperative outcomes and surgical-pathological measurements. BJOG. 2010;117:746–51.
18. Possover M, Stöber S, Plaul K, Schneider A. Identification and preservation of the motoric innervation of the bladder in radical hysterectomy type III. Gynecol Oncol. 2000;79(2):154–7.
19. Liang Z, Chen Y, Xu H, Li Y, Wang D. Laparoscopic nerve-sparing radical hysterectomy with fascia space dissection technique for cervical cancer: description of technique and outcomes. Gynecol Oncol. 2010; 119(2):202–7.
20. Park NY, Chong GO, Hong DG, Cho YL, Park IS, Lee YS. Oncologic results and surgical morbidity of laparoscopic nerve-sparing radical hysterectomy in the treatment of FIGO stage IB cervical cancer: long-term follow-up. Int J Gynecol Cancer. 2011;21(2):355–62.
21. Koler C, Tozzi R, Possover M, Schneider A. Explorative laparoscopy prior to exenterative surgery. Gynecol Oncol. 2002;86(3):311–5.
22. Martínez A, Filleron T, Vitse L, Querleu D. Laparoscopic pelvic exenteration for gynaecological malignancy: is there any advantage? Gynecol Oncol. 2011;120:374–9.
23. Puntambekar S, Kudchadkar RJ, Gurjar AM, Sathe RM, Chaudhari YC, Agarwal GA, Rayate NV. Laparoscopic pelvic exenteration for advanced pelvic cancers: a review of 16 cases. Gynecol Oncol. 2006;102(3):513–6.
24. Magrina JF, Kho RM, Weaver AL. Robotic radical hysterectomy: comparison with laparoscopy and laparotomy. Gynecol Oncol. 2008;109(1):86–91.
25. Maggioni A, Minig L, Zanagnolo V, Peiretti M, Sanguineti F, Bocciolone L, Colombo N, Landoni F, Roviglione G, Vélez JI. Robotic approach for cervical cancer: comparison with laparotomy: a case control study. Gynecol Oncol. 2009;115(1):60–4.
26. Boggess JF, Gehrig PA, Cantrell L, Shafer A, Ridgway M, Skinner EN, Fowler WC. A case-control study of robot-assisted type III radical hysterectomy with pelvic lymph node dissection compared with open radical hysterectomy. Am J Obstet Gynecol. 2008;199(4):357.
27. Kruijdenberg CBM, Van Den Einden LCG, Hendriks JCM, Zusterzeel PLM, Bekkers RLM. Robot-assisted versus total laparoscopic radical hysterectomy in early cervical cancer, a review. Gynecol Oncol. 2011;120(2011):334–9.
28. Chong GO, Lee YH, Hong DG, Cho YL, Park IS, Lee YS. Robot versus laparoscopic nerve-sparing radical hysterectomy for cervical cancer: a comparison of the intraoperative and perioperative results of a single surgeon's initial experience. Int J Gynecol Cancer. 2013;23(6):1145–9.
29. Magrina JF, Pawlina W, Kho RM, Magtibay PM. Robotic nerve-sparing radical hysterectomy: feasibility and technique. Gynecol Oncol. 2011;121(3): 605–9.
30. Gil-Ibáñez B, Díaz-Feijoo B, Pérez-Benavente A, Puig-Puig O, Franco-Camps S, Centeno C, Xercavins J, Gil-Moreno A. Nerve sparing technique in robotic-assisted radical hysterectomy: results. Int J Med Robot. 2013;9(3):339–44.
31. Nick AM, Frumovitz MM, Soliman PT, Schmeler KM, Ramirez PT. Fertility sparing surgery for treatment of early-stage cervical cancer: open vs. robotic radical trachelectomy. Gynecol Oncol. 2012;124(2):276–80.
32. Persson J, Imboden S, Reynisson P, Andersson B, Borgfeldt C, Bossmar T. Reproducibility and accuracy of robot-assisted laparoscopic fertility sparing radical trachelectomy. Gynecol Oncol. 2012;127: 484–8.
33. Lambaudie E, Narducci F, Bannier M, Jauffret C, Pouget N, Leblanc E, Houvenaeghel G. Role of robot-assisted laparoscopy in adjuvant surgery for locally advanced cervical cancer. Eur J Surg Oncol. 2010;36(4):409–13.
34. Lim PC. Robotic assisted total pelvic exenteration: a case report. Gynecol Oncol. 2009;115(2):310–1.
35. Davis MA, Adams S, Eun D, Lee D, Randall TC. Robotic-assisted laparoscopic exenteration in recurrent cervical cancer Robotics improved the surgical experience for 2 women with recurrent cervical cancer. Am J Obstet Gynecol. 2010;202(6):663.
36. Lambaudie E, Narducci F, Leblanc E, Bannier M, Houvenaeghel G. Robotically-assisted laparoscopic anterior pelvic exenteration for recurrent cervical cancer: report of three first cases. Gynecol Oncol. 2010;116(3):582–3.
37. Hahn HS, Kim YW. Single-port laparoscopic pelvic lymph node dissection with modified radical vaginal hysterectomy in cervical cancer. Int J Gynecol Cancer. 2010;20(8):1429–32.
38. Cancer Research UK. Ovarian cancer statistics 2009. http://info.cancerresearchuk.org.
39. George JP. Presentation and management of laparoscopic incisional hernias. J Am Assoc Gynecol Laparosc. 1994;1:S12.
40. Franchi M, Ghezzi F, Buttarelli M, Tateo S, Balestreri D, Bolis P. Incisional hernia in gynaecologic oncology patients: a 10 year study. Obstet Gynecol. 2001;97: 696–700.
41. Zivanovic O, Sonoda Y, Diaz JP, Levine DA, Brown CL, et al. The rate of port-site metastases after 2251 laparoscopic procedures in women with underlying malignant disease. Gynecol Oncol. 2008;111:431–7.

42. Young RC, Decker DG, Wharton JT, et al. Staging laparotomy in early ovarian cancer. J Am Med Assoc. 1983;250:3072–6.
43. Soper JT, Johnson P, Johnson J, Berchuk A, Clarke-Pearson DL. Comprehensive restaging laparotomy in women with apparent early ovarian carcinoma. Obstet Gynecol. 1992;80:949–53.
44. Vergote I, De Brabanter I, Fyles A, Bertelsen K, Einhorn N, Sevelda P, et al. Prognostic importance of degree of differentiation and cyst rupture in stage I invasive epithelial ovarian carcinoma. Lancet. 2001; 357:176–82.
45. Sevelda P, Dittrich C, Salzer H. Prognostic value of the rupture of the capsule in stage I epithelial ovarian carcinoma. Gynecol Oncol. 1989;35:321–2.
46. Dembo AJ, Davy M, Stenwig AE, Berle EJ, Bush RS, Kjorstad K. Prognostic factors in patients with stage I epithelial ovarian cancer. Obstet Gynecol. 1990;75:263–72.
47. Wenzl R, Lehner R, Husslein P, Sevelda P. Laparoscopic surgery in cases of ovarian malignancies: an Austria-wide surgery. Gynecol Oncol. 1996;63:57–61.
48. Canis M, Rabischong B, Botchorishvili R, Tamburro S, Wattiez A, Mage G, et al. Risk of spread of ovarian cancer after laparoscopic surgery. Curr Opin Obstet Gynecol. 2001;13:9–14.
49. Brockbank EC, Harry V, Kolomainen D, Mukhopadhyay D, Sohaib A, Bridges JE, Nobbenhuis MA, Shepherd JH, Ind TE, Barton DP. Laparoscopic staging for apparent early stage ovarian or fallopian tube cancer. First case series from a UK cancer centre and systematic literature review. Eur J Surg Oncol. 2013;39(8):912–7.
50. Schreuder HW, Pattij TO, Zweemer RP, van Baal MW, Verheijen RH. Increasing experience in laparoscopic staging of early ovarian cancer. Gynecol Surg. 2012;9(1):89–96.
51. Magrina JF, Zanagnolo V, Noble BN, et al. Robotic approach for ovarian cancer: perioperative and survival results and comparison with laparoscopy and laparotomy. Gynecol Oncol. 2011;121:100–5.
52. Fanning J, Yacoub E, Hojat R. Laparoscopic-assisted cytoreduction for primary advanced ovarian cancer: success, morbidity and survival. Gynecol Oncol. 2011;123:47–9.
53. Jemal A, Siegel R, Xu J, Ward E. Cancer statistics, 2010. CA Cancer J Clin. 2010;60:277–300.
54. Jemal A, Bray F, Center MM, Ferlay J, Ward W, Forman D. Global cancer statistics. CA Cancer J Clin. 2011;61:69–90.
55. Rowlands IJ, Weinstein P, Nagle CM, et al. Season of birth and risk of endometrial cancer. Asian Pac J Cancer Prev. 2011;12:1193–6.
56. El-Nashar SA, Mariani A. Uterine carcinosarcoma. Clin Obstet Gynecol. 2011;54:292–304.
57. Salani R, Backes FJ, Fung MF, et al. Posttreatment surveillance and diagnosis of recurrence in women with gynecologic malignancies: society of Gynecologic Oncologists recommendations. Am J Obstet Gynecol. 2011;204:466–78.
58. Manchana T. Long-term lower urinary tract dysfunction in gynecologic cancer survivors. Asian Pac J Cancer Prev. 2011;12:285–8.
59. Carter JR. Laparoscopy or laparotomy for endometrial cancer? A review of three prospective randomised trials. Aust N Z J Obstet Gynaecol. 2011;51:387–92.
60. Frumovitz M, Escobar P, Ramirez PT. Minimally invasive surgical approaches for patients with endometrial cancer. Clin Obstet Gynecol. 2011;54:226–34.
61. Fram KM. Laparoscopically assisted vaginal hysterectomy versus abdominal hysterectomy in stage I endometrial cancer. Int J Gynecol Cancer. 2002; 12(1):57–61.
62. Janda M, Gebski V, Brand A, Hogg R, Jobling TW, Land R, et al. Quality of life after total laparoscopic hysterectomy versus total abdominal hysterectomy for stage I endometrial cancer (LACE): a randomised trial. Lancet Oncol. 2010;11(8):772–80.
63. Malzoni M, Tinelli R, Consentino F, Perone C, Rasile M, Iuzzolino D, et al. Total laparoscopic hysterectomy vs. abdominal hysterectomy with lymphadenectomy for early stage endometrial cancer: a prospective randomized study. Gynecol Oncol. 2009;112:126–33.
64. Tozzi R, Malur S, Koehler C, Schneider A. Laparoscopy versus laparotomy in endometrial cancer: first analysis of survival of a randomized prospective study. J Minim Invasive Gynecol. 2005;12(2):130–6.
65. Walker JL, Piedmonte M, Spirtos N, Eisenkop S, Schlaerth JB, Mannel RS, Spiegel G, Barakat R, Pearl ML, Sharma SK. Laparoscopy compared with laparotomy for comprehensive surgical staging of uterine cancer: Gynecologic Oncology Group Study LAP2. J Clin Oncol. 2009;27:5331–6.
66. Mourits MJ, Bijen CB, Arts HJ, Ter Brugge HG, Van der Sidje R, Paulsen L, et al. Safety of laparoscopy versus laparotomy in early-stage endometrial cancer: a randomised trial. Lancet Oncol. 2010;11(8):763–71.
67. Zorlu CG, Simsek T, Seker AE. Laparoscopy or laparotomy for the management of endometrial cancer. J Soc Laparoendosc Surg. 2005;9:442–6.
68. Zullo F, Palomba S, Falbo A, Russo T, Mocciaro R, Tartaglia E, et al. Laparoscopic surgery vs laparotomy for early stage endometrial cancer: long-term data of a randomized controlled trial. Am J Obstet Gynecol. 2009;200(3):e1–9.
69. Yu X, Lum D, Kiet TK, Fuh KC, Orr J, Brooks RA, Ueda SM, Chen LM, Kapp DS, Chan JK. Utilization of and charges for robotic versus laparoscopic versus open surgery for endometrial cancer. J Surg Oncol. 2013;107(6):653–8.
70. Coronado PJ, Herraiz MA, Magrina JF, Fasero M, Vidart JA. Comparison of perioperative outcomes and cost of robotic-assisted laparoscopy, laparoscopy and laparotomy for endometrial cancer. Eur J Obstet Gynecol Reprod Biol. 2012;165(2):289–94.
71. Peiretti M, Zanagnolo V, Bocciolone L, Landoni F, Colombo N, et al. Robotic surgery: changing the surgical approach for endometrial cancer in a referral cancer center. J Minim Invasive Gynecol. 2009;16(4):427–31.
72. Fagotti A, Boruta DM, Scambia G, Fanfani F, Paglia A, Escobar PF. First 100 early endometrial cancer cases treated with laparoendoscopic single-site surgery: a multicentric retrospective study. Am J Obstet Gynecol. 2012;206(4):353.e1–6.

Sentinel Lymph Node Mapping for Endometrial Cancer

29

Nadeem R. Abu-Rustum

29.1 Mapping Techniques

Radioactive Tracer ^{99m}Tc

Radiolabeled colloid, typically the metastable nuclear isomer of technetium-99, symbolized as ^{99m}Tc, is used for sentinel lymph node (SLN) detection [1]. After intracervical injection, colloid enters the lymphatic capillaries and is transported with lymph to SLNs. There are particles of different size, and size affects the quickness and intensity of spread in the lymphatic system. Smaller particles, less than 50 nm, show quick transport to secondary nodes. This radioactive tracer partly enters the systematic circulation and is caught by the reticuloendothelial system (liver and spleen). Different radiopharmaceuticals are registered for use in lymphoscintigraphy in the Unites States, Europe, and Asia.

Doses and Timing of Application

In "long" protocols, radiocolloid is injected 20–24 h before surgery. Doses that are used in these "long" protocols are higher by 2.0–4 mci (74–148 MBq) because half-time of degradation is 6 h, and after 24 h we measure only residual activity. "Short" protocols are used more often. In "short" protocols, radiocolloid is injected 2–4 h before surgery and lymphoscintigraphy is performed 20–30 min after injection. The usual doses are between 0.2 and 1.0 mci (7.4–37 MBq).

Technique of Application

Different administration techniques of the colloid have been reported via the cervical injection route: all these require a **submucosal** (superficially-subepithelial) injection of 0.1–1.0 ml volume.

Stroma of the cervix (10–15 mm deep—slow injection from the deepest point of needle to the subepithelial point, in 1–2 ml volume) is usually reserved to colored dye injections. The injection is given directly into the cervix using a needle with a small diameter: the 22 G Potocky needle (Cooper Surgical), or a spinal needle can be used. Injections at the 3 and 9 o'clock positions are the most common injection sites at our institution (Fig. 29.1).

29.2 Lymphoscintigraphy

A preoperative planar lymphoscintigram is obtained after the injection (Fig. 29.2). Two series of pictures are obtained: immediate "dynamic images" and subsequent "static

N.R. Abu-Rustum, MD, FACOG, FACS
Gynecology Service, Department of Surgery,
Memorial Sloan Kettering Cancer Center,
New York, NY, USA
e-mail: abu-rusn@mskcc.org

H.R.H. Patel et al. (eds.), *Pelvic Cancer Surgery: Modern Breakthroughs and Future Advances*,
DOI 10.1007/978-1-4471-4258-4_29, © Springer-Verlag London 2015

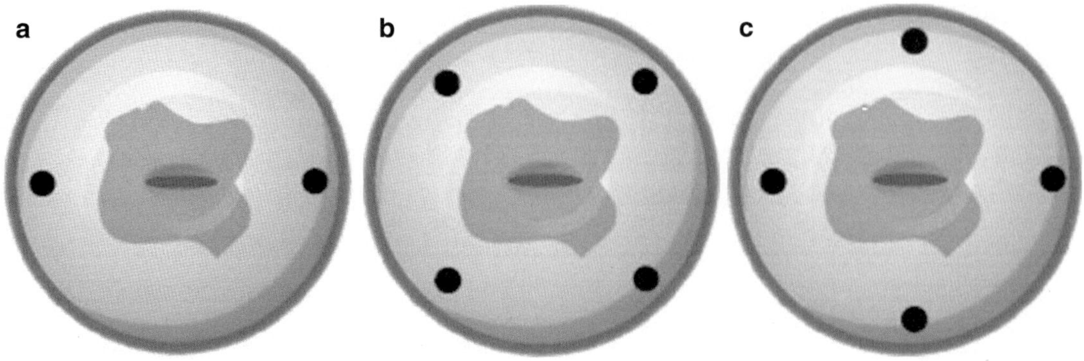

Fig. 29.1 Three different options for direct cervical injection: four-quadrant options (**b**, **c**) and a two-sided option (**a**) (Courtesy Abu-Rustum NR, Rob L. Atlas of Procedures in Gynecologic Oncology, 2013)

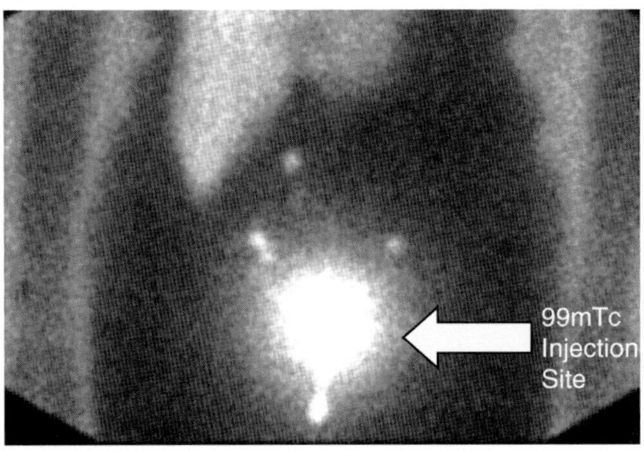

Fig. 29.2 Lymphoscintigraphy. A preoperative planar lymphoscintigram in a 70-year-old woman with endometrial serous cancer is obtained after the cervical injection

images" to localize the nodes. Some departments prefer single-photon emission computed tomography (SPECT/CT), which allows for enhanced three-dimensional localization of "hot" nodes.

29.3 Colored Dye

Several commercially available colored dyes are available throughout the world (Fig. 29.3a–d). The technique of cervical application is the same as the application of radioactive tracer. A spinal needle or Potocky needle is used to inject a total of 2–4 ml of blue dye directly into the cervical submucosa and stroma. A tenaculum can be used to assist in the stromal injection (Fig. 29.4). The injections can be given at the 3 and 9 o'clock positions, which correspond more to the parametria and avoid blue dye staining of the bladder flap secondary to the 12 o'clock injection. It is paramount to apply the blue Dye very slowly, at a rate of 5–10 s for each quadrant. After the injection, the patient is prepped and draped in the usual sterile fashion.

Some of the adverse effects of isosulfan blue or Patente blue include allergic reactions (<1 % of patients). Examples of such include localized swelling and pruritus of the hands, feet, abdomen, and neck. Severe reactions, including edema of the face and glottis, respiratory distress, and shock, have been occasionally reported with other similar compounds. In some instances, isosulfan blue can cause a transient drop in oxygen saturation as measured by the anesthesiologist's pulse oximetry. Blue dyes will turn the urine blue-green for up to 24 h following injection. Contraindications include known hypersensitivity to these compounds.

The injection of isosulfan blue (Lymphazurin®) (Fig. 29.3a), Methylene Blue (Fig. 29.3b) or Patente–Blue (Blue Patente V sodique®) (Fig. 29.3c), or ICG (Fig. 29.3d) is given in the operating room at the time of the examination while the patient is under anesthesia. Isosulfan blue is a sterile aqueous solution packaged in 5 ml vials. No preparation is needed, and it can be stored at room temperature. Patente–Blue 2.5 % is a sterile solution that comes in 2 ml vials and is often diluted in 2 ml of Saline solution. Methylene blue is available in 10 ml vials

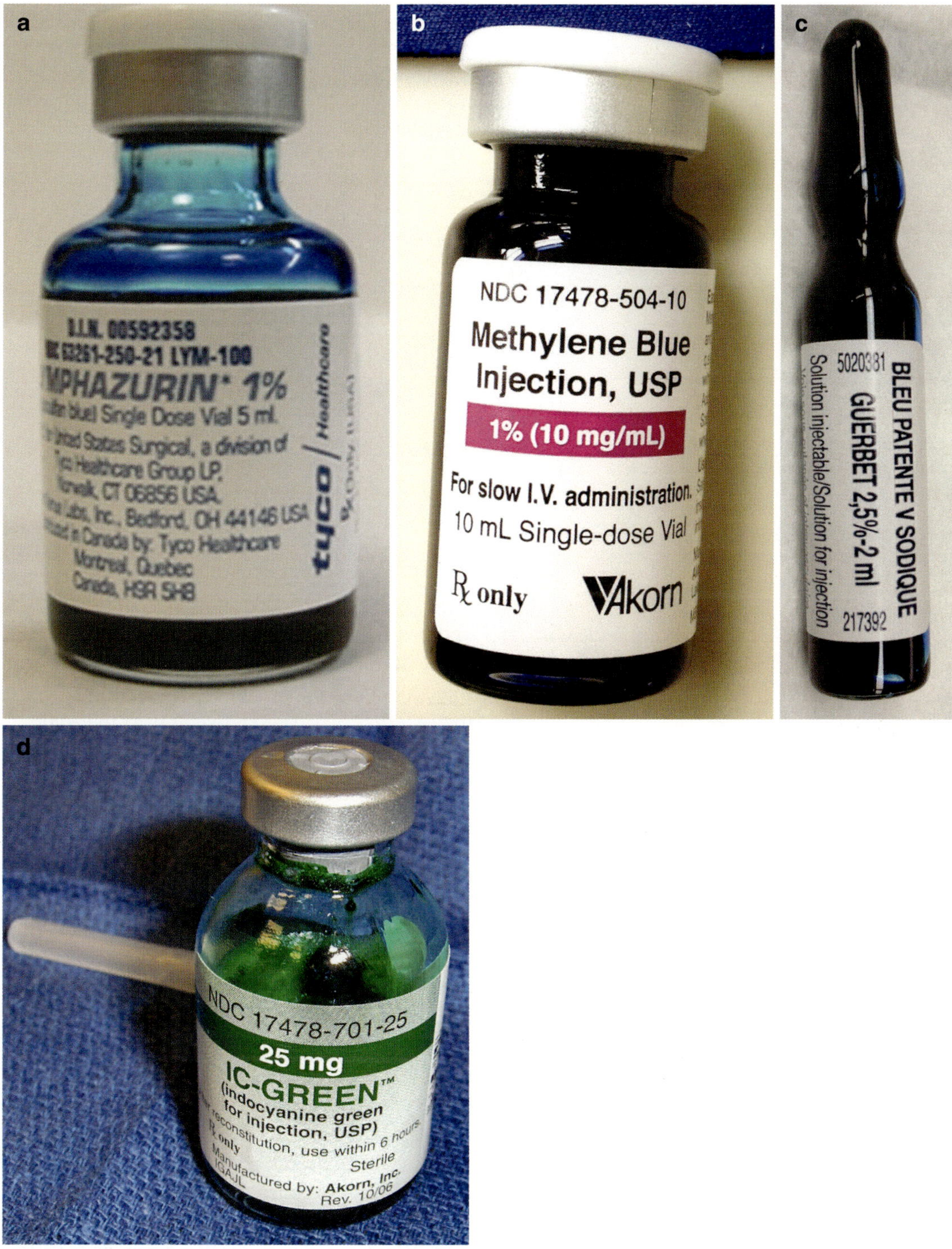

Fig. 29.3 (**a–d**) Isosulfan blue 1 %, methylene blue 1 %, patente blue 2.5 % sodium, and indocyanine green (ICG)

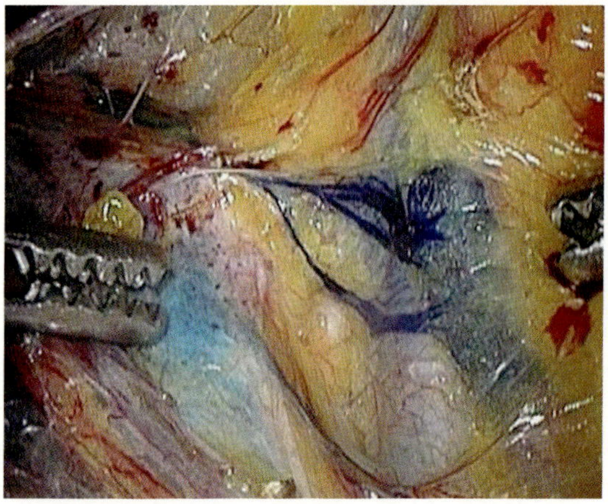

Fig. 29.4 Shows a blue right sentinel external iliac lymph node using methylene blue; blue channels can be seen leading to the lymph node

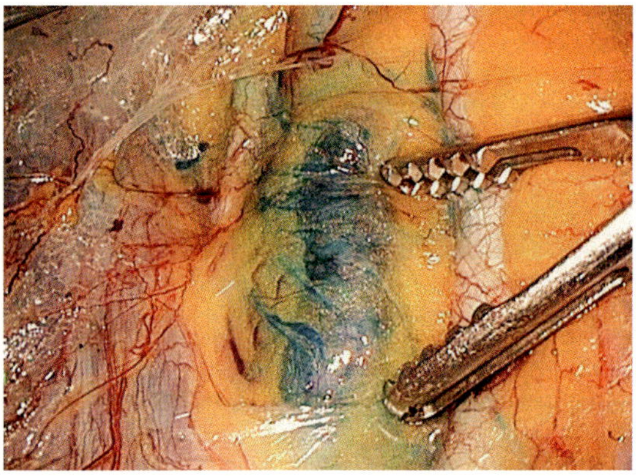

Fig. 29.5 Shows blue lymphatic channels leading into a right external iliac sentinel lymph node

at 10 mg/ml and can be injected without any preparation or dilution. ICG recently emerged as a very useful and safe dye for interstitial cervical injection and requires a near-infrared camera for visualization. ICG comes in a 25-mg dry powder vial and is mixed with 10–20 ml of sterile water in a 25-mg vial, and up to 5 mg is used directly into the cervix as well.

Figure 29.4 shows a blue right sentinel external iliac lymph node using Methylene Blue; blue channels can be seen leading to the lymph node. Figure 29.5 shows a blue right external lymph node using Isosulfan blue. Figure 29.6 shows blue lymphatic channels from the left parametria

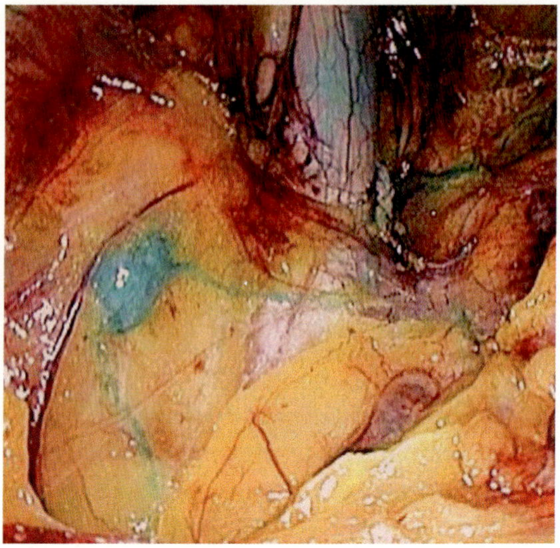

Fig. 29.6 Shows afferent and efferent blue lymphatic channels with a blue left external iliac sentinel lymph node medial to the iliac artery

and broad ligament leading to a blue SLN in the left external iliac region. Following a cervical injection, most pelvic SLNs are located medial to the external iliac vessels, ventral to the internal iliac system, and in the superior part of the obturator space.

29.4 Discussion

The optimal technique of SLN mapping in uterine corpus cancer continues to be the subject of much debate. A cervical, hysteroscopic, and a fundal serosal injection can be utilized [2]. The cervical injection is described above, and although it may not appear rational to some surgeons to only inject the dye into the cervix when dealing with uterine cancer, it has been repeatedly demonstrated that a superficial and deep injection into the uterine cervix provides excellent dye penetration to the region of the uterine vessels and main lymphatic trunks that condenses in the parametria in the majority of cases (Fig. 29.7). The cervical injection technique is easy to utilize and has gained more acceptance in recent years. The combination of a superficial (1–3 mm) and deep (1–2 cm) cervical injection can lead to dye delivery to the main

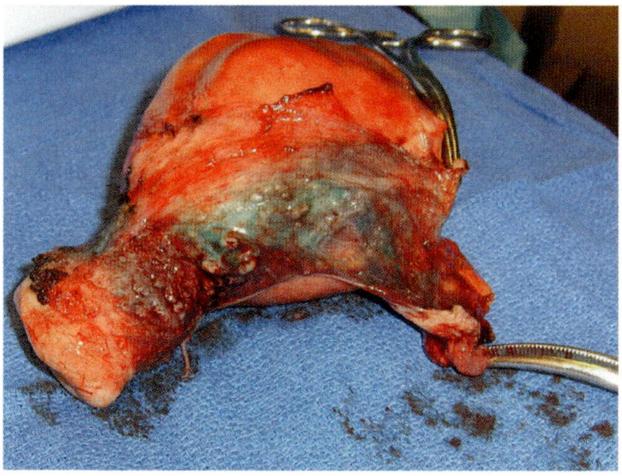

Fig. 29.7 Sentinel lymph node mapping for uterine cancer. A superficial and deep injection into the uterine cervix provides excellent dye penetration to the region of the uterine vessels and main lymphatic trunks that condenses in the parametria in the majority of cases

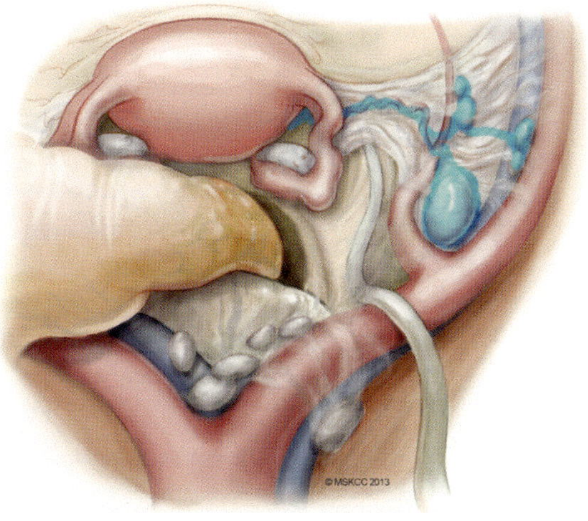

Fig. 29.8 Most common mapping topography following cervical injection of dye (©2013, Memorial Sloan Kettering Cancer Center)

three layers of lymphatic channel origins in the cervix and corpus, namely the superficial subserosal, intermediate stromal, and deep submucosal lymphatic sites of origin [3, 4]. The dye commonly condenses around the parametria and appears in the main lymph trunks in the broad ligament and parametria and leads to pelvic and occasionally paraaortic nodes. Figure 29.8 demonstrates the most common location of SLNs after a cervical injection. Figure 29.9 demonstrates a less common location, usually seen when the

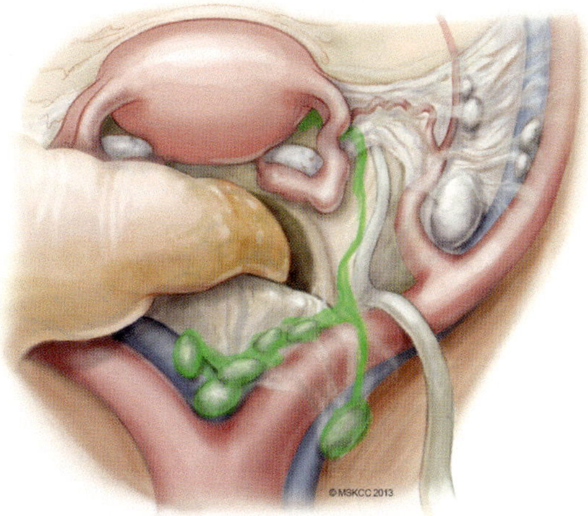

Fig. 29.9 Less common mapping topography. If the lymphatic trunks do not cross laterally over the umbilical ligament, as seen in the previous diagram, but instead drain cephalad and located in the mesoureter, this usually indicates that the sentinel lymph node will be located in the common iliac and presacral regions (©2013, Memorial Sloan Kettering Cancer Center)

lymph trunks do not cross over the obliterated umbilical and move cephalad following the mesoureter. Figure 29.10 demonstrates an example of an SLN identified by ICG during endometrial cancer surgery.

Another technique is the submucosal injection under hysteroscopic control. This technique is difficult, adds cost, and may not be useful in the larger tumors. The next technique is image-guided subserosal peritumoral injections; in this technique the blue dye and Tc are injected peritumorally based on ultrasound or MRI findings. Lastly, multiple subserous injections from eight subserosal (front and back) sites that concern lymphatic drainage of whole uterine corpus may be utilized. The same radioactive tracers are used as in cervical injection. Similarly, the same blue dyes may be utilized (Isosulfan Blue 1 %, Methylene Blue 1 %, and Patent Blue 2.5 % sodium).

29.5 Summary of Study Results

In 2009 Abu-Rustum reported on 42 patients with a preoperative diagnosis of grade 1 endometrial carcinoma treated from 3/06 to 8/08 [3, 5].

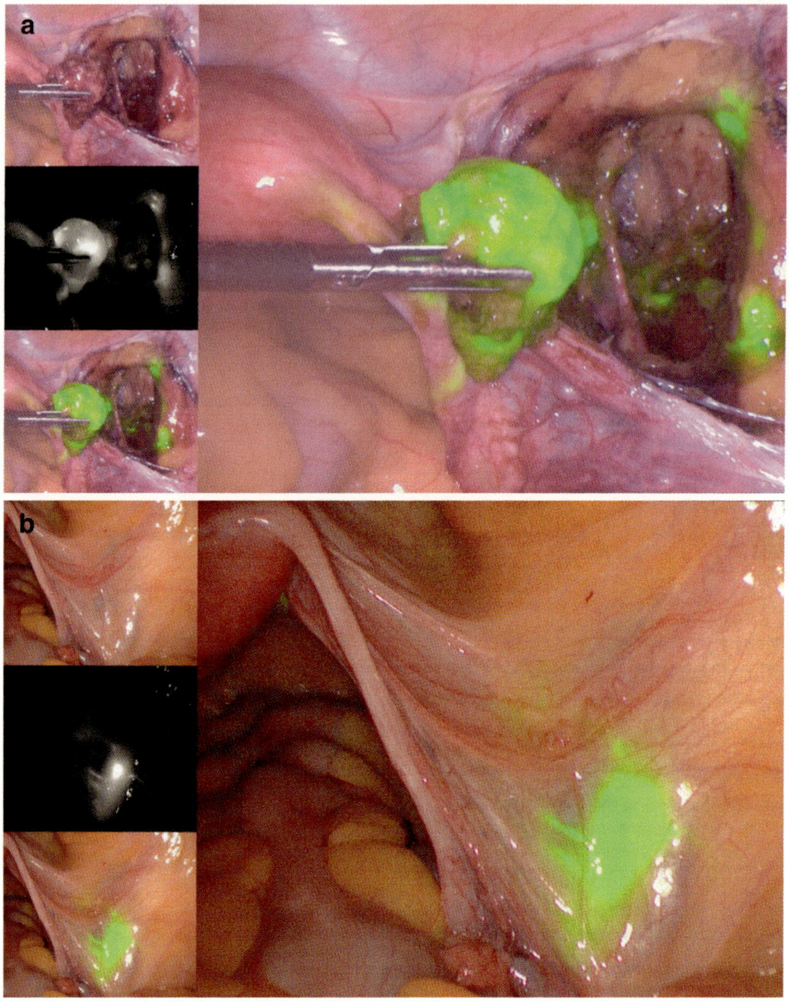

Fig. 29.10 (**a**, **b**) Two examples of sentinel lymph node detection in the right iliac region after indocyanine green (ICG) intracervical injection with near-infrared imaging (NIR) visualization during laparoscopy

Preoperative lymphoscintigraphy visualized SLNs in 30 patients (71 %); intraoperative localization of the SLN was possible in 36 patients (86 %). A median of 3 SLNs (range, 1–14) and 14.5 non-SLNs (range, 4–55) were examined. In all, 4/36 (11 %) had positive SLNs–3 seen on H&E and 1 as cytokeratin-positive cells on immunohistochemistry (IHC). All node-positive cases were picked up by the SLN; there were no false-negative cases. The sensitivity of the SLN procedure in the 36 patients who had an SLN identified was 100 %. The authors concluded that SLN mapping using a cervical injection with combined Tc and blue dye is feasible and accurate in patients with grade 1 endometrial cancer and may be a reasonable option for this select group of patients. Regional lymphadenectomy remains the gold standard in many practices, particularly for the approximately 15 % of cases with failed SLN mapping.

This was followed by another report in 2009 on 115 patients with endometrial cancer [4]. The cervix was the only site of injection in 82 cases (71 %), while a combined cervical and fundal injection was performed in 33 cases (29 %). Overall, SLN detection was achieved in 98 (85 %)

cases. In the initial 27 months of the study, an SLN was identified in 50 of 64 cases (78 %), with 2 falsenegative cases. In the subsequent 15 months, successful mapping was achieved in 48 of 51 cases (94 %) with no falsenegative cases. When examining an individual provider's performance, after the first 30 cases, the rate of successful mapping significantly increased from 77 to 94 % ($P=0.033$). The authors stressed that SLN mapping in uterine cancer requires a dedicated effort to achieve high detection rates. Surgeons should determine their individual detection rates and falsenegative rates. These data demonstrate that high SLN detection rates can be achieved in women with uterine cancer, and increasing surgical volume (30 cases) is associated with significantly increased detection rates.

As far as lowvolume metastasis to SLNs, our team investigated the effect of uterine manipulation on isolated tumor cells (ITCs) and micrometastasis (MM) to SLNs and Frimer in 2010 [6] reported on 175 patients who had successful SLN mapping. Of these, 145 (83 %) had negative nodes, 11 (6 %) had positive nodes, and 19 (11 %) met the criteria for MM and ITCs. The uterine procedure used to diagnose endometrial cancer, type of hysterectomy, tumor grade, histology, positive pelvic washings, and type of uterine manipulator utilized did not appear to be associated with MM/ITCs. However, the presence of lymphovascular invasion ($P<0.001$) and the depth of myometrial invasion ($P=0.01$) were significantly higher in the MM/ITC group. These data demonstrated that the presence of MM and ITCs in SLNs of endometrial cancer patients is not an artifact of uterine manipulation or instrumentation. Rather, it is a real pathologic finding likely associated with lymphovascular invasion and depth of myoinvasion.

A later report by Khoury-Collado et al. from 2011 [7] described 266 patients with endometrial cancer who underwent lymphatic mapping. SLN identification was successful in 223 (84 %) cases. Positive nodes were diagnosed in 32/266 (12 %) patients. Of those, 8/266 patients (3 %) had metastasis detected only by additional section or IHC as part of SLN ultrastaging. Excluding the eight cases with positive SLNs on ultrastaging only, 24/801 (3 %) SLNs and 30/2698 (1 %) non-SLNs were positive for metastatic disease ($p=0.0003$). These data demonstrated that using a cervical injection for mapping, metastatic cells from endometrial cancer are three times as likely to be detected in SLNs than in the non-SLNs. This finding strongly supports the concept of lymphatic mapping in endometrial cancer to fine tune the nodal dissection topography. By adding SLN mapping to our current surgical staging procedures we may increase the likelihood of detecting metastatic cancer cells in regional lymph nodes. An additional benefit of incorporating pathologic ultrastaging of SLNs is the detection of micrometastasis, which may be the only evidence of extrauterine spread.

In 2012 Barlin [8] reported on 498 patients who received a blue dye cervical injection for SLN mapping. At least one lymph node was removed in 95 % of cases (474/498); at least one SLN was identified in 81 % (401/498). SLNs correctly diagnosed 40/47 patients with nodal metastases who had at least one SLN mapped, resulting in a 15 % false-negative rate. After applying the Memorial algorithm, the false-negative rate dropped to 2 %. Only one patient, whose lymph node spread would not have been caught by the algorithm, had an isolated positive right paraaortic lymph node with a negative ipsilateral SLN and pelvic lymph node dissection. These results stressed that satisfactory SLN mapping in endometrial cancer requires adherence to a surgical SLN algorithm and goes beyond just the removal of blue SLNs. Removal of any suspicious node along with side-specific lymphadenectomy for failed mapping are an integral part of the Memorial SLN algorithm. Further validation of the false-negative rate of this algorithm is necessary. The Memorial algorithm is shown in Fig. 29.11.

Most recently, in 2013 Leitao [9] identified a total of 507 cases of endometrial cancer treated with minimally invasive surgery and SLN mapping over a 3-year period. The distribution of cases was 143 in year 1 (Y1), 190 in year 2 (Y2), and 174 in year 3 (Y3). Tumor grade and high-risk

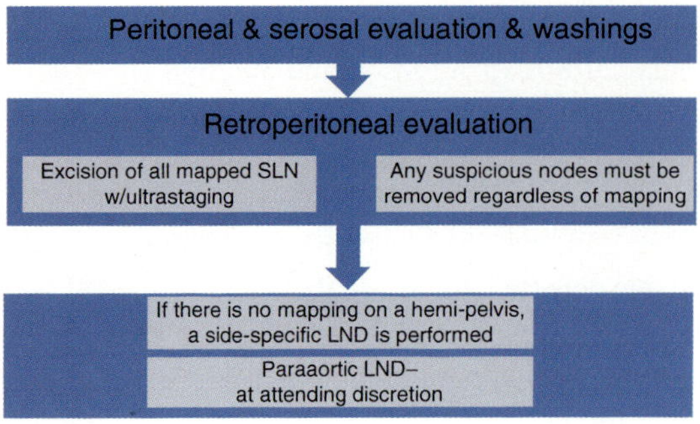

Fig. 29.11 Sentinel lymph node mapping algorithm

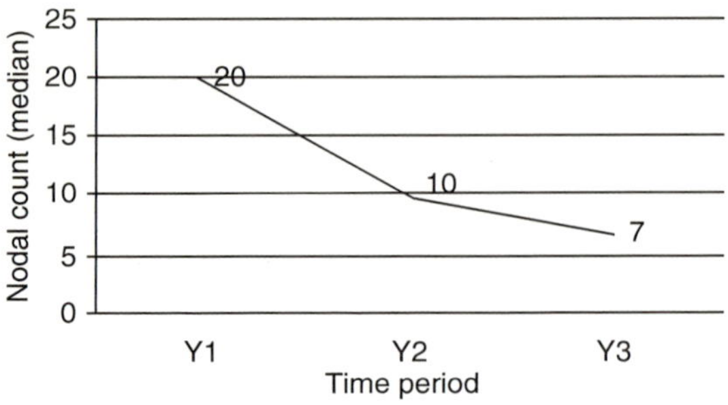

Fig. 29.12 Total number of nodes removed over a 3-year period

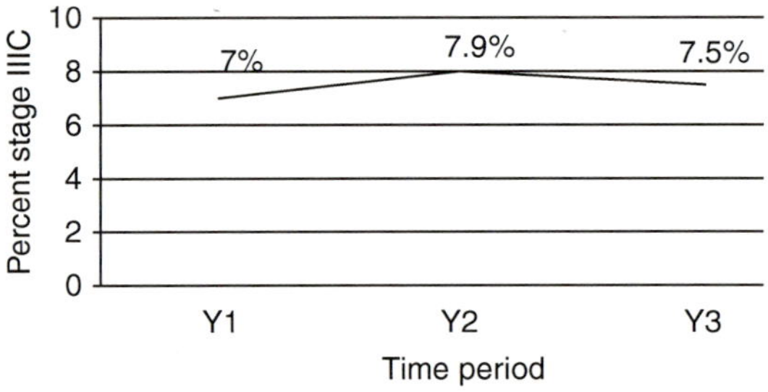

Fig. 29.13 The detection rate of stage IIIC disease

histologies did not differ during the three time periods. A standard staging procedure was performed in the following cases: Y1 (93/143; 65 %), Y2 (66/166; 35 %), and Y3 (40/164; 23 %) ($P<0.001$). Median operative times were as follows: Y1 (218 min), Y2 (198 min), and Y3 (176.5 min) ($P<0.001$). The median numbers of total lymph nodes removed among cases with at least one node retrieved were: Y1 (20); Y2 (10); Y3 (7) ($P<0.001$) (Fig. 29.12). Cases diagnosed as stage IIIC were as follows: Y1 (10/143; 7 %), Y2 (15/166; 7.9 %), and Y3 (13/164; 7.5 %) ($P=1.0$) (Fig. 29.13). The authors concluded that the incorporation of a modified staging approach utilizing the SLN mapping algorithm reduces the need for standard lymphadenectomy and does not appear to adversely affect the rate of stage IIIC detection. The emergence and utility of intracervical ICG injection as a powerful dye for SLN mapping was recently reported by Jewell et al. in 2014 and clearly demonstrated that ICG alone is sufficient for SLN mapping, with high (95 %) SLN detection rates and high (79 %) bilateral localization of SLNs [10].

Key Points

- Following a cervical injection of dye, sentinel lymph nodes (SLNs) are three times more likely to harbor disease than non-SLNs.
- With immunohistochemical "ultrastaging," pathologists were able to detect an additional 3–8 % of micrometastasis to SLNs, which may have been otherwise missed by routine hematoxylin and eosin staining.
- The optimal technique of SLN mapping in uterine corpus cancer continues to be the subject of much debate; a cervical, hysteroscopic, or fundal serosal injection can be used. A cervical injection is the most validated, easiest, and most reproducible technique.
- The cervical injection may not appear to some clinicians as a rational strategy for detection in uterine cancer, but a superficial and deep injection into the cervix has repeatedly shown excellent dye penetration to the region of the uterine vessels and main lymphatic trunks that condenses in the parametria in most cases.
- Regional lymphadenectomy remains the gold standard in many practices, particularly for the approximately 15 % of cases with failed SLN mapping (no SLNs seen).

- Increasing surgical volume of SLN cases (30 cases) is associated with significantly increased SLN detection rates.
- The presence of micrometastases and isolated tumor cells in SLNs of endometrial cancer patients is not an artifact of uterine manipulation or instrumentation; it is a real pathologic finding likely associated with lymphovascular invasion and depth of myoinvasion.
- Satisfactory SLN mapping in endometrial cancer requires adherence to a surgical SLN algorithm developed by Memorial Sloan Kettering Cancer Center and goes beyond just the removal of blue SLNs.
- Removal of any suspicious node along with side-specific lymphadenectomy for cases of failed mapping are an integral part of the Memorial SLN algorithm.
- Incorporation of a modern staging approach utilizing the Memorial SLN mapping algorithm reduces the need for standard lymphadenectomy and does not appear to adversely affect the rate of stage IIIC detection.

References

1. Pandit-Taskar N, Gemignani ML, Lyall A, Larson SM, Barakat RR, Abu-Rustum NR. Single photon emission computed tomography SPECT-CT improves sentinel node detection and localization in cervical and uterine malignancy. Gynecol Oncol. 2010;117(1): 59–64.
2. Abu-Rustum NR. The increasing credibility of sentinel lymph node mapping in endometrial cancer. Ann Surg Oncol. 2013;20(2):353–4.
3. Abu-Rustum NR, Khoury-Collado F, Pandit-Taskar N, Soslow RA, Dao F, Sonoda Y, Levine DA, Brown CL, Chi DS, Barakat RR, Gemignani ML. Sentinel lymph node mapping for grade 1 endometrial cancer: is it the answer to the surgical staging dilemma? Gynecol Oncol. 2009;113(2):163–9.
4. Khoury-Collado F, Glaser GE, Zivanovic O, Sonoda Y, Levine DA, Chi DS, Gemignani ML, Barakat RR, Abu-Rustum NR. Improving sentinel lymph node detection rates in endometrial cancer: how many cases are needed? Gynecol Oncol. 2009;115(3): 453–5.
5. Abu-Rustum NR, Gomez JD, Alektiar KM, Soslow RA, Hensley ML, Leitao Jr MM, Gardner GJ, Sonoda Y, Chi DS, Barakat RR. The incidence of isolated paraaortic nodal metastasis in surgically staged endometrial cancer patients with negative pelvic lymph nodes. Gynecol Oncol. 2009;115(2):236–8.
6. Frimer M, Khoury-Collado F, Murray MP, Barakat RR, Abu-Rustum NR. Micrometastasis of endometrial cancer to sentinel lymph nodes: is it an artifact of uterine manipulation? Gynecol Oncol. 2010;119(3): 496–9.
7. Khoury-Collado F, Murray MP, Hensley ML, et al. Sentinel lymph node mapping for endometrial cancer improves the detection of metastatic disease to regional lymph nodes. Gynecol Oncol. 2011;122: 251–4.
8. Barlin JN, Khoury-Collado F, Kim CH, Leitao Jr MM, Chi DS, Sonoda Y, Alektiar K, Delair DF, Barakat RR, Abu-Rustum NR. The importance of applying a sentinel lymph node mapping algorithm in endometrial cancer staging: beyond removal of blue nodes. Gynecol Oncol. 2012;125(3): 531–5.
9. Leitao Jr MM, Khoury-Collado F, Gardner G, Sonoda Y, Brown CL, Alektiar KM, Hensley ML, Soslow RA, Barakat RR, Abu-Rustum NR. Impact of incorporating an algorithm that utilizes sentinel lymph node mapping during minimally invasive procedures on the detection of stage IIIC endometrial cancer. Gynecol Oncol. 2013;129(1):38–41.
10. Jewell EL, Huang JJ, Abu-Rustum NR, Gardner GJ, Brown CL, Sonoda Y, Barakat RR, Levine DA, Leitao Jr MM. Detection of sentinel lymph nodes in minimally invasive surgery using indocyanine green and near-infrared fluorescence imaging for uterine and cervical malignancies. Gynecol Oncol. 2014;133(2): 274–7.

Treatment of Endometrial Cancer

30

Patricia J. Eifel

30.1 Introduction

Although endometrial cancer is the most common gynecologic malignancy diagnosed in developed nations, high-risk endometrial cancer is relatively rare. Because simple hysterectomy alone is curative in 70–80 % of patients with endometrial cancer, the margin for improvement with additional therapy is small, and the addition of potentially toxic adjuvant treatments must be considered very carefully.

Clinicopathologic studies demonstrate that most of the recurrence risk is concentrated in a minority of patients whose endometrial cancers exhibit two or more disease-related risk factors, including high grade, deep muscle invasion, lymph-vascular space invasion, and large tumor size. Recurrence also appears to be independently correlated with advanced patient age. Serous carcinomas are associated with a relatively high recurrence risk and are more likely than endometrioid cancers to recur with intra-abdominal carcinomatosis [1]. In general, patients without two or more of these risk factors have such a small margin for improvement with adjuvant treatment that the risks of such treatment, even if small, are likely to exceed the benefit. However, patients who have cancers demonstrating two or more risk factors or who have evidence of regional metastasis do have a sufficiently high likelihood of local or distant recurrence to justify the addition of effective adjuvant treatment.

The challenges for clinicians have been to identify effective adjuvant treatments, define the subgroups of patients for whom the benefit of adjuvant treatments exceeds the risks, and design and complete trials that document a survival benefit from adjuvant treatments. During the past 30 years, numerous phase III trials have been conducted in an effort to define the value of adding lymphadenectomy, chemotherapy, or radiation therapy to hysterectomy. Although these trials provide some hints, the body of evidence has yet to definitively demonstrate that any of these treatments improves the overall survival rate of women with uterine cancer.

30.2 Lymphadenectomy

Before the mid-1980s, lymphadenectomy was rarely included in the initial surgical management of uterine cancer. However, in 1988, following prospective trials that confirmed the prognostic importance of lymph node involvement, the International Federation of Gynecology and Obstetrics (FIGO) staging system was changed to include histologic information about lymph node metastasis. In subsequent years, lymphadenectomy was increasingly performed with hysterectomy in patients undergoing surgery for newly diagnosed uterine cancer.

P.J. Eifel, MD
Department of Radiation Oncology,
MD Anderson Cancer Center, Houston, TX, USA
e-mail: peifel@mdanderson.org

H.R.H. Patel et al. (eds.), *Pelvic Cancer Surgery: Modern Breakthroughs and Future Advances*,
DOI 10.1007/978-1-4471-4258-4_30, © Springer-Verlag London 2015

Although many clinicians considered lymphadenectomy to be primarily a diagnostic tool that could guide the use of other adjuvant treatments, some investigators argued that surgical removal of the regional lymph nodes might also play a direct curative role via surgical elimination of regional metastases [2]. Other clinicians argued that there was no actual proof of a survival benefit to justify the added cost and operative morbidity associated with lymphadenectomy. It was not until 2008–2009 that two randomized trials examined the potential survival benefit of lymphadenectomy directly [3, 4]. In both trials, patients were randomized to have hysterectomy with or without pelvic lymphadenectomy. Neither study demonstrated an improvement in overall survival for patients who had lymphadenectomy; in one study, patients who underwent lymphadenectomy actually had a significantly poorer relapse-free survival than those who underwent hysterectomy alone.

These trials have been criticized on several grounds, including the inclusion of patients with relatively low recurrence risk, failure to evaluate para-aortic nodes, and inconsistent use of subsequent adjuvant treatments. Of course, inconsistent use of subsequent adjuvant treatments could influence the trial results only if the differences were substantial and if the adjuvant treatments were themselves effective.

Lymphadenectomy adds to the cost, operative time, and perioperative morbidity of endometrial cancer surgery. Several studies have demonstrated that the rate of post-irradiation bowel complications is increased in patients who have had lymphadenectomy [5], although there are few data indicating the magnitude of risk for patients whose pre-irradiation surgery was performed laparoscopically. Mariani et al. [6] have suggested a method of intraoperative triage that would avoid lymphadenectomy in patients who have a very low likelihood of node metastases; however, the value of this approach has not been tested prospectively. Others have investigated the use of sentinel node evaluation as a means of improving diagnostic accuracy without the morbidity of full lymphadenectomy [7].

Although the results of lymphadenectomy may guide use of other adjuvant treatments, lymphadenectomy also adds to the overall morbidity of treatment. Ultimately, the risk-benefit ratio for lymphadenectomy must be considered in the context of other multidisciplinary treatment preferences.

30.3 Adjuvant Radiation Therapy

Although hysterectomy and radiation therapy were first combined to treat uterine cancers in the early 1900s, only one phase III trial testing the efficacy of adjuvant radiation therapy was published during the entire twentieth century [8]. However, beginning in the year 2000, a series of new randomized phase III trials in patients with variably defined "intermediate-risk" cancers assessed the value of adjuvant pelvic radiation therapy by comparing it either with no adjuvant treatment or with vaginal brachytherapy alone [9–13]. For the most part, these trials concluded that although pelvic radiation therapy improved local control, it provided little or no survival benefit. However, the low-risk profiles of many of the patients entered in the trials, the resulting relatively small number of events, and the heterogeneity of the study populations made it impossible to rule out clinically significant benefit for the patients with multiple risk factors who had the most to gain from adjuvant treatment.

In the first of these recent trials, PORTEC 1, which originated in the Netherlands, patients characterized as having intermediate-risk disease were randomized after hysterectomy to receive either pelvic radiation therapy or no further treatment. Patients who were randomized to receive pelvic radiation therapy had a significantly lower pelvic recurrence rate (5 % vs. 14 %, $P<0.001$), but this did not translate into an improved overall survival rate. The study had several limitations. Most patients were operated on by community surgeons and did not have surgical staging of lymph nodes. Deeply invasive grade 3 cancers were excluded. Also, there were problems with pathologic classification of tumors. Initial eligibility and the final statistical analysis were based

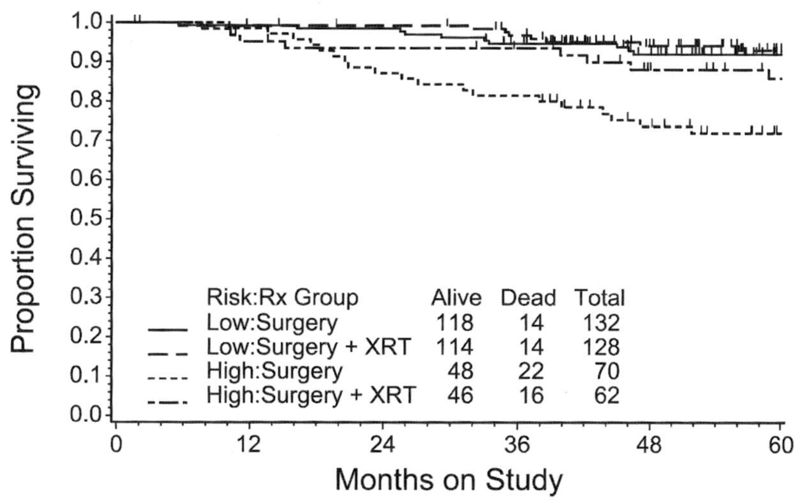

Fig. 30.1 Overall survival rates for patients treated with or without adjuvant pelvic radiation therapy for low-intermediate-risk or high-intermediate-risk endometrial cancer on Gynecologic Oncology Group trial GOG-99 (Reprinted from Keys et al. [11], Copyright 2004, with permission from Elsevier)

on pathology reports from the operating centers. However, a subsequent central review of about 80 % of cases demonstrated that the percentage of patients with grade 1 disease, initially thought to be 21 %, was actually 69 %. In retrospect, 24 % of patients had low-risk cancers that did not meet the trial eligibility criteria, and most of the remaining patients had low-intermediate-risk cancers. This translated to an endometrial cancer-related death rate of only 10 % at 10 years, leaving a very small margin for improvement with adjuvant treatment [14].

In 2009, Blake et al. and the ASTEC/EN.5 Study Group published pooled results of two similar trials. Results were similar to those of PORTEC-1. The trials that were pooled had some of the same limitations as PORTEC-1, with a low event rate, and are somewhat difficult to interpret because of variations in staging and treatment assignments, including the uncontrolled use of vaginal brachytherapy in many patients randomized to the "observation" arm.

In 2003, the Gynecologic Oncology Group published the results of GOG-99. This trial had a randomization scheme similar to that of PORTEC-1, but GOG-99 required somewhat higher-risk intrauterine features, used pre-randomization pathology review to confirm patient eligibility, and required "selective bilateral pelvic and paraaortic lymphadenectomy," excluding patients from analysis if they had "incomplete staging." Despite this, most patients still had relatively low-risk disease (58 % had <50 % invasion and 28 % had grade 1 disease). Like PORTEC-1, GOG-99 demonstrated a significant reduction in the rate of recurrence; however, with only 34 disease-related deaths, the trial was insufficiently powered to reliably detect a survival difference. As expected, most of the recurrences in the no-further-treatment arm of this trial occurred in a small subgroup of 70 patients who had multiple risk factors (Fig. 30.1). Within this group of patients with high-intermediate-risk cancers, patients treated with pelvic radiation therapy appeared to have a substantially lower death rate (hazard ratio=0.73, 90 % confidence interval, 0.43–1.26). However, because the trial had not originally been stratified for these subgroups, the authors did not test for the statistical significance of this comparison. The overall 5-year survival rate of patients with low-intermediate-risk tumors was >90 % in both arms.

The authors of these trials discouraged the use of adjuvant radiation therapy, particularly for patients with low-intermediate-risk disease, for whom the acute and late effects of radiation could not be justified by the negligible benefit. In addition, analysis of recurrence patterns demonstrated that the greatest difference between the treatment arms of these trials was a higher rate of vaginal recurrences, some of which were cured with salvage radiation therapy.

Several studies have evaluated whether vaginal cuff irradiation alone could prevent local recurrences without the added morbidity of pelvic irradiation. A Norwegian trial conducted during the 1970s [8] demonstrated no survival difference in a comparison of pelvic irradiation with vaginal cuff irradiation only. However, the overall favorable profile of the patients and subsequent changes in staging, histologic classification, and treatment technique make it difficult to generalize the results of this trial. Two recent trials revisited this question [12, 13]. In both studies, overall survival was similar for patients treated with pelvic radiation therapy and those treated with vaginal radiation therapy, but as for earlier trials, the power to detect differences was limited by the favorable risk profile of the patients entered. PORTEC-2 [12] was intended to limit enrollment to patients with high-intermediate-risk disease. However, post-analysis pathologic review again demonstrated that patients had much more favorable disease than anticipated, and the event rate was similar to that for PORTEC-1. A second recent trial [13] had approximately twice as many endometrial cancer-related deaths in patients treated with vaginal brachytherapy only, but this was balanced by a higher number of intercurrent deaths in the pelvic radiation therapy arm in a trial that had few events overall.

In summary, available data clearly demonstrate that patients who have low-risk disease (minimally invasive grade 1 and 2 disease) rarely if ever require adjuvant treatment after hysterectomy. Patients with intermediate-risk disease have a vaginal recurrence risk that ranges between 5 and 20 %, depending on the individual findings. These patients may benefit from adjuvant vaginal cuff radiation treatment. Adjuvant irradiation undoubtedly reduces the risk of local recurrence in higher-risk patients; however, available trials do not provide sufficient information about the influence of pelvic irradiation on survival to permit generalizable conclusions. Data from PORTEC-1 [10] indicate a strong correlation between grade and vaginal recurrence risk, which may be >20 % for grade 3 tumors, even minimally invasive ones. These data, combined with the relatively poor salvage rate for high-grade vaginal recurrences [15], provide a strong rationale for giving at least vaginal radiation therapy even for minimally invasive grade 3 tumors. Results of GOG-99 [11] suggest that pelvic radiation therapy may improve survival for patients with high-intermediate-risk disease, but high-quality trials focused on this group are still needed to answer this question with confidence. In the meantime, many practitioners continue to consider pelvic radiation therapy to be standard for patients with high-intermediate-risk disease.

In all cases, the decision to treat should be made after weighing the risks and benefits for an individual patient. For patients whose tumor grade and depth of invasion indicate borderline risk, other risk factors, such as lymph-vascular space invasion and large tumor size, may suggest a greater risk of recurrence and margin for improvement with adjuvant treatment. On the other hand, previous lymphadenectomy (particularly through an open approach) increases the risk of postirradiation complications, and if no positive lymph nodes were found, this probably indicates a decreased likelihood of benefit from pelvic irradiation. Patients who have very thin body habitus, history of pelvic infection, or heavy smoking may have a greater risk of postirradiation complications, shifting the risk-benefit ratio. However, modern radiation therapy techniques that reduce the dose to central pelvic structures (Fig. 30.2) may reduce short- and long-term side effects and increase the potential for gain with adjuvant radiation therapy.

30.4 Adjuvant Radiation Therapy and Chemotherapy for Patients with High-Risk Disease

In discussions of the prognosis of patients with endometrial cancer, the term "high risk" is usually used to designate a group that includes patients with FIGO stage III disease (e.g., having involvement

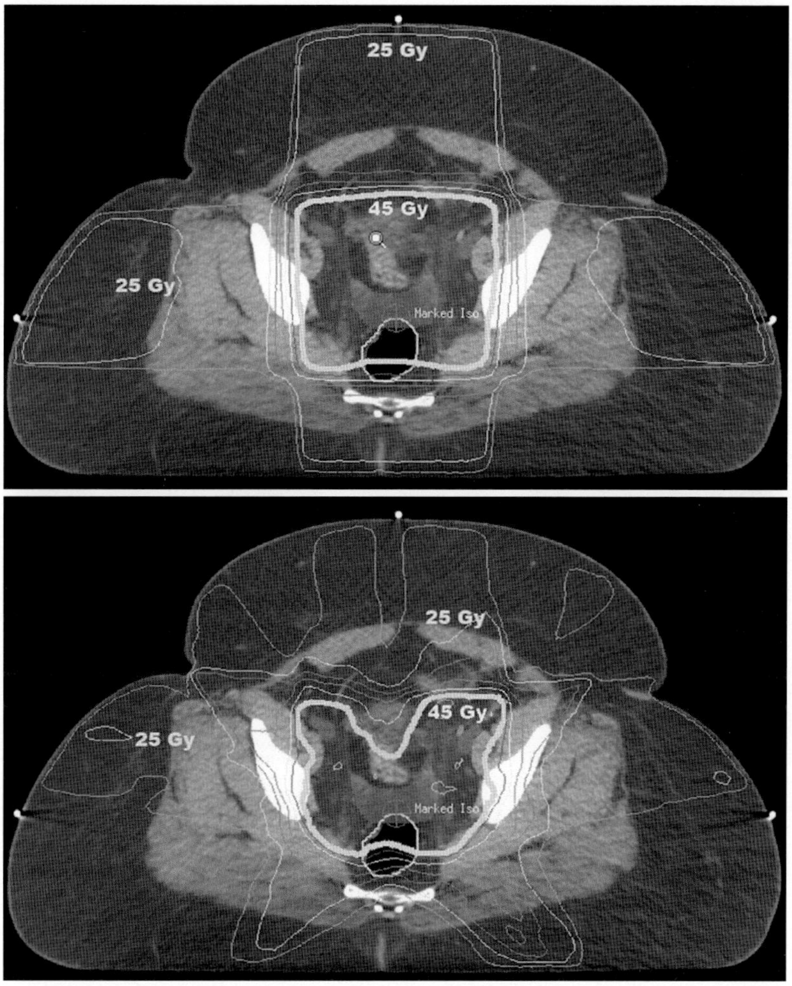

Fig. 30.2 Radiation isodose distributions in a patient treated with postoperative pelvic radiation therapy for high-intermediate-risk endometrial cancer. The *top image* shows the dose distribution achieved using a traditional four-field technique. The *bottom image* shows the dose distribution achieved using an intensity-modulated radiation therapy (IMRT) technique. With IMRT, central pelvic structures receive a lower dose of radiation, as do peripheral soft tissues

of lymph nodes, uterine serosa, adnexa, or vagina). Some trials have included patients with positive peritoneal cytology, although this is no longer considered to be an important independent predictor of prognosis. Sometimes patients with serous cancers or deeply invasive grade 3 cancers are included in the high-risk category. Some trials have admixed high-risk patients with those having advanced disease (stage IV) or high-intermediate-risk disease. The heterogeneity and variable definitions of this category complicate interpretation of trials that evaluated the roles of radiation therapy and chemotherapy in the management of high-risk cancers.

Before 2006, pelvic radiation therapy was generally considered to be the standard treatment for patients with high-risk disease, and the prevailing opinion was that chemotherapy had a very limited role in the adjuvant treatment of uterine cancer. However, in that year, the Gynecologic Oncology Group published the results of GOG-122 [16], the first major trial that compared adjuvant chemotherapy alone with adjuvant radiation therapy. That trial randomly compared adjuvant doxorubicin and cisplatin with adjuvant whole-abdominal radiation therapy (Table 30.1) in patients with "high-risk" disease. The eligibility criteria were very broad—patients who had stage III or IV disease after total abdominal hysterectomy and bilateral salpingo-oophorectomy were eligible if they had no evidence of hematogenous or extra-abdominal disease, had no residual disease >2 cm in diameter, had reasonable performance status, and had received no prior chemotherapy or radiation

Table 30.1 Randomized trials evaluating the roles of adjuvant treatments in patients with endometrial cancer

Author(s) (trial name or country)	Eligibility	Study arms	No. of pts.	LRR rate (%)	DFS rate (%)	OS rate (%)	No. of endometrial cancer-related deaths	Median F/U time, mo	Comments
Trials evaluating the role of lymphadenectomy									
Kitchener et al. (MRC ASTEC) [3]	Endometrial carcinoma clinically confined to corpus	Pelvic lymphadenectomy	704	–	73[a]	82		37	Median number nodes dissected =12
		No lymphadenectomy	704	–	79[a]	81			
Benedetti et al. (Italy) [4]	Endometrioid or adenosquamous carcinoma clinically confined to the corpus	Pelvic lymphadenectomy	264		82	86	42 (total)	49	Median number nodes dissected =12
		No lymphadenectomy	250		82	90			
Trials evaluating the role of adjuvant RT for intermediate-risk disease									
Aalders et al. (Norway) [8]	Clinical stage I (FIGO)	Pelvic RT + VBC	260			89	28	>60	
		VBC	277			91	25		
Creutzberg et al. (PORTEC-1) [10]	FIGO I with: G1, >50 % myometrial invasion, G2, any invasion, or G3, <50 % invasion	Pelvic RT	354	4[a,c]		81	23	52	Lymph node staging not required; no pre-entry pathology review
		No adjuvant treatment	361	14[a,c]		85	18		
Keys et al. (GOG-99) [11]	G2–3 + LVSI + >2/3 invasion	Pelvic RT	190	1.6[a]		92[d]	19	69	
	≥50 years old with two of these features								
	≥70 years old with any of these features	No adjuvant treatment	202	7.4[a]		86[d]	15		
Blake et al. (MRC ASTEC/NCIC CTG EN.5) [9]	FIGO (1988) I or IIA with ither G3 (including serous) or >50 % myometrial invasion	Pelvic RT	452			84	37	58	Lymph node staging not required; no pre-entry pathology review; VCB given to 53 % in "observation" arm
		Observation	453			84	41		
Nout et al. (PORTEC-2) [12]	FIGO (1988) I or IIA and: G1–2, >60 years old, <50 % invasion or	Pelvic RT	214	0.5	83	80	10	45	Lymph node staging not required; no pre-entry pathology review
	G3 with <50 % invasion or								
	IIA, G1–2 or G3, <50 % invasion	VCB	213	1.5	78	85	15		

Sorbe et al. (Sweden) [13]	FIGO (1988) stage I endometrioid carcinoma and nuclear grade 1–2 with FIGO G3, ≥50 % invasion, or DNA aneuploidy	Pelvic RT + VBC	224	1.5		89	15	62	
		VCB	223	5		90	27		
Trials evaluating the roles of adjuvant chemotherapy and radiation therapy in high-risk disease									
Randall et al. (GOG-122) [16]	FIGO III-IV, maximum residual disease ≤2 cm, no hematogenous metastases	RT (whole abdomen and pelvis)	202		38	42[b]	100	74	See text; node sampling optional for patients who met other eligibility criteria
		Chemotherapy (AP)	194		42	53[b]	78		
Susumu et al. (Japan) [18]	FIGO (1988) IC-IIIC with >50 % myometrial invasion	Pelvic RT	193	7	84	85	21	60	77 % had extended or radical hysterectomy; 96 % had nodal staging
		Chemotherapy (CAP)	192	7	82	87	13		
Maggi et al. (Italy) [17]	FIGO I-II with >50 % myometrial invasion or IIIC; high-risk histologies excluded	Pelvic RT	166	11		69		95	
		Chemotherapy (CAP)	177	14	63	66			
Kuoppala et al. (Finland) [19]	FIGO (1988) IA-B, G3, or IC-IIIA	Pelvic RT	72	3		85[e]	26 (total)		
		Pelvic RT + sequential chemotherapy (CEP)	84	3		82[e]			
Hogberg et al. (NSGO/EORTC and MaNGO) [20]	NSGO/EORTC: FIGO IA-C with "risk profile that qualified for adjuvant treatment," IIA, IIIA, IIIC (pelvic) with no gross residual	Pelvic RT	267		69[a]	74[a]			High-risk histologic types eligible for NSGO/EORTC but not MaNGO
	MaNGO: FIGO 1988 IIB-IIIC (pelvic)	Pelvic RT + sequential chemotherapy (various)	267		80[a]	84[a]			

AP doxorubicin and cisplatin, *CAP* cyclophosphamide, doxorubicin, and cisplatin, *CEP* cyclophosphamide, epirubicin, and cisplatin, *DFS* disease-free survival, *EORTC* European Organization for Research and Treatment of Cancer, *F/U* follow-up, *FIGO* International Federation of Gynecology and Obstetrics *G* grade, *LRR* local-regional recurrence, *LVSI* lymph-vascular space invasion, *MaNGO* Mario Negri Gynecologic Oncology group, *NSGO* Nordic Society of Gynecologic Oncology, *OS* overall survival, *pts.* patients, *RT* radiation therapy, *VCB* vaginal cuff brachytherapy

[a]Difference between treatment arms, $P<0.05$

[b]Difference between treatment arms, $P<0.05$ after adjustment for stage imbalance between arms

[c]Calculated at 2 years follow-up

[d]Calculated at 4 years follow-up

[e]Disease-specific survival

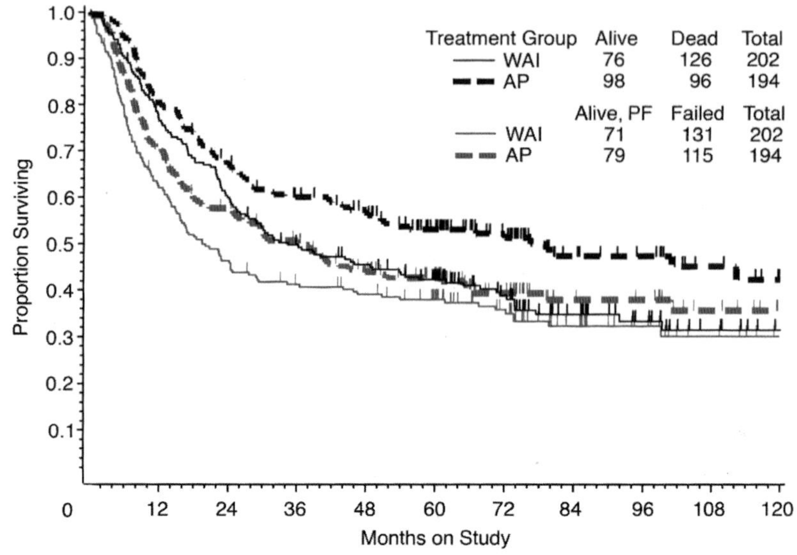

Fig. 30.3 Progression-free survival (*gray*) and overall survival (*black*) for patients treated with either whole-abdominal radiation therapy (*WAI*) or chemotherapy (doxorubicin and cisplatin; AP) on Gynecologic Oncology Group trial GOG-122. In this illustration, the curves have been superimposed to highlight the relationships between progression-free and overall survival rates for the two arms (Adapted from Randall et al. [16], with permission from Elsevier)

therapy. Although patients were supposed to have surgical staging, many did not undergo node dissection. Tomographic imaging was not routinely performed before or after surgery to verify the completeness of surgical resection. When the trial opened in 1992, neither of the treatments could have been considered "standard" for this diverse group of patients, although both treatment approaches had their advocates. By the time the trial was published 14 years later, it was generally understood that the dose of radiation used in GOG-122 was inadequate to control gross residual disease, that the volume irradiated was inappropriate for many subsets, and that patients whose only risk factor was positive peritoneal cytology probably did not require adjuvant treatment at all.

In their report of GOG-122, the authors concluded, "chemotherapy significantly improved progression-free and overall survival compared with whole-abdominal radiation" [16]. Although this conclusion profoundly influenced opinions about the value of chemotherapy as an adjuvant treatment and led to its much broader use in the community, the trial has a number of flaws that raise doubts about the generalizability of the results. The difference in the primary endpoint, progression-free survival, was only significant after the authors employed a statistical adjustment for an apparent imbalance in FIGO (1988) stage; the validity of such adjustment can be questioned in a study that did not require consistent surgical staging methods. The most notable finding from this trial was the relatively high overall survival rate of patients in the chemotherapy arm. However, patients in the chemotherapy arm had an overall survival rate that was also substantially better than the progression-free survival rate (Fig. 30.3), suggesting that at least some of the difference between the two arms may have reflected more effective salvage of treatment failures in the chemotherapy arm. Although the radiation given to patients in this trial was frequently inadequate to control residual disease (60 % of recurrences were confined to sites within the radiation fields), it was enough to prevent future delivery of definitive radiation therapy to sites of recurrence or progression. For patients in the chemotherapy arm, though, definitive radiation therapy would still have been a viable option for localized disease recurrences. It is notable that most of the benefit seen with chemotherapy was in patients with endometrioid cancers, which tend to have confined local recurrences; patients with serous tumors, which tend to recur in a more disseminated fashion, did not benefit from chemotherapy in subset analysis.

These issues would be less important if more recent trials had provided more evidence of benefit from chemotherapy. However, two subsequent trials comparing pelvic radiation therapy with chemotherapy demonstrated no difference in outcome (Table 30.1) [17, 18]. A small trial comparing adjuvant radiation therapy and sequential chemotherapy in an unusual split-course schedule also demonstrated no improvement with chemotherapy [19]. One of the most encouraging reports, a pooled analysis of two randomized trials involving several European multi-institutional groups, was published by Hogberg et al. [20] in 2010. The treatment groups involved radiation therapy with or without various combinations of sequential chemotherapy. Overall, the trial demonstrated significantly better progression-free survival for patients who received chemotherapy ($P=0.009$), but the difference in overall survival was not statistically significant.

Although randomized trials comparing radiation therapy with no treatment have included very few patients with stage IIIC disease, retrospective studies suggest that regional radiation therapy to the pelvis or pelvis and para-aortic nodes can be curative in such patients, particularly for patients with endometrioid cancers. In one of the larger published series, Klopp et al. [21] reported a 5-year disease-specific survival rate of 81 % for 31 patients treated with regional radiation therapy for grade 1–2 stage IIIC disease. Seventeen patients with grade 3 cancers had a somewhat poorer outcome ($P=0.06$): disease-specific survival rates were 67 and 40 % at 5 and 10 years, respectively. The overall rate of pelvic disease control was 98 % for patients treated with pelvic radiation therapy, compared with only 61 % in a group of 18 patients who had chemotherapy with or without vaginal brachytherapy ($P=0.001$). Of interest, several of the patients treated with chemotherapy had locoregional recurrences that were salvaged with localized radiation therapy.

Several investigators have advocated use of combined chemotherapy and radiation therapy to maximize local and distant disease control in patients with high-risk disease. Secord et al. [22] have advocated an alternating "sandwich" approach with three cycles of chemotherapy followed by radiation therapy and then three additional courses of chemotherapy. Although this schedule has become very popular, updated analyses [23] by the group failed to demonstrate any advantage of sequential chemotherapy and radiation therapy over radiation therapy alone for stage IIIC disease. However, patients treated with chemotherapy alone had a high local-regional recurrence rate and poorer survival than those treated with radiation. An alternative approach has been to give initial concurrent chemoradiation followed by four to six courses of chemotherapy [24, 25]. Phase II trials have demonstrated that this approach, which avoids delays in administration of postoperative radiation therapy, is generally well tolerated. However, prospective trials will be needed to demonstrate the relative value of this approach in high-risk disease.

30.5 Summary

Most patients with endometrial cancer are cured with hysterectomy alone. For patients who have low-grade and minimally invasive cancers, adjuvant treatment is rarely if ever indicated. Depending on the specific findings, tumors that demonstrate multiple risk factors, such as high grade, deep muscle invasion, large size, or lymph-vascular space invasion, may have a higher recurrence risk that suggests the need for adjuvant therapies. For patients with intermediate-risk disease, vaginal brachytherapy may be sufficient to prevent recurrence in the upper vagina, the most common type of recurrence. For patients with higher-risk disease, particularly those with high-grade, deeply invasive cancers, high-risk subtypes (such as serous carcinoma), or stage III disease, adjuvant regional irradiation or chemotherapy may be indicated. Regional radiation therapy consistently reduces the risk of local recurrence. Radiation therapy has not been proven to improve survival, but most trials have included too many low-risk patients to yield useful information about the impact of radiation therapy in patients with higher-risk disease. Trials have yielded conflicting results about the value of adjuvant chemotherapy. However, clinicians are increasingly turning to cytotoxic agents in an effort to reduce the risk of distant metastases in patients with high-risk disease. In all patients, the potential benefits must be balanced against the possible toxic effects of adjuvant treatments.

Key Points

- Most patients with endometrial cancer are cured with hysterectomy alone.
- Lymphadenectomy may help clinicians to guide posthysterectomy adjuvant treatment but also contributes to treatment-related side effects and has not been proven to improve survival.
- Among patients with cancer confined to the uterus, most recurrences are seen in those who have two or more of the following risk factors: high grade, deep myometrial invasion, lymph-vascular space invasion, or age >60–70 years. These patients are often described as having "high intermediate risk."
- Other factors, such as tumor size and DNA ploidy, also may be predictive of recurrence risk.
- Patients with low-risk endometrial cancer (minimally invasive grade 1 or 2 disease) derive little or no benefit from adjuvant treatment.
- For patients with intermediate-risk disease, the most frequent site of recurrence is the vagina. These patients may benefit from vaginal brachytherapy.
- For patients with high-intermediate-risk disease, adjuvant pelvic radiation therapy reduces the risk of recurrence but has not been demonstrated to improve survival. Subset analysis of Gynecologic Oncology Group trial GOG-99 hinted at a survival benefit in higher-risk patients, but that trial and most other trials of adjuvant radiation therapy included patients with a relatively favorable prognosis, leaving little margin for improvement.
- Regional radiation therapy can be curative in 70–80 % of patients with grade 1–2 and 30–40 % of patients with grade 3, stage IIIC endometrioid cancers.
- The results of trials evaluating the benefit of adjuvant chemotherapy have been mixed. However, patients with high-risk endometrial cancer (including grade 3 disease, serous cancers and stage III cancers) have a relatively high rate of distant metastasis and may benefit from adjuvant chemotherapy.
- Chemotherapy alone has generally been associated with a high rate of local recurrence. Combinations of chemotherapy and regional radiation therapy have been demonstrated to be tolerable, but the optimal integration of these treatments has not yet been determined.

References

1. Hendrickson M, et al. Uterine papillary serous carcinoma: a highly malignant form of endometrial adenocarcinoma. Am J Surg Pathol. 1982;6(2):93–108.
2. Kilgore LC, et al. Adenocarcinoma of the endometrium: survival comparisons of patients with and without pelvic node sampling. Gynecol Oncol. 1995; 56(1):29–33.
3. Kitchener H, et al. Efficacy of systematic pelvic lymphadenectomy in endometrial cancer (MRC ASTEC trial): a randomised study. Lancet. 2009; 373(9658):125–36.
4. Benedetti Panici P, et al. Systematic pelvic lymphadenectomy vs. no lymphadenectomy in early-stage endometrial carcinoma: randomized clinical trial. J Natl Cancer Inst. 2008;100(23):1707–16.
5. Corn BW, et al. Impact of improved irradiation technique, age and lymph node sampling on the severe complication rate of surgically staged endometrial cancer patients: a multivariate analysis. J Clin Oncol. 1994;12:510–5.
6. Mariani A, et al. Prospective assessment of lymphatic dissemination in endometrial cancer: a paradigm shift in surgical staging. Gynecol Oncol. 2008; 109(1):11–8.
7. How J, et al. Accuracy of sentinel lymph node detection following intra-operative cervical injection for endometrial cancer: a prospective study. Gynecol Oncol. 2012;127(2):332–7.
8. Aalders J, et al. Postoperative external irradiation and prognostic parameters in stage I endometrial carcinoma: clinical and histopathologic study of 540 patients. Obstet Gynecol. 1980;56(4):419–27.
9. Blake P, et al. Adjuvant external beam radiotherapy in the treatment of endometrial cancer (MRC ASTEC and NCIC CTG EN.5 randomised trials): pooled trial results, systematic review, and meta-analysis. Lancet. 2009;373(9658):137–46.

10. Creutzberg CL, et al. Outcome of high-risk stage IC, grade 3, compared with stage I endometrial carcinoma patients: the postoperative radiation therapy in endometrial carcinoma trial. J Clin Oncol. 2004;22(7):1234–41.
11. Keys HM, et al. A phase III trial of surgery with or without adjunctive external pelvic radiation therapy in intermediate risk endometrial adenocarcinoma: a Gynecologic Oncology Group Study. Gynecol Oncol. 2004;92(3):744–51.
12. Nout RA et al. Vaginal brachytherapy versus external beam pelvic radiotherapy for high-intermediate risk endometrial cancer: results of the randomized PORTEC-2 trial. Proceedings of the 44th Annual Meeting of the American Society of Clinical Oncology, 2008: p. 181.
13. Sorbe B, et al. External pelvic and vaginal irradiation versus vaginal irradiation alone as postoperative therapy in medium-risk endometrial carcinoma—a prospective randomized study. Int J Radiat Oncol Biol Phys. 2012;82(3):1249–55.
14. Scholten AN, et al. Postoperative radiotherapy for stage 1 endometrial carcinoma: long-term outcome of the randomized PORTEC trial with central pathology review. Int J Radiat Oncol Biol Phys. 2005;63(3):834–8.
15. Jhingran A, Burke TW, Eifel PJ. Definitive radiotherapy for patients with isolated vaginal recurrence of endometrial carcinoma after hysterectomy. Int J Radiat Oncol Biol Phys. 2003;56(5):1366–72.
16. Randall ME, et al. Randomized phase III trial of whole-abdominal irradiation versus doxorubicin and cisplatin chemotherapy in advanced endometrial carcinoma: a Gynecologic Oncology Group Study. J Clin Oncol. 2006;24(1):36–44.
17. Maggi R, et al. Adjuvant chemotherapy vs radiotherapy in high-risk endometrial carcinoma: results of a randomised trial. Br J Cancer. 2006;95(3):266–71.
18. Susumu N, et al. Randomized phase III trial of pelvic radiotherapy versus cisplatin-based combined chemotherapy in patients with intermediate- and high-risk endometrial cancer: a Japanese Gynecologic Oncology Group Study. Gynecol Oncol. 2008;108(1):226–33.
19. Kuoppala T, et al. Surgically staged high-risk endometrial cancer: randomized study of adjuvant radiotherapy alone vs. sequential chemo-radiotherapy. Gynecol Oncol. 2008;110(2):190–5.
20. Hogberg T, et al. Sequential adjuvant chemotherapy and radiotherapy in endometrial cancer—results from two randomised studies. Eur J Cancer. 2010;46(13):2422–31.
21. Klopp AH, et al. Node-positive adenocarcinoma of the endometrium: outcome and patterns of recurrence with and without external beam irradiation. Gynecol Oncol. 2009;115(1):6–11.
22. Secord AA, et al. A multicenter evaluation of sequential multimodality therapy and clinical outcome for the treatment of advanced endometrial cancer. Gynecol Oncol. 2009;114(3):442–7.
23. Secord AA, et al. A multicenter evaluation of adjuvant therapy in women with optimally resected stage IIIC endometrial cancer. Gynecol Oncol. 2013;128(1):65–70.
24. Greven K, et al. Final analysis of RTOG 9708: adjuvant postoperative irradiation combined with cisplatin/paclitaxel chemotherapy following surgery for patients with high-risk endometrial cancer. Gynecol Oncol. 2006;103(1):155–9.
25. Jhingran A, et al. A prospective phase II study of chemoradiation followed by adjuvant chemotherapy for FIGO stage I-IIIA (1988) uterine papillary serous carcinoma of the endometrium. Gynecol Oncol. 2013;129(2):304–9.

Management of Advanced Endometrial Cancer and Inhibitors of the PI3K/AKT/mTOR Pathway

31

Michael J. Flynn and Rebecca Kristeleit

31.1 Introduction

Endometrial cancer is the most common gynaecological malignancy in the industrialised world and the seventh most common cause of cancer death in women in western Europe [1]. More than 90 % of cases occur in women over 50 years of age and the incidence is rising [2, 4, 5, 16]. Mortality is also increasing, particularly in older patients [16, 22]. As endometrial cancer is a disease related to lifetime oestrogen exposure in many cases [23, 24], the rise in incidence has been predominantly attributed to increasing obesity, life expectancy, and adjuvant Tamoxifen use for breast cancer [3].

Although most patients with endometrial cancer present with early stage disease amenable to potentially curative surgery, approximately 20 % subsequently relapse and die from their disease [25, 26]. A further estimated 15 % of patients present de novo with inoperable advanced or metastatic disease [6, 25, 26]. In one series, patients who presented with FIGO stage IIIc1 or IIIc2 endometrial cancer relapsed, despite surgery followed by chemotherapy and/or radiotherapy in approximately 40 % of cases [27].

M.J. Flynn, MD • R. Kristeleit, MD, PhD (✉)
Department of Oncology, University College London, London, UK
e-mail: r.kristeleit@ucl.ac.uk

There is no established standard of care for advanced, inoperable endometrial cancer. Chemotherapy and endocrine therapy are often used despite limited efficacy or OS benefit [8–10, 28, 29]. Patient co-morbidity further limits treatment options in many cases [30–32].

Historically, endometrial cancers have been designated Type I (typically well-differentiated, low grade, endometrioid histology) or Type II (typically poorly differentiated, high grade, serous or clear cell histology) based on clinicopathologic features [25]. This classification is of limited utility for predicting prognosis or response to treatment although there is a tendency for Type II cancers to have a more aggressive clinical course [25, 33, 34]. The majority of clinical trials in advanced endometrial cancer have not stratified outcome or selected patients according to Type I or Type II designation. As a result, endometrial carcinomas regardless of type are managed with the same chemotherapy regimens despite biological differences. Whilst certain molecular lesions predominate in each type of endometrial cancer (Table 31.1), there is significant overlap. The integration of molecular profiling with the clinicopathologic classification is likely to have greater discriminatory value for predicting prognosis and response [34–36].

In order to improve outcomes, patient selection according to histologic morphology, even with the known limitation of diagnostic reproducibility [37–39], may be a better approach whilst

H.R.H. Patel et al. (eds.), *Pelvic Cancer Surgery: Modern Breakthroughs and Future Advances*,
DOI 10.1007/978-1-4471-4258-4_31, © Springer-Verlag London 2015

Table 31.1 Estimated frequency of selected molecular lesions in Type I and Type II endometrial cancer [33]

Molecular lesion	Type I (%)	Type II (%)	References
PIK3CA			
Mutation	30	20	[20, 81–83, 122]
Amplification	2–14	46	[42, 122]
KRAS mutation	11–26	2	[119, 123, 124]
AKT mutation	3	Undetected	[85]
PTEN functional loss	50–83	5	[73, 74]
FGFR2 mutation	12–16	1	[117, 119, 125]
TP53 mutation	20	90	[82, 124, 126]
Microsatellite instability	20–45	<5	[127, 128]
HER2			
Overexpression	3–10	32	[129, 130]
Amplification	1	17	[131]

developing an understanding of the predominant molecular drivers in endometrial malignancy that predict prognostic or therapeutic outcome.

There remains currently a significant unmet need for tolerable, effective therapy to treat patients with advanced endometrial cancer. Due to the relatively poor results with chemotherapy regimens, many classes of novel targeted therapy are being explored in this indication. These include anti-angiogenics, EGFR inhibitors, HER2 inhibitors and most extensively, drugs targeting the PI3K/AKT/mTOR pathway [14, 15, 19, 21, 33, 40, 41].

The PTEN/PI3K/AKT/mTor axis is the most commonly disrupted signaling pathway in endometrial cancer and as a result has received the greatest amount of clinical attention in terms of drug development [33, 42]. Several drugs targeting this signaling pathway are currently being evaluated in the setting of advanced disease and some trials have reported results [19, 41, 43, 44]. The current experience, status, limitations and future directions of novel therapeutics targeting the PTEN/PI3K/AKT/mTor pathway in endometrial cancer will be explored. The importance of continuously evaluating our understanding of endometrial tumour biology and integrating predictive biomarker identification and development with the clinical development of these agents to improve outcomes by directing patient selection will be discussed.

31.2 Strategies for the Medical Management of Advanced Endometrial Cancer

Chemotherapy

There is currently no standard first line chemotherapy in advanced or recurrent disease [1, 8, 10–15, 28, 29, 33]. Although Phase II trials have demonstrated activity with doxorubicin, paclitaxel and platinum compounds, only paclitaxel-containing regimens have consistently shown a response rate (RR) >20 % in advanced disease [1, 45, 46]. Consideration of alternative schedules of chemotherapy may help to improve response rates, with weekly carboplatin-paclitaxel being the most promising with RR up to 71 % in one study and an acceptable toxicity profile [47–50]. Combination chemotherapeutic regimens are generally more active in endometrial cancer than monotherapies, but this is at the expense of greater toxicity. One systematic review of eight randomized controlled trials (RCT) showed that treatment consisting of 'more' chemotherapy was associated with longer OS and progression free survival (PFS) [29] although no definitive recommendation could be made for a specific regimen [8, 29]. The GOG177 trial showed that combination of cisplatin/paclitaxel/doxorubicin had significantly greater RR (57 % vs 34 %) and OS (15.3 months vs 12.3 months) compared to doxorubicin/cisplatin but the utility of this regimen is compromised by significant toxicity [51]. Three meta-analyses conclude there is currently no statistically significant evidence to suggest one particular doublet chemotherapy over any other doublet, or a particular single-agent chemotherapy over another [8, 28, 29]. However, data for making comparisons is limited [8, 28, 29]. In view of the substantial side-effect profile of three drug regimens, recurrent endometrial cancer is most commonly treated with a combination of carboplatin/paclitaxel and less commonly, a doxorubicin-containing doublet [40].

Endocrine Therapy

A systematic review of the use of endocrine therapy for the management of endometrial cancer concluded that there is insufficient evidence that hormonal treatment improves the survival of patients with advanced or recurrent disease [9]. However, the authors concede the conclusions are limited by the small patient numbers on RCT which limit the ability to prove a significant benefit [9]. GOG153, a Phase II trial evaluating patients receiving MPA (medroxyprogesterone acetate) alternating with tamoxifen, reported meaningful activity where RR was observed to be 27 % and OS 14 months [52].

Biological Therapy

Preliminary data for several molecular targeted agents in endometrial cancer are emerging [14, 15, 19, 21, 33, 40, 41]. Although a number of established drug targets are expressed in endometrial cancer, therapeutic targeting of several of these in an unselected endometrial cancer population has not yielded much activity. The epidermal growth factor receptor (EGFR) is frequently expressed in normal endometrium as well as endometrial cancer [53] but use of the EGFR inhibitor erlotinib was associated with a RR of only 13 % [54]. Similarly, although HER-2 is overexpressed or amplified in a proportion of endometrial cancers [55], there were no objective responses to trastuzumab in a phase II trial of a selected population of HER-2 positive endometrial cancer patients [56]. Evidence suggests that angiogenesis and vascular endothelial growth factor (VEGF) signaling have a key role in endometrial cancer progression [57]. Two Phase II clinical trials have shown very encouraging activity of bevacizumab monotherapy in advanced or recurrent endometrial cancer [58, 59] making this one of the most promising novel targets for monotherapy in endometrial cancer. Several trials with bevacizumab in endometrial cancer are continuing [40]. A Phase II trial of the antiangiogenic agent sorafenib, an oral, multitargeted tyrosine kinase inhibitor showed disappointing activity in the endometrial population [60]. More recent trials are tending to select an appropriate patient population based on prospective mutational status of a molecular target, e.g. FGFR2 (dovitinib) or PI3K (PF-04691502) when targeting specific pathways (Table 31.2), a practice that is likely to increase.

Table 31.2 Selected current trials of PI3K/AKT/mTOR pathway inhibitors as monotherapy and in combination for endometrial cancer

Drug	Target	Phase	clinicaltrials.gov identifier
BKM120	PI3K	II	NCT01289041
XL147	PI3K	II	NCT01013324
PF-05212384	Dual mTor/PI3K	II	NCT01420081
GDC-0980	Dual mTor/PI3K	II	NCT01455493
DS7423	Dual mTor/PI3K	I	NCT01364844
MK2206	Akt inhibitor	II	NCT01307631
Temsirolimus	mTOR	II	NCT01460979
Ridaforolimus	mTOR	II	NCT00122343
Everolimus	mTOR	II	NCT00087685
Temsirolimus/bevacizumab	mTOR/VEGF	II	NCT01010126
Temsirolimus/carboplatin/paclitaxel	mTOR/DNA/microtubules	II	NCT00977574
Temsirolimus/R04929097	mTOR/gamma-secretase	I	NCT01198184
Temsirolimus/pegylated liposomal doxorubicin	mTOR/DNA	I	NCT00982631
Everolimus/letrozole	mTOR/aromatase inhibitor	II	NCT01068249
Dovitinib	FGFR2, VEGF	II	NCT01379534
Trastuzumab/carboplatin/paclitaxel	HER2/DNA/microtubules	II	NCT01367002

31.3 PTEN/PI3K/AKT/mTor Signalling

The PI3K pathway (Fig. 31.1) plays an important role in key cellular functions such as cell growth, proliferation, metabolism and survival [19, 41, 61–63]. Oncogenic dysregulation of the pathway is common in solid tumours due to several different mechanisms of genetic disruption including PIK3CA mutation and PTEN loss [19, 41, 61–63]. Aberrant signalling through the PI3K cascade has also been implicated in chemoresistance in a number of tumour types [19, 41, 61–63]. Within the pathway there are several targets that have been identified for development of novel targeted therapies including mTOR (mammalian

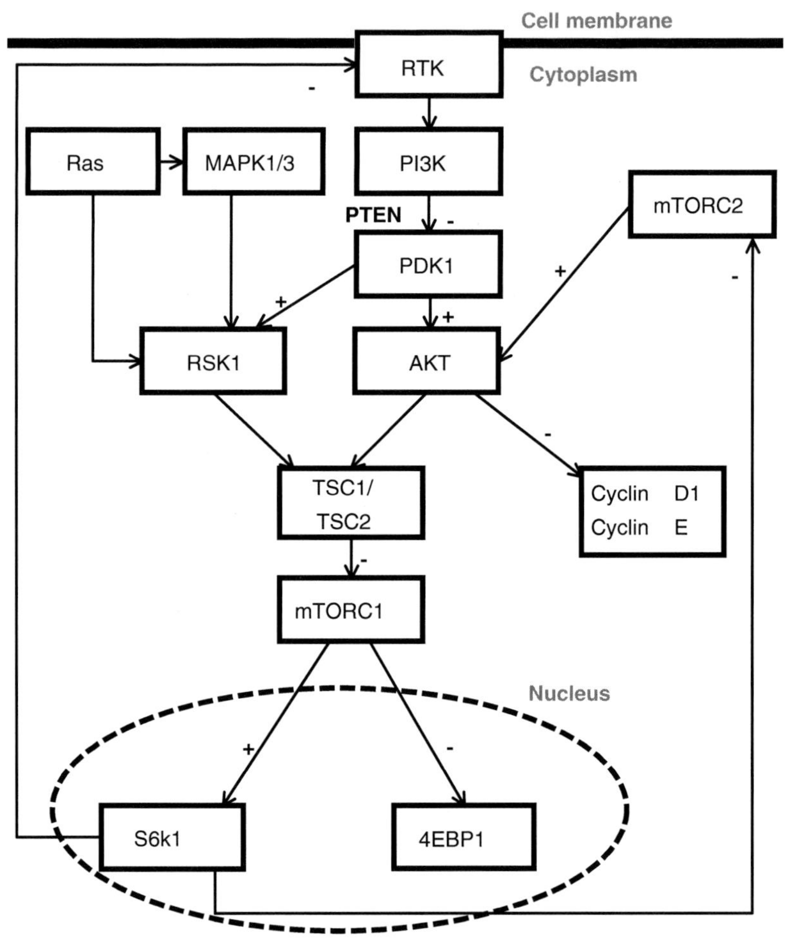

Fig. 31.1 Schematic of the PI3K/mTor pathway. Receptor tyrosine kinases (RTKs) signal through PI3K to activate phosphoinositide-dependent protein kinase-1 (PDK1). PDK1 phosphorylates AKT and ribosomal S6 kinase (RSK1), all of which require a second activating phosphorylation, e.g. by mTORC1, mTORC2, and MAPK3 [133–136]. Thus, PI3K and mTOR pathways act together to promote cell growth, division, and survival [70–72]. TSC1/2 (Tuberous Sclerosis 1/2) functions as a molecular hub, integrating growth factor and energy-sensing pathways to regulate mTOR/Raptor activity [137–141]. The inhibition of mTORC1 does reduce feedback inhibition on upstream regulators and this may be relevant in molecular targeting [132]. High levels of AKT activation leads to survival signals by phosphorylation of several targets including mTORC1 and mTORC2 [132, 142]. mTOR drives cancer growth by activating the lipid and protein biosynthesis needed for robust tumour expansion. This occurs via the resulting hyperactivation of the critical mTORC1 effectors S6K1 (serine 6 kinase 1) and 4EBP1. Oncogenic mTORC1 and mTORC2 activation also drives cell proliferation via increases in cyclin D1 and cyclin E [132, 143, 144]

target of rapamycin) and PI3K (Fig. 31.1). PTEN (phosphatase and tensin homolog) acts as a suppressor of pathway activation.

There are three classes of phosphoinositide 3-kinase (PI3K) each with distinct structure and function. Class IA PI3K heterodimers are the most studied, encoded by the PIK3CA and PIK3R1/PIK3R2 genes for the catalytic (p110) and regulatory (p85) subunits respectively [61, 64, 65]. PTEN is a lipid phosphatase that cleaves phosphoinostides, negatively regulating PI3K-dependent signalling [61, 64, 65]. Phosphorylation of PI3K substrates activates signalling through AKT which initiates a cascade of downstream events [61, 62, 64, 65]. mTOR complex 1 (mTORC1) is one of the main effectors of AKT signaling, mediating lipid and protein synthesis, whilst mTORC2 is part of a positive feedback loop that activates AKT [65–67] which can be problematic in therapeutic targeting of mTORC1 [68, 69].

In summary, oncogenic PI3K/AKT/mTOR signaling promotes cell growth, division, survival and maintenance of the oncogenic phenotype [64–72].

31.4 The PI3K Pathway and Endometrial Cancer

Alterations in the PTEN/PI3K/AKT/mTor pathway are frequent in Type I and Type II endometrial cancers, often co-exist and are involved in pathogenesis of the disease [20, 33, 42, 73].

One of the most important mechanisms of endometrial carcinogenesis is functional inactivation of PTEN which is often present in precancers suggesting a central role in pathogenesis [73]. PTEN loss is associated with improved prognosis in endometrial malignancy [74, 75] and occurs as a result of various mechanisms including gene mutation, promoter methylation and protein degradation [33, 76, 77]. Although inactivation is rare in normal endometrium, it is present in 20 % of endometrial hyperplasia, 35–50 % of endometrioid endometrial cancer (EEC), and 10 % of non-endometrioid endometrial cancer (NEEC) [20, 25, 26, 33, 63, 76–79].

Activating PIK3CA mutations are estimated to be present in approximately 30 % of EEC and 15 % of NEEC and are frequently coexistent with dysfunctional PTEN [20, 33, 80, 81]. Mutation of the PIK3CA gene is associated with poor survival and an aggressive disease course [42, 82, 83]. The PIK3R1 and PIK3R2 genes encoding for p85α[alpha] and p85β[beta] respectively, regulatory subunits of PI3K, have been found to be amplified and mutated in endometrial cancer, the latter sometimes in the absence of PTEN loss [75, 84]. Novel activating mutations continue to be identified [76].

Other less frequent mutations of this signalling pathway in endometrial malignancy include somatic mutation of AKT1 estimated at 2 % of EEC [85]. Mutations in TSC1/TSC2 have been recently described in endometrial cancer suggesting a novel upstream disruption of mTORC1 activity [86].

31.5 Therapeutics Targeting the PI3K/AKT/mTor Pathway in Endometrial Cancer

There are four main categories of novel drug that target different proteins in the PTEN/PI3K/AKT/mTor pathway (Fig. 31.2) with varying amounts of clinical experience for each: mTor inhibitors, PI3K inhibitors, dual PI3K/mTor inhibitors, AKT inhibitors. Combination therapies with these agents are also being clinically explored.

mTOR Inhibitors

Of all drugs targeting the PI3K pathway, the first generation mTor inhibitors (rapamycin analogues) have been the most extensively evaluated in endometrial cancer. Second generation compounds targeting mTor catalytic function through the mTor kinase domain, inhibit mTorc1/mTorc2 simultaneously and demonstrate greater potency [87–89]. Dual targeting of mTorc1 and mTorc2 circumvents the unwanted positive feedback loop where uninhibited mTorc2 stimulates AKT activation as can occur with the rapalogs [68, 69].

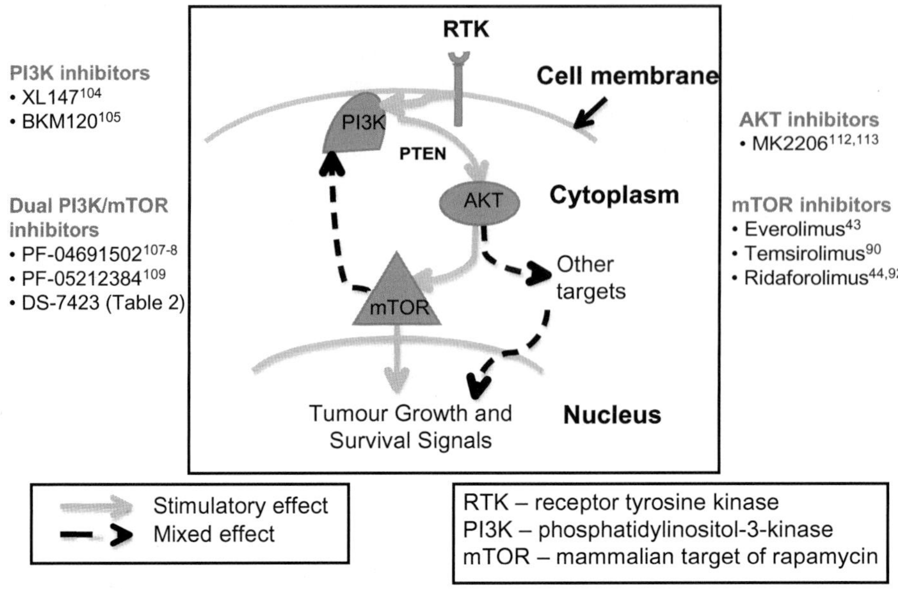

Fig. 31.2 PI3K/mTOR therapeutic agents in endometrial cancer

Temsirolimus [90], ridaforolimus [44, 91, 92] and everolimus [43] have been evaluated as monotherapy in unselected patients with inoperable advanced or metastatic endometrial cancer. Objective response rates were 14 % (temsirolimus [90]) and 4.4–7.7 % (ridaforolimus [91, 92]) with no objective response obtained with everolimus [43]. Many patients within these Phase II studies, however, benefited from long term disease stabilisation and those with no prior therapy for advanced disease benefited more [43, 91, 92]. A randomized Phase II ridaforolimus trial demonstrated a statistically significant benefit in progression free survival for ridaforolimus over more standard treatment [44]. Common adverse events were fatigue, rash, mucositis, hyperglycaemia (defined as on-target toxicity) and pneumonitis with hypertriglyceridaemia being less common [43, 44, 90–92]. Neither PTEN nor PIK3CA status correlated with response to temsirolimus [90] and analysis is ongoing for ridaforolimus [92]. Studies examining the relationship of PTEN and PIK3CA mutation as predictors of response to everolimus also found no correlation with outcome [93, 94].

The mechanism of the greater efficacy and potency of second generation mTOR catalytic site inhibitors may be due to their ability to inhibit the rapamycin-resistant mTorc1 functions rather than the additional inhibition of mTorc2 [95, 96]. It was established, however, that inhibition of mTorc2 prevented phosphorylation of Akt [96]. However, these agents had minimal effects on the phosphorylation state of several Akt substrates despite effectively inhibiting Akt S473 phosphorylation, suggesting they may not disable all components of Akt signalling [96, 97]. Other pathways of activation may remain unblocked allowing feedback activation still to occur which may result in hyperactivation of Akt-independent effectors of PI3K signalling [96–98]. mTor kinase inhibitors in early phase trial for solid tumours that include endometrial cancer are AZD2014, OSI-027 and INK128 (clinicaltrials.gov).

PI3K Inhibitors

PI3K inhibitors can be divided into isoform-specific inhibitors or pan-PI3K inhibitors which target all four Class I PI3Ks. Isoform-specific inhibitors are potentially more tumour-specific and have a better side effect profile due to their specificity. For example, p110α[alpha]-specific inhibitors may effectively shut off PI3K–Akt signalling in cancers with PIK3CA mutations [98]. A p110β[beta]-specific inhibitor has shown promise in preventing PI3K signalling in PTEN-deficient cancers [99–102]. However, even in cancers that seem to be specifically reliant on either p110α[alpha] or p110β[beta], there is the concern that other non-targeted p110 isoforms might eventually compensate for decreased activity of the targeted isoform [98]. Given the prevalence of PTEN loss and PIK3CA mutation in endometrial cancers, the isoform-specific inhibitors, e.g. INK1117, NVP-BYL719 and GSK2636771 may be beneficial in this patient population. However, this depends on these genetic mutations predicting for response which has not been the case for mTor inhibition [90, 93, 94].

Phase 2 clinical trials are ongoing with the pan-PI3K inhibitors NVP-BKM120 and XL147 in endometrial cancer (clinicaltrials.gov). The side effect profile of these agents has been tolerable in Phase I studies mainly with nausea, vomiting and g-i upset and manageable hyperglycaemia [103, 104]. The results from the endometrial cancer trials are awaited with interest. Consistent with its mechanism of action, NVP-BKM120 decreases the cellular levels of p-Akt and preferentially inhibits tumour cells bearing PIK3CA mutations, in contrast to either KRAS or PTEN mutant models [105]. NVP-BKM120 behaves synergistically when combined with either targeted agents such as MEK or HER2 inhibitors or with cytotoxic agents such as docetaxel or temozolomide [105]. These findings may impact future development of this class of drugs.

Dual PI3K/mTOR Inhibitors

Most of the dual PI3K-mTOR inhibitors target the Class I PI3K isoforms (p110α[alpha], p110β[beta] and p110δ[delta] predominantly) as well as mTORC1 and mTORC2 in order to maximally inhibit PI3K pathway signaling. This approach may also minimize the feedback activation of PI3K signaling observed with mTorc1 inhibitors and generate greater therapeutic benefit [68, 106]. This class of inhibitors might also be effective in cancers with Akt mutations or amplifications [98]. The potential advantages of these compounds over other agents targeting the PI3K cascade are being established as the drugs progress through clinical development.

PF-04691502 and PF-05212384 are dual PI3K/mTor inhibitors being investigated in a second line Phase 2 trial in endometrial cancer. In PIK3CA-mutant and PTEN-deleted cancer cell lines, PF-04691502 reduced phosphorylation of AKT inhibited cell proliferation via mTORC1 activity inhibition [107]. In the first in human, Phase I studies both PF-04691502 and PF-05212384 had been well tolerated with the most common treatment-related adverse events being fatigue, nausea, vomiting, decreased appetite, rash, and hyperglycaemia, similar to pan-PI3K inhibitors [108, 109]. GDC-0980 is another dual PI3K/mTor inhibitor [110] found to be tolerable in Phase I [111], also being evaluated in endometrial cancer with results awaited (Table 31.2).

Akt Inhibitors

Although Akt mutation is uncommon in endometrial cancer, this target is being pursued in this indication with MK2206 (Table 31.2). Cancers with AKT1 mutations and AKT1 and AKT2 amplifications might be expected to be more sensitive to Akt inhibitors [98]. MK2206 is a potent inhibitor of Akt 1, 2 and 3, with broad preclinical antitumor activity and tolerability as well as clinical activity in Phase I trial [112, 113]. Common drug-related toxicities include hyperglycemia, skin rash, nausea, fatigue, and diarrhoea [112].

Combination Trials

In an attempt to reduce resistance and enhance efficacy of the various drugs targeting the PI3K pathway, trials investigating combinations with mechanistically diverse agents are underway (clinicaltrials.gov, Table 31.2). The main limitation for this approach is increased toxicity. The role of overactive PI3K signaling in chemoresistance supports the combination of PI3K pathway targeting agents with chemotherapeutics (temsirolimus, carboplatin, paclitaxel) as well as endocrine therapy (letrozole and everolimus) [19]. In addition, combinations of mechanistically complementary agents both with activity in endometrial cancer for example bevacizumab and temsirolimus, are being evaluated.

Limitations of PI3K/mTOR Pathway Inhibitors in Endometrial Cancer

Despite a high incidence of molecular disruption in the PTEN/PI3K/AKT/mTor axis in endometrial cancers, only a small percentage of patients have responded to this class of drugs. One possible reason for this is the lack of patient selection and a tendency towards including patients with mutations in this pathway in clinical trials of PI3K/AKT/mTOR inhibitors has gained some momentum [115]. However, even though these are targeted agents, it is not clear which patients are most likely to benefit as the presence of PIK3CA mutation and PTEN loss have not so far been predictive of clinical benefit [90, 93, 94]. One recent report suggests a subtype of PIK3CA mutation, H1047R, may be predictive of response to drugs targeting this pathway but warrants further investigation [116]. This is likely to be a reflection of the complexity of the signalling networks and the multiplicity of feedback loops within and around the pathway [98]. Possibly, these drugs should be investigated in the first line/adjuvant setting, before resistance is established.

Further understanding of the molecular events and drivers in endometrial cancer through initiatives such as The Cancer Genome Project (TCGA) will help to inform biomarker development in order that patients can be appropriately selected for treatment [17, 18]. Validating assays for biomarker assessment and finding cost-effective measures to roll-out testing of samples in a directed way is becoming more important.

The specific toxicity of these drugs has limitations within this patient population. Whilst on the whole they are fairly well-tolerated and orally administered, the potential for hyperglycaemia will be problematic for a proportion of endometrial cancer patients due to pre-existing insulin resistance associated with obesity. Optimal absorption of oral preparations may be impeded by intra-abdominal disease. Other considerations are general ill-health of patients presenting with advanced disease due to other co-morbidities [32]. If used in combination regimens with other drugs toxicity may be enhanced.

31.6 Future Directions

The future of novel agents targeting this molecular pathway in endometrial cancer will depend on the ability to define a sensitive patient population for monotherapy and finding effective, tolerable combination strategies.

Studies have shown that inhibition of mTORC1 also leads to activation of the ERK signalling pathway [114], raising concerns that crosstalk could mitigate the effectiveness of PI3K pathway inhibitors. An increasing amount of preclinical data suggest that activating KRAS mutations may predict resistance [94, 114]. In the latter case, combined inhibition of the RAS/RAF/MEK and PI3K/AKT/mTOR pathways has been suggested as a therapeutic strategy. In addition, the PI3K/AKT/mTOR pathway has been implicated in conferring resistance to conventional therapies, and so PI3K/AKT/mTOR pathway inhibitors in combination with hormonal and/or cytotoxic agents are being evaluated.

Frequent mutations in fibroblast growth factor receptor 2 (FGFR2) in EEC (12 %) also point to the importance of receptor tyrosine kinase (RTK) signalling in the aetiology of this disease [117]. In vitro studies have shown that endometrial cancer cell lines with activating FGFR2 mutations are selectively sensitive to a pan-FGFR inhibitor, PD173074. Several agents with activity against FGFRs are currently in clinical trials [118, 119]. These are also potential therapeutics to consider in combination with PI3K pathway inhibitors although combination toxicity may be problematic.

Angiogenesis is a key component of tumour growth, and metastasis and angiogenic growth factors, such as vascular endothelial growth factor (VEGF), are highly expressed in endometrial carcinomas [57, 120]. VEGF expression has been correlated with poor prognostic factors such as lymphovascular space invasion (LVSI), nodal metastasis and poor survival [120, 121]. Anti-angiogenic agents such as bevacizumab show clinical promise [58] and are being combined with mTor inhibitors in endometrial cancer (Table 31.2).

The first line treatment of disease with biologics is a development direction that may be warranted. In response to evidence supporting combination regimens with cytotoxic and targeted agents, many trials are underway to demonstrate superior efficacy in the first line. One example is the GOG phase II trial, GOG 86P that compares the current standards (carboplatin and a taxol plus bevacizumab or temsirolimus) with carboplatin, bevacizumab and ixebepilone in the first-line treatment of advanced endometrial cancer [14].

31.7 Summary

Drugs targeting the PI3K axis are showing promise in endometrial cancer but are not without toxicity. Understanding how to molecularly select patients for these treatments is likely to improve their clinical benefit. Combination regimens may also broaden their activity for the treatment of endometrial cancer.

Key Points

- Endometrial cancer is the most common gynaecological cancer in the industrialized world and incidence is increasing
- The PI3K signaling pathway is the most commonly disrupted in endometrial cancer and implicated in pathogenesis
- Loss of the tumour suppressor function of PTEN frequently occurs in endometrial cancer which can activate the PI3K pathway
- Type I and Type II histological subtypes have significant overlap in molecular profile of PI3K pathway disruption
- Inhibitors of mTor, PI3K, PI3K/mTor and AKT are in Phase II clinical trial in endometrial cancer as monotherapies
- Clinical trials of mTor inhibitors have reported clinical benefit (response and stable disease) in endometrial cancer
- Toxicity is manageable and includes rash, hyperglycaemia and gastrointestinal side effects
- Phase II trials are yet to definitively conclude whether the presence or absence of PIK3CA mutations or PTEN loss correlate with efficacy and whether they should be used for patient selection
- Appropriate patient selection once a validated biomarker profile is identified may increase the clinical benefit of these agents as monotherapies
- Combination strategies of PI3K pathway targeting drugs with standard chemotherapeutics, hormonal agents and other targeted biologics will be part of ongoing development

References

1. Colombo N, Preti E, Landoni F, Carinelli S, Colombo A, Marini C, Sessa C, ESMO Guidelines Working Group. Endometrial cancer: ESMO Clinical Practice Guidelines for diagnosis, treatment and follow-up. Ann Oncol. 2011;22(Supp 6):vi35–9.
2. Jemal A, Bray F, Center MM, Ferlay J, Ward E, Forman D. Global cancer statistics. CA Cancer J Clin. 2011;61(2):69–90.
3. Bray F, Dos Santos SI, Moller H, Weiderpass E. Endometrial cancer incidence trends in Europe: underlying determinants and prospects for prevention. Cancer Epidemiol Biomarkers Prev. 2005;14(5):1132–42.
4. Evans T, Sany O, Pearmain P, Ganesan R, Blann A, Sundar S. Trends in the rising incidence of endometrial cancer by type: data from a UK population-based registry from 1994 to 2006. Br J Cancer. 2011;104(9):1505–10.
5. National Cancer Institute: Surveillance Epidemiology and End Results. SEER cancer statistics review 1975–2009 (Vintage 2009 populations) 2012 Apr (updated 20 Aug 2012; cited 2 Dec 2012). Available from: http://seer.cancer.gov/csr/1975_2009_pops09/.

6. Lindahl B, Ranstam J, Willén R. Relapse of endometrial carcinoma: follow-up of 272 patients with relapse. Anticancer Res. 2012;32(8):3391–5.
7. Greer BE, Koh WJ, Abu-Rustum N, Bookman MA, Bristow RE, Campos SM, Cho KR, Copeland L, Crispens MA, Eifel PJ, Huh WK, Jaggernauth W, Kapp DS, Kavanagh JJ, Lurain 3rd JR, Morgan M, Morgan RJ, Powell CB, Remmenga SW, Reynolds RK, Alvarez Secord A, Small Jr W, Teng N. Uterine neoplasms. Clinical Practice Guidelines in Oncology. J Natl Compr Canc Netw. 2009;7(5):498–531.
8. Vale CL, Tierney J, Bull SJ, Symonds PR. Chemotherapy for advanced, recurrent or metastatic endometrial carcinoma. Cochrane Database Syst Rev. 2012;(8):CD003915.
9. Kokka F, Brockbank E, Oram D, Gallagher C, Bryant A. Hormonal therapy in advanced or recurrent endometrial cancer. Cochrane Database Syst Rev. 2010;(12):CD007926.
10. Pectasides D, Pectasides E, Economopoulos T. Systemic therapy in metastatic or recurrent endometrial cancer. Cancer Treat Rev. 2007;33(2):177–90.
11. Dizon DS. Treatment options for advanced endometrial carcinoma. Gynecol Oncol. 2010;117(2):373–81.
12. Dellinger TH, Monk BJ. Systemic therapy for recurrent endometrial cancer: a review of North American trials. Expert Rev Anticancer Ther. 2009;9(7):905–16.
13. Ray M, Fleming G. Management of advanced-stage and recurrent endometrial cancer. Semin Oncol. 2009;36(2):145–54.
14. Hill EK, Dizon DS. Medical therapy of endometrial cancer: current status and promising novel treatments. Drugs. 2012;72(5):705–13.
15. Tsoref D, Oza AM. Recent advances in systemic therapy for advanced endometrial cancer. Curr Opin Oncol. 2011;23(5):494–500.
16. Jemal A, Siegel R, Ward E, Hao Y, Xu J, Murray T, Thun MJ. Cancer statistics. CA Cancer J Clin. 2008; 58(2):71–96.
17. National Cancer Institute: The Cancer Genome Atlas. Uterine Corpus Endometrial Cancer. [Internet] 2012 (updated 14 May 2012; cited 2 Dec 2012). Available from: http://cancergenome.nih.gov/cancersselected/endometrial.
18. Liang H, Cheung LW, Li J, Ju Z, Yu S, Stemke-Hale K, Dogruluk T, Lu Y, Liu X, Gu C, Guo W, Scherer SE, Carter H, Westin SN, Dyer MD, Verhaak RG, Zhang F, Karchin R, Liu CG, Lu KH, Broaddus RR, Scott KL, Hennessy BT, Mills GB. Whole-exome sequencing combined with functional genomics reveals novel candidate driver cancer genes in endometrial cancer. Genome Res. 2012;22(11):2120–9.
19. Slomovitz BM, Coleman RL. The PI3K/AKT/mTOR pathway as a therapeutic target in endometrial cancer. Clin Cancer Res. 2012;18(21): 5856–64.
20. Oda K, Stokoe D, Taketani Y, McCormick F. High frequency of coexistent mutations of PIK3CA and PTEN genes in endometrial carcinoma. Cancer Res. 2005;65(23):10669–73.
21. Dedes KJ, Wetterskog D, Ashworth A, Kaye SB, Reis-Filho JS. Emerging therapeutic targets in endometrial cancer. Nat Rev Clin Oncol. 2011;8(5):261–71.
22. Ferlay J, Shin HR, Bray F, Forman D, Mathers C, Parkin DM. Estimates of worldwide burden of cancer in 2008: GLOBOCAN 2008. Int J Cancer. 2010; 127(12):2893–917.
23. Carlson MJ, Thiel KW, Yang S, Leslie KK. Catch it before it kills: progesterone, obesity, and the prevention of endometrial cancer. Discov Med. 2012;14(76):215–22.
24. Cramer DW. The epidemiology of endometrial and ovarian cancer. Hematol Oncol Clin North Am. 2012;26(1):1–12.
25. Hecht JL, Mutter GL. Molecular and pathologic aspects of endometrial carcinogenesis. J Clin Oncol. 2006;24(29):4783–91.
26. Amant F, Moerman P, Neven P, Timmerman D, Van Limbergen E, Vergote I. Endometrial cancer. Lancet. 2005;366(9484):491–505.
27. Gadduci A, Cosio S, Fabrini MG, Guerrieri ME, Greco C, Genazzani AR. Analysis of failures in patients with FIGO stage IIIc1-IIIc2 endometrial cancer. Anticancer Res. 2012;32(1):201–5.
28. Carey MS, Gawlik C, Fung-Kee-Fung M, Chambers A, Oliver T, Cancer Care Ontario Practice Guidelines Initiative Gynecology Cancer Disease Site Group. Systematic review of systemic therapy for advanced or recurrent endometrial cancer. Gynecol Oncol. 2006;101(1):158–67.
29. Humber CE, Tierney JF, Symonds RP, Collingwood M, Kirwan J, Williams C, Green JA. Chemotherapy for advanced, recurrent or metastatic endometrial cancer: a systematic review of Cochrane collaboration. Ann Oncol. 2007;18(3):409–20.
30. Truong PT, Kader HA, Lacy B, Lesperance M, MacNeil MV, Berthelet E, McMurtie E, Alexander S. The effects of age and comorbidity on treatment and outcomes in women with endometrial cancer. Am J Clin Oncol. 2005;28(2):157–64.
31. Modesitt SC, Van Nagell Jr JR. The impact of obesity on the incidence and treatment of gynecologic cancers: a review. Obstet Gynecol Surv. 2005;60(10):683–92.
32. Kitchener HC. Survival from endometrial cancer in England and Wales up to 2001. Br J Cancer. 2008;99 Suppl 1:S68–9.
33. Salvesen HB, Haldorsen IS, Trovik J. Markers for individualised therapy in endometrial carcinoma. Lancet Oncol. 2012;13(8):e353.
34. McMeekin DS, Filiaci VL, Thigpen JT, Gallion HH, Fleming GF, Rogers WH, Gynecologic Oncology Study Group Study. The relationship between histology and outcome in advanced and recurrent endometrial cancer patients participating in first- line chemotherapy trials: a Gynecologic Oncology Group study. Gynecol Oncol. 2007;106(1):16–22.
35. Levan K, Partheen K, Osterberg L, Olsson B, Delle U, Eklind S, Horvath G. Identification of a gene expression signature for survival prediction in type I endometrial carcinoma. Gene Expr. 2010;14:361–70.

36. Samarnthai N, Hall K, Yeh IT. Molecular profiling of endometrial malignancies. Obstet Gynecol Int. 2010;2010:162363.
37. Fadare O, Parkash V, Dupont WD, Acs G, Atkins KA, Irving JA, Pirog EC, Quade BJ, Quddus MR, Rabban 3rd JT, Vang R, Hecht JL. The diagnosis of endometrial carcinomas with clear cells by gynecologic pathologists: an assessment of interobserver variability and associated morphologic features. Am J Surg Pathol. 2012;36(8):1107–18.
38. Scholten AN, Smit VT, Beerman H, van Putten WL, Creutzberg CL. Prognostic significance and interobserver variability of histologic grading systems for endometrial carcinoma. Cancer. 2004;100(4):764–72.
39. Kwon JS, Francis JA, Qiu F, Weir MM, Ettler HC. When is a pathology review indicated in endometrial cancer? Obstet Gynecol. 2007;110(6): 1224–30.
40. Wright JD, Barrena Medel NI, Sehouli J, Fujiwara K, Herzog TJ. Contemporary management of endometrial cancer. Lancet. 2012;379(9823):1352–60.
41. Diaz-Padilla I, Duran I, Clarke BA, Oza AM. Biologic rationale and clinical activity of mTOR inhibitors in gynecological cancer. Cancer Treat Rev. 2012;38(6):767–75.
42. Salvesen HB, Carter SL, Mannelqvist M, Dutt A, Getz G, Stefansson IM, Raeder MB, Sos ML, Engelsen IB, Trovik J, Wik E, Greulich H, Bø TH, Jonassen I, Thomas RK, Zander T, Garraway LA, Oyan AM, Sellers WR, Kalland KH, Meyerson M, Akslen LA, Beroukhim R. Integrated genomic profiling of endometrial carcinoma associates aggressive tumors with indicators of PI3 kinase activation. Proc Natl Acad Sci U S A. 2009;106(12):4834–9.
43. Slomovitz BM, Lu KH, Johnston T, Coleman RL, Munsell M, Broaddus RR, Walker C, Ramondetta LM, Burke TW, Gershenson DM, Wolf J. A phase 2 study of the oral mammalian target of rapamycin inhibitor, everolimus, in patients with recurrent endometrial carcinoma. Cancer. 2010;116(23):5415–9.
44. Oza A, Poveda A, Clamp R, Pignata S, Scambia G, Del Campo JM, McCormack M, Sevcik L, Schwartz BM, Guan S, Lee R, Cheng JD, Haluska FD. A randomized phase II (RP2) trial of ridaforolimus (R) compared with progestin (P) or chemotherapy (C) in female adult patients with advanced endometrial carcinoma [abstract 5009]. Proceedings of the ASCO annual meeting 3–7 Jun 2011, Chicago.
45. Lincoln S, Blessing JA, Lee RB, Roceroto TF. Activity of paclitaxel as second-line chemotherapy in endometrial carcinoma: a Gynecologic Oncology Group study. Gynecol Oncol. 2003;88(3):277–81.
46. Homesley HD, Meltzer NP, Nieves L, Vaccarello L, Lowendowski GS, Elbendary AA. A phase II trial of weekly 1-hour paclitaxel as second-line therapy for endometrial and cervical cancer. Int J Clin Oncol. 2008;13(1):62–5.
47. Vandenput I, Vergote I, Leunen K, Berteloot P, Neven P, Amant F. Leuven dose-dense paclitaxel/carboplatin regimen in patients with primary advanced or recurrent endometrial carcinoma. Int J Gynecol Cancer. 2009;19(6):1147–51.
48. Secord AA, Havrilesky LJ, Carney ME, Soper JT, Clarke-Pearson DL, Rodriguez GC, Berchuck A. Weekly low-dose paclitaxel and carboplatin in the treatment of advanced or recurrent cervical and endometrial cancer. Int J Clin Oncol. 2007;12(1): 31–6.
49. Ito K, Tsubamoto H, Itani Y, Kuroboshi H, Fujita H, Nobunaga T, Coleman RL. A feasibility study of carboplatin and weekly paclitaxel combination chemotherapy in endometrial cancer: a Kansai Clinical Oncology Group study (KCOG0015 trial). Gynecol Oncol. 2011;120(2):193–7.
50. Vandenput I, Vergote I, Neven P, Amant F. Weekly paclitaxel-carboplatin regimen in patients with primary advanced or recurrent endometrial carcinoma. Int J Gynecol Cancer. 2012;22(4):617–22.
51. Fleming GF, Brunetto VL, Cella D, Look KY, Reid GC, Munkarah AR, Kline R, Burger RA, Goodman A, Burks RT. Phase III trial of doxorubicin plus cisplatin with or without paclitaxel plus filgrastim in advanced endometrial carcinoma: a Gynecologic Oncology Group Study. J Clin Oncol. 2004;22: 2159–66.
52. Fiorica VL, Hanjani P, Lentz SS, Mannel R, Andersen W, Gynecologic Oncology Group. Phase II trial of alternating courses of megestrol acetate and tamoxifen in advanced endometrial carcinoma: a Gynecologic Oncology Group study. Gynecol Oncol. 2004;92(1):10–4.
53. Khalifa MA, Mannel RS, Haraway SD, Walker J, Min KW. Expression of EGFR, HER-2/neu, P53, and PCNA in endometrioid, serous papillary, and clear cell endometrial adenocarcinomas. Gynecol Oncol. 1994;53(1):84–92.
54. Oza AM, Eisenhauer EA, Elit L, Cutz JC, Sakurada A, Tsao MS, Hoskins PJ, Biagi J, Ghatage P, Mazurka J, Provencher D, Dore N, Dancey J, Fyles A. Phase II study of erlotinib in recurrent or metastatic endometrial cancer: NCIC IND-148. J Clin Oncol. 2008;26(26):4319–25.
55. Grushko TA, Filiaci VL, Mundt AJ, Ridderstrale K, Olopade OI, Fleming GF, Gynecologic Oncology Group. An exploratory analysis of HER-2 amplification and overexpression in advanced endometrial carcinoma: a Gynecologic Oncology Group study. Gynecol Oncol. 2008;108(1):3–9.
56. Fleming GF, Sill MW, Darcy KM, McMeekin DS, Thigpen JT, Adler LM, Berek JS, Chapman JA, DiSilvestro PA, Horowitz IR, Fiorica JV, Gynecologic Oncology Group. Phase II trial of trastuzumab in women with advanced or recurrent, HER2-positive endometrial carcinoma: a Gynecologic Oncology Group study. Gynecol Oncol. 2010;116(1):15–20.
57. Kamat AA, Merritt WM, Coffey D, Lin YG, Patel PR, Broaddus R, Nugent E, Han LY, Landen Jr CN, Spannuth WA, Lu C, Coleman RL, Gershenson DM, Sood AK. Clinical and biological significance of

vascular endothelial growth factor in endometrial cancer. Clin Cancer Res. 2007;13(24):7487–95.
58. Aghajanian C, Sill MW, Darcy KM, Greer B, McMeekin DS, Rose PG, Rotmensch J, Barnes MN, Hanjani P, Leslie KK, Gynecologic Oncology Group. Phase II trial of bevacizumab in recurrent or persistent endometrial cancer: a Gynecologic Oncology Group study. J Clin Oncol. 2011;29(16):2259–65.
59. Wright JD, Powell MA, Rader JS, Mutch DG, Gibb RK. Bevacizumab therapy in patients with recurrent uterine neoplasms. Anticancer Res. 2007;27(5B):3525–8.
60. Nimeiri HS, Oza AM, Morgan RJ, Huo D, Elit L, Knost JA, Wade 3rd JL, Agamah E, Vokes EE, Fleming GF. A phase II study of sorafenib in advanced uterine carcinoma/carcinosarcoma: a trial of the Chicago, PMH, and California Phase II Consortia. Gynecol Oncol. 2010;117(1): 37–40.
61. Bunney TD, Katan M. Phosphoinositide signalling in cancer: beyond PI3K and PTEN. Nat Rev Cancer. 2010;10(5):342–52.
62. Bartholomeusz C, Gonzalez-Angulo AM. Targeting the PI3K signaling pathway in cancer therapy. Expert Opin Ther Targets. 2012;16(1):121–30.
63. Naumann RW. The role of the phosphatidylinositol 3-kinase (PI3K) pathway in the development and treatment of uterine cancer. Gynecol Oncol. 2011;123(2):411–20.
64. Grant S. Cotargeting survival signaling pathways in cancer. J Clin Invest. 2008;118(10):3003–6.
65. Luo J, Manning BD, Cantley LC. Targeting the PI3K-Akt pathway in human cancer: rationale and promise. Cancer Cell. 2003;4(4):257–62.
66. Engelman JA, Luo J, Cantley LC. The evolution of phosphatidylinositol 3-kinases as regulators of growth and metabolism. Nat Rev Genet. 2006;7(8): 606–19.
67. Courtney KD, Corcoran RB, Engelman JA. The PI3K pathway as drug target in human cancer. J Clin Oncol. 2010;28(6):1075–83.
68. O'Reilly KE, Rojo F, She QB, Solit D, Mills GB, Smith D, Lane H, Hofmann F, Hicklin DJ, Ludwig DL, Baselga J, Rosen N. mTOR inhibition induces upstream receptor tyrosine kinase signaling and activates AKT. Cancer Res. 2006;66(3):1500–8.
69. Dibble CC, Asara JM, Manning BD. Characterization of rictor phosphorylation sites reveals direct regulation of mTOR complex 2 by S6K1. Mol Cell Biol. 2009;29(21):5657–70.
70. Frodin M, Gammeltoft S. Role and regulation of 90kDa ribosomal S6 kinase (RSK) in signal transduction. Mol Cell Endocrinol. 1999;151(1–2): 65–77.
71. Manning BD, Cantley LC. AKT/PKB signaling; navigating downstream. Cell. 2007;129(7):1261–74.
72. Tessier M, Woodgett JR. Serum and glucocorticoid-regulated protein kinases: variations on a theme. J Cell Biochem. 2006;98(6):1391–407.
73. Mutter GL, Lin MC, Fitzgerald JT, Kum JB, Baak JP, Lees JA, Weng LP, Eng C. Altered PTEN expression as a diagnostic marker for the earliest endometrial precancers. J Natl Cancer Inst. 2000;92(11):924–30.
74. Risinger JI, Hayes K, Maxwell GL, Carney ME, Dodge RK, Barrett JC, Berchuck A. PTEN mutation in endometrial cancers is associated with favorable clinical and pathologic characteristics. Clin Cancer Res. 1998;4(12):3005–10.
75. Mackay HJ, Gallinger S, Tsao MS, McLachlin CM, Tu D, Keiser K, Eisenhauer EA, Oza AM. Prognostic value of microsatellite instability (MSI) and PTEN expression in women with endometrial cancer: results from studies of the NCIC Clinical Trials Group (NCIC CTG). Eur J Cancer. 2010;46(8): 1365–73.
76. Cheung LW, Hennessy BT, Li J, Yu S, Myers AP, Djordjevic B, Lu Y, Stemke-Hale K, Dyer MD, Zhang F, Ju Z, Cantley LC, Scherer SE, Liang H, Lu KH, Broaddus RR, Mills GB. High frequency of PIK3R1 and PIK3R2 mutations in endometrial cancer elucidates a novel mechanism for regulation of PTEN protein stability. Cancer Discov. 2011;1(2):170–85.
77. Sun H, Enomoto T, Fujita M, Wada H, Yoshino K, Ozaki K, Nakamura T, Murata Y. Mutational analysis of the PTEN gene in endometrial carcinoma and hyperplasia. Am J Clin Pathol. 2001;115(1):32–8.
78. Kanamori Y, Kigawa J, Itamochi H, Shimada M, Takahashi M, Kamazawa S, Sato S, Akeshima R, Terakawa N. Correlation between loss of PTEN expression and Akt phosphorylation in endometrial carcinoma. Clin Cancer Res. 2001;7(4):892–5.
79. Quddus MR, Ologun BA, Sung CJ, Steinhoff MM, Lawrence WD. Utility of PTEN expression of endometrial "surface epithelial changes" and underlying atypical endometrial hyperplasia. Int J Gynecol Pathol. 2009;28(5):471–6.
80. Velasco A, Bussaglia E, Pallares J, Dolcet X, Llobet D, Encinas M, Llecha N, Palacios J, Prat J, Matias-Guiu X. PIK3CA gene mutations in endometrial carcinoma: correlation with PTEN and K-RAS alterations. Hum Pathol. 2006;37(11):1465–72.
81. Hayes MP, Douglas W, Ellenson LH. Molecular alterations of EGFR and PIK3CA in uterine serous carcinoma. Gynecol Oncol. 2009;113(3):370–3.
82. Catasus L, Gallardo A, Cuatrecasas M, Prat J. Concomitant PI3K-AKT and p53 alterations in endometrial carcinomas are associated with poor prognosis. Mod Pathol. 2009;22(4):522–9.
83. Catasus L, Gallardo A, Cuatrecasas M, Prat J. PIK3CA mutations in the kinase domain (exon 20) of uterine endometrial adenocarcinomas are associated with adverse prognostic parameters. Mod Pathol. 2008;21(2):131–9.
84. Urick ME, Rudd ML, Godwin AK, Sgroi D, Merino M, Bell DW. PIK3R1 (p85alpha) is somatically mutated at high frequency in primary endometrial cancer. Cancer Res. 2011;71(12):4061–7.

85. Shoji K, Oda K, Nakagawa S, Hosokawa S, Nagae G, Uehara Y, Sone K, Miyamoto Y, Hiraike H, Hiraike-Wada O, Nei T, Kawana K, Kuramoto H, Aburatani H, Yano T, Taketani Y. The oncogenic mutation in the pleckstrin homology domain of AKT1 in endometrial carcinomas. Br J Cancer. 2009;101(1):145–8.
86. Tanwar PS, Kaneko-Tarui T, Zhang L, Tanaka Y, Crum CP, Teixeira JM. Stromal liver kinase B1 [STK11] signaling loss induces oviductal adenomas and endometrial cancer by activating mammalian target of rapamycin complex 1. PLoS Genet. 2012;8(8):1–14.
87. Zhang YJ, Duan Y, Zheng XF. Targeting the mTOR kinase domain: the second generation of mTOR inhibitors. Drug Discov Today. 2011; 16(7–8):325–31.
88. Vilar E, Perez-Garcia J, Tabernero J. Pushing the envelope in the mTOR pathway: the second generation of inhibitors. Mol Cancer Ther. 2011;10(3): 395–403.
89. Dancey J. mTOR signalling and drug development in cancer. Nat Rev Clin Oncol. 2010;7(4):209–19.
90. Oza AM, Elit L, Tsao MS, Kamel-Reid S, Biagi J, Provencher DM, Gotlieb WH, Hoskins PJ, Ghatage P, Tonkin KS, Mackay HJ, Mazurka J, Sederias J, Ivy P, Dancey JE, Eisenhauer EA. Phase II study of temsirolimus in women with recurrent or metastatic endometrial cancer: a trial of the NCIC Clinical Trials Group. J Clin Oncol. 2011;29(24):3278–85.
91. Colombo N, McMeekin S, Schwartz P, Kostka J, Sessa C, Gehrig P, Holloway R, Braly P, Matei D, Einstein M. A phase II trial of the mTOR inhibitor AP23573 as a single agent in advanced endometrial cancer [abstract 5516]. 2007 ASCO annual meeting proceedings; 20 Jun 2007, Chicago.
92. Mackay H, Welch S, Tsao MS, Biagi JJ, Elit L, Ghatage P, Martin LA, Tonkin KS, Ellard S, Lau SK, McIntosh L, Eisenhauer EA, Oza AM. Phase II study of oral ridaforolimus in patients with metastatic and/or locally advanced recurrent endometrial cancer [abstract 5013]; 2011 ASCO annual meeting proceedings; 3–7 Jun 2011, Chicago.
93. Trédan O, Treilleux I, Wang Q, Gane N, Pissaloux D, Bonnin N, Petit T, Cretin J, Bonichon-Lamichhane N, Priou F, Lavau-Denes S, Mari V, Freyer G, Lebrun D, Alexandre J, Ray-Coquard I. Predicting everolimus treatment efficacy in patients with advanced endometrial carcinoma: a GINECO group study. Target Oncol. 2012;13:243.
94. Shoji K, Oda K, Kashiyama T, Ikeda Y, Nakagawa S, Sone K, Miyamoto Y, Hiraike H, Tanikawa M, Miyasaka A, Koso T, Matsumoto Y, Wada-Hiraike O, Kawana K, Kuramoto H, McCormick F, Aburatani H, Yano T, Kozuma S, Taketani Y. Genotype-dependent efficacy of a dual PI3K/mTOR inhibitor, NVP-BEZ235, and an mTOR inhibitor, RAD001, in endometrial carcinomas. PLoS One. 2012;7(5):1230.
95. Thoreen CC, Kang SA, Chang JW, Liu Q, Zhang J, Gao Y, Reichling LJ, Sim T, Sabatini DM, Gray NS. An ATP-competitive mammalian target of rapamycin inhibitor reveals rapamycin- resistant functions of mTORC1. J Biol Chem. 2009; 284(12):8023–32.
96. Feldman ME, Apsel B, Uotila A, Loewith R, Knight ZA, Ruggero D, Shokat KM. Active-site inhibitors of mTOR target rapamycin-resistant outputs of mTORC1 and mTORC2. PLoS Biol. 2009;7(2):371.
97. Jacinto E, Facchinetti V, Liu D, Soto N, Wei S, Jung SY, Huang Q, Qin J, Su B. SIN1/MIP1 maintains rictor–mTOR complex integrity and regulates Akt phosphorylation and substrate specificity. Cell. 2006;127(1):125–37.
98. Engelman JA. Targeting PI3K signalling in cancer: opportunities, challenges and limitations. Nat Rev. 2009;9(8):550–62.
99. Ni J, Liu Q, Xie S, Carlson C, Von T, Vogel K, Riddle S, Benes C, Eck M, Roberts T, Gray N, Zhao J. Functional characterization of an isoform-selective inhibitor of PI3K-p110β[beta] as a potential anticancer agent. Cancer Discov. 2012;2(5):425–33.
100. Jia S, Zhenning L, Zhang S, Liu P, Zhang L, Lee SH, Zhang J, Signoretti S, Loda M, Roberts TM, Zhao JJ. Essential roles of PI(3)K–p110 in cell growth, metabolism and tumorigenesis. Nature. 2008;454: 776–9.
101. Wee S, Wiederschain D, Maira SM, Loo A, Miller C, de Beaumont R, Stegmeier F, Yao YM, Lengauer C. PTEN-deficient cancers depend on PIK3CB. Proc Natl Acad Sci U S A. 2008;105(35):13057–62.
102. Torbett NE, Luna-Moran A, Knight ZA, Houk A, Moasser M, Weiss W, Shokat KM, Stokoe D. A chemical screen in diverse breast cancer cell lines reveals genetic enhancers and suppressors of sensitivity to PI3K isoform-selective inhibition. Biochem J. 2008;415(1):97–110.
103. Bendell JC, Rodon J, Burris HA, de Jonge M, Verweij J, Birle D, Demanse D, De Buck SS, Ru QC, Peters M, Goldbrunner M, Baselga J. Phase I, dose-escalation study of BKM120, an oral pan-class I PI3K inhibitor, in patients with advanced solid tumors. J Clin Oncol. 2012;30(3):282–90.
104. Edelman G, Bedell C, Shapiro G, Pandya SS, Kwak EL, Scheffold C,et al. A phase I dose-escalation study of XL147 (SAR245408), a PI3K inhibitor administered orally to patients (pts) with advanced malignancies [abstract 3004]. 2010 ASCO annual meeting proceedings; 4–8 Jun 2010, Chicago.
105. Maira SM, Pecchi S, Huang A, Burger M, Knapp M, Sterker D, Schnell C, Guthy D, Nagel T, Wiesmann M, Brachmann S, Fritsch C, Dorsch M, Chène P, Shoemaker K, De Pover A, Menezes D, Martiny-Baron G, Fabbro D, Wilson CJ, Schlegel R, Hofmann F, García-Echeverría C, Sellers WR, Voliva CF. Identification and characterization of NVP-BKM120, an orally available pan-class I PI3-kinase inhibitor. Mol Cancer Ther. 2012;11(2):317–28.
106. Fan QW, Cheng CK, Nicolaides TP, Hackett CS, Knight ZA, Shokat KM, Weiss WA. A dual phosphoinositide-3-kinase/mTOR inhibitor cooperates with blockade of epidermal growth factor receptor in PTEN-mutant glioma. Cancer Res. 2007;67(17):7960–5.

107. Yuan J, Mehta PP, Yin MJ, Sun S, Zou A, Chen J, Rafidi K, Feng Z, Nickel J, Engebretsen J, Hallin J, Blasina A, Zhang E, Nguyen L, Sun M, Vogt PK, McHarg A, Cheng H, Christensen JG, Kan JL, Bagrodia S. PF-04691502, a potent and selective oral inhibitor of PI3K and mTOR kinases with antitumor activity. Mol Cancer Ther. 2011;10(11): 2189–99.
108. Millham R, Houk B, Borzillo G, LoRusso P, Marburg L, Britten C, Wainberg Z, Adjei A, Dy G. Abstract B163: first-in-patient study of PF-04691502, a small molecule intravenous dual inhibitor of PI3K and mTOR in patients with advanced cancer: Update on safety, efficacy, and pharmacology. Proceedings of the AACR-NCI-EORTC international conference: Molecular Targets and Cancer Therapeutics; 12–16 Nov 2011, San Francisco.
109. Millham R, Houk B, Borzillo G, Tabernero J, Bell-McGuinn K, Bendell J, Molina J, Eunice Kwak E, Shapiro G. First-in-patient study of PF-05212384, a small molecule intravenous dual inhibitor of PI3K and mTOR in patients with advanced cancer: update on safety, efficacy, and pharmacology. Proceedings of the AACR-NCI-EORTC international conference: Molecular Targets and Cancer Therapeutics; 12–16 Nov 2011, San Francisco.
110. Wallin JJ, Edgar KA, Guan J, Berry M, Prior WW, Lee L, Lesnick JD, Lewis C, Nonomiya J, Pang J, Salphati L, Olivero AG, Sutherlin DP, O'Brien C, Spoerke JM, Patel S, Lensun L, Kassees R, Ross L, Lackner MR, Sampath D, Belvin M, Friedman LS. GDC-0980 is a novel class I PI3K/mTOR kinase inhibitor with robust activity in cancer models driven by the PI3K pathway. Mol Cancer Ther. 2011;10(12):2426–36.
111. Wagner AJ, Bendell JC, Dolly S, Morgan JA, Ware JA, Fredrickson J, Mazina KE, Lauchle JO, Burris HA, De Bono JS. A first-in-human phase I study to evaluate GDC-0980, an oral PI3K/mTOR inhibitor, administered QD in patients with advanced solid tumors. Proceedings of the 2011 ASCO annual meeting; 3–7 Jun 2011, Chicago.
112. Yap TA, Yan L, Patnaik A, Fearen I, Olmos D, Papadopoulos K, Baird RD, Delgado L, Taylor A, Lupinacci L, Riisnaes R, Pope LL, Heaton SP, Thomas G, Garrett MD, Sullivan DM, de Bono JS, Tolcher AW. First-in-man clinical trial of the oral pan-AKT inhibitor MK-2206 in patients with advanced solid tumors. J Clin Oncol. 2011; 29(35):4688–95.
113. Hirai H, Sootome H, Nakatsuru Y, Miyama K, Taguchi S, Tsujioka K, Ueno Y, Hatch H, Majumder PK, Pan BS, Kotani H. MK-2206, an allosteric Akt inhibitor, enhances antitumor efficacy by standard chemotherapeutic agents or molecular targeted drugs in vitro and in vivo. Mol Cancer Ther. 2010;9(7):1956–67.
114. Carracedo A, Ma L, Teruya-Feldstein J, Rojo F, Salmena L, Alimonti A, Egia A, Sasaki AT, Thomas G, Kozma SC, Papa A, Nardella C, Cantley LC, Baselga J, Pandolfi PP. Inhibition of mTORC1 leads to MAPK pathway activation through a PI3K-dependent feedback loop in human cancer. J Clin Invest. 2008;118(9):3065–74.
115. Janku F, Wheler JJ, Westin SN, Moulder SL, Naing A, Tsimberidou AM, Fu S, Falchook GS, Hong DS, Garrido-Laguna I, Luthra R, Lee JJ, Lu KH, Kurzrock R. PI3K/AKT/mTOR inhibitors in patients with breast and gynecologic malignancies harboring PIK3CA mutations. J Clin Oncol. 2012;30(8):777–82.
116. Janku F, Wheler JJ, Naing A, Falchook GS, Hong DS, Stepanek V, Fu S, Piha-Paul SA, Lee JJ, Luthra R, Tsimberidou AM, Kurzrock R. PIK3CA mutation H1047R is associated with response to PI3K/AKT/mTOR signaling pathway inhibitors in early phase clinical trials. Cancer Res. 2012;12:765.
117. Dutt A, Salvesen HB, Chen TH, Ramos AH, Onofrio RC, Hatton C, Nicoletti R, Winckler W, Grewal R, Hanna M, Wyhs N, Ziaugra L, Richter DJ, Trovik J, Engelsen IB, Stefansson IM, Fennell T, Cibulskis K, Zody MC, Akslen LA, Gabriel S, Wong KK, Sellers WR, Meyerson M, Greulich H. Drug-sensitive FGFR2 mutations in endometrial carcinoma. Proc Natl Acad Sci U S A. 2008;105(25):8713–7.
118. Byron SA, Pollock PM. FGFR as a molecular target in endometrial cancer. Future Oncol. 2009;5(1): 27–32.
119. Byron SA, Gartside MG, Wellens CL, Mallon MA, Keenan JB, Powell MA, Goodfellow PJ, Pollock PM. Inhibition of activated fibroblast growth factor receptor 2 in endometrial cancer cells induces cell death despite PTEN abrogation. Cancer Res. 2008;68(17):6902–7.
120. Hirai M, Nakagawara A, Oosaki T, Hayashi Y, Hirono M, Yoshinora T. Expression of vascular endothelial growth factors (VEGF-A/VEGF-1 and VEGF-C/VEGF-2) in postmenopausal uterine endometrial carcinoma. Gynecol Oncol. 2001;80(2):181–8.
121. Yokoyama Y, Sato S, Futagami M, Fukushi Y, Sakamoto T, Umemoto M, Saito Y. Prognostic significance of vascular endothelial growth factor and its receptors in endometrial carcinoma. Gynecol Oncol. 2000;77(3):413–8.
122. Miyake T, Yoshino K, Enomoto T, Takata T, Ugaki H, Kim A, Fujiwara K, Miyatake T, Fujita M, Kimura T. PIK3CA gene mutations and amplifications in uterine cancers, identified by methods that avoid confounding by PIK3CA pseudogene sequences. Cancer Lett. 2008;261(1):120–6.
123. Koul A, Willén R, Bendahl PO, Nilbert M, Borg A. Distinct sets of gene alterations in endometrial carcinoma implicate alternate modes of tumorigenesis. Cancer. 2002;94(9):2369–79.
124. Lax SF, Kendall B, Tashiro H, Slebos RJ, Hedrick L. The frequency of p53, K-ras mutations, and microsatellite instability differs in uterine endometrioid and serous carcinoma: evidence of distinct molecular genetic pathways. Cancer. 2000;88(4):814–24.

125. Pollock PM, Gartside MG, Dejeza LC, Powell MA, Mallon MA, Davies H, Mohammadi M, Futreal PA, Stratton MR, Trent JM, Goodfellow PJ. Frequent activating FGFR2 mutations in endometrial carcinomas parallel germline mutations associated with craniosynostosis and skeletal dysplasia syndromes. Oncogene. 2007;26(50):7158–62.
126. Jia L, Liu Y, Yi X, Miron A, Crum CP, Kong B, Zheng W. Endometrial glandular dysplasia with frequent p53 gene mutation: a genetic evidence its precancer nature for endometrial serous carcinoma. Clin Cancer Res. 2008;14(8):2263–9.
127. MacDonald ND, Salvesen HB, Ryan A, Iversen OE, Akslen LA, Jacobs IJ. Frequency and prognostic impact of microsatellite instability in a large population-based study of endometrial carcinomas. Cancer Res. 2000;60(6):1750–2.
128. Basil JB, Goodfellow PJ, Rader JS, Mutch DG, Herzog TJ. Clinical significance of microsatellite instability in endometrial carcinoma. Cancer. 2000; 89(8):1758–64.
129. Fadare O, Zheng W. Insights into endometrial serous carcinogenesis and progression. Int J Clin Exp Pathol. 2009;2(5):411–32.
130. Morrison C, Zanagnolo V, Ramirez N, Cohn DE, Kelbick N, Copeland L, Maxwell GL, Fowler JM. HER-2 is an independent prognostic factor in endometrial cancer: association with outcome in a large cohort of surgically staged patients. J Clin Oncol. 2006;24(15):2376–85.
131. Konecny GE, Santos L, Winterhoff B, Hatmal M, Keeney GL, Mariani A, Jones M, Neuper C, Thomas B, Muderspach L, Riehle D, Wang HJ, Dowdy S, Podratz KC, Press MF. HER2 gene amplification and EGFR expression in a large cohort of surgically staged patients with nonendometrioid (type II) endometrial cancer. Br J Cancer. 2009;100(1):89–95.
132. Wander SA, Hennessy BT, Slingerland JM. Next-generation mTOR inhibitors in clinical oncology: how pathway complexity informs therapeutic strategy. J Clin Investig. 2011;121(4):1230–41.
133. Sarbassov DD, Guertin DA, Ali SM, Sabatini DM. Phosphorylation and regulation of Akt/PKB by the rictor-mTOR complex. Science. 2005;307(5712): 1098–101.
134. Hresko RC, Mueckler M. mTOR.RICTOR is the Ser473 kinase for Akt/protein kinase B in 3T3-L1 adipocytes. J Biol Chem. 2005;280(49):40406–16.
135. Hong F, Larrea MD, Doughty C, Kwiarkowski DJ, Squillate R, Slingerland JM. mTOR-raptor binds and activates SGKl to regulate p27 phosphorylation. Mol Cell. 2008;30(6):701–11.
136. Garcia-Marrinez JM, Alessi DR. mTOR complex 2 (mTORC2) controls hydrophobic motif phosphorylation and activation of serum- and glucocorticoid-induced protein kinase 1 (SGKl). Biochem J. 2008;416(3):375–85.
137. Tee AR, Manning BD, Roux PP, Cantley LC, Blenis J. Tuberous sclerosis complex gene products, tuberin and hamartin, control mTOR signaling by acting as a GTPase-activating protein complex toward Rheb. Curr Biol. 2003;13(15):1259–68.
138. Kim DH, Sarbassoy DD, Ali SM, King JE, Latek RR, Erdiument-Bromage H, Tempst P, Sabatini DM. mTOR interacts with raptor to form a nutrient-sensitive complex that signals to the cell growth machinery. Cell. 2002;110(2):163–75.
139. Potter CJ, Pedraza LG, Xu T. Akt regulates growth by directly phosphorylating Tsc2. Nat Cell Biol. 2002;4(9):658–65.
140. Manning BD, Tee AR, Logsdon MN, Blenis J, Cantley LC. Identification of the tuberous sclerosis complex-2 tumor suppressor gene product tuberin as a target of the phosphoinositide 3-kinase/akt pathway. Mol Cell. 2002;10(1):151–62.
141. Inoki K, Li Y, Zhu T, Wu J, Guan KL. TSC2 is phosphorylated and inhibited by Akt and suppresses mTOR signalling. Nat Cell Biol. 2002;4(9): 648–57.
142. Darb-Esfahani S, Faggad A, Noske A, Weichert W, Buckendahl AC, Müller B, Budczies J, Röske A, Dietel M, Denkert C. Phospho-mTOR and phospho-4EBP1 in endometrial adenocarcinoma: association with stage and grade in vivo and link with response to rapamycin treatment in vitro. J Cancer Res Clin Oncol. 2009;135:933–41.
143. Liang J, Slingerland JM. Multiple roles of the PI3K/PKB (Akt) pathway in cell cycle progression. Cell Cycle. 2003;2(4):339–45.
144. Zhou BP, Liao Y, Xia W, Spohn B, Lee MH, Hung MC. Cytoplasmic localization of p21Cip1/WAFl by Akt-induced phosphorylation in HER-2/neu-over-expressing cells. Nat Cell Biol. 2001; 3(3):245–52.

32 Fertility Preservation in Early Cervical Cancer

John H. Shepherd and Emily S. Shepherd

32.1 Introduction

Over half a million women are affected by cervical cancer worldwide every year. Screening programs have reduced the incidence of invasive cancer dramatically with a consequent increase in the number of small early stage tumours and pre-invasive lesions. Treatment by either chemo radiotherapy or radical hysterectomy in early stage disease has cure rates of over 90 % but with the inevitable morbidity of compromised fertility. As women especially in the developed world, have delayed child bearing there has been an increasing demand for fertility sparing techniques to be developed.

Vaginal cervicectomy (trachelectomy) was first described in 1948 by Franz Novak [1]. Aburel [2] in 1956 described an abdominal approach for uterine conservation, neither technique gained much support as hysterectomy proved to be a simpler safer procedure with successful outcomes. In 1977, Burghardt [3] recognized that radical hysterectomy with parametrectomy unnecessarily removed the body of the uterus in many cases of early small cervical cancer.

J.H. Shepherd, FRCS, FRCOG, FACOG
Department of Gynaecological Oncology,
The Royal Marsden Hospital, London, England, UK

E.S. Shepherd, MBBS, BMedSci, DRCOG (✉)
Department of Obstetrics and Gynaecology,
St Mary's Hospital Imperial College NHS Trust,
London, UK
e-mail: eshepherd@doctors.org.uk

Dargent [4] in 1994 performed a radical vaginal excision of the cervix conserving the corpus uteri with a simultaneous laparoscopic pelvic node dissection. Shepherd [5] in London modified this technique and Roy [6] in Quebec reported successful pregnancies after such surgical treatment. The principal that these three authors advocated was that a wide local excision of the primary tumour could be performed with surrounding paracervical and vaginal tissue as described for the lower part of a Schauta Radical Vaginal Hysterectomy with laparoscopic assistance to remove the pelvic lymph nodes. In 2005 Ungar [7] reported an abdominal approach as an alternative option for radical cervical excision initially described by Smith [8].

As a result of these approaches be they abdominal or vaginal, it was realized that even more conservative surgery by large cone biopsy with or without a pelvic node dissection might be suitable for certain small tumours confined to the lower and central cervix when surrounded by uninvolved stroma. The key to successful conservative treatment is careful selection after histopathology review and magnetic resonance imaging.

32.2 Patient Selection

Patients present with an abnormal smear or irregular, perhaps post-coital bleeding. A suspicious lesion as seen on examination, necessitates the

H.R.H. Patel et al. (eds.), *Pelvic Cancer Surgery: Modern Breakthroughs and Future Advances*,
DOI 10.1007/978-1-4471-4258-4_32, © Springer-Verlag London 2015

need for colposcopy and biopsy. It is important to gain an accurate assessment of depth and diameter in order to adequately stage the tumour.

The majority of lesions are squamous cell carcinomas (scc) but an increasing number are adenocarcinomas of glandular origin and rarely small cell (neuroendocrine) tumours. The reduction of scc is probably due to the screening out of these tumours by early detection as pre-invasive intra-epithelial neoplasia which is then successfully treated.

32.3 Imaging

Having made a diagnosis, magnetic resonance imaging (MRI) is used to measure the lesion and assess its location and distance from the isthmus (Fig. 32.1), Sadhev et al. [9]. The use of an endovaginal coil has improved the accuracy of imaging [10] (Fig. 32.2).

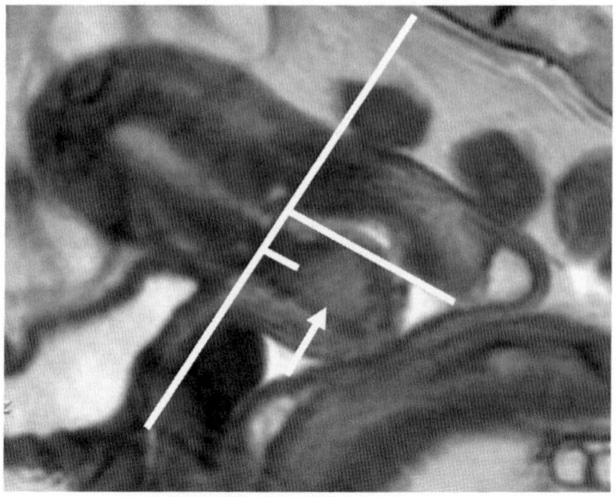

Fig. 32.1 Sagittal MRI indentifying tumour and length of endocervical canal, with distance from isthmus

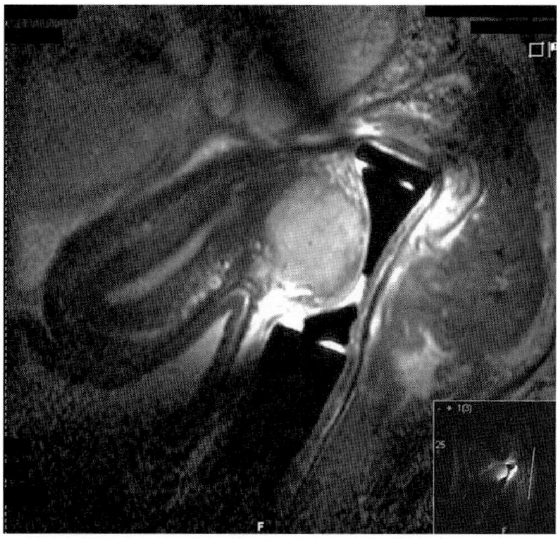

Fig. 32.2 Endovaginal coil MRI scan identifying tumour

32.4 Staging

The traditional method of staging is by clinical examination under anesthesia (staging EUA). Applying FIGO staging [11] (Table 32.1) enables a decision to be made as to the best form of treatment. Stages IAI and IAII may be adequately treated by cone biopsy ensuring that an adequate margin of clearance is obtained. Risk of lymph node involvement for a stage IAI tumour is 1 % increasing up to 7–8 % in stage IAII [12]. With lympho-vascular space invasion (LVSI), a pelvic node dissection is required and the incidence of this in stages IAI and IAII is between 3 and 4 %. The incidence of lymph node involvement, with metastases increases to 16–18 % with stage IB tumours. These lesions require a thorough pelvic node dissection with a Wertheim's radical hysterectomy.

Pelvic node dissection may be carried out by laparoscopy with or without robotic assistance. This is part of the overall staging procedure but whether the removal of microscopically negative lymph nodes as an en bloc dissection is therapeutic, is debatable. Improving imaging perhaps with PET scanning or sentinel node assessment may change this.

32.5 Radical Trachelectomy: Selection of Method

There is debate as to which surgical approach should be undertaken; vaginal or abdominal. Abdominal surgery may be open, laparoscopic or with robotic assistance. Careful patient selection will result in low morbidity with low recurrence rates and acceptably high pregnancy rates. The risk of significant prematurity may be decreased if it is possible to conserve a small portion of the

Table 32.1 International Federation of Gynaecology and Obstetrics (FIGO) staging [11]

TNM	FIGO	Surgical-pathologic findings
Categories	*Stages*	
TX		Primary tumour cannot be assessed
T0		No evidence of primary tumour
Tis		Carcinoma in situ (pre-invasive carcinoma)
T1	I	Cervical carcinoma confined to the cervix (disregard extension to the corpus)
T1a	IA	Invasive carcinoma diagnosed only by microscopy; stromal invasion with a maximum depth of 5.0 mm measured from the base of the epithelium and a horizontal spread of 7.0 mm or less; vascular space involvement, venous or lymphatic, does not affect classification
T1a1	IA1	Measured stromal invasion ≤3.0 mm in depth and ≤7.0 mm in horizontal spread
T1a2	IA2	Measured stromal invasion >3.0 mm and ≤5.0 mm with a horizontal spread ≤7.0 mm
T1b	IB	Clinically visible lesion confined to the cervix or microscopic lesion greater than T1a/IA2
T1b1	IB1	Clinically visible lesion ≤4.0 cm in greatest dimension
T1b2	IB2	Clinically visible lesion >4.0 cm in greatest dimension
T2	II	Cervical carcinoma invades beyond uterus but not to pelvic wall or to lower third of vagina
T2a	IIA	Tumour without parametrial invasion
T2a1	IIA1	Clinically visible lesion ≤4.0 cm in greatest dimension
T2a2	IIA2	Clinically visible lesion >4.0 cm in greatest dimension
T2b	IIB	Tumour with parametrial invasion
T3	III	Tumour extends to pelvic wall and/or involves lower third of vagina and/or causes hydronephrosis or nonfunctional kidney
T3a	IIIA	Tumour involves lower third of vagina, no extension to pelvic wall
T3b	IIIB	Tumour extends to pelvic wall and/or causes hydronephrosis or nonfunctional kidney
T4	IV	Tumour invades mucosa of bladder or rectum and/or extends beyond true pelvis (bullous oedema is not sufficient to classify a tumour as T4)
T4a	IVA	Tumour invades mucosa of bladder or rectum (bullous oedema is not sufficient to classify a tumour as T4)
T4b	IVB	Tumour extends beyond true pelvis
Regional lymph nodes (N)		
NX	Regional lymph nodes cannot be assessed	
N0	No regional lymph node metastasis	
N1	Regional lymph node metastasis	
Distant metastasis (M)		
M0	No distant metastasis	
M1	Distant metastasis (including peritoneal spread; involvement of supraclavicular, mediastinal, or para-aortic lymph nodes; and lung, liver, or bone)	

upper (proximal) cervix at the isthmus depending on the exact position of the tumour and the ability to obtain an adequate, clear margin.

Most authorities agree that the upper limit in size for suitability is 2 cm in diameter. However the overall volume needs to be taken into account. Radical vaginal trachelectomy involves the first or bottom part of a Schauta radical hysterectomy. This can be challenging to perform, hence some oncological surgeons have opted for the abdominal approach. Practice with the vaginal technique allows adequate vaginal and para-cervical resection which may be tailored to the needs of the tumour. The difficulty that some may have is in mobilizing the ureter which they may feel more comfortable dealing with abdominally. Whilst potential complications maybe the same, there is a reduced hospital stay and less inconvenience to the patient, making the vagina the favoured approach to the authors.

32.6 Pelvic Node Dissection

This is carried out laparoscopically either at the time of the staging EUA or in conjunction with the vaginal trachelectomy. The advantage of the former is that patients with positive lymph node metastases are identified before definitive surgery to the cervix is undertaken. A four portal approach is employed using a Hasson direct entry technique. The abdominal and pelvic cavity is thoroughly inspected not only to look for possible metastatic disease especially involving the pelvic peritoneum and Pouch of Douglas but also to look for other pathology such as endometriosis or chronic pelvic inflammation.

The pelvic side walls are exposed with a T shaped incision into the peritoneum overlying the external iliac vessels, just proximal to the round ligaments. The infundibulo-pelvic ligament is identified and separated from the ureter. The nodes are removed from the lower common iliac, internal and external iliac and obturator regions. The obturator nerve is exposed and conserved. The paravesical space is identified and opened. Care is taken to avoid aberrant obturator vessels.

The procedure is repeated on the contralateral side resulting in a harvest of approximately 30–40 lymph nodes.

32.7 Radical Vaginal Trachelectomy (RVT)

An extended lithotomy position is used to expose the cervix which is infiltrated with 0.25 % Bupivacaine and 1 in 200,000 adrenaline. The technique is well described by Shepherd [13] utilizing a circumcervical incision including a 2 cm cuff of vagina with cutting diathermy. Sharp dissection mobilizes the bladder anteriorly, identifying the bladder pillars by opening the paravesical space on either side. Posteriorly the uterosacral ligaments and rectovaginal septum are identified. The harmonic scalpel (ultracision Eithicon endoscopy LLC) is used for dissection and haemostasis. The bladder pillar is transected and the descending branch of the uterine artery supplying the cervix is isolated and divided after cauterization. The ureteric tunnel is identified and the ureter reflected cranially and laterally. The dissection continues laterally dividing the lateral (cardinal) ligaments the utero-sacral ligaments posterolaterally. As much paracervical and paravaginal tissue as necessary depending on the size of the tumour, should be resected (Fig. 32.3). To give an adequate 1–2 cm clearance of tumour-free tissue. The rectovaginal septum is incised and the tissue posteriorly pushed by blunt dissection cranially. It is not necessary to open the Pouch of Douglas and by keeping this closed possible sepsis spreading to the pelvis is avoided. If the peritoneal cavity is opened, this may be easily closed with absorbable sutures. The dissection is performed on both sides thus mobilizing the central cervix including a 2 cm cuff of vagina. A no. 6 Hegar dilator is placed into the endocervical canal which may then be transected using cutting diathermy (Fig. 32.4). The isthmus is easily identified by visualizing where the peritoneum is reflected anteriorly, above the uterovesical ligament and posteriorally at the reflection of the Pouch of Douglas. An individual decision

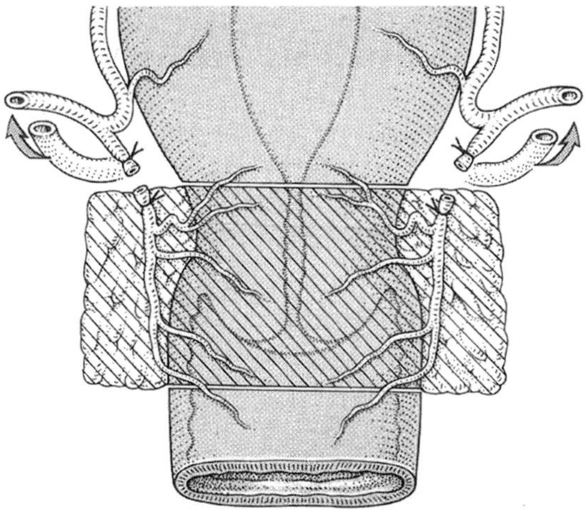

Fig. 32.3 Tissue to be resected

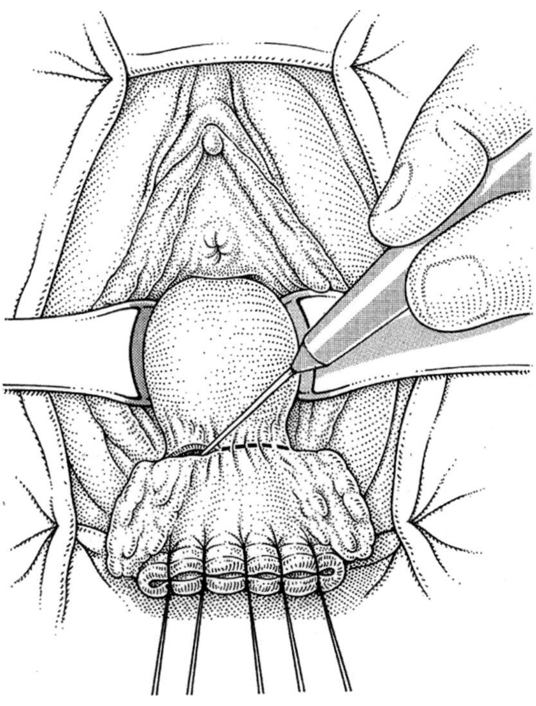

Fig. 32.4 Transecting isthmus with cutting diathermy

is taken as to whether a complete trachelectomy removing all the cervix is required or whether it is possible to conserve a small cuff of proximal upper cervix depending on the exact location of the tumour.

32.8 Isthmic Cerclage

An isthmic cerclage using monofilament, non-absorbable material, such as No 1 nylon or prolene, is inserted with four large bites around the isthmus, through the stroma of the cervix. Care is taken not to occlude the isthmic os by keeping the Hegar dilator in situ during this procedure. The knot is tied anteriorly around this dilator. This will allow normal menstruation to occur and passage of a cannula for any future necessary procedures.

32.9 Vagino-Isthmic Anastomosis

Holding the cerclage suture for identification and traction, the vaginal margins are grasped and anastomosed to the isthmus using four interrupted mattress sutures with no 1 Vicryl (Polyglactin, Ethicon). Care is taken to avoid closing the isthmic and endocervical canal by leaving the Hegar 6 dilator in situ whilst inserting the sutures. Two or three further mattress sutures are placed on either side to close the angles of the lateral fornices (Fig. 32.5).

The Hegar dilator is removed and replaced with a size 12 Foley catheter into the uterine cavity. The balloon is distended using 3 mls of water and left in situ for 72 h to discourage synechiae developing and prevent isthmic stenosis. A bladder catheter is required to drain the bladder for 5 days. A vaginal pack is inserted and removed after 24 h. Blood loss on average is between 50 and 100 mls.

32.10 Post Operative Care

Prophylactic broad spectrum antibiotics are administered intraoperatively and continued for 24 h. The patient is able to mobilize the next day once the vaginal pack has been removed. The uterine catheter remains until the third day when she may be discharged home with her bladder catheter for a further 48 h. The patient returns on day 5 for removal of this and bladder scans are used to confirm adequate voiding. Pelvic floor

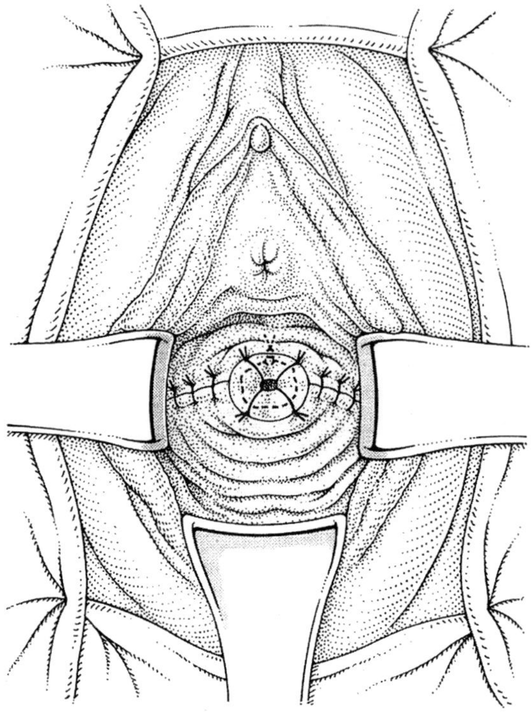

Fig. 32.5 Vagino-isthmic anastamosis and cerclage

exercises and bladder drill are commenced as retention of urine or hesitancy occurs in approximately 5 % of patients.

32.11 Follow Up Management

The patient returns for a discussion regarding the pathology after 2 weeks and to confirm adequate voiding. Contraception is advised for at least 6 months. Continuing follow up is at three monthly intervals for a year, four monthly for the second year and six monthly up to 5 years. This decreases to yearly for 10 years before returning to the national screening program.

At each visit a careful clinical examination is carried out with vaginal vault and isthmic smears taken. Colposcopy and assessment by MRI is carried out at 6, 12 and 24 months. If the patient is disease free and anxious to conceive she may do so after 6 months and is encouraged to sooner rather than later.

32.12 Abdominal Radical Trachelectomy (ART)

This may be undertaken either by open surgery [8] or by laparoscopy [14] with or without robotic assistance [15]. The procedure comprises the lower part of a radical abdominal hysterectomy.

The paravesical spaces are opened once the lymph node dissection has been completed and the uterine vessels identified. It is not necessary to divide the uterine artery as it is the cervical branches that supply the cervix. The ureters are reflected laterally and descending uterine artery branches (the cervical branches) are divided. The pararectal spaces are opened enabling adequate paracervical and paravaginal tissue to be dissected including the lateral and uterosacral ligaments with a 2 cm cuff of vagina. The bladder is reflected anteriorly and the rectum posteriorly. Having removed the specimen, a vagino-isthmic anastomosis is performed and isthmic cerclage inserted. This is more accurately and easily performed under robotic guidance than laparoscopically.

32.13 Results

At the corresponding author's institution, 224 patients have undergone radical vaginal trachelectomy with laparoscopic pelvic node dissection. The mean age of the women was 30.6 years with the majority (96 %) having stage IBI tumours. A small number have IAII or stage IIA lesions. Careful individualization and planning is essential to identify suitable patients. Four rare tumours including clear cell carcinoma and a neuroendocrine tumour have been operated on. The largest tumour measured 5–6 cm but was exophytic. 21 (10 %) patients had lesions larger than 2 cm. Three patients were pregnant (16, 10 and 6 weeks) at the time of surgery. All carried successful pregnancies, the first delivered prematurely (by caesarean section).

Twenty-four patients (12 %) have required completion treatment due to adverse prognostic factors such as either positive lymph node involvement or close margins. By carrying out a lymphadenectomy first as part of the staging

EUA, this number has been reduced, thus avoiding unnecessary surgery as further treatment is by chemo radiotherapy.

Elective hysterectomy on completion of childbearing has been abandoned as careful follow up has shown that outcomes are good. In three women where this was performed, the surgery was complicated by excessive adhesions and scarring from the previous surgery.

32.14 Complications

Ten percent of women have experienced some form of complication, the most significant being ureteric damage with fistulae. These occurred in the first 50 patients operated on, two of whom had extensive microscopic disease beyond the cervix making dissection difficult. One also had unexpected positive lymph nodes. Extension of tumour therefore may have compromised surgical excision. There were also three uterine perforations probably related to excessive handling of the uterine corpus during the trachelectomy. These were not significant with only one requiring a laparoscopic suture. There is a 6 % isthmic stenosis rate: hence the introduction of a uterine catheter postoperatively. Two port site hernias have developed, both through 5 mm ports, which possibly were enlarged by rotation and manipulation of instruments.

32.15 Recurrence

There have been 8 recurrences out of the 221 patients, 5 of whom had tumours larger than 2 cm, 4 had lymphovascular space invasion. None had other adverse prognostic factors on the final histopathology that would have necessitated further treatment.

32.16 Pregnancy and Reproductive Outcome

Fertility rates have been shown to be high [13]. In the author's current series there have been 131 pregnancies with 76 live births. There has been one stillbirth which was arguably preventable. The number of first trimester miscarriages is not greater than would have been expected (27 in 21 women) although the mid-trimester losses are increased (19 in 14 women) (Table 32.2).

Prematurity is a significant risk due to premature rupture of the membranes and ascending chorio-amnionitis, resulting from the lack of a cervical mucus plug. Failure of the cerclage does not appear to be a factor in premature labour, although five have cut out. There have been 14 significantly premature births between 24 and 32 weeks. Delivery should be by classical caesarean section, either electively at 37–38 weeks or at the onset of labour. If any proximal cervix was retained at the time of the trachelectomy then it may be possible to assess if a measurable lower segment has formed and to consider a transverse uterine incision. However, one woman had an attempted lower segment caesarean section with an almost fatal laceration extending into the broad ligament, severing the uterine artery. If the whole cervix has been removed at trachelectomy then there will be no lower segment therefore this should not be attempted.

Obstetric supervision should be in experienced feto-maternal units with adequate resources to deal with prematurity. Vaginal progesterone is advocated by some obstetricians to help prolong pregnancy and it is advisable to limit activity and to take measures to avoid infection. Consideration should be given to either vaginal antibiotic

Table 32.2 Pregnancies amongst 224 women who were selected for radical trachelectomy

Live births	76 in 54 woman
Stillbirths	1 in 1 woman
Neonatal deaths	0
Miscarriages <14/40	27 in 21 women
Miscarriages >=14/40	19 in 14 women
Terminations	2 in 2 women
Ectopic pregnancy	1 woman
Ongoing pregnancy	3 women
Surrogate live pregnancy	3 women
Total pregnancies	131

Pregnancy and reproductive outcome figures from St Bartholomew's and The Royal Marsden Hospitals 1994–2013

Table 32.3 Worldwide data radical vaginal trachelectomy

Center	Number	Pregnancies	Live births	<32 weeks	Recurrences	Deaths
London Shepherd [12]	224	131(3)	75	14	8	5
Toronto Covens	121	45	34	6	7	4
Quebec Roy/Plante [6]	125	106	49	3	6	2
Jena /Berlin/Cologne Schneider/Hertel	100	18	12	3	4	2
Lyon Dargent/Methevet	118	61 (3)	34	5	7	5
Los Angeles Roman/Burnett/Shlaerth	69	8	6	1	2	0
New York Abu-Rustam	41	3 (3)	3	0	0	0
Toulouse Querlou	29	4	4	0	1	0
Copenhagen Svane	24	N/A	N/A	N/A	0	0
Beijing Shen	16	N/A	N/A	N/A	1	0
Stockholm Hellberg	8	6	4	0	0	0
Total	875	382	221	32 (15 %)	36 (4 %)	18 (2 %)

Table 32.4 Worldwide data for abdominal radical trachelectomy

Author	Number	Pregnancies	Live births	<32 weeks
Ungar	81	13	6 (3)	1
Nishio	57	4	2	2
Cibula	17	6	5	2
Abu Rustum	15	2	0 (1)	0
Pajera	14	3	3	1
Duska	10	4	2 (1)	1
Wang	13	3	3	0
Total	207	35	21 (5)	7

applications or prophylactic oral antibiotics at times of particular risk which appear to be 16–18 weeks and 22–24 weeks.

32.17 Worldwide Experience

This is summarized in Tables 32.3 and 32.4 [16, 17]. There have been approximately 1,000 reported radical vaginal trachelectomies and approximately 400 abdominal procedures. Recurrence rates by either technique are approximately 4 % (4.2 % after RVT [16], 3.8 % after AVT [17]) with 2 % deaths (2.9 % RVT, 0.4 % AVT). All reporting authors agree that in general tumours of less than 2 cm are suitable as recurrence is more common with larger lesions. These figures do represent a better cure rate than for other patients with similar stage disease. This is not because the treatment is superior but confirms that the selection process is good. Fertility rates appear to be better using the vaginal approach where there is more data in the literature. Prematurity rates appear to be similar in the two approaches.

32.18 Summary

It may be concluded that fertility sparing surgery is a realistic option for young women with a small early stage cervical cancer. This is suitable for tumours of less than 2 cm in diameter although on an individual basis, larger tumours maybe resected with uterine conservation. The route chosen depends on the surgical skills and facilities available. Recurrence rates are acceptable. Fertility rates are encouraging although prematurity is a risk. Careful patient selection is of paramount importance.

Key Points

- Absolute desire for fertility preservation
- Early stage, <2 cm diameter cervical cancer
- Individualization of treatment after careful counseling
- Thorough histopathological review and careful MRI assessment of the size and location of the tumour
- Surgical approach depends on the experience of the surgeon remembering that there may be a limited place for large cone biopsy with or without laparoscopic pelvic node dissection in certain small tumours
- Laparoscopic pelvic node dissection is part of surgical staging
- If the abdominal route is chosen then robotic surgery may be the most appropriate
- Careful follow up is by clinical examination, colposcopy, cytology and MRI scans
- Experienced antenatal supervision in view of the risk of premature rupture of the membranes is essential
- Delivery should be by a classical caesarean section, using a low vertical uterine incision, either at the onset of labour or electively at 37–38 weeks

References

1. Novak F. Radical abdominal subcorporeal extirpation of the cervix with bilateral pelvic lymph nodes dissection in cancer in-situ of the cervix uteri. Acta Med Lugosl. 1952;6(1):59–71.
2. Aburel E. In Chirurgia Gineccologica technical, si tactica op-eratiorie (1956), vol II sub redaetia Panait Sirbu. 2nd edn. Bucharest, Romania: Editura Medicola Bucuresti; 1976.
3. Burghardt E, Holzer E. Diagnosis and treatment of micro-invasive carcinoma of the cervix uteri. Obstet Gynecol. 1977;49:641–53.
4. Dargent D, Brun JL, Roy M, Mathevet P. La trachelectomie élargie: uné alternative á l'hystérectomie. Radicale dansu traitment des cancers in filtrants. JOBGYN. 1994;2:285–92.
5. Shepherd JH, Crawford RAF, Oram DH. Radical trachelectomy: a way to preserve fertility in the treatment of early cervical cancer? Br J Obstet Gynecol. 1998;105:912–6.
6. Roy M, Plant M. Pregnancies after radical vaginal trachelectomy for early stage cervical cancer. Am J Obstet Gynecol. 1998;179:1491–6.
7. Ungar L, Palfalvi L, Hogg R, Sirló S, Boyle DCM, Del Priore G, et al. Abdominal radical trachelectomy. A sparing option for women with early cervical cancer. BJOG. 2005;112:366–9.
8. Smith JR, Boyle DC, Corless DJ, Ungar AD, Lawson AD, et al. Abdominal radical trachelectomy: a new surgical technique for the conservative management of cervical carcinoma. Br J Obstet Gynecol. 1997;104:1196–200.
9. Sadhev A, Sohaib SA, Shepherd JH, Reznek RH. Magnetic resonance imaging in gynaecological malignancies. Cancer Imaging. 2005;5:539. Downey et al (MRI).
10. Charles—Edwards E, Morgan V, Attygale A, Giles S, Ind TE, Davies M, Shepherd JH, McWhinneey N, de Souza NM. Endovaginal magnetic resonance imaging stage Ia/Ibi cervical cancer with a T2 and diffusion weighted magnetic resonance technique: effect of lesion size and previous cone biopsy on tumour detectabilty. Gynecol Oncol. 2011;120:368–73.
11. Pecorelli S. Revised FIGO staging for carcinoma of the vulva, cervix, and endometrium. Int J Gynaecol Obstet. 2009;105(2):103–4.
12. Sevin BU, Nadji M, Averette H, Hilsenbeck S, Smith D, et al. Micro-invasive carcinoma of the cervix. Cancer. 1992;70:2121–8.
13. Shepherd JH, Spencer C, Herod J, Ind TEJ. Radical vaginal trachelectomy asa fertility-sparing procedure in women with early-stage cervical cancer—cumulative pregnancy rate in a series of 123 women. BJOG. 2006;113:719–24.
14. Abu-Rustum NR, Sonoda Y, Black D, Levine DA, Chi DS, Barrakat KR. Fertility-sparing radical abdominal trachelectomy for cervical cancer: technique and review of the literature. Gynecol Oncol. 2006;103:807–13.
15. Persson J, Kannisto P, Bossmar T. Robot-assisted abdominal laparoscopic radical trachelectomy. Gynecol Oncol. 2008;111(3):564–71. Robotic ART.
16. Ribeiro CAF, Ferreira CJI, Costa MF, Branco AP. Fertility-sparing surgery for early-stage cervical cancer. Int J Surg Oncol. 2012;2012:936534.
17. Pareja R, Rendon GJ, Sanz-Lomana CM, Monzon O, Ramirez PT. Surgical, oncological and obstetrical outcomes after abdominal radical trachelectomy—a systematic literature review. Gynecol Oncol. 2013;131:77–82.

Radical Hysterectomy in Cervical Cancer

33

David Cibula

33.1 Introduction

Radical hysterectomy, with its 100-year history, is a basic procedure in gynecological oncology. Yet none of the other surgical procedures has more varieties in its performance as well as in array of its classification. Inconsistent terminology, classification, anatomic landmarks as well as the procedure performance as such have a negative impact on the harmonization of current clinical practice, international cooperation, training of the young generation and surgical data comparison. For this reason the following chapter is going to deeply focus on the proper terminology as well as the classification system.

It should be emphasized that the approach to the surgical treatment of cervical cancer has developed enormously in recent years thanks to influence from a large number of factors. Probably the most crucial factor is the refinement of clinical staging, which used to be based on an inaccurate physical examination. The quality of current imaging methods enables us carry out local staging with high accuracy, including not only identification of parametrial involvement, but also size of the tumor and its localization in the cervix. MRI has become the golden standard, however in recent years arguments supporting the use of ultrasound have grown as it is a comparable or even more precise method that is less economically demanding, faster and broadly available [16, 18, 49]. Abandonment of surgery due to intra-operatively detected inoperability should be considered as a major failure of preoperative staging. Detailed data about local tumor extent allow planning for much better treatment strategy including the type of performed hysterectomy.

Progress in pelvic anatomy knowledge is another significant factor that has influenced surgical treatment. Studies on cadavers as well as intra-operative studies have enabled us to describe pelvic anatomy in greater detail, mainly the course of autonomic nerves when damage to them may cause severe postoperative morbidity [17].

Another considerable factor is the development and evolution in surgical technologies. New possibilities in tissue dissection (bipolar coagulation, harmonic scalpel) offer safe hemostasis with minimal lateral thermal spread. Endoscopic approach, both laparoscopic and robotic, enables a synoptic and enlarged view at the operation field even in hardly accessible regions of the pelvis.

33.2 History

The first attempts to surgically treat cervical cancer date back to the first half of the nineteenth century. The majority of these patients

D. Cibula, MD, PhD
Department of Obstetrics and Gynecology,
Gynecologic Oncology Center,
General University Hospital, First Medical School,
Charles University, Prague, Czech Republic
e-mail: d_cibula@yahoo.com

H.R.H. Patel et al. (eds.), *Pelvic Cancer Surgery: Modern Breakthroughs and Future Advances*,
DOI 10.1007/978-1-4471-4258-4_33, © Springer-Verlag London 2015

died during or shortly after the surgery [56]. Early recurrences prevailing in the vaginal cuff in patients who did not die encouraged surgeons to increase radicality of the surgery [20]. The first hysterectomy with the resection of lateral parametria was described in 1895 by Clark [13]. Lymphadenectomy was not part of this procedure. Only 3 years later E. Wertheim performed the first radical hysterectomy in combination with pelvic lymph node removal in Vienna [68]. Mortality oscillated around 30 % at the beginning and decreased quickly in time with his increasing skill to as low as 10 % (as early as 1911 he reported 500 operations). Just a couple of years later Schauta developed a technique of vaginal radical hysterectomy that was first published in 1908 [57]. The mortality in Schauta' s group fluctuated around 10 % as well. Both operative techniques, abdominal and vaginal, have become the foundation for the radical surgical treatment of cervical cancer. The principles were modified during the twentieth century by many other personalities: vaginal approach primarily by Amreich (1960); abdominal Wertheim's procedure by his successor Werner; W. Latzko [34] and mainly Okabayashi [41], who further increased the radicality of parametria resection. An American, Joe V. Meigs [39], earned his place in history thanks to his abdominal approach promoting technique modification and increased lymphadenectomy radicality.

33.3 Indication

The opinions on the indications for radical hysterectomy are currently far from being uniform; the main controversial areas are the following: choice of radical versus simple hysterectomy in early stages, use of primary radiotherapy versus radical hysterectomy in locally advanced tumors, performing a radical hysterectomy or abandoning the surgery and referring the patient to radiotherapy in case of intra-operative detection of positive lymph nodes. Another controversy is in the choice of the type and radicality of radical hysterectomy depending on the stage of the disease and presence of risk factors. Data from controlled studies from all the above mentioned fields are lacking.

Among commonly accepted indication is the early stage FIGO IB. Even this stage, however, comprises a broad spectrum of tumors of various sizes (from invasion above 5 mm up to size of 4 cm), depth of the invasion into stroma and different localization of the tumor in the cervix (e.g. exophytic growth, along the endocervix or towards the pericervical fascia) (Fig. 33.1). It is very probable that the risk of

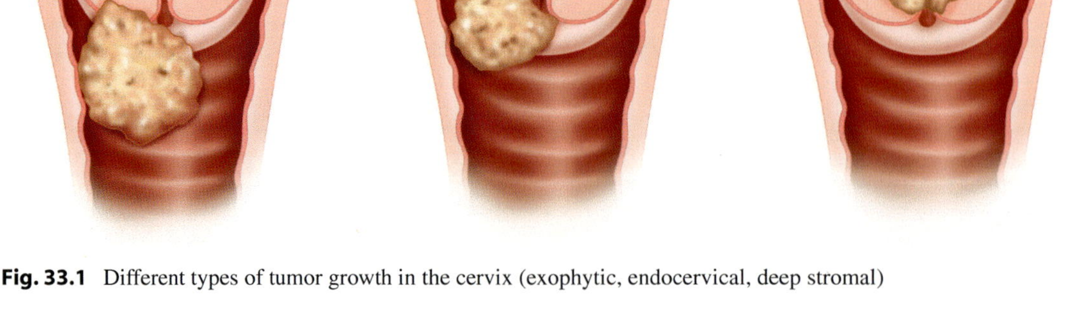

Fig. 33.1 Different types of tumor growth in the cervix (exophytic, endocervical, deep stromal)

lymph nodes involvement, as they are the most significant prognostic parameter, will vary in equally large tumors depending on their position in the cervix, even though the significance of these factors has never been proven prospectively.

Early Stages

Patients with micro invasive carcinoma stage FIGO IA (stromal invasion ≤5 mm; horizontal extension ≤7 mm) have an excellent prognosis and, not surprisingly, minimal risk of parametrial invasion [1, 27, 65]. Simple extrafascial hysterectomy is an appropriate surgery in this case. In recent years a number of reports show that satisfactory outcomes can be achieved even in selected patients (largest tumor size ≤2 cm, stromal invasion ≤2/3; negative pelvic lymph nodes) with IB stage when parametrectomy is not performed [21, 50]. These reports are supported by arguments from retrospective series substantiating low risk of parametria involvement in this very group of patients [21, 63]. However, these retrospective series are limited by standard parametrial pathological processing which does not enable small size metastasis detection, particularly tumor emboli in lymphatic channels. Therefore the standard surgical procedure in stage IB should, according to current knowledge, be radical hysterectomy, which means including parametria removal. Any change in the guidelines should be preceded by the confirmation of oncological safety in ongoing prospective trials (SHAPE—Simple Hysterectomy and Pelvic Node Dissection in Early Stage Low Risk Cervical Cancer).

Locally Advanced Staged

A broad range of alternatives is currently applied in the management of locally advanced stages (IB2, IIA, IIB): (a) Primary chemoradiation, (b) neoadjuvant chemotherapy followed by radical hysterectomy, (c) neoadjuvant radiotherapy followed by simple or radical hysterectomy, or (d) upfront radical surgery with or without adjuvant radiotherapy or chemotherapy. It is necessary to emphasize that as a result of the massive improvement of imaging diagnostics (MRI, ultrasound, PET) clinical staging, including the assessment of parametrial, paracolpial or pelvic lymph nodes involvement, has become much more accurate. It can be assumed that the spectrum of patients classified into stage IB2 or IIB is currently much more accurate compared to 5 or 10 years ago.

Primary surgical treatment of large tumors or tumors with initial parametrial invasion is feasible and it has, according to available data, a satisfactory oncological outcome comparable with radiotherapy [10, 26]. Surgical approach has two main limitations though. Extensive parametrectomy (type C2 or D) must be performed due to anatomical conditions in patients with massive tumors, a high risk of parametrial metastatic involvement in stage IB2 or the presence of parametrial invasion in patients with stage IIB. Furthermore, the proportion of patients referred to adjuvant treatment for lymph node involvement is high in these stages, reaching up to 40 % [12]. Postoperative morbidity increases in a large number of patients due to the accumulation of two different treatment modalities—extensive surgical procedure and adjuvant radiotherapy. Prospective studies are necessary to refine the management of locally advanced stages, as they would compare oncological outcome and their impacts on quality of life in each treatment modality.

33.4 Terminology

The unification of terminology describing the key anatomical structures is crucial for international understanding and comprehension. One of the key structures for radical hysterectomy is the parametrium, which has three components on both sides of the cervix: the ventral parametrium (including vesico-uterine and vesico-vaginal ligaments), the lateral parametrium (paracervix or cardinal ligament), and the dorsal parametrium (including recto-uterine and recto-vaginal

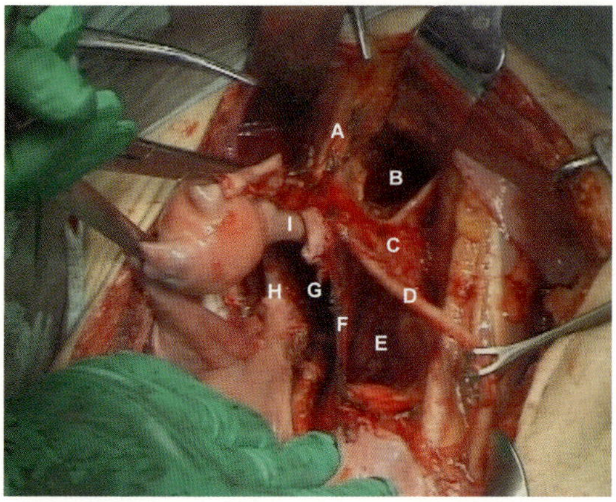

Fig. 33.2 Intra-operative picture of the ventral, lateral and dorsal parametrium. *A* Ventral parametrium, *B* paravesical space, *C* lateral parametrium, *D* ureter, *E* pararectal space (lateral pararectal space), *F* dorsal parametrium, *G* sacro-uterine space (medial pararectal space), *H* rectum, *I* cervix

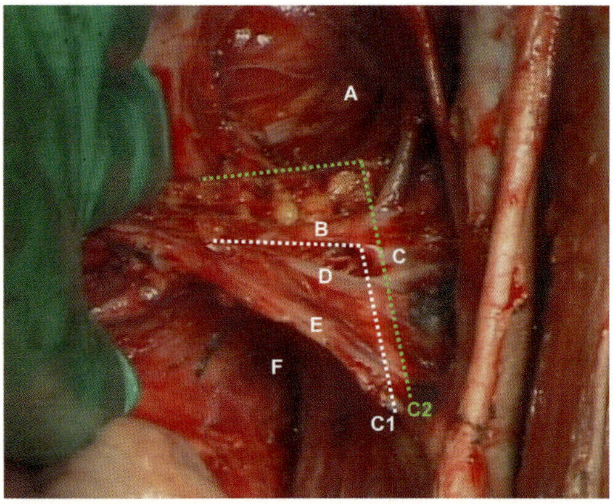

Fig. 33.3 Intra-operative picture of resection lines on the lateral parametrium *A* paravesical space, *B* deep uterine vein (vaginal vein), *C* internal iliac vein, *D* uterine vein, *E* uterine artery, *F* pararectal space. *C1, C2* resection lines on the lateral parametrium for types C1 and C2 radical hysterectomy

ligaments) (Fig. 33.2). The term "mesoureter" describes the lateral laminar part of the dorsal parametria, which is stretched dorsally and caudally from the ureter and contains the inferior hypogastric plexus [62].

Two parts of the ventral parametria are recognized in sagittal plane—cranial (above the ureter) and caudal (below the ureter), divided by the course of the ureter. Two different spaces are described dorsally—the sacro-uterine space (medial pararectal space) between the rectum and the dorsal parametrium, and the pararectal space between the dorsal parametrium and iliac vessels (Fig. 33.2). The deep uterine vein (vaginal vein) is an important landmark in the lateral parametrium (Fig. 33.3). In most cases there is not only one but a few veins in the lateral parametrium, and it is the largest one which is called the vaginal vein, usually located about 1–2 cm below the uterine artery and vein.

33.5 Classification

Different classifications are currently used to describe individual types of radical hysterectomy. Most historical classification systems do not include an unambiguous and precise description and specification of anatomical landmarks. As a consequence, the extent of the parametria resection varies substantially among institutions and surgeons, even if the same terminology is used. In many institutions, one type of "universal" or "classical" radical hysterectomy is used even though it is unclear with what kind of parametria resection it corresponds.

Principles of Classification

Modern classification of radical hysterectomy should be based on the following principles:

(a) The key and sole parameter for differentiation between types of radical hysterectomy is the extent of parametria resection. The resection or removal of other organs or structures (i.e. urinary bladder, ureter, rectum, pelvic floor muscle) is not included in the classification system. Also, the size of the removed vaginal cuff is not a decisive parameter for type of procedure.

(b) The extent of resection should be precisely defined for all three parts of the parametria (ventral, lateral, dorsal) in all three planes (sagittal, frontal and transverse). The resection margins in the vertical (deep parametrial) dimension determine long term morbidity due to the location of autonomic nerves.

(c) Although the classification system is usually proposed for radical hysterectomy, it is applicable to the radical trachelectomy and the radical parametrectomy.

(d) Surgical margins should be defined by stable anatomical landmarks. There are a few of such structures eligible in the pelvis, such as urinary bladder, rectum, ureter, large vessels, and nerves.

(e) The classification system must be sufficiently comprehensible and simple to allow for easy reproducibility.

ABCD Classification System

The classification system described in this chapter was first published by Querleu and Morrow in 2008 [52], and later extended into a 3D model [11]. Five types of the procedure (A, B, C1, C2, D) correspond to other common historical types of radical hysterectomy (Table 33.1). The new classification system has some exceptional aspects to it: (a) recognizes the size and type of parametria resection as the crucial and sole parameter for classification, (b) includes new type of nerve sparing procedure, (c) uses stable anatomical landmarks for description of surgical resection margins, (d) identifies surgical landmarks in three planes—frontal, sagittal and transverse.

Table 33.1 ABCD classification system and corresponding historical types of radical hysterectomy

New classification system	Corresponding types
A	Extrafascial hysterectomy
B	Modified radical hysterectomy Type II radical hysterectomy
C1	Nerve sparing radical hysterectomy
C2	Type III radical hysterectomy Classical/standard radical hysterectomy
D	Laterally extended parametrectomy

Type A corresponds to the extrafascial hysterectomy, the main principle of which is pericervical tissue removal up to the attachment of vaginal fornices. The ureter does not need to be identified or dissected in the parametrium, parametria are not resected and autonomic nerves remain fully preserved.

Type B corresponds mostly to the modified radical hysterectomy. Ureter is the major resection margin ventrally and laterally (Fig. 33.4). It must be identified in the parametrium, its course is unroofed, dissected from the cervix and displaced laterally, but not dissected from the lateral or ventral parametria. Such extent of distal ureteral dissection enables the resection of only a small initial part of the ventral and lateral parametria. Identification of autonomic nerves is not required, and the hypogastric plexus remains hidden in a deeper part of the parametria, thus remaining fully preserved.

There are significant differences, particularly in the vertical (deep parametrial) dimension, between type C1, which corresponds to the nerve-sparing procedure, and type C2, which aims for a complete parametrial resection. In type C1 the ureter is unroofed, dissected from the cervix and lateral parametria, but only partially from the ventral parametria, while type C2 requires complete dissection of the

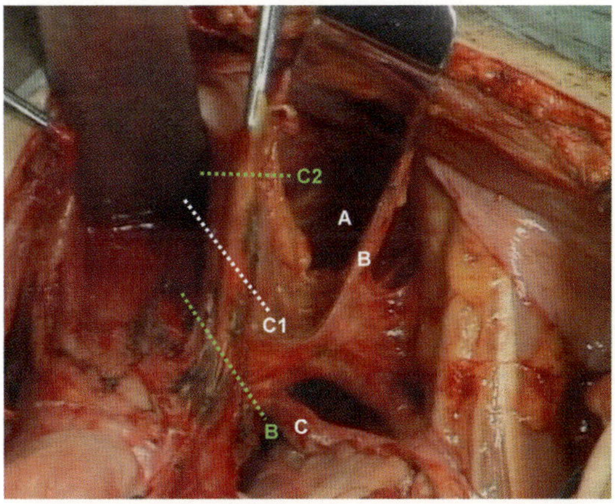

Fig. 33.4 Intra-operative picture of horizontal resection lines on the ventral parametrium *A* paravesical space, *B* umbilical ligament, *C* ureter. *B*, *C1*, *C2* resection lines on the ventral parametrium for types B, C1 and C2 radical hysterectomy

ureter from the ventral parametria up to the urinary bladder wall. Laterally, resection margins in a transverse plane are identical for both types, formed by the medial aspect of the internal iliac vein (Fig. 33.4). In type C1 the deep parametrial resection margin on the lateral parametria is formed by the deep uterine vein (vaginal vein), which is a large vein located about 1–2 cm below the uterine artery and vein (Fig. 33.3). As such the caudal part of the lateral parametria containing the splanchnic nerves is preserved. In type C2 the resection line continues alongside the medial aspect of the internal iliac vessels up to the sacral bone (Fig. 33.3). Such deep resection allows for greater mobility of the lateral parametria, facilitating its complete removal. Ventrally, in type C1 a partial dissection of the ureter from the ventral parametria allows for limited resection in a sagittal plane of 1–2 cm of the ventral parametria (Fig. 33.5). Even more important is a vertical resection margin on the ventral parametria, which must be at the level of ureter to preserve bladder branches of the hypogastric plexus localized below the course of the ureter [29, 30]. In type C2, a complete dissection of the ureter from the ventral parametria is required, which allows for complete resection of the ventral parametria up to the urinary bladder wall (Fig. 33.5). Bladder branches of the hypogastric plexus are sacrificed. Dorsally, type C1 requires separation of two parts of the dorsal parametria: the medial part, which is composed by the recto-uterine and recto-vaginal ligaments, and the lateral laminar structure, which contains the hypogastric plexus, also called the mesoureter (Fig. 33.6). Main branches of the hypogastric plexus are preserved on the lateral part (mesoureter), while recto-uterine and recto-vaginal ligaments can be resected at the level of its rectal attachment. Type C2 aims to a complete resection of the dorsal parametria deeply below the rectal attachment, so that separation of major branches of the hypogastric plexus is not needed and these nerves are sacrificed (Fig. 33.6).

Type D differs from type C2 only in a lateral extent of the lateral parametria resection. Ureteral dissection and resection of both dorsal and ventral parametria is identical to type C2. Laterally, however, it requires ligation and removal of internal iliac artery and vein, together with their branches, including gluteal, internal pudendal and obturator vessels. Lateral resection line is formed by the lumbosacral nerve plexus, piriformis muscle and obturator internal muscle.

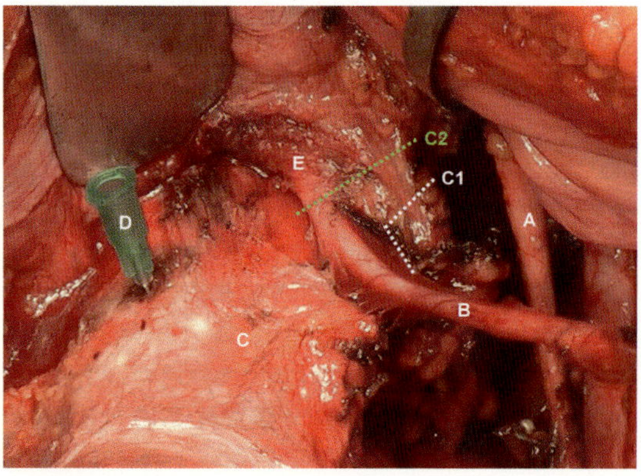

Fig. 33.5 Intra-operative picture of resection lines on the ventral parametrium (ureter unroofed) *A* umbilical ligament, *B* ureter, *C* cervix, *D* needle indicating level of vaginal fornix, *E* distal ureteral entrance into the bladder. *C1*, *C2* resection lines on the ventral parametrium for types C1 and C2 radical hysterectomy

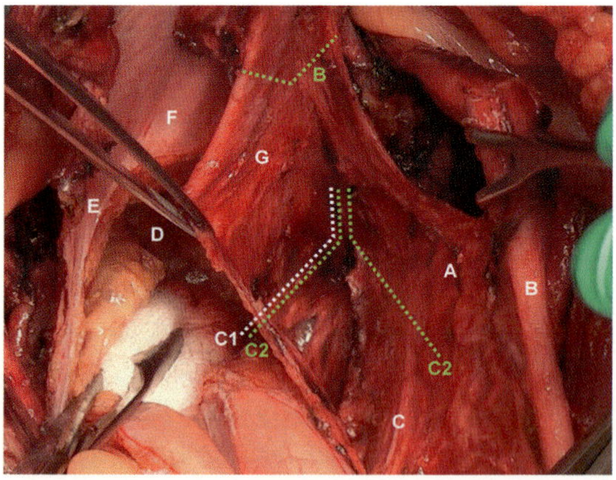

Fig. 33.6 Intra-operative picture of resection lines on the dorsal parametrium *A* mesoureter; *B* ureter, *C* branches of the hypogastric plexus (*white strips*), *D* rectovaginal space, *E* left dorsal parametrium (mesoureter not yet dissected from recto-uterine ligament), *F* cervix, *G* recto-uterine ligament. *B*, *C1*, *C2* resection lines on the dorsal parametrium for types B, C1 and C2 radical hysterectomy

33.6 Procedure Performance

Procedure performance depends mostly on the type of radical hysterectomy. The sequence of each procedure step can vary according to surgeon's preference. Pelvic lymphadenectomy, which is typically part of the procedure, is preferably performed at the beginning as it enables better pelvic structure identification. The entire procedure can be divided into a few steps:

Lateral Dissection

Round ligament is identified at the beginning of the procedure, cut through and the retroperitoneum is broadly exposed above the external iliac vessels. Paravesical and lateral pararectal spaces are opened by blind dissection and the lateral parametrium remains revealed between these two spaces. Umbilical ligament is dissected from the ventral parametria and preserved. The origin of the uterine artery is identified on the medial aspect of internal iliac artery; at this point it is interrupted, usually together with the uterine vein, localized below the artery. Now the lateral parametrium can be dissected from the pelvic side wall—lateral resection margin is formed by the medial aspect of internal iliac vein—caudal margin depends on the type of radical hysterectomy, formed by the deep uterine vein in type C1, while dissection continues up to the sacral bone in type C2. Type D requires ligation and resection of both internal iliac vessels.

Distal Dissection of the Ureter

Ureter is identified on the posterior leaf of broad ligament; it is sharply mobilized up to its entrance to lateral parametria. Mobilization of the distal ureter requires caudal dissection of the urinary bladder from the cervix and proximal vagina. Ureteral tunnel in the lateral parametrium is blindly opened; parametria resected above the ureter and the ureter is completely mobilized from the cervix and ventrally from the upper vagina. Such dissection of distal ureter is adequate for type B, while type C1 requires complete mobilization of the ureter from lateral parametria, whereas for type C2 additional complete dissection from ventral parametria up to its entrance into the urinary bladder is necessary.

Ventral Dissection

The extent of urinary bladder caudal dissection is determined by the projected size of vaginal cuff removal. The extent of ventral parametrial resection depends on the type of radical hysterectomy: ventral parametria are not resected in type B, while about 2 cm of proximal part located above the ureter is removed in type C1. In type C2 and D after the ureter has been fully dissected, ventral parametrium is resected completely at the bladder wall.

Dorsal Dissection

The rectovaginal peritoneal flap is cut and rectum is caudally dissected from the vagina and lateral parametria. Dorsal parametria are resected in the extent of 1–2 cm in type B. Type C1 requires separation of two parts of the dorsal parametria—hypogastric plexus is preserved in laterally separated part (mesoureter) while sacrouterine and sacrovaginal ligaments can be resected at the level of its attachment into the rectum. Separation of two parts of the dorsal parametrium is not required for type C2 or D as dorsal parametria are completely resected and hypogastric plexus is inevitably sacrificed.

Final Specimen Removal

Finally the paracolpium is interrupted in transverse plane at the level of intended vaginal resection, the vagina is resected and vaginal cuff sutured, preferably by submucosal closure which allows for further complete visualization of the upper vagina during the follow-up.

33.7 Choice of Radical Hysterectomy Type

The type of radical hysterectomy is determined by a number of prognostic factors: tumor size, depth of stromal invasion, presence of LVSI (lymphovascular invasion), or lymph node status. Indication criteria for C2 resection are not uniform, these procedures are typically performed in bulky tumors with their size bigger than 4 cm, also when two-thirds of cervical stroma is involved, when tumors invade into uterine isthmus and also in tumors of stage IIB with initial invasion into parametria. Type B or C1 should be preferred in small size tumors with negative lymph nodes with the intention to decrease post-operative morbidity thanks to autonomic nerve preservation. From the above description it is obvious that type B hysterectomy only enables a small part of parametria removal—it is a task for future studies to prove if this extent of parametrectomy brings any benefit for oncological outcome or if an identical outcome can be achieved in the same size tumors when simple hysterectomy is performed. Type D radical hysterectomy is done rarely, mostly for central pelvic recurrences or locally advanced tumors [42].

33.8 Pre-operative Procedure Description

An accurate surgical plan should be determined conclusively before every single procedure. Considering the above-mentioned principles of radical hysterectomy classification it is obvious that the type of radical hysterectomy purely describes the radicality of the surgery performed on parametria. For an adequate description of the procedure performance, the following parameters should be specified pre-operatively: (a) procedure on the adnexa (i.e. salpingo-oophorectomy; ovarian transposition.); (b) type of lymph node dissection (i.e. sentinel node biopsy, pelvic lymphadenectomy and its type, paraaortic lymphadenectomy and its cranial extent); (c) size of the vagina removal; (d) type of the procedure (radical hysterectomy, radical parametrectomy, radical trachelectomy), and (e) extent of parametria removal (classification system—type A–D).

33.9 Surgical Approach

An alternative to classical radical hysterectomy performed by laparotomy is an endoscopic approach. These procedures can be performed fully by laparoscopy or robotically or in combination with vaginal approach (LARVH—laparoscopic assisted radical vaginal hysterectomy; VALRH—vaginal assisted laparoscopic radical hysterectomy). Feasibility of both minimally invasive approaches, laparoscopic or robotic surgery, were well proven in early stages, locally advanced stages, old patients, obese patients, or for nerve sparing type (type C1) of radical hysterectomy [14, 23, 25, 31, 38, 40, 43, 44, 61].

Endoscopic approach is associated with less blood loss and shorter hospital stays, but, on the other hand, longer operation times when compared with open approach. All these parameters relate to short term morbidity. More significant data concerning the quality of life with a longer interval after the surgery are unfortunately still lacking. Even though many studies substantiated comparable oncological outcome, these are typically experiences from single institutions and retrospective design, short follow up and small cohorts to evaluate their prognosis. Attention should be paid to recent reports on atypical port-site metastasis after robotic or laparoscopic radical hysterectomy in cervical cancer patients, or higher number of local recurrences after robotic surgery in cervical cancer patients [32, 58, 59].

Oncological outcome after endoscopic surgery should be evaluated in multicenter randomized trials, especially in patients with higher risk of recurrence, in whom achievement of proper radicality can be crucial.

33.10 Radical Parametrectomy

The resection of parametria, the tissue that surrounds the cervix, is the main principle of radical hysterectomy. Parametrectomy can also be carried out as a separate procedure, should a simple hysterectomy have been performed previously for a different diagnosis, and cervical cancer was identified afterwards in the histological specimen. Most frequently a simple hysterectomy had been performed for precancerous lesions (CIN) in these patients who were not preoperatively adequately examined. Pelvic radiotherapy represents an alternative to radical parametrectomy. The aim of this surgery is to amend the procedure as if an adequate surgical procedure had been performed, typically in combination with pelvic lymphadenectomy and proximal vaginal resection [35].

This procedure is substantiated mainly in cases when there is a high probability that the surgery is a definite treatment and adjuvant radiotherapy will not be required: free surgical margins in the hysterectomy specimen, absence of clinically evident residual tumor, absence of lymph nodes suspicious from metastatic involvement. It is important to emphasize that no prospective study that would compare morbidity and oncological outcomes of radiotherapy versus radical parametrectomy has been carried out.

Feasibility of laparoscopic and robotic approach has been proven in small studies from single institutions [5, 24, 54]. Technical performance is surely more demanding due to the absence of uterus, postoperative adhesions, mainly the bladder to the vaginal cuff, and postoperative fibrosis in retroperitoneum and parametria. As a consequence, a higher risk of intra-operative complications, especially urinary bladder and ureteral injuries, can be expected [35, 36]. The same principles of classification are asserted for radical parametrectomy as well as for radical hysterectomy.

33.11 Postoperative Morbidity and Mortality

Mortality after radical hysterectomy in the original works of Wertheim and Shauta oscillated around 10 % [67]. Currently the mortality is minimal, the most frequent cause of death after radical hysterectomy being anesthesiological complications, rarely vascular injury, early postoperative bleeding or pulmonary embolism.

Most studies that showed postoperative morbidity focus unfortunately on the short interval a few months after the surgery. It is well documented that the morbidity corresponds with the radicality of hysterectomy, in particular with the extent of parametrial resection [19, 33, 53]. The most significant symptom in the early postoperative period is the impairment of spontaneous voiding. Voiding recovery varies in the literature from 4 to 31 days [6, 22, 33, 48, 51]. Such a broad range is mostly a consequence of different radicality of parametrectomy [17]. Pathophysiology remains insufficiently explained, yet it is hypothesized that perivesical edema, autonomic denervation and loss of urinary bladder support play their role.

Urinary bladder dysfunctions are also the most frequent and best documented type of late morbidity after radical hysterectomy. The most frequently reported symptoms include urinary incontinence, impairment of bladder sensation or voiding with abdominal straining [3, 7, 9, 46, 69]. These symptoms can persist even 12 months after the surgery. The preservation of autonomic nerves does not eliminate the symptoms but it significantly decreases the severity and frequency of their manifestation [55]. Much less attention is paid to anorectal dysfunctions, which typically are not common but negatively influence quality of life [2, 8, 60, 64]. Among the most frequent symptoms are constipation and flatulence incontinence, mainly in cases with extensive resection of dorsal parametria or extensive vaginectomy. The third area of late morbidity entails sexual dysfunctions. Their etiology is multifactorial, psychological, functional and anatomical changes all play a role. Shortening of the vagina has a negative effect on the quality of postoperative vaginal intercourse, surgical menopause as a consequence of BSO is associated with climacteric symptoms reducing libido, insufficient lubrication and dyspareunia, and cancer diagnosis as such is associated with anxiety and fear that sexual activity can cause disease recurrence. The main sexual dysfunctions after radical hysterectomy are sexual desire disorder, objective arousal disorder and dyspareunia [4, 15, 28, 37, 45, 47, 66]. It has been shown that the majority of patients do not require intensive sexuological care, however sufficient conversation about sexuality is an important preventive measure, which should entail preoperative information about potential sexual problems after the surgery. Other frequent symptoms, such as the presence of lymphedema or lymphocele, is rather a consequence of simultaneous lymphadenectomy.

33.12 Summary

Despite the progress in radiotherapy, introduction of neoadjuvant chemotherapy and surgical radicality reduction in small size tumors, radical hysterectomy remains the basic procedure in gynecological oncology in treatment of the early stages of cervical cancer. Procedure performance has evolved throughout its more-than-100-year history and until today discrepancies in terminology, classification, performance, and attitude to radicality have endured. It is important to emphasize that radical hysterectomy is not one universal procedure but the extent of parametrial removal can differ significantly in both horizontal and vertical planes. The extent of parametrectomy should be precisely scheduled pre-operatively according to well-known prognostic parameters. Broad acceptance of uniform terminology and classification is a basis for result sharing, collaboration, research and postgraduate training in the future. The key parameter for radical hysterectomy classification is the extent of parametria resection. The ABCD classification system recognizes four types of the procedure (B, C1, C2, D), including nerve sparing modification. It uses stable anatomical landmarks, defines surgery extent in all three parts of the parametria in three dimensions all of which enable to achieve adequate reproducibility. Different radicality of parametrectomy is crucial for the frequency and severity of early and long term morbidity. The most frequent symptom in early postoperative period is impairment of spontaneous voiding. Most often late morbidities entail urinary bladder dysfunctions, particularly urinary incontinence, and impairment of bladder sensation. Quality of life can also be compromised due to less frequent symptoms such as anorectal dysfunctions and sexual dysfunctions.

Key Points

- Radical hysterectomy is indicated for treatment of IB stage of cervical cancer; in locally advanced tumors (stages IB2 and selected IIB cases) it represents a method of choice together with primary chemoradiotherapy.
- Radical hysterectomy does not represent one universal procedure, but the extent of parametria removal can vary substantially.
- The main parameter for radical hysterectomy classification is the extent of parametria resection.
- Each type of radical hysterectomy should be clearly defined using stable anatomical landmarks.
- The description of every type of radical hysterectomy should include instructions for distal ureter dissection and the extent of the removal of all three parametrial parts (ventral, lateral, and dorsal) in three planes (frontal, sagittal, horizontal).
- The extent of parametrial resection, mainly in vertical dimension, significantly influences the postoperative morbidity, mostly the risk and severity of bladder dysfunctions but also anorectal dysfunctions.
- Type of lymph node surgical staging, type of radical hysterectomy (extent of parametrial resection) and extent of vaginal resection are variables that must be defined before the surgery.
- The ABCD classification system differentiates 4 types of radical hysterectomy (B, C1, C2, D), includes nerve sparing modification and meets all criteria for modern classification.
- Radical parametrectomy is a method of choice in patients after inadequate simple hysterectomy for previously unrevealed cervical cancer; its aim is

parametrial resection and proximal vaginectomy, and it uses the same surgical technique and classification as in radical hysterectomy.

- The type of radical hysterectomy should correspond with the stage of the disease and the presence of risk factors; greater parametrectomy extent (type C2) in locally advanced tumors, while less radical performance enabling preservation of autonomic nerves (Type B or C1) should be preferred in small tumors with negative lymph nodes.

Acknowledgement This work was supported by Charles University in Prague (UNCE 204024 and PRVOUK-P27/LF1/1).

References

1. Baalbergen A, Smedts F, Helmerhorst TJ. Conservative therapy in microinvasive adenocarcinoma of the uterine cervix is justified: an analysis of 59 cases and a review of the literature. Int J Gynecol Cancer. 2011;21(9):1640–5.
2. Barnes W, Waggoner S, Delgado G, Maher K, Potkul R, Barter J, Benjamin S. Manometric characterization of rectal dysfunction following radical hysterectomy. Gynecol Oncol. 1991;42:116–9.
3. Benedetti-Panici P, Zullo MA, Plotti F, Manci N, Muzii L, Angioli R. Long-term bladder function in patients with locally advanced cervical carcinoma treated with neoadjuvant chemotherapy and type 3–4 radical hysterectomy. Cancer. 2004; 100:2110–7.
4. Bergmark K, Avall-Lundqvist E, Dickman PW, Henningsohn L, Steineck G. Vaginal changes and sexuality in women with a history of cervical cancer. N Engl J Med. 1999;340(18):1383–9.
5. Buda A, Pellegrino A, Vitobello D, Meroni MG, Recalcati D, Perego P. Total laparoscopic radical parametrectomy, partial colpectomy, and pelvic lymphadenectomy in patients with occult cervical cancer. Int J Gynaecol Obstet. 2009;107(1):73–6.
6. Charoenkwan K, Srisomboon J, Suprasert P, Tantipalakorn C, Kietpeerakool C. Nerve-sparing class III radical hysterectomy: a modified technique to spare the pelvic autonomic nerves without compromising radicality. Int J Gynecol Cancer. 2006;16:1705–12.
7. Charoenkwan K, Pranpanas S. Prevalence and characteristics of late postoperative voiding dysfunction in early-stage cervical cancer patients treated with radical hysterectomy. Asian Pac J Cancer Prev. 2007;8:387–9.
8. Cibula D, Sláma J, Velechovská P, Fischerova D, Zikán M, Pinkavová I, Hill M. Factors affecting spontaneous voiding recovery after radical hysterectomy. Int J Gynecol Cancer. 2010;20(4):685–90.
9. Cibula D, Velechovska P, Sláma J, et al. Late morbidity following nerve-sparing radical hysterectomy. Gynecol Oncol. 2010;116(3):506–11.
10. Cibula D, Abu-Rustum NR, Benedetti-Panici P, et al. New classification system of radical hysterectomy: emphasis on a three-dimensional anatomic template for parametrial resection. Gynecol Oncol. 2011;122(2):264–8.
11. Cibula D, Pinkavova I, Dusek L, et al. Local control after tailored surgical treatment of early cervical cancer. Int J Gynecol Cancer. 2011;21(4):690–8.
12. Cibula D, Abu-Rustum NR, Dusek L, et al. Prognostic significance of low volume sentinel lymph node disease in early-stage cervical cancer. Gynecol Oncol. 2012;124(3):496–501.
13. Clark JG. A more radical method of performing hysterectomy for cancer of the uterus. Bull Johns Hopkins Hosp. 1895;6:120.
14. Ditto A, Martinelli F, Hanozet F, et al. Class III NSRH: oncological outcome in 170 cervical cancer patients. Gynecol Oncol. 2010;119:192–7.
15. Donovan KA, Taliaferro LA, Alvarez EM, Jacobsen PB, Roetzheim RG, Wenham RM. Sexual health in women treated for cervical cancer: characteristics and correlates. Gynecol Oncol. 2007;104(2):428–34.
16. Epstein E, Testa A, Gaurilcikas A, et al. Early-stage cervical cancer: tumor delineation by magnetic resonance imaging and ultrasound—a European multicenter trial. Gynecol Oncol. 2013;128(3):449–53.
17. Ercoli A, Delmas V, Gadonneix P, Fanfani F, Villet R, Paparella P, Manusco S, Scambia G. Classical and nerve-sparing radical hysterectomy: an evaluation of the risk of injury to the autonomous pelvic nerves. Surg Radiol Anat. 2003;25:200–6.
18. Fischerova D, Cibula D, Stenhova H, et al. Transrectal ultrasound and magnetic resonance imaging in staging of early cervical cancer. Int J Gynecol Cancer. 2008;18(4):766–72.
19. Fotiou S, Tserkezoglou A, Hatzieleftheriou G, Apostolikas N. Class III vs. class II radical hysterectomy in stage IB cervical carcinoma: a comparison of morbidity and survival. Int J Gynecol Cancer. 1997;7:17–21.
20. Freund WA. Eine neue methode der exstirpation des ganten uterus. Zentralbl Gynakol. 1878;10:222.
21. Frumovitz M, Sun CC, Schmeler KM, Deavers MT, Dos Reis R, Levenback CF, Ramirez PT. Parametrial involvement in radical hysterectomy specimens for women with early-stage cervical cancer. Obstet Gynecol. 2009;114(1):93–9.
22. Fujii S, Takakura K, Matsumura N, Higuchi T, Yura S, Mandai M, Baba T, Yoshika S. Anatomic identification and functional outcomes of the nerve sparing Okabayashi radical hysterectomy. Gynecol Oncol. 2007;107:4–13.

23. Geetha P, Nair MK. Laparoscopic, robotic and open method of radical hysterectomy for cervical cancer: a systematic review. J Minim Access Surg. 2012;8(3):67–73.
24. Geisler JP, Orr C, Manahan KJ. Robotically-assisted laparoscopic radical parametrectomy and radical vaginectomy. Eur J Gynaecol Oncol. 2011;32(6):674–6.
25. Gil-Ibáñez B, Díaz-Feijoo B, Pérez-Benavente A, Puig-Puig O, Franco-Camps S, Centeno C, Xercavins J, Gil-Moreno A. Nerve sparing technique in robotic-assisted radical hysterectomy: results. Int J Med Robot. 2013;9:339–44.
26. Höckel M, Horn LC, Manthey N, Braumann UD, Wolf U, Teichmann G, Frauenschläger K, Dornhöfer N, Einenkel J. Resection of the embryologically defined uterovaginal(Müllerian) compartment and pelvic control in patients with cervical cancer: a prospective analysis. Lancet Oncol. 2009;10(7): 683–92.
27. Hou J, Goldberg GL, Qualls CR, Kuo DY, Forman A, Smith HO. Risk factors for poor prognosis in microinvasive adenocarcinoma of the uterine cervix (IA1 and IA2): a pooled analysis. Gynecol Oncol. 2011;121(1):135–42.
28. Jensen PT, Groenvold M, Klee MC, Thranov I, Petersen MA, Machin D. Early-stage cervical carcinoma, radical hysterectomy, and sexual function. A longitudinal study. Cancer. 2004;100(1):97–106.
29. Katahira A, Niikura H, Ito K, Takano T, Nagase S, Murakami G, Yaegashi N. Vesicouterine ligament contains abundant autonomic nerve ganglion cells: the distribution in histology concerning nerve-sparing radical hysterectomy. Int J Gynecol Cancer. 2008;18:193–8.
30. Kato T, Murakami G, Yabuki Y. Does the cardinal ligament of the uterus contain a nerve that should be preserved in radical hysterectomy? Anat Sci Int. 2002;77:161–8.
31. Koehler C, Gottschalk E, Chiantera V, Marnitz S, Hasenbein K, Schneider A. From laparoscopic assisted radical vaginal hysterectomy to vaginal assisted laparoscopic radical hysterectomy. BJOG. 2012;119(2):254–62.
32. Kohlberger PD, Edwards L, Collins C, Milross C, Hacker NF. Laparoscopic port-site recurrence following surgery for a stage IB squamous cell carcinoma of the cervix with negative lymph nodes. Gynecol Oncol. 2000;79(2):324–6.
33. Landoni F, Maneo A, Cormio G, Perego P, Milani R, Caruso O. Class II versus class III radical hysterectomy in stage IB—IIA cervical cancer: a prospective randomised study. Gynecol Oncol. 2001;80:3–12.
34. Latzko W, Schiffmann J. Klinisches and anatomisches zur radikaloperation des gebarmutterkrebses. Zentralbl Gynakol. 1919;43:715.
35. Leath 3rd CA, Straughn JM, Bhoola SM, Partridge EE, Kilgore LC, Alvarez RD. The role of radical parametrectomy in the treatment of occult cervical carcinoma after extrafascial hysterectomy. Gynecol Oncol. 2004;92(1):215–9.
36. Li J, Xu H, Chen Y, Wang D, Li Y, Liang Z. Laparoscopic nerve-sparing radical parametrectomy for occult early-stage invasive cervical cancer after simple hysterectomy. Int J Gynecol Cancer. 2012;22(8):1383–8.
37. Maas CP, ter Kuile MM, Laan E, Tuijnman CC, Weijenborg PT, Trimbos JB, Kenter GG. Objective assessment of sexual arousal in women with a history of hysterectomy. BJOG. 2004;111(5):456–62.
38. Magrina JF, Magtibay PM. Robotic nerve-sparing radical parametrectomy: feasibility and technique. Int J Med Robot. 2012;8(2):206–9.
39. Meigs JV. The Wertheim operation for carcinoma of the cervix. Am J Obstet Gynecol. 1945;49:542.
40. Naik R, Jackson KS, Lopes A, Cross P, Henry JA. Laparoscopic assisted radical vaginal hysterectomy versus radical abdominal hysterectomy—a randomised phase II trial: perioperative outcomes and surgicopathological measurements. BJOG. 2010;117(6):746–51.
41. Okabayashi H. Radical abdominal hysterectomy for cancer of the cervix uteri. Surg Gynecol Obstet. 1921;33:335.
42. Pálfalvi L, Ungár L. Laterally extended parametrectomy (LEP), the technique for radical pelvic side wall dissection: feasibility, technique and results. Int J Gynecol Cancer. 2003;13(6):914–7.
43. Park JY, Kim DY, Kim JH, Kim YM, Kim YT, Nam JH. Laparoscopic versus open radical hysterectomy for elderly patients with early-stage cervical cancer. Am J Obstet Gynecol. 2012;207(3):195.e1–8.
44. Park JY, Kim DY, Kim JH, Kim YM, Kim YT, Nam JH. Laparoscopic compared with open radical hysterectomy in obese women with early-stage cervical cancer. Obstet Gynecol. 2012;119(6):1201–9.
45. Park SY, Bae DS, Nam JH, et al. Quality of life and sexual problems in disease-free survivors of cervical cancer compared with the general population. Cancer. 2007;110(12):2716–25.
46. Pieterse QD, Maas CP, Ter Kuile MM, Lowik M, Van Eijkeren MA, Trimbos JBMZ, Kenter GG. An observational longitudinal study to evaluate miction, defecation, and sexual function after radical hysterectomy with pelvic lymhadenectomy for early-stage cervical cancer. Int J Gynecol Cancer. 2006;16:1119–29.
47. Pieterse QD, Ter Kuile MM, Deruiter MC, Trimbos JB, Kenter GG, Maas CP. Vaginal blood flow after radical hysterectomy with and without nerve sparing. A preliminary report. Int J Gynecol Cancer. 2008;18(3):576–83.
48. Pikaart DP, Holloway RW, Ahmad S, Finkler NJ, Bigsby GE, Ortiz BH, DeNardis SA. Clinical-pathologic and morbidity analyses of types 2 and 3 abdominal radical hysterectomy for cervical cancer. Gynecol Oncol. 2007;107:205–10.
49. Pinkavova I, Fischerova D, Zikan M, et al. Transrectal ultrasound and magnetic resonance imaging in the evaluation of tumor size after application of neoadjuvant chemotherapy for locally advanced cervical cancer. Ultrasound Obstet Gynecol. 2013;42(6):705–12.

50. Pluta M, Rob L, Charvat M, Chmel R, Halaska Jr M, Skapa P, Robova H. Less radical surgery than radical hysterectomy in early stage cervical cancer: a pilot study. Gynecol Oncol. 2009;113(2):181–4.
51. Possover M, Stober S, Plaul K, Schneider A. Identification and preservation of the motoric innervation of the bladder in radical hysterectomy type III. Gynecol Oncol. 2000;79:154–7.
52. Querleu D, Morrow CP. Classification of radical hysterectomy. Lancet Oncol. 2008;9:297–303.
53. Ralph G, Winter R, Michelitsch L, Tamussino K. Radicality of parametrial resection and dysfunction of the lower urinary tract after radical hysterectomy. Eur J Gynaecol Oncol. 1991;12:27–30.
54. Ramirez PT, Schmeler KM, Wolf JK, Brown J, Soliman PT. Robotic radical parametrectomy and pelvic lymphadenectomy in patients with invasive cervical cancer. Gynecol Oncol. 2008;111(1):18–21.
55. Raspagliesi F, Ditto A, Fontanelli R, et al. Type II versus type III nerve sparing radical hysterectomy: comparison of lower urinary tract dysfunctions. Gynecol Oncol. 2006;102:256–62.
56. Sauter, Johann Nepomuk. Die gänzliche Extirpation der carcinomatösen Gebärmutter: ohne selbst entstandenen oder künstlich bewirkten Vorfall vorgenommen und glücklich vollführt. Constanz: W. Wallis, 1822. 188 s.
57. Schauta F. Die erweiterte vaginale Totalexstirpation des Uterus beim Kollumkarzinom. Wien: Verlag von J. Safar; 1908.
58. Sert B. Robotic port-site and pelvic recurrences after robot-assisted laparoscopic radical hysterectomy for a stage IB1 adenocarcinoma of the cervix with negative lymph nodes. Int J Med Robot. 2010;6(2):132–5.
59. Sert MB, Abeler V. Robot-assisted laparoscopic radical hysterectomy: comparison with total laparoscopic hysterectomy and abdominal radical hysterectomy; one surgeon's experience at the Norwegian Radium Hospital. Gynecol Oncol. 2011;121(3):600–4.
60. Sood AK, Nygaard I, Shahin MS, Sorosky JI, Lutgendorf SK, Rao SSC. Anorectal dysfunction after surgical treatment for cervical cancer. J Am Coll Surg. 2002;195:513–9.
61. Tinelli R, Malzoni M, Cosentino F, Perone C, Fusco A, Cicinelli E, Nezhat F. Robotics versus laparoscopic radical hysterectomy with lymphadenectomy in patients with early cervical cancer: a multicenter study. Ann Surg Oncol. 2011;18(9):2622–8.
62. Trimbos JB, Maas CP, Deruiter MC, Peters AA, Kenter GG. A nerve-sparing radical hysterectomy: guidelines and feasibility in Western patients. Int J Gynecol Cancer. 2001;11:180–6.
63. Schmeler KM, Frumovitz M, Ramirez PT. Conservative management of early stage cervical cancer: is there a role for less radical surgery? Gynecol Oncol. 2011;120(3):321–5.
64. van Dam JH, Gosselink MJ, Drogendijk AC, Hop WCJ, Schouten WR. Changes in bowel function after hysterectomy. Dis Colon Rectum. 1997; 40:1342–7.
65. van Meurs H, Visser O, Buist MR, Ten Kate FJ, van der Velden J. Frequency of pelvic lymph node metastases and parametrial involvement in stage IA2 cervical cancer: a population-based study and literature review. Int J Gynecol Cancer. 2009;19(1):21–6.
66. Vrzackova P, Weiss P, Cibula D. Sexual morbidity following radical hysterectomy for cervical cancer. Expert Rev Anticancer Ther. 2010;10(7): 1037–42.
67. Wertheim E. The extended abdominal operation for carcinoma uteri (based on 500 operative cases). Am J Obstet Dis Women Child. 1912;66:169–232.
68. Wertheim E. Zur frag der radikaloperation beim uteruskrebs. Arch Gynakol. 1900;61:627.
69. Zullo MA, Manci N, Angioli R, Muzii L, Benedetti-Panici P. Vesical dysfunctions after radical hysterectomy for cervical cancer: a critical review. Crit Rev Oncol Hematol. 2003;48:287–93.

34 Sentinel Lymph Node Mapping in the Management of Cervical Cancer

Lukas Rob

34.1 Introduction

Cancer of the cervix is the third most common life-threatening cancer in women worldwide, with over 530,000 incident cases and the fourth leading cause of cancer mortality in women. In Europe, we observe an East-West gradient, where there is a higher incidence occurring in post-communistic countries [1]. These variations are possible to explain in terms of assorted screening strategies and different levels of health care. The importance of cervical cancer becomes even more apparent in light of the evidence that >54 % of women diagnosed with this disease are <50 years of age [2, 3]. For treatment of early cervical cancer, surgery remains the preferred treatment option, especially in younger women. Nevertheless, well-performed radical hysterectomy with systematic pelvic lymphadenectomy can be accompanied by early and late postoperative morbidity [4–6]. Attention in the past two decades has largely centered on risk factors for cervical cancer that allow for individualized therapy and selection of patients for optimal treatment (nerve-sparing surgery, less radical fertility-sparing surgery or chemoradiotherapy). Management of the most common squamous cell cancer and adenocarcinoma is not performed differently and it is important to exclude only neuroendocrine carcinomas, which require a different management approach. Treatment in these cases would start with chemotherapy [7]. Development of imaging methods, particularly magnetic resonance imagining (MRI) and ultrasonography (US), allows not only exact tumor measurement but also helps to determine tumor volume, determination of the extent of infiltration of the cervical stroma and the amount of healthy stroma [8–10]. In early cervical cancer, the status of regional lymph nodes is a critical factor in determining prognosis. Systematic pelvic lymph node dissection is routinely performed as part of standard surgical therapy, except stage IA1 [11]. Systematic pelvic lymphadenectomy is associated with short- and long- term morbidities, such as increased blood loss, neurovascular injury, lymphocyst formation and infection, and lower-limb lymphedema [3]. During the past 15 years, considerable efforts have been undertaken to develop preoperative and intraoperative methods to identify nodal involvement. Although lymphangiography, computed tomography (CT) and MRI are commonly used for lymph node assessment, a systematic review and meta-analysis of the literature on diagnostic accuracy suggest low sensitivity and specificity in detecting lymph node metastasis, particularly in early stage cervical cancer [12]. Large expectations were projected on 18F-fluorodeoxyglucose positron emission CT (PET-CT). This imaging tool is the

L. Rob, MD, PhD (✉)
Department of Obstetrics and Gynecology, 2nd Medical Faculty, Charles University, Prague, Czech Republic
e-mail: lukas.rob@fnmotol.cz

H.R.H. Patel et al. (eds.), *Pelvic Cancer Surgery: Modern Breakthroughs and Future Advances*, DOI 10.1007/978-1-4471-4258-4_34, © Springer-Verlag London 2015

most accurate preoperative evaluation but has low sensitivity as well as poor positive predictive value for pretreatment lymph node staging [12–14]. The main difficulty in patients with early cervical cancer is that lymph node metastases <7 mm are not detectable by current preoperative, noninvasive imaging techniques, including PET-CT.

The technique of sentinel lymph node mapping (SLNM) was studied in cancers that spread by the lymphatic system. The sentinel lymph node (SLN) is the first lymph node that receives drainage directly from the primary tumor and is therefore useful in detecting lymph nodes with the highest metastatic risk. The number of publications concerning SLN biopsy (SLNB) and cervical cancer has increased dramatically in the past 15 years [15–23]. This interest in SLNB in relation to cervical cancer is logical because early stages of the most common histological types of squamous and adenocarcinoma metastasize primarily to lymph nodes. Hematogenous spread is rare, often occurring late in the disease process, except for neuroendocrine tumors. Currently, the SLNM procedure has been incorporated into cervical cancer fertility-sparing surgery and individually tailored surgery in many centers worldwide. A number of studies have confirmed that SLNM is feasible and highly accurate in predicting the status of regional lymph nodes in early cervical cancer [16–20]. This chapter is a critical review of the literature and a summary of our experience over the past 15 years with SLNM in cervical cancer patients.

34.2 Mapping Techniques

Colorimetric Technique

The first procedure to localize SLNs in patients with cervical cancer involved the use of blue dye. The injection of isosulfan blue dye (Lymphazurin®), Methylene Blue (B) or Patente Blue (Bleu Patente V sodique®) is administered to the patient in the operating room just before surgery in the general anesthesia. Two blue dye techniques have been reported in the detection of SLN in cervical cancer. Most authors use a four-quadrant technique, which involves injecting 0.5–1 ml of blue dye into each quadrant of the cervix peritumorally. Some surgical teams prefer to dilute 2 ml blue with 2 ml saline solution [17, 20, 21, 24]. In patients who have undergone prior cone biopsy the injection is given around of the cone [17–20]. A less frequent technique is to inject the blue dye at the 3 and 9 o'clock positions [22]. Two techniques of injection are used: very superficial, submucosal peritumoral injection and injection into the cervical stroma (10–15 mm deep, very slow injection from the deepest point of the needle to the subepithelial point). Our team prefers the four-quadrant technique with injection into the cervical stroma. One adverse effect of blue dye involves severe allergic reactions (0.3–1.8 %), but no deaths have been reported. Three severe allergic reactions (0.6 %) were mentioned by our group of 525 women who were given blue dye injection. A more frequent adverse effect is less serious localized swelling or pruritus (2–4 %), but >95 % of the patients have been observed with a bluish coloring of the skin, mucosa and urine [17, 23–25]. Preventive antiallergic measures have generally not been recommended. Another adverse effect of blue dye injection is the transient decrease in pulse oximetry reading, which typically occurs between 2 and 10 min after blue dye application. Reduction in pulse oximetry readings is not accompanied by a decrease in arterial oxygen saturation and thus represents only colorimetric interference [26]. SLNM with blue dye is clearly inferior to SLNM with a radio-isotopic method alone or in combination with a blue dye plus a radio-isotopic method for sensitivity, detection rate (DR) and site-specific DR (SSDR) [17, 23]. Blue dye in combination with a radioisotope versus a radioisotope alone slightly increases SLN detection (DR 1–4 % and SSDR 2–7 %). The major advantage of blue dye in combination with a radioisotope is the possibility to identify individual blue lymphatic channels as well as identifying SLNs in the medial part of the paracervix (between the cervical fascia and the obliterated umbilical artery). In this area in vivo identification only by blue dye is possible because radioactivity is very high near the cervix [17, 23, 27]. The combination of blue dye and a radioisotope decreases the risk of parametrial SLNs going undetected and increases the safety of fertility-sparing surgery and less radical procedures. Identification of blue channels also allows easy identification of SLNs in unusual locations (e.g., the parametrial or presacral area). Blue lymphatic channels that terminate near the enlarged lymph node decrease the risk of omission of fully infiltrated lymph nodes. Injections of both blue dye and a radioisotope are popular in Europe, the USA and Canada. In Asia, it is more common to use a radioisotope alone.

Radioisotope Technique

Different sizes of radiolabeled colloids (typically technetium Tc99) are used to detect SLNs in cervical cancer. The ideal tracer should combine rapid and predictable transport from the cervix towards the sentinel node (SN) with persistent retention in the first nodes. After intracervical application, colloid enters the lymphatic capillaries and is transported by lymph vessels to the first lymph nodes. Particles of different sizes spread in the lymphatic system at different speeds. The smallest particles (<50 nm) are quickly transported to secondary nodes. The particles are possible to divide according to size into Nanocolloids Tc99 (95 % of the particles have a size from 8 to 80 nm). The size of the particles depends on the final filtration. The second group of particles is radioisotopes with the majority of particles in the range of 100–600 nm. Our team found this particle size to be optimal. The largest particles that can be used are the Tc 99m phytate (150–1,500 nm), which is mostly applied in Asia. Different doses and timing are currently employed in detecting SLNs. In many centers "long" (2-days) protocols are used when radiocolloid is injected 1 day (i.e., 20–24 h) before surgery. Lymphoscintigraphy is performed 1–3 h after injection. The doses used in these "long" 2-day protocols are very high (2.0–4 mci, 74–148 MBq) because the half time of degradation is 6 h and after 24 h only residual activity is measured (average 10–15 %) [19, 27–29]. However, short "1-day" protocols are increasingly employed. Doses between 0.2 and 1.0 mci (7.4–37 MBq) are commonly used [23, 30, 31]. Radiocolloid in these protocols is injected 2–4 h before surgery and lymphoscintigraphy is performed 20–30 min after injection. Some departments do not perform preoperative lymphoscintigraphy and use only intraoperative gamma probe detection. The third timing interval involves "ultra-short" protocols: radiocolloid in doses of 0.4–0.55 mci (14.8–20 MBq) is injected in the operating theater in the beginning of general anesthesia before injection of the blue dye. Injection is easier and more accurate in general anesthesia. Detection of SLNs is performed after 15–20 min of the injection by a hand-held gamma probe without lymphoscintigraphy [17, 21, 27]. Exclusion of preoperative lymphoscintigraphy and use of only intraoperative detection of SLNs by a hand-held or laparoscopic gamma probe are not thought to decrease the DR of SLNs. Management without lymphoscintigraphy is simple and less expensive [17, 21, 27, 31–33]. We prefer ultra-short protocols without lymphoscintigraphy.

Techniques used in the application of radiocolloid are identical to those of blue dye: submucosally (superficially-subepithelially) in 0.1–1.0 ml volume or peritumorally into the stroma of the cervix 10–15 mm deep, followed by slow injection from the deepest point of the needle to the subepithelial layer in 0.5–1 ml volume in each quadrant. No adverse effects of radiolabeled colloids were described in literature. Using an ultra-short protocol, all tampons and needles must be returned to the Department of Nuclear Medicine. Recent data show that intraoperative detection using a hand-held gamma or laparoscopic probe is a more sensitive instrument (i.e., results in higher detection) than lymphoscintigraphy [17, 21, 32]. Lymphoscintigraphy the day before surgery is poorly correlated to surgical intraoperative mapping [33]. An increasing number of surgical teams have abandoned preoperative lymphoscintigraphy and instead opted for intraoperative detection only, which is both cost-effective and offers uncomplicated management.

34.3 Detection of Intraoperative SLNs

The cervix is a midline structure whose lymphatic drainage is bilateral and thus the DR per patient is less accurate. Thus, DR must be interpreted using the SSDR method [17, 23, 34, 35]. The most important factor in SLNM is the timing between the radioactive isotope and blue dye injection into the cervix. Direct visualization of the pelvis allows the surgeon to identify the blue-colored lymphatic channels and blue nodes. Optimal time for identification of the blue channels and nodes is 5–20 min [23, 27, 34]. After identification of the blue-colored lymphatic channels and nodes, the next step is to identify the radioactive nodes (hot nodes) with a hand-held or laparoscopic gamma probe. SLN nodes need minimal radioactivity of three to ten times more than the baseline activity. Most authors recommend control over the radioactivity of the removed SLNs outside the surgery field. It is necessary to verify the presence of residual radioactivity in the pelvic and paraaortic regions after removal of the hot nodes. Identification of SLNs in the medial part of the lateral parametrium (between the cervical fascia and obliterated umbilical artery) is possible in vivo, but only by blue dye because radioactivity is very high near the cervix. An important component in identifying SLNs is the detection of suspect, bulky lymph nodes. Fully infiltrated lymph nodes can have lower radioactivity and may not appear blue in that the blue dye and tracer may bypass these nodes. These lymph nodes should not be called SLNs. Bulky nodes have to be extirpated and sent for frozen section (FS). In the event that positive enlarged nodes are detected it is necessary to terminate identification of SLNs and perform debulking with complete pelvic lymphadenectomy and paraaortic lymphadenectomy with or without radical hysterectomy, or to abandon surgery as a treatment option and have the patient undergo chemoradiotherapy.

34.4 Distribution of SLNs

Due to small numbers of patients and the lack of standardization of surgical anatomical landmarks, huge differences have been observed between studies. For example, presacral SLNs are less often diagnosed during laparoscopic surgery. This observation may be explained in terms of technical difficulties and that some authors classify the presacral lymph nodes as belonging to the paraaortal [35] or internal iliac area [18]. Paraaortal lymph nodes were often detected during the 2-day protocols, which used ultra-small particles (<100 nm). The smallest particles show quick transport to the secondary nodes. The lack of a clear surgically based classification and landmark underlines the difficulties in comparing pelvic SN localization data. For pelvic lymphadenectomy, it is important to use uniform terminology with clear and simple landmarks. Figure 34.1 displays the terminology we use, which describes clear landmarks for pelvic lymphadenectomy. Figure 34.2 depicts the distribution of 1,120 SLNs in 372 women with early cervical cancer in our series in which a combination of radiocolloid and blue dye was used. Figure 34.3 portrays the distribution of 77 positive SLNs in 59 women.

34.5 Histopathological Procedure in SLN

We divided tumor deposits of SLNs in patients with cervical cancer into three categories: macrometastasis (diameter >2 mm), micrometastasis (diameter >0.2 mm but not >2 mm) and isolated tumor cells (ITCs, diameter ≤0.2 mm). The presence of macrometastatic or micrometastastatic disease in SLNs is described as positive nodes in the N category of the tumor, node, metastasis (TNM) staging system for cervical cancer. Although the extent of involvement of lymph

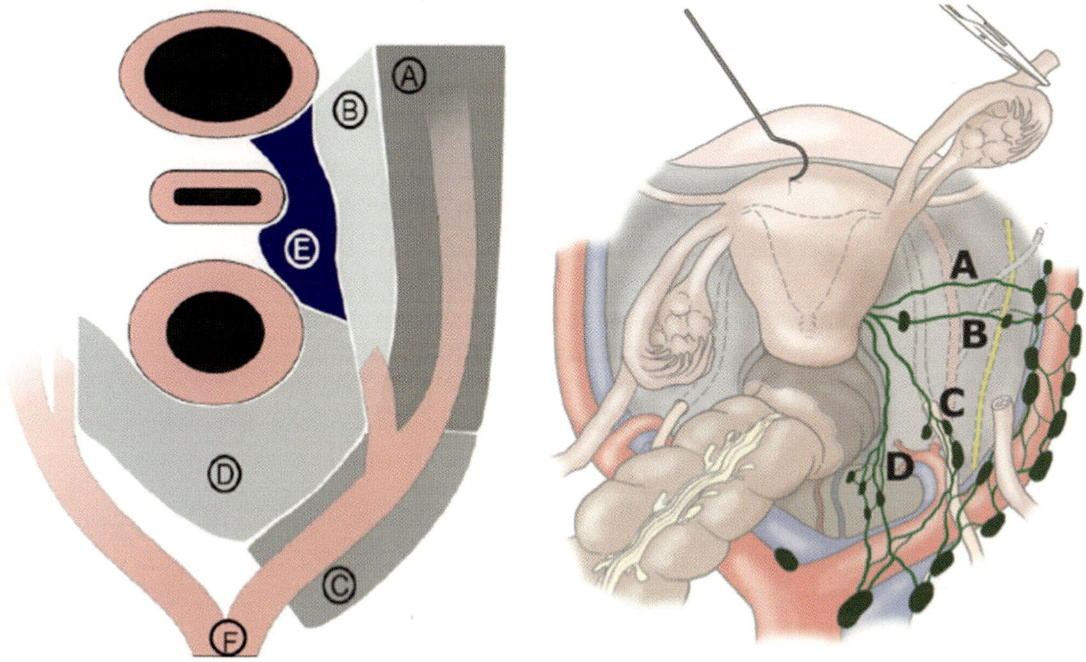

Fig. 34.1 *A* External iliac artery region: lymph nodes that are attached to the external iliac artery and vein from the bifurcation till groin; *B* Obturator region: lymph nodes around internal iliac artery and vein, medial border by obliterated umbilical chord, lateral border pelvic side wall, caudally femoral canal; *C* Common iliac artery and vein region: lymph nodes that are attached to the vessels, between aortal bifurcation and iliac bifurcation; *D* Presacral region lymph nodes between common iliac arteries and veins, not in the attachment with the vessels; *E* Paracervical region: lymph nodes between cervix, umbilical chord, and internal iliac vessels; *F* Low paraaortal region: lymph nodes along aorta and vena cava inferior, between aortal bifurcation and a. mesenterica inferior

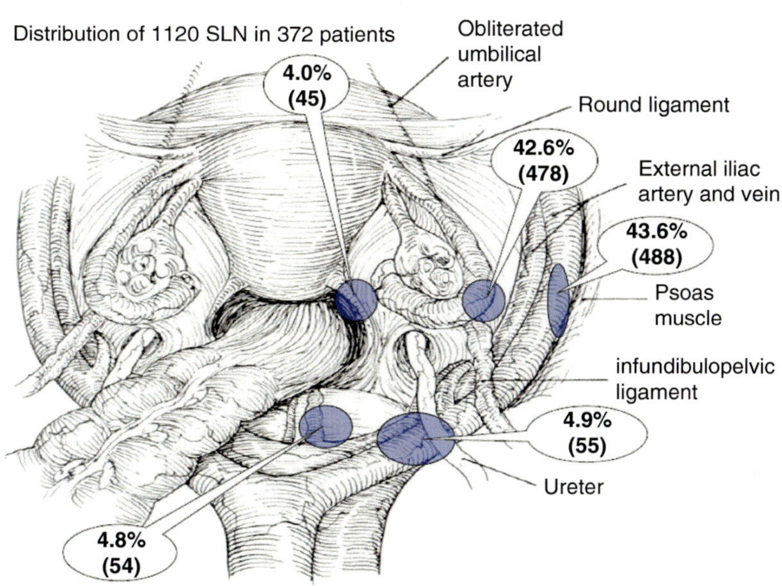

Fig. 34.2 Distribution of 1,120 SLN in 372 patients (From Rob et al. [17]. Used with permission from Elsevier)

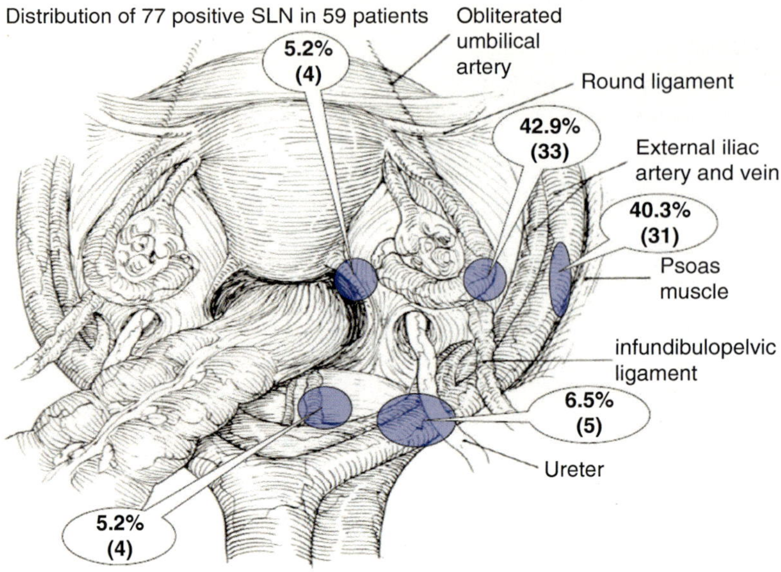

Fig. 34.3 Distribution of 77 positive SLN in 59 patients (From Rob et al. [17]. Used with permission from Elsevier)

nodes is an important prognostic factor, it still has not been validated in the literature. In cervical cancer surgery we have less extensive data though a recent multicenter study confirmed the prognostic significance of micrometastatic lymph node involvement [36]. However, the clinical significance of ITCs is still unknown. The identification of most micrometastases requires serial sectioning. We have no consensus about optimal leveling; however, in routine clinical practice 150–250 μm leveling seems acceptable.

A major controversy concerns FS biopsy of SLNs, including its benefits and limitations. The intraoperative assessment of SLNs potentially modifies the surgical procedure and subsequent treatment management. Despite the obvious benefits of FS examination for the patient, this technique has serious limitations in the microscopic evaluation of selected portions of tissue. Intraoperative serial cutting of the entire SLN is not applicable because of the prolongation of the operating time, technical limitations of the processing of frozen material and loss of tissue for postoperative evaluation. Presently, no standardization for the number of levels taken from each tissue block is available. Our algorithm of tissue sectioning in FS enables the disclosure of macrometastatic tumor deposits. However, it leads to reduced sensitivity in detecting micrometastases and may result in false negatives [17]. Using a good diagnostic tool such as FS allows reliable detection of clinically important metastases in lymph nodes (metastases >2 mm), but will miss a significant proportion of patients with micrometastatic disease (<2 mm) and ITCs [11, 23, 24, 27, 37–39]. Importantly, if there were negative SLNs in the hemipelvis in early cervical cancer, it is extremely rare to have metastasis in non-SLNs [16–19, 22, 23, 27–31, 40]. Further, if there were micrometastases in final ultrastaging of SLNs that were missed by FS, it is extremely rare to have metastasis in non-SLNs [39, 41–43]. Selection of patients with macrometastatic positive SLNs allows preoperative modifications of the treatment. In contrast, negative FS of SLN biopsy for early cervical cancer is an important adjunct of individually tailored less radical treatment options [43–47].

34.6 Identification of SLNs: Detection Rate

The cervix is a midline structure where the DR per patient is less accurate than the DR per hemipelvis (SSDR). General agreement has

Table 34.1 Results of the "prague fn motol protocol"

Stage	Number of patients	DR (%)	SSDR (%)
IB1 <20 mm	182	98.4	95.6
IB1 >20 mm	92	94.6	91.3
IB2 (NAC)	98	90.8	86.7

372 patients (385 patients included, 13 patients excluded for bulky lymph nodes, 2 false negative cases)

been emerging that optimal mapping implies identification of at least one SLN on each side. It is evident that Tc 99m or Tc 99m with blue dye is superior to blue dye alone. During the past decade, studies on SLNM have used different patient selection criteria, application methods, radiocolloid particles and timing of SLNM. In the literature the DR in tumors with small tumor volume (<2 cm) was 93.8–100 % and 58–87.8 % in tumors with large tumor volume (>2 cm). The SSDR, a more important measure, was 69.4–95.6 % in tumors with small tumor volume and 41.9–69.5 % in tumors with large tumor volume. Concerning clinical practice, the sensitivity and negative predictive value (NPV) for endpoints are also of importance. Sensitivity in the group of patients with small tumor volume was 99–100 % versus 84–100 % in the group with large tumor volume. Table 34.1 summarizes the results of our FN Motol ultra-short protocol.

34.7 Summary

In the past two decades considerable attention has been directed toward optimal surgical management of early cervical cancer. Although enormous efforts have been made in developing exact preoperative methods to identify nodal involvement, diagnostic accuracy is still limited in terms of low sensitivity and specificity in detecting lymph node metastasis, especially in early cervical cancer. Several studies have confirmed that SLNM is a feasible and accurate technique in predicting the status of pelvic nodes in early cervical cancer patients. Using SLNM, we found that 15 % of the SLNs from "unusual' locations could be identified. SLN biopsy and serial sectioning allowed precise histopathological evaluation of the "high-risk" nodes because serial sectioning and ultrastaging of whole lymph nodes were not possible. There are sufficient data to suggest that SLNM with 99mTc plus blue dye in the hands of an experienced surgeon should prove important in fertility-sparing and individually tailored surgery for cervical cancer.

Key Points

- Sufficient data are available to suggest that SLNM mapping with a combination of 99mTc and blue dye should prove to be an important component in fertility-sparing and individually tailored surgery.
- A number of studies confirm that SLNM is feasible and highly accurate in predicting the status of regional lymph nodes in small volume cervical cancer (<2 cm and less than one-half stromal invasion).
- Uncommon lymphatic drainage has been reported in 15 % of cervical cancer patients.
- Recent data establish that intraoperative detection is more sensitive than preoperative lymphoscintigraphy. A question for thought is whether the added benefit of preoperative lymphoscintigraphy for SLNM detection in cervical cancer is justified.
- The cervix is a midline structure whose lymphatic drainage is bilateral and therefore DR must be interpreted per side (SSDR).
- Bilateral SLN detection with histopathology ultrastaging is more sensitive than systematic pelvic lymphadenectomy.

References

1. Arbyn M, Castellsague X, Sanjose S, Bruni L, Saraiya M, Bray F, et al. Worldwide burden of cervical cancer in 28. Ann Oncol. 2011;22:2675–86.

2. Watson M, Saraiya M, Benard V. Burden of cervical cancer in the United States, 1998–2003. Cancer. 2008;113 Suppl 10:2855–64.
3. Rob L, Skapa P, Robova H. Fertility–sparing surgery in patients with cervical cancer. Lancet Oncol. 2011;12:192–200.
4. Rob L, Halaska M, Robova H. Nerve—sparing and individually tailored surgery for cervical cancer. Lancet Oncol. 2010;11(3):292–301.
5. Undurraga M, Loubeyre P, Dubuisson JB, Schneider D, Petignat P. Early-stage cervical cancer: is surgery better than radiotherapy? Expert Rev Anticancer Ther. 2010;10(3):451–60.
6. Vrzackova P, Weiss P, Cibula D. Sexual morbidity following radical hysterectomy for cervical cancer. Expert Rev Anticancer Ther. 2010;10(7):1037–42.
7. Zivanovic O, Leitao MM, Park JK, Zhao H, Diaz JP, Konner J, et al. Small cell neuroendocrine carcinoma of the cervix: analysis of outcome, recurrence pattern and the impact of platinum-based combination chemotherapy. Gynecol Oncol. 2009;112(3):590–3.
8. De Souza NM, Dina R, McIndoe GA, Soutter WP. Cervical cancer: value of an endovaginal coil magnetic resonance imaging technique in detecting small volume disease and assessing parametrial extension. Gynecol Oncol. 2006;102(1):80–5.
9. Sahdev A, Sohaib SA, Wenaden AE, Shepard JH, Reznek RH. The performance of magnetic resonance imaging in early cervical carcinoma: a long-term experience. Int J Gynecol Cancer. 2007;17(3):629–36.
10. Fischerova D, Cibula D, Stehnova H, Vondrickova H, Calda P, Zikan M, et al. Transrectal ultrasound and magnetic resonance imaging in staging of early cervical cancer. Int J Gynecol Cancer. 2008;18:766–72.
11. Rob L, Robova H, Chmel R, Komar M, Halaska M, Skapa P. Surgical options in early cervical cancer. Int J Hyperthermia. 2012;28(6):489–500.
12. Selman TJ, Mann C, Zamora J, Appleyard TL, Khan K. Diagnostic accuracy of test for lymph node status in primary cervical cancer: a systematic review and meta-analysis. CMAJ. 2008;178(7):855–62.
13. Wright JD, Dehdashti F, Herzog TJ, Much DG, Huettner PC, Rader JS, et al. Preoperative lymph node staging of early—stage cervical carcinoma by /18F/–fluoro-2-deoxy-D-glucose-positron emission tomography. Cancer. 2005;104(11):2484–91.
14. Signorelli M, Guerra L, Montanelli L, Crivellaro C, Buda A, Dell AT, et al. Preoperative staging of cervical cancer: is 18-FDG-PET/CT really effective with early stage disease? Gynecol Oncol. 2011;123:236–40.
15. Levenback CF, van der Zee AG, Rob L, Plante M, Covens A, Schneider A, et al. Sentinel lymph node biopsy in patients with gynaecologic cancers. Expert panel statement from the International Sentinel Node Society Meeting, February 21, 2008. Gynecol Oncol. 2009;114:151–6.
16. Plante M, Renaud MC, Tetu B, Harel F, Roy M. Laparoscopic sentinel node mapping in early- stage cervical cancer. Gynecol Oncol. 2003;91(3):494–503.
17. Rob L, Strnad P, Robova H, Charvat M, Pluta M, Schlegerova D, et al. Study of lymphatic mapping and sentinel node identification in early stage cervical cancer. Gynecol Oncol. 2005;98:281–8.
18. Marnitz S, Köhler C, Bongardt S, Braig U, Hertel H, Schneider A. Topographic distribution of sentinel lymph nodes in patients with cervical cancer. Gynecol Oncol. 2006;103:35–44.
19. Altgassen C, Hertel H, Brandstädt A, Kohler C, Durst M, Schneider A. Multicenter validation study of the sentinel lymph node concept in cervical cancer: AGO study group. J Clin Oncol. 2008;26:2943–51.
20. Lécuru F, Mathevet P, Querleu D, Leblanc E, Mirice P, Darai E. Bilateral negative sentinel nodes accurately predict absence of lymph node metastasis in early cervical cancer: results of the SENTICOL study. J Clin Oncol. 2011;29(13):1686–91.
21. Slama J, Dundr P, Dusek L, Fischerova D, Pinkavova I, Zikan M, et al. Sentinel lymph node status in patients with locally advanced cervical cancers and impact of neoadjuvant chemotherapy. Gynecol Oncol. 2012;125(2):303–6.
22. Cormier B, Diaz JP, Shih K, Samson RM, Sonoda Y, Park KJ, et al. Establishing a sentinel lymph node mapping algorithm for the treatment of early cervical cancer. Gynecol Oncol. 2011;122(2):275–80.
23. Roy M, Bouchard-Fortier G, Popa I, Grégorie J, Renaud MC, Tetu B, et al. Value of sentinel node mapping in cancer of the cervix. Gynecol Oncol. 2011;122(2):269–74.
24. Euscher ED, Malpica A, Atkinson EN, Lavenback CF, Frumovitz M, Deavers MT. Ultrastaging improves detection of metastases in sentinel lymph nodes of uterine cervix squamous cell carcinoma. Am J Surg Pathol. 2008;32(9):1336–43.
25. Bricou A, Barranger E, Uzan S, Darai E. Anaphylactic shock during the sentinel lymph node procedure for cervical cancer. Gynecol Oncol. 2009;114(2):375–6.
26. Vieira SC, Sousa RB, Tavares MB, Abreu BA, Ibia Pina JO, Sousa Oliveira AK. Changes in pulse oximetry after patent blue dye injection into the uterine cervix. Ann Surg Oncol. 2008;15(10):2862–6.
27. Pluta M, Rob L, Charvat M, Chmel R, Halaska M, Skapa P, et al. Less radical surgery than radical hysterectomy in early stage cervical cancer: a pilot study. Gynecol Oncol. 2009;113(2):181–4.
28. Darlin L, Persson J, Bossmar T, Lindahl B, Kannisto P, Masback A, et al. The sentinel node concept in early cervical cancer performs well in tumors smaller than 2 cm. Gynecol Oncol. 2010;117(2):266–9.
29. Kato H, Todo Y, Minobe S, Suzuki Y, Nakatani M, Ohba Y, et al. Previous conization on patient eligibility of sentinel lymph node detection for early invasive cervical cancer. Int J Gynecol Cancer. 2011;21(8):1491–4.
30. Gortzak-Uzan L, Jimenez W, Nofech-Mozes S, Ismiil N, Khalifa MA, Dubé V, et al. Sentinel lymph node biopsy vs. pelvic lymphadenectomy in early stage cervical cancer: is it time to change the gold standard? Gynecol Oncol. 2010;116(1):28–32.

31. Bats AS, Lavoué V, Rouzier R, Coutant C, Kerrou K, Darai E. Limits of day-before lymphoscintigraphy to localize sentinel nodes in women with cervical cancer. Ann Surg Oncol. 2008;15(8):2173–9.
32. Bats AS, Lavoué V, Barranger E, Daraï E. Is preoperative lymphoscintigraphy for sentinel node in cervical cancer required? Am J Obstet Gynecol. 2007;197(1):116.
33. Vieira SC, Sousa RB, Tavares MB, Silva JB, Abreu BA, Santos LG, et al. Preoperative pelvic lymphoscintigraphy is of limited usefulness for sentinel lymph node detection in cervical cancer. Eur J Obstet Gynecol Reprod Biol. 2009;145(1):96–9.
34. Gien LT, Covens A. Quality control in sentinel lymph node biopsy in cervical cancer. J Clin Oncol. 2008;26(18):2930–1.
35. Devaja O, Mehra G, Coutts M, Montalto SA, Donaldson J, Kodampur M, et al. A prospective single-center study of sentinel lymph node detection in cervical carcinoma: is there a place in clinical practice? Int J Gynecol Cancer. 2012;22(6):1044–9.
36. Cibula D, Abu-Rustum NR, Dusek L, Zikan M, Zaal A, Sevcik L, et al. Prognostic significance of low volume sentinel lymph node disease in early-stage cervical cancer. Gynecol Oncol. 2012;124(3):496–501.
37. Bats AS, Buénerd A, Querleu D, Leblanc E, Darai E, Morice P, et al. SENTICOL collaborative group. Diagnostic value of intraoperative examination of sentinel lymph node in early cervical cancer: a prospective, multicenter study. Gynecol Oncol. 2011; 123(2):230–5.
38. Fader AN, Edwards RP, Cost M, Kanbour-Shakir A, Kelley JL, Schwartz B, et al. Sentinel lymph node biopsy in early-stage cervical cancer: utility of intraoperative versus postoperative assessment. Gynecol Oncol. 2008;111(1):13–7.
39. Okamoto S, Niikura H, Yoshinaga K, Satoshi MT, Hitoshi MD, Kosuke MD, et al. Detection of micrometastases in cervical cancer with a system that evaluates both sentinel and nonsentinel lymph nodes. Int J Gynecol Cancer. 2009;19(4):708–11.
40. Wydra D, Sawicki S, Wojtylak S, Bandurski T, Emerich J. Sentinel node identification in cervical cancer patients undergoing transperitoneal radical hysterectomy: a study of 100 cases. Int J Gynecol Cancer. 2006;16:649–54.
41. Horn LC, Hentschel B, Fischer U, Peter D, Bilek K. Detection of micrometastases in pelvic lymph nodes in patients with carcinoma of the cervix uteri using step sectioning: frequency, topographic distribution and prognostic impact. Gynecol Oncol. 2008;111(2): 276–81.
42. Popa I, Plante M, Renaud MC, Roy M, Tetu B. Negative sentinel lymph node accurately predicts negative status of pelvic lymph nodes in uterine cervix carcinoma. Gynecol Oncol. 2006;103(2):649–53.
43. Rob L, Pluta M, Skapa P, Robova H. Advances in fertility-sparing surgery for cervical cancer. Expert Rev Anticancer Ther. 2010;10(7):1101–14.
44. Rob L, Charvat M, Robova H, Pluta M, Strnad P, Hrehorcak M, et al. Less radical fertility-sparing surgery than radical trachelectomy in early cervical cancer. Int J Gynecol Cancer. 2007;17(1):304–10.
45. Rob L, Pluta M, Strnad P, Hrehorcak M, Chmel R, Skapa P, et al. A less radical treatment option to the fertility-sparing radical trachelectomy in patients with stage I cervical cancer. Gynecol Oncol. 2008;111:S116–20.
46. Daraï E, Lavoué V, Rouzier R, Coutant C, Barranger E, Bats AS. Contribution of the sentinel node procedure to tailoring the radicality of hysterectomy for cervical cancer. Gynecol Oncol. 2007;106(1):251–6.
47. Frumovitz M, Ramirez PT, Levenback CF. Lymphatic mapping and sentinel lymph node detection in women with cervical cancer. Gynecol Oncol. 2008;110 (3 Suppl 2):S17–20.

Neoadjuvant Chemotherapy in the Management of Cervical Carcinoma

35

Gemma K.D. Eminowicz and Mary McCormack

35.1 Introduction

Cervical carcinoma is the third most common cancer in women worldwide and remains a significant health burden [1]. In 2008, 530,000 women across the world were diagnosed with cervical cancer, with more than 80 % of these cases being diagnosed in the developing world. The worldwide incidence varies from 15.3 per 100,000 population to 10.1 per 100,000 in the United Kingdom (UK) [2]. The fall in incidence in the UK and other western countries is largely due to the introduction of national screening programs. The screening program introduced in the UK in 1988, by detecting and treating pre-invasive disease, has led to a fall in the number of invasive cancers diagnosed from 4,082 in 1988 to 2,851 in 2010 [2].

The majority of these cases are locally advanced FIGO stage IB2-IVA [3].

For more than a decade the standard of care for women with locally advanced disease has been chemo-radiotherapy (CRT). This followed the publication in 1999 of a number of large randomized trials demonstrating a significant survival advantage with the addition of concurrent platinum based chemotherapy to radiotherapy [4, 5]. These trials led to the National Cancer Institute (NCI) issuing an alert recommending the use of concurrent cisplatin-based chemotherapy with radiotherapy in women undergoing treatment with curative intent [6]. This practice was widely adopted in the UK [7].

More recently, an individual patient data meta-analysis based on 18 trials from 11 countries confirmed the benefit of chemo-radiotherapy with a 6 % improvement in 5-year overall survival (OS) from 60 to 66 %, HR 0.81, and an 8 % improvement in disease-free survival (DFS) from 50 to 58 % [8]. Whilst the benefits were seen across all stages regardless of age, histology and grade they appeared to be lower in patients with more advanced disease. We will return to this later in the chapter.

35.2 Neoadjuvant Chemotherapy

Over the years, various investigators have focused on the additional role of chemotherapy given before (neoadjuvant, NACT) radical radiotherapy or surgery. Most of these trials were conducted in the pre CRT era. This chapter will address this approach to treatment.

The administration of chemotherapy before definitive therapy (either surgery or radiotherapy) may help to reduce the tumor burden which may in turn render inoperable tumors operable or improve the tumor oxygenation [9]. Furthermore, the use of systemic treatment may also eliminate micrometastatic disease and therefore potentially

G.K.D. Eminowicz, MBChB, MRCP, MSc, FRCR •
M. McCormack, BSc, MSc, PhD, MBBS, FRCR (✉)
Department of Oncology, University College London Hospital, London, UK
e-mail: Mary.mccormack@uclh.nhs.uk

H.R.H. Patel et al. (eds.), *Pelvic Cancer Surgery: Modern Breakthroughs and Future Advances*,
DOI 10.1007/978-1-4471-4258-4_35, © Springer-Verlag London 2015

improve survival. More recently, this approach has been used in an attempt to preserve fertility [10]. There is evidence suggesting response to NACT can predict longer term outcomes and may therefore be a useful biological marker [11]. Despite these possible benefits of NACT there are concerns that NACT causes unnecessary delays in the definitive radical treatment, therefore potentially jeopardizing efficacy of radical treatment. It has also been postulated that pre-treatment with chemotherapy may lead to accelerated tumor repopulation thereby compromising the effectiveness of a course of radiotherapy [12].

35.3 Neoadjuvant Chemotherapy Before Surgery

This approach has been the subject of several trials spanning more than two decades. A meta-analysis of randomized trials conducted between 1975 and 1998 was undertaken and the findings published in 2003 [13]. This identified seven trials that compared NACT plus surgery (+/− radiotherapy) versus radiotherapy alone. On further review five trials fulfilled the pre-specified criteria for inclusion. The number of patients randomized varied from 50 to 441 and included patients with bulky FIGO IB to IIIB disease. Platinum based combination chemotherapy was used in various doses and schedules and for a minimum of three and a maximum of seven cycles. However, the cycle durations were in general less than 10 days (i.e. dose- dense). The radiation doses in the control arms were similar across the trials. In some trials up to 90 % of patients received adjuvant radiotherapy in the surgery arms. Nevertheless, despite the relatively small number of patients and the heterogeneity between the trials, the findings suggested a highly significant effect of NACT. The HR of 0.65 indicates a 14 % absolute overall improvement in 5-year survival (see Fig. 35.1).

In 2007 the Gynecologic Oncology Group (GOG) published the results of GOG-141. This trial randomized 288 patients (over 5 years) with stage IB2 cervical cancer to NACT using three cycles of cisplatin and vincristine given every 10 days followed by surgery or surgery alone. This trial was closed early due to poor accrual and frequent off protocol use of post operative radiotherapy (45 % of NACT patients and 52 % of surgery alone). Response rates as defined by 'clinical objective response' to NACT were 52 % but no significant differences were seen in pathological findings, progression free survival (PFS) or overall survival [14].

Mossa et al. demonstrated similar results having randomized 288 patients with FIGO stage IB to III cervical cancer to NACT with three cycles of cisplatin, vincristine and bleomycin versus conventional treatment (surgery or radiotherapy alone). For the vast majority of these patients (258) the conventional treatment was surgery and the remaining 30 were stage III patients who received radiotherapy (6 in NACT group, 24 in conventional group). At 7 year follow up no statistically significant benefit in disease free or overall survival was seen but the trend was favoring NACT, OS 70.4 % NACT versus 65.9 %, DFS 65.4 % versus 53.5 % [15].

More recently two randomized trials, SNAP-01 and SNAP-02, showed that paclitaxel containing regimens are associated with improved response rates. Paclitaxel/ifosfamide/cisplatin (TIP) or paclitaxel/epirubicin/cisplatin (TEP) yielded optimal response rates (no residual or <3 mm stromal invasion) of 42–48 % but at the expense of significant hematological toxicity [9].

A number of phase two studies have investigated the platinum/paclitaxel doublet given in a dose dense schedule (cycles <10 days) to patients with FIGO stage IB-IIB disease prior to surgery [16, 17]. Although these are small trials response rates of up to 90 % were observed with a short course of dose dense chemotherapy without the significant toxicity observed in the Italian studies above.

Three cycles of neoadjuvant carboplatin and paclitaxel given every 21 days was used by Duenas-Gonzalez et al. with even more impressive response rates of 95 % in 43 patients with FIGO IB2-IIIB cervical cancer, but this was assessed by clinical response rather than MRI [18].

In 2010 a Cochrane review comparing NACT and surgery versus surgery alone in FIGO stage

Trial	Neoad CT (no. events/no. entered)	No Neoad CT	O-E	Variance
Sardi, 1996	25/53	41/54	−13.81	15.65
Sardi, 1998	22/80	33/74	−9.33	13.34
Kigawa, 1996	10/25	15/25	−3.00	6.21
Benedetti, 2002	88/227	101/214	−15.65	46.60
Chang, 2000	21/68	12/52	2.61	8.12
Total	166/453	202/419	−39.17	89.92

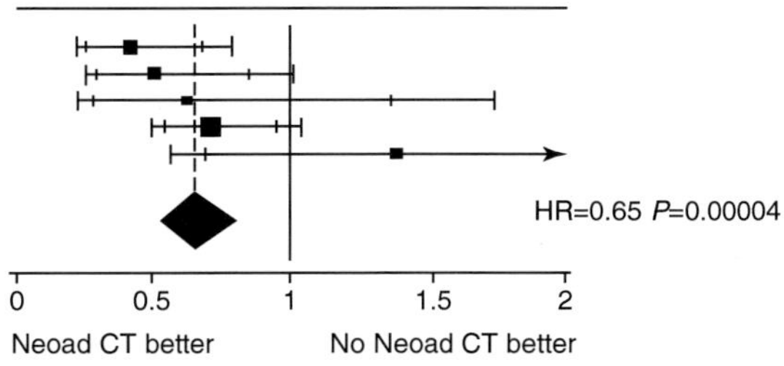

Fig. 35.1 Overall survival comparison for NACT in surgical setting from NACCMA Collaboration meta-analysis (From Tierney et al. [13]; used with permission from Elsevier)

IB to III was published. Six randomized controlled trials involving over 1,000 women were identified and whilst data for PFS was available for all trials, overall survival, resection rates and pathological response data was not available for one trial. Recurrence data was only available for three trials. Therefore the final analysis was limited to five trials with 604 women. This review concluded that NACT before surgery was associated with an improvement in PFS (HR 0.76 p=0.01) whilst there was a trend towards an improvement in overall survival this did not reach statistical significance (HR 0.85, p=0.17). Once again, these trials were very heterogeneous and results were confounded by the frequent use of radiotherapy in addition to the chemotherapy and surgery [19].

A further meta-analysis of five randomized controlled trials and four observational studies involving 1,784 patients with FIGO IB1 to IIA was published in 2013 [20]. The authors concluded that NACT, whilst decreasing tumor bulk and lymph node metastases, did not improve survival. They did note that postoperative radiotherapy was less frequently indicated. However, these findings need to be interpreted with caution due to the limitations of the review and the inclusion of observational studies.

The ongoing European Organization for Research and Treatment of Cancer (EORTC 55994) randomized phase three trial may help to define the role, if any, of NACT in early stage disease. This compares the use of NACT followed by surgery with concurrent chemo-radiotherapy for FIGO stage IB2-IIB cervical squamous cell carcinoma, adenosquamous or adenocarcinoma. The NACT regimen typically consists of three cycles of 21 day cisplatin based combination chemotherapy. Overall survival is the primary endpoint with PFS, toxicity, and Quality of Life as secondary endpoints. However the trial has been open to recruitment since 2002 and accrual has been slow (Table 35.1).

35.4 Neoadjuvant Chemotherapy Before Radiotherapy/Chemo-Radiotherapy

A meta-analysis of individual patient data from 21 randomized trials comparing NACT before radiotherapy versus radiotherapy alone was published in 2003 [13]. The final analysis included data from 18 trials with a total of 2,074 patients. Overall the analysis concluded that NACT had no significant impact on overall survival. However, heterogeneity in chemotherapy cycle length and platinum dose intensity were identified as important factors in determining outcome. Trials using a short cycle length (<14 days) gave a pooled HR of 0.83, equivalent to a 7 % improvement (45–52 %) in 5 year survival (see Fig. 35.2). In contrast, those trials that used longer cycle lengths (>14 days) gave a pooled HR of 1.25 equivalent to an absolute detriment in survival of 8 % (45–37 %) at 5 years. Platinum dose intensities >25 mg/m^2 were also associated with better outcomes. Furthermore, there was significant

Table 35.1 Summary of trials investigating NACT in the surgical setting

Author	Year	No of pts	NACT regimen	Outcome
Sardi et al.	1997	210	3× cisplatin 50 mg/m², vincristine 1 mg/m², bleomycin 25 mg/m² (day 1–3) q10	At 67 months DFS 80 % vs 61 %
Eddy et al.	2007	288	3× cisplatin 50 mg/m², vincristine 1 mg/m², q10	Clinical objective RR 52 % No sig diff in path, PFS, OS
Mossa et al.	2010	288	3× cisplatin 50 mg/m², vincristine 1 mg/m² bleomycin 25 mg/m²	At 7 years OS 70.4 % vs 65.9 % (not sig) DFS 65.4 % vs 53.5 %(not sig)
Park et al.	2004	43	3× cisplatin 60 mg/m², paclitaxel 60 mg/m² q10	Clin response 90.7 % (MRI&exam) Path downstaging 72.1 %
Mori et al.	2008	30	6× carboplatin AUC2, paclitaxel 60 mg/m² q7	Objective RR 87 % (MRI&exam)
Duenas Gonzalez et al.	2003	43	3× carboplatin AUC6, paclitaxel 175 mg/m² q21	Clinical RR 95 % (MRI)

Trial	Neoad CT (no. events/no. entered)	No Neoad CT (no. events/no. entered)	O-E	Variance
>14 day cycles				
Chauvergne, 1993	57/92	54/90	−0.47	27.66
Souhami, 1991	29/48	31/55	7.64	13.64
Tattersall, 1992	20/34	18/37	2.17	9.41
Herod, 2001	68/89	62/88	2.60	32.39
Cardenas, 1991	7/13	9/18	0.37	3.84
Cardenas, 1993	12/14	8/16	2.16	4.91
Chiara, 1994	22/32	16/32	4.68	9.33
Sundfor, 1996	31/48	35/48	−3.41	16.40
CCSG AOCOA	38/129	28/131	8.08	16.31
Kumar, 1998	49/88	34/85	7.43	20.73
LGOG	9/15	2/12	3.61	2.73
Sub-total	342/602	297/612	34.85	157.36
≤14 day cycles				
Sardi, 1997	19/104	32/106	−7.97	12.69
Sardi, 1998	30/73	33/74	−4.61	15.56
Sardi, 1996	34/54	41/54	−10.61	17.89
PMB	9/16	15/19	−2.68	5.94
Symonds, 2000	68/105	76/110	−5.86	35.84
Leborgne, 1997	32/48	28/49	2.98	14.94
MRC CeCa	19/24	9/24	7.86	6.64
Sub-total	211/424	234/436	−20.89	109.48
Total	553/1026	531/1048	13.96	266.85

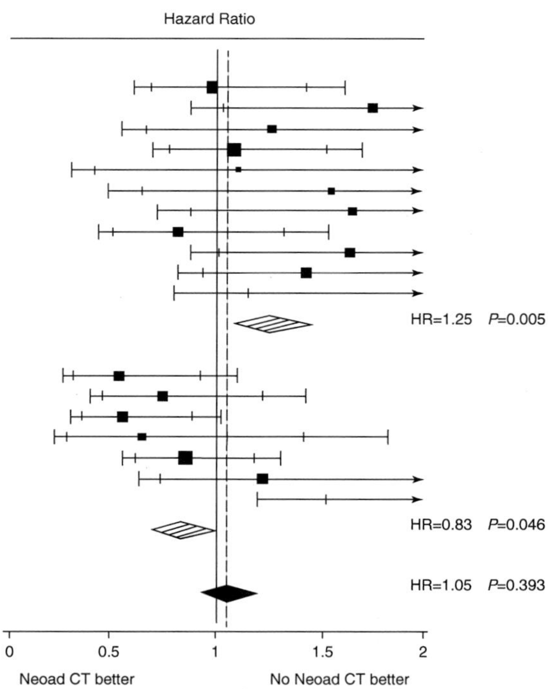

Fig. 35.2 Forrest plot demonstrating overall survival by planned chemotherapy cycle length from NACCMA Collaboration meta-analysis (From Tierney et al. [13]; used with permission from Elsevier)

variation in radiation dose (both external beam and brachytherapy with the total doses delivered in the range 55–80 Gy) and the interval between completing chemotherapy and commencing radiotherapy. It is possible that the detrimental effect of longer chemotherapy cycle length is due to accelerated tumor regrowth in a tumor that is known to have a high growth fraction and proliferation rate. It is also important to note that this meta-analysis excluded trials using concurrent chemo-radiotherapy which is now the standard of care (Table 35.2).

Table 35.2 Summary of trials investigating NACT in the radiotherapy setting

Author	Year	No of pts	NACT regimen	RT details	Outcome
Souhami et al.	1991	103	BOMP	50 Gy/25#	5 years OS
			3× Bleomycin 120U, vincristine 1 mg/m^2, mitomycin 10 mg/m^2, cisplatin 50 mg/m^2 q21	40 Gy intracavity	23 % (NACT) vs 39 % (RT) $p=0.02$
Sardi et al.	1996	155	Modified VBP:	50–60 Gy/28–30#	OS at 4 years
			3× vincristine 1 mg/m^2, cisplatin 50 mg/m^2, bleomycin 25 mg/m^2 q10	25–35 Gy intracavity	RT 37 %
					NACT&RT 53 %
					NACT&surg 63 %
McCormack et al.	2013	46	6× carboplatin AUC2, paclitaxel 80 mg/m^2 q7	50.4 Gy/28# +cisplatin 40 mg/m^2	Observed RR 70 %
				15 Gy/2# HDR intracavity	3 years PFS 68 %
					3 years OS 67 %

In 2009, the initial findings from a phase two trial, CXII, using dose dense weekly carboplatin (AUC2) and paclitaxel (80 mg/m^2) for 6 weeks followed immediately by conventional chemo-radiotherapy were presented [21]. The final results have recently been published [22]. This study recruited 46 patients with locally advanced cervical cancer and included patients with positive lymph nodes. The majority (72 %) of the patients had squamous cell cancers. Response to this NACT regimen was assessed by MRI using the RECIST criteria at the end of the sixth and final week of chemotherapy. Overall response was assessed, again with MRI, 12 weeks after completion of all chemo-radiation treatment. Seventy percent of patients achieved a complete or partial response at the end of NACT and 85 % at the end of chemo-radiotherapy. Nine patients (20 %) experienced grade 3 or 4 toxicity with this NACT regimen, the majority of which was hematological and easily managed. Overall survival rates at 3 and 5 years were 67 % with no deaths or progression between 3 and 5 years (see Fig. 35.3). Three out of the five patients with positive para-aortic lymph nodes were alive with no evidence of disease. This highlighted, despite the small numbers, a possible patient group who may derive significant benefit from this treatment approach. This trial confirmed that this dose dense approach was feasible without compromising the CRT with 96 % of the patients completing the course within 50 days. These findings have been used to design an international randomized multicenter phase III trial (clinicaltrials.gov NCT01566240 INTERLACE) to determine whether this treatment strategy leads to a significant improvement in survival.

Conclusion

The role of NACT in the treatment of cervical cancer remains to be defined. It is hoped that the current trials will determine the benefits or otherwise of this treatment approach.

Key Points

- Locally advanced cervical carcinoma is the third most common cancer in women in the world.
- The incidence of cervical cancer has decreased in the United Kingdom, with the screening program estimated to save up to 5,000 lives per year.
- Concurrent chemo-radiotherapy is standard of care for management of locally advanced cervical carcinoma.
- Platinum is a key component of chemotherapy regimes in the treatment of cervical carcinoma.
- Chemotherapy before radical surgery (neoadjuvant) may downstage tumors to increase operability.

(continued)

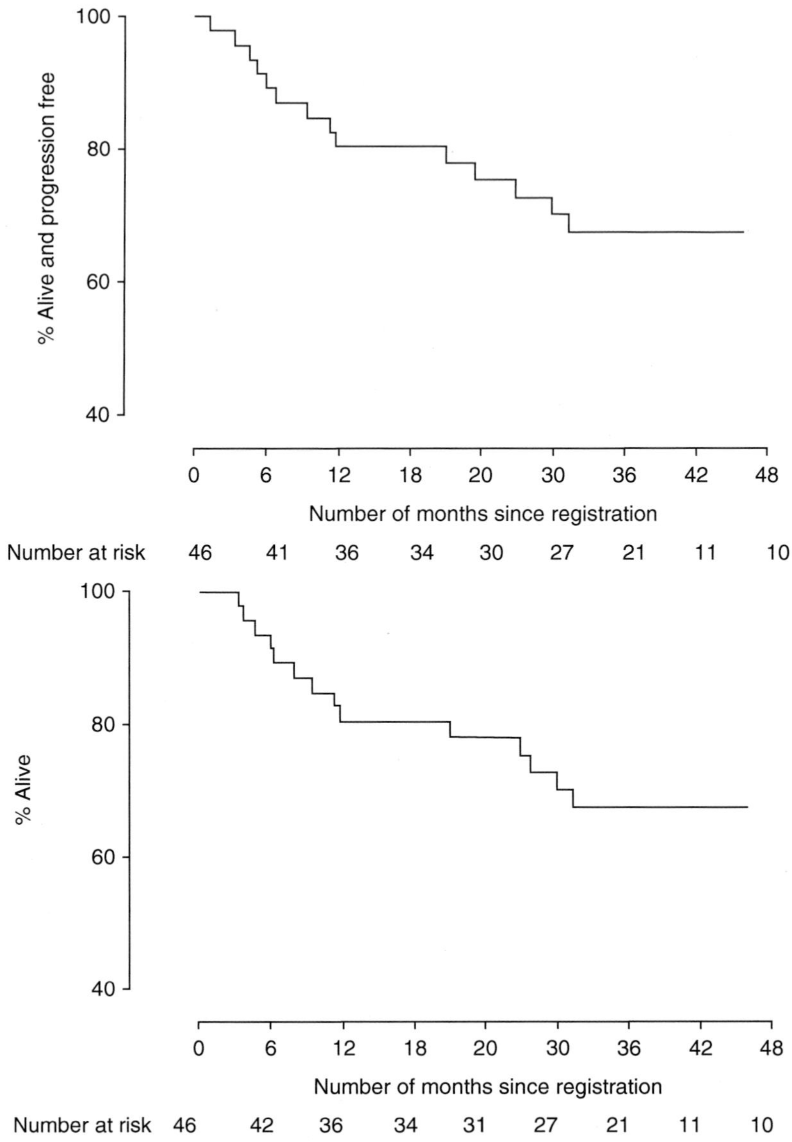

Fig. 35.3 Kaplan-Meier plots for Progression Free Survival (*PFS* upper) and overall survival (*OS* lower) for the 46 patients in the CXII trial (Reprinted by permission from Macmillan Publishers Ltd: McCormack et al. [22])

- Chemotherapy before radical (chemo-) radiotherapy (induction) may have radiobiological advantages of decreased tumor bulk leading to decreased hypoxic fraction and therefore increased radiosenstitivity.
- NACT before radiotherapy shows survival advantages if short cycle platinum dose intense regimens are used.

- INTERLACE is an international randomized multicenter phase III trial comparing 6 weeks of induction carboplatin and paclitaxel chemotherapy followed by standard chemo-radiotherapy with chemo-radiotherapy alone in women with FIGO stage IB2 to IVA.
- EORTC 55994 is a randomized phase III trial comparing NACT (typically

(continued)

3 cycles of platinum based chemotherapy on a 21 day schedule) followed by surgery with standard chemo-radiotherapy in FIGO stage IB2-IIB cervical cancer.

- The role or otherwise of NACT in the treatment of cervical cancer will only be determined through large well conducted randomized clinical trials and patients should be encouraged to participate.

References

1. GLOBOCAN. Cancer fact sheet: cervical cancer incidence, mortality and prevalence worldwide in 2008. 2008 [cited 2013 April 20]; Available from: http://globocan.iarc.fr/factsheet.asp.
2. ONS. Office for National Statistics: Cancer Registrations. 2013 [cited 2013 April 20]; Available from: http://www.ons.gov.uk/ons/search/index.html?newquery=cancer+registrations.
3. Pecorelli S, Zigliani L, Odicino F. Revised FIGO staging for carcinoma of the cervix. Int J Gynecol Obstet. 2009;105:107–8.
4. Rose PG, Bundy BN, Watkins EB, Thigpen JT, Deppe G, Maiman MA, Clarke-Pearson DL, Insalaco S. Concurrent cisplatin-based radiotherapy and chemotherapy for locally advanced cervical cancer. N Engl J Med. 1999;340(15):1144–53.
5. Keys HM, Bundy BN, Stehman FB, Muderspach LI, Chafe WE, Suggs CL, Walker JL, Gersell D. Cisplatin, radiation and adjuvant hysterectomy compared with radiation and adjuvant hysterectomy for bulky stage IB cervical carcinoma. N Engl J Med. 1999;340(15):1154–61.
6. NCI. NCI issues clinical announcement on cervical cancer: chemotherapy plus radiation improves survival. NIH News Advisory 1999 [updated cited 22 Feb 1999]; Available from: http://www.nih.gov/news/pr/feb99/nci-22.htm.
7. McCormack M, Brown RSD, Birtle AJ. A national audit of chemo-radiation practice for cervical carcinoma in the United Kingdom. Royal College of Radiologists Annual Scientific Meeting 2001. Clin Oncol. 2001;13:318–9.
8. CCCMAC. Reducing uncertainties about the effects of chemoradiotherapy for cervical cancer: a systematic review and meta-analysis of individual patient data from 18 randomised trials. Chemoradiotherapy for Cervical Cancer Meta-Analysis Collaboration. J Clin Oncol. 2008;26:5802–12.
9. Lissoni AA, Colombo N, Pellegrino A, Parma G, Zola P, Katsaros D, Chiari S, Buda A, Landoni F, Peiretti M, Dell'anna T, Fruscio R, Signorelli M, Grassi R, Floriani I, Fossati R, Torri V, Rulli E. A phase II, randomized trial of neo-adjuvant chemotherapy comparing a three-drug combination of paclitaxel, ifosfamide, and cisplatin (TIP) versus paclitaxel and cisplatin (TP) followed by radical surgery in patients with locally advanced squamous cell cervical carcinoma: the Snap-02 Italian Collaborative Study. Ann Oncol. 2009;20(4):660–5.
10. Eiriksson L, Covens A. Advancing fertility-sparing treatments in cervical cancer: where is the limit? Gynecol Oncol. 2012;126(3):317–8.
11. Li R, Lu S, Si J, Liu B, Wang H, Mei Y, Linghu H. Prognostic value of responsiveness of neoadjuvant chemotherapy before surgery for patients with stage IB2/IIA2 cervical cancer. Gynecol Oncol. 2013;128(3):524–9.
12. Gonzalez-Martin A, Gonzalez-Cortijo L, Carballo N, Garcia JF, Lapuente F, Rojo A, Chiva LM. The current role of neoadjuvant chemotherapy in the management of cervical carcinoma. Gynecol Oncol [Meta-Analysis Review]. 2008;110(3 Suppl 2):S36–40.
13. Tierney JF, Stewart LA, Parmar MKB. Neoadjuvant chemotherapy for locally advanced cervical cancer meta-analysis collaboration. Neoadjuvant chemotherapy for locally advanced cervical cancer: a systematic review and meta-analysis of individual patient data from 21 randomised trials. Eur J Cancer. 2003;39(17):2470–86.
14. Eddy GL, Bundy BN, Creasman WT, Spirtos NM, Mannel RS, Hannigan E, O'Connor D. Treatment of ("bulky") stage IB cervical cancer with or without neoadjuvant vincristine and cisplatin prior to radical hysterectomy and pelvic/para-aortic lymphadenectomy: a phase III trial of the gynecologic oncology group. Gynecol Oncol. 2007;106(2):362–9.
15. Mossa B, Mossa S, Corosu L, Marziani R. Follow-up in a long term randomized trial with neoadjuvant chemotherapy for squamous cell cervical carcinoma. Eur J Gynaecol Oncol. 2010;31(5):497–503.
16. Park D. Phase II, trial of neoadjuvant paclitaxel and cisplatin in uterine cervical cancer. Gynecol Oncol. 2004;92(1):59–63.
17. Mori T, Hosokawa K, Kinoshita Y, Watanabe A, Honjo H. Neoadjuvant chemotherapy with weekly carboplatin and paclitaxel for locally advanced cervical carcinoma. Int J Gynecol Cancer. 2008;18:85–9.
18. Dueñas-Gonzalez A, López-Graniel C, González-Enciso A, Cetina L, Rivera L, Mariscal I, Montalvo G, Gómez E, de la Garza J, Chanona G, Mohar A. A phase II study of multimodality treatment for locally advanced cervical cancer: neoadjuvant carboplatin and paclitaxel followed by radical hysterectomy and adjuvant cisplatin chemoradiation. Ann Oncol. 2003;14(8):1278–84.
19. Rydzewska L, Tierney J, Vale CL, Symonds PR. Neoadjuvant chemotherapy plus surgery versus surgery for cervical cancer. Cochrane Database Syst Rev. 2010 Jan 20;(1):CD007406. doi:10.1002/14651858.CD007406.pub2.

20. Kim HS, Sardi JE, Katsumata N, Ryu HS, Nam JH, Chung HH, Park NH, Song YS, Behtash N, Kamura T, Cai HB, Kim JW. Efficacy of neoadjuvant chemotherapy in patients with FIGO stage IB1 to IIA cervical cancer: an international collaborative meta-analysis. Eur J Surg Oncol. 2013;39(2):115–24.
21. McCormack M, Ledermann JA, Hall-Craggs MA, Symonds RP, Warwick V, Simonds H, Fernando I, Hackshaw A. A phase II study of weekly neoadjuvant chemotherapy followed by radical chemoradiation for locally advanced cervical cancer. J Clin Oncol. 2009;27(15s):5586.
22. McCormack M, Kadalayil L, Hackshaw A, Hall-Craggs MA, Symonds RP, Warwick V, Simonds H, Fernando I, Hammond M, James L, Feeney A, Ledermann J. A phase II study of weekly neoadjuvant chemotherapy followed by radical chemoradiation for locally advanced cervical cancer. Br J Cancer. 2013;108:2464–9.

Chemoradiation for Cervical Cancer

36

Haider Mahdi and Peter G. Rose

36.1 Introduction

Although radiation therapy is the primary effective modality for treatment of locally advanced cervical cancer, the cure rate is still low with potential room for improvement. A positive correlation between tumor size and dose of radiation therapy essential for tumor control was demonstrated by Fletcher et al. in 1970s [1]. As a result, approximately two-thirds of patients with locally advanced cervical cancer treated with radiation therapy alone fail locally in the pelvis within the field of radiation therapy. In large cervical tumors, the required radiation dose cannot be delivered because it exceeds the maximum tolerated dose by adjacent normal tissues. Further, pelvic control rates decline with increasing tumor size and FIGO stage. Therefore, many efforts have been directed to investigate the role of other treatment modalities to augment the effect of radiation therapy like hyperthermia, heavy particle radiation and chemotherapy. As tumor cells progress through different phases of cell cycles, their sensitivity to radiation therapy vary significantly. Cells are most radiosensitive in late G2 or M phases and least radiosensitive in G1 and S phases [2]. Chemotherapy given with radiation therapy may complement the effect of radiation therapy by inducing cell synchrony, inhibiting repair of radiation induced damage and direct cytotoxicity. In cervical cancer, the addition of chemotherapy to radiation therapy has been introduced in two schedules. The first is where chemotherapy is given before radiation therapy (neoadjuvant chemotherapy) and the second is where chemotherapy and radiation therapy are given concurrently.

36.2 Neoadjuvant Chemotherapy Followed by Radiation Therapy

The concept of utilizing chemotherapy to reduce tumor size before radiation therapy is attractive. However, the results of randomized clinical trials comparing neo-adjuvant chemotherapy followed by radiation therapy and radiation therapy alone in locally advanced cervical cancer has been disappointing with no survival difference [3–12]. In fact, two randomized clinical trials showed a worse survival when chemotherapy is given prior to radiation therapy [6, 8]. Further, a meta-analysis of 18 clinical trials involving 2,074 patients did not show an improvement in outcome with neoadjuvant chemotherapy followed by radiation therapy compared to radiation alone. However, this metaanalysis is limited by the heterogeneity between the trials in term of chemotherapy regimens, schedules and number of chemotherapy cycles [13]. The exact explanation

H. Mahdi, MD • P.G. Rose, MD (✉)
Women's Health Institute/Gynaecologic Oncology Division, Cleveland Clinic Health System, Cleveland, OH, USA
e-mail: rosep@ccf.org

H.R.H. Patel et al. (eds.), *Pelvic Cancer Surgery: Modern Breakthroughs and Future Advances*, DOI 10.1007/978-1-4471-4258-4_36, © Springer-Verlag London 2015

for the lack of survival benefit with neoadjuvant chemotherapy preceding radiation therapy is not clear. However, many theories have been postulated including: altering tumor biology by induction of accelerated repopulation of tumor cells that are resistant to radiation therapy, prolonging radiation therapy schedule, and cross-resistance between chemotherapy and radiation therapy [14, 15].

36.3 Cisplatin-Based Concurrent Chemo-Radiation Therapy

The promising result of the five randomized clinical trials [16–20] investigating the role of concurrent chemoradiation therapy stands in stark contrast to the disappointing results of neoadjuvant chemotherapy trials. Due to the compelling evidence of these five clinical trials, the National Cancer Institute issued clinical bulletin recommending concurrent cisplatin-based chemotherapy for patients requiring radiation therapy. These five randomized trials of cisplatin based chemoradiation therapy used slightly different regimens and are conducted in patients with different clinical scenario: from early stage disease with high risk factors (positive pelvic lymph nodes, positive margins or parametrial extension) following radical hysterectomy and pelvic lymphadenectomy (GOG109), bulky stage IB2 (GOG 123) before performing adjuvant simple hysterectomy to locally advanced disease where chemoradiation therapy was the primary treatment (GOG85, RTOG9001 and GOG120). In each of these trials, platinum-based chemoradiation therapy has led to an increase in relative progression free survival and relative survival of 30–50 % (Fig. 36.1). Currently, the most widely acceptable regimen is using six cycles of weekly cisplatin (40 mg/m^2) given during external pelvic radiation therapy and brachytherapy.

Early Stage Non-bulky Disease

Patients with an early stage non-bulky cervical cancer (IA2, IB1 and IIA) are often treated with radical hysterectomy and pelvic lymphadenectomy. However, some patients remain at high risk of recurrence and have worse survival outcomes. Patients with positive pelvic nodes, positive margins or parametrial involvement have the highest risk. The Southwestern Oncology group enrolled 243 patients with early stage disease (IA2, IB1 or IIA) who underwent radical hysterectomy with pelvic lymphadenectomy and were found to have one of the following high risk factors: positive pelvic lymph nodes (~85 %), parametrial extension (~34 %) and positive margins (~5 %). Patients were randomized to either external pelvic radiation therapy (49.3 Gy) alone or combined with concurrent chemotherapy with four cycles of cisplatin 70 mg/m^2 and 5-fluouracil 1 g/m^2/day as 96-h infusion on week 1, 4, 7 and 11 (Table 36.1). Patients with positive

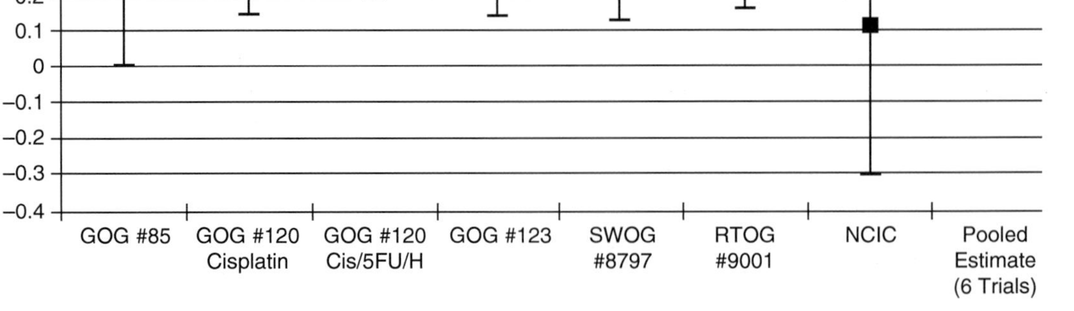

Fig. 36.1 Reduction in the risk (1 – relative risk) of death from six chemoradiation clinical trials in cervix cancer. (■) Risk reduction, (—) 95 % confidence interval, *Cis* cisplatin, *5FU* fluorouracil, *SWOG* Southwest Oncology Group, *H* hydroxyurea

Table 36.1 Clinical trials investigating the role of chemoradiation therapy in cervical cancer including ongoing clinical trials

Clinical trial name	Chemotherapeutic agents	Regimen	Median duration of radiation therapy	Radiation dose
SWOG-8797/ GOG-109	Cisplatin 70 mg/m^2 5-FU 1 g/m^2/day as 96-h infusion	Week 1, 4, 7, 11	41–43 days	Pelvic RT: 49.3 Gy 45 GY to para-aortic field when positive high common iliac nodes No brachytherapy
GOG-123	Cisplatin 40 mg/m^2	Weekly × 6	50 days	EBRT: 45 Gy Brachytherapy: 30 Gy
GOG-85	Arm1: cisplatin 50 mg/m^2+5-FU 1 g/m^2/day as a 96-h infusion Arm2: hydroxyurea 80 mg/kg	Day 1 and 29 Twice weekly	9.1 weeks	EBRT: 40.8 Gy for stage IIB and 51 Gy for stage III–IV Brachytherapy: 40 Gy for stage IIB and 30 Gy for stage III–IV
RTOG 90-01	Cisplatin 70 mg/m^2 and 5-FU 1 g/m^2/day as a 96-h infusion	3 cycles (day 1, 29 and during brachytherapy)	58 days	EBRT: 45 Gy with extended field in the radiation only arm Low dose brachytherapy allowed Total dose point A: 85 Gy
GOG-120	Arm 1: weekly cisplatin 40 mg/m^2 Arm 2: cisplatin (50 mg/m^2) with 5-FU (1 g/m^2/day as a 96-h infusion) on day 1 and 29 with twice weekly oral hydroxyurea 2 g/m^2 Arm 3: oral hydroxyurea 3 g/m^2 twice weekly		8.9–9.3 weeks	EBRT: 40.8 Gy for stage IIB and 51 Gy for stage III–IV Brachytherapy: 40 Gy for stage IIB and 30 Gy for stage III–IV Total dose point A: 80.8 Gy for stage IIB and 81.0 Gy for stage III–IV
NCIC-Pearcey et al.	Cisplatin 40 mg/m^2	Weekly for 5 weeks		EBRT 45 Gy Brachytherapy: LDR 35 gy or MDR 27 Gy or HDR 24 Gy
RTOG/GOG 0724	Arm1: cisplatin 40 mg/m^2 Arm2: cisplatin 40 mg/m^2 Carboplatin AUC 5 and paclitaxel 135 mg/m^2 after completing chemoradiation therapy	Weekly × 5–6 cycles Weekly × 5–6 cycles 4 cycles q21 days		EBRT: 45–50.4 Gy IMRT is optional
KGOG/GOG263	Cisplatin 40 mg/m^2	Weekly ×6 cycles		EBRT: 50.4 Gy IMRT is optional
ANZGOG 0902/ GOG-0274/ RTOG 1174, OUTBACK trial	Arm1: cisplatin 40 mg/m^2 Arm2: cisplatin 40 mg/m^2 Carboplatin AUC 5 and placlitaxel 155 mg/m^2 after completing chemoradiation therapy	Weekly ×5 cycles Weekly ×5-cycles 4 cycles q21 days		EBRT: 45–50.4 Gy

Table 36.2 Rate of pelvic and distant failures, acute and late toxicities in chemoradiation trials in cervical cancer

	Local (pelvic)	Distant	Acute toxicities	Late toxicities
SWOG8797/GOG109	5.5 % vs. 17.2 %	7 % vs.11.2 %	G4: 22.1 % vs. 3.5 %	One late death RT-CT arm
GOG-123	9 % vs. 21 %	11 % vs. 15 %	G3/4: 35 % vs. 13 %	3.8 % vs. 3.2 %
GOG-85	25 % vs. 30 %	Lung: 6 % vs. 9 % Distant except lung: 11 % vs. 12 %	G3/4: 4 % vs. 24 %	16.2 % vs. 16.5 %
RTOG90-01	14 % vs. 33 %	19 % vs. 35 %	G3/4: 44 % vs. 4 %	12 % vs. 11 %
GOG-120	19 %, 20 %, 30 %	Lung: 3 %, 4 %, 10 %	G3/4: 19 %, 20 %, 30 %	4.7 %, 0.9 %, 2.6 %
NCIC-Pearcey	27 % vs. 33 %	–	G ≥ 3: 31 % vs. 3 %	6 % vs. 0 %

high common iliac lymph nodes received radiation to para-aortic field (45 Gy) [16]. No brachytherapy was allowed in this study. After median follow up of 42 months, the projected progression free survival and overall survival was significantly higher for patients received concurrent chemoradiation therapy compared to patients received radiation alone (4-year PFS 80 % vs. 63 %, 4-year survivals 81 % vs. 71 % respectively). The rate of pelvic and extra-pelvic recurrence was less frequent in patients received concurrent chemotherapy. However there was no significant difference in the pattern of recurrence between the two treatment arms (Table 36.2). This study established chemoradiation therapy as the standard adjuvant therapy in patients with high risk factors early stage disease after radical surgery. An updated follow-up was released showing that after a median follow-up of 5.2 years, the estimated 5-year survival was 80 % vs. 66 % favoring the chemoradiation group [21]. Because chemotherapy was given both during radiation and for two additional cycles, this study raised an important question as whether the chemotherapy was effective as a radiosensitizer only or as adjuvant chemotherapy or both. Currently, there is an ongoing intergroup study (RTOG/GOG 0724) evaluating the impact of adding four cycles of adjuvant chemotherapy with carboplatin and paclitaxel after completing chemoradiation therapy with concurrent cisplatin (Table 36.1). Interestingly this trial also showed that patients with adenocarcinoma or adenosquamous carcinoma who received radiation alone had worse prognosis compared to squamous cell carcinoma case. In contrast, this difference disappeared in patients who received chemoradiation therapy with improved survival in both groups. These data raise the question whether patients with adenocarcinoma or adenosquamous carcinoma will benefit more from concurrent chemoradiation therapy and even adjuvant chemotherapy compared to patients with squamous cell carcinoma. Further studies are needed to answer this question.

A second question is raised is whether there is a role for chemoradiation therapy as an adjuvant therapy for patients with early stage disease who were found to have intermediate risk factors after radical hysterectomy (large clinical tumor size, deep >1/3 stromal invasion and lymphovascular space invasion). The Gynecologic Oncology study by Sedlis et al. evaluated the impact of adjuvant radiation therapy versus postoperative observation in 277 patients with stage IB with at least two of the three intermediate risk factors. Patients received adjuvant radiation therapy had significant reduction in recurrence rate and disease progression but not a significant difference in overall survival [22, 23]. This study established radiation therapy as the standard treatment after radical hysterectomy in patients with early stage disease who were found to have intermediate risk factors. Currently, there is an ongoing intergroup trial (GOG263/KGOG) evaluating the role of chemoradiation therapy with concurrent cisplatin in patients with stage I–IIA disease with two or more intermediate risk factors after radical hysterectomy and pelvic lymphadenectomy (Table 36.1).

Bulky Stage IB Disease

Large tumor >4 cm in size is well established as a poor prognostic factor in patients with stage IB disease with higher recurrence rate compared with smaller tumor. This led to the FIGO definition of IB1 (≤4 cm) and 1B2 (>4 cm). A variety of treatment schemas including surgery, radiation, and chemotherapy have been used to treat stage IB2 cervical cancer. A Gynecologic Oncology Group study performed prior to the chemoradiation era (GOG 71) demonstrated that adjuvant extrafascial hysterectomy did reduce the rate of pelvic recurrences [24]. Therefore to evaluate the impact of chemoradiation, the Gynecologic Oncology Group enrolled 369 patients with stage IB2 cervical cancer into a trial comparing radiation therapy to radiation therapy combined with concurrent weekly cisplatin followed in all patients by adjuvant hysterectomy (GOG#123) (Table 36.1). Patients who received concurrent weekly cisplatin had more frequent pathologic clearance in the hysterectomy specimen (52 % vs. 41 %), and decreased recurrence rate (21 % vs. 37 %) compared to patients received radiation therapy alone (Table 36.2). Significant improvement in both progression free survival (relative risk 0.51) and overall survival (relative risk 0.54) was noted favoring chemoradiation therapy group. With a median follow up of 36 months, the estimated 3-year survival was 83 % for chemoradiation therapy group compared with 74 % in the radiation only group. On the other hand, more grade 3 or 4 toxicities mainly hematologic and gastrointestinal toxicities were noted in the chemoradiation therapy group but these were transient with no serious consequences [17, 25] (Table 36.2). At 72 months of follow-up, the difference in progression-free survival and overall survival remained significant favoring the chemoradiation group compared to the radiation only group (PFS 71 % vs. 60 % and 78 % vs. 63 % respectively) [25]. With mature follow up on GOG 71 it was found that adjuvant hysterectomy did not improve survival. The authors of the study concluded that chemoradiation alone would be adequate therapy. A retrospective study of 49 patients treated for stage IB2 cervical cancer with chemoradiation alone found similar survivals to chemoradiation and adjuvant hysterectomy [26].

Locally Advanced Disease

Three randomized clinical trials were conducted in patients with locally advanced cervical cancer (stage IIB-IVA) comparing chemoradiation therapy with radiation alone. In GOG#85, 368 patients with locally advanced cervical cancer (stage IIB-IV) were randomly assigned to receive either chemoradiation therapy with concurrent cisplatin (50 mg/m^2) and 5-fluorouracil (1 g/m^2/day for 4 days) on day 1 and 29 versus hydroxyurea orally 80 mg/kg twice weekly (Table 36.1). Patients in the cisplatin and 5-fluorouracil containing arm had significant improvement in progression free survival and overall survival compared to hydroxyurea arm. After a median follow-up of 8.7 years, 43 % vs. 57 % had disease progression and 45 % vs. 57 % had died in 5-fluouracil/cisplatin and hydroxyurea containing arms respectively. Grade 3 and 4 toxicities mainly hematologic and gastrointestinal were more prominent in patient received hydoxyurea compared to those who received cisplatin and 5-fluorouracil (26 % vs. 4 %, Table 36.2) [18].

In a subsequent randomized clinical trial, the Radiation Oncology Group (RTOG) enrolled 388 patients with stage IB/IIA (≥5 cm clinical tumor size or positive pelvic lymph nodes, 34 % in each arm)-IVA cervical cancer comparing chemoradiation therapy with concurrent cisplatin (75 mg/m^2) and 5- fluorouracil (1 g/m^2/day as a 96-h infusion) for three cycles versus extended field radiation therapy (Table 36.1). Para-aortic lymph nodes were assessed by either lymphangiography or surgical staging. Chemoradiation therapy with cisplatin and 5-FU showed superior outcome in term of recurrence rate, progression free survival and overall survival. The estimated 5-year progression free survival and overall survival were 67 % vs. 40 % and 73 % vs. 58 % respectively for chemoradiation arm and extended field radiation arm [19]. The rate of locoregional and distant metastasis were significantly lower in the cisplatin/5-FU containing arm compared to extended field radiation arm (14 % vs. 33 % and 19 % vs. 35 % respectively) (Table 36.2). Patients received combined chemoradiation therapy had more frequent grade 3 and 4 toxicities compared to extended field radiation (44 % vs. 4 %). However, these effects were self-limited and there was no significant difference in late serious effects between the two groups (12 % vs. 11 %) (Table 36.2). Updated report after median follow-up of 6.6 years confirmed persistent advantage of chemoradiation therapy over extended field radiation with median survival of 67 % versus 41 % at 8 years respectively and 51 % reduction in risk of recurrence [27]. Interestingly, subgroup analysis showed that patients with stage III–IV who received chemoradiation therapy had significant improvement in progression free survival and trend toward improved survival with no significant difference. However, the trial was not powered to detect difference in outcome in this subgroup of patients.

A third randomized trial conducted by the GOG involving 526 patients with stage IIB–IVA cervical cancer and negative para-oartic nodes by extra-peritoneal staging (GOG-120). Patients in this study were randomized to receive radiation therapy combined with one of three chemotherapy regimens: weekly cisplatin (40 mg/m^2) vs. combined cisplatin (50 mg/m^2) followed by 5-FU (1 g/m^2/day as 96-h infusion) on day 1 and 29 with twice weekly oral hydroxyurea 2 g/m^2 for 6 weeks vs. oral hydroxyurea (3 g/m^2 twice weekly) (Table 36.1). This study demonstrated superior progression free survival and overall survival favoring the two platinum containing regimens compared to hydroxyurea only regimen. Furthermore, the rate of pelvic recurrence was significantly lower among platinum containing groups compared to only hydroxyurea group (19–20 % vs. 30 % respectively) (Table 36.2). Patients received cisplatin containing therapy had lower rate of lung metastasis than those who had only hydroxyurea therapy (3–4 % vs. 10 %) respectively. The rate of grade 3 or 4 toxicities was the highest among patients who received the three drug regimen compared to the other two regimens. The cisplatin only regimen was associated with the least severe toxicity [20] (Table 36.2). However, late grade 3 and 4 gastrointestinal and urologic toxicities were not different between treatment groups (4.7 % vs. 0.9 % vs. 2.6 %) (Table 36.2). After median follow-up of 106 months, improvement in PFS and OS continued to be evident in the two cisplatin containing regimen compared with hydroxyurea only regimen. PFS rates at 10 years for the three arms (cisplatin, cisplatin/5-FU/hydroxyurea and hydroxyurea alone) were 46, 43 and 26 % respectively. Similarly, overall survival at 10 years was 53, 53 and 34 % respectively [28]. Further, subgroup analysis was performed to evaluate the impact of cisplatin based chemoradiation therapy on stage IIB and III individually. In each of these stages, progression free survival and overall survival significantly improved with cisplatin based chemoradiation therapy compared to hydroxyurea alone.

After this clinical announcement by the NCI, a sixth clinical trial was released by the National Cancer Institute of Canada (NCIC). This trial enrolled 253 patients with stage IB2/IIA (>5 cm or positive pelvic nodes)-IVA disease and randomly assigned them to receive radiation therapy alone or radiation with concurrent weekly cisplatin (40 mg/m^2) for 5 weeks (Table 36.1). After median follow up of 82 months, the study showed no significant difference in progression free survival and overall survival between the two treatment groups. At 3 and 5 years, survival was not significantly different (69 % vs. 66 %, and 62 % vs. 58 %) for chemoradiation and radiation only groups respectively. However, the rate of pelvic recurrence was lower in patients received chemoradiation therapy compared to those receive radiation alone (27 % vs. 33 %). The rate of acute grade 3 or 4 toxicities was higher in the chemoradiation arm but it was not serious enough to cause treatment delay. Further, there was no significant difference in rate of late toxicities (Table 36.2) [29].

This trial has several strengths including: a multicenter prospective randomized trial, included cisplatin with appropriate dosing, and optimal dose and schedule of radiation therapy (~80 Gy to point A over around 48–51 days).

However, it was limited by several factors including: small number of patients enrolled (n=253) with large confidence intervals with potential statistical underpower to detect improvement in survival. In contrast to prior trials in advanced stage cervical cancer, in which surgical staging was performed to exclude para-aortic lymph nodes metastasis, patients in this trial were staged by computed tomography with potential inclusion of patients with extrapelvic metastasis in either treatment arms. This further decreases the power of the study to estimate the relative effect of chemoradiation therapy. Lastly, the proportion of patients received chemoradiation therapy had significantly greater anemia compared to those who received radiation alone.

Recently, a meta-analysis was released involving 13 clinical trials comparing chemoradiation therapy with radiation therapy alone. The meta-analysis showed a 6 % improvement in absolute survival and 8 % improvement in progression free survival favoring chemoradiation therapy. Further, chemoradiation reduced the rate of local and distant recurrence compared to radiation therapy alone [30]. However this metaanalysis did not include data from GOG-120 and GOG-85 because hydroxyurea was included in the radiation arm and RTOG-9001 because radiation therapy was extended to the para-aortic filed in the radiation alone arm.

36.4 Non-platinum Based Concurrent Chemoradiation Therapy

Other radiation sensitizing agents that have been studied in the past include mitomycin C and 5-fluorouracil. However, these agents have not been shown to have superior effect compared to cisplatin-based chemoradiation therapy. In a retrospective study comparing the rate of grade 3 late bowel toxicity in locally advanced cervical cancer cases treated with chemoradiation protocol containing 5-fluorouracil with and without mitomycin C, the addition of mitomycin C was associated with significant increase in the rate of grade 3 late bowel toxicity (25 % vs. 10 %) compared to those who did not receive it with no significant improvement in overall survival [31].

The Gynecologic Oncology Group conducted a clinical trial comparing weekly cisplatin (40 mg/m^2) with 5-fluorouracil in a continuous infusion (225 mg/m^2/day for 5 days) for six cycles (GOG-165). The planned interim analysis showed that the risk of disease progression was 35 % higher in the 5-fluorouracil arm compared to the cisplatin arm. The study was closed prematurely because significant improvement in progression free survival in 5-fluorouracil arm compared to cisplatin arm were not able to be achieved even if the study was completed [32].

Carboplatin, another platinum agent, represents an interesting alternative to cisplatin in platinum based chemoradiation therapy. Theoretically, carboplatin has similar efficacy to cisplatin with less toxicity especially gastrointestinal, renal and neurologic toxicities but greater myelosuppression. In a phase I trial using weekly carboplatin (AUC of 2) concurrent with radiation therapy in 32 patients with stage IB–IV cervical cancer, no cases of grade 3 or 4 gastrointestinal, renal or neurologic toxicities were reported with 2 % grade 3 hematologic toxicities. The Objective complete response rate was 90 % with median follow-up of 12 months [33]. In another small pilot study, using carboplatin as radiation sensitizer twice weekly was not associated with late gastrointestinal, renal or grade 4 toxicities [34]. However, there is no prospective randomized trial comparing carboplatin vs. cisplatin as a radiation sensitizer in treatment of cervical cancer.

36.5 Adjuvant Chemotherapy After Chemoradiation Therapy

There is no strong evidence whether adjuvant chemotherapy given after chemoradiation therapy has a survival advantage in term of overall survival or progression free survival. The Southwestern Oncology group trial (SWOG 8797) evaluated the impact of concurrent and adjuvant chemotherapy in patients with stage IA2–IB1 with high risk factors after radical hysterectomy [16]. In the experimental arm, patients received four cycle of cisplatin and 5-fluorouracil. The first two cycles were given concurrently with radiation therapy followed by two additional cycles. Among patients received chemoradiation therapy, having more cycles of chemotherapy were favorably associated with progression free survival and overall survival. Currently, there is an ongoing trial conducted by the Radiation Oncology Group (RTOG/GOG 0724) to evaluate the impact of adjuvant chemotherapy with carboplatin and taxol for four cycles after chemoradiation therapy in patients with stage IA2–IB1 cervical cancer with high risk factors after radical hysterectomy.

Another trial conducted by Duenas-Gonzalez et al. studied the effect of adding gemcitabine as a concurrent and adjuvant chemotherapy with cisplatin on survival of patients with locally advanced cervical cancer. Five hundred and 15 patients with stage IIB–IV disease were enrolled and randomized into two arms: the experimental Arm A of weekly cisplatin 40 mg/m^2 with gemcitabine 125 mg/m^2 weekly for 6 weeks concurrent with radiation therapy then followed by adjuvant chemotherapy of cisplatin 50 mg/m^2 on day 1 and gemcitabine 1,000 mg/m^2 on day 1 and 8 every 3 weeks for two cycles, or the control Arm B of standard weekly cisplatin 40 mg/m^2 concurrent with radiation therapy for 6 weeks. Compared to the control arm, significant improvement in overall PFS and OS was noted for the experimental arm. Progression free survival at 3 year was 74.4 % for the experimental arm vs. 65.0 % for the control arm. However, grade 3 and 4 toxicities were more frequent in experimental arm 86.5 % vs. 46.4 % [35].

In locally advanced cervical cancer, Lorvidhaya conducted a randomized clinical trial comparing radiation alone with concurrent chemotherapy and adjuvant chemotherapy using mitomycin C and 5-fluorouracil. In this trial, patients with stage IIB–IV disease were randomized into four arms: radiation therapy alone (arm 1), radiation therapy with adjuvant chemotherapy (arm 2), radiation therapy with concurrent chemotherapy (arm 3) and radiation therapy with both concurrent and adjuvant chemotherapy (arm 4). There was significant improvement in overall survival with concurrent chemotherapy but not with adjuvant chemotherapy compared to radiation therapy alone. Additionally, there was no difference in overall survival between those who received concurrent chemotherapy and those who received both concurrent and adjuvant chemotherapy [36].

Currently, an international trial is being conducted to investigate the impact of adjuvant chemotherapy with carboplatin and paclitaxel for four cycles following chemoradiation therapy with concurrent weekly cisplatin in patients with locally advanced cervical cancer (stage IB 1 with positive nodes or stage IB2–IV) (ANZGOG 0902/GOG-0274/RTOG 1174, OUTBACK trial) (Table 36.1).

36.6 Biologic Agents Concurrent with Cisplatin Based Chemoradiation Therapy

Biologic agents have different mechanism of action and adverse effects which make their use as a radiation sensitizer either alone or with cisplatin promising.

Tirapazamine is a compound with selective cytotoxicity toward hypoxic cells. At low oxygen level, tirapazamine forms highly reactive radicals that are capable of causing DNA damage resulting in cell death. In a phase I study, tirapazamine was added to weekly cisplatin and radiation therapy in 11 patients with locally advanced cervical cancer (stage IB2–IV). Tirapazamine (290 mg/m^2) was associated with significant toxicity requiring reduction in the dose of both cisplatin (30 mg/m^2) and tirapazamine (260 mg/m^2) [37]. The Gynecologic oncology group conducted a phase III randomized trial comparing cisplatin (60 mg/m^2) and tirapazamine administered on day 1, 15 and 29 concurrent with radiation therapy versus weekly cisplatin concurrent with radiation therapy in patients with locally advanced cervical cancer (stage IB 2, IIA2, IIB, IIIB and IVA) (GOG-0219). This study was closed prematurely in September 2009 due to lack of Tirapazamine supply. After median follow-up of 27.5 months, progression free survival and overall survival were similar in both arms. 3-year progression free survival 66 and 63.5 % respectively (p=0.64) and 3-year overall survival on both arms were 72 and 71.5 % respectively (p=0.82) [38].

Cetuximab is a monoclonal antibody that specifically binds to epidermal growth factor receptor (EGFR) leading to inhibition of cell signaling and ultimately cell cycle arrest and cell death. EGFR has been found to be over-expressed in cervical cancer [39]. In patients with locally advanced squamous cell carcinoma of head and neck, patients were randomly assigned to receive either radiation therapy alone or radiation therapy with concurrent weekly cetuximab followed by seven doses of weekly cetuximab. Patients who received cetuximab and radiation therapy had significant improvement in locoregional control and overall survival compared to radiation therapy alone [40, 41]. A phase I trial was conducted by the GOG to investigate the role of cetuximab in combination with cisplatin and radiation therapy in treating locally advanced cervical cancer (GOG-9918). In this study, cetuximab with a loading dose of 400 mg/m^2 followed by weekly dose of 250 mg/m^2 combined with weekly cisplatin 30 mg/m^2 was feasible if combined with whole pelvic radiation therapy, however it was not feasible if combined with extended field radiation therapy due to increased toxicities mainly gastrointestinal and metabolic [42].

Bevacizumab is a humanized monoclonal antibody which specifically binds to vascular endothelial growth factor (VEGF) preventing binding of VEGF to its receptor thereby inhibiting angiogenesis. Bevacizumab has been studied in recurrent and metastatic cervical cancer. However, there is limited data about its efficacy as a radiation sensitizer. Recently, the RTOG released the result of a phase II trial where bevacizumab (10 mg/kg) every other week was added to weekly cisplatin and radiation therapy in patients with bulky stage IB–IIIB tumors (RTOG 0417) [43]. In this study, no serious adverse events were reported. Thirty-one percent (15/49) developed treatment related adverse events, most of which were hematologic. This study showed that addition of bevacizumab to chemoradiation therapy of cervical cancer is safe and feasible as 76 % of patients were able to receive cisplatin and bevacizumab as outlined per the protocol [43]. The efficacy of Bevacizumab as a radiation sensitizer needs to be explored in future randomized trials.

References

1. Fletcher GH. Clinical dose-response curves of human malignant epithelial tumours. Br J Radiol. 1973;46:1–12.
2. Terasima T, Tolmach LJ. X-ray sensitivity and DNA synthesis in synchronous populations of HeLa cells. Science. 1963;140:490–2.
3. Chauvergne J, Rohart J, Heron JF, Ayme Y, Berlie J, Fargeot P, George M, Lebrun-Jezekova D, Pigneux J, Chenal C, et al. Randomized trial of initial chemotherapy in 151 locally advanced carcinoma of the cervix (T2b-N1, T3b, MO). Bull Cancer. 1990;77:1007–24.
4. Chauvergne J, Lhomme C, Rohart J, Heron JF, Ayme Y, Goupil A, Fargeot P, David M. Neoadjuvant chemotherapy of stage IIb or III cancers of the uterine cervix. Long-term results of a multicenter randomized trial of 151 patients. Bull Cancer. 1993;80:1069–79.
5. Kumar L, Kaushal R, Nandy M, Biswal BM, Kumar S, Kriplani A, Singh R, Rath GK, Kochupillai V. Chemotherapy followed by radiotherapy versus radiotherapy alone in locally advanced cervical cancer: a randomized study. Gynecol Oncol. 1994; 54:307–15.
6. Souhami L, Gil RA, Allan SE, Canary PC, Araujo CM, Pinto LH, Silveira TR. A randomized trial of chemotherapy followed by pelvic radiation therapy in stage IIIB carcinoma of the cervix. J Clin Oncol. 1991;9:970–7.
7. Tattersall MH, Ramirez C, Coppleson M. A randomized trial comparing platinum-based chemotherapy followed by radiotherapy vs. radiotherapy alone in patients with locally advanced cervical cancer. Int J Gynecol Cancer. 1992;2:244–51.
8. Tattersall MH, Lorvidhaya V, Vootiprux V, Cheirsilpa A, Wong F, Azhar T, Lee HP, Kang SB, Manalo A, Yen MS, et al. Randomized trial of epirubicin and cisplatin chemotherapy followed by pelvic radiation in locally advanced cervical cancer. Cervical Cancer Study Group of the Asian Oceanian Clinical Oncology Association. J Clin Oncol. 1995;13:444–51.
9. Kumar L, Grover R, Pokharel YH, Chander S, Kumar S, Singh R, Rath GK, Kochupillai V. Neoadjuvant chemotherapy in locally advanced cervical cancer: two randomised studies. Aust N Z J Med. 1998;28:387–90.
10. Leborgne F, Leborgne JH, Doldan R, Zubizarreta E, Ortega B, Maisonneuve J, Musetti E, Hekimian L, Mezzera J. Induction chemotherapy and radiotherapy

of advanced cancer of the cervix: a pilot study and phase III randomized trial. Int J Radiat Oncol Biol Phys. 1997;37:343–50.
11. Sundfor K, Trope CG, Hogberg T, Onsrud M, Koern J, Simonsen E, Bertelsen K, Westberg R. Radiotherapy and neoadjuvant chemotherapy for cervical carcinoma. A randomized multicenter study of sequential cisplatin and 5-fluorouracil and radiotherapy in advanced cervical carcinoma stage 3B and 4A. Cancer. 1996;77:2371–8.
12. Chiara S, Bruzzone M, Merlini L, Bruzzi P, Rosso R, Franzone P, Orsatti M, Vitale V, Foglia G, Odicino F, et al. Randomized study comparing chemotherapy plus radiotherapy versus radiotherapy alone in FIGO stage IIB-III cervical carcinoma. GONO (North-West Oncologic Cooperative Group). Am J Clin Oncol. 1994;17:294–7.
13. Neoadjuvant Chemotherapy for Locally Advanced Cervical Cancer Meta-analysis Collaboration. Neoadjuvant chemotherapy for locally advanced cervical cancer: a systematic review and meta-analysis of individual patient data from 21 randomised trials. Eur J Cancer. 2003;39:2470–86.
14. Withers HR, Taylor JM, Maciejewski B. The hazard of accelerated tumor clonogen repopulation during radiotherapy. Acta Oncol. 1988;27:131–46.
15. Ozols RF, Masuda H, Hamilton TC. Mechanisms of cross-resistance between radiation and antineoplastic drugs. NCI Monogr. 1988;6:159–65.
16. Peters 3rd WA, Liu PY, Barrett 2nd RJ, Stock RJ, Monk BJ, Berek JS, Souhami L, Grigsby P, Gordon Jr W, Alberts DS. Concurrent chemotherapy and pelvic radiation therapy compared with pelvic radiation therapy alone as adjuvant therapy after radical surgery in high-risk early-stage cancer of the cervix. J Clin Oncol. 2000;18:1606–13.
17. Keys HM, Bundy BN, Stehman FB, Muderspach LI, Chafe WE, Suggs 3rd CL, Walker JL, Gersell D. Cisplatin, radiation, and adjuvant hysterectomy compared with radiation and adjuvant hysterectomy for bulky stage IB cervical carcinoma. N Engl J Med. 1999;340:1154–61.
18. Whitney CW, Sause W, Bundy BN, Malfetano JH, Hannigan EV, Fowler Jr WC, Clarke-Pearson DL, Liao SY. Randomized comparison of fluorouracil plus cisplatin versus hydroxyurea as an adjunct to radiation therapy in stage IIB-IVA carcinoma of the cervix with negative para-aortic lymph nodes: a Gynecologic Oncology Group and Southwest Oncology Group study. J Clin Oncol. 1999;17:1339–48.
19. Morris M, Eifel PJ, Lu J, Grigsby PW, Levenback C, Stevens RE, Rotman M, Gershenson DM, Mutch DG. Pelvic radiation with concurrent chemotherapy compared with pelvic and para-aortic radiation for high-risk cervical cancer. N Engl J Med. 1999;340:1137–43.
20. Rose PG, Bundy BN, Watkins EB, Thigpen JT, Deppe G, Maiman MA, Clarke-Pearson DL, Insalaco S. Concurrent cisplatin-based radiotherapy and chemotherapy for locally advanced cervical cancer. N Engl J Med. 1999;340:1144–53.
21. Monk BJ, Wang J, Im S, Stock RJ, Peters 3rd WA, Liu PY, Barrett 2nd RJ, Berek JS, Souhami L, Grigsby PW, Gordon Jr W, Alberts DS. Rethinking the use of radiation and chemotherapy after radical hysterectomy: a clinical-pathologic analysis of a Gynecologic Oncology Group/Southwest Oncology Group/Radiation Therapy Oncology Group trial. Gynecol Oncol. 2005;96:721–8.
22. Sedlis A, Bundy BN, Rotman MZ, Lentz SS, Muderspach LI, Zaino RJ. A randomized trial of pelvic radiation therapy versus no further therapy in selected patients with stage IB carcinoma of the cervix after radical hysterectomy and pelvic lymphadenectomy: a Gynecologic Oncology Group Study. Gynecol Oncol. 1999;73:177–83.
23. Rotman M, Sedlis A, Piedmonte MR, Bundy B, Lentz SS, Muderspach LI, Zaino RJ. A phase III randomized trial of postoperative pelvic irradiation in Stage IB cervical carcinoma with poor prognostic features: follow-up of a gynecologic oncology group study. Int J Radiat Oncol Biol Phys. 2006; 65:169–76.
24. Keys HM, Bundy BN, Stehman FB, Okagaki T, Gallup DG, Burnett AF, Rotman MZ, Fowler Jr WC. Radiation therapy with and without extrafascial hysterectomy for bulky stage IB cervical carcinoma: a randomized trial of the Gynecologic Oncology Group. Gynecol Oncol. 2003;89:343–53.
25. Stehman FB, Ali S, Keys HM, Muderspach LI, Chafe WE, Gallup DG, Walker JL, Gersell D. Radiation therapy with or without weekly cisplatin for bulky stage 1B cervical carcinoma: follow-up of a Gynecologic Oncology Group trial. Am J Obstet Gynecol. 2007;197:503.e1–6.
26. Goksedef BP, Kunos C, Belinson JL, Rose PG. Concurrent cisplatin-based chemoradiation international federation of gynecology and obstetrics stage IB2 cervical carcinoma. Am J Obstet Gynecol. 2009;200:175.e1–5.
27. Eifel PJ, Winter K, Morris M, Levenback C, Grigsby PW, Cooper J, Rotman M, Gershenson D, Mutch DG. Pelvic irradiation with concurrent chemotherapy versus pelvic and para-aortic irradiation for high-risk cervical cancer: an update of radiation therapy oncology group trial (RTOG) 90–01. J Clin Oncol. 2004;22:872–80.
28. Rose PG, Ali S, Watkins E, Thigpen JT, Deppe G, Clarke-Pearson DL, Insalaco S. Long-term follow-up of a randomized trial comparing concurrent single agent cisplatin, cisplatin-based combination chemotherapy, or hydroxyurea during pelvic irradiation for locally advanced cervical cancer: a Gynecologic Oncology Group Study. J Clin Oncol. 2007;25: 2804–10.
29. Pearcey R, Brundage M, Drouin P, Jeffrey J, Johnston D, Lukka H, MacLean G, Souhami L, Stuart G, Tu D. Phase III trial comparing radical radiotherapy with and without cisplatin chemotherapy in patients with advanced squamous cell cancer of the cervix. J Clin Oncol. 2002;20:966–72.

30. Chemoradiotherapy for Cervical Cancer Meta-Analysis Collaboration. Reducing uncertainties about the effects of chemoradiotherapy for cervical cancer: a systematic review and meta-analysis of individual patient data from 18 randomized trials. J Clin Oncol. 2008;26:5802–12.
31. Rakovitch E, Fyles AW, Pintilie M, Leung PM. Role of mitomycin C in the development of late bowel toxicity following chemoradiation for locally advanced carcinoma of the cervix. Int J Radiat Oncol Biol Phys. 1997;38:979–87.
32. Lanciano R, Calkins A, Bundy BN, Parham G, Lucci 3rd JA, Moore DH, Monk BJ, O'Connor DM. Randomized comparison of weekly cisplatin or protracted venous infusion of fluorouracil in combination with pelvic radiation in advanced cervix cancer: a gynecologic oncology group study. J Clin Oncol. 2005;23:8289–95.
33. Higgins RV, Naumann WR, Hall JB, Haake M. Concurrent carboplatin with pelvic radiation therapy in the primary treatment of cervix cancer. Gynecol Oncol. 2003;89:499–503.
34. Muderspach LI, Curtin JP, Roman LD, Gebhardt JA, Klement V, Qian D, Morrow CP, Felix JC, Formenti SC, Muggia FM. Carboplatin as a radiation sensitizer in locally advanced cervical cancer: a pilot study. Gynecol Oncol. 1997;65:336–42.
35. Duenas-Gonzalez A, Zarba JJ, Patel F, Alcedo JC, Beslija S, Casanova L, Pattaranutaporn P, Hameed S, Blair JM, Barraclough H, Orlando M. Phase III, open-label, randomized study comparing concurrent gemcitabine plus cisplatin and radiation followed by adjuvant gemcitabine and cisplatin versus concurrent cisplatin and radiation in patients with stage IIB to IVA carcinoma of the cervix. J Clin Oncol. 2011;29:1678–85.
36. Lorvidhaya V, Chitapanarux I, Sangruchi S, Lertsanguansinchai P, Kongthanarat Y, Tangkaratt S, Visetsiri E. Concurrent mitomycin C, 5-fluorouracil, and radiotherapy in the treatment of locally advanced carcinoma of the cervix: a randomized trial. Int J Radiat Oncol Biol Phys. 2003;55:1226–32.
37. Rischin D, Narayan K, Oza AM, Mileshkin L, Bernshaw D, Choi J, Hicks R, McClure B, Fyles A. Phase 1 study of tirapazamine in combination with radiation and weekly cisplatin in patients with locally advanced cervical cancer. Int J Gynecol Cancer. 2010;20:827–33.
38. DiSilvestro PA, Ali S, Craighead PS, Lucci JA, Lee YC, Cohn D, Spirtos NM, Tewari K, Muller C, Steinhoff MM. A Gynecologic Oncology Group phase III randomized trial of weekly cisplatin and radiation versus cisplatin and tirapazamine and radiation in stage IB2, IIA, IIIB and IVA cervical carcinoma limited to the pelvis. Gynecol Oncol. 2012;125(s1) (SGO #2): S3. (Abstract). 12012.
39. Kim JW, Kim YT, Kim DK, Song CH, Lee JW. Expression of epidermal growth factor receptor in carcinoma of the cervix. Gynecol Oncol. 1996;60:283–7.
40. Bonner JA, Harari PM, Giralt J, Cohen RB, Jones CU, Sur RK, Raben D, Baselga J, Spencer SA, Zhu J, Youssoufian H, Rowinsky EK, Ang KK. Radiotherapy plus cetuximab for locoregionally advanced head and neck cancer: 5-year survival data from a phase 3 randomised trial, and relation between cetuximab-induced rash and survival. Lancet Oncol. 2010;11:21–8.
41. Bonner JA, Harari PM, Giralt J, Azarnia N, Shin DM, Cohen RB, Jones CU, Sur R, Raben D, Jassem J, Ove R, Kies MS, Baselga J, Youssoufian H, Amellal N, Rowinsky EK, Ang KK. Radiotherapy plus cetuximab for squamous-cell carcinoma of the head and neck. N Engl J Med. 2006;354:567–78.
42. Moore KN, Sill MW, Miller DS, McCourt C, De Geest K, Rose PG, Cardenes HR, Mannel RS, Farley JH, Schilder RJ, Fracasso PM. A phase I trial of tailored radiation therapy with concomitant cetuximab and cisplatin in the treatment of patients with cervical cancer: a gynecologic oncology group study. Gynecol Oncol. 2012;127:456–61.
43. Schefter TE, Winter K, Kwon JS, Stuhr K, Balaraj K, Yaremko BP, Small Jr W, Gaffney DK. A phase II study of bevacizumab in combination with definitive radiotherapy and cisplatin chemotherapy in untreated patients with locally advanced cervical carcinoma: preliminary results of RTOG 0417. Int J Radiat Oncol Biol Phys. 2012;83:1179–84.

37 (Laterally) Extended Endopelvic Resection for the Treatment of Locally Advanced and Recurrent Cervical Cancer

Michael Höckel

37.1 Introduction

For selected patients with persistence or pelvic recurrence of cervicovaginal cancer, particularly after radiotherapy, and those with locally advanced primary cancer not suitable for radiation, pelvic exenteration is a treatment option with curative potential. The surgical principles of pelvic exenteration introduced more than 60 years ago have remained essentially unchanged [1]. This "ultraradical" operation aims at excising the tumor by resection of the female genital tract en bloc with adjacent pelvic organs such as the distal urinary tract (urethra, bladder, ureters) and/or the anorectum. Several types of pelvic exenteration have been defined to tailor the multivisceral surgery for the individual tumor situation [2]. Significant improvements have been achieved in the reconstruction of the pelvic organ functions [3]. However, despite the progress in pelvic imaging exenteration is still aborted or leads to intralesional resection in up to 50 % of the cases [4, 5]. These failures spoil patients' hopes and waste considerable resources.

We have proposed the compartment theory of locoregional spread for malignant tumors and provided several lines of evidence that a new principle of surgical radicality, namely the resection of developmental compartments, is superior to the conventional treatment concepts extirpating tissues according to their function [6–8]. These insights have also been translated into procedures for the surgical therapy of locally advanced and recurrent cancer of the lower female genital tract termed (Laterally) Extended Endopelvic Resection (L)EER [9–12]. (L)EER achieves R0 resection and locoregional tumor control not only in patients which are regarded suitable candidates for conventional pelvic exenteration but also in patients with pelvic side wall disease currently excluded from surgical treatment either pre- or intraoperatively.

M. Höckel, MD, PhD
Department of Gynecology, Women's and Children's Center, University of Leipzig, Leipzig, Germany
e-mail: michael.hoeckel@uniklinik-leipzig.de

37.2 Ontogenetic Anatomy of the Female Pelvis

Prerequisite for the performance of (L)EER is the knowledge of the developmental anatomy of the pelvis in the human female which will be briefly outlined here, supplemented by Table 37.1 and Fig. 37.1. For further reading I refer to textbooks and monographs [13–17].

The pelvic ground plan is laid down in the fourth developmental week through migration, proliferation and specific interaction of cell lineages from the three germ layers—endoderm, mesoderm, ectoderm—establishing four *primitive pelvic metacompartments* for which I suggest the terms endopelvis, mesopelvis, ectopelvis and pelvic orifice. Interaction of cell populations from

H.R.H. Patel et al. (eds.), *Pelvic Cancer Surgery: Modern Breakthroughs and Future Advances*,
DOI 10.1007/978-1-4471-4258-4_37, © Springer-Verlag London 2015

Table 37.1 Ontogenetic anatomy of the female pelvis: compartments

Mature metacompartment	Building blocks	Primitive metacompartment	Developmental domains with fixed topological relations to each other	Mature ontogenetic compartments
Endopelvis	Endoderm	Cloaca and allantois	Primitive bladder	Bladder
	Splanchnopleuric mesoderm		Internal UGS	Internal UGS compartment[a]
			Hindgut	Rectum and mesorectum
Ectopelvis	Ectoderm	Primitive pelvic walls and tail with sacral and coccygeal somites	Pelvic integumental primordium	Pelvic integument
	Somatopleuric mesoderm			
	Paraxial mesoderm			Pelvic fascia, muscles and bones
	Caudal eminence mesoderm		Pelvic fascio-musculo-skeletal blastema	Pelvic parietal peritoneum
	Intermediate mesoderm		Pelvic coelom	
Mesopelvis		Urogenital ridges with mesonephroi	Primordial gonads	Ovaries and mesovars
			Paramesonephric-mesonephric complex	Müllerian compartment[b]
	Splanchnopleuric mesoderm			Pelvic ureters
			Metanephric complex	Definitive UGM[c]
	Somatopleuric mesoderm		Primordial UGM	
Pelvic orifice	Ectoderm	Cloacal membrane and folds	External UGS	External UGS compartment[d]
	Endoderm			
	Extraembryonic mesoderm			

UGS urogenital sinus, *UGM* urogenital mesentery

[a]Internal UGS compartment contains the urethra, distal vagina and distal rectovaginal septum

[b]Müllerian compartment contains the Fallopian tubes, uterus, proximal vagina, proximal mesometrium and mesocolpium

[c]Definitive UGM contains the infundibulopelvic ligament, mesureter, distal bladder mesentery, distal mesometrium, mesocolpium and mesopelvic fascia and suspensorium

[d]External UGS compartment contains the vulva (except labia majora), meatus urethrae, perineum and ventral anus

different primitive metacompartments during the following embryonic development (weeks 5–8) results in the formation of distinct epithelial-mesenchyme complexes that finally occupy domains with invariable topographical relations to each other. These epithelial-mesenchyme complexes are spatially defined by robust boundaries which prevent the mixing with cells of adjacent domains during further differentiation and maturation. They represent developmental (ontogenetic) compartments with fixed determination acting as modules of development independent from each other. Generally, within each compartment various subcompartments are formed during later development.

Synchronous with the formation of the pelvic developmental compartments three networks for their support are established from central primordia: the pelvic vascular system from the dorsal aorta, the pelvic lymphatic system from the posterior cardinal veins and the pelvic nervous system from the spinal neural tube, the spinal neural crest and the neural cord derived from the caudal eminence. Each support system can be regarded as a metacompartment in itself, and support compartments can be defined as mature differentiation products of the corresponding regional primordia. As an example, the lymphatic system of the pelvis can be divided into distal mesenteric, iliac and inguinal lymph compartments [18].

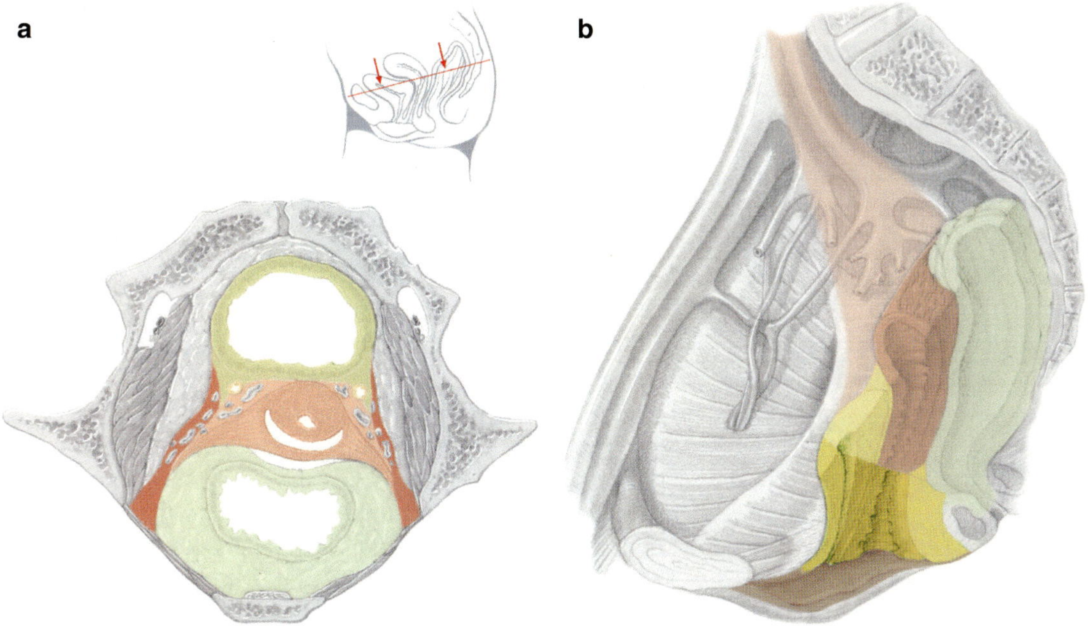

Fig. 37.1 Ontogenetic anatomic mapping of the adult female pelvis indicating developmental compartments. (**a**) Transverse section at the level indicated by the inset. (**b**) Midsagittal section with hollow organs transected transversely, visceral branches of the internal iliac vessels and lymph fatty tissue removed. Uncolored, ectopelvis; *yellow*, endopelvis; *red*, mesopelvis; *brown*, pelvic orifice (Modified from Höckel et al. [12])

The distal parts of the support system, e.g. the lymph capillaries, interact with their recipient compartments and adopt features specific for that particular tissue. The proximal parts are conduction structures which transit other compartments within defined corridors.

Differentiation of the pelvic compartments during the fetal period is gender specific.

The female *endopelvic compartments*, hindgut, bladder primordium and internal urogenital sinus (UGS), develop into the rectum with its mesorectum, the bladder, and the internal UGS compartment. The latter forms the urethra, distal vagina and distal rectovaginal septum as described in detail elsewhere [19]. Dorsally, the internal UGS compartment is attached to the anterior rectum and merges caudally with the external UGS compartment (see below).

The *mesopelvic compartments* bridge the ectopelvis and the endopelvis. The gonadal primordia, paramesonephric-mesonephric complex and the metanephric complex are bilaterally connected to the ectopelvis by the primitive urogenital mesentery. These primordia differentiate in the female pelvis into the ovaries with mesovars, Müllerian compartment, pelvic ureters and the definitive pelvic urogenital mesentery. The structurally complex Müllerian compartment is described in detail elsewhere [7, 8]. The ureters sprout from the distal mesonephric ducts at the site of the junction with the primitive bladder. The resulting short common nephric duct is then incorporated into the bladder primordium undergoing apoptosis and fusing the ureter orifice to the bladder epithelium. Further differentiation and growth of this bladder region produce the trigone and shift the ureterovesical junction ventralward [20]. The ureter tip interacts with the metanephric blastema forming the early kidney which ascends outside of the pelvis. Thus, in the mature pelvis only the pelvic ureter is left from the metanephric system. The mature *pelvic urogenital mesentery* derived from its primitive precursor consists of fibrofatty tissue providing the corridors for the ureter, the visceral branches of the internal iliac vessel system, the lymph collectors and eventually intercalated lymph nodes from the Müllerian, bladder and UGS compartments [18]. The urogenital mesentery also fixes these compartments to the ectopelvis with a "mesopelvic fascia" anteriorly and a structurally complex "mesopelvic suspensorium" posteriorly. Using the ureter as landmark the pelvic urogenital mesentery can be formally divided into a supraureteral peritoneal part and an infraureteral retroperitoneal part. Below the level of the obliterated umbilical artery the retroperitoneal part proceeds into the subperitoneal part. Inferolaterally, the subperitoneal urogenital mesentery is attached to the pubo- and iliococcygeus muscles anteriorly at the site of the arcus tendineus fasciae pelvis and to the coccygeus muscles/sacrospinous ligament close to the sciatic spine posteriorly. Superolaterally, the subperitoneal urogenital mesentery abuts the internal iliac vessel system, the proximal sciatic nerve and sacral plexus. Medially, it is separated by the plexus hypogastricus inferior from the ligamentous mesometria and mesocolpia which are parts of the Müllerian and internal UGS compartments. The peritoneal part of the pelvic urogenital mesentery corresponds to the distal broad ligament.

The *ectopelvic compartments* are represented by the pelvic epidermis, dermis, hypodermis, fasciae and musculoskeletal structures as well as the parietal peritoneum. Of particular relevance is the ectopelvic origin of the dorsolateral perineal complex which differentiates into the "Dartos fat pads" and overlying dermis providing the bulk of the labia majora and into the striated muscles of the superficial and deep perineum. The dorsolateral perineal complex has to be distinguished from the external UGS compartment derived from the pelvic orifice metacompartment which provides all other morphological structures of the vulva as well as the gynecologic perineum and the ventral anal segment [21].

(Laterally) Extended Endopelvic Resection

Extended Endopelvic Resection based on ontogenetic anatomy aims to resect multiple pelvic developmental (ontogenetic) compartments instead of tissues related to functions, i.e. multiple pelvic viscera. The Müllerian compartment is resected en bloc with the bladder compartment and eventually with the hindgut compartment. Integrated into these multicompartment resections is the *proximal* part of the pelvic urogenital mesentery. The resection can be caudally expanded by including the internal and external UGS compartments. In the latter case the procedure has to be performed both from the abdominal and perineal routes, whereas otherwise solely the abdominal approach is adequate (Fig. 37.2).

Laterally Extended Endopelvic Resection (*LEER*) includes the *distal* parts of the urogenital mesentery. In order to assure the completeness of its caudal resection the pubo-, ilio- and coccygeus muscles together with the mesopelvic fascia and suspensorium are included in the specimen. Rostral resection of the distal subperitoneal urogenital mesentery necessitates the inclusion of the internal iliac vessel system. Whereas the merging area of the caudal subperitoneal urogenital mesentery with the ectopelvis is defined by the smooth surface of the striated pelvic muscles, the spatial transition of the rostral subperitoneal urogenital mesentery to the internal iliac vessel system and the sacral plexus is complex (Fig. 37.3). Consequently, cervicovaginal tumors fixed to the pelvic wall below the sciatic notch level can be reliably resected by the inclusion of these pelvic floor and wall muscles into the en bloc specimen. However, if clinical symptoms or imaging indicate tumor involvement of the ectopelvis at the sciatic foramen, tumor control can no longer be accomplished with LEER.

A uniform nomenclature system describes the specific procedure within the spectrum of (L) EER: Total endopelvic resection designates the inclusion of the bladder compartment and the hindgut compartment, anterior endopelvic resection and posterior endopelvic resection indicate the inclusion of solely the bladder compartments or the hindgut compartment.

The abdominal procedure contains the complete Müllerian compartment or its remains following prior surgery. The abdominoperineal procedure includes both the Müllerian and the internal UGS compartments and may also integrate the external UGS compartment. The lateral

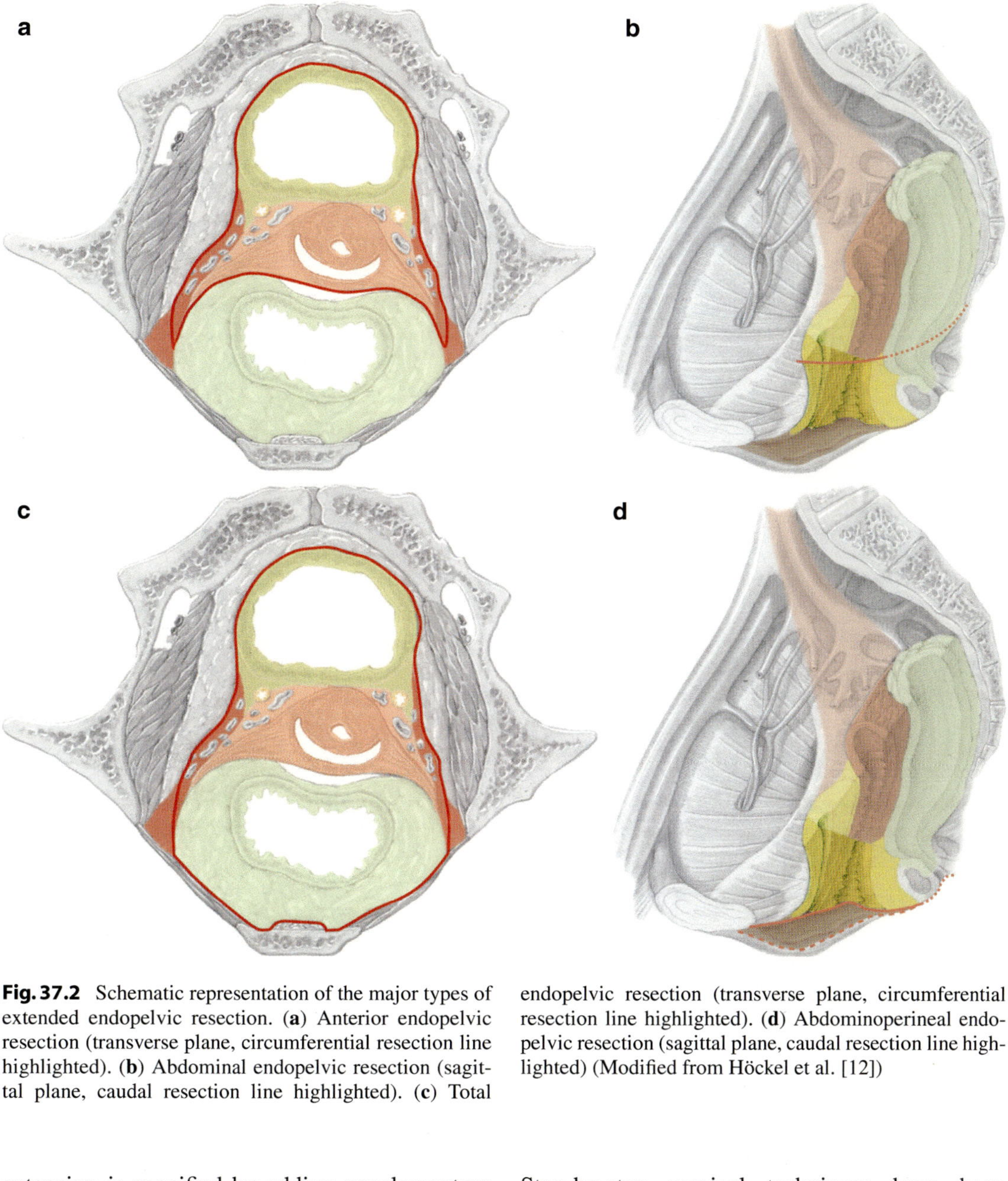

Fig. 37.2 Schematic representation of the major types of extended endopelvic resection. (**a**) Anterior endopelvic resection (transverse plane, circumferential resection line highlighted). (**b**) Abdominal endopelvic resection (sagittal plane, caudal resection line highlighted). (**c**) Total endopelvic resection (transverse plane, circumferential resection line highlighted). (**d**) Abdominoperineal endopelvic resection (sagittal plane, caudal resection line highlighted) (Modified from Höckel et al. [12])

extension is specified by adding supplementary information, r = right, 1 = left, c = caudal, r = rostral part of the distal subperitoneal urogenital mesentery. For example: Abdominoperineal laterally [rcr] extended anterior endopelvic resection designates the en bloc extirpation of the Müllerian, internal UGS, and bladder compartments with the complete pelvic urogenital mesentery, ilio- and pubococcygeus muscles and internal iliac vessel system on the right side. Step-by-step surgical techniques have been described elsewhere [22].

Therapeutic Lymph Node Dissection

For regional tumor control (L)EER is supplemented by therapeutic lymph node dissection (tLND) based on ontogenetic anatomy as described for early cervical carcinoma [18]. tLND is performed in all

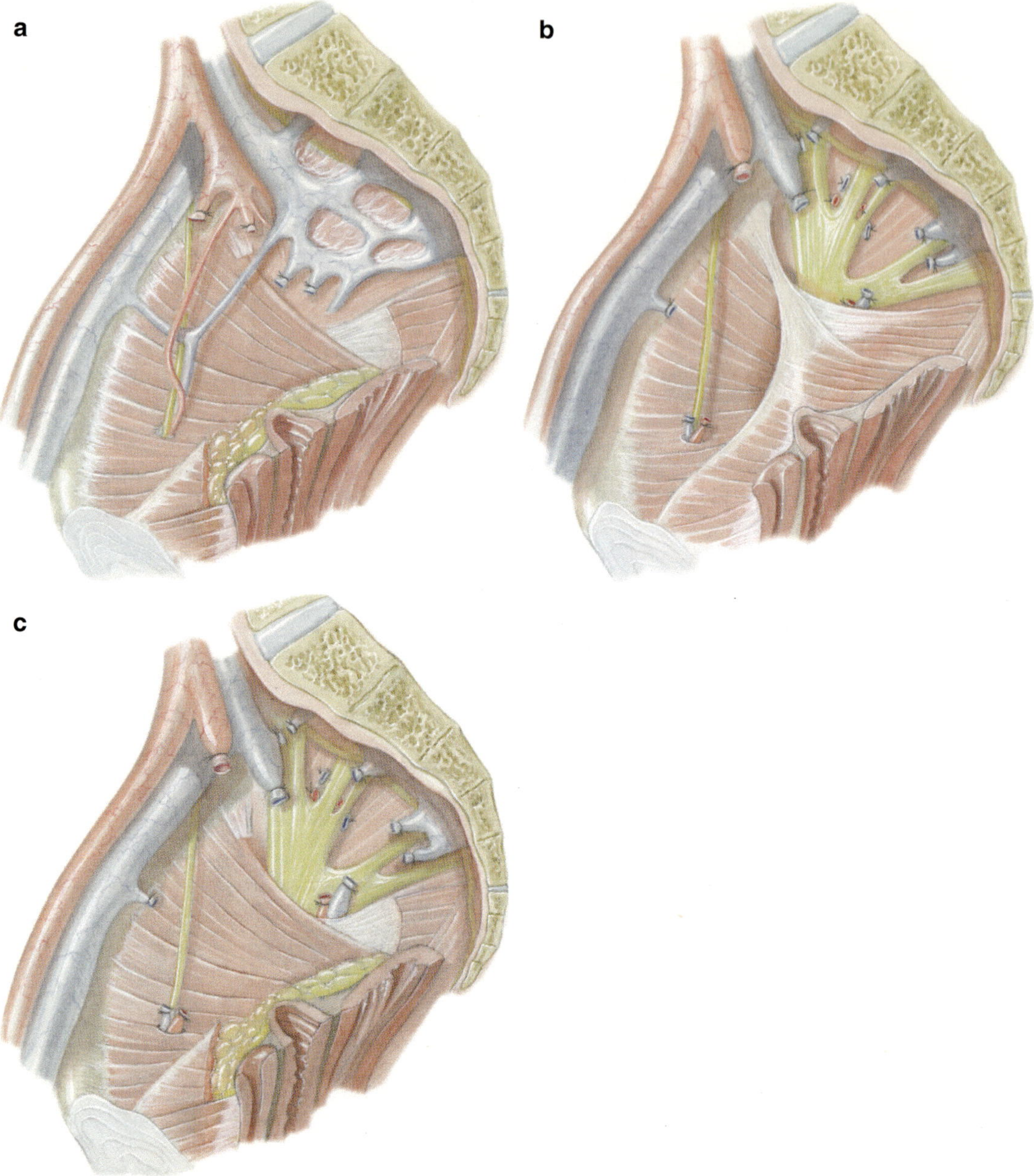

Fig. 37.3 The three types of lateral extension of endopelvic resection demonstrated at the right pelvic side wall. (**a**) Dissection of the caudal part of the distal urogenital mesentery including the pubo-, ilio- and coccygeus muscles into the LEER specimen. (**b**) Dissection of the rostral part of the urogenital mesentery including the internal iliac vessels into the LEER specimen. (**c**) Dissection of the complete urogenital mesentery including the pubo-, ilio- and coccygeus muscles and the internal iliac vessels into the LEER specimen (Modified from Höckel et al. [12])

patients who had not undergone surgical and/or radiotherapeutic therapy of the lymph node regions before and in those whose previous treatment for lymph node metastases has been incomplete.

The surgical procedure involves the complete stripping of the adventitia of all iliac vessels along with the lymph vessels and nodes mobilizing the vessels against each other, towards the peripheral nerves and towards the parietal muscles and fasciae. The paravisceral fat pad is resected completely, the presacral one to S2. The genitofemoral and obturator nerves, the lumbosacral trunk and the proximal sciatic nerve are exposed. The superior hypogastric plexus and the hypogastric nerves are mobilized and preserved. Parietal branches of the internal iliac vessels are sealed and cut to remove the gluteal lymph nodes. The external iliac and paravisceral fractions are intraoperatively assessed by frozen section. If metastases are diagnosed, lymph node dissection is extended downstream to the paraaortic region.

For paraaortic tLND the adventitia of the vena cava and of the aorta is stripped off caudocranially followed by the removal of the paracaval, interaortocaval and paraaortal fatty tissue. The large vessels are then lifted with elastic loops to remove all dorsal lymph fatty tissue thus exposing the spine. Lumbar vessels may have to be sealed and cut for the thoroughness of the lymph node dissection, however, the sympathetic trunk and its ganglia are preserved. Unless encased by nodal conglomerates the lumbar splanchnic nerves are isolated and spared. Paraaortic lymph node dissection is performed first to the level of the inferior mesenteric artery, and the surgical specimen is again histopathologically examined using frozen sections. If no metastases are detected, the procedure is terminated, otherwise dissection proceeds further cranially in the same manner up to the level of the left renal vein.

Pelvic Reconstruction

Vital organ functions lost by the resective procedure are reconstructed or substituted adhering to the following principles:

- Choosing the optimal procedure from several reconstructive options considering the patient's preference,
- Setting surgical safety over patient comfort in case of doubt,
- Strictly avoiding irradiated tissue for reconstruction.

This topic is dealt with in depth in Chap. 38.

Patient Evaluation and Selection

Patients with a persistence and recurrence of cervicovaginal cancer after radiotherapy and patients with advanced primary disease suffering from fistulae between the genital and urinary tracts and/or anorectum are candidates for (L) EER if the following conditions are met preoperatively:

- Exclusion of distant metastases,
- No ectopelvic tumor involvement at the site of the sciatic foramen,
- Patient's physical and mental fitness is adequate for the extensive nature of the surgery.

Patients with locally advanced disease without fistulae and patients with post-surgical pelvic recurrence in an unirradiated pelvis are primarily considered for chemoradiation. They may be evaluated for (L)EER, however, if the radiotherapist votes for or the patient requests surgical treatment. In patients with locally advanced and recurrent cervicovaginal cancer selected according to these criteria (L)EER achieved a 100 % R0 resection rate without abortion of any procedure during the resection phase [12]. R0 resection has been proven to be the most important factor for pelvic tumor control and cure [4, 5, 23]. Locoregional tumor control of 90 % and overall survival of 60 % have been obtained in the treatment of locally advanced and recurrent cancer, the majority of which were tumors fixed to the pelvic side wall which are usually not considered for exenterative treatment at all. R0 resection and locoregional tumor control rates of (L)EER treatment prove the principle of cancer surgery based on ontogenetic anatomy for advanced compartment- transgressing tumor states and at the same time question the traditional concept and practice of pelvic exenteration.

37.3 Summary

Pelvic exenteration designating the en bloc resection of multiple pelvic organs is a time-honored salvage operation for a subset of patients with persistent and recurrent cervicovaginal cancer. The procedure which is based on conventional surgical anatomy can also cure locally advanced primary disease not suitable for radiotherapy. However, high operative abortion and intralesional tumor resection rates significantly limit its clinical benefit. To overcome these weaknesses procedures termed (Laterally) Extended Endopelvic Resection ((L)EER) have been developed. Extended Endopelvic Resection extirpates multiple ontogenetic developmental instead of functional anatomical units such as the Müllerian, bladder, urogenital sinus compartments as well as the proximal urogenital mesentery. If indicated, the hindgut compartment can be included into the abdominal resection. To integrate the external urogenital sinus compartment, the procedure has to be performed abdominoperineally. Resection of the distal urogenital mesentery—necessary for the surgical treatment of disease fixed to the pelvic walls—mandates the inclusion of the internal iliac vessel system and/or pelvic wall and floor muscles. These procedures are termed Laterally Extended Endopelvic Resection (LEER).

(L)EER reliably achieves R0 resection in patients with locally advanced and recurrent cervicovaginal cancer if tumor fixation at the region of the sciatic foramen and peritoneal spread can be excluded.

Key Points

- Pelvic exenteration designates the en bloc resection of multiple pelvic organs; the time-honored operation is based on functional anatomy.
- Locally extended and recurrent cervicovaginal cancer can be cured with pelvic exenteration.
- A high abortion rate and frequent intralesional tumor resection with traditional exenteration limit the clinical benefit of pelvic exenteration.
- Tumors spread locally in permissive developmental (ontogenetic) compartments.
- Ontogenetic anatomy maps developmental compartments and their subcompartments within distinct body regions. It differs from traditional anatomy which uses structure as a tool to comprehend function.
- Compartment resection based on ontogenetic anatomy defines a new principle of surgical radicality achieving maximum local tumor control at minimum morbidity.
- (Laterally) Extended Endopelvic Resection ((L)EER) extirpates multiple pelvic ontogenetic compartments.
- Various types of (L)EER adjust the procedure to the extent of the disease.
- (L)EER reliably achieves R0 resection in patients with locally advanced and recurrent cervicovaginal cancer.
- LEER controls both central tumors and tumors fixed to the pelvic sidewall except those involving the region of the sciatic foramen.

References

1. Brunschwig A. Complete excision of pelvic viscera for advanced carcinoma. Cancer. 1948;1:177–83.
2. Magrina JF. Types of pelvic exenterations: a reappraisal. Gynecol Oncol. 1990;37:363–6.
3. Salorn EM, Mendez LE, Schey D, Lambrou N, Kassira N, Gomez-Marin O, Averette H, Penalver M. Continent ileocolonic urinary reservoir (Miami pouch): the University of Miami experience over 15 years. Am J Obstet Gynecol. 2004;190:994–1000.
4. Höckel M, Dornhöfer N. Pelvic exenteration for gynaecologic tumours: achievements and unanswered questions. Lancet Oncol. 2006;7:837–47.
5. Schmidt A-M, Imesch P, Fink D, Egger H. Indications and long-term clinical outcomes in 282 patients with pelvic exenteration for advanced or recurrent cervical cancer. Gynecol Oncol. 2012;125:604–9.
6. Höckel M. Cancer permeates locally within ontogenetic compartments: clinical evidence and implications for cancer surgery. Future Oncol. 2012;8:29–36.

7. Höckel M, Horn L-C, Fritsch H. Association between the mesenchymal compartment of uterovaginal organogenesis and local tumour spread in stage IB-IIB cervical carcinoma: a prospective study. Lancet Oncol. 2005;6:751–6.
8. Höckel M, Horn L-C, Manthey N, Braumann U-D, Wolf U, Teichmann G, Frauenschläger K, Dornhöfer N, Einenkel J. Resection of the embryologically defined uterovaginal (Müllerian) compartment and pelvic control in patients with cervical cancer: a prospective analysis. Lancet Oncol. 2009;10:683–92.
9. Höckel M. Laterally extended endopelvic resection: surgical treatment of infrailiac pelvic wall recurrences of gynecologic malignancies. Am J Obstet Gynecol. 1999;180:306–12.
10. Höckel M. Laterally extended endopelvic resection: novel surgical treatment of locally recurrent cervical carcinoma involving the pelvic side wall. Gynecol Oncol. 2003;91:369–77.
11. Höckel M. Laterally extended endopelvic resection (LEER)—principles and practice. Gynecol Oncol. 2008;111:S13–7.
12. Höckel M, Horn L-C, Einenkel J. (Laterally) extended endopelvic resection: surgical treatment of locally advanced and recurrent cancer of the uterine cervix and vagina based on ontogenetic anatomy. Gynecol Oncol. 2012;127:297–302.
13. Sadler TW. Langman's medical embryology. 9th ed. Philadelphia: Lippincott, Williams & Wilkins; 2004.
14. Larsen WJ. Human embryology. 3rd ed. Philadelphia: Churchill Livingstone; 2001.
15. O'Rahilly R, Müller F. Human embryology and teratology. 3rd ed. New York: Wiley-Liss; 2001.
16. Keibel F. Zur Entwicklungsgeschichte des menschlichen Urogenitalapparates. Leipzig: Archiv für Anatomie und Physiologie; 1896. p. 55–156.
17. Van der Putte SCJ. The development of the perineum in the human. In: Advances in anatomy, embryology and cell biology, vol. 177. New York: Springer; 1975.
18. Höckel M, Horn L-C, Tetsch E, Einenkel J. Pattern analysis of regional spread and therapeutic lymph node dissection in cervical cancer based on ontogenetic anatomy. Gynecol Oncol. 2012;125:168–74.
19. Höckel M, Horn L-C, Illig R, Dornhöfer N, Fritsch H. Ontogenetic anatomy of the distal vagina: relevance for local tumor spread and implications for cancer surgery. Gynecol Oncol. 2011;122:313–8.
20. Batourina E, Tsai S, Lambert S, Sprenkle P, Viana R, Dutta S, Hensle T, Wang F, Niederreither K, McMahon AP, Carroll TJ, Medlesohn CL. Apoptosis induced by vitamin A signaling is crucial for connecting the ureters to the bladder. Nat Genet. 2005;37:1082–9.
21. Höckel M, Schmidt K, Bornmann K, Horn L-C, Dornhöfer N. Vulvar field resection: novel approach to the surgical treatment of vulvar cancer based on ontogenetic anatomy. Gynecol Oncol. 2010;119:106–13.
22. Höckel M. Laterally extended endopelvic resection. In: Smith JR, DelPriore G, Coleman PL, Monaghan JM, editors. An atlas of gynecologic oncology investigation and surgery. 3rd ed. London: Informa Medical Books; 2009. p. 120–6.
23. Andikyan V, Khoury-Collado F, Sonoda Y, Gerst SR, Alektyar KM, Sandhu JS, Bochner BH, Barakat RR, Boland PJ, Chi DS. Extended pelvic resections for recurrent or persistent uterine and cervical malignancies: an update on out of the box surgery. Gynecol Oncol. 2012;125:404–8.

Reconstruction in Exenterative Surgery

38

Luis M. Chiva, Fernando Lapuente, Sonsoles Alonso, and Matias Jurado

38.1 Introduction

Exenterative surgery in gynecologic oncology includes a number of surgical procedures necessary to eliminate a primary or recurrent gynecologic tumor that infiltrates the bladder, the rectum or both organs. The classical concept of pelvic exenteration is typically applied to the surgical operation that extirpates recurrent radiated neoplasias, most frequently recurrent cervical cancer [1]. In other circumstances such as advanced ovarian carcinoma invading the rectum or untreated cases of advanced cervical or endometrial tumors, an exenterative procedure might be indicated as the main initial treatment.

Since the original operation was first described by Alexander Brunschwig in 1948 [2], hundreds of cases has been reported in the literature showing the benefit of this surgical approach in selected cases of primary or recurrent gynecologic tumors.

Academically, pelvic exenteration is denominated to every pelvic operation that removes the bladder or the rectum along with the gynecologic neoplasia.

L.M. Chiva, MD, PhD (✉) • F. Lapuente, MD
S. Alonso, MD
Department of Gynecologic Oncology, MD Anderson Cancer Center, Madrid, Spain
e-mail: lchiva@mdanderson.es

M. Jurado
Department of Gynecology, University of Navarre, Pamplona, Spain

Magriña suggested a useful classification to understand the extension of the different types of pelvic exenteration [3]. He categorizes the procedure depending on the removed organs in: anterior, posterior or total exenteration. Regarding the depth of resection he proposes to divide this operation in supra or infralevator exenteration with or without vulvectomy.

During last 60 years of experience with this procedure many surgical modifications have been suggested in order to improve not only the survival but also the quality of life of these patients.

Therefore this chapter will focus on the surgical techniques required to reconstruct the urinary tract, the bowel, as well as sexual function when possible.

38.2 Urinary Reconstruction

The anatomy of the low urinary tract and its close connection with gynecological organs makes it vulnerable to be affected by gynecological tumors or adjuvant local treatment such as pelvic radiation. For this reason, in gynecologic oncology there are different circumstances where the disease involves urinary organs. Typically in such situations, especially if the pelvis has received a complete dose of radiation, a cystectomy must be accomplished along with the tumor (Fig. 38.1a, b).

These oncologic situations include primary advanced gynecological tumors, but more

H.R.H. Patel et al. (eds.), *Pelvic Cancer Surgery: Modern Breakthroughs and Future Advances*,
DOI 10.1007/978-1-4471-4258-4_38, © Springer-Verlag London 2015

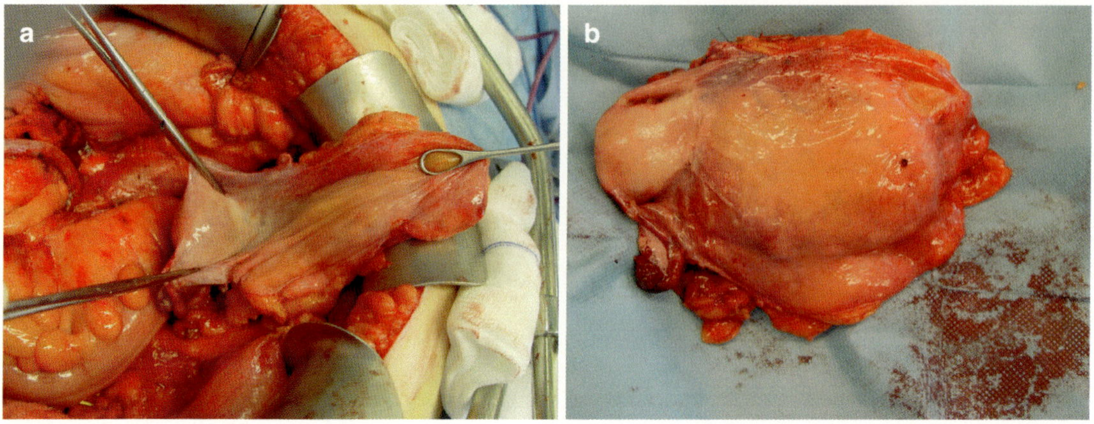

Fig. 38.1 (**a**, **b**) Specimen of anterior exenteration, including the uterus and the bladder

frequently recurrent pelvic disease, in patients who have already received radiation therapy. In those cases, the preservation of healthy bladder tissue to obtain safe oncological and functional results is very complicated. All these patients will need a urinary diversion. Furthermore, sequelae from radiotherapy such as vesicovaginal fistula, patients with disabling urinary incontinence due to contracted bladder and ureteral stricture are also indications for a urinary reconstruction.

In most of these cases a total infralevator pelvic exenteration is required to eliminate the tumor and the entire urethra needs to be removed. Nevertheless, in a select number of patients undergoing pelvic exenteration the urethra may be preserved. These highly selected cases include patients who undergo a supralevator exenteration where the urethra could be free of any tumor involvement. In these patients, we may consider the option of an orthotopic bladder reconstruction, which spares the patient from the need of a urostomy or external appliance, with the consequent improvement in quality of life.

The goals of urinary diversion after cystectomy have evolved from simple diversion and protection of the renal units to a functioning and anatomic reconstitution as close as possible to the physiologic preoperative state.

Initially, first procedures of reconstruction were done diverting the ureters through the rectum or exteriorizing them directly to the skin.

More recently, the evolution of urinary diversion has developed throughout three different routes: incontinent diversion (conduit); continent cutaneous diversion (pouch); and, most recently, continent urinary diversion to the intact native urethra (neobladder, orthotopic reconstruction).

Urinary Diversion via the Rectum

Ureterosigmoidostomy was the initial procedure used to divert the urine. The ureters were implanted in an anti-reflux fashion into the rectosigmoid colon [4]. The result is an output mixture of urine with feces either throughout the rectum or through a wet stoma. Contraindications for urinary diversion via the rectum are renal failure, pathologic conditions of the rectosigmoid colon such as diverticulosis, completed or planned radiotherapy of the pelvis and an incompetent anal sphincter.

The benefits are the avoidance of a stoma, acceptable continence, and the short duration of the procedure.

Complications include stricture of the ureteral anastomosis, periodic ascending urinary tract infections and severe metabolic acidosis. Incontinence is rare but requires conversion to a different type of urinary diversion. This urinary diversion increases the risk of developing an adenocarcinoma at the site of the ureterointestinal anastomosis [5]. For this reason, the follow-up after should include annual colonoscopy. In the daily basis this approach is rarely used in the gynecologic setting since many of the circumstances for urinary diversion are indicated within a radiated field.

Incontinent Diversion

Ureterocutaneostomy

The exteriorization of the ureters through the skin is the simplest form of urinary diversion, which can be done without performing bowel surgery. This maneuver has a high complications rate, especially ureteral stenosis, obliging patients to catheterize the stoma. Indications for ureterocutaneostomy include palliative treatment, serious comorbidities, reduced life expectancy, previous or intended radiotherapy of the intestine, or other conditions of the bowel (ulcerative colitis, Crohn's disease) that require the use of bowel to be avoided [6].

Ileal or Colon Conduit

Since Bricker first described his procedure in 1950, the ileal conduit or Briker's procedure has been for many years the gold standard for urinary diversions after cystectomy for bladder cancer or after exenteration for gynecologic malignancies [7]. The Bricker's ileal conduit is still performed by many cancer surgeons around the world. There is a global perception that the ileal conduit is a safer procedure because of its technical simplicity.

The ileal conduit is still the most commonly used type of urinary diversion (33–63 %). An ileal segment of about 15 cm is detached and laterally brought out as a stoma from the lower abdomen. The ureters are anastomosed into the ileum segment; the urine can flow back into the kidney from the conduit Fig. 38.2a, b. Creating an ileal conduit is technically easier and the procedure takes less time than any other diversion. Furthermore, less of the bowel is resected when an ileal conduit is created. Complications reported in the long term include deterioration in renal function, problems with the stoma, recurring urinary tract infections, ureteral stenosis with development of renal atrophy and calculi. An ileal conduit can be created even in patients with severe renal failure (serum creatinine >2 mg/dL) as well as in those patients who are physically or mentally frail [8].

In specific circumstances when the terminal ileum shows severe post radiation changes, a segment of colon, typically transverse colon can be used as conduit.

Continent Diversion (Pouch)

This form of urinary diversion is a continent alternative to the incontinent conduit. However, it is essential for patients to be intellectually and physically able to catheterize the reservoir. Contraindications include renal failure, liver function disorders, and intestinal disorders.

Usually, a reservoir is created from an ileal or ileocecal segment, which is evacuated by self-catheterization through a permanent stoma. The continence mechanism usually relies on a submucosally surrounded appendix [9], an ileum invagination nipple [10], or a Yang-Monti procedure [11].

Complications that are specific to urinary diversion that should be cited include formation of calculi in the reservoir, voiding injuries of the reservoirs subsequent to stoma stenosis and stenosis of the ureteral anastomosis. Incontinence requiring revision surgery is rare, at <5 % [12]. Since the terminal ileum is used to form the reservoirs, patients may develop metabolic acidosis, as well as vitamin B12 deficiency and chlorogenic diarrhea.

Orthotopic Reconstruction (Neobladder)

The rationale for recommending orthotopic neobladder reconstruction includes the fact that sparing the urethra in selected cases might not compromise the oncologic outcome as evidenced by the literature in patients with bladder cancer.

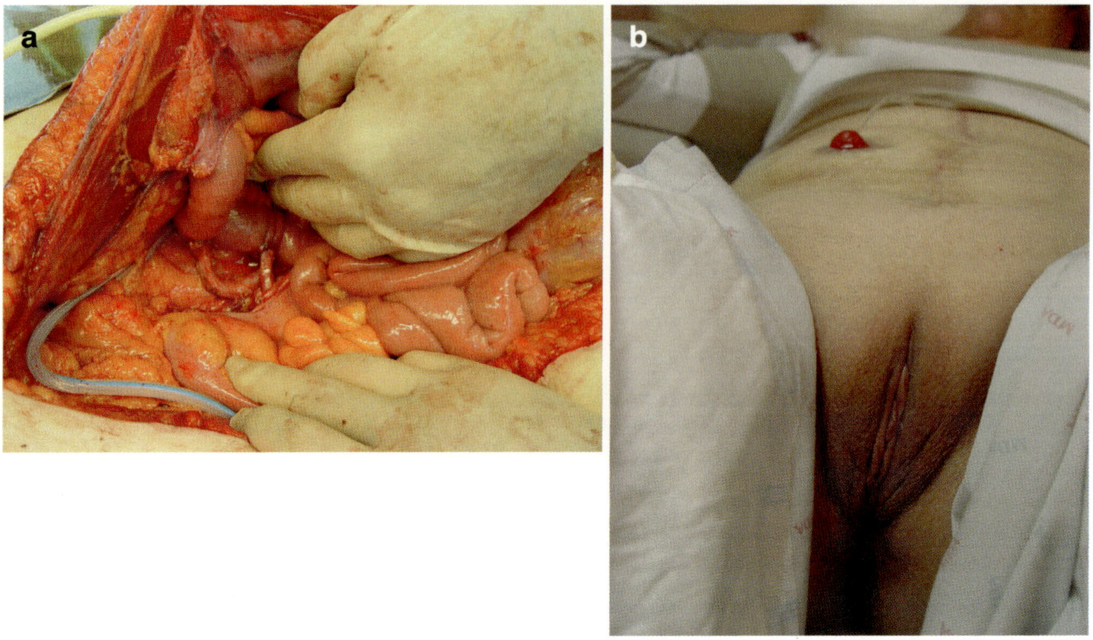

Fig. 38.2 (**a**, **b**) Ileal conduit and urinary stoma

According to a consensus conference on bladder cancer that reviewed the literature on urinary diversion, the orthotopic bladder replacement and continent urinary diversion constituted up to 70 % of all procedures [13]. But this review did not show any superiority of orthotopic neobladder over the other options of transposed intestinal segment surgery in regard of quality of life, and the committee's decision relied heavily on expert opinion and single-institution retrospective series.

The orthotopic bladder reconstruction is associated with an approximately 80 % rate of urinary continence [14, 15].

However there is virtually no experience in developing the urinary neobladder in gynecologic oncology. There are a number of reasons that explain this fact. First, there are only few situations where is possible to preserve the urethra at the time of a pelvic exenteration without compromising the oncological outcome. Second, most of the indications for pelvic exenteration include patients that have been previously radiated and therefore we must expect worse functional and surgical results than in non-irradiated patients.

With orthotopic urinary reconstruction it is possible to achieve a functional lower urinary tract. But this advantage can be counteracting by an increased rate of complications because of the major technical complexity of these operations. For some authors, complication of neobladders are actually similar or lower than the true rates after conduit formation, in contrast to the popular view that conduits are simple and safe [16].

In gynecologic oncology, there is limited experience with orthotopic reconstruction of the bladder. Ungar and Palfalvi published the first large series of gynecological cancer patients with anterior or total pelvic exenteration reconstructed without external urinary diversion [17]. These authors described their experience with a colonic orthotopic neobladder in 13 women who underwent an exenteration after irradiation for cervical cancer, 30 % of patients suffered a fistula formation, and 70 % achieved adequate daytime continence.

Since 2005, our group has acquired some experience in neobladder after pelvic exenteration. We have developed a modified technique of Fontana's reservoir, that is create by performing a

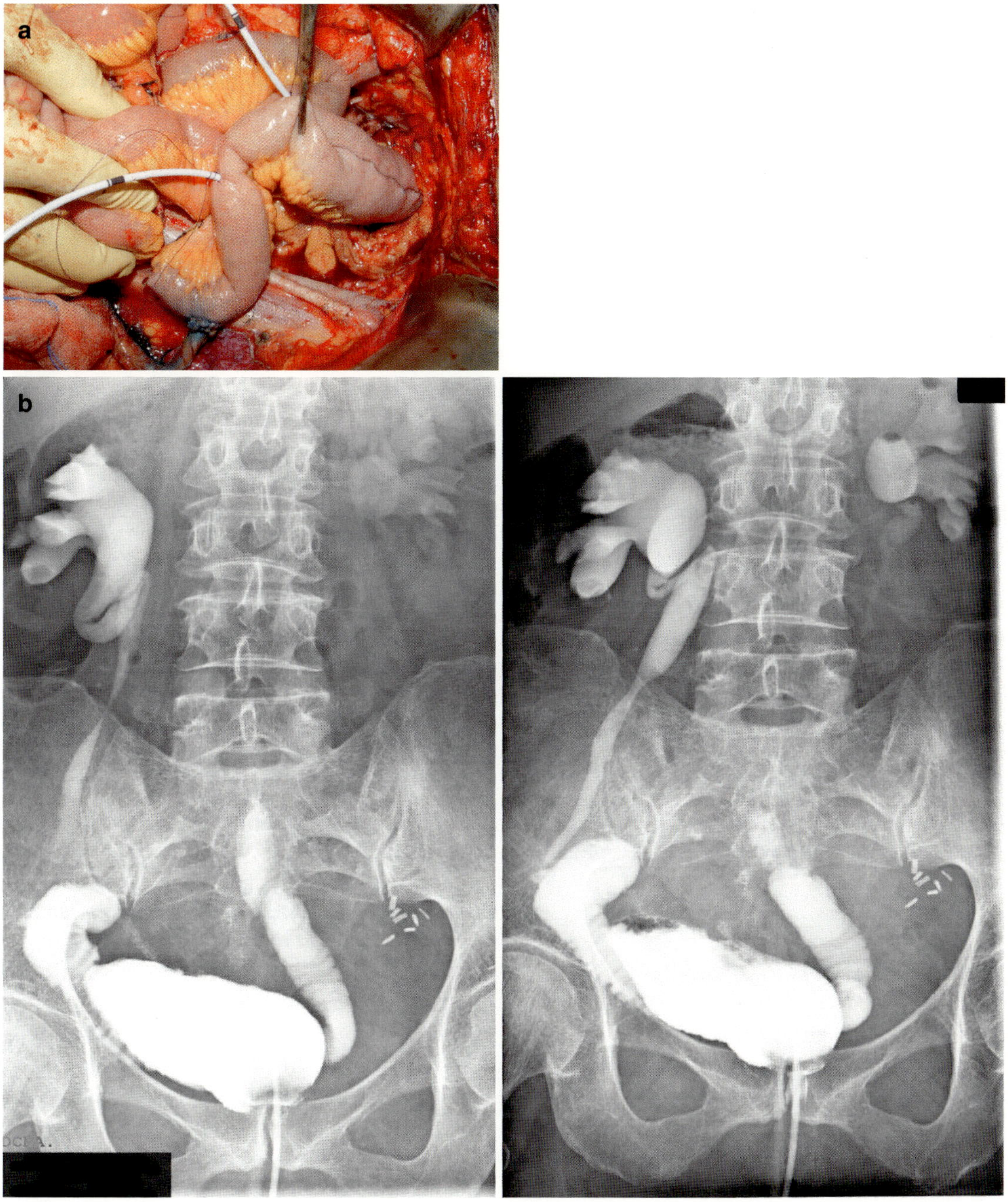

Fig. 38.3 (**a**, **b**) Ileal "Y" shaped orthotopic neobladder and postoperative cystogram

"Y" shaped ileal neobladder connected to the urethra Fig. 38.3a, b. Up to the present time, 14 cases have been accomplished. The rate urinary continence was 60 %, and the rate of fistula formation was 25 % [18].

In summary, nowadays, reconstruction of the urinary tract after pelvic exenteration have allowed many patients to improved their quality of life even after undergoing an incontinent diversion.

38.3 Colorectal Reconstruction

Colorectal resection has become an indispensable tool within the armamentarium of gynecologic oncology surgery. In pelvic exenteration, commonly performed in local recurrence of cervical or endometrial cancer, this procedure is habitually part of the pelvic viscera resection [19, 20]. In ovarian cancer, since the recognition that complete tumor cytoreduction is the best independent prognostic factor for survival, this procedure is performed more often as part of the "en bloc" removal of the pelvic disease [21].

In fact as can be observed in the literature, one out three patients with advanced ovarian cancer needs a colorectal resection to obtain complete exeresis of the tumor [22].

The development of specific devices for mechanical anastomosis have allowed an easier, safer and faster procedure even more important for a low or very low anastomosis that would help for the restoration of the intestinal continuity as well as its natural function, both important in these woman's quality of life. Although colorectal surgeons developed these techniques, it is important to emphasize the specific behavior of gynecologic malignancies and their previous treatments.

Performing the Anastomosis

Care must be taken to ensure that the anterior longitudinal muscle layer of the rectum is included in the anastomosis because it tends to be cut during the dissection and retract distally. It is of particular importance that low rectal anastomosis is performed without tension. This will usually require mobilization of the splenic flexure. Although the anastomosis can be hand sewn or stapled, automatic stapling devices make the procedure easier to perform and are probably superior to the hand-sewn techniques in terms of outcome.

Out of the several techniques described, the most frequently used is the end-to-end anastomosis with the circular stapling device inserted through the anus. The largest circular stapler that will fit the bowel segments should be used because of the proclivity of these anastomoses to develop stenosis (Fig. 38.4a–c).

After completing the anastomosis, it is checked for viability and integrity. First, the tissue donuts around the cartridge shaft are checked for defects. Second, the proximal bowel segment to the anastomosis is occluded, and the anastomosis distended by methylene blue. Water can be placed in the pelvis and air placed via the rectum to check for air leaks. If any leakage is presented, the defect in the staple line is reinforced with some sutures. If the leak is inaccessible for repair, the anastomosis must be redone or a proximal diverting stoma is performed. The anastomosis can be wrapped in an omental pedicle if available but no definitive advantage has been demonstrated.

Other options for rectal anastomoses include the end-to-side EEA, functional end-to-end GIA, and side-to-side GIA with the bowel ends overlapping. It is believed that the end-to side and side-to-side anastomoses have a somewhat better blood supply. Furthermore, the end-to-side and anastomoses and functional end-to-end anastomoses sometimes conform better to the natural curve in the sigmoid colon. Patients with low colorectal anastomosis (less than 7 cm from the anal verge) commonly suffer from frequent stools, urgency, and soiling. The colonic reservoir or J-pouch provides a reservoir when all or most of the rectum has been removed but not all the sigmoid colon [23].

Predisposing patient factors that have been reported to increase the risk for complications from bowel surgery are advanced age, gender, chronic steroid use, diabetes mellitus, arteriosclerosis, chronic inflammatory bowel disease, prior radiation therapy or chemotherapy, extensive adhesions, poor nutrition (low serum albumin), anemia, renal failure, malignancy, bowel obstruction before surgery, sepsis (abscess, peritonitis), surgery duration, number of blood units transfused, and hypotension.

The most important common complications of the bowel surgery are anastomotic leak, stenosis, and hemorrhage [24].

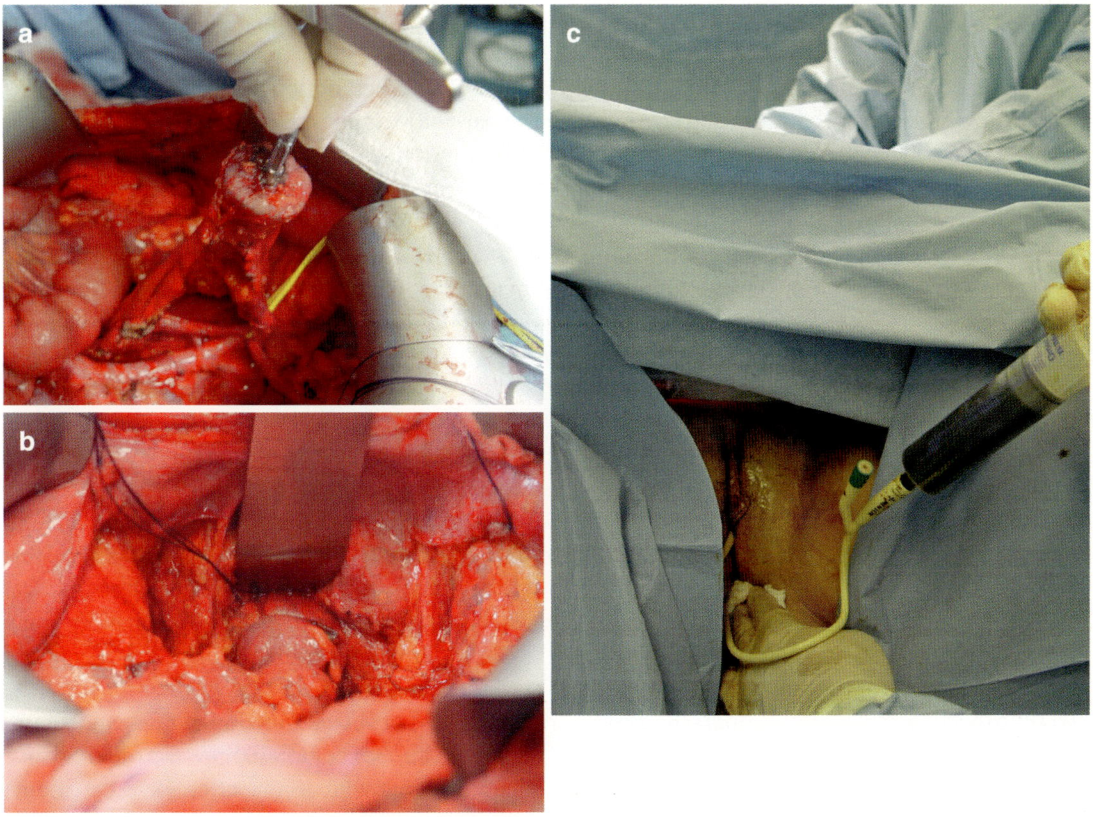

Fig. 38.4 (**a–c**) Colorectal anastomosis: introducing the trocar, firing the device and checking the anastomosis with methylene blue

Technical factors that might be related to the risk for complications include: failure to observe the general principles of bowel surgery (i.e., avoiding tension and ischemia, ensuring good hemostasis, making an adequate-size anastomotic ring, and checking the integrity of the anastomosis; the specific technique of the anastomosis (i.e., stapled or hand sewn, single or double layer) and the bowel involved in the anastomosis (i.e., small bowel, colon or rectum, intraperitoneal or retroperitoneal) [25].

The anastomotic leak frequency reported in the literature varies from 0 to 30 % for clinical leaks and up to 50 % when routine postoperative water-soluble contrast studies have been performed at 10–14 days postoperatively. Leaks may occur from 3 to 45 days postoperatively and the diagnosis is made >30 days after surgery in 12 % of patients [26].

Below 6–7 cm from the anal verge, the incidence of anastomotic leak becomes significantly higher and the more distal the anastomosis is the higher the risk of fistula. The main reasons for this may be related to technical difficulties in accessing the deepest part of the pelvis and the poorer blood supply. Reported rates of anastomotic leak in the gynecologic oncology vary from 2.1 to 53.8 % depending on the type of tumor, with the lowest average rate (2.1 %) for ovarian cancer and the highest (14–53.8 %) when series include cervix, vaginal or uterine cancers, particularly after radiation therapy [20].

Management of anastomotic leak has to be individualized according to morbidity seriousness, comorbidity and features of every patient, and size of dehiscence. According to several authors, conservative treatment could be considered for every patient with general good condition and a small anastomotic defect [27]. Guided drainage of a collection seen on CT scanning can help resolve fever. If fever persists despite guided drainage of a collection, or if vaginal fecal drainage persists for more than 2 weeks, a defunctioning colostomy should be considered.

The role of proximal diversion for preventing anastomotic breakdown has been widely discussed in the literature about colorectal cancer surgery and current data show a benefit (67 % reduction) in terms of clinical anastomotic leak and reoperation reduction. No prospective studies have addressed this issue in gynecologic oncology [28].

In cases with a history of radiotherapy, the evidence is not conclusive but most gastrointestinal surgeons recommend diversion with a low rectal anastomosis [24]. In gynecologic oncology surgery, data on the issue of previous radiotherapy as a risk factor for anastomotic leak are scarce and retrospective, and do not support the systematic use of a proximal diversion [29]. There is no consensus on the best defunctioning procedure, thus a loop ileostomy or a loop colostomy may be used [28].

Pelvic abscess can result from an anastomotic leak, an inadequate preparation with intraoperative spill of feces, or from a post-operative hematoma. Its frequency is not well reported in the literature but may be around 5 %. It is mainly influenced by the presence of anastomotic leak and previous radiotherapy [20].

Anastomotic hemorrhage is not often reported and in colorectal surgery for rectal cancer varies from 0.5 to 1 % after stapled anastomosis. It might be expected in this group because the staples are not hemostatic, but it is not reported to be a problem. This risk is also increased in patients with any impairment of coagulation including antithrombotic prophylaxis [30].

The incidence of stenosis after colorectal anastomosis occurs between 0 and 30 %, but with clinical relevance is not more frequent than 2–3 %. This complication is exceptional in anastomosis proximal to the rectum [31].

38.4 Vaginal Reconstruction

Vaginal and pelvic floor reconstruction is being performed with increasing frequency after pelvic exenteration for cervical cancer. After this ultra radical surgery, the resulting perineal defect is so large, especially in patients who have undergone a total pelvic infralevator exenteration, that many gynecologic oncologists have judged it necessary to fill the defect with well-vascularized tissue. Moreover, after an infralevator total pelvic exenteration, the pelvic floor is frequently exposed and denuded, predisposing it to gastrointestinal fistulas. Several studies have reported that pelvic reconstruction with a vascularized flap decreases complications in patients after pelvic exenteration, compared with patients who do not have this type of reconstruction [32]. Furthermore, radical resection of recurrent gynecologic cancers may involve partial or total resection of the vagina and levator muscles.

The loss of sexual function in this patient population can be demoralizing, especially since many patients with recurrent cervical carcinoma are young. Therefore, reconstructive operations, particularly the creation of a neovagina, are advisable in patients who undergo such extensive extirpative procedures. The effect of vaginal reconstruction on a patient's quality of life and body image has been stressed in numerous publications. A number of surgical techniques have been developed to fill the pelvic hollow and to create a neovagina after radical pelvic surgery. The initial attempts involved omentum or peritoneum stretched over a pelvic mold to allow epithelialization or the use of skin grafting to the omentum and/or peritoneum. McCraw et al. were the first to report vaginal reconstruction using the classic gracilis myocutaneous flap concurrently with radical surgery [33]. Since then, a variety of fasciocutaneous and myocutaneous flaps have been reported for vaginal reconstruction.

The superior rectus abdominis myocutaneous (RAM) flap is probably the most widely used among gynecologic oncologists [34]. The RAM flap, deriving its blood supply from the inferior mammary artery, was first used for breast

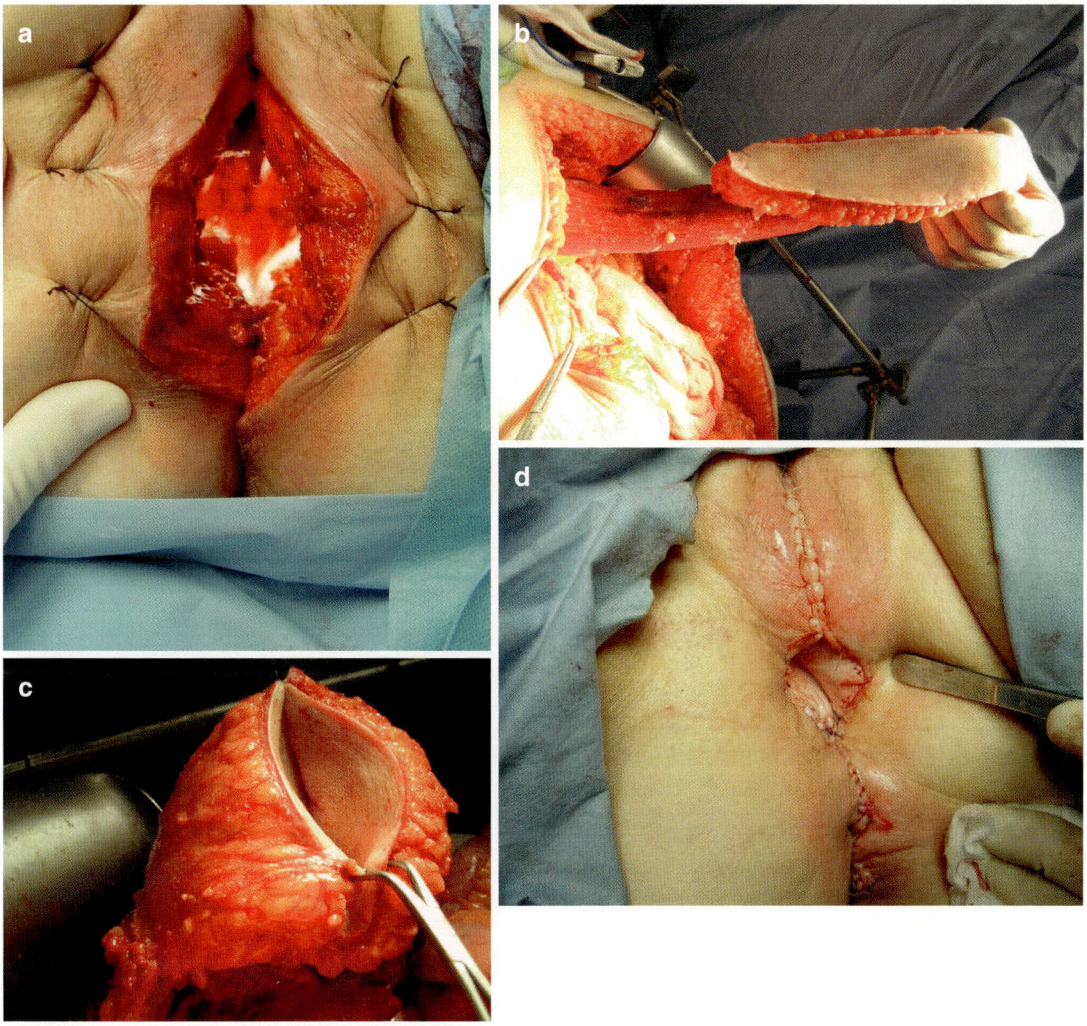

Fig. 38.5 Creation of neovagina with a RAM flap: (**a**) Perineal defect after total infralevator exenteration. (**b**) RAM Flap has been dissected. (**c**) The neovagina is developed. (**d**) Neovagina in situ after final suturing

reconstruction. For vaginal reconstruction, the inferior or distal RAM flap, supplied by the deep inferior epigastric vessels, is optimal. We typically use a modified RAM flap with a longitudinal rotation (instead of the typical transverse rotation); this flap allows us to give the neovagina a very natural shape and fits easily into the perineal defect (Fig. 38.5).

However, the thickness of this flap makes its application difficult when the pelvic defect is not large or when a supralevator exenteration with colorectal anastomosis has been carried out. Techniques such as the Singapore flap are better suited to such cases. This neurovascular pudendal thigh flap was described for vaginal reconstruction by Wee in 1989 and modified by Woods in 1991 [35]. This procedure provides well-vascularized tissue to the area, being thin and flexible and can be inserted easily into the rectovaginal space to seal the repair. This flap's vascular supply is reliable and robust. The Singapore flap has certain advantages over conventional muscle flaps in this situation. It avoids bulkiness while still providing good vascular coverage. In addition, the donor-site morbidity is low, with minimal postoperative scarring. Furthermore, this flap retains the original innervation, so partial sensation is potentially present. It is a good, consistent option for small and medium defects.

Omental Flap

The omental flap or omental carpet provide a non irradiated vascular pedicle flap able to fill a surgical defect, to wrap any anastomosis throughout the abdomen or to provide vascularized tissue surrounding a fistula repair.

Habitually, many indications for pelvic exenteration are for patients in whom the greater omentum has not been removed.

This flap is very versatile and very manageable, and aside from thin patients, it provides a large amount of vascularized tissue that can cover or fill any dead space in the pelvis. This maneuver is important since small bowel loops trend to adhere to the deepest and denudated pelvic areas, resulting in intestinal fistulas.

38.5 Summary

Pelvic recurrence especially after radiation therapy is probably one of the most complicated challenges that a gynecologic oncologist has to face. Since Brunschwig published his preliminary experience with pelvic exenteration, the literature has demonstrated improving understanding of the surgical indications with lower morbidity and mortality rates. In addition, important achievements have been in the reconstructive part of pelvic exenteration. During the last few years, a number of publications have appeared demonstrating different ways to rebuild the urinary tract, to anastomose the colon more safely, and to create a neovagina using very different surgical techniques. In many cases, these efforts have increased patients' quality of life. However, these maneuvers prolong the operating time and may increase postoperative complications.

Key Points

- Pelvic exenteration is currently the only therapeutic approach with reasonable survival, morbidity, and perioperative mortality rates that can be offered to patients with recurrent gynecologic cancer who have undergone irradiation.
- In carefully selected patients, more than 40 % will survive longer than 5 years.
- During the past 60 years, a number of outstanding improvements have been achieved—not only in surgical outcomes, but also in quality of life owing to new reconstructive approaches.
- The incontinent ileal conduit (or Bricker's procedure) remains the gold standard for urinary diversion after anterior exenteration.
- Continent conduits are currently considered feasible and safe and theoretically may improve the quality of life of these patients. Further studies are needed to demonstrate similar long term outcomes to ileal conduits.
- In carefully selected patients where the urethra can be preserved an orthotopic neobladder may be indicated. The patient should be informed of the risks of complications after radiation including high rates of fistulae.
- Colorectal resection is feasible in patients who underwent a pelvic exenteration with sphincter preservation. Since most of them are radiated the expected leakage and fistula rate is high.
- The closer is the anastomosis to the anal verge the higher is the risk of disruption.
- Typically, in radiated patients placing a protecting temporary loop ileostomy must be considered.
- In some patients, creation of a neovagina can be planned. This is especially indicated in those with a total infralevator exenteration where filling the pelvis with a neo-vascularized flap may diminish the rate of complications.

References

1. Chiva LM, Lapuente F, González-Cortijo L, González-Martín A, Rojo A, García JF, Carballo N. Surgical treatment of recurrent cervical cancer: state of the art and new achievements. Gynecol Oncol. 2008;110(3 Suppl 2):S60–6.
2. Brunschwig A. Complete excision of pelvic viscera for advanced carcinoma. Cancer. 1948;1:177.
3. Magrina JF. Types of pelvic exenterations: a reappraisal. Gynecol Oncol. 1990;37:363–6.
4. Tollefson MK, Elliott DS, Zincke H, Frank I. Long-term outcome of ureterosigmoidostomy: an analysis of patients with >10 years of follow-up. BJU Int. 2010;105:860–3.
5. Kalble T, Hofmann I, Riedmiller H, Vergho D. Tumor growth in urinary diversion: a multicenter analysis. Eur Urol. 2011;60:1081–6.
6. Kilciler M, Bedir S, Erdemir F, Zeybek N, Erten K, Ozgok Y. Comparison of ileal conduit and transureteroureterostomy with ureterocutaneostomy urinary diversion. Urol Int. 2006;77(3):245–50.
7. Bricker EM. Bladder substitution after pelvic evisceration. Surg Clin N Am. 1950;30:1511.
8. Hautmann RE, Hautmann SH, Hautmann O. Complications associated with urinary diversion. Nat Rev Urol. 2011;8(12):667–77.
9. Stein JP, Daneshmand S, Dunn M, Garcia M, Lieskovsky G, Skinner DG. Continent right colon reservoir using a cutaneous appendicostomy. Urology. 2004;63:577–80.
10. Salom EM, Mendez LE, Schey D, Lambrou N, Kassira N, Gómez-Marn O, et al. Continent ileocolonic urinary reservoir (Miami pouch): the University of Miami experience over 15 years. Am J Obstet Gynecol. 2004;190:994–1003.
11. Monti PR, Lara RC, Dutra MA, de Carvalho JR. New techniques for construction of efferent conduits based on the Mitrofanoff principle. Urology. 1997;49:112.
12. Urh A, Soliman PT, Schmeler KM, Westin S, Frumovitz M, Nick AM, Fellman B, Urbauer DL, Ramirez PT. Postoperative outcomes after continent versus incontinent urinary diversion at the time of pelvic exenteration for gynecologic malignancies. Gynecol Oncol. 2013;129(3):580–5.
13. Hautmann RE, Abol-Enein H, Hafez K, et al. World Health Organization (WHO) consensus conference on bladder cancer. Urinary diversion. Urology. 2007;69(1 Suppl):17–49. Review.
14. Hautmann RE. 15 years experience with the ileal neobladder: what have we learned? Urologe A. 2001;40:360–7.
15. Stenzl A, Höltl L. Orthotopic bladder reconstruction in women—what we have learned over the last decade. Crit Rev Oncol Hematol. 2003;47(2):147–54.
16. Hautmann RE. Urinary diversion: ileal conduit to neobladder. J Urol. 2003;169:834–42.
17. Ungar L, Palfalvi L. Pelvic exenteration without external urinary or fecal diversion in gynecological cancer patients. Int J Gynecol Cancer. 2006;16:364–8.
18. Chiva LM, Lapuente F, Núñez C, Ramirez PT. Ileal orthotopic neobladder after pelvic exenteration for cervical cancer. Gynecol Oncol. 2009;113:47–51.
19. Hatch KD, Gelder MS, Soong SJ, Baker VV, Shingleton HM. Pelvic exenteration with low rectal anastomosis: survival, complications, and prognostic factors. Gynecol Oncol. 1990;38:462–7.
20. Jurado M, Alcazar JL, Baixauli J, Hernandez-Lizoain JL. Low colorectal anastomosis after pelvic exenteration for gynecologic malignancies risk factors analysis for leakage. Int J Gynecol Cancer. 2011;21:397–402.
21. Bristow RE, Puri I, Chi DS. Cytoreductive surgery for recurrent ovarian cancer: a meta-analysis. Gynecol Oncol. 2009;112(1):265–74.
22. Peiretti M, Bristow RE, Zapardiel I, Gerardi M, Zanagnolo V, Biffi R, Landoni F, Bocciolone L, Aletti GD, Maggioni A. Rectosigmoid resection at the time of primary cytoreduction for advanced ovarian cancer. A multi-center analysis of surgical and oncological outcomes. Gynecol Oncol. 2012; 126(2):220–3.
23. Slieker JC, Daams F, Mulder IM, Jeekel J, Lange JF. Systematic review of the technique of colorectal anastomosis. JAMA Surg. 2013;148(2):190–201.
24. Kingham TP, Pachter HL. Colonic anastomotic leak: risk factors, diagnosis, and treatment. J Am Coll Surg. 2009;208:269–78.
25. Karanjia ND, Corder AP, Bearn P, Heald RJ. Leakage from stapled low anastomosis after total mesorectal excision for carcinoma of the rectum. Br J Surg. 1994;81:1224–6.
26. Vignali A, Fazio VW, Lavery IC, Milsom JW, Church JM, Hull TL, Strong SA, Oakley JR. Factors associated with the occurrence of leaks in stapled rectal anastomoses: a review of 1,014 patients. J Am Coll Surg. 1997;185:105–13.
27. Phitayakorn R, Delaney CP, Reynolds HL, Champagne BJ, Heriot AG, Neary P, Senagore AJ. Standardized algorithms for management of anastomotic leaks and related abdominal and pelvic abscesses after colorectal surgery. International anastomotic leak study group. World J Surg. 2008;32:1147–56.
28. Rondelli F, Reboldi P, Rulli A, Barberini F, Guerrisi A, Izzo L, Bolognese A, Covarelli P, Boselli C, Becattini C, Noya G. Loop ileostomy versus loop colostomy for fecal diversion after colorectal or coloanal anastomosis: a meta-analysis. Int J Color Dis. 2009;24(5):479–88.
29. Berek JS, Howe C, Lagasse LD, Hacker NF. Pelvic exenteration for recurrent gynecologic malignancy: survival and morbidity analysis of the 45-year experience at UCLA. Gynecol Oncol. 2005;99:153–9.
30. Martínez-Serrano MA, Parés D, Pera M, Pascual M, Courtier R, Egea MJ, Grande L. Management of lower gastrointestinal bleeding after colorectal resection and stapled anastomosis. Tech Coloproctology. 2009;13(1):49–53.
31. Bannura GC, Cumsille MA, Barrera AE, Contreras JP, Melo CL, Soto DC. Predictive factors of stenosis after stapled colorectal anastomosis: prospective

analysis of 179 consecutive patients. World J Surg. 2004;28(9):921–5.
32. Jurado M, Bazán A, Alcázar JL, Garcia-Tutor E. Primary vaginal reconstruction at the time of pelvic exenteration for gynecologic cancer: morbidity revisited. Ann Surg Oncol. 2009;16(1):121–7.
33. McCraw JB, Massey FM, Shanklin KD, Horton CE. Vaginal reconstruction with gracilis myocutaneous flaps. Plast Reconstr Surg. 1976;58:176–83.
34. Soper JT, Havrilesky LJ, Secord AA, Berchuck A, Clarke-Pearson DL. Rectus abdominis myocutaneous flaps for neovaginal reconstruction after radical pelvic surgery. Int J Gynecol Cancer. 2005;15: 542–8.
35. Wee JT, Joseph VT. A new technique of vaginal reconstruction using neurovascular pudendal-thigh flaps: a preliminary report. Plast Reconstr Surg. 1989;83:701–9.

Treatment of Early Ovarian Cancer

39

Francesco Raspagliesi, Antonino Ditto, Fabio Martinelli, and Domenica Lorusso

39.1 Introduction

Ovarian cancer is the second most common gynecologic malignancy and the most common cause of death among women with gynecologic cancer [1]. Lifetime risk is about 1.6 %, but women with affected first-degree relatives have a 5 % risk. Women with a mutated BRCA1 or BRCA2 gene carry a risk between 25 and 60 % depending on the specific mutation [2].

Epithelial ovarian cancer kills more women than all other gynecologic malignancies combined because of our inability to detect early-stage disease. Unfortunately, attempts to develop screening programs for epithelial ovarian cancer using pelvic imaging or tumor markers have not yet been successful [3].

Early stages of the disease are potentially curable. In early epithelial ovarian cancer (eEOC) the 5-years survival ranges from 50 to 95 %. These wide ranges are due to the heterogeneity of the literature data, which are based on small series, with different procedures of staging and different postsurgical treatments [4–7].

In spite of the generally favorable outcome of eEOC there is considerable 20–50 % risk of recurrence. The largest retrospective study in stage I epithelial ovarian cancer, which included a total of 1,545 women, concluded that the most important independent prognostic factors were degree of differentiation followed by rupture before surgery, rupture during surgery, FIGO substage IB versus IA, and age [8]. According to these prognostic factors patients are divided into risk groups [9]. The excellent prognosis of patients with low-risk stage IA grade 1 tumor treated with complete surgery alone is widely recognized [10]: they have a very good prognosis with approximately 95 % 5-year OS [11] and do not need any adjuvant treatment. Many centers include stage IB grade 1 tumors in this low risk group [12].

F. Raspagliesi, MD (✉) • A. Ditto, MD
F. Martinelli, MD • D. Lorusso, MD
Department of Gynecologic Oncology,
National Cancer Institute of Milan, Milan, Italy
e-mail: francesco.raspagliesi@istitutotumori.mi.it

39.2 Surgical Treatment of Early Stage Ovarian Cancer

FIGO surgical stage is the most relevant prognostic factor for disease free and overall survival of apparent eEOC patients. A thorough surgical staging is crucial to address appropriate treatment and guarantee optimal survival. Comprehensive surgical staging consisting in extrafascial hysterectomy, bilateral adhenaxectomy, omentectomy, random multiple biopsy, multiple site peritoneal washing and para-aortic and pelvic lymph node dissection. Less extensive surgical procedures may fail to detect the exact spread of the disease. Several papers reported on the risk of unrecognized occult disease, with a 30 % likelihood of upstaging on repeated surgery [13, 14]. The

H.R.H. Patel et al. (eds.), *Pelvic Cancer Surgery: Modern Breakthroughs and Future Advances*,
DOI 10.1007/978-1-4471-4258-4_39, © Springer-Verlag London 2015

results of the literature showed that re-staging, detects either the patients who need chemotherapy and/or who can be proposed for surgery only. The mini-invasive techniques seems to be an acceptable and safe procedure to perform restaging of eEOC [15].

Lymph node evaluation is recommend in the surgical treatment of eEOC according to FIGO criteria; however, the radicality of the lymphadenectomy remains unclear [16, 17]. Literature data reported nodal involvement in 4–25 % of patients with tumor apparently confined to the ovaries. Evaluating only data from systematic lymph node dissection, the mean rate of retroperitoneal metastases was 16 % ranging from 13 to 25 % [18–25]. The data of a prospective study [26] are similar to those reported by other single institution series and comparable to those reported in a recent literature review by Kleppe [27, 28]. Fourteen studies were included in this analysis reporting a mean incidence of lymph node metastases in clinical stages I–II EOC of 14.2 % (range 6.1–29.6 %), of which 46.9 % only in the para-aortic basin, 23.2 % only in the pelvic basin, and 29.9 % both in the para-aortic and pelvic region. An higher node positivity rate (22 %) was reported in the systematic lymphadenectomy arm of an Italian randomized study [29]. Literature data reported that serous carcinoma is characterized by the highest incidence of node metastases [30], endometrioid, clear cell, and undifferentiated tumors behave similarly [30] while no lymph node metastases were found in mucinous histotype in literature data independently of grading [31]. Concerning the grading of cancer, several studies have reported node metastases in more than 30 % of Grade 3 patients with eEOC [29].

Lymph node evaluation should always be integrated in comprehensive staging of eEOC because in patients with lymph node metastases, the systematic lymphadenectomy has a prognostic and potentially therapeutic role. In addition, an upstaging warrants adjuvant treatments, while a thorough surgical staging could avoid any further medical treatment, according to the ICON-ACTION trial [6, 31, 32].

Considering the very good prognosis following an adequate surgical staging in eEOC, the Fertility-sparing surgery (FSS) for women of childbearing age has become an argument of debate in the last decades. Twenty-five percent of EOCs are diagnosed in early stages. About 14 % of those early stage patients are under the age of 40 at the time of diagnosis, about half of which are FIGO stage I. These women are potentially interested in preserving their fertility [33–35].

Literature data, even if based on retrospective series, confirm the likelihood to consider conservative surgery for eEOC in young patients [36–38]. However, there is still a lack of consensus about the selection criteria to deem patients suitable for FSS. Some authors [39] use restrictive criteria, for example IAG1–2 FIGO stage, to admit patients to FSS, while others [11, 40] consider all stage I EOC patients eligible for conservative treatment. More controversial is whether or not to address patients with high risk EOC (≥IA G3) for FSS.

Data on obstetrical outcome showed encouraging results (Table 39.1). Because patients undergone to FSS, not always attempt to conceive, the selection criteria have to be very restrictive and the patients should be thoroughly counseled and highly motivated. A large study has been reported by Japanese GOG [37] on a total of 211 patients (stage IA, n 126; stage IC, n 85) from 30 institutions underwent FSS. Authors concluded that FSS is a safe treatment for stage IA patients with favorable histology. They suggest, also, that stage IA patients with clear cell histology and stage IC patients with favorable histology can be candidates for fertility-sparing surgery followed by adjuvant chemotherapy. Another study based on SEER data [6] evaluated 1,186 women aged 50 years with stage IA or IC EOC, of which 754 (64 %) underwent radical treatment with bilateral salpingo-oophorectomy, and 432 (36 %) underwent FSS. The comparison of data revealed that the FSS was safe in young women who had stage IA and IC EOC. Recently, a large Italian retrospective study [38] evaluated 240 patients with malignant eEOC treated with FSS. At a median follow-up of 9 years, 27 patients had relapsed (11 %) and 11 (5 %) had died of progressive disease. Multivariate analysis found only grade 3 negatively affected the

Table 39.1 Obstetrical outcome, literature review

Author	Nr. patients	Nr.of pts having pregnancies	Nr. of pts with term deliveries	Nr. of pts with abortion
Colombo [66]	24	7	6	–
Zanetta [65]	56	20	17 babies	4 (2 ectopic preg)
Raspagliesi [40]	10	3	3	–
Morice [39]	34	9 (10 preg)	7	1
Colombo [66]	24	7	6	–
Park [34]	62	–	22	2
Anchezar [67]	18	6 (7 preg)	6	–
Kajiyama [68]	60	13	10	3
Satoh [37]	211	55 (76 preg)	53 (66 babies)	
Fruscio [38]	240	84	68 (93 babies)	16
Ditto [26]	18	7	5 (5 babies)	2

More recent case series may include previously published data from the same group

prognosis of patients. Of the 105 patients (45 %) who tried to become pregnant, 84 (80 %) were successful. The authors concluded that conservative treatment can be proposed to all young patients when tumor is limited to the ovaries, as ovarian recurrences can always be managed successfully. Patients with G3 tumors are more likely to have distant recurrences and should be closely monitored.

In literature, there are many retrospective data and three large studies designed to investigate the role of FSS have confirmed the safety of FSS in a select group of young patients with eEOC. According to literature data, a conservative surgery should be considered in the treatment of young women with stage IA, grade 1 and 2. FSS in clear cell cancer and high risk patient with FIGO stage ≥IA G3 is still under debate. Anyway, an accurate surgical staging, including pelvic and para-aortic lymphadenectomy, is mandatory in this subset of patients.

39.3 Adjuvant Chemotherapy

The optimal adjuvant therapy for intermediate risk group (FIGO stage IA G2, IB and IC G1) and high-risk group (FIGO stage IAG3, IB G2-G3, IC G2-G3 and clear cell) had not yet been established until 2003 when solid scientific proof of the clinical effectiveness of adjuvant chemotherapy was provided. In 2003, in fact, two large prospective randomized trial (ICON 1 and ACTION) and two meta-analyses including five trials [41] on 1,234 patients addressing the positive role of adjuvant chemotherapy (AC) in reducing the risk of progression and death in eEOC were published. Until that no studies in eEOC had shown the effect, if any, of adjuvant treatment (using either radiotherapy or chemotherapy) but all the trials have insufficient power to detect any difference between treatments because too few patients were randomly assigned and insufficient surgical staging was performed [42–44].

ICON1 [45] was a pragmatic trial in which 477 women with FIGO stage I–II ovarian cancer for which clinicians had some uncertainty of the need of adjuvant chemotherapy (AC) were randomized to receive adjuvant platinum-based chemotherapy or observation. Recommended surgical staging was less stringent than in the ACTION trial [5], with the minimum requirement being the removal of all visible disease. The majority of women in the treatment group (87 %) received carboplatin AUC 5 for six cycles. The authors reported a significant benefit for chemotherapy in terms of both OS (Hazard Ratio, HR 0.66) and PFS (HR 0.65). Update results after 9.2 years follow up confirmed survival advantage for chemotherapy treated patients (72 % vs 64 %; HR 0.74) [46]. The trial also reported the results of a sub group analysis on the effect of AC by level of risk: among the high- risk women (IA G3, IB or IC G2 or G3, clear cell), those who received AC had significantly better OS and RFS than those who did not receive chemotherapy (HR 0.48 and HR 0.52 respectively), whereas among low/medium- risk women (IA G1 and G2, IB or IC G1) there was no significant difference in survival outcomes between treatment arms (HR 0.96 and HR 0.96 respectively). Given that the analysis were not pre-planned and the number of patients in each sub group not provided, these results must be evaluated with caution and need to be confirmed.

ACTION [5] was a RCT run by the European Organization for Research and Treatment of Cancer (EORTC) which recruited 448 FIGO stage IA and IB G2-G3, all stage IC and stage IIA women. Surgical staging procedures were specified and recommended, nevertheless only 34 % of patients received optimal surgical staging. Patients were randomized to receive platinum based chemotherapy (47 % had cisplatin in combination with cyclophosphamide and 33 % had single-agent carboplatin) for at least four cycles versus no further treatment. The authors reported a significant benefit of chemotherapy in terms of RFS (HR 0.63) and a non significant benefit in terms of OS (HR 0.69). In a preplanned sub group analysis the effect of AC with respect to surgical staging adequacy was evaluated: among the 295 sub-optimally staged women, those who received adjuvant chemotherapy had significantly better OS and RFS than those who did not, whereas among the 151 optimally staged women, there was no significant difference in survival outcomes. A similar phenomenon was seen for RFS. Moreover in the suboptimally staged patients, the salvage rates at the time of recurrence in the observation arm and the AC arm were super imposable, whereas in the optimally staged patients, salvage chemotherapy treatment at the time of recurrence did well in the observation arm than in the AC arm. Although the number of patients involved in this sub group analysis was small, it is of interest that the same difference in the effectiveness of salvage chemotherapy treatment in optimally staged patients not receiving AC was found in the Bolis trial [43]. However we should consider that ACTION trial was not designed to compare different surgical staging procedures, nor were women prospectively stratified by these categories; in addition, the number of participants in the 'optimally staged' subgroup was small and the number of events even lesser (18 events) so that some benefit of AC in optimally staged disease cannot be excluded. For this reason, almost all the authors support the practice of offering adjuvant chemotherapy to optimally staged women, who have other risk factors coming from histology [47]. Moreover, given that even inside a randomized controlled clinical trial with recommended staging procedures only one third of patients received optimal staging, it appears reasonable to consider that suboptimally staged patients represent the "real word" and the results of these two trial may be applied to all eEOC patients.

Since the two largest ICON 1 and ACTION trial were conducted in parallel and spanned the same 10 years period, their results were matched. The analysis of the combined trials [48], on 925 patients, showed better OS for patients in the AC arm than for patients in the observation arm (82 % versus 74 %, respectively). RFS was also better for patients in the AC arm (76 % versus 65 %, respectively). A systematic review of 5 RCTs, enrolling 1,277 women, was published and subsequently updated [41, 47]: meta-analysis of three trials, assessing 1,008 women, indicated that women who received adjuvant platinum-based chemotherapy had better OS than those who did not (HR 0.71); meta-analysis of four trials, on 1,170 women, indicated that women who received AC had better PFS than those who did not (HR 0.67). This review would seem the definitive proof of the benefit of platinum based AC for all patient with intermediate and high risk eEOC, but unfortunately many questions need to be answered.

Type of Chemotherapy

Although only 6 % of women in the combined analysis of ICON-ACTION trials received taxanes, given the reported activity of paclitaxel in advanced ovarian cancer, the benefit of taxane treatments have been translated in early stage disease. At least three retrospective trials comparing platinum monotherapy vs platinum paclitaxel combination in eEOC [49–51] did not report any significant advantage in terms of recurrence and death rate for the combination treatment at the prize of higher toxicity. All the trials have however several limitations: they are retrospective in nature, account very limited numbers of patients, and surgical staging was incomplete for most part of patients. In the light of these considerations, according to the recently published conclusions of the 4th Ovarian Cancer Consensus Conference [52], Carboplatin-Paclitaxel remains the standard of care also for early stage disease. Carboplatin monotherapy is an attractive alternative for patients with poor performance status and, probably, for intermediate risk disease.

Duration of Treatment

The optimal duration of AC in eEOC is unclear: the ACTION and ICON trials used four and six courses of platinum based chemotherapy respectively, leading to the same conclusions on the benefit of treatment. In order to better clarify the appropriate number of chemotherapy courses GOG carried out GOG 157 trial [53] on 427 EOC patients (69 % stage I) comparing three versus six cycles of platinum-paclitaxel chemotherapy. The toxicities from treatment were statistically significantly higher in the six-cycle arm and also less patients complete treatment in the six cycles arm (83 % vs 96 % respectively). The recurrence rate after six cycles was 24 % non statistically significant lower (HR 0.761) than that after three cycles, and also the overall death rate was similar for both arms (HR 1.02). The authors concluded that three cycles of carboplatin-paclitaxel chemotherapy could be considered an appropriate treatment for eEOC. An explorative non pre-planned sub-group analysis of GOG 157 [54] reported that serous tumors showed a significantly decreased risk of recurrence after six cycles of chemotherapy compared to three cycles (HR 0.33), while the benefit of 3 additional chemotherapy courses disappeared in non serous tumors.

Mannel et al. [55] recently published the results of a GOG RCT comparing three cycles of Carboplatin-Paclitaxel followed by either maintenance paclitaxel at 40 mg/m^2/week × 24 weeks or observation in a population of 542 eEOC patients. The authors reported no difference in terms of RFS (HR 0.807) or OS between the two treatment arms.

Perspectives

According to Winter-Roach et al. [47] between 9 and 100 women have to be treated with AC to prevent one death and between 7 and 33 women have to be treated with AC to prevent one disease recurrence. The real goal for the future should be to identify patients who can be spared unnecessary AC. A high priority for upcoming studies will be to use molecular markers, gene expression and microarray profiles [56], DNA ploidy [57] or serum protein patterns [58] to further separate poor from good prognosis early stage patients who do not require additional therapy. In this context, retrospective and prospective studies on DNA ploidy in stage I disease [57, 59–61] have shown that ploidy is the second most important independent prognostic factor after degree of differentiation so that some authors propone to include diploid FIGO stage IA G2 tumors inside the low risk subgroup of EOC [62].

Given the apparent lack of efficacy of contemporary adjuvant chemotherapy in clear cell carcinoma [63] and the discouraging bad prognosis of subsets of high grade serous tumor which recur and die despite optimal AC, other therapeutic options are urgently needed. ICON7 trial [64] is a RTC in 1,528 patients with high-risk, early-stage (FIGO stage I or IIA clear cell or grade 3 carcinoma) or advanced-stage epithelial ovarian carcinoma, evaluating the addition of anti VEGF monoclonal antibody bevacizumab to standard chemotherapy in combination and in maintenance for 12 months. The trial reported a significant increase of PFS for the experimental arm (HR 0.87); no different impact of the addition of Bevacizumab treatment with respect to FIGO stage appeared at exploratory analysis.

39.4 Summary

Comprehensive surgical staging with para-aortic and pelvic lymph node dissection is mandatory in eEOC. A group of patients with eEOC and no other risk factors will not benefit from further treatment if fully staged, while those with undetected metastases risk to be undertreated if not surgically evaluated. However, a tailored approach should always be kept in mind; based on literature data, omitting a systematic lymphadenectomy can be considered in mucinous tumors regardless of grade.

The Literature data demonstrate the feasibility of FSS in eEOC. FSS in eEOC underwent comprehensive surgical staging is safe with oncological results comparable to radical surgery group. The opportunity to extent the indication to conservative surgery to women with more advanced disease is highly controversial and needs further investigations. Clearer data are warranted by prospective controlled studies.

In spite of the generally favorable outcome of early stage disease there is considerable 20–50 % risk of recurrence.

Platinum-based adjuvant chemotherapy has reported to increase progression-free and overall survival in intermediate risk and high-risk ovarian cancer patients.

A high priority for upcoming studies will be to use molecular markers, gene expression and microarray profiles, to further separate poor from good prognosis early stage patients who do not require additional therapy.

Key Points

- The exact cause of ovarian cancer remains unknown.
- Ovarian cancer is the second most common gynecologic malignancy and the most common cause of death among women with gynecologic cancer.
- Lifetime risk is about 1.6 %, but women with affected first-degree relatives have a 5 % risk. Women with a mutated BRCA1 or BRCA2 gene carry a risk between 25 and 60 % depending on the specific mutation.
- Comprehensive staging is mandatory in the treatment of early epithelial ovarian cancer
- Lymphadenectomy is indicated even if not based on high level evidence of medicine
- Re-staging is indicated even if not based on high level evidence of medicine. Laparoscopic approach should be addressed.
- Fertility-sparing surgery is a safe treatment for stage IA patients with favorable histology. Stage IA patients with clear cell histology and stage IC patients with favorable histology can be candidates for fertility-sparing surgery followed by adjuvant chemotherapy.
- Patients with low-risk stage IA grade 1 tumor do not need adjuvant treatment.
- Platinum-based adjuvant chemotherapy has reported to increase progression-free and overall survival in intermediate and high-risk ovarian cancer patients.
- The real goal for the future should be to identify patients who can be spared unnecessary adjuvant chemotherapy: molecular biology, gene expression and microarray profiles may help in this selection

References

1. Lowe KA, Chia VM, Taylor A, et al. An international assessment of ovarian cancer incidence and mortality. Gynecol Oncol. 2013;130(1):107–14. doi:10.1016/j.ygyn0.2013.03.026. Epub 2013 Apr 2.
2. Mavaddat N, Peock S, Frost D, et al. Cancer risks for BRCA1 and BRCA2 mutation carriers: results from prospective analysis of EMBRACE. J Natl Cancer Inst. 2013;105(11):812–22. Epub 2013 Apr 29.
3. Reade CJ, Riva JJ, Busse JW, Goldsmith CH, Elit L. Risks and benefits of screening asymptomatic women for ovarian cancer: a systematic review and meta-analysis. Gynecol Oncol. 2013. doi:10.1016/j.ygyn0.2013.06.029.
4. Heintz AP, Odicino F, Maisonneuve P, Beller U, Benedet JL, Creasman WT, Ngan HY, Pecorelli S. Carcinoma of the ovary. Int J Gynaecol Obstet. 2003;83 Suppl 1:135–66.

5. Trimbos JB, Vergote I, Bolis G, Vermorken JB, Mangioni C, Madronal C, Franchi M, Tateo S, Zanetta G, Scarfone G, Giurgea L, Timmers P, Coens C, Pecorelli S, EORTC-ACTION collaborators. European Organisation for Research and Treatment of Cancer-Adjuvant ChemoTherapy in Ovarian Neoplasm. Impact of adjuvant chemotherapy and surgical staging in early-stage ovarian carcinoma: European Organisation for Research and Treatment of Cancer-Adjuvant ChemoTherapy in Ovarian Neoplasm trial. J Natl Cancer Inst. 2003;95(2): 113–25.
6. Trimbos B, Timmers P, Pecorelli S, Coens C, Ven K, van der Burg M, Casado A. Surgical staging and treatment of early ovarian cancer: long-term analysis from a randomized trial. J Natl Cancer Inst. 2010;102(13): 982–7.
7. Cancer Facts & Figure 2013. http://www.cancer.org/acs/groups/content/@epidemiologysurveilance/documents/document/acspc-036845.pdf.
8. Vergote I, De Brabanter J, Fyles A, Bertelsen K, Einhorn N, Selvelda P, et al. Prognostic importance of degree of differentiation and cyst rupture in stage 1 invasive epithelial carcinoma. Lancet. 2001;357:176–82.
9. Vergote I, Amant F. Time to include high-risk early ovarian cancer in randomized phase III trials of advanced ovarian cancer. Gynecol Oncol. 2006;102: 415–7.
10. Ozols RF. Chemotherapy for ovarian cancer. Semin Oncol. 1999;26(6 suppl 18):34–40.
11. Schilder JM, Thompson AM, DePriest PD, Ueland FR, Cibull ML, Kryscio RJ, Modesitt SC, Lu KH, Geisler JP, Higgins RV, Magtibay PM, Cohn DE, Powell MA, Chu C, Stehman FB, van Nagell J. Outcome of reproductive age women with stage IA or IC invasive epithelial ovarian cancer treated with fertility-sparing therapy. Gynecol Oncol. 2002;87(1): 1–7.
12. Kobel M, Kalloger SE, Santos JL, et al. Tumor type and sub stage survival in stage I and II ovarian carcinoma: insights and implications. Gynecol Oncol. 2010;116:50–6.
13. Young RC, Decker DG, Wharton JT, et al. Staging laparotomy in early ovarian cancer. JAMA. 1983; 250(22):3072–6.
14. Di Re F, Baiocchi G. Value of lymph node assessment in ovarian cancer: status of the art at the end of the second millennium. Int J Gynecol Cancer. 2000; 10(6):435–42.
15. Leblanc E, Querleu D, Narducci F, Occelli B, Papageorgiou T, Sonoda Y. Laparoscopic restaging of early stage invasive adnexal tumors: a 10-year experience. Gynecol Oncol. 2004;94(3):624–9.
16. Bergman F. Carcinoma of the ovary. A clinicopathological study of 86 autopsied cases with special reference to mode of spread. Acta Obstet Gynecol Scand. 1966;45(2):211–31.
17. Di Re F, Fontanelli R, Raspagliesi F, di Re E. Pelvic and para-aortic lymphadenectomy in cancer of the ovary. In: Burghardt E, Monaghan JM, editors. Bailliere's clinical obstetrics and gynecology, vol. 3. Philadelphia: Saunders; 1989. p. 131–42. No. 1.
18. Knapp RC, Friedman EA. Aortic lymph node metastases in early ovarian cancer. Am J Obstet Gynecol. 1974;119:1013–7.
19. Chen SS, Lee L. Incidence of para-aortic and pelvic node metastases in epithelial carcinoma of the ovary. Gynecol Oncol. 1983;16:95–100.
20. Pickel H, Lahousen M, Stettner H, Girardi F. The spread of ovarian cancer. In: Burghardt E, Monaghan JM, editors. Clinical obstetrics and gynecology, vol. 3. London: Bailliere Tindall; 1989. p. 3–12.
21. Burghardt E, Girardi F, Lahousen M, Tamussino K, Stettner H. Patterns of pelvic and paraaortic lymph node involvement in ovarian cancer. Gynecol Oncol. 1991;40:103–6.
22. Benedetti-Panici P, Greggi S, Maneschi F, et al. Anatomical and pathological study of retroperitoneal nodes in epithelial ovarian cancer. Gynecol Oncol. 1993;51:150–4.
23. Petru E, Lahousen M, Tamussino K, et al. Lymphadenectomy in stage I ovarian cancer. Am J Obstet Gynecol. 1994;170:656–62.
24. Onda T, Yoshikawa H, Yokota H, Yasugi T, Taketani Y. Assessment of metastases to aortic and pelvic lymph nodes in epithelial ovarian carcinoma. Cancer. 1996;78:803–8.
25. Carnino F, Fuda G, Ciccone G, et al. Significance of lymph node sampling in epithelial carcinoma of the ovary. Gynecol Oncol. 1997;65:467–72.
26. Ditto A, Martinelli F, Reato C, Kusamura S, Solima E, Fontanelli R, Haeusler E, Raspagliesi F. Systematic para-aortic and pelvic lymphadenectomy in early stage epithelial ovarian cancer: a prospective study. Ann Surg Oncol. 2012;19(12):3849–55. doi:10.1245/s10434–012–2439–7. Epub 2012 Jun 16.
27. Powless CA, Aletti GD, Bakkum-Gamez JN, Cliby WA. Risk factors for lymph node metastasis in apparent early-stage epithelial ovarian cancer: implications for surgical staging. Gynecol Oncol. 2011;122(3): 536–40.
28. Kleppe M, Wang T, Van Gorp T, Slangen BF, Kruse AJ, Kruitwagen RF. Lymph node metastasis in stages I and II ovarian cancer: a review. Gynecol Oncol. 2011;123(3):610–4.
29. Maggioni A, Benedetti Panici P, Dell'Anna T, et al. Randomised study of systematic lymphadenectomy in patients with epithelial ovarian cancer macroscopically confined to the pelvis. Br J Cancer. 2006;95(6): 699–704.
30. Schmeler KM, Tao X, Frumovitz M, Deavers MT, Sun CC, Sood AK, Brown J, Gershenson DM, Ramirez PT. Prevalence of lymph node metastasis in primary mucinous carcinoma of the ovary. Obstet Gynecol. 2010;116(2 Pt 1):269–73.
31. Chan J, Fuh K, Shin J, et al. The treatment and outcomes of early-stage epithelial ovarian cancer: have we made any progress? Br J Cancer. 2008;98(7): 1191–6.

32. Trimbos JB, Vergote I, Bolis G, EORTC-ACTION collaborators. European Organisation for Research and Treatment of Cancer-Adjuvant ChemoTherapy in Ovarian Neoplasm, et al. Impact of adjuvant chemotherapy and surgical staging in early-stage ovarian carcinoma: European Organisation for Research and Treatment of Cancer-Adjuvant ChemoTherapy in Ovarian Neoplasm trial. Natl Cancer Inst. 2003;95(2):113–25.
33. Duska LR, Chang YC, Flynn CE, Chen AH, Goodman A, Fuller AF, Nikrui N. Epithelial ovarian carcinoma in the reproductive age group. Cancer. 1999; 85(12):2623–9.
34. Park JY, Kim DY, Suh DS, Kim JH, Kim YM, Kim YT, Nam JH. Outcomes of fertility-sparing surgery for invasive epithelial ovarian cancer: oncologic safety and reproductive outcomes. Gynecol Oncol. 2008;110(3):345–53.
35. McHale MT, DiSaia PJ. Fertility-sparing treatment of patients with ovarian cancer. Compr Ther. 1999; 25(3):144–50.
36. Wright JD, Shah M, Mathew L, Burke WM, Culhane J, Goldman N, Schiff PB, Herzog TJ. Fertility preservation in young women with epithelial ovarian cancer. Cancer. 2009;115(18):4118–26.
37. Satoh T, Hatae M, Watanabe Y, Yaegashi N, Ishiko O, Kodama S, Yamaguchi S, Ochiai K, Takano M, Yokota H, Kawakami Y, Nishimura S, Ogishima D, Nakagawa S, Kobayashi H, Shiozawa T, Nakanishi T, Kamura T, Konishi I, Yoshikawa H. Outcomes of fertility-sparing surgery for stage I epithelial ovarian cancer: a proposal for patient selection. J Clin Oncol. 2010;28(10):1727–32.
38. Fruscio R, Corso S, Ceppi L, Garavaglia D, Garbi A, Floriani I, Franchi D, Cantù MG, Bonazzi CM, Milani R, Mangioni C, Colombo N. Conservative management of early-stage epithelial ovarian cancer: results of a large retrospective series. Ann Oncol. 2013; 24(1):138–44.
39. Morice P, Leblanc E, Rey A, Baron M, Querleu D, Blanchot J, Duvillard P, Lhommé C, Castaigne D, Classe JM, Bonnier P, GCCLCC and SFOG. Conservative treatment in epithelial ovarian cancer: results of a multicentre study of the GCCLCC (Groupe des Chirurgiens de Centre de Lutte Contre le Cancer) and SFOG (Société Francaise d'Oncologie Gynécologique). Hum Reprod. 2005;20(5):1379–85.
40. Raspagliesi F, Fontanelli R, Paladini D, di Re EM. Conservative surgery in high-risk epithelial ovarian carcinoma. J Am Coll Surg. 1997;185(5):457–60.
41. Winter-Roach B, Hooper L, Kitchener H. Systematic review of adjuvant therapy for early stage (epithelial) ovarian cancer. Int J Gynecol Cancer. 2003;13(4):395–404.
42. Young RC, Walton LA, Ellenberg SS, Homesley HD, Wilbanks GD, Decker DG, et al. Adjuvant therapy in stage I and stage II epithelial ovarian cancer. Results of two prospective randomized trials. N Engl J Med. 1990;322(15):1021–7.
43. Bolis G, Colombo N, Pecorelli S, Torri V, Marsoni S, Bonazzi C, et al. Adjuvant treatment for early epithelial ovarian cancer: results of two randomised clinical trials comparing cisplatin to no further treatment or chromic phosphate (32P). G.I.C.O.G.: Gruppo Interregionale Collaborativo in Ginecologia Oncologica. Ann Oncol. 1995;6(9):887–93.
44. Trope C, Kaern J, Hogberg T, Abeler V, Hagen B, Kristensen G, et al. Randomized study on adjuvant chemotherapy in stage I high-risk ovarian cancer with evaluation of DNA ploidy as prognostic instrument. Ann Oncol. 2000;11(3):281–8.
45. Colombo N, Guthrie D, Chiari S, Parmar M, Qian W, Swart AM, et al. International Collaborative Ovarian Neoplasm trial 1: a randomized trial of adjuvant chemotherapy in women with early-stage ovarian cancer. J Natl Cancer Inst. 2003;95(2):125–32.
46. Swart AC, ICON collaborators. Long-term follow-up of women enrolled in a randomized trial of adjuvant chemotherapy for early stage ovarian cancer (ICON1). J Clin Oncol. 2007;25(18S):5509.
47. Winter-Roach B, Kitchener H, Lawrie TA. Adjuvant post surgery chemotherapy for early stage epithelial ovarian cancer. Int J Gynecol Cancer. 2012;3:1–33.
48. Trimbos JB, Parmar M, Vergote I, Guthrie D, Bolis G, Colombo N, et al. International collaborative ovarian neoplasm trial 1 and adjuvant ChemoTherapy in ovarian neoplasm trial: two parallel randomized phase III trials of adjuvant chemotherapy in patients with early-stage ovarian carcinoma. J Natl Cancer Inst. 2003;95(2):105–12.
49. Adams GJ, Wong ZH, Walking J, Greena JA. Platinum-based adjuvant chemotherapy for early-stage epithelial ovarian cancer: single or combination chemotherapy? Gynecol Oncol. 2010;10:1459–67.
50. Skirnisdottir I, Lindborg K, Sorbe B. Adjuvant chemotherapy with carboplatin and taxane compared with single drug carboplatin in early stage epithelial ovarian carcinoma. Oncol Rep. 2007;18:1249–56.
51. Garcia-Saenz JA, Casado J, Puente J, et al. Twenty years treating early-stage epithelial ovarian carcinoma patients with adjuvant platinum-based chemotherapy. A single institution's experience. J Clin Oncol. 2005;23:5167.
52. Stuart GC, Kitchener H, Bacon M, participants of 4th Ovarian Cancer Consensus Conference (OCCC); Gynecologic Cancer Intergroup. 2010 Gynecologic Cancer InterGroup (GCIG) consensus statement on clinical trials in ovarian cancer: report from the Fourth Ovarian Cancer Consensus Conference. Int J Gynecol Cancer. 2011;21(4):750–5. doi:10.1097/IGC.0b013e31821b2568. Review.
53. Bell J, Brady MF, Young RC, Walker JL, Look KY, Rose GS, et al. Randomised phase III trial of three versus six cycles of adjuvant carboplatin and paclitaxel in early stage epithelial ovarian carcinoma: a Gynecologic Oncology Group study. Gynecol Oncol. 2006;102(3):432–9.
54. Chan JK, Tian C, Fleming GF. The potential benefit of 6 vs. 3 cycles of chemotherapy in subsets of women with early-stage high-risk epithelial ovarian cancer: an exploratory analysis of a Gynecologic Oncology Group study. Gynecol Oncol. 2010;116:301–6.

55. Mannel RS, Brady MF, Kohn EC, Hanjani P, Hiura M, Lee R, et al. A randomized phase III trial of IV carboplatin and paclitaxel × 3 courses followed by observation versus weekly maintenance low-dose paclitaxel in patients with early-stage ovarian carcinoma: a Gynecologic Oncology Group Study. Gynecol Oncol. 2011;122(1):89–94.
56. Mok SC, Chao J, Skates S, Wong K, Yiu GK, Muto MG, et al. Prostasin, a potential serum marker for identification through microarray technology. J Natl Cancer Inst. 2001;93:1458–64.
57. Kristensen GB, Kildal W, Abeler VM, et al. Large-scale genomic instability predicts long-term outcome for women with invasive stage I ovarian cancer. Ann Oncol. 2003;14:1494–500.
58. Petricoin EF, Ardekani AM, Hitt BA, Levin PJ, Fusaro VA, Steinberg SM, et al. Use of proteomic patterns in serum to identify ovarian cancer. Lancet. 2002;359:572–7.
59. Schueler JA, Trimbos JB, van der Burg M, et al. DNA index reflects the biological behavior of ovarian carcinoma stage I-IIa. Gynecol Oncol. 1996;62:59–66.
60. But I, Gorisek B. DNA-ploidy as an independent prognostic factor in patients with serous ovarian carcinoma. Int J Gynaecol Obstet. 2000;71:259–62.
61. Skirnisdo' ttir I, Sorbe B, Karlsson M, et al. Prognostic importance of DNA ploidy and p53 in early stages of epithelial ovarian carcinoma. Int J Oncol. 2001;19:1295–302.
62. Trope C, Kaern J. Adjuvant chemotherapy for early stage ovarian cancer: review of the literature. J Clin Oncol. 2007;25:2909–20.
63. Sugiyama T, Kamura T, Kigawa J, et al. Clinical characteristics of clear cell carcinoma of the ovary: a distinct histologic type with poor prognosis and resistance to platinum-based chemotherapy. Cancer. 2000;88:2584–9.
64. Perren TJ, Swart AM, Pfisterer J, et al. A phase 3 trial of bevacizumab in ovarian cancer. N Engl J Med. 2011;365:2484–96.
65. Zanetta G, Chiari S, Rota S, et al. Conservative surgery for stage I ovarian carcinoma in women of childbearing age. Br J Obstet Gynaecol. 1997;104(9):1030–5.
66. Colombo N, Chiari S, Maggioni A, et al. Controversial issues in the management of early epithelial ovarian cancer: conservative surgery and role of adjuvant therapy. Gynecol Oncol. 1994;55(3 Pt 2):S47–51. Review.
67. Anchezar JP, Sardi J, Soderini A. Long-term follow-up results of fertility sparing surgery in patients with epithelial ovarian cancer. J Surg Oncol. 2009;100(1):55–8. doi:10.1002/jso.21297.
68. Kajiyama H, Shibata K, Mizuno M, et al. Long-term survival of young women receiving fertility-sparing surgery for ovarian cancer in comparison with those undergoing radical surgery. Br J Cancer. 2011;105(9):1288–94. doi:10.1038/bjc.2011.394. Epub 2011 Oct 4.

Extended Surgery for Advanced Ovarian Cancer

40

Eric L. Eisenhauer and Dennis S. Chi

40.1 Introduction

Worldwide, ovarian cancer is diagnosed in approximately 225,000 women each year and is responsible for 140,000 deaths [1]. Stage remains the strongest predictor of survival, and the majority of women will have advanced stage disease at diagnosis. Despite best initial therapy, most of these women will recur, and only 20–25 % will be long-term survivors [2].

Advances in chemotherapy have continued to improve response and extend survival, but the effectiveness of primary therapy has remained linked to the ability to surgically remove visible metastatic disease. As cytoreductive surgery has evolved, the tenets provided by Hoskins and colleagues in two essential ancillary data studies of Gynecologic Oncology Group (GOG) protocols 52 and 97 have continued to hold true: [1] there is an inverse correlation between maximal diameter of residual disease and overall survival [2], there is a threshold diameter of residual disease above which surgical debulking provides no survival benefit, and [3] survival is ultimately linked to multiple factors including age, stage, chemotherapy, effectiveness of surgery, and tumor biology [3, 4]. Multiple single institution and cooperative group trial series have demonstrated an association between cytoreduction to no visible residual disease and improved survival, shifting the goal of ovarian cancer surgery to removal of all visible metastases [5–11]. In our current treatment era, the apparent benefit of effective surgical therapy is further magnified beyond the demonstrated association between less residual disease and improved survival. Women who have undergone maximal cytoreduction are candidates to receive intraperitoneal chemotherapy, a modality that has repeatedly been shown to extend survival over standard intravenous therapy [8, 12, 13]. As regional therapy has advanced to extend survival times overall, the degree to which complete cytoreduction provides an advantage over minimal but visible disease is more pronounced [14].

"Extended surgery" for advanced ovarian cancer refers to a series of procedures that can be performed to remove metastatic ovarian cancer beyond the "standard" surgical hysterectomy, salpingo-oophorectomy, omentectomy, and lymph node dissection. In essence, these procedures are a natural extension of the rationale for performing any cytoreduction, as it is debatable whether "tumor biology" has any bearing on whether a metastatic ovarian cancer cell implants on the diaphragm instead of the omentum. Because

E.L. Eisenhauer, MD (✉)
Gynecologic Oncology, Department of Obstetrics and Gynecology, University of Cincinnati College of Medicine, Cincinnati, OH, USA
e-mail: eric.eisenhauer@uc.edu

D.S. Chi, MD
Gynecology Service, Pelvic Reconstructive Surgery, Department of Surgery, Memorial Sloan Kettering Cancer Center, New York, NY, USA
e-mail: chid@mskcc.org

H.R.H. Patel et al. (eds.), *Pelvic Cancer Surgery: Modern Breakthroughs and Future Advances*,
DOI 10.1007/978-1-4471-4258-4_40, © Springer-Verlag London 2015

procedures requiring resection of the diaphragm, pancreas, porta hepatis, and other upper abdominal structures are outside the scope of standard gynecologic pelvic and mid-abdominal surgery, they may not be part of standard gynecologic cancer surgery training, and may require additional post-fellowship experience. As these procedures require a different anatomic and technical understanding in order to not delay primary chemotherapy, it is appropriate that they are recognized as an "extended" skill set. Experts differ as to whether segmental bowel or colon resections should be considered "extended surgery" since they may be performed in as many as 30 % of women with advanced ovarian cancer [15, 16]. A recent Cochrane analysis of "ultra-radical surgery" for ovarian cancer excluded all studies in which bowel resection was not considered "ultra-radical," and so such bowel surgery has been included as an "extended" surgical procedure here [17].

40.2 Cytoreduction

Ovarian cancer spreads throughout the entire peritoneal cavity, and the procedures frequently required to achieve complete cytoreduction have been organized by abdominal region. We cannot emphasize enough the need to examine the entire abdomen and pelvis before proceeding with radical cytoreduction, in order to ensure resectability of other sites of disease. Moreover, patient selection is critical, and we recommend that gynecologic surgeons track their patient outcomes in order to better understand when major complications occur. While experienced surgeons generally report good outcomes and acceptable complication rates from these procedures, these cannot be unilaterally applied for all cases.

Radical Pelvic Resection

Ovarian cancer frequently involves the lateral pelvic peritoneum and rectosigmoid colon, and the posterior cul de sac is often obliterated. En bloc posterior pelvic resection has been increasingly applied to clear tumor from this region, and is referred to by several different designations: radical oophorectomy, modified posterior pelvic exenteration, and en bloc rectosigmoid colectomy. When performed en bloc, the retroperitoneal spaces are opened laterally and posteriorly, the ureters are mobilized laterally, the bladder is dissected down to the mid-vagina, and the upper vagina is divided to open the rectovaginal septum and identify the rectum below the posterior cul de sac (Fig. 40.1). Even with extensive peritoneal involvement, the superior rectal artery can be identified and divided in the rectal mesentery, and the presacral space developed. The rectum is divided with a TA or contour stapler and the uterus, adnexa, parametria, pelvic peritoneum, posterior cul de sac, and rectosigmoid colon are removed en bloc (Fig. 40.2). Anatomic considerations include the length of remaining proximal colon, as well as the distance from the anal verge to the peritoneal reflection in the posterior cul de sac, since the rectum will be stapled below this point (Fig. 40.3). As there is generally >5 cm of distal rectum remaining, a primary anastomosis with or without a diverting loop ileostomy may be performed, and end colostomy is rarely required.

Series of patients undergoing en bloc posterior pelvic resection have been reported from multiple centers with acceptable complication rates, and are listed in Table 40.1 [16, 18–26]. In patients undergoing several separate cytoreductive procedures, the "per procedure" complication rate can be difficult to determine. In these series, the procedure-related complication rate was generally 2–6 %, the most common of which was anastomotic leak or fistula. Houvenaeghel and colleagues reported the combined experience of nine French centers, in which 168 patients underwent modified posterior exenteration in the primary setting with a low rate of protective stoma [25]. The total perioperative complication rate was 27 %, with a low rate of fistula/abscess.

Extrapelvic Bowel Resection

Outside of the pelvis, the two most common sites of bowel involvement are the ileocecum and the

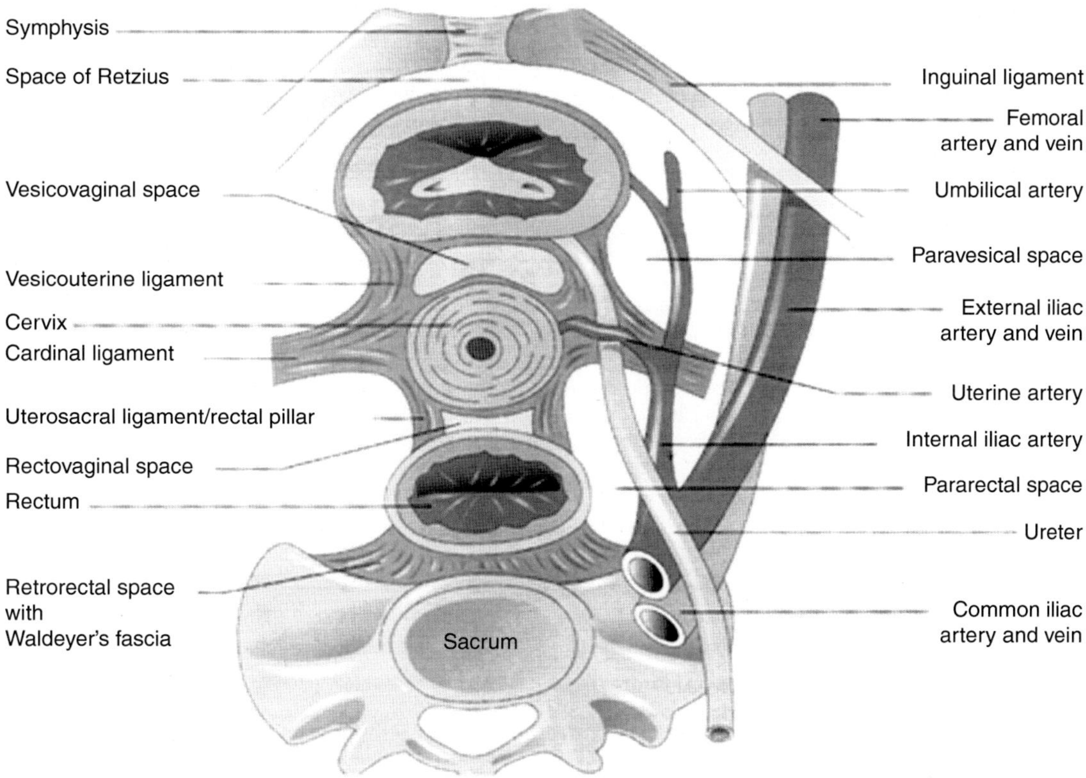

Fig. 40.1 Eight potential spaces of the pelvis: retropubic space of Retzius, paravesicle spaces (2), vesicovaginal space, pararectal spaces (2), rectovaginal space, and presacral space (Reprinted with permission from: Bristow et al. [55])

transverse colon. Anatomic considerations when considering resection in these areas are primarily due to vascular supply. Variability in watershed areas, and the degree of communication between the ileocolic, right colic, and middle colic arteries need to be considered so that resultant anastomoses have adequate supply.

Perhaps because of this, or because patients with extrapelvic bowel involvement have more extensive disease, the reported procedure-related complication rate of approximately 8 % is slightly higher than after en bloc pelvic resection (see Table 40.2) [27–34]. In Hoffman's series of 144 patients with advanced ovarian cancer, 36 % had extensive bowel involvement outside the pelvis, with a 6 % risk of procedure-related complication [28]. Silver and colleagues reported their series of 19 patients undergoing extended left colon resection, with a low overall complication rate and detailed analysis of relevant vascular considerations when rotating the remaining right colon around the ileocolic artery pedicle [33].

Right Upper Quadrant Resection

The right upper quadrant is frequently involved due to the pooling of ascites containing metastatic cells in the right subphrenic space; this pooling is caused by gravity and the falciform ligament. Up to 40 % of women with advanced ovarian cancer present with bulky metastatic disease to the diaphragm, and diaphragm implants have been described as one of the most common factors precluding optimal cytoreduction [35]. The ability to safely remove these diaphragm lesions is an essential component of the comprehensive approach to surgical cytoreduction, which has been associated with improved survival in these patients [15]. The extent of resection

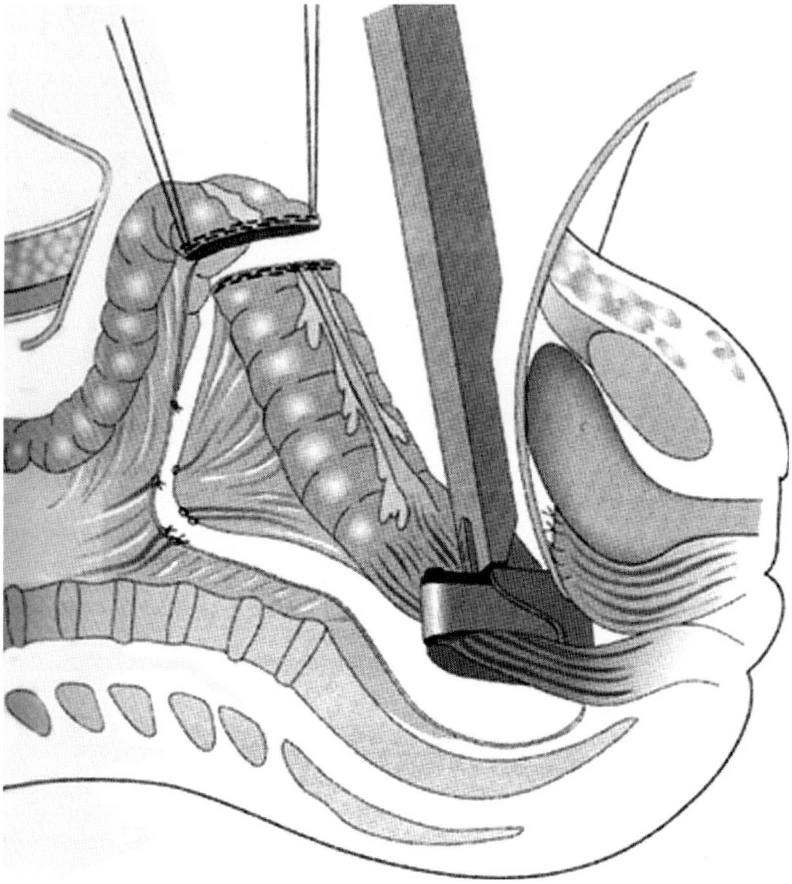

Fig. 40.2 Radical oophorectomy: type II modification. The rectum is divided between a TA stapler and proximal bowel clamp to complete the resection. (Reprinted with permission from: Bristow et al. [55])

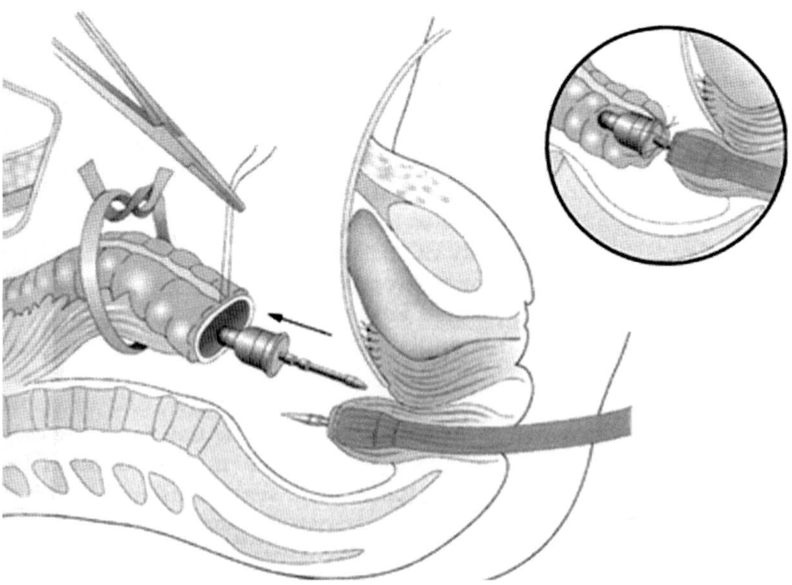

Fig. 40.3 Circular end-to-end stapled anastomosis using the automated CEEA stapler. The CEEA anvil is introduced into the proximal colon and the purse-string suture tied with the notch on the anvil shaft; the main CEEA instrument is passed transanally and the trochar advanced through the rectal stump. The trochar is removed and the anvil shaft inserted into the cartridge shaft of the main CEEA instrument (*inset*). *Abbreviation*: *CEEA*, circular end-to-end anastomosis. (Reprinted with permission from: Bristow et al. [55])

Table 40.1 Literature on feasibility of radical pelvic resection (radical oophorectomy, modified posterior exenteration, or en bloc rectosigmoid colectomy)

			Complications (%)		
Study	Year	Patients	Overall	Procedure-related	Mortality
Soper et al. [18]	1991	21	NA	NA	NA
Scarabelli et al. [19]	2000	66	13 (20)	1 (1)	0
Obermair et al. [20]	2001	65	19 (29)	3 (5)	1 (1)
Clayton et al. [21]	2002	129	38 (30)	3 (2)	4 (3)
Bristow et al. [22]	2003	31	4 (13)	1 (3)	0
Mourton et al. [23]	2005	70	22 (31)	4 (6)	1 (1)
Aletti et al. [16]	2006	57	NA	1 (2)	0
Park et al. [24]	2006	46	15 (33)	2 (4)	0
Houvenaeghel [25]	2009	168	45 (27)	NA	NA
Tixier et al. [26]	2010	41	14 (34)	4 (10)	3 (7)

NA, not available

Table 40.2 Literature on feasibility of bowel resection

			Complications (%)		
Study	Year	Patients	Overall	Procedure-related	Mortality
Gillette-Cloven et al. [27]	2001	105	18 (17)	10 (10)	6 (6)
Hoffman et al. [28]	2005	144	23 (16)	9 (6)	0
Estes et al. [29]	2006	48	5 (10)	4 (8)	2 (4)
Bidzinski et al. [30]	2007	39	8 (20)	5 (13)	0
Salani et al. [31]	2007	125	30 (24)	11 (9)	2 (2)
Bristow et al. [32]	2008	33	NA	NA	1 (3)
Silver [33]	2009	19	3 (16)	NA	1 (5)
Song et al. [34]	2009	22	7 (32)	0	0

NA, not available

required is determined by the surface area involved and the presence of muscular invasion. Primary anatomic considerations include the relevant hepatic attachments and the underlying central vasculature, as the right liver must be mobilized medially in order to gain access to the entire right diaphragm [36]. The coronary ligaments reflect off the liver capsule and delineate the posterior extent of the diaphragm peritoneum. The right hepatic vein drains into the inferior vena cava at the medial portion of the right coronary ligament, and additional caution is essential during this part of the dissection to avoid injury to this vessel. In addition, the right phrenic nerve penetrates the central tendon of the diaphragm but is usually not encountered until the right coronary ligament is divided and the base area of the liver is exposed.

Diaphragm peritonectomy and/or resection (Figs. 40.4 and 40.5) are generally well tolerated, and the reported complication rates vary somewhat between series, as shown in Table 40.3 [37–44]. This variability appears to depend on how pleural effusions were scored as complications, and whether a chest tube was placed as a prophylactic measure at the time of surgery. One series evaluating 59 patients in whom intraoperative chest tubes were not placed after diaphragm surgery and who had daily postoperative chest imaging showed a 58 % incidence of ipsilateral effusions; 15 % required postoperative drainage [42]. Chereau and colleagues recently reported their series in which 144 patients underwent diaphragm surgery for primary, interval, or recurrent disease; 35 % of the patients had chest tubes placed intraoperatively and 43 % developed pulmonary complications [44].

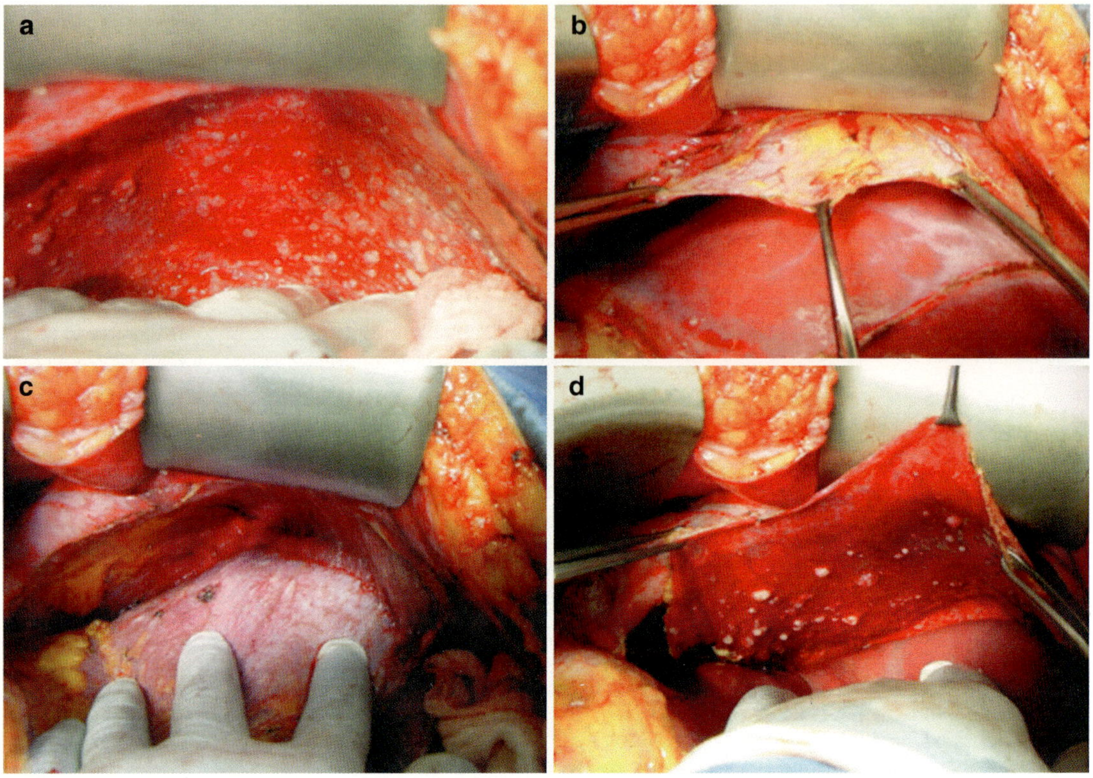

Fig. 40.4 Diaphragm peritonectomy. (**a**) The self-retaining retractor has been positioned to provide maximal elevation of the costal margin. (**b**) The diaphragm peritoneum is incised along the costal margin, developing a broad front of dissection in the subperitoneal plane. (**c**) The diaphragm peritoneum is placed on downward traction, exposing the plane of dissection at the interface with the muscular surface. (**d**) The dissection is carried posteriorly to the peritoneal reflection of the coronary and right triangular ligaments. (Reprinted with permission from: Bristow et al. [55])

Resection of metastatic disease from the celiac lymph nodes or porta hepatis can be difficult due to anatomic variations in the vascular anatomy and proximity to the hepatic and gastric vessels. Lymphadenectomy in this region is performed by surgical oncologists and hepatobiliary surgeons for staging or resection of some gastric, biliary, or hepatic cancers. Anatomic considerations in this region are multiple, including the celiac axis, portal triad, pancreas, and duodenum. Two recent series report successful ovarian cancer cytoreduction in this region with a low complication rate when performed with a multidisciplinary team including surgical oncologists, as shown in Table 40.3 [45, 46].

Left Upper Quadrant

Left upper quadrant structures are most frequently involved near the splenic hilum where tumor from the lateral edge of the omentum may involve the spleen, splenic hilum, and distal pancreas. Anatomic considerations include the splenic vascular anatomy and left adrenal gland, as well as the proximity of the distal pancreas from the splenic hilum, and will be encountered differently whether an anterior or posterior approach is used. Bulky anterior or hilar disease is best approached via a posterior approach, where the splenic flexure is mobilized, the lienorenal ligament divided, and the spleen elevated

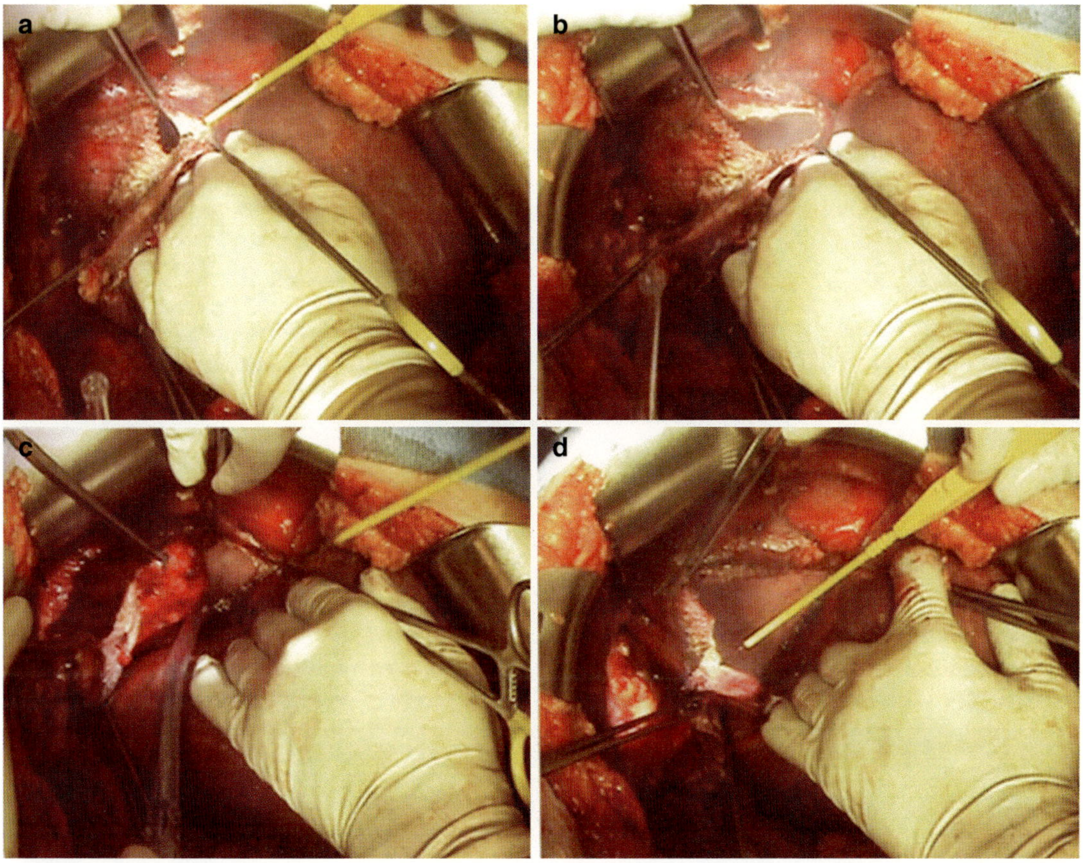

Fig. 40.5 Full-thickness resection of the diaphragm. (**a**) The diaphragm muscle is incised with electrocautery and the pleural space entered. (**b**) The pleural space is explored to define the extent of resection. (**c**) The resection is carried posterior and laterally along the upper margin of the bare area of the liver. (**d**) The specimen is everted and the diaphragmatic pleura and muscle resected en bloc. (Reprinted with permission from: Bristow et al. [55])

Table 40.3 Literature on feasibility of right upper quadrant resection

			Complications (%)		
Study	Year	Patients	Overall	Procedure-related	Mortality
Diaphragm peritonectomy, resection or ablation					
Montz et al. [37]	1989	14	NA	1 (7)	0
Silver et al. [38]	2004	7	0	0	0
Cliby et al. [39]	2004	41	8 (20)	6 (15)	0
Eisenhauer et al. [42]	2006	59	NA	9 (15)	0
Chereau et al. [40]	2009	18	5 (28)	4 (22)	0
Einekel et al. [41]	2009	30	14 (47)	11 (37)	1 (3)
Gouy et al. [43]	2010	63	11 (17)	6 (10)	0
Chereau et al. [44]	2011	144	99 (69)	62 (43)	2 (3)
Celiac axis or porta hepatis resection					
Song et al. [45]	2011	2	0	0	0
Martinez et al. [46]	2011	28	10 (36)	1 (3)	0

NA, not available

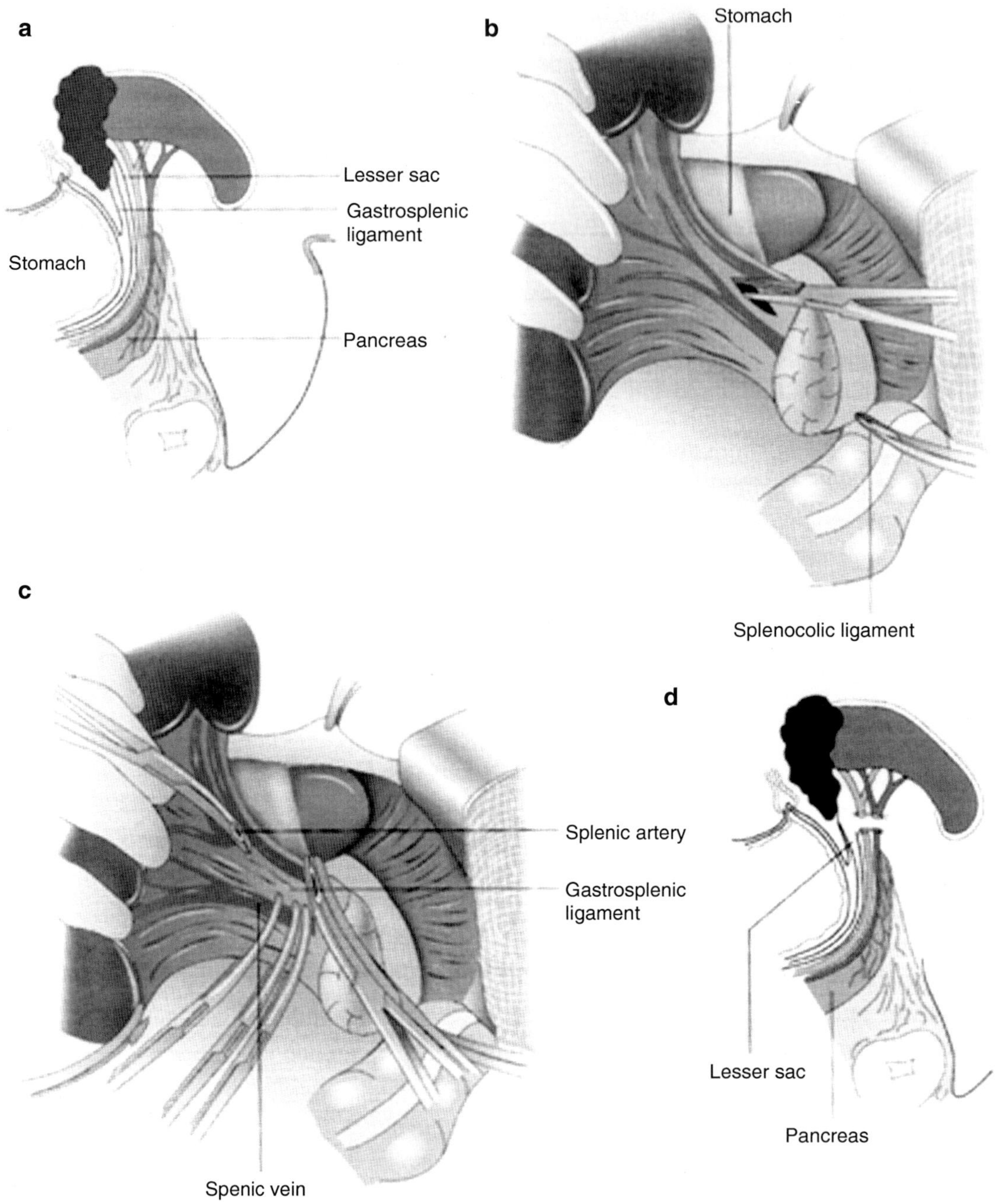

Fig. 40.6 Splenectomy-posterior approach. (**a**) Tumor obscures the gastrosplenic ligament and anterior access to the splenic hilum; the spleen is drawn medially to expose the lienorenal ligament. (**b**) The lienorenal ligament is incised and the splenic artery and vein are identified within the areolar tissue. (**c**) The splenic artery and vein are clamped, divided, and ligated. (**d**) After division of the vasculature, the lesser sac can be properly developed, any remaining tumor attachments to the gastrosplenic ligament are taken down, and the specimen is removed. (Reprinted with permission from: Bristow et al. [55])

medially (Fig. 40.6). From this position, the splenic vessels can be divided and the distal pancreas divided or dissected free. In the presence of bulky posterior or left diaphragm disease, surgeons take an anterior approach through the omentum into the lesser sac to divide the gastrosplenic ligament and short gastric arteries and expose the splenic vessels. After dividing the

Table 40.4 Literature on feasibility of left upper quadrant resection (splenectomy, distal pancreatectomy, en bloc left upper quadrant resection)

			Complications (%)		
Study	Year	Patients	Overall	Procedure-related	Mortality
Sonnendecker et al. [47]	1989	6	5 (83)	NA	1 (17)
Ayhan et al. [48]	2004	34	10 (29)	NA	3 (9)
Yildirim et al. [49]	2005	6	4 (67)	1 (17)	0
Eisenkop et al. [50]	2006	49	20 (41)	3 (6)	1 (2)
Hoffman et al. [51]	2007	6	3 (50)	2 (33)	0
Kehoe et al. [52]	2009	17	NA	4 (24)	0

NA not available

vessels and the lienorenal ligament, distal pancreas can be dissected free or divided. The distal pancreas is generally divided with a vascular stapler and reinforced with permanent suture. Elective ligation of the pancreatic duct may reduce the incidence of pancreatic leak, and a drain may be left in the dissection bed.

Several groups have reported their experience with left upper quadrant resection, with variable complication rates depending on whether splenectomy was performed alone, or as a combined procedure with either distal pancreatectomy or en bloc left upper quadrant resection, as shown in Table 40.4 [47–52]. Pancreatic resection is associated with a noted increase in complication rate, and consultation with a pancreatic surgeon or surgical oncologist may be justified.

Feasibility of Changing Institutional Surgical Approach

Many centers have incorporated an increasingly extensive approach to ovarian cancer cytoreduction, and several have detailed both the process and results of this change [7, 53, 54]. Generally, these have incorporated both a desire to improve complete cytoreduction rates, as well as the ability to work with other surgical services to learn additional skills and limit complication rates. In 2009, Chi and associates reported their experience and outcomes following a paradigm shift towards more extensive surgical cytoreduction at Memorial Sloan Kettering Cancer Center from 1996 to 2004 [53]. By incorporating extensive upper abdominal procedures during an era when standard primary chemotherapy was the same, the complete cytoreduction rate increased from 11 to 27 %, the optimal cytoreduction rate increased from 46 to 80 %, and the medial survival improved from 43 to 54 months. In Europe, Harter and colleagues reported the results of introducing a surgical quality management program to improve ovarian cancer cytoreduction [54]. During the period of the study, the rate of extended surgical procedures increased from 0 to 43 %, and complete cytoreduction increased from 33 to 62 %, with an improvement in median overall survival from 26 to 45 months. These studies demonstrate that cytoreduction rates at an institution can be improved, and that a concerted multidisciplinary effort toward complete cytoreduction is an achievable goal.

40.3 Summary

For women with advanced ovarian cancer, there is substantial evidence that cytoreduction of all visible metastatic disease is associated with the best survival outcomes. Moreover, only patients with optimal residual disease are candidates for intraperitoneal chemotherapy, which has been shown to give the longest survival benefit. "Extended surgery" for ovarian cancer is the surgical approach that allows more patients to realize this benefit, but it requires care in terms of adequate surgical preparation and patient selection. The ability to perform radical removal of pelvic and upper abdominal metastases for the majority of women with advanced ovarian cancer is both reasonable and feasible. As more centers adopt an approach toward complete cytoreduction, it is clear that an institutional commitment and a dedicated approach can improve patient outcomes.

Key Points

- As regional therapy has advanced to extend survival times overall, the degree to which complete cytoreduction provides an advantage over minimal but visible disease is more pronounced.
- "Extended surgery" for advanced ovarian cancer refers to a series of procedures that can be performed to remove metastatic ovarian cancer beyond the "standard" surgical hysterectomy, salpingo-oophorectomy, omentectomy, and lymph node dissection.
- As these procedures require a different anatomic and technical understanding in order to not delay primary chemotherapy, it is appropriate that they are recognized as an "extended" skill set.
- We cannot emphasize enough the need to examine the entire abdomen and pelvis before proceeding with radical cytoreduction, in order to ensure resectability of other sites of disease.
- While experienced surgeons generally report good outcomes and acceptable complication rates from these procedures, these cannot be unilaterally applied for all cases.
- Ovarian cancer frequently involves the lateral pelvic peritoneum and rectosigmoid colon, and the posterior cul de sac is often obliterated; en bloc posterior pelvic resection has been increasingly applied to clear tumor from this region.
- Outside of the pelvis, the two most common sites of bowel involvement are the ileocecum and the transverse colon.
- Up to 40 % of women with advanced ovarian cancer present with bulky metastatic disease to the diaphragm, and diaphragm implants have been described as one of the most common factors precluding optimal cytoreduction.
- Pancreatic resection is associated with a noted increase in complication rate, and consultation with a pancreatic surgeon or surgical oncologist may be justified.
- Several studies demonstrate that cytoreduction rates at an institution can be improved, and that a concerted multidisciplinary effort toward complete cytoreduction is an achievable goal.

References

1. Jemal A, Bray F, Center MM, Ferlay J, Ward E, Forman D. Global cancer statistics. CA Cancer J Clin. 2011;61(2):69–90.
2. Ozols RF. Treatment goals in ovarian cancer. Int J Gynecol Cancer. 2005;15 Suppl 1:3–11.
3. Hoskins WJ, Bundy BN, Thigpen JT, Omura GA. The influence of cytoreductive surgery on recurrence-free interval and survival in small-volume stage III epithelial ovarian cancer: a Gynecologic Oncology Group study. Gynecol Oncol. 1992;47(2):159–66.
4. Hoskins WJ, McGuire WP, Brady MF, Homesley HD, Creasman WT, Berman M, et al. The effect of diameter of largest residual disease on survival after primary cytoreductive surgery in patients with suboptimal residual epithelial ovarian carcinoma. Am J Obstet Gynecol. 1994;170(4):974–9; discussion 979–80.
5. Eisenkop SM, Spirtos NM, Friedman RL, Lin WC, Pisani AL, Perticucci S. Relative influences of tumor volume before surgery and the cytoreductive outcome on survival for patients with advanced ovarian cancer: a prospective study. Gynecol Oncol. 2003;90(2):390–6.
6. Chi DS, Eisenhauer EL, Lang J, Huh J, Haddad L, Abu-Rustum NR, et al. What is the optimal goal of primary cytoreductive surgery for bulky stage IIIC epithelial ovarian carcinoma (EOC)? Gynecol Oncol. 2006;103(2):559–64.
7. Aletti GD, Dowdy SC, Gostout BS, Jones MB, Stanhope CR, Wilson TO, et al. Aggressive surgical effort and improved survival in advanced-stage ovarian cancer. Obstet Gynecol. 2006;107(1):77–85.
8. Armstrong DK, Bundy B, Wenzel L, Huang HQ, Baergen R, Lele S, et al. Intraperitoneal cisplatin and paclitaxel in ovarian cancer. N Engl J Med. 2006;354(1):34–43.
9. Winter 3rd WE, Maxwell GL, Tian C, Carlson JW, Ozols RF, Rose PG, et al. Prognostic factors for stage III epithelial ovarian cancer: a Gynecologic Oncology Group Study. J Clin Oncol. 2007;25(24):3621–7.
10. du Bois A, Reuss A, Pujade-Lauraine E, Harter P, Ray-Coquard I, Pfisterer J. Role of surgical outcome as prognostic factor in advanced epithelial ovarian cancer: a combined exploratory analysis of 3 prospectively randomized phase 3 multicenter trials: by the Arbeitsgemeinschaft Gynaekologische Onkologie Studiengruppe Ovarialkarzinom (AGO-OVAR) and

the Groupe d'Investigateurs Nationaux Pour les Etudes des Cancers de l'Ovaire (GINECO). Cancer. 2009;115(6):1234–44.
11. Wimberger P, Wehling M, Lehmann N, Kimmig R, Schmalfeldt B, Burges A, et al. Influence of residual tumor on outcome in ovarian cancer patients with FIGO stage IV disease: an exploratory analysis of the AGO-OVAR (Arbeitsgemeinschaft Gynaekologische Onkologie Ovarian Cancer Study Group). Ann Surg Oncol. 2010;17(6):1642–8.
12. Alberts DS, Liu PY, Hannigan EV, O'Toole R, Williams SD, Young JA, et al. Intraperitoneal cisplatin plus intravenous cyclophosphamide versus intravenous cisplatin plus intravenous cyclophosphamide for stage III ovarian cancer. N Engl J Med. 1996;335(26):1950–5.
13. Markman M, Bundy BN, Alberts DS, Fowler JM, Clark-Pearson DL, Carson LF, et al. Phase III trial of standard-dose intravenous cisplatin plus paclitaxel versus moderately high-dose carboplatin followed by intravenous paclitaxel and intraperitoneal cisplatin in small-volume stage III ovarian carcinoma: an intergroup study of the Gynecologic Oncology Group, Southwestern Oncology Group, and Eastern Cooperative Oncology Group. J Clin Oncol. 2001;19(4):1001–7.
14. Chang SJ, Bristow RE. Evolution of surgical treatment paradigms for advanced-stage ovarian cancer: redefining 'optimal' residual disease. Gynecol Oncol. 2012;125(2):483–92.
15. Eisenhauer EL, Abu-Rustum NR, Sonoda Y, Levine DA, Poynor EA, Aghajanian C, et al. The addition of extensive upper abdominal surgery to achieve optimal cytoreduction improves survival in patients with stages IIIC-IV epithelial ovarian cancer. Gynecol Oncol. 2006;103(3):1083–90.
16. Aletti GD, Podratz KC, Jones MB, Cliby WA. Role of rectosigmoidectomy and stripping of pelvic peritoneum in outcomes of patients with advanced ovarian cancer. J Am Coll Surg. 2006;203(4):521–6.
17. Ang C, Chan KK, Bryant A, Naik R, Dickinson HO. Ultra-radical (extensive) surgery versus standard surgery for the primary cytoreduction of advanced epithelial ovarian cancer. Cochrane Database Syst Rev. 2011(4):CD007697.
18. Soper JT, Couchman G, Berchuck A, Clarke-Pearson D. The role of partial sigmoid colectomy for debulking epithelial ovarian carcinoma. Gynecol Oncol. 1991;41(3):239–44.
19. Scarabelli C, Gallo A, Franceschi S, Campagnutta E, De G, Giorda G, et al. Primary cytoreductive surgery with rectosigmoid colon resection for patients with advanced epithelial ovarian carcinoma. Cancer. 2000;88(2):389–97.
20. Obermair A, Hagenauer S, Tamandl D, Clayton RD, Nicklin JL, Perrin LC, et al. Safety and efficacy of low anterior en bloc resection as part of cytoreductive surgery for patients with ovarian cancer. Gynecol Oncol. 2001;83(1):115–20.
21. Clayton RD, Obermair A, Hammond IG, Leung YC, McCartney AJ. The Western Australian experience of the use of en bloc resection of ovarian cancer with concomitant rectosigmoid colectomy. Gynecol Oncol. 2002;84(1):53–7.
22. Bristow RE, del Carmen MG, Kaufman HS, Montz FJ. Radical oophorectomy with primary stapled colorectal anastomosis for resection of locally advanced epithelial ovarian cancer. J Am Coll Surg. 2003;197(4):565–74.
23. Mourton SM, Temple LK, Abu-Rustum NR, Gemignani ML, Sonoda Y, Bochner BH, et al. Morbidity of rectosigmoid resection and primary anastomosis in patients undergoing primary cytoreductive surgery for advanced epithelial ovarian cancer. Gynecol Oncol. 2005;99(3):608–14.
24. Park JY, Seo SS, Kang S, Lee KB, Lim SY, Choi HS, et al. The benefits of low anterior en bloc resection as part of cytoreductive surgery for advanced primary and recurrent epithelial ovarian cancer patients outweigh morbidity concerns. Gynecol Oncol. 2006; 103(3):977–84.
25. Houvenaeghel G, Gutowski M, Buttarelli M, Cuisenier J, Narducci F, Dalle C, et al. Modified posterior pelvic exenteration for ovarian cancer. Int J Gynecol Cancer. 2009;19(5):968–73.
26. Tixier H, Fraisse J, Chauffert B, Mayer F, Causeret S, Loustalot C, et al. Evaluation of pelvic posterior exenteration in the management of advanced-stage ovarian cancer. Arch Gynecol Obstet. 2010;281(3):505–10.
27. Gillette-Cloven N, Burger RA, Monk BJ, McMeekin DS, Vasilev S, DiSaia PJ, et al. Bowel resection at the time of primary cytoreduction for epithelial ovarian cancer. J Am Coll Surg. 2001;193(6):626–32.
28. Hoffman MS, Griffin D, Tebes S, Cardosi RJ, Martino MA, Fiorica JV, et al. Sites of bowel resected to achieve optimal ovarian cancer cytoreduction: implications regarding surgical management. Am J Obstet Gynecol. 2005;193(2):582–6; discussion 586–8.
29. Estes JM, Leath 3rd CA, Straughn Jr JM, Rocconi RP, Kirby TO, Huh WK, et al. Bowel resection at the time of primary debulking for epithelial ovarian carcinoma: outcomes in patients treated with platinum and taxane-based chemotherapy. J Am Coll Surg. 2006; 203(4):527–32.
30. Bidzinski M, Derlatka P, Kubik P, Ziolkowska-Seta I, Danska-Bidzinska A, Gmyrek L, et al. The evaluation of intra- and postoperative complications related to debulking surgery with bowel resection in patients with FIGO stage III-IV ovarian cancer. Int J Gynecol Cancer. 2007;17(5):993–7.
31. Salani R, Zahurak ML, Santillan A, Giuntoli 2nd RL, Bristow RE. Survival impact of multiple bowel resections in patients undergoing primary cytoreductive surgery for advanced ovarian cancer: a case-control study. Gynecol Oncol. 2007;107(3):495–9.
32. Bristow RE, Peiretti M, Zanagnolo V, Salani R, Giuntoli 2nd RL, Maggioni A. Transverse colectomy in ovarian cancer surgical cytoreduction: operative technique and clinical outcome. Gynecol Oncol. 2008;109(3):364–9.
33. Silver DF, Bou Zgheib N. Extended left colon resections as part of complete cytoreduction for ovarian

cancer: tips and considerations. Gynecol Oncol. 2009;114(3):427–30.
34. Song YJ, Lim MC, Kang S, Seo SS, Park JW, Choi HS, et al. Total colectomy as part of primary cytoreductive surgery in advanced Mullerian cancer. Gynecol Oncol. 2009;114(2):183–7.
35. Eisenkop SM, Spirtos NM. What are the current surgical objectives, strategies, and technical capabilities of gynecologic oncologists treating advanced epithelial ovarian cancer? Gynecol Oncol. 2001;82(3): 489–97.
36. Eisenhauer EL, Chi DS. Liver mobilization and diaphragm peritonectomy/resection. Gynecol Oncol. 2007;104(2 Suppl 1):25–8.
37. Montz FJ, Schlaerth JB, Berek JS. Resection of diaphragmatic peritoneum and muscle: role in cytoreductive surgery for ovarian cancer. Gynecol Oncol. 1989;35(3):338–40.
38. Silver DF. Full-thickness diaphragmatic resection with simple and secure closure to accomplish complete cytoreductive surgery for patients with ovarian cancer. Gynecol Oncol. 2004;95(2):384–7.
39. Cliby W, Dowdy S, Feitoza SS, Gostout BS, Podratz KC. Diaphragm resection for ovarian cancer: technique and short-term complications. Gynecol Oncol. 2004;94(3):655–60.
40. Chereau E, Ballester M, Selle F, Cortez A, Pomel C, Darai E, et al. Pulmonary morbidity of diaphragmatic surgery for stage III/IV ovarian cancer. BJOG. 2009;116(8):1062–8.
41. Einenkel J, Ott R, Handzel R, Braumann UD, Horn LC. Characteristics and management of diaphragm involvement in patients with primary advanced-stage ovarian, fallopian tube, or peritoneal cancer. Int J Gynecol Cancer. 2009;19(7):1288–97.
42. Eisenhauer EL, D'Angelica MI, Abu-Rustum NR, Sonoda Y, Jarnagin WR, Barakat RR, et al. Incidence and management of pleural effusions after diaphragm peritonectomy or resection for advanced Mullerian cancer. Gynecol Oncol. 2006;103(3):871–7.
43. Gouy S, Chereau E, Custodio AS, Uzan C, Pautier P, Haie-Meder C, et al. Surgical procedures and morbidities of diaphragmatic surgery in patients undergoing initial or interval debulking surgery for advanced-stage ovarian cancer. J Am Coll Surg. 2010; 210(4):509–14.
44. Chereau E, Rouzier R, Gouy S, Ferron G, Narducci F, Bergzoll C, et al. Morbidity of diaphragmatic surgery for advanced ovarian cancer: retrospective study of 148 cases. Eur J Surg Oncol. 2011;37(2):175–80.
45. Song YJ, Lim MC, Kang S, Seo SS, Kim SH, Han SS, et al. Extended cytoreduction of tumor at the porta hepatis by an interdisciplinary team approach in patients with epithelial ovarian cancer. Gynecol Oncol. 2011;121(2):253–7.
46. Martinez A, Pomel C, Mery E, Querleu D, Gladieff L, Ferron G. Celiac lymph node resection and porta hepatis disease resection in advanced or recurrent epithelial ovarian, fallopian tube, and primary peritoneal cancer. Gynecol Oncol. 2011;121(2):258–63.
47. Sonnendecker EW, Guidozzi F, Margolius KA. Splenectomy during primary maximal cytoreductive surgery for epithelial ovarian cancer. Gynecol Oncol. 1989;35(3):301–6.
48. Ayhan A, Al RA, Baykal C, Demirtas E, Ayhan A, Yuce K. The influence of splenic metastases on survival in FIGO stage IIIC epithelial ovarian cancer. Int J Gynecol Cancer. 2004;14(1):51–6.
49. Yildirim Y, Sanci M. The feasibility and morbidity of distal pancreatectomy in extensive cytoreductive surgery for advanced epithelial ovarian cancer. Arch Gynecol Obstet. 2005;272(1):31–4.
50. Eisenkop SM, Spirtos NM, Lin WC. Splenectomy in the context of primary cytoreductive operations for advanced epithelial ovarian cancer. Gynecol Oncol. 2006;100(2):344–8.
51. Hoffman MS, Tebes SJ, Sayer RA, Lockhart J. Extended cytoreduction of intraabdominal metastatic ovarian cancer in the left upper quadrant utilizing en bloc resection. Am J Obstet Gynecol. 2007;197(2):209 e1–4. discussion 209e.4–5.
52. Kehoe SM, Eisenhauer EL, Abu-Rustum NR, Sonoda Y, D'Angelica M, Jarnagin WR, et al. Incidence and management of pancreatic leaks after splenectomy with distal pancreatectomy performed during primary cytoreductive surgery for advanced ovarian, peritoneal and fallopian tube cancer. Gynecol Oncol. 2009;112(3):496–500.
53. Chi DS, Eisenhauer EL, Zivanovic O, Sonoda Y, Abu-Rustum NR, Levine DA, et al. Improved progression-free and overall survival in advanced ovarian cancer as a result of a change in surgical paradigm. Gynecol Oncol. 2009;114(1):26–31.
54. Harter P, Muallem ZM, Buhrmann C, Lorenz D, Kaub C, Hils R, et al. Impact of a structured quality management program on surgical outcome in primary advanced ovarian cancer. Gynecol Oncol. 2011;121(3):615–9.
55. Bristow RE, Karlan BY, Chi DS, editors. Surgery for ovarian cancer, principles and practice. 2nd ed. New York: Informa Healthcare; 2010.

Neoadjuvant and Adjuvant Chemotherapy for Advanced Ovarian Cancer, Including Biological Agents

41

Shelize S. Khakoo and Susana Banerjee

41.1 Introduction

The worldwide incidence of ovarian cancer is estimated to be 225, 000 cases per year [1]. In Europe, there are approximately 65, 697 new cases and 41, 448 ovarian cancer-related deaths per year [1]. While women with disease confined to the ovaries (stage I) usually have a good outlook (5-year survival of >90 %), due to the lack of well-defined symptoms, the vast majority (75–80 %) unfortunately present with more advanced disease (FIGO III-IV) and little prospect of cure, with a 5 year survival rate of approximately 40 % [2]. Around 90 % of ovarian carcinomas are epithelial in origin whereas the remainder arise from germ cells or stromal cells. The principles of the initial management of epithelial ovarian cancer has remained largely unchanged over the years and consists of attempted maximal cytoreductive surgery and platinum-based chemotherapy. Improvements in surgical techniques and chemotherapy strategies have led to improved clinical outcomes. However, disease recurrence and drug resistance continue to pose persistent management challenges. Advances in our knowledge of the molecular biology underlying ovarian cancer coupled with development of novel agents offers promise. A number of clinical trials address the optimal schedule, mode of administration of established chemotherapy drugs and the integration of targeted agents. This chapter provides an overview of the initial management of advanced ovarian cancer and the integration of targeted therapies in this setting.

S.S. Khakoo, MBChB, BSc, MRCP
S. Banerjee, MA, MBBS, MRCP, PhD (✉)
Department of Medicine, Royal Marsden
NHS Foundation Trust, Sutton, London, UK
e-mail: susana.banerjee@rmh.nhs.uk

41.2 Systemic Therapy for the Initial Management of Advanced Ovarian Cancer

The current international standard of care for advanced ovarian cancer is either initial or interval optimal cytoreductive surgery (no residual disease) and a total of six cycles of three-weekly intravenous (IV) chemotherapy with carboplatin (area under the curve [AUC] 5–7.5) given in combination with paclitaxel (175 mg/m^2) [3]. Chemotherapy given following surgery is termed 'adjuvant' and upfront chemotherapy followed by interval debulking surgery is referred to as 'neo-adjuvant.' The recommendation of a platinum/paclitaxel combination is based on a series of phase III studies over the last two decades which address type of platinum, combination therapy, dosage and scheduling [4–7] (see Table 41.1). The results of the Gynecologic Oncology Group (GOG) 111 trial demonstrated the importance of incorporating taxanes into first line chemotherapy

H.R.H. Patel et al. (eds.), *Pelvic Cancer Surgery: Modern Breakthroughs and Future Advances*,
DOI 10.1007/978-1-4471-4258-4_41, © Springer-Verlag London 2015

Table 41.1 Key first line adjuvant trials for the treatment of advanced epithelial ovarian cancer

Study	N	Study population	Treatment arms	PFS (months)	OS (months)
GOG 111	410	Stage III with residual disease >1 cm after initial surgery or stage IV disease	Cisplatin (75 mg/m^2)/Cyclophosphamide (750 mg/m^2)	13	24
			Cisplatin (75 mg/m^2)/Paclitaxel (135 mg/m^2 over 24 h)	18 (p<0.001)	38 (p<0.001)
EORTC-NCIC OV-10	680	FIGO stage IIB-IV with either ≤1 cm residual disease or >1 cm residual disease after initial surgery	Cisplatin (75 mg/m^2)/Cyclophosphamide (750 mg/m^2)	11.5	25.8
			Cisplatin (75 mg/m^2)/Paclitaxel (175 mg/m^2 over 3 h)	15.5 (p<0.0005)	35.6 (p=0.0016)
GOG 132	648	Stage III with residual disease >1 cm after initial surgery or stage IV disease	Cisplatin (100 mg/m^2)	16.4	30.2
			Paclitaxel (200 mg/m^2 over 24 h)	10.8	25.9
			Cisplatin (75 mg/m^2)/Paclitaxel (135 mg/m^2 over 24 h)	14.1 (p=0.002)	26.3 (p=0.310)
ICON 3	2,074	All FIGO stages irrespective of optimal or sub-optimal debulking surgery	CAP* or Carboplatin (AUC5 or 6)	16.1	35.4
			Carboplatin (AUC5 or 6)/Paclitaxel (175 mg/m^2 over 3 h)	17.3 (p=0.16)	36.1 (p=0.74)
AGO-OVAR-3	798	FIGO stage IIB-IV	6 cycles of Carboplatin (AUC6)/Paclitaxel (185 mg/m^2 over 3 h)	17.2	43.3
			6 cycles of Cisplatin (75 mg/m^2)/Paclitaxel (185 mg/m^2 over 3 h)	19.1 NS	44.1 NS
GOG-158	792	FIGO stage III with ≤1 cm residual disease after initial surgery	6 cycles of Carboplatin (AUC7.5)/Paclitaxel (175 mg/m^2 over 3 h)	20.7***	57.4***
			6 cycles of Cisplatin (75 mg/m^2)/Paclitaxel (135 mg/m^2 over 24 h)	19.4	48.7
Dutch-Danish Intergroup study	208	FIGO stage IIB-IV	≥6 cycles of Carboplatin (AUC5)/Paclitaxel (175 mg/m^2 over 3 h)	N/A	32
			≥6 cycles of Cisplatin ((75 mg/m^2)/Paclitaxel (175 mg/m^2 over 3 h)		30 (HR1.07; 95 CI, 0.78-0.48)
GOG 218	1,873	FIGO stage III or stage IV	6 cycles Carboplatin (AUC6)/Paclitaxel (175 mg/m^2), placebo with cycles 2–22	10.3	N/A
			Carboplatin (AUC6)/Paclitaxel (175 mg/m^2), bevacizumab (15 mg/Kg) with cycles 2–6 followed by placebo cycles 7–22	11.2 (p=0.16)	
			Carboplatin (AUC6)/Paclitaxel (175 mg/m^2), bevacizumab (15 mg/Kg) with cycles 2–22	14.1 (p<0.001)	

Table 41.1 (continued)

Study	N	Study population	Treatment arms	PFS (months)	OS (months)
ICON 7	1,528	High risk early stage disease (FIGO stage I OR IIA and clear cell or grade 3 tumors) or advanced ovarian cancer (FIGO IIB-IV)	6 cycles of Carboplatin (AUC 5 or 6)/ Paclitaxel (175 mg/m^2)	17.3	28.8**
			6 cycles Carboplatin (AUC 5 or 6)/ Paclitaxel (175 mg/m^2)/bevacizumab (7.5 mg/Kg) +12 cycles bevacizumab maintenance or until disease progression	19 (p=0.004)	36.6** (p=0.002)
Intraperitoneal (IP) chemotherapy studies					
GOG 104	546	Stage III with debulking surgery to a size of ≤2 cm residual	6 cycles of 3-weekly IV cyclophosphamide (600 mg/m^2)/IV Cisplatin (100 mg/m^2)		41
			6 cycles of 3-weekly IV cyclophosphamide (600 mg/m^2)/IP Cisplatin (100 mg/m^2)		49 (p=0.02)
GOG 114	462	Stage III with ≤1 cm residual disease after debulking surgery	6 cycles of 3-weekly IV paclitaxel (135 mg/m^2)/ IV Cisplatin (75 mg/m^2)	22	52
			2 cycles of 4-weekly IV Carboplatin (AUC 9) followed by 6 cycles of 3-weekly IV paclitaxel (135 mg/m^2)/IP Cisplatin (100 mg/m^2)	28 (p=0.01)	63 (p=0.05)
GOG 172	415	Stage III with ≤1 cm residual disease after debulking surgery	6 cycles of 3-weekly IV paclitaxel (135 mg/m^2)/ IV Cisplatin (75 mg/m^2)	18.3	49.7
			6 cycles of 3-weekly IV paclitaxel (135 mg/m^2)/IP Cisplatin (100 mg/m^2) on day 2 and IP paclitaxel (60 mg/m^2) on day 8	23.8 (p=0.05)	65.6 (p=0.03)

**CAP* cyclophosphamide (500 mg/m^2), doxorubicin (50 mg/m^2) and cisplatin (50 mg/m^2), **OS from pre-planned analysis in patients at highest risk of progression (stage III with >1 cm residual disease or stage IV), final OS data NS, ***Relative risk (RR) of progression 0.88(95 % CI 0.75–1.03, RR of death 0.84(95 % CI 0.70–1.02), *NS* not statistically significant, *HR* hazard ratio

with platinum [4]. Four hundred and ten women with advanced ovarian cancer and residual masses larger than 1 cm after initial surgery were randomized to receive cisplatin (75 mg/m^2) with either cyclophosphamide (750 mg/m^2) or paclitaxel (135 mg/m^2 over 24 h). Progression free survival (PFS), (median, 18 vs. 13 months, p<0.001) and overall survival (OS), (median 38 vs. 24 months, p<0.001) were significantly longer in the cisplatin/paclitaxel arm compared to cisplatin/cyclophosphamide in women with sub-optimally debulked ovarian cancer.

The results of the European and Canadian Intergroup trial (EORTC-NCIC OV-10) provided confirmatory evidence for cisplatin and paclitaxel as the standard regimen in advanced ovarian cancer [5]. Compared to GOG-111, this study had a broader selection of patients by also including patients with optimally debulked stage III or IV disease, as well as those having FIGO stage IIB or IIC disease and allowed recruitment of patients who had undergone interval debulking surgery. Additionally, the dose of paclitaxel was higher (175 mg/m^2 vs. 135 mg/m^2) with a shorter infusion time of 3 h, instead of 24 h, as this strategy had previously been found to be more convenient, produce less neutropenia, as well as confer a PFS advantage. After a median follow-up of 38.5 months, a longer PFS (15.5 vs. 11.5 months, p=0.0005) and OS (35.6 vs. 25.8 months, p=0.0016) was observed in the cisplatin and paclitaxel arm compared to the cisplatin and cyclophosphamide arm.

However, the GOG-132 trial which compared cisplatin (100 mg/m^2) or paclitaxel (200 mg/m^2 24 h infusion) monotherapy with the cisplatin (75 mg/m^2) and paclitaxel (135 mg/m^2) combination therapy in suboptimally debulked stage III or IV ovarian cancer did not find any difference in PFS or OS in the combination arm compared to either of the monotherapy arms [6]. Similarly, the International collaborative ovarian neoplasm (ICON)-3 group study which compared carboplatin (AUC5, if glomerular filtration rate (GFR) used and AUC6, if Cockcroft Gault equation used) and paclitaxel (175 mg/m^2 over 3 h) against either single agent carboplatin (AUC5 or 6) or a combination of cyclophosphamide (500 mg/m^2), doxorubicin (50 mg/m^2) and cisplatin (50 mg/m^2) (CAP) also failed to show an OS advantage for the carboplatin/paclitaxel arm [7]. A likely explanation for the lack of survival advantage seen in GOG-132 and ICON3 is that a significant proportion of patients crossed over prior to progression (>20 %) thereby diminishing any potential survival benefit in the platinum/paclitaxel arms. A possible interpretation of the results is that sequential treatment with platinum/paclitaxel is equivalent to the combination.

Once the role of paclitaxel in combination with a platinum agent was established, the AGO-OVAR-3, GOG-158 and Dutch-Danish Intergroup studies concluded that first line chemotherapy with carboplatin and paclitaxel was at least as effective and associated with a better toxicity profile than the cisplatin combination [8–10].

41.3 Optimizing First-Line Combination Chemotherapy

Following the adoption of carboplatin in combination with paclitaxel every 3 weeks for six cycles as the international standard of care, issues including choice of taxane, triple therapy, chemotherapy scheduling and mode of delivery to further improve outcome have been evaluated. However, many questions regarding the optimization of chemotherapy in this setting remain unclear and the results of ongoing studies are awaited.

Choice of Chemotherapy

The Scottish Randomised Trial in Ovarian Cancer (SCOTROC)-1 established that the substitution of paclitaxel (175 mg/m^2) with docetaxel (75 mg/m^2) was not inferior in terms of survival or clinical response and was associated with less neurotoxicity, at the expense of increased grade 3/4 neutropenia [11]. Carboplatin in combination with docetaxel may be an acceptable alternative to carboplatin/paclitaxel for some patients where neurotoxicity is a particular concern.

Several phase III trials have addressed the addition of a third cytotoxic agent to carboplatin/paclitaxel [12–14]. The GOG0182-ICON5 was a randomized, phase III trial containing five arms which incorporated gemcitabine, liposomal doxorubicin, or topotecan compared with carboplatin and paclitaxel [14]. The addition of a third cytotoxic agent has not been shown to improve long-term clinical outcomes and is associated with increased hematological toxicity.

Scheduling of Carboplatin/Paclitaxel

The standard of care is a three-weekly schedule of carboplatin and paclitaxel. However, it has suggested that a dose-fractionated schedule may enhance antitumor activity leading to improved survival. A Japanese study JGOG3016 set out to address this. The study compared six cycles of dose dense weekly paclitaxel (80 mg/m^2, given IV over 1 h) in addition to 3-weekly carboplatin (AUC6) against 3-weekly carboplatin (AUC 6) and paclitaxel (180 mg/m^2 IV over 3 h) in patients with advanced ovarian cancer [15]. Despite higher rates of myelosuppression, delays and dose modifications in the dose dense group, at the median follow up period of 76.8 months, the median PFS (28.2 months vs. 17.5 months, P=0.004) and median OS (100.5 months vs. 62.2 months, P=0.039) was longer in the dose dense group compared to the conventional group [16]. The outcome of this study could lead to change in standard of care and confirmation of the findings of the JGOG study in different study populations is required. Results of the MITO-7 study comparing 3-weekly carboplatin (AUC6) and paclitaxel (175 mg/m^2) against weekly carboplatin (AUC2) and weekly paclitaxel (80 mg/m^2) did not demonstrate a significant benefit in PFS with weekly administration compared to standard carboplatin/paclitaxel every 3 weeks, but was associated with better QoL and toxicity [17]. The ongoing ICON-8 trial is a randomized, phase III, three arm, study evaluating dose fractionation schedules (3 weekly carboplatin/paclitaxel vs 3 weekly carboplatin/weekly paclitaxel vs weekly carboplatin/paclitaxel) following immediate surgery or as part of delayed primary surgery.

Maintenance Chemotherapy

Despite surgery and first-line chemotherapy, at least 65 % of women who achieve a complete response will eventually relapse, at which stage the condition is deemed incurable. Maintenance chemotherapy after initial therapy has been explored as a possible strategy to prevent or delay relapse. In the phase III SWOG 9701/GOG 178 study, patients with advanced ovarian cancer who had achieved complete clinical response were randomly assigned to receive 3 or 12 additional cycles of 4-weekly paclitaxel. Based on an interim analysis which reported a significant improvement in PFS of 7 months (21 vs 28 months) in the 12 cycle arm, the study was stopped prematurely [18]. However, no OS advantage was demonstrated [19]. Potential reasons for a lack of OS benefit include the effect of subsequent therapies, crossover of patients from 3 cycles to 12 cycles and reduced sample size due to the closure of the study. The Italian Cooperative Group After-6 phase III trial evaluated six cycles of 3-weekly paclitaxel as maintenance therapy compared with observation. No significant difference in PFS (34 vs 30 months) or OS (2 year survival rate: 87 % vs 90 %) between the paclitaxel and observation arms was seen following an interim futility analysis and the study closed early [20]. The ongoing GOG-0212 study is evaluating paclitaxel or polyglutamate paclitaxel or observation in women with stage III/IV ovarian cancer who achieve a complete clinical response to primary platinum/paclitaxel chemotherapy.

41.4 The Role of Neoadjuvant Chemotherapy

Primary surgery aims to achieve complete tumor resection with no residual disease because it has been shown that the volume of residual disease following surgery is an independent prognostic indicator.

In some cases of advanced ovarian cancer including stage IV disease, complete cytoreductive surgery with no residual disease may not realistically be achievable. In addition, a proportion of patients may be too unwell at presentation to undergo such major, radical surgery. This has led to debate regarding whether primary surgery or neoadjuvant chemotherapy followed by interval debulking surgery after three to four cycles of chemotherapy is the preferred option [21–23]. Cytoreductive surgery is an integral component in the management of ovarian cancer, there are some concerns that delaying surgery for patients to have chemotherapy may impact on overall outcome. In addition, some subtypes of epithelial ovarian cancer, such as low-grade serous carcinomas do not respond well to chemotherapy and in such cases there is an argument for primary surgery. The European Organisation for Research and Treatment of Cancer (EORTC) 55971 trial recruited potentially operable patients with stage IIIc or IV disease and randomized them to receive either primary debulking surgery and chemotherapy or neoadjuvant chemotherapy followed by interval debulking surgery [24]. The PFS and OS were similar in the two arms but in the neoadjuvant chemotherapy arm 80.6 % had $\leq$1 cm residual tumor remaining compared to only 41.6 % of patients in the primary surgery arm, where post-operative morbidity was more common. The recent results of the phase III CHORUS study [25] support the findings of the EORTC 55971 trial.

As more patients are likely to be receiving neoadjuvant chemotherapy followed by interval debulking surgery, it is important that this strategy is recognized and incorporated into future trial designs of advanced ovarian cancer. At present, the decision regarding whether neoadjuvant chemotherapy followed by interval debulking surgery or primary surgery should be made on a case by case basis in a multidisciplinary setting. Upfront surgery is the preferred option in fit patients where it is believed that cytoreduction with no residual disease can be achieved. However, neoadjuvant therapy can achieve equivalent therapeutic outcomes and may be associated with less morbidity for patients with bulky disease [24].

Time to Initiate Chemotherapy Following Primary Surgery

In patients undergoing primary surgery, the optimal time to initiate chemotherapy is an important issue. While it can be argued that chemotherapy should be initiated as soon as possible to prevent metastatic re-growth, patients who have been optimally debulked may have required invasive surgery including liver and/or bowel resection, as well as diaphragmatic stripping. In an analysis of prospective phase III trials, the median time to chemotherapy was 19 days (range 1–56) and a delayed start to chemotherapy was associated with decreased OS ($p=0.038$) in optimally debulked patients whereas in patients with residual disease, a longer time to initiate chemotherapy had no effect on OS ($p=0.452$) [26]. This analysis provides evidence to support an earlier start to initiate chemotherapy in optimally debulked patients.

Intraperitoneal Chemotherapy

Intra-peritoneal (IP) chemotherapy is another strategy that has been investigated in an attempt to improve outcomes in ovarian cancer. The rationale behind its use stems from the concept that advanced ovarian cancer predominantly affects peritoneal surfaces. Delivering cytotoxic agents directly to the peritoneum therefore increases dose intensity while preventing systemic toxicity.

Three randomized trials provided evidence for a survival advantage with IP chemotherapy compared to IV administration in women with optimally debulked (to <0.5 cm) stage III epithelial ovarian cancer [27–29]. The GOG 104 study compared six cycles of three-weekly IV cyclophosphamide (600 mg/m^2) combined with either IV or IP cisplatin (100 mg/m^2) [27]. The IP arm had a significantly longer median survival, (49 vs. 41 months, $P=0.02$) but at the expense of more frequent moderate to severe abdominal pain. The GOG 114 trial incorporated a taxane into the treatment arms and provided further support for IP chemotherapy [29]. Six cycles of IV paclitaxel (135 mg/m^2) and cisplatin (75 mg/m^2) every 3 weeks was compared with IV carboplatin (AUC 9) every 28 days for two cycles followed by six cycles of IV paclitaxel (135 mg/m^2) and IP cisplatin (100 mg/m^2) every 3 weeks in patients with stage III optimally debulked ovarian cancer. Median PFS was longer in the IP arm (28 months vs. 22 months, $P=0.01$) and median OS was increased in this arm (63 months vs. 52 months, $P=0.05$) but again patients in the IP arm experienced increased toxicity and 18 % of patients received less than two courses of IP chemotherapy as a consequence. In GOG 172, 415 patients with optimally debulked stage III ovarian cancer were randomized to receive 63 weekly cycles of IV paclitaxel (135 mg/m ^{2} over 24 h) followed by either IV cisplatin (75 mg/m^2) on day 2 or IP cisplatin (100 mg/m^2) on day 2 plus IP cisplatin (60 mg/m^2) on day 8 [28]. The median survival data was impressive and again in favor of the IP arm (65.6 months vs. 49.7 months, $P=0.03$). Despite the results of all three trials appearing to support the role of IP chemotherapy, it has not become routine clinical practice internationally. This is in part largely due to the increased toxicity (abdominal discomfort, infection, bowel injury, catheter-related problems, fatigue, hematological, gastrointestinal and neurological events) in the IP arms. It has been argued that the favorable outcome in GOG 114 [29] may be influenced by the increased amount of chemotherapy delivered in the IP arm (eight cycles). Furthermore, in GOG 172, the control arm did not receive the current standard of care i.e., IV carboplatin and paclitaxel and the dose and schedule of cisplatin and paclitaxel was different in the two arms of the study [28]. Therefore the higher dose of chemotherapy in the IP arm may have played a significant part in the survival benefit seen rather than the mode of delivery itself. Finally, the analysis was not a true intention-to-treat analysis and therefore it is feasible for minor imbalances in the number of excluded patients impacting on the statistical significance.

Combined data from the GOG114 and GOG172 demonstrated a significant improvement in median OS with IP administration, compared with IV administration (61.8 vs 51.4 months; P=0.048) [30]. A subset analysis of 393 patients within the GOG172 study suggested that the survival advantage of IP chemotherapy was limited to a subset of patients with low BRCA1 expression as measured by immumohistochemistry (84 months IP vs 47 months IV; p=0.0002) and that low BRCA1 expression was an independent prognostic factor for better survival in women randomized to IP therapy (hazard ratio (HR)=0.67 p=0.032) [31].

Several trials of IP chemotherapy are ongoing and include GOG-252, NCIC-CTG OV21/NCRI-PETROC and JGOG 3109. Issues addressed include the use of carboplatin/paclitaxel as the control arm, incorporating dose-dense scheduling of paclitaxel, bevacizumab and IP administration of carboplatin.

41.5 Novel Biological Agents

Novel biologically targeted agents aim to target tumor cells and/or the microenvironment by exploiting specific molecular abnormalities in the tumor leading to greater selectivity and a better toxicity profile than traditional chemotherapy [32]. Epithelial ovarian cancer has previously been treated as a single disease. It is recognized that ovarian cancer is a heterogenous disease rather than a single entity, made up of several histological subtypes with distinct clinical outcomes and molecular aberrations (high grade serous- p53, BRCA, homologous recombination deficiency; low grade serous- BRAF, KRAS, NRAS, HER2); clear cell-PIK3CA, PTEN; endometrioid PIK3CA, PTEN; and mucinous- KRAS, HER2). Multiple molecules involved in critical, signalling pathways which drive growth and progression of ovarian cancer can now be targeted with novel drugs [32]. Angiogenesis inhibitors and PARP inhibitors are the most developed in ovarian cancer.

41.6 Angiogenesis Inhibitors

Angiogenesis is the formation of new blood vessels and is a critical component of cancer growth and metastasis. Vascular endothelial growth factor (VEGF) is a key promoter in the process of angiogenesis in epithelial ovarian cancer. Strategies to target either the ligand or the receptor have been explored. Bevacizumab is a humanized monoclonal antibody that targets VEGF-A and prevents it from binding to VEGF receptors and subsequent downstream signalling. Two randomized, phase III trials, the Gynecologic Oncology Group (GOG) trial 0218 [33] and ICON-7 trial [34], set out to evaluate the addition of bevacizumab to the combination of carboplatin/paclitaxel followed by maintenance therapy as first-line treatment for advanced ovarian cancer. The GOG-0218 study was a three arm, double blind placebo-controlled trial enrolling 1,873 patients with either stage III or stage IV epithelial ovarian cancer who had undergone debulking surgery [33]. The study participants were randomized to receive either standard treatment with IV carboplatin and paclitaxel for six cycles every 3 weeks followed by placebo every 3 weeks for cycles 7–22 or standard treatment with the addition of bevacizumab (15 mg/kg) from cycle 2 until cycle 22 (a total of 15 months) or standard treatment with the addition of bevacizumab (15 mg/kg) from cycle 2–6 followed by placebo for cycles 7–22. Patients in the bevacizumab throughout arm had a significant improvement in PFS compared to the control arm (14.1 vs. 10.3 months HR 0.717; P<0.001). The IOCN-7 study was an open label study that assigned 1,528 patients to either carboplatin and paclitaxel with concurrent bevacizumab (7.5 mg/kg) followed by maintenance bevacizumab for 12 cycles (or until disease progression) or carboplatin and paclitaxel alone [34]. This study confirmed an improvement in PFS with the addition of bevacizumab (19.0 vs. 17.3 months; HR 0.81; P=0.004). A pre-planned analysis of the patients at highest risk of progression (stage III with >1 cm residual disease or stage IV disease), showed that bevacizumab conferred a greater magnitude of benefit in this sub-population (restricted means 18.1 vs. 14.5 months; HR 0.73; P=0.002). Furthermore, early analyses demonstrated a significant improvement in OS in the high risk group (28.8 vs. 36.6 months HR=0.64, 95 % CI 0.48–0.85; P=0.002). However, the final OS data from the ICON-7 study showed no benefit from the addition of bevacizumab and an OS benefit was not evident in GOG-0218. In ICON-7, in a pre-specified sub-group analysis of poor prognosis patients, a benefit of 4.8 months in the restricted means survival time was observed [35].

In both studies, the addition of bevacizumab was relatively well-tolerated with adverse effects as expected for angiogenesis inhibitors [36]-(≥grade 2, ICON-7 18 % (bevacizumab arm) vs 2 % (chemotherapy)), thromboembolism (≥grade 3, ICON-7 7 % (bevacizumab arm) vs 3 % (chemotherapy)). Recognized complications of bevacizumab include gastrointestinal (GI) perforation and fistula formation. However, in ICON-7 and GOG-0218, the reported rates of GI perforation are low (≥grade 3 ICON-7 1 % bevacizumab arm; <3 % in GOG 218 and 1 %). The results of these studies led to the European Medicines Agency (EMA) approval of bevacizumab to be used in combination with carboplatin and paclitaxel in the front line setting of patients with advanced ovarian cancer (FIGO stage IIIB, IIIC and IV).

The role of bevacizumab has also been investigated in recurrent ovarian cancer. The OCEANS study, a double-blind, placebo-controlled trial evaluated the addition of bevacizumab (15 mg/kg) to carboplatin (AUC 4) and gemcitabine (1,000 mg/m2 on day 1 and day 8) continued until progression in women with first relapse platinum-sensitive ovarian cancer [37]. This study provided evidence for bevacizumab in the platinum sensitive setting with an improvement in PFS (12.4 vs 8.4 months, P<0.0001). In addition, the AURELIA study provided support for the use of bevacizumab (15 mg/kg) in the platinum resistant setting [38]. Bevacizumab in combination with paclitaxel, topotecan or liposomal doxorubicin led to a significant improvement in PFS (6.7 vs. 3.4 months; HR 0.48, P<0.001) but no statistically significant improvement in OS.

It is currently not known whether bevacizumab should be used in the first line setting or reserved for platinum-sensitive or platinum-resistant relapse. Ongoing trials of bevacizumab address the role of bevacizumab with IP chemotherapy, dose dense chemotherapy, extending the duration of maintenance therapy and the continuation of bevacizumab beyond progression. Preliminary data from the GOG-262 trial, evaluating bevacizumab in combination with dose dense chemotherapy suggests that bevacizumab does not confer any additional benefit to dose dense treatment [39].

VEGF receptor tyrosine kinase inhibitors (TKIs) inhibit downstream VEGF signalling and other pro-angiogenic molecules such as platelet derived growth factor (PDGFR) and fibroblast growth factor (FGFR). VEGFR TKIs is a potential strategy to help overcome some mechanisms of resistance to antiangiogenic therapy [40]. The AGO-OVAR 16 trial is a phase III randomized, double-blind study which involved 940 patients with FIGO stage II to IV ovarian, fallopian tube, or primary peritoneal cancer who had been initially treated with surgery and chemotherapy to receive 800 mg of pazopanib or placebo daily for up to 24 months [41]. There was a significant improvement in median PFS (17.9 months vs 12.3 months; HR 0.788, p=0.002). However, 58 % of patients in the treatment arm required a dose reduction compared with 14 % of patients in the placebo arm and the most frequent grade 3 or

4 toxicity was hypertension (31 % vs 6 %). Nevertheless, this is the first study of a targeted agent administered as maintenance therapy only, showing a meaningful PFS benefit. The OS data remain immature. The results of the AGO-OVAR12, a phase III trial of nintedanib (BIBF1120), an inhibitor of VEGFR, FGFR and PDGFR in combination with carboplatin/paclitaxel followed by maintenance therapy in the first-line setting, showed a modest PFS benefit in the nintedanib arm (17.3 vs. 16.6 months, p=0.024). The most significant PFS benefit with nintedanib was seen in the low risk group with low volume disease following surgery (27.1 vs. 20.8 months, p=0.005) suggesting its role in maintenance treatment in such patients [42].

Cediranib, an oral pan-VEGFR kinase inhibitor has been evaluated in relapsed platinum sensitive disease in combination with chemotherapy followed by maintenance in the ICON-6 trial. Cediranib is the first TKI to demonstrate a statistically significant OS benefit (2.7 months) [43].

Most recently, the results of TRINOVA-1, a double blind placebo controlled phase III trial using Trebananib to target the angiopoietin axis as an alternative anti-angiogenic strategy, have been published. Trebananib is an Fc fusion protein that binds to the angiopoietins, Ang1 and Ang2 and prevents their interaction with the Tie2 receptor. Patients that had been treated with ≤ three previous regimens and had a platinum free interval of <12 months were enrolled to receive weekly paclitaxel with IV Trebananib or placebo. Median PFS was longer in the Trebananib group (7.2 vs. 5.4 months, p<0.0001) although Trebananib was related to more adverse event-related treatment discontinuation [44].

41.7 PARP Inhibitors

Women with mutations in the *BRCA* genes (*BRCA1* or *BRCA2*) have an increased risk of developing ovarian cancer due to defects in DNA repair pathways (called homologous recombination). Tumors in patients with a *BRCA* mutation are particularly susceptible to drugs called PARP inhibitors which generate specific DNA lesions that require functional BRCA1 and BRCA2 for DNA repair [45]. PARP inhibitors in clinical trials of ovarian cancer include olaparib, rucaparib and niraparib. Encouraging response rates were seen in patients with heavily pre-treated ovarian cancer that harbor a germline BRCA mutation (57.6 % RECIST and CA–125 criteria) [46, 47]. Based on the observation that up to 50 % of high-grade serous, sporadic ovarian cancers may have homologous recombination defects (including somatic BRCA mutations, BRCA methylation) which confer sensitivity to PARP inhibition, a randomized phase II trial of maintenance therapy with olaparib was performed [48]. In this study, olaparib extended PFS by almost 4 months (median 8.4 months vs. 4.8 months; HR 0.35, P<0.001), in patients with platinum-sensitive, relapsed, high-grade serous ovarian cancer with or without *BRCA1* or *BRCA2* germline mutations. The improvement in PFS was greater in *BRCA* mutation carriers (median: 11.2 vs 4.1 months; HR, 0.17; P<0.001) [49].

A phase III trial of maintenance olaparib or placebo in patients who have responded to first-line chemotherapy is currently recruiting.

41.8 Other Targeted Agents

Epidermal growth factor receptor (EGFR) inhibition has been investigated as maintenance therapy following first-line chemotherapy. Maintenance erlotinib, an EGFR inhibitor, did not improve PFS or OS in the EORTC55041/OV07 [50]. A randomized trial of oregovomab monotherapy (monoclonal antibody directed against CA-125) maintenance post first-line therapy also failed to show an improvement in clinical outcome [51].

Folate receptors are overexpressed in epithelial ovarian cancer but not in normal tissues therefore anti-folate receptor antibodies and folate chemotherapy-conjugates have been investigated as treatment strategies. Farletuzumab, a monoclonal antibody that binds to folate receptorα has been investigated in a double blind placebo-controlled phase III trial in combination with carboplatin and taxane chemotherapy in patients with first platinum sensitive relapse [52]. The results were disappointing as the study did not meet its primary end point of PFS. Vintafolide (EC145), is a folic acid-desacetylvinblastine conjugate that binds to the folate receptor. Etarfolatide is a folate receptor targeted imaging agent thought to be helpful in selecting patients likely to benefit from vintafolide. A phase II study investigated vintafolide in combination with pegylated liposomal doxorubicin (PLD) compared to PLD alone in platinum resistant patients and showed an improvement in PFS (5 vs. 2.7 months, p=0.031) [53]. The encouraging results from this study prompted a randomized, double blind, phase III trial in platinum resistant ovarian cancer, the PROCEED study which was terminated early. The results are awaited.

Many other targeted agents are under investigation in recurrent ovarian cancer and include targeting the RAS/Raf/MEK pathway and PI3 kinase/AKT/mTOR pathway [32]. Successful strategies in recurrent ovarian cancer are likely to be developed in the first-line setting as has been the case with bevacizumab and olaparib.

Conclusion

Advanced ovarian cancer remains an incurable disease for the majority of patients. Improvements in first-line systemic therapies delivered in the neoadjuvant and/or adjuvant settings have the potential to prevent or at least delay disease relapse. Carboplatin in combination with paclitaxel remains the standard of care worldwide. Bevacizumab is approved in Europe as part of first line treatment and other angiogenesis inhibitors such as pazopanib may follow suit. PARP inhibitors appear promising and a trial as first-line maintenance is planned in *BRCA* mutation carriers. The successful integration of targeted therapy with chemotherapy will depend on the identification of the correct patient population, managing new toxicities, utilizing biomarkers to guide management and overcoming drug resistance.

Key Points

- The majority of women present with advanced ovarian cancer and the OS is around 40 %
- 'Adjuvant' refers to chemotherapy given following surgery. 'Neoadjuvant' refers to upfront chemotherapy followed by interval debulking surgery (followed by chemotherapy)
- The international standard of care for advanced ovarian cancer is either upfront or interval attempted optimal cytoreductive surgery and six cycles of carboplatin in combination with paclitaxel
- Neoadjuvant chemotherapy followed by interval debulking surgery is a valid treatment option for patients with bulky stage IIIC or IV ovarian carcinoma
- IP chemotherapy is a promising approach. It is not considered standard of care. Further clinical trials are ongoing.
- Bevacizumab in combination with first line chemotherapy followed by maintenance therapy improves PFS
- There is an OS benefit from bevacizumab when given in the first line setting to women at high risk of disease progression (>1 cm residual disease or stage IV)
- Anti-angiogenic agents improve clinical outcome in the first line and recurrent (platinum sensitive and platinum resistant) setting
- PARP inhibitors as maintenance therapy following chemotherapy for platinum-sensitive relapse significantly improve PFS. Phase III clinical trials are underway
- BRCA mutation carriers derive the most benefit from PARP inhibitors

Acknowledgments We acknowledge support from the National Institute of Health Research (NIHR) Biomedical Research Centre.

References

1. Ferlay J, Shin HR, Bray F, Forman D, Mathers C, Parkin DM. Estimates of worldwide burden of cancer in 2008: GLOBOCAN 2008. Int J Cancer. 2010;127(12):2893–917. PubMed PMID: 21351269. Epub 2011/02/26. eng.
2. CRUK. Cancer Research UK ovarian incidence statistics. 2010 http://info.cancerresearchuk.org/cancerstats/incidence/risk/. Accessed 2013.
3. du Bois A, Quinn M, Thigpen T, Vermorken J, Avall-Lundqvist E, Bookman M, et al. 2004 consensus statements on the management of ovarian cancer: final document of the 3rd International Gynecologic Cancer Intergroup Ovarian Cancer Consensus Conference (GCIG OCCC 2004). Ann Oncol. 2005;16 Suppl 8:viii 7–12. PubMed PMID: 16239238.
4. McGuire WP, Hoskins WJ, Brady MF, Kucera PR, Partridge EE, Look KY, et al. Cyclophosphamide and cisplatin compared with paclitaxel and cisplatin in patients with stage III and stage IV ovarian cancer. N Engl J Med. 1996;334(1):1–6. PubMed PMID: 7494563.
5. Piccart MJ, Bertelsen K, James K, Cassidy J, Mangioni C, Simonsen E, et al. Randomized intergroup trial of cisplatin-paclitaxel versus cisplatin-cyclophosphamide in women with advanced epithelial ovarian cancer: three-year results. J Natl Cancer Inst. 2000;92(9):699–708. PubMed PMID: 10793106.
6. Muggia FM, Braly PS, Brady MF, Sutton G, Niemann TH, Lentz SL, et al. Phase III randomized study of cisplatin versus paclitaxel versus cisplatin and paclitaxel in patients with suboptimal stage III or IV ovarian cancer: a gynecologic oncology group study. J Clin Oncol. 2000;18(1):106–15. PubMed PMID: 10623700.
7. Group. ICON. Paclitaxel plus carboplatin versus standard chemotherapy with either single-agent carboplatin or cyclophosphamide, doxorubicin, and cisplatin in women with ovarian cancer: the ICON3 randomised trial. Lancet. 2002;360(9332):505–15. PubMed PMID: 12241653. Epub 2002/09/21. eng.
8. du Bois A, Luck HJ, Meier W, Adams HP, Mobus V, Costa S, et al. A randomized clinical trial of cisplatin/paclitaxel versus carboplatin/paclitaxel as first-line treatment of ovarian cancer. J Natl Cancer Inst. 2003;95(17):1320–9. PubMed PMID: 12953086.
9. Ozols RF, Bundy BN, Greer BE, Fowler JM, Clarke-Pearson D, Burger RA, et al. Phase III trial of carboplatin and paclitaxel compared with cisplatin and paclitaxel in patients with optimally resected stage III ovarian cancer: a Gynecologic Oncology Group study. J Clin Oncol. 2003;21(17):3194–200. PubMed PMID: 12860964.
10. Neijt JP, Engelholm SA, Tuxen MK, Sorensen PG, Hansen M, Sessa C, et al. Exploratory phase III study of paclitaxel and cisplatin versus paclitaxel and carboplatin in advanced ovarian cancer. J Clin Oncol. 2000;18(17):3084–92. PubMed PMID: 10963636.
11. Vasey PA, Jayson GC, Gordon A, Gabra H, Coleman R, Atkinson R, et al. Phase III randomized trial of docetaxel-carboplatin versus paclitaxel-carboplatin as first-line chemotherapy for ovarian carcinoma. J Natl Cancer Inst. 2004;96(22):1682–91. PubMed PMID: 15547181.
12. Kristensen GB, Vergote I, Stuart G, Del Campo JM, Kaern J, Lopez AB, et al. First-line treatment of ovarian cancer FIGO stages IIb-IV with paclitaxel/epirubicin/carboplatin versus paclitaxel/carboplatin. Int J Gynecol Cancer. 2003;13 Suppl 2:172–7. PubMed PMID: 14656276.
13. du Bois A, Weber B, Rochon J, Meier W, Goupil A, Olbricht S, et al. Addition of epirubicin as a third drug to carboplatin-paclitaxel in first-line treatment of advanced ovarian cancer: a prospectively randomized gynecologic cancer intergroup trial by the Arbeitsgemeinschaft Gynaekologische Onkologie Ovarian Cancer Study Group and the Groupe d'Investigateurs Nationaux pour l'Etude des Cancers Ovariens. J Clin Oncol. 2006;24(7):1127–35. PubMed PMID: 16505432.
14. Bookman MA, Brady MF, McGuire WP, Harper PG, Alberts DS, Friedlander M, et al. Evaluation of new platinum-based treatment regimens in advanced-stage ovarian cancer: a phase III trial of the Gynecologic Cancer Intergroup. J Clin Oncol. 2009;27(9):1419–25. PubMed PMID: 19224846. Pubmed Central PMCID: 2668552.
15. Katsumata N, Yasuda M, Takahashi F, Isonishi S, Jobo T, Aoki D, et al. Dose-dense paclitaxel once a week in combination with carboplatin every 3 weeks for advanced ovarian cancer: a phase 3, open-label, randomised controlled trial. Lancet. 2009;374(9698):1331–8. PubMed PMID: 19767092.
16. Katsumata N, Yasuda M, Isonishi S, Takahashi F, Michimae H, Kimura E, et al. Long-term results of dose-dense paclitaxel and carboplatin versus conventional paclitaxel and carboplatin for treatment of advanced epithelial ovarian, fallopian tube, or primary peritoneal cancer (JGOG 3016): a randomised, controlled, open-label trial. Lancet Oncol. 2013;14(10):1020–6. PubMed PMID: 23948349.
17. Pignata S, Scambia G, Katsaros D, Gallo C, Pujade-Lauraine E, De Placido S, et al. Carboplatin plus paclitaxel once a week versus every 3 weeks in patients with advanced ovarian cancer (MITO-7): a randomised, multicentre, open-label, phase 3 trial. Lancet Oncol. 2014;15(4):396–405. PubMed PMID: 24582486.
18. Markman M, Liu PY, Wilczynski S, Monk B, Copeland LJ, Alvarez RD, et al. Phase III randomized trial of 12 versus 3 months of maintenance paclitaxel in patients with advanced ovarian cancer after complete response to platinum and paclitaxel-based chemotherapy: a Southwest Oncology Group and Gynecologic Oncology Group trial. J Clin Oncol. 2003;21(13):2460–5. PubMed PMID: 12829663.
19. Markman M, Liu PY, Moon J, Monk BJ, Copeland L, Wilczynski S, et al. Impact on survival of 12 versus 3 monthly cycles of paclitaxel (175 mg/m2) adminis-

tered to patients with advanced ovarian cancer who attained a complete response to primary platinum-paclitaxel: follow-up of a Southwest Oncology Group and Gynecologic Oncology Group phase 3 trial. Gynecol Oncol. 2009;114(2):195–8. PubMed PMID: 19447479. Epub 2009/05/19. eng.
20. Pecorelli S, Favalli G, Gadducci A, Katsaros D, Panici PB, Carpi A, et al. Phase III trial of observation versus six courses of paclitaxel in patients with advanced epithelial ovarian cancer in complete response after six courses of paclitaxel/platinum-based chemotherapy: final results of the after-6 protocol 1. J Clin Oncol. 2009;27(28):4642–8. PubMed PMID: 19704064. Epub 2009/08/26. eng.
21. Bristow RE, Chi DS. Platinum-based neoadjuvant chemotherapy and interval surgical cytoreduction for advanced ovarian cancer: a meta-analysis. Gynecol Oncol. 2006;103(3):1070–6. PubMed PMID: 16875720.
22. Kumar L, Hariprasas R, Kumar S. Neoadjuvant chemotherapy (NACT) followed by interval debulking surgery versus upfront surgery followed by chemotherapy (CT) in advanced epithelial ovarian carcinoma (EOC): a prospective randomized study – interim results. J Clin Oncol. 2007;25(18S):abstr 5531.
23. van der Burg ME, van Lent M, Buyse M, Kobierska A, Colombo N, Favalli G, et al. The effect of debulking surgery after induction chemotherapy on the prognosis in advanced epithelial ovarian cancer. Gynecological Cancer Cooperative Group of the European Organization for research and treatment of cancer. N Engl J Med. 1995;332(10):629–34. PubMed PMID: 7845426. Epub 1995/03/09. eng.
24. Vergote I, Trope CG, Amant F, Kristensen GB, Ehlen T, Johnson N, et al. Neoadjuvant chemotherapy or primary surgery in stage IIIC or IV ovarian cancer. N Engl J Med. 2010;363(10):943–53. PubMed PMID: 20818904.
25. Kehoe S, Hook J, Nankivell M, Jayson G, Kitchener H, Lopes T, et al. Chemotherapy or upfront surgery for newly diagnosed advanced ovarian cancer: results from the MRC CHORUS trial. J Clin Oncol. 2013;31(Suppl):abstr 5500.
26. Mahner S, Eulenburg C, Staehle A, Wegscheider K, Reuss A, Pujade-Lauraine E, et al. Prognostic impact of the time interval between surgery and chemotherapy in advanced ovarian cancer: analysis of prospective randomised phase III trials. Eur J Cancer. 2013;49(1):142–9. PubMed PMID: 22921185.
27. Alberts DS, Liu PY, Hannigan EV, O'Toole R, Williams SD, Young JA, et al. Intraperitoneal cisplatin plus intravenous cyclophosphamide versus intravenous cisplatin plus intravenous cyclophosphamide for stage III ovarian cancer. N Engl J Med. 1996;335(26):1950–5. PubMed PMID: 8960474.
28. Armstrong DK, Bundy B, Wenzel L, Huang HQ, Baergen R, Lele S, et al. Intraperitoneal cisplatin and paclitaxel in ovarian cancer. N Engl J Med. 2006;354(1):34–43. PubMed PMID: 16394300.
29. Markman M, Bundy BN, Alberts DS, Fowler JM, Clark-Pearson DL, Carson LF, et al. Phase III trial of standard-dose intravenous cisplatin plus paclitaxel versus moderately high-dose carboplatin followed by intravenous paclitaxel and intraperitoneal cisplatin in small-volume stage III ovarian carcinoma: an intergroup study of the Gynecologic Oncology Group, Southwestern Oncology Group, and Eastern Cooperative Oncology Group. J Clin Oncol. 2001;19(4):1001–7. PubMed PMID: 11181662.
30. Tewari D, Java J, Salani R, Armstrong D, Markman M, Herzog T, et al. Long-term survival advantage of intraperitoneal chemotherapy treatment in advanced ovarian cancer: an analysis of a Gynecologic Oncology Group ancillary data study. Gynecol Oncol. 2013;130:e4.
31. Lesnock JL, Darcy KM, Tian C, Deloia JA, Thrall MM, Zahn C, et al. BRCA1 expression and improved survival in ovarian cancer patients treated with intraperitoneal cisplatin and paclitaxel: a Gynecologic Oncology Group Study. Br J Cancer. 2013;108(6):1231–7. PubMed PMID: 23462720. Pubmed Central PMCID: 3619264. Epub 2013/03/07. eng.
32. Banerjee S, Kaye SB. New strategies in the treatment of ovarian cancer: current clinical perspectives and future potential. Clin Cancer Res. 2013;19(5):961–8. PubMed PMID: 23307860. Epub 2013/01/12. eng.
33. Burger RA, Brady MF, Bookman MA, Fleming GF, Monk BJ, Huang H, et al. Incorporation of bevacizumab in the primary treatment of ovarian cancer. N Engl J Med. 2011;365(26):2473–83. PubMed PMID: 22204724. Epub 2011/12/30. eng.
34. Perren TJ, Swart AM, Pfisterer J, Ledermann JA, Pujade-Lauraine E, Kristensen G, et al. A phase 3 trial of bevacizumab in ovarian cancer. N Engl J Med. 2011;365(26):2484–96. PubMed PMID: 22204725. Epub 2011/12/30. eng.
35. Oza A, Perren T, Swart A, Schroder W, Pujade-Lauraine E, Havsteen H, et al. ICON7: final overall survival results in the GCIG phase III randomized trial of bevacizumab in women with newly diagnosed ovarian cancer. Eur J Cancer. 2013;49 Suppl 3:abstr 6.
36. Stone RL, Sood AK, Coleman RL. Collateral damage: toxic effects of targeted antiangiogenic therapies in ovarian cancer. Lancet Oncol. 2010;11(5):465–75. PubMed PMID: 20226736. Pubmed Central PMCID: 3199129. Epub 2010/03/17. eng.
37. Aghajanian C, Blank SV, Goff BA, Judson PL, Teneriello MG, Husain A, et al. OCEANS: a randomized, double-blind, placebo-controlled phase III trial of chemotherapy with or without bevacizumab in patients with platinum-sensitive recurrent epithelial ovarian, primary peritoneal, or fallopian tube cancer. J Clin Oncol. 2012;30(17):2039–45. PubMed PMID: 22529265.
38. Pujade-Lauraine E, Hilpert F, Weber B, Reuss A, Poveda A, Kristensen G, et al. Bevacizumab combined with chemotherapy for platinum-resistant recurrent ovarian cancer: the AURELIA open-label randomized phase III trial. J Clin Oncol. 2014;32(13):1302–8. PubMed PMID: 24637997.
39. Chan J, Brady M, Penson R, Monk B, Boente M, Walker J, et al., editors. Phase III trial of every-3-

weeks paclitaxel versus dose dense weekly paclitaxel with carboplatin+/−bevacizumab in epithelial ovarian, peritoneal, fallopian tube cancer: GOG 262 (NCT0116712). Oral presentation at the 18th International Meeting of the European Society of Gynecological Oncology, Liverpool, UK; 2013.
40. Bottsford-Miller JN, Coleman RL, Sood AK. Resistance and escape from antiangiogenesis therapy: clinical implications and future strategies. J Clin Oncol. 2012;30(32):4026–34. PubMed PMID: 23008289. Pubmed Central PMCID: 3488272. Epub 2012/09/26. eng.
41. Andreas Du Bois AF, Kim JW, Rau J, Del Campo JM, Friedlander M, Pignata S, Fujiwara K, Vergote I, Colombo C, Mirza MR, Monk BJ, Wimberger P, Ray-Coquard I, Zang R, Diaz-Padilla I, Baumann KH, Kim JH, Harter P. Randomized, double-blind, phase III trial of pazopanib versus placebo in women who have not progressed after first-line chemotherapy for advanced epithelial ovarian, fallopian tube, or primary peritoneal cancer (AEOC): results of an international intergroup trial (AGO-OVAR16). J Clin Oncol. 2013;31(Suppl):abstr LBA5503.
42. Du Bois A, Kristensen G, Ray-Coquard I, Reuss A, Pignata S, Colombo N, et al., editors. Ago-ovar 12: a randomized placebo-controlled gcig/engot-intergroup phase iii trial of standard frontline chemotherapy plus/-nintedanib for advanced ovarian cancer. Int J Gynecol Cancer; 2013: Philadelphia: Lippincott Williams & Wilkins. 23(8 Suppl 1)7–8.
43. Ledermann J, Perren T, Raja F, et al. Randomised double-blind phase III trial of cediranib (AZD 2171) in relapsed platinum sensitive ovarian cancer: results of the ICON6 trial. European Society for Medical Oncology Congress 2013; September 27–October 1, 2013; Amsterdam, The Netherlands. Abstract 10
44. Monk BJ, Poveda A, Vergote I, Raspagliesi F, Fujiwara K, Bae DS, et al. Anti-angiopoietin therapy with trebananib for recurrent ovarian cancer (TRINOVA-1): a randomised, multicentre, double-blind, placebo-controlled phase 3 trial. Lancet Oncol. 2014;15(8):799–808. PubMed PMID: 24950985.
45. Ashworth A. A synthetic lethal therapeutic approach: poly(ADP) ribose polymerase inhibitors for the treatment of cancers deficient in DNA double-strand break repair. J Clin Oncol. 2008;26(22):3785–90. PubMed PMID: 18591545. Epub 2008/07/02. eng.
46. Fong PC, Boss DS, Yap TA, Tutt A, Wu P, Mergui-Roelvink M, et al. Inhibition of poly(ADP-ribose) polymerase in tumors from BRCA mutation carriers. N Engl J Med. 2009;361(2):123–34. PubMed PMID: 19553641. Epub 2009/06/26. eng.
47. Fong PC, Yap TA, Boss DS, Carden CP, Mergui-Roelvink M, Gourley C, et al. Poly(ADP)-ribose polymerase inhibition: frequent durable responses in BRCA carrier ovarian cancer correlating with platinum-free interval. J Clin Oncol. 2010;28(15):2512–9. PubMed PMID: 20406929. Epub 2010/04/22. eng.
48. Ledermann J, Harter P, Gourley C, Friedlander M, Vergote I, Rustin G, et al. Olaparib maintenance therapy in platinum-sensitive relapsed ovarian cancer. N Engl J Med. 2012;366(15):1382–92. PubMed PMID: 22452356. Epub 2012/03/29. eng.
49. Jonathan A, Ledermann PH, Gourley C, Friedlander M, Vergote I, Rustin GJS, Scott GL, Meier W, Shapira-Frommer R, Safra T, Matei T, Fielding A, Macpherson E, Dougherty B, Jürgensmeier JM, Orr M, Matulonis U. Olaparib maintenance therapy in patients with platinum-sensitive relapsed serous ovarian cancer (SOC) and a BRCA mutation (BRCAm). J Clin Oncol. 2013;31(Suppl):abstr 5505.
50. Vergote IB, Joly F, Katsaros D, Corneel Coens AR, Marcia H, Steer CB, Nicoletta C, Anne L, Antonio C, Edgar P, John G, Martin B, Isabelle Laure R-C, Annamaria F, Laure F, Nicholas R, Herve C, Jimeno A, Pujade-Lauraine E. Randomized phase III study of erlotinib versus observation in patients with no evidence of disease progression after first-line platin-based chemotherapy for ovarian carcinoma: a GCIG and EORTC-GCG study. J Clin Oncol. 2012;30(Suppl):abstr LBA5000.
51. Berek J, Taylor P, McGuire W, Smith LM, Schultes B, Nicodemus CF. Oregovomab maintenance monoimmunotherapy does not improve outcomes in advanced ovarian cancer. J Clin Oncol. 2009;27(3):418–25. PubMed PMID: 19075271. Epub 2008/12/17. eng.
52. Vergote J, Armstrong D, Scambia G, Fujiwara K, Gorbunova V, Schweizer C. Phase III double-blind, placebo-controlled study of weekly farletuzumab with carboplatin/taxane in subjects with platinum-sensitive ovarian cancer in first relapse. Int J Gynecol Cancer. 2013;23(8 Suppl 1):11.
53. Naumann RW, Coleman RL, Burger RA, Sausville EA, Kutarska E, Ghamande SA, et al. PRECEDENT: a randomized phase II trial comparing vintafolide (EC145) and pegylated liposomal doxorubicin (PLD) in combination versus PLD alone in patients with platinum-resistant ovarian cancer. J Clin Oncol. 2013;31(35):4400–6. PubMed PMID: 24127448.

Part IV

Colorectal

Anatomy of the Rectum and Anus

42

Nelya Melnitchouk and Martin R. Weiser

42.1 Pelvic Anatomy

The pelvis is enclosed by rigid bony, ligamentous and vascular walls, creating a funnel-shaped cavity that contains nerves and viscera. Precise dissection within the confines of this complex anatomical space presents a challenge, even to the most experienced clinician. For the colorectal, urologic or gynecologic surgeon, a detailed knowledge of pelvic anatomy is essential.

42.2 Bony Pelvis

The bony pelvis comprises four bones creating a strong ring: two hip bones laterally and anteriorly, and the sacrum and coccyx posteriorly. Together, these support the body's weight.

The hip bones are formed by a fusion of three bones at puberty: the ilium, ischium and pubis. The ilium articulates with the sacrum, forming the sacroiliac joints posteriorly. Two pubic bones join by cartilaginous attachment anteriorly, forming the symphysis pubis. All three bones fuse to form the acetabulum, which articulates with the head of the femur. The pelvis is angled posteriorly from the abdominal cavity; the anterior superior iliac spine and anterior aspect of the pubic symphysis form one vertical plane.

The bony pelvis is divided into the greater (false) and lesser (true) pelvis by an oblique plane that passes from the sacral promontory posteriorly, and the terminal lines laterally and anteriorly.

42.3 Ligaments

Ligaments connect the bones of the pelvis, contributing to pelvic stability. The anterior and posterior sacrococcygeal ligaments stabilize the articulation between sacrum and coccyx. The sacrospinous ligament extends from the lateral border of the sacrum to the ischial spine to enclose the lesser sciatic notch, forming the lesser sciatic foramen.

Several structures pass through the lesser sciatic foramen: the tendon of the obturator internus, the nerve to the obturator internus, the pudendal nerve, and the internal pudendal artery. The sacrotuberous ligament extends from the dorsum, the lateral border of the sacrum, and the posterior surface of the ilium to the ischial tuberosity, enclosing and forming the greater sciatic foramen.

Several structures pass through the greater sciatic foramen: the piriformis muscle; the sciatic nerve; the inferior gluteal artery and nerve; the

N. Melnitchouk, MD
Department of Surgery, Memorial Sloan Kettering Cancer Center, New York, NY, USA

M.R. Weiser, MD (✉)
Colorectal Service, Department of Surgery, Memorial Sloan Kettering Cancer Center and Weill Cornell Medical College,
1275 York Avenue, Room C-1075, New York, NY 10065, USA
e-mail: weiser1@mskcc.org

H.R.H. Patel et al. (eds.), *Pelvic Cancer Surgery: Modern Breakthroughs and Future Advances*,
DOI 10.1007/978-1-4471-4258-4_42,

internal pudendal artery, nerve, and vein; the nerves to the obturator internus; the quadratus femoris; and the posterior cutaneous nerve of the thigh [1]. The obturator foramen is enclosed by the obturator membrane and forms the obturator canal superiorly, through which the obturator artery, vein and nerve exit the pelvis.

42.4 Pelvic Walls, Muscles and Floor

The pelvic walls are referred to as anterior, lateral and posterior. The anterior wall is formed by the pubic bones and pubic symphysis. The lateral wall is formed by the hip bone, obturator membrane and obturator internus muscle. The obturator internus passes through the lesser sciatic foramen, attaching to the greater trochanter of the femur. The posterior wall is formed by the sacrum and coccyx, adjacent parts of the ilia, and the sacroiliac joints and ligaments. The piriformis muscle covers the wall posterolaterally, exiting the pelvis through the greater sciatic foramen to attach to the upper border of the greater trochanter of the femur. Medial to the piriformis muscle are the nerves of the sacral plexus.

The pelvic floor, or diaphragm, is formed by the levator ani and coccygeus muscles, and the fascia covering them. The levator ani comprises three parts: the pubococcygeus, puborectalis and iliococcygeus [2]. The pubococcygeus comprises a major part of the levator, arising from the posterior aspect of the body of the pubis and passing back horizontally to the coccyx. The right and left puborectalis unite behind the anorectal junction to form a U-shaped muscular sling [3]. The iliococcygeus muscle is often poorly developed. Damage to the pelvic floor as a result of surgery or child bearing can lead to incontinence and pelvic organ prolapse.

42.5 Major Arterial Supply

Blood supply to the major pelvic organs is provided by the major branches of the distal abdominal aorta. The inferior mesenteric artery (IMA) gives the superior hemorrhoidal (rectal) branch, crossing the left common iliac vessels and descending to the mesorectum, in the sigmoid mesocolon. In most cases, it bifurcates into a right and a left branch at the level of S3; in a small percentage of cases, multiple branches are present [4].

The superior hemorrhoidal artery anastomoses with the middle hemorrhoidal arteries. The middle hemorrhoidal arteries vary in size and number; in some anatomical dissections, they present in only a minority of specimens [4, 5].

The inferior hemorrhoidal arteries arise from the pudendal arteries in Alcock's canal, traversing the ischioanal fossa to supply the anal canal and external sphincter muscles [4]. The inferior and superior hemorrhoidal arteries form connections in the walls of the rectum and the anal canal [6].

The aorta bifurcates at the level of L3–L4 into the right and left common iliac arteries. These arteries course along the pelvic sidewall, bifurcating at the level of L5-S1 into external and internal (hypogastric) branches. At this point, the hypogastric artery is transversed by the ureter. The hypogastric arteries dive deep into the pelvis, descending posteriorly to the greater sciatic foramen and supplying branches to pelvic viscera and muscles. The external iliac artery is medial to the psoas muscle, giving several branches in the pelvis: the inferior epigastric artery, the recurrent obturator artery, and the superior vesical artery.

The hypogastric artery branches into two divisions at the superior edge of the greater sciatic foramen. The anterior division gives rise to the uterine, superior vesical, obturator, vaginal, middle rectal, inferior gluteal, and internal pudendal arteries. The posterior division travels toward the ischial spine, giving rise to the lateral sacral, iliolumbar, and superior gluteal arteries.

In surgery for locally recurrent rectal cancer, dissection of the hypogastric branches is frequently necessary when operating outside the parietal layer of the endopelvic fascia. In exenteration with sacrectomy, it is critical.

The median sacral artery originates directly from the aorta, just superior to the aortic bifurcation, and travels downward. Reaching the pelvis, it forms a few anastomotic loops, gives off small branches to the posterior rectal wall, and forms connections with lateral sacral arteries. This can be a source of bleeding during rectal mobilization [4].

The ovarian arteries originate from the abdominal aorta, inferior to the renal arteries. They travel downward along the medial aspect of the psoas muscle, through infundibulopelvic ligaments, in close proximity to the ureter. During surgical division of the infundibulopelvic ligament as it enters the pelvis, the ureter is vulnerable to damage [7].

42.6 Major Venous Drainage

The pelvis is drained by both the portal and systemic venous systems. With the exception of the rectum, the majority of pelvic viscera drain into systemic circulation via the internal iliac vein and its tributaries. The superior rectal vein drains the rectum and upper anal canal into the portal system via the inferior mesenteric vein. The middle rectal veins drain the lower part of the rectum and upper part of the anal canal into systemic circulation, via the internal iliac veins. The inferior rectal veins drain the lower part of the anal canal via the internal pudendal veins, which empty into the internal iliac veins.

The internal iliac veins are posteroinferior to the internal iliac arteries. With the exception of the umbilical artery, the tributaries are similar to the branches of the internal iliac arteries. The presacral plexus, anterior to the sacrum, is a major source of pelvic bleeding intraoperatively.

The presacral venous plexus is formed by anastomoses between the lateral and medial sacral veins, which reside on the anterior aspect of the body of the sacrum [8]. These thin-walled vessels without valves are generally not directly visible during rectal surgery; consequently, they are a potential source of injury and substantial bleeding [9].

The venous drainage pattern of rectal cancer explains patterns of distant recurrence. Mid and distal rectal cancers drain via both the systemic and portal systems. Not surprisingly, the majority of distal rectal cancers recur in the lung rather than the liver [10].

42.7 Lymphatic Drainage

Lymphatic drainage follows the course of the pelvic vessels. Lymph from the upper rectum drains almost exclusively upward, to the inferior mesenteric nodes. Lymphatic drainage from the lower one-third of the rectum occurs not only along the superior hemorrhoidal vessels but laterally, along the middle hemorrhoidal vessels, to the internal iliac lymph nodes.

In the anal canal, the dentate line is a landmark for two different systems of lymphatic drainage: above, to the IMA and internal iliac nodes; and below, to the superficial inguinal nodes (or, less frequently, along the inferior hemorrhoidal arteries).

The lymphatic drainage of the uterus and upper two-thirds of the vagina is to the obturator and internal and external iliac lymph nodes, and ultimately to the common iliac lymph nodes. The distal one-third of the vagina, urethra and vulva drains to the inguinal nodes. The lymphatic drainage of the ovaries travels along the ovarian vessels to the paraaortic lymph nodes.

The lymphatic drainage of the rectum and anus explains the pattern of recurrence observed in rectal and anal cancers. Mid and distal rectal cancer metastasizes to nodal basins in the pelvic sidewall via the internal iliac vessels, which are not normally resected during TME. Distal rectal and anal cancers frequently drain to the inguinal lymph nodes. In anal cancer this is considered locoregional recurrence rather than distant metastasis.

42.8 Innervation

Both the somatic and autonomic nervous systems are present in the pelvis. The somatic nerves of the pelvis originate from the lumbar and sacral plexus. The roots of the lumbar plexus (L1–L4) are associated with the psoas muscle. The genitofemoral and ilioinguinal nerves derive from L1 and supply the cremaster muscle, the skin on the anterolateral aspect of the scrotum/labia, and the skin over the mons pubis and anterior aspect of the scrotum or labia, respectively.

The femoral and obturator nerves arise from L2, L3, and L4. The femoral nerve travels underneath the inguinal ligament and, in the pelvis, gives motor branches to the iliopsoas muscle. The obturator nerve traverses the lesser pelvis, exiting via the obturator canal.

The sacral plexus (L4-S4) lies within the pelvis on the anterior surface of the piriformis muscle, deep to the main branches of the internal iliac vessels and presacral fascia. It has both somatic and parasympathetic components. The somatic component includes nerves to the levator ani and coccygeus (S3, S4), the piriformis nerve (S1, S2), the pudendal nerve (S2, S3, S4), the superior gluteal nerve (L4, L5, S1), the inferior gluteal nerve (L5, S1, S2), and the sciatic nerve (L4, L5, S1, S2, S3). The sciatic nerve emerges from the pelvis below the piriformis, entering the thigh between the ischial tuberosity and greater trochanter.

Sympathetic innervation to the pelvis is provided by the superior hypogastric plexus. The superior hypogastric plexus (presacral nerve) is the unpaired continuation of the lower end of the aortic plexus, below the aortic bifurcation. The hypogastric nerves form a wishbone-like pattern as they exit the inferior aspect of the superior hypogastric plexus in the midline, descending into the pelvis along the mesorectal fascia 1–2 cm medial to the ureters. Careful dissection of these nerves away from the mesorectum, especially at the sacral promontory, is essential to prevent injury during rectal mobilization [11]. Injury to the sympathetic nerves results in retrograde ejaculation in males, and bladder dysfunction in both sexes [11].

Parasympathetic innervation to the pelvis derives from the sacral plexus. Branches from the ventral rami of S2–S4 travel to their respective side's inferior hypogastric plexus. The inferior hypogastric plexus, located anterolateral to the rectum, appears as a rhomboid-like plate on the pelvic sidewall [11]. It is formed by the interdigitating fibers of the hypogastric and sacral nerves, and has both sympathetic and parasympathetic components. The hypogastric plexus then forms the nervi erigentes, innervating the pelvic organs. The parasympathetic nerves are extremely vulnerable to injury during dissection of the rectum and mesorectum laterally in the pelvis, anteriorly along the seminal vesicles and prostate in a male, and along the vagina in a female [12]. Injury results in erectile dysfunction in males, and dyspareunia and failure to achieve sexual arousal/orgasm in women. In both sexes, injury to the parasympathetic fibers can result in serious bladder dysfunction (inability to empty the bladder) [13].

In sacrectomy, the level of bony division predicts the consequent neurologic deficit. As a crude rule of thumb, division at S1 results in denervation and atrophy of the medial gastrocnemius muscle; at S2, sexual dysfunction; at S3, bowel and bladder dysfunction.

42.9 Pelvic Viscera

Ureters, Bladder, Urethra

The ureters connect the kidneys and the urinary bladder, transporting urine between these two organs. The ureters are retroperitoneal structures, traversing the pelvic brim and bifurcation of the common iliac arteries as they enter the pelvis and running postero-inferiorly on the lateral pelvic walls. They are external to the peritoneum and anterior to the internal iliac arteries, curving antero-medially superior to the levator to enter the bladder. In males, the ureters are posterolateral to the vas deferens, entering the bladder just superior to the seminal vesicles. In females, the uterine artery crosses over the ureter lateral to the cervix. The ureters enter the bladder at the trigone. Ureteral injury during hysterectomy can occur when dividing the infundibulopelvic ligament parametria [7].

The bladder is a muscular organ that lies in the lesser pelvis when empty, posterior to the pubic bones. It is separated from the pubic bones by the extraperitoneal space of Retzius (the retropubic space). The dome of the bladder is covered by the peritoneum. The bladder neck is fixed by the puboprostatic ligament in males, and by the pubovesical ligament in females.

The internal urethral opening is at one of the angles of the trigone of the bladder. The urethra is a muscular tube that transports urine from the internal to the external urethral opening. In males it is divided into four parts, according to location: the pre-prostatic urethra, the prostatic urethra, the membranous urethra and the spongy urethra. The female urethra is shorter and lies anterior to the vagina.

Female Pelvis: Ovaries, Uterus and Vagina

The uterus, a muscular organ located between the bladder and the rectum, incorporates the uterine corpus and cervix. The cervix is a tubular structure serving as a conduit between the endometrial cavity and the vagina. The anterior cervix lies posterior to the bladder, forming the anterior boundary of the posterior cul-de-sac (the Pouch of Douglas).

The uterosacral/cardinal ligament suspends the uterus and upper vagina. The uterine vessels course mostly within the cardinal ligaments that connect the upper vagina and cervix to the pelvic sidewall. The uterosacral ligaments attach to the ischial spine and sacrum. The round ligaments begin at the uterine fundus anteriorly and inferior to the fallopian tubes, traveling retroperitoneally through the layers of broad ligament and entering the inguinal canal. This broad ligament comprises the visceral and parietal peritoneum, and is located lateral to the uterine corpus and cervix.

The ovaries are suspended laterally and posteriorly to the uterus. The utero-ovarian ligament attaches the ovary to the uterus; the infundibulopelvic ligament attaches the ovary to the pelvic sidewall and contains the ovarian vessels. The fallopian tubes arise from the uterine corpus posteriorly and superiorly to the round ligament and travel to the ovary, supported by the broad ligament.

Male Pelvis: Prostate and Seminal Vesicles, Vas Deferens

The vas deferens begins at the tail of the epididymis, ascending in the spermatic cord through the inguinal canal, exiting through the internal inguinal ring, and crossing over the external iliac vessels to enter the pelvis. There, it travels along the lateral pelvic wall, joining the duct of the seminal vesicles to form the ejaculatory duct.

The seminal vesicles are elongated structures located between the fundus of the bladder and the rectum. The superior aspects of the seminal vesicles lie posterior to the ureters. The prostate surrounds the prostatic urethra and has a dense, fibrous capsule. The base of the prostate corresponds to the neck of the bladder; its posterior surface is corresponds to the rectal ampulla.

42.10 Rectum and Anus

The rectum is a continuation of the colon, beginning at the level of the sacral promontory where the taeniae coli spread out. Measuring 12–15 cm in length, it descends along the curvature of the sacrum and coccyx, passing through the levator ani muscles before turning postero-inferiorly to form the anal canal. The rectum has three lateral curves (or folds): an upper and a lower curve on the right, and a middle curve on the left. On their inner aspects, these transverse folds are known as Houston's valves. The middle fold generally corresponds to the peritoneal reflection.

The anal canal begins where the rectum passes through the puborectalis muscle. Measuring approximately 4 cm in length, it terminates at the anal verge. The anal canal is surrounded by the internal and external anal sphincter. The internal anal sphincter is a continuation of the muscularis propria of the rectum. Therefore, when performing an ultra-low anterior resection, the internal anal sphincter can be removed (intersphincteric resection) to gain additional distal margin.

The mucosa of the anal canal is lined by columnar epithelium in the upper part, and by squamous epithelium in the lower part. The dentate line marks the junction between these two epithelia. Above the dentate line, innervation is provided by the autonomic nervous system; below the dentate line, somatic innervation is present. Anal crypts connect to the anal glands above the dentate line. If these glands become obstructed, perianal abscesses or fistula may occur. The anal glands are the site of origin of primary anal canal adenocarcinoma.

42.11 Pelvic Fascia and Spaces

The pelvic fascia, a connective tissue, occupies all the spaces between the peritoneum, pelvic walls and pelvic floor that are not occupied by the pelvic organs. It is traditionally described as having parietal and visceral components, with endopelvic layer in between. The parietal fascia covers the pelvic surfaces of the obturator internus, piriformis, coccygeus, levator ani, and a portion of sphincter urethrae muscle. The visceral pelvic fascia covers the extraperitoneal surface of the pelvic organs.

The sacrum and coccyx are covered with a layer of parietal fascia known as presacral or Waldeyer's fascia [14]. Waldeyer's fascia covers the median sacral vessels. The recto sacral fascia extends from the periosteum of the fourth sacral segment to the posterior rectal wall, and must be divided during rectal mobilization. The supralevator space lies below the recto sacral fascia and above the levators.

Anteriorly, the rectum is separated from the seminal vesicles and the prostate or vagina by Denonvilliers' fascia. The extraperitoneal surfaces of the rectum are covered by the investing fascia (fascia propria) of the rectum.

The posterior cul-de-sac, or pouch of Douglas, is located between the anterior surface of the rectum and the posterior vaginal wall and cervix. The space of Retzius is between the anterior bladder wall and symphysis pubis.

In rectal dissection, a complete understanding of the many different fascial planes of the pelvis is critical. The mesorectal plane, popularized by Heald in his seminal 1982 publication [15], is now the standard for primary resection of rectal cancer. Dissection proceeds between the visceral and parietal layers of the endopelvic fascia. This ensures complete and total mesorectal excision (TME) [15, 16]. Because low-lying rectal cancer has the potential to spread to lateral lymph nodes, extended lateral lymph node dissection should also be considered. Takahashi describes three planes of rectal cancer dissection: the inner plane, corresponding to the TME plane; the intermediary plane, corresponding to the parietal fascia; and the outer plane, located outside of the internal iliac arteries and including the obturator space [17]. When operating on locally recurrent rectal cancer, these planes are crucial. In the setting of recurrent cancer after TME, dissection should proceed in a lateral plane (either the intermediate or outer) to include the parietal layer of the endopelvic fascia.

References

1. Moore KL, Agur, AM, Dalley AF, editors. Ch 6. Pelvis and Perineum. In: Clinically oriented anatomy. 4th ed. Wolters-Kluwer/Lippincott Williams & Wilkins, Philadelphia. 2010.
2. Kearney R, Sawhney R, DeLancey JO. Levator ani muscle anatomy evaluated by origin-insertion pairs. Obstet Gynecol. 2004;104(1):168–73.
3. Shafik A. New concept of the anatomy of the anal sphincter mechanism and the physiology of defecation. II. Anatomy of the levator ani muscle with special reference to puborectalis. Investig Urol. 1975;13:175–82.
4. Ayoub SF. Arterial supply to the human rectum. Acta Anat (Basel). 1978;100(3):317–27.
5. Sato K, Sato T. The vascular and neuronal composition of the lateral ligament of the rectum and the rectosacral fascia. Surg Radiol Anat. 1991;13(1):17–22.
6. Griffiths JD. Surgical anatomy of the blood supply of the distal colon. Ann R Coll Surg Engl. 1956;19(4):241–56.
7. Daly JW, Higgins KA. Injury to the ureter during gynecologic surgical procedures. Surg Gynecol Obstet. 1988;167(1):19–22.
8. Baqué P, Karimdjee B, Iannelli A, Benizri E, Rahili A, Benchimol D, Bernard JL, Sejor E, Bailleux S, de Peretti F, Bourgeon A. Anatomy of the presacral venous plexus: implications for rectal surgery. Surg Radiol Anat. 2004;26(5):355–8.
9. Church JM, Raudkivi PJ, Hill GL. The surgical anatomy of the rectum—a review with particular relevance to the hazards of rectal mobilisation. Int J Color Dis. 1987;2(3):158–66.
10. Ding P, Liska D, Tang P, Shia J, Saltz L, Goodman K, Downey RJ, Nash GM, Temple LK, Paty PB, Guillem JG, Wong WD, Weiser MR. Pulmonary recurrence predominates after combined modality therapy for rectal cancer: an original retrospective study. Ann Surg. 2012;256(1):111–6.
11. Guillem JG, Lee-Kong SA. Autonomic nerve preservation during rectal cancer resection. J Gastrointest Surg. 2010;14(2):416–22.

12. Moszkowicz D, Alsaid B, Bessede T, Penna C, Nordlinger B, Benoît G, Peschaud F. Where does pelvic nerve injury occur during rectal surgery for cancer? Color Dis. 2011;13(12):1326–34.
13. Delacroix Jr SE, Winters JC. Voiding dysfunction after pelvic colorectal surgery. Clin Colon Rectal Surg. 2010;23(2):119–27.
14. Crapp AR, Cuthbertson AM. William Waldeyer and the rectosacral fascia. Surg Gynecol Obstet. 1974;138(2):252–6.
15. Heald RJ, Husband EM, Ryall RD. The mesorectum in rectal cancer surgery-the clue to pelvic recurrence? Br J Surg. 1982;69:613–6.
16. Heald RJ. The "holy plane" of rectal surgery. J R Soc Med. 1988;81:503–8.
17. Takahashi T, Ueno M, Azekura K, Ohta H. Lateral node dissection and total mesorectal excision for rectal cancer. Dis Colon Rectum. 2000; 43:S59–68.

Training Surgeons for Rectal Cancer Surgery: Clinical and Simulation

43

Danilo Miskovic and Hugh Mackenzie

43.1 Introduction

Rectal cancer surgery is complex and notoriously difficult to learn. The margins for surgical error are narrow and may have dramatic consequences for the patient, such as anastomotic leak or cancer recurrence. Despite the high level of surgical complexity (or maybe because of it), little has been done to tackle educational challenges, and most training is delivered in a traditional apprenticeship model. With technological advances, such as minimally-invasive surgery, additional challenges have been added and the traditional apprenticeship model may not be sufficient for effective training. Historical data from self-taught laparoscopic colorectal surgeons demonstrate an alarmingly long learning curve of up to 150 procedures before stable clinical outcomes were achieved [1] Fig. 43.1. We believe that this learning curve has been significantly reduced when surgeons follow a structured, supervised curriculum. In this chapter we discuss some basic educational theory, the challenges as well as possible solutions and considerations when designing training programs for rectal cancer surgery.

D. Miskovic, PhD, MD, FRCS (✉)
The John Goligher Colorectal Unit, St James University Hospital, University of Leeds, Beckett Street, Leeds, West Yorkshire LS9 8DX, UK
e-mail: d.miskovic@leeds.ac.uk

H. Mackenzie, MBBS, BSc, MRCS
Department of Surgery and Cancer, Imperial College London, Paddington, London, UK

43.2 Educational Challenges in Rectal Cancer Surgery

Rectal cancer surgery conveys training challenges on an anatomical, technological and oncological level:

Anatomy: the pelvic anatomy is compact, complex and difficult to conceptualize. Anatomical landmarks of the oncological TME (total mesorectal excision) planes are subtle and failure in recognizing them can have a significant impact on outcome [2]. The three dimensional relationship of visible and hidden structures in the pelvis requires a high degree of spatial imagery. The understanding of anatomical variations (e.g. gender-specific configuration of the pelvis) can significantly increase the surgical complexity of a case. *Surgical anatomy teaching for rectal cancer surgery needs to embrace spatial learning methods.*

Technology: Minimally-invasive surgery is increasingly accepted as the standard approach for colorectal cancer surgery. Laparoscopic surgery is particularly difficult in the pelvis due to the limited range of movements of the long rigid instruments in a narrow space. Training in rectal surgery must acknowledge the progression of technology since recent developments in robotic, single-port and trans-anal surgery may require specific training modalities. *Psychomotor skill training is essential in rectal cancer surgery.*

H.R.H. Patel et al. (eds.), *Pelvic Cancer Surgery: Modern Breakthroughs and Future Advances*,
DOI 10.1007/978-1-4471-4258-4_43, © Springer-Verlag London 2015

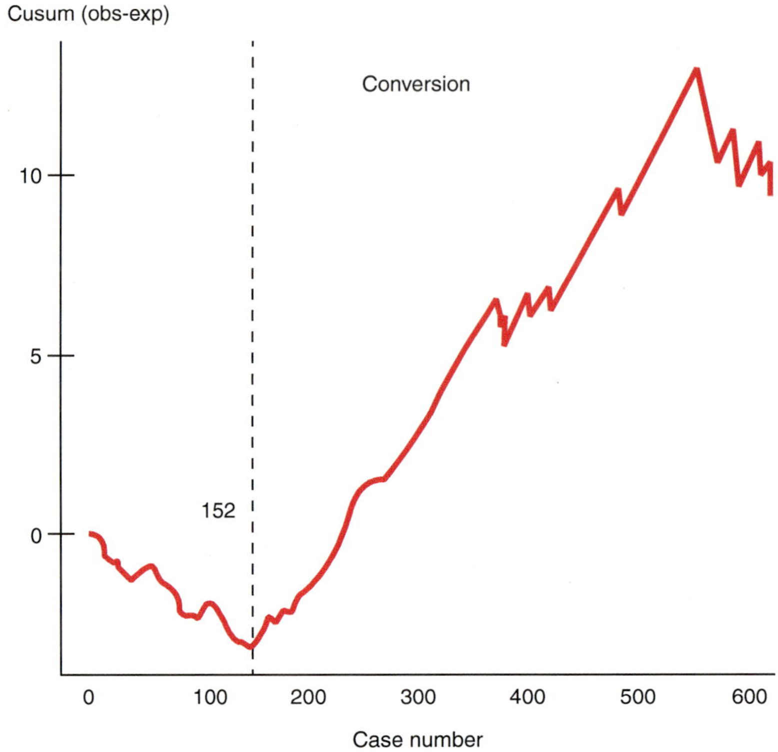

Fig. 43.1 The learning curve for self-taught laparoscopic colorectal surgery is up to 150 procedures (Adapted from Miskovic et al. [1])

Clinical and oncology: Rectal cancer surgery is high-risk surgery. Outcomes are related to surgical performance. This implies ethical considerations when training surgeons on patients which have hardly been addressed to date. Oncological outcome (cancer recurrence) is directly linked to the quality of surgical resection. Assessment of surgical specimens has been successfully correlated with long-term oncological outcomes. *Training rectal cancer surgery requires a thorough auditing and assessment process.*

These factors have an impact on shaping training programs for rectal cancer surgery. In order to enhance the training quality and effectiveness a multimodal approach using cognitive training, simulation, direct supervision and assessment is required. Despite this seemingly obvious statement, most training in rectal cancer surgery is still based on a very basic apprenticeship model and the evidence of comprehensive, multimodal and multifocal training programs is sparse.

43.3 On How We Learn

Traditionally, surgeons show very little interest into educational theories which may be surprising to an outside person as surgeons have a reputation of being talented teachers. However, surgeons are pragmatic people with a short attention span and a tendency to angry irritation when bored with information on seemingly meaningless theory. Nevertheless, understanding some very basic principles and educational theories on how we learn are useful when shaping a training program. This is by far not a comprehensive discussion of educational principles but a summary of some examples that hopefully stimulate the interested reader to explore further.

Observations on Deliberate Practice

The aim of surgical training is to gain expertise in knowledge, decision making, communication and technical skills. Previously, expertise has been thought to be closely linked to volume of experience. However, extensive experience alone has been shown to be a poor predictor of expert performance. Instead it is achieved by undertaking deliberate practice; carrying out repetitive tasks, with a clear goal and constructive feedback, in order to improve a specific skill [3]. The accumulated amount of deliberate practice is closely related to attained performance, taking at least 10 years or 10,000 repetitions to become expert. Therefore the progression of learning, although influenced by talent and innate ability, is primarily due to deliberate practice. It is unlikely that a surgeon would carry out the same operation 10,000 times in a lifetime, and it would be wrong to assume that deliberate practice can only be employed in the operating room (OR). Simulating specific parts of a procedure or certain skills can replace 'practicing' on a real patient. The relationship of deliberate practice and OR performance in surgery equates to rehearsal and stage performance for a musician. Experts within their field, be it surgery, sport, music or chess have used repetition to not only accrue knowledge, but also organize this information so that it can be rapidly and consistently accessed [3].

A Journey to Expertise

The brothers Hubert and Stuart Dreyfus have described a popular model for the acquisition of expertise. The Dreyfus model of skill acquisition contains five stages; novice, advanced beginner, competent, proficient and finally expert (Table 43.1). These stages define how an individual progresses from learning knowledge without context to analyzing situations holistically and making decisions intuitively. An important part of this development is reflection on failures and successes in order to learn from one's experiences [4].

Construction Work: Proximal Development and Scaffolding

The learning of surgical knowledge and skill can be enhanced by using certain educational strategies. An example is the concept of the 'zone of proximal development' introduced by the Russian psychologist Lev Vygotsky [5, 6]. This describes the potential difference in development between problem solving, individually and with guidance from a more capable colleague. Although this was initially described for childhood development it is equally applicable to surgery and describes the difference in learning curves between self-taught and supervised training surgeons. This concept can be further extended into the theory of scaffolding; which explains the process of the more competent trainer providing the skills necessary for individual problem solving and the revoking of assistance when the trainee becomes independent [6, 7]. The transfer of information is also influenced by the teaching modality. Some training methods are more effective than others and this has been detailed in Edgar Dale's Cone of Experience and more recently in the Miller's Learning Pyramid [8] (Fig. 43.2). Although the actual retention rates have been contested it would seem prudent when learning technical skills to utilize active rather than passive training methods.

43.4 Training Modalities

Research in Surgical Education has a relative short history and flourished recently with the introduction of novel simulation technologies. Providing evidence for clinical effectiveness of a training method or a whole training curriculum is more difficult than assumed and randomized controlled trials are often impractical and impose ethical dilemmas. Although evidence on simulation technology makes a high proportion of research, a good training program should not rely solely on expensive simulation technology but also make use of other resources—learning opportunities within a clinical setting are readily available but often grossly underused. In the

Table 43.1 The progression of knowledge and skill level from novice to expert [4]

	Knowledge	Standard of work	Autonomy	Coping with complexity	Perception of context
Novice	Minimal knowledge without connection to practice	Unsatisfactory unless closely supervised	Needs close supervision	Little or no concept of dealing with complexity	Sees actions in isolation
Advanced beginner	Working knowledge of key aspects of practice	Straightforward tasks completed to an acceptable standard	Some steps achieved using own judgement but supervision needed for overall task	Appreciates complex situations but only able to achieve partial resolution	Sees actions as a series of steps
Competent	Good working and background knowledge of area of practice	Fit for purpose, may lack refinement	Able to achieve most tasks using own judgement	Copes with complex situations through deliberate analysis	Sees actions at least partly in terms of longer-term goals
Proficient	Depth of understanding of discipline and area of practice	Fully acceptable standard achieved routinely	Takes full responsibility for own work	Deals with complex situations holistically, decision making more confident	Sees overall picture and how individual actions fit within it
Expert	Authoritative knowledge of discipline and deep tacit understanding across area of practice	Excellence achieved with relative ease	Able to take responsibility for going beyond existing standards and creating own interpretations	Holistic grasp of complex situations, moves between intuitive and analytical approaches with ease	Sees overall picture and alternative approaches; vision of what may be possible

following section we discuss the effectiveness and opportunities of different training modalities and their relevance to rectal cancer surgical training.

Cognitive Training and Mental Practice

According to the Learning Pyramid by Miller the acquisition of knowledge through textbook reading or lectures is highly inefficient. How can we increase the efficiency of cognitive training? A good example of changing a classically passive training domain into an active learning opportunity is mental practice. Mental practice is nothing novel or fancy, in fact most surgeons consciously or more often unconsciously use mental practice methods. This may include mental imagery of certain steps of a procedure or perioperative requirements several days or just minutes before a challenging operation. Just think of that operation you are doing tomorrow or next week and you are already performing mental practice—you are rehearsing the procedure in your mind. Nevertheless, despite this natural behavior, the opportunities of this potentially very effective training method have been poorly studied and insufficiently exploited for surgical training. Other high complexity performers, such as athletes or musicians, have implemented mental practice as an integral part of their training and rehearsing techniques [9]. Current evidence of mental practice in surgical training is based on low complexity procedures (laparoscopic cholecystectomy) for relatively junior trainees demonstrating a potential benefit [10, 11]. Rectal surgery with all its complexities described above lends itself for mental practice. Mental practice can not only be enhanced by using mental practice protocols such as a task analysis of the procedure (breakdown of the procedure into steps) but could be extended to radiologist-guided reviews of CT or MRI scans, review of (interactive) teaching videos and anatomy rehearsals using virtual

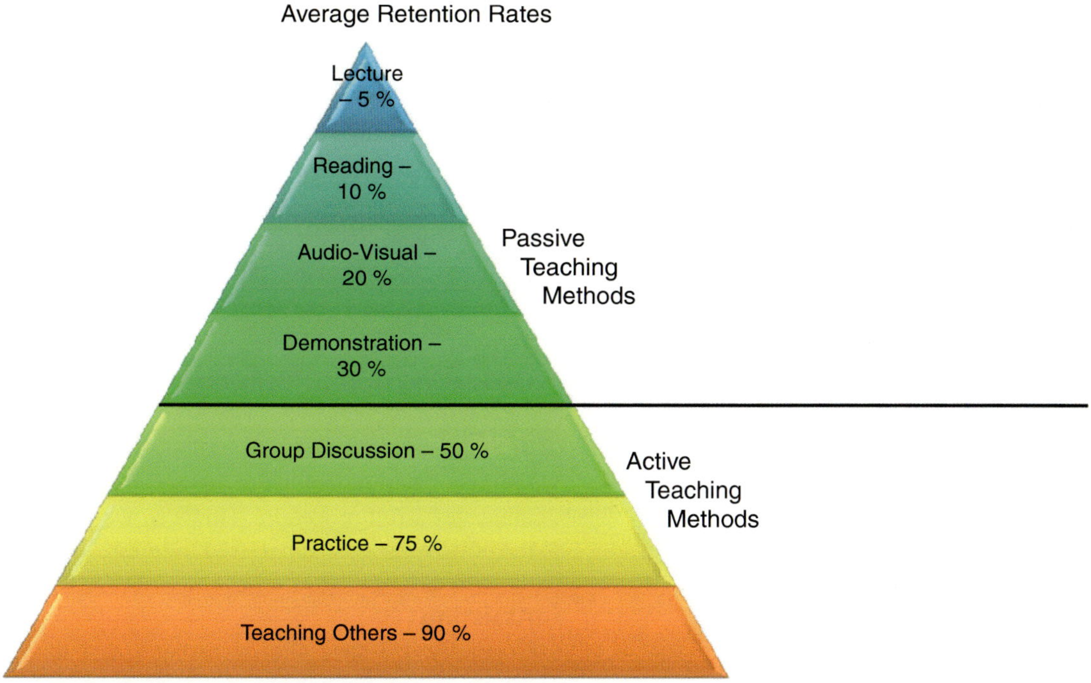

Fig. 43.2 The learning pyramid: active learning styles are more efficient than passive ones (Adapted from National Training Laboratories. Bethel, Maine; with kind permission)

computer technology. Several techniques have been described previously in parts or as isolated interventions, but there is no consensus on a combined, integrated approach using a multitude of these methods.

Simulation

Surgical simulation has often been compared with commercial or combat pilot training. Nevertheless, the two professions are very dissimilar and the fidelity, realism, controllability and observability of surgical simulation lacks far behind aviation training. So, what surgical skills can be trained through simulation and what simulation modalities are available?

The value of surgical simulation has been increasingly studied over the past 20 years. Advancements in simulation technology have opened new avenues using virtual and augmented reality. However, before purchasing the latest and most sophisticated virtual surgical simulator, it is worth taking a step back to ask the question what is the purpose of simulation. Should it be used for the acquisition of some basic manual skills, for the training of a full procedure or certain steps of it, or can it be used to train whole operating teams?

Skills Training

There is pretty compelling evidence of the effectiveness of simulation training programs for the development of basic laparoscopic skills. The most widely studied such curriculum is the Fundamentals of Laparoscopic Surgery (FLS), which was designed to train basic laparoscopic skills [12, 13]. It is a box trainer system with a competency-based curriculum for five different tasks. This program has been shown to reduce the learning curve and is widely accepted for teaching and assessing laparoscopic skills [12, 13]. Similar results can be achieved with other simulation modalities, such as virtual reality or augmented reality simulations (Fig. 43.3).

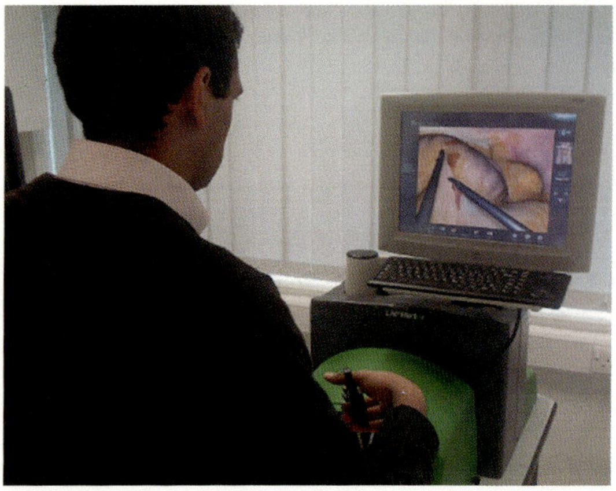

Fig. 43.3 Example of a virtual reality simulator. The trainee is using a robotic interface that translates the movements of the surgeon into motion within a virtual reality environment. Haptic feedback to the instruments can enhance the perceived level of reality

Procedural Training

Currently there is no simulation model available for the training of rectal cancer surgery. There have been attempts to construct a low cost model using cheap materials and a virtual reality simulation model, but no commercialized product has emerged yet. Several training centers use animal models and human cadavers for training. Anesthetized, living animals (usually pigs) have the advantage of providing perfused and realistic tissues, however the anatomy is significantly different and the purpose of full procedural training is questionable. Ethical questions arise whether it is necessary to use animals solely for training standard surgical procedures. Trainees and faculty have rated human cadavers to be better in terms of anatomy and training value [14]. The disadvantage of a lacking bloodstream was not considered to be a major disadvantage for training. Special embalming techniques reduce unpleasant smells without compromising the tissue properties [15].

Team Simulation Training

Full OR team simulations can be used to teach team behavior and communication skills. These so-called "non-technical" skills are probably an underestimated entity with a significant impact on surgical outcome. Nevertheless, it may be questionable if the high level of complexity, manpower and investment required to run full theater team simulations is justified for rectal cancer surgery. However, the concept of team simulations could also be applied to other aspects in the area of rectal cancer, such as decision-making exercises for multidisciplinary teams; an example within the UK is the national training program in low rectal cancer surgery (Lorec).

Operating Room Training

The OR provides a variety of teaching opportunities, ranging from assistance to independent performance of a full procedure. How can we improve the effectiveness of supervised training?

Assisting

Hopefully, we have already demonstrated that a variety of other training modalities can be applied to efficiently acquire all necessary skills. So, is there a place for assisting in the OR in a modern curriculum for rectal cancer surgery? The answer, of course, is yes. Not a single simulation technology can reproduce the experience of a real case. Again, the trainer should attempt to change the traditionally passive role of an assistant into an active learning experience. The assistant needs to be involved in the decision-making process and discussions on the current activity should be encouraged.

Modular Training

Historically new surgical techniques have been learnt at the patients' expense with a temporary increase in morbidity and mortality. The presence of an expert trainer ("mentor") has been shown to be effective to reduce negative clinical outcomes significantly. A structured, modular approach to teach in the OR has been shown to be practical. There is evidence that competency in the different operative task areas of a procedure are achieved at different rates (Fig. 43.4). Hence, the operation should be broken down into separate tasks and learnt in a modular fashion, teaching the easier tasks first and when achieving competency stepping up to the more complex ones [16–18]. This modular approach can be used efficiently by

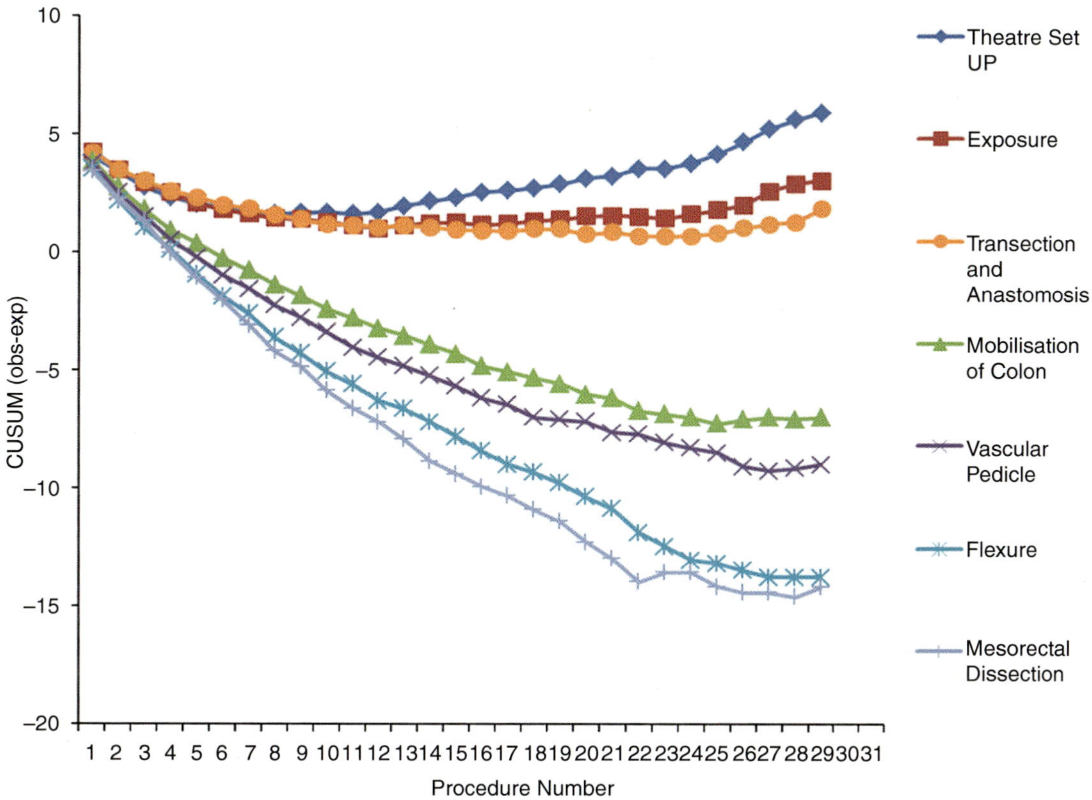

Fig. 43.4 Different parts of an operation are learnt at different speeds. The curves level out when the trainee achieves a level of competence

training two trainees of different levels on the same case, with the less experienced performing the straightforward tasks whilst an experienced trainee completes the more difficult tasks. This has been used effectively whilst training in laparoscopic colorectal surgery, with effective training and good clinical outcomes [18].

Case Selection

Poor case selection increases morbidity and mortality during self-taught laparoscopic colorectal surgery. Even with an expert mentor present during the operation the effect of selecting a poor case for training is still present with an increase in complication and mortality rates. Poor case selection not only affects clinical outcomes but also the training performance. Training performance in the most complex task areas, such as dissection of the mesorectum, is affected the most by poor training case selection. The ideal patient for starting training on rectal resection is a slim female, American Society of Anesthesiology (ASA) grade 1 or 2 and should not have had prior abdominal surgery. More specifically for rectal cancer, cases with T-stage of 3 or 4 and those with long course radiotherapy should also be avoided at the beginning of training. However, although learning at the patients' expense is unacceptable, overzealous case selection may be impractical due to the unavailability of the ideal patient [19]. Especially as patients with a BMI of <25 m^2/kg are increasingly rare in a Western society with the rising obesity problem. The problem of stringent case selection can be addressed by using the modular training approach [18]. A patient with a high T stage tumor may still have an appropriate IMA dissection for training, after which the expert trainer can perform the

Table 43.2 Six point teaching strategy to resolve a difficult training situation

1	Stop!	Stop the trainee's manual activity
2	Identify the problem	What is the problem? "Why are you struggling?"
3	Explain	What are possible solutions to the problem? Discuss different solutions
4	Instruct	What is the best plan to proceed?
5	Check understanding	Has the trainee understood the problem and the solution?
6	Judge capability	Is the trainee capable of progressing safely?

Adapted from Lapco TT

Table 43.3 The SHARP framework for structured debriefing in the OR

Before the procedure	**S**et learning objectives	"What would you like to get out of this case?"
	How did it go?	"What went well?" "Why did it go well?"
	Address concerns	"What did not go well?" "Why did it not go well?"
After the procedure	**R**eview learning points	"Did you meet the learning objectives for this case?" "What did you learn about your technical skills?" "What did you learn about your teamwork skills?"
	Plan ahead	"What actions can you take to improve your future practice?"

Adapted from Ahmed et al. [20] used with permission

TME. On the other hand an obese, female patient may have a complex dissection around the vascular pedicle but a relatively straight forward TME.

Faculty Training

Successful mentored training not only relies upon a motivated trainee and an appropriate training case but also on a skilled and enthusiastic trainer. The English National Training Program for laparoscopic colorectal surgery (Lapco) has developed a dedicated training course for faculty trainers. In essence, a three stage approach to training laparoscopic colorectal surgery is taught; (i) Set—Introduction, align agendas, set objectives and lay ground rules, (ii) Dialogue—the 'training' using clear, concise and consistent language, (iii) Closure—Summary of the case, feedback, take home message and objectives for the next case. In the 'Dialogue' strategies to tackle difficult situations are provided. If a trainee is stuck at a certain point during the procedure, the trainer applies a six point plan to engage the trainee to resolve the problem, by identifying the issue and discussing and applying the most practical solution (Table 43.2). Following the course an immediate benefit is seen in the quality of training; in particular the trainers use a more structured approach to training and increase the time and detail within the 'Set'.

Feedback and Assessment

Traditionally assessment of quality of surgery has been achieved by looking at clinical outcomes. This technique is flawed as it relies on injury to patients to identify poor quality surgery. Assessment can be categorized into formative and summative assessment.

Formative Assessment

Formative assessment is the type of feedback that aims to improve performance at the next training episode by discussing positive and negative points and agreeing on learning objectives. A simple framework to follow is outlined in Table 43.3 and it gives the trainees the opportunity to reflect on their performance, followed by a discussion on details of the procedure before agreeing on learning points and a plan for the next training episode [20]. Such a discussion should take place after each training procedure and can be highly efficient without taking too much time. Structured assessment forms can facilitate formative feedback. The Lapco program is using a simple task-breakdown as a basis for discussion (Table 43.4) [21]; other structured assessment forms have been developed based on OSATS (Objective structured assessment of technical skill)

Table 43.4 Example of the formative assessment form (GAS form) used in the national training program for laparoscopic colorectal surgery in England

Task area	Task	Description	Score 1–6
Exposure	Theater setup	Position of surgeons, scrub nurse, drapes, instruments	
	Patient positioning	Adequate positioning of patient	
	Laparoscopic access	Open or close techniques to gain pneumoperitoneum, and insertion of ports)	
	Exposure of operating field	Exposure of operating field (moving of omentum, small bowel etc.)	
Vascular pedicle dissection	Pedicle transection	Incision of peritoneum, creation of window below and above, and dissection with stapler, clips, ultrasound dissection tool or other techniques	
	Mesocolic mobilization	Retrocolic dissection of mesentery (right side towards hepatic flexure, left side towards splenic flexure)	
	Landmarks	Identification of landmark (right side: duodenum, left side: left ureter)	
Mobilization	Flexure	Dissection of flexure (right side: hepatic, left side: splenic)	
	Mesorectal mobilization	Mesorectal dissection (including total mesorectal excision (TME), only for rectal resections)	
	Dissection of bowel	Transection, using stapler other similar device	
Anastomosis	Extraction of specimen	Incision, extraction of specimen, completion of resection	
	Anastomosis	Anastomosis (intra- or extra-corporeal)	

Scores
0 – Not applicable
1 – Not performed, step had to be done by trainer
2 – Partly performed, step had to be partly done by trainer
3 – Performed, with substantial verbal support
4 – Performed with minor verbal support
5 – Competent performance, safe (without guidance)
6 – Proficient performance, couldn't be better

[22, 23]. To date, there is no dedicated assessment form for rectal cancer surgery.

Summative Assessment

The aim of summative assessment is to test someone's competence of performance, without focusing on the improvement of skills. It is basically an examination, rather than a feedback exercise. There has to be a structure and ideally a validated assessment tool to provide a fair and valid judgment of performance. Summative assessments are a sensitive but necessary topic to discuss, especially in times where revalidation and relicensing is already or about to be implemented in many countries. For rectal surgery two modalities are practical: firstly, direct observation of operative skills. This is ideally performed by blinded assessors, evaluating operating videos. For laparoscopic surgery, videos are easy to obtain. Lapco and the Japanese National Training Program both use structured assessment forms [24]. Alternatively, video assessment methods can be applied to gather more detailed information on error performance (OCHRA—observational clinical human reliability assessment) [25]. Secondly, the quality of the end product can be assessed using metrics to measure the quality of the specimens. The TME specimen provides an opportunity to measure surgical quality. Pathologists are able to assess the quality of resection and an assessment of a 'complete mesorectum' has a positive impact on overall and local recurrence rates [26].

43.5 The Implementation of a Multimodal and Multifocal Rectal Cancer Training Program

There are a few examples for comprehensive training programs for rectal and laparoscopic colorectal training programs. The Japanese National Training Program for laparoscopic colorectal surgery has been in place for several years. It focuses on summative assessment at the end of training but the type of training and training modalities are not prescribed and depend on the individual training facility. Lapco provides a curriculum, including course training (cadaveric or animal lab), OR supervision by trainers that underwent faculty training and a comprehensive formative and summative assessment structure. The program and data collection are still ongoing but preliminary results demonstrate that the learning curve has been significantly reduced. A randomized controlled trial comparing traditional training in laparoscopic colonic surgery with a curriculum incorporating cognitive training, virtual reality simulation and cadaveric training for laparoscopic colorectal surgery demonstrated a significant improvement of theater performance for the intervention group [27]. Recently, a National Program for low rectal cancer surgery (Lorec) has been established in the UK. This program is dedicated not only to improve operative skills through technical skills courses but enhance the performance of whole multidisciplinary teams by training decision making processes. All examples demonstrate, that rectal cancer training can be improved by implementing different training modalities. An ideal training program in rectal cancer surgery should also focus on different training targets, including decision-making, team performance and of course operative competence.

All good examples of training programs are competency-based rather than limited by time or case number. Inter-individual performance varies and what might be right for one trainee could be too much or too little for the other. Therefore, focusing on competency aims, rather than a set number of cases is a more efficient and economical way of running a training program.

There is evidence that high volume centers achieve better outcomes in rectal surgery [28, 29]. It makes sense that these centers of excellence should be identified and encouraged to deliver training programs for rectal cancer surgery as they can provide volume, manpower, financial investment and expertise required. A training program director, ideally with educational support should be appointed to provide quality control and implementation of the program. Networks and collaborations between different training sites should be facilitated.

The future belongs to comprehensive multimodal, multifocal and multi-site training programs. Simply providing a 1-day course on rectal cancer surgery is not a sustainable strategy to provide high quality training.

Key Points

- The acquisition of some basic educational principles is useful before designing training programs
- Rectal cancer surgery bears anatomical, technological and clinic-oncological complexities
- Cognitive training and mental practice can be trained and are likely to improve performance
- Simulation training includes skills, procedural training and team training—all modalities can be useful for rectal cancer surgery
- A realistic and validated simulator for rectal cancer surgery has yet to be developed
- Educational effectiveness of supervision in the OR can be improved by faculty training and application
- Assessment and feedback should be essential components of a training program in rectal cancer surgery

- A training program should focus on various targets and employ several training modalities
- A competency-based curriculum is more effective than a number- or time-based program
- Training centers of excellence should be identified and interconnected into national or regional training networks

References

1. Miskovic D, et al. Learning curve and case selection in laparoscopic colorectal surgery – an international multi-centre analysis of 4852 cases. Dis Colon Rectum. 2012;55:1300–10.
2. Targarona EM, et al. Can we predict immediate outcome after laparoscopic rectal surgery? Multivariate analysis of clinical, anatomic, and pathologic features after 3-dimensional reconstruction of the pelvic anatomy. Ann Surg. 2008;247(4):642–9.
3. Ericsson KA. Deliberate practice and acquisition of expert performance: a general overview. Acad Emerg Med. 2008;15(11):988–94.
4. Dreyfus HL, Dreyfus SE. Expertise in real world contexts. Organ Stud. 2005;26(5):779–92.
5. Vygotsky LS. Interaction between learning and development, in Mind in society: The development of higher psychological processes1978. Cambridge, MA: Harvard University Press; 1978. p. 79–91.
6. Kneebone RL, et al. Simulation and clinical practice: strengthening the relationship. Med Educ. 2004;38(10):1095–102.
7. Wood D, Bruner JS, Ross G. Role of tutoring in problem-solving. J Child Psychol Psychiatry. 1976;17(2):89–100.
8. Miller RH, Lalley JP. The learning pyramid: does it point teachers in the right direction? Educ Inf Technol. 2007;128(1):64–79.
9. Rogers RG. Mental practice and acquisition of motor skills: examples from sports training and surgical education. Obstet Gynecol Clin North Am. 2006; 33(2):297–304, ix.
10. Arora S, et al. Mental practice enhances surgical technical skills: a randomized controlled study. Ann Surg. 2011;253(2):265–70.
11. Immenroth M, et al. Mental training in surgical education: a randomized controlled trial. Ann Surg. 2007;245(3):385–91.
12. Fried GM, et al. Proving the value of simulation in laparoscopic surgery. Ann Surg. 2004;240(3):518–25; discussion 525–8.
13. Okrainec A, et al. Trends and results of the first 5 years of Fundamentals of Laparoscopic Surgery (FLS) certification testing. Surg Endosc. 2011;25(4):1192–8.
14. Wyles SM, et al. Analysis of laboratory-based laparoscopic colorectal surgery workshops within the English national training programme. Surg Endosc. 2010;5:1559–66.
15. Giger U, et al. Laparoscopic training on Thiel human cadavers: a model to teach advanced laparoscopic procedures. Surg Endosc. 2008;22(4):901–6.
16. Stolzenburg JU, et al. Modular surgical training for endoscopic extraperitoneal radical prostatectomy. BJU Int. 2005;96(7):1022–7.
17. Lund L, Dubrowski A, Carnahan H. A modular approach for training urologists in laparoscopy. BJU Int. 2007;100(6):1216–8.
18. Hemandas A, et al. Modular training in laparoscopic colorectal surgery maximizes training opportunities without clinical compromise. World J Surg. 2011; 35(2):409–14.
19. Leong S, et al. Considerations on the learning curve for laparoscopic colorectal surgery: a view from the bottom. Int J Colorectal Dis. 2007;22(9):1109–15.
20. Ahmed M, et al. Identifying best practice guidelines for debriefing in surgery: a tri-continental study. Am J Surg. 2012;203(4):523–9.
21. Miskovic D, et al. Development, validation and implementation of a monitoring tool for training in laparoscopic colorectal surgery in the English National Training Program. Surg Endosc. 2011;25(4): 1136–42.
22. Palter VN, MacRae HM, Grantcharov TP. Development of an objective evaluation tool to assess technical skill in laparoscopic colorectal surgery: a Delphi methodology. Am J Surg. 2011;201(2): 251–9.
23. Sarker SK, Kumar I, Delaney C. Assessing operative performance in advanced laparoscopic colorectal surgery. World J Surg. 2011;34(7):1594–603.
24. Miskovic D, et al. Is competency assessment at the specialist level achievable? A study for the national training programme in laparoscopic colorectal surgery in England. Ann Surg. 2013;257(3): 476–82.
25. Miskovic D, et al. Observational clinical human reliability analysis (OCHRA) for competency assessment in laparoscopic colorectal surgery at the specialist level. Surg Endosc. 2012;26(3):796–803.
26. Nagtegaal ID, et al. Macroscopic evaluation of rectal cancer resection specimen: clinical significance of the pathologist in quality control. J Clin Oncol. 2002;20(7):1729–34.
27. Palter VN, et al. Validation of a structured training and assessment curriculum for technical skill acquisition in minimally invasive surgery: a randomized controlled trial. Ann Surg. 2013;257(2):224–30.
28. Archampong D, Borowski DW, Dickinson HO. Impact of surgeon volume on outcomes of rectal cancer surgery: a systematic review and meta-analysis. Surgeon. 2010;8(6):341–52.
29. Baek JH, et al. The association of hospital volume with rectal cancer surgery outcomes. Int J Colorectal Dis. 2013;28(2):191–6.

Perioperative Care for Patients Undergoing Major Pelvic Operations

44

Ian D. White and Robin H. Kennedy

44.1 Introduction

The last two decades have seen dramatic changes in colorectal surgery leading to improved outcomes. One of the most important was pioneered by Henrik Kehlet in the 1990s. He asked the question 'why does the patient need to stay in hospital for more than 2–3 days after colorectal resection?' His publications in 2000 [1, 2] reporting stays of 2–3 days for colonic resection heralded the concept known as 'Fast-Track' or 'Enhanced Recovery' care, which has transformed perioperative care worldwide. This approach involves a multimodal program of largely evidence based improvements in care that both reduces complications and shortens hospital stay (Fig. 44.1). It is important to stress that there is a reduction in complications as shown by the meta-analysis from Varadhan and colleagues (Figs. 44.2 and 44.3) [3] and that this change is not designed merely to shorten hospital stay for economic reasons. At the time of these publications in 2000, median hospital stay in England after laparoscopic colonic resection was around 7 days and median stay generally was approximately 10 days [4], clarifying further Kehlets contribution.

Perioperative care consists of pre-, intra- and postoperative interventions. This chapter will subdivide the interventions based on the chronological order in the patient's journey.

Throughout this chapter the information is based on published evidence which has been summarized in Table 44.1 [5, 6].

44.2 Pre-operative Care

Health Optimization: Prediction of Risk

Although some specialties will not undertake surgery in people with reversible risk, e.g. smoking or obesity, this is often not possible in patients coming for cancer interventions due to the short time frame. Risk should however be predicted and minimized by optimization of the preoperative health status e.g. stopping smoking [7] and excess alcohol intake [8] for at least 4 weeks prior to surgery, when time allows. We would routinely ensure that anyone with significant cardiac comorbidity undergoes examination using stress echocardiography, and if necessary, angiographic evaluation. Those people with compromised respiratory function would also have appropriate assessment of their respiratory capacity in order to ensure the anesthetist is fully informed regarding any limitation and, when possible, to improve

I.D. White, MB BS
Surgery B, Meir General Hospital, Kfar Saba, Israel

R.H. Kennedy, MB, BS, MS, FRCS (✉)
Department of Surgery, St. Mark's Hospital, Harrow, Middlesex, UK
e-mail: Robin.Kennedy@nhs.net

H.R.H. Patel et al. (eds.), *Pelvic Cancer Surgery: Modern Breakthroughs and Future Advances*, DOI 10.1007/978-1-4471-4258-4_44, © Springer-Verlag London 2015

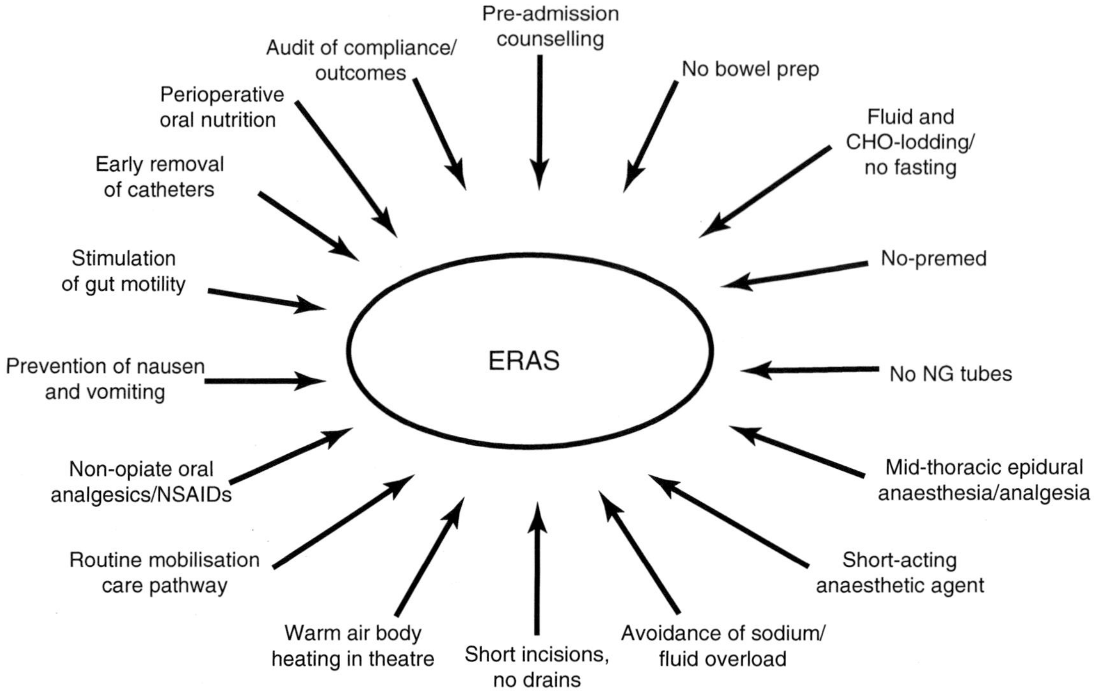

Fig. 44.1 Main elements of the ERAS protocol (Reprinted from Fearon et al. [59]; with permission from Elsevier)

Study or Subgroup	ERAS Events	ERAS Total	TC Events	TC Total	Weight	Risk Ratio M-H, Random, 95% CI
Anderson 2003[10]	4	14	5	11	6.0%	0.63[0.22, 1.80]
Delaney 2003[20]	7	31	10	33	9.6%	0.75[0.32, 1.71]
Gatt 2005[21]	9	19	15	20	23.1%	0.63[0.37, 1.08]
Khoo 2007[22]	9	35	16	35	14.9%	0.56[0.29, 1.10]
Muller 2009[3]	16	76	37	75	37.5%	0.43[0.26, 0.70]
Serclova 2009[4]	11	51	25	52	18.8%	0.43[0.25, 0.81]
Total (95% CI)		**226**		**226**	**100.0%**	**0.53 [0.41, 0.69]**
Total events	56		108			

Heterogeneity: $Tau^2 = 0.00$; $Chi^2 = 2.26$, df = 5 (P = 0.81); $I^2 = 0\%$
Test for overall effect: Z = 4.81 (P < 0.00001)

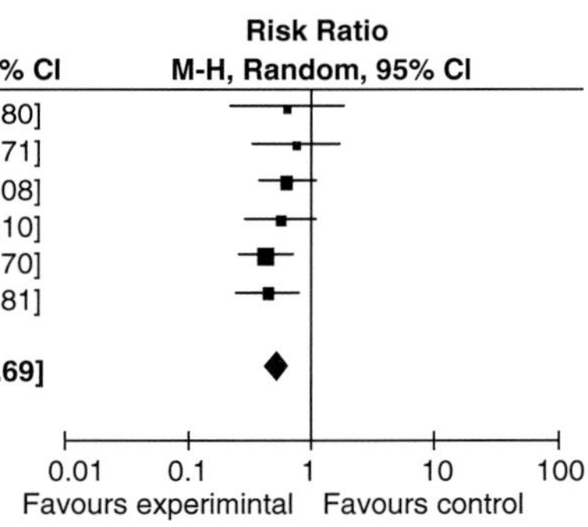

Fig. 44.2 Complications within an eras program. Forest plot of comparison: ERAS (experimental group), Traditional Care (Control) (Reprinted from Varadhan et al. [3]; with permission from Elsevier)

Study or Subgroup	ERAS Mean	ERAS SD	ERAS Total	TC Mean	TC SD	TC Total	Weight	Mean Difference IV, Random, 95% CI
Anderson 2003[19]	4	1.8	14	7	2.1	11	19.3%	−3.00 [−4.56, −1.44]
Delaney 2003[20]	5.2	2.5	31	5.8	3	33	21.7%	−0.60 [−1.95, 0.75]
Gatt 2005[21]	6.6	4.4	19	1	4.6	20	9.6%	−2.40 [−5.22, 0.42]
Khoo 2007[22]	5	8.5	35	7	14.75	35	3.1%	−2.00 [−7.64, 3.34]
Muller 2009[8]	6.7	4.84	76	10.3	4.97	75	19.2%	−3.60 [−5.17, −2.03]
Serdova 2009[4]	7.4	1.3	51	10.4	3.1	52	21.1%	−3.00 [−3.92, −2.08]
Total (95% CI)			**226**			**226**	**100.0%**	**2.51 [−3.54, −1.47]**

Heterogeneity; $Tau^2 = 0.80$; $chi^2 = 11.04$,df = 5 (P =0.05); $I^2 = 55\%$
Test for overall effect; Z = 4.76 (P< 0.00001)

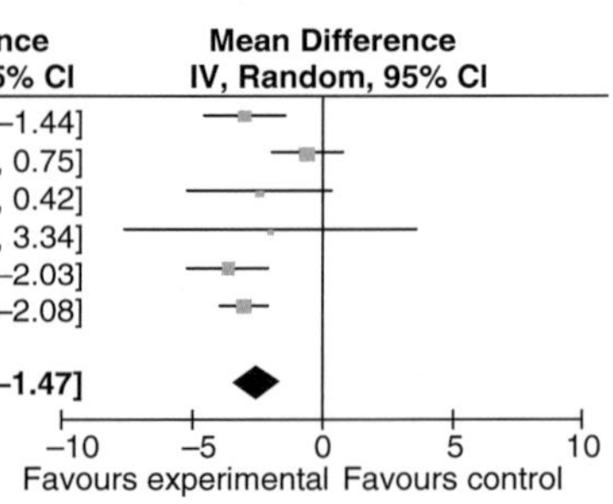

Fig. 44.3 Length of hospital stay (days) within an eras program. Forest plot of comparison: ERAS (experimental group), Traditional Care (Control) (Reprinted from Varadhan et al. [3]; with permission from Elsevier)

Table 44.1 Guidelines for perioperative care in elective rectal/pelvic surgery: Enhanced Recovery After Surgery (ERAS) society recommendations

Item	Recommendation	Evidence level	Recommendation guide
Preoperative information, education and counseling	Patients should routinely receive dedicated preoperative counseling	Low	Strong
Preoperative optimization	Preoperative optimization of medical conditions (e.g., anemia), cessation of smoking and alcohol intake 4 weeks before rectal surgery is recommended. Increasing exercise preoperatively may be of benefit. Preoperative specialized nutritional support should be considered for malnourished patients	Medical optimization: moderate Pre-habilitation: very low Cessation of smoking: moderate Cessation of excess consumption of alcohol: low	Medical optimization: strong Pre-habilitation: no Cessation of smoking: Strong Cessation of excess consumption of alcohol: strong
Preoperative bowel preparation	In general, MBP should not be used in pelvic surgery. However, when a diverting ileostomy is planned, MBP may be necessary (although this needs to be studied further)	Anterior resection: (no MBP) high Total mesorectal excision (TME) with diverting stoma: (use MBP) low	Anterior resection: strong TME with diverting stoma: weak
Preoperative fasting	Intake of clear fluids up to 2 h and solids up to 6 h prior to induction of anesthesia	Moderate	Strong
Preoperative treatment with carbohydrates	Preoperative oral carbohydrate loading should be administered to all non-diabetic patients	Reduced postop insulin resistance: moderate Improved clinical outcomes: low	Strong
Preanesthetic medication	No advantages in using long-acting benzodiazepines Short-acting benzodiazepines can be used in young patients before potentially painful interventions (insertion of spinal or epidural, arterial catheter), but they should not be used in the elderly (age >60 years)	Moderate	Strong
Prophylaxis against thromboembolism	Patients should wear well-fitting compression stockings, and receive pharmacological prophylaxis with LMWH. Extended prophylaxis for 28 days should be considered in patients with colorectal cancer or other patients with increased risk of VTE	High	Strong
Antimicrobial prophylaxis	Patients should receive antimicrobial prophylaxis before skin incision in a single dose. Repeated doses may be necessary depending on the half-life of drug and duration of surgery	High	Strong

(continued)

Item	Recommendation	Evidence level	Recommendation guide
Skin preparation	A recent RCT has shown that skin preparation with a scrub of chlorhexidine-alcohol is superior to povidone-iodine in preventing surgical-site infections	Moderate	For skin preparation in general: strong Specific choice of preparation: weak
Standard anesthetic protocol	To attenuate the surgical stress response, intraoperative maintenance of adequate hemodynamic control, central and peripheral oxygenation, muscle relaxation, depth of anesthesia, and appropriate analgesia is strongly recommended	Epidural: moderate IV lidocaine: low Remifentanil: low High oxygen concentration: high	Epidural: strong IV lidocaine: weak Remifentanil: strong High oxygen concentration: strong
PONV	Prevention of PONV should be included as standard in ERAS protocols. More specifically, a multimodal approach to PONV prophylaxis should be adopted in all patients with two or more risk factors undergoing major colorectal surgery. If PONV is present, treatment should be via a multimodal approach	High-risk patients: high In all patients: low	Strong
Laparoscopic resection of benign disease	With proven safety and at least equivocal disease-specific outcomes, laparoscopic proctectomy and proctocolectomy for benign disease can be carried out by an experienced surgeon within an ERAS protocol with the goals of reduced perioperative stress (manifested by decreased postoperative ileus), decreased LOSH, and fewer overall complications	Low	Strong
Laparoscopic resection of rectal cancer	Laparoscopic resection of rectal cancer is currently not generally recommended outside of a trial setting (or specialized center with ongoing audit) until equivalent oncologic outcomes are proven	Moderate	Strong
Nasogastric intubation	Postoperative nasogastric tubes should not be used routinely	High	Strong
Preventing intraoperative hypothermia	Patients undergoing rectal surgery need to have their body temperature monitored during and after surgery. Attempts should be made to avoid hypothermia because it increases the risk of perioperative complications	High	Strong
Perioperative fluid management	Fluid balance should be optimized by targeting cardiac output and avoiding overhydration. Judicious use of vasopressors is recommended with arterial hypotension. Targeted fluid therapy using the oesophageal Doppler system is recommended	Moderate	Strong
Drainage of peritoneal cavity	Pelvic drains should not be used routinely	Low	Weak
Transurethral catheter	After pelvic surgery with a low estimated risk of postoperative urinary retention, the transurethral bladder catheter may be safely removed on postoperative day 1, even if epidural analgesia is used	Low	Weak
Suprapubic catheter	In patients with an increased risk of prolonged postoperative urinary retention, placement of a suprapubic catheter is recommended	Prolonged catheterization: low	Weak

Chewing gum	A multimodal approach to optimizing gut function after rectal resection should involve chewing gum	Moderate	Strong
Postoperative laxatives and prokinetics	A multimodal approach to optimizing gut function after rectal resection should involve oral laxatives	Low	Weak
Postoperative analgesia	TEA is recommended for open rectal surgery for 48–72 h in view of the superior quality of pain relief compared with systemic opioids. Intravenous administration of lidocaine has also been shown to provide satisfactory analgesia, but the evidence in rectal surgery is lacking. If a laparoscopic approach is used, epidural or intravenous lidocaine, in the context of ERAS, provides adequate pain relief and no difference in the duration of LOSH and return of bowel function. Rectal pain can be of neuropathic origin, and needs to be treated with multimodal analgesic methods. There is limited evidence for the routine use of wound catheters and continuous TAP blocks in rectal surgery	Epidural for open surgery: high Epidural for laparoscopy: low Intravenous lidocaine: moderate Wound infiltration and TAP blocks: low	Epidural for open surgery: strong Epidural for laparoscopy: weak Intravenous lidocaine: weak Wound infiltration and TAP blocks: weak
Early oral intake	An oral ad libitum diet is recommended 4 h after rectal surgery	Moderate	Strong
Oral nutritional supplements	In addition to normal food intake, patients should be offered ONS to maintain adequate intake of protein and energy	Low	Strong
Postoperative glucose control	Maintenance of perioperative blood sugar levels within an expert-defined range results in better outcomes. Therefore, insulin resistance and hyperglycemia should be avoided using stress-reducing measures, or if already established by active treatment. The level of glycemia to target for intervention at the ward level remains uncertain, and is dependent upon local safety aspects	Use of stress-reducing measures: moderate Level of glycemia for insulin treatment: low	Use of stress-reducing treatments: strong Insulin treatment (non- diabetics) at the ward level: weak
Early mobilization	Patients should be nursed in an environment that encourages independence and mobilization. A care plan that facilitates patients being out of bed for 2 h on the day of surgery and 6 h thereafter is recommended	Low	Strong

Reprinted from: Nygren et al. [6]; used with permission

MBP Mechanical bowel preparation, *PONV* Postoperative nausea and vomiting, *TEA* Thoracic epidural analgesia, *LOSH* Length of stay in hospital function. Other comorbidities such as renal function should be assessed and all factors taken into consideration when planning whether to operate, what operation to perform and what risk of mortality and morbidity to state when taking consent.

In order to improve risk prediction and allow comparison between populations, the Physiological & Operative Severity Score for the enumeration of mortality and morbidity (POSSUM) was devised. It uses 12 physiological and six surgical parameters in order to calculate the risk of intervention. An adaptation for colorectal surgery, the ColoRectal POSSUM (CR-POSSUM) use only six physiological parameters and four operative measures for prediction of morbidity [9]. Their accuracy is limited but their major disadvantage is that they require intraoperative data for their calculation. The use of cardiopulmonary exercise (CPEx) testing provides a combined assessment of cardiac and respiratory fitness following exercise and will provide the team and, more importantly the patient, with an objective assessment of the risk of intervention. Swart and Carlisle [10] have used CPEx testing and risk assessment preoperatively and identified factors which independently influence subsequent year on year mortality. They showed that attending a consultant lead preoperative clinic and admission to a perioperative critical care unit reduce adverse outcomes [11]. A 6 min walking test has been well validated [12] for the prediction of risk and is a relatively straight forward assessment. That and other approaches such as comorbidity measurement and frailty testing [13] have the potential to impact on outcome by altering the approach to surgery or choice of operation, but to date have been routinely used in very few centers.

Conditioning of Expectation and Pre-assessment

Sir David Cuthbertson (1900–1989), a biochemist working in Glasgow during the 1920s, was one of the first scientists to uncover the link between the physiological (neuro-hormonal) stress response and the negative impact it can have on outcomes. We have built on that principle by providing explicit preoperative information including goal setting, which facilitates postoperative recovery, pain control and discharge [14]. A clear explanation of expectations prior to and during hospitalization facilitates adherence to the care pathway, allowing patients to feel part of and to expedite their recovery. The knowledge of targets including nutrition, mobilization and other tasks provides encouragement and positive reinforcement, leading to earlier recovery and discharge[5]. Our standard approach to this is the provision of written and oral information 1–2 weeks preoperatively by a dedicated preadmission nurse for all patients undergoing elective rectal resection. This usually takes 30—40 min and is performed with a family member or friend present in order to aid discharge planning. It will be scheduled earlier and with medical assessment when patients have certain comorbidities in order to correctly identify them, thus allowing time for optimization if possible.

Pre-operative Preparation

1. There are few reasons now to admit patients the day before surgery as when admitted on the day of surgery they will experience decreased levels of stress and have less chance of acquiring resistant organisms.
2. It is not advantageous to administer preoperative long acting sedatives or relaxants since they will delay postoperative recovery and mobilization [15].
3. The use of mechanical bowel preparation in colorectal surgery has been shown to increase anastomotic leakage in randomized trials, as well as increasing dehydration and electrolyte abnormalities, especially in the elderly and renally impaired [16, 17]. The French Greccar III Multicenter Single-Blinded RT of low anterior resection for rectal cancer did however link those without mechanical bowel preparation to higher overall and infectious morbidity, but without any significant increase in anastomotic leak rate [18]. This was not proven in a multicenter RCT assessing anastomotic leakage and septic complications below the peritoneal verge [19]. This study, when

examining covering ileostomies, in a subgroup analysis, found no difference when assessing complications in patients without MBP both with and without a diverting ileostomy. Platell [20] however argues that if the pelvic abscesses reported in this study plus those of Jung [21] (another large clinical trial) are included as 'anastomotic leaks' there is a significant benefit to those who receive MBP. Furthermore, Matthiesson [22] as well as a Cochrane study [23] (which included Matthiesson's data) have demonstrated that total mesorectal excision (TME) without a covering stoma is associated with increased leak rates and the consequences of leakage.

For these reasons we perform a defunctioning loop stoma when performing TME. In order to avoid a column of stool between the stoma and the anastomosis which might worsen morbidity if leakage occurs, we currently still administer mechanical bowel preparation for TME surgery. We merely use a phosphate enema preoperatively in patients undergoing abdominoperineal excision (APE) of the rectum or high anterior resection (PME).

4. Preoperative pharmacological prophylaxis is recommended to reduce symptomatic venous thromboembolism (VTE), without increasing side effects such as bleeding. Additionally, compression stockings reduce the incidence of VTE. Both in hospital prophylaxis and 4 week post operative continued prophylaxis has been associated with significantly reduced VTE, without an increase in postoperative bleeding complications or other side effects. We currently only administer heparin preoperatively and during the hospital stay due to the low incidence of VTE in our practice. Care should be taken if an epidural analgesic protocol is to be used and we administer prophylactic heparin not less than 12 h before the planned procedure. Low molecular weight heparin (LMWH) is preferable due to its once daily administration and a lower risk of heparin induced thrombocytopenia [6].
5. Fasting from midnight, previously a universal recommendation, is unnecessary and hinders the elective patient's recovery. Anesthesia guidelines now should recommend fasting for only 2 h for clear fluids and 6 for solids, particulate fluids and those containing fat. Multiple RCTs plus a Cochrane review reveal no resultant increase in complications [24]
6. Preoperative metabolic stress is reduced in the 'fed' patient, leading to decreased postoperative insulin resistance. Preoperative carbohydrate loading with specifically formulated iso-osmolar solutions of 12.5 % dextrose, 2–3 h preoperatively, can reduce post-operative thirst, hunger and anxiety [25]. They result in earlier return of gut function and reduce post-operative hospital stay, especially when compared to fasting [26, 27]. No increase in pulmonary aspiration has been found as gastric emptying is similar to that with water. Postoperative insulin resistance is analogous to a type II diabetic state and is induced by starvation, major stress and immobilization. Thus enhanced recovery care is directed towards avoiding all these triggers [5, 6, 28].

44.3 Intraoperative Factors

Antibiotics

Single dose prophylactic antibiotic administration is as effective as multiple pre- and post-surgical administrations. Publications have compared a variety of drug combinations and protocols, reporting that surgical site infection as well as postoperative infection is significantly reduced after administration of appropriate antibiotics within 30–60 min prior to incision. Follow up doses are recommended for prolonged surgery although a specific length of time is not commonly agreed upon [29, 30].

Fluids

Lobo [31] and Brandstrup [32] have shown a 3–6 kg increase in weight after colorectal surgery when too much sodium or too great a volume of fluid is administered. They demonstrated an increase in postoperative ileus and other complications, resulting in longer hospital stays. They hypothesized that salt and water overload results in increased gut permeability, decreased mesenteric blood flow and tissue oxygenation, impaired wound healing and adverse outcomes. With a daily requirement of 0.9–1.2 mmol/kg of sodium the average 70 kg person would require 63–84 mmol/day. It must be remembered that 'normal saline' contains 154 mmol of sodium/l and 'Hartmann's Solution' 131 mmol/l. Therefore patients will be overloaded with sodium if attention is not paid to this. Once excess sodium is given, this results in excess water retention and the consequences described above. Initially authors referred to a 'restrictive' postoperative fluid regime but it is more correctly described as euvolemic fluid replacement. It is important to stress that in people with renal impairment fluid restriction is potentially dangerous and for this reason we analyze urea and creatinine in all patients on a daily basis to avoid this possibility. Allowing patients to drink water until 2 h prior to surgery and using carbohydrate loading helps avoid preoperative dehydration. When oral bowel preparation is given appropriate rehydration should be emphasized, or if patients are unfit, preoperative intravenous fluids administered the night before surgery. Intraoperative 'goal directed' fluid therapy (GDT) guides fluid administration against a measure of cardiac output—one method of doing this is to use an esophageal Doppler probe which analyzes aortic flow. By using aliquots of fluid one can maximize the patient's stroke volume without causing fluid overload, which leads to improved outcomes with reduced complications and hospital stay [33, 34]. This approach will become more refined as recently a randomized trial from New Zealand [35] did not identify a benefit to GDT when patients are already being treated within an enhanced recovery protocol.

Intraoperative Analgesia

The avoidance of intraoperative stress has been a feature of publications on enhanced recovery care and the use of thoracic epidural analgesia during surgery was proposed in order to block the stress response [6]. By inserting the epidural at the T7–8 level, postoperatively motor block in the lower limbs is also avoided, allowing 'dynamic' pain relief. In addition this minimizes gut paralysis. No ideal anesthetic method has been established although short acting medications such as propofol and remifentinil are preferred to longer acting agents such as opiates, in order to reduce side effects. Nausea and vomiting after surgery can be extremely distressing, but mid thoracic (T7/8) epidural using a combination of opiate and local anesthetic is superior to opiates in terms of analgesia, avoidance of nausea and improvement in pulmonary function [5, 6]. With the increased use of laparoscopic surgery clinicians have questioned the necessity for postoperative epidural analgesia and various studies have supported its avoidance. Delaney and colleagues have provided evidence that it can be avoided [36] and more recently Rockall's group [37] have proposed the use of spinal opiate injection at surgery, supplemented postoperatively by patient controlled intravenous opiate analgesia (PCA). In a randomized trial of spinal opiate plus PCA, versus PCA alone, or a third arm of thoracic epidural alone, the spinal + PCA group were improved by comparison with PCA alone. The worst outcomes were in the epidural group in terms of hospital stay and fluid retention after laparoscopic colorectal resection. Many clinicians have now moved towards alternatives to intra and postoperative epidural usage although, if a good thoracic epidural service is available with a low failure rate, it provides excellent analgesia.

Incisions

Various authors have reported that transverse incisions are beneficial, reducing pain and complications with less postoperative opiate usage, less impairment of respiratory function and decreased rates of post operative hernias as well as cosmetic superiority [38, 39]. This approach might apply best to colonic surgery as the use of a transverse lower abdominal incision for rectal surgery generally provides inferior access when compared to a lower midline incision, particularly when performing complex procedures.

The Use of Laparoscopy

The short-term benefits of laparoscopic versus open surgery for colorectal cancer have been well established in the literature to date and include reduced post-operative morbidity, earlier passage of flatus, less narcotic analgesic requirements and a shorter length of stay [40]. The evidence of benefit from laparoscopy specifically in rectal surgery is less established, but two recently published randomized trials have reported improvements in outcome following laparoscopic resection [41, 42]. Analysis of our data shows that we use laparoscopy in 90 % of our population [43], but individual surgeons must audit their own data in order to ensure they are not disadvantaging patients due to the technical challenges of laparoscopic rectal surgery.

Normothermia

Preserving intra-operative normothermia reduces endocrine-metabolic responses and sympathetic reflexes, and changes the fibrinolytic-coagulatory balance, resulting in reduced bleeding. This can be achieved using an upper-body forced-air heating system and keeping the theater at appropriate temperatures. It leads to reduced bleeding, subsequent transfusion requirements, wound infections and cardiac complications. Extending systemic warming to 2 h before and after surgery has been reported to have additional benefits [5, 6, 44].

Antiemetics

The routine use of an antiemetic before the end of surgery has been shown to decrease postoperative nausea and vomiting and it is reported that this can be improved further with the addition of dexamethasone [45, 46].

Abdominal/Pelvic Drains

A Cochrane Review published in 2004 [47] did not find anastomotic drainage following colorectal surgery reduced anastomotic leakage. Bretagnol and colleagues undertook a meta-analysis examining three randomized trials looking specifically at rectal surgery and also found that leakage was unaffected by drainage [48]. Despite this data, if surgeons feel uncomfortable not draining a potential pelvic hematoma, in case it becomes infected and discharges into the rectum, then leaving a drain is unlikely to worsen outcome provided it is removed early the day after surgery, thus not impeding mobilization.

44.4 Postoperative Factors

Nasogastric Tubes and Nutrition

A 2010 updated Cochrane meta-analysis [49] of 37 studies with over 5,700 patients confirmed that postoperative nasogastric tubes are ineffective in achieving their goals, and in fact significant benefit may be obtained by avoidance of prolonged intubation, only selective tube insertion being recommended. A nasogastric tube may reduce vomiting postoperatively but because of the adverse outcomes we advise tubes are removed before the patient leaves theater.

Multiple randomized controlled trials have shown that there is no advantage in keeping patients "nil by mouth" after surgery, versus early feeding. Early feeding reduces the risk of infection, length of hospital stay, anastomotic dehiscence and even death. Early feeding is dependant however on other issues such as good pain control to reduce nausea, avoidance of opiates (except in epidurals), correct fluid replacement and appropriate antiemetic usage [5, 6].

Oral nutritional supplements help patients to reach their recommended calorie and protein intakes early after surgery, resulting in better nitrogen balance, and less insulin resistance. When possible foods should be given in preference to supplements as sometimes the latter cause nausea [5, 6].

Chewing gum has been shown to be safe and beneficial in reducing time to first bowel movement by one day after open gastrointestinal surgery [50], although there is no conclusive data regarding use after laparoscopy.

Various ERAS programs have reported on the efficacy of oral laxatives post operatively. Whilst appearing to have some benefit, little has been addressed in regard to anastomotic leakage [6]. Our protocol includes routine treatment—unless an ileostomy has been formed—with postoperative oral laxative to decrease time to first flatus and bowel movement.

Intravenous Fluids, Analgesia and Mobilization

George H Evans already published in *JAMA* in 1911 that "One cannot fail to be impressed with the danger . . . (of) the utter recklessness with which salt solution is frequently prescribed, particularly in the postoperative period . . ." The use of excess sodium and/or intravenous fluid has been shown to cause ileus and increase complications—provided oral intake is satisfactory on the morning following surgery the intravenous infusion is discontinued (see above).

A multimodal approach to analgesia is routine in our practice. Combining paracetamol and a non steroidal anti-inflammatory drug (NSAID) such as ibuprofen is an effective opiate sparing strategy in order to minimize nausea and ensure one can continue to rely on the oral route of administration. Recently, the possibility that NSAID's may increase anastomotic leakage has been examined with mixed findings including no significance in a meta-analysis [51], therefore we currently only use ibuprofen (with daily creatinine monitoring) which seems unlikely to cause leakage [52]. As described above, epidural analgesia postoperatively has been considered the gold standard, but increasingly with laparoscopic surgery, we are using PCA—with or without an intraoperative spinal opiate injection—which is usually discontinued on day 1.

Mobilization is vital in the postoperative period. Getting the patient out of bed early reduces ileus, thromboembolism, muscle wasting, insulin resistance and pulmonary complications, whilst improving tissue oxygenation [53]. The enhanced recovery protocol advises that the patient should be out of bed for 2 h on the day of surgery, provided the operation has been early enough in the day, and at least 6 h per day thereafter. We also encourage walking to a specific dining area for meals and four 60 m walks per day. Analgesia should aid this goal and facilitate mobilization. To further liberate patients, if a urethral catheter has been placed it will be removed on day 1 when upper rectal surgery has been performed and in low rectal surgery on day 2 or 3—in case any nerve damage results in retention. Although several studies have demonstrated a reduction in morbidity with suprapubic catheterization we usually employ urethral catheters and remove them early to avoid complications [54, 55]. The routine removal of all attachments as soon as possible, including oxygen when saturation levels are normal, will facilitate mobilization, reducing metabolic stress and complications. For APE all drains are abdominal for comfort and to decrease the possibility of subsequent perineal discharge.

Discharge Criteria

Although there were high rates of readmission during the development of enhanced recovery care this has not persisted. Once a patient is mobile, eating and drinking and has good pain control using oral medication, they can be safely discharged. Awaiting the first bowel movement is usually unnecessary. Stoma training is commenced preoperatively and, particularly in patients having laparoscopic surgery, can progress rapidly enough to allow discharge as early as day 3 in certain individuals. Suitable solutions to social problems such as patients living alone will have been discussed pre-operatively in order facilitate discharge. Monitoring CRP daily helps detect problems early [56, 57] and if patients who have undergone laparoscopic rectal resection are not progressing towards discharge within 3–4 days of surgery CT scanning is undertaken, in order to detect an occult anastomotic leak.

Patients prosper when discharge is directed and discussed both preoperatively, as well as daily after surgery. A carefully directed, goal orientated plan, engaging the patient and the whole team, leads to improved results (see above). Early review in the outpatient clinic is now usually possible at 10–14 days after laparoscopic surgery when it is performed within an enhanced recovery program. In addition written advice is provided on recovery after discharge, particularly providing hospital contact numbers to facilitate immediate hospital review should there be problems within 2 weeks of surgery, rather than seeing a community/general practitioner.

Post Operative Outcomes

In order to analyze outcome, audit and data collection are vital. An enhanced recovery facilitator, usually a senior nurse, is required to set up and run the program and data collection can now be facilitated by bespoke packages such as that marketed by the ERAS group [58].

44.5 Summary

Perioperative care in major colorectal pelvic surgery has seen dramatic changes over the last 20 years due to the introduction of Enhanced Recovery programs. These consist of multimodal, evidence-based improvements which reduce complications, attenuate the response to stress, speed recovery and shorten hospital stay.

Preassessment which involves health optimization, risk prediction, conditioning of expectation, reduction in preoperative fasting and avoidance of mechanical bowel preparation, results in healthier patients and a decrease in metabolic stress. The provision of preoperative information conditions expectation and facilitates adherence to the care pathway. Anesthetic improvements involve avoidance of long acting sedatives, the use of short acting anesthetic agents, goal directed fluid therapy, a reduction in opiate use, and a multimodal approach to postoperative analgesia—all of these benefit the patient whilst assisting the recovery process.

Superior outcomes are achieved by using laparoscopic surgery, improved fluid management with avoidance of excess sodium administration and reduced nasogastric tube and abdominal drain usage. Post-operative goal orientated plans involve early feeding and mobilization along with the removal of unnecessary intervention such as urinary catheters, intravenous cannulae and all superfluous tubes.

Finally, data collection and audit are required for analysis in order to monitor and improve outcomes.

Key Learning Points

- Enhanced recovery programs consist of multimodal, evidence-based improvements which reduce complications, speed recovery and shorten hospital stay, generally by reducing peri-operative stress.
- Conditioning of expectation during preoperative counseling is essential to increase patient compliance.
- Preoperative interventions reduce metabolic stress and include health optimization, improved nutrition, carbohydrate loading, reduction of preoperative fasting and avoidance of mechanical bowel preparation when appropriate.
- Intra-operative elements include the use of short acting anesthetic agents, laparoscopic surgery, meticulous surgical technique, and the avoidance of opiates, excess fluid and sodium, drains and nasogastric tubes.
- Reduced insulin resistance is achieved through decreased pre-operative fasting, carbohydrate loading, minimizing the traumatic surgical insult and early post-operative feeding.

(continued)

- Goal-directed fluid therapy optimizes fluid balance especially avoiding overhydration.
- Laparoscopic surgery reduces complications, reduces the duration of recovery and shortens hospital stay.
- Multimodal analgesia with minimal use of opiates decreases complications, improving nutrition and mobilization.
- Reduced insulin resistance and metabolic stress is enhanced by early postoperative nutrition and mobilization, early removal of catheters, intravenous lines and drains.
- Appropriate data collection and audit are required in order to monitor and improve outcomes.

References

1. Bardram L, Funch-Jensen P, Kehlet H. Rapid rehabilitation in elderly patients after laparoscopic colonic resection. Br J Surg. 2000;87(11):1540–5.
2. Basse L, Hjort Jakobsen D, Billesbølle P, Werner M, Kehlet H. A clinical pathway to accelerate recovery after colonic resection. Ann Surg. 2000;232(1):51–7.
3. Varadhan KK, Neal KR, Dejong CH, Fearon KC, Ljungqvist O, Lobo DN. The enhanced recovery after surgery (ERAS) pathway for patients undergoing major elective open colorectal surgery: a meta-analysis of randomized controlled trials. Clin Nutr. 2010;29(4):434–40.
4. Faiz O, Warusavitarne J, Bottle A, Tekkis PP, Darzi AW, Kennedy RH. Laparoscopically assisted vs. open elective colonic and rectal resection: a comparison of outcomes in English National Health Service Trusts between 1996 and 2006. Dis Colon Rectum. 2009;52(10):1695–704.
5. Lassen K, Soop M, Nygren J, Cox PB, Hendry PO, Spies C, von Meyenfeldt MF, Fearon KC, Revhaug A, Norderval S, Ljungqvist O, Lobo DN, Dejong CH. Consensus review of optimal perioperative care in colorectal surgery. Enhanced Recovery After Surgery (ERAS) Group recommendations. Arch Surg. 2009;144(10):961–9.
6. Nygren J, Thacker J, Carli F, Fearon KC, Norderval S, Lobo DN, Ljungqvist O, Soop M, Ramirez J. Enhanced recovery after surgery society. Guidelines for perioperative care in elective rectal/pelvic surgery: Enhanced Recovery After Surgery (ERAS®) Society recommendations. Clin Nutr. 2012;31(6):801–16.
7. Mastracci TM, Carli F, Finley RJ, Muccio S, Warner DO. Effect of preoperative smoking cessation interventions on postoperative complications. J Am Coll Surg. 2011;212(6):1094–6.
8. Tonnesen H, Nielsen PR, Lauritzen JB, Moller AM. Smoking and alcohol intervention before surgery: evidence for best practice. Br J Anaesth. 2009;102(3):297e306.
9. Tekkis PP, Prytherch DR, Kocher HM, et al. Development of a dedicated riskadjustment scoring system for colorectal surgery (colorectal POSSUM). Br J Surg. 2004;91(9):1174–82.
10. Swart M, Carlisle JB. Case-controlled study of critical care or surgical ward care after elective open colorectal surgery. BJS. 2012;99:295–9.
11. Carlisle J, Swart M, Dawe EJC, Chadwick M. Factors associated with survival after resection of colorectal adenocarcinoma in 314 patients. BJA. 2012;108(3):430–5.
12. Moriello C, Mayo NE, Feldman L, Carli F. Validating the six-minute walk test as a measure of recovery after elective colon resection surgery. Arch Phys Med Rehabil. 2008;89(6):1083–9.
13. Tan KY, Kawamura YJ, Tokomitsu A, Tang T. Assessment for frailty is useful for predicting morbidity in elderly patients undergoing colorectal cancer resection whose comorbidities are already optimized. Am J Surg. 2012;204(2):139–43.
14. Wilmore D. From cuthbertson to fast-track surgery:70 years of progress in reducing stress in surgical patients. Ann Surg. 2002;236(5):643–8.
15. Smith AF, Pittaway AJ. Premedication for anxiety in adult day surgery [update of: Cochrane Database Syst Rev. 2000;(3):CD002192]. Cochrane Database Syst Rev. 2003;(1):CD002192.
16. Holte K, Nielsen KG, Madsen JL, Kehlet H. Physiologic effects of bowel preparation. Dis Colon Rectum. 2004;47(8):1397–402.
17. Bucher P, Gervaz P, Morel P. Should preoperative mechanical bowel preparation be abandoned? Ann Surg. 2007;245:662.
18. Bretagnol F, Panis Y, Rullier E, Rouanet P, Berdah S, Dousset B, Portier G, Benoist S, Chipponi J, Vicaut E, French Research Group of Rectal Cancer Surgery (GRECCAR). Rectal cancer surgery with or without bowel preparation: The French GRECCAR III multicenter single-blinded randomized trial. Ann Surg. 2010;252(5):863–8.
19. Contant CME, Hop WCJ, van't Sant HP, et al. Mechanical bowel preparation for elective colorectal surgery: outcome of a multicenter randomised study. Lancet. 2007;370:2112–7.
20. Platell C, Hall J. Mechanical bowel preparation before colorectal surgery? Lancet. 2007;370(9605):2073–5.
21. Jung B, Påhlman L, Nyström PO, Nilsson E, Mechanical Bowel Preparation Study Group. Multicentre randomized clinical trial of mechanical bowel preparation in elective colonic resection. Br J Surg. 2007;94(6):689–95.

22. Matthiessen P, Hallböök O, Rutegård J, Simert G, Sjödahl R. Defunctioning stoma reduces symptomatic anastomotic leakage after low anterior resection of the rectum for cancer: a randomized multicenter trial. Ann Surg. 2007;246(2):207–14.
23. Montedori A, Cirocchi R, Farinella E, Sciannameo F, Abraha I. Covering ileo- or colostomy in anterior resection for rectal carcinoma. Cochrane Database Syst Rev. 2010;(5).
24. Soreide E, Ljungqvist O. Modern preoperative fasting guidelines: a summary of the present recommendations and remaining questions. Best Pract Res Clin Anaesthesiol. 2006;20(3):483e91.
25. Hausel J, Nygren J, Lagerkranser M, et al. A carbohydrate-rich drink reduces preoperative discomfort in elective surgery patients. Anesth Analg. 2001;93(5):1344–50.
26. Nygren J, Thorell A, Ljungqvist O. Preoperative oral carbohydrate nutrition: an update. Curr Opin Clin Nutr Metab Care. 2001;4(4):255–9.
27. Noblett SE, Watson DS, Huong H, Davison B, Hainsworth PJ, Horgan AF. Pre-operative oral carbohydrate loading in colorectal surgery: a randomized controlled trial. Color Dis. 2006;8(7):563–9.
28. Nygren J. The metabolic effects of fasting and surgery. Best Pract Res Clin Anaesthesiol. 2006;20(3): 429–38.
29. Bratzler DW, Houck PM. Antimicrobial prophylaxis for surgery: an advisory statement from the National Surgical Infection Prevention Project. Clin Infect Dis. 2004;38(12):1706e15.
30. Nelson RL, Glenny AM, Song F. Antimicrobial prophylaxis for colorectal surgery. Cochrane Database Syst Rev. 2009;21(1):CD001181.
31. Lobo DN, Bostock KA, Neal KR, Perkins AC, Rowlands BJ, Allison SP. Effect of salt and water balance on recovery of gastrointestinal function after elective colonic resection: a randomised controlled trial. Lancet. 2002;359(9320):1812–8.
32. Brandstrup B, Tonnesen H, Beier-Holgersen R, Danish Study Group on Perioperative Fluid Therapy, et al. Effects of intravenous fluid restriction on postoperative complications: comparison of two perioperative fluid regimens: a randomized assessor-blinded multicenter trial. Ann Surg. 2003;238(5):641–8.
33. Giglio MT, Marucci M, Testini M, Brienza N. Goal-directed haemodynamic therapy and gastrointestinal complications in major surgery: a meta-analysis of randomized controlled trials. Br J Anaesth. 2009;103(5):637e46.
34. Wakeling HG, McFall MR, Jenkins CS, et al. Intraoperative oesophageal Doppler guided fluid management shortens postoperative hospital stay after major bowel surgery. Br J Anaesth. 2005;95(5):634–42.
35. Srinivasa S, Taylor MH, Singh PP, Yu TC, Soop M, Hill AG. Randomized clinical trial of goal-directed fluid therapy within an enhanced recovery protocol for elective colectomy. Br J Surg. 2013;100(1): 66–74.
36. Delaney CP, Zutshi M, Senagore AJ, et al. Prospective, randomized, controlled trial between a pathway of controlled rehabilitation with early ambulation and diet and traditional postoperative care after laparotomy and intestinal resection. Dis Colon Rectum. 2003;46(7):851–9.
37. Levy BF, Scott MJ, Fawcett W, Fry C, Rockall TA. Randomized clinical trial of epidural, spinal or patient-controlled analgesia for patients undergoing laparoscopic colorectal surgery. Br J Surg. 2011;98(8):1068–78.
38. Brown SR, Goodfellow PB. Transverse verses midline incisions for abdominal surgery. Cochrane database of systematic reviews 2005;(4):CD005199.
39. Bickenbach KA, Karanicolas PJ, Ammori JB, Jayaraman S, Winter JM, Fields RC, Govindarajan A, Nir I, Rocha FG, Brennan MF. Up and down or side to side? A systematic review and meta-analysis examining the impact of incision on outcomes after abdominal surgery. Am J Surg. 2013;206(3):400–9.
40. Abraham NS, Byrne CM, Young JM, Solomon MJ. Meta-analysis of non-randomized comparative studies of the short-term outcomes of laparoscopic resection for colorectal cancer. ANZ J Surg. 2007;77(7):508–16.
41. Kang SB, Park JW, Jeong SY, Nam BH, Choi HS, Kim DW, Lim SB, Lee TG, Kim DY, Kim JS, Chang HJ, Lee HS, Kim SY, Jung KH, Hong YS, Kim JH, Sohn DK, Kim DH, Oh JH. Open versus laparoscopic surgery for mid or low rectal cancer after neoadjuvant chemoradiotherapy (COREAN trial): short-term outcomes of an open-label randomised controlled trial. Lancet Oncol. 2010;11(7):637–45.
42. van der Pas MH, Haglind E, Cuesta MA, Fürst A, Lacy AM, Hop WC, Bonjer HJ. Colorectal cancer Laparoscopic or Open Resection II (COLOR II) Study Group. Laparoscopic versus open surgery for rectal cancer (COLOR II): short-term outcomes of a randomised, phase 3 trial. Lancet Oncol. 2013;14(3):210–8.
43. Buchanan GN, Malik A, Parvaiz A, Sheffield JP, Kennedy RH. Laparoscopic resection for colorectal cancer. Br J Surg. 2008;95(7):893–902.
44. Wong PF, Kumar S, Bohra A, Whetter D, Leaper DJ. Randomized clinical trial of perioperative systemic warming in major elective abdominal surgery. Br J Surg. 2007;94(4):421–6.
45. Wallenborn J, Gelbrich G, Bulst D, et al. Prevention of postoperative nausea and vomiting by metoclopramide combined with dexamethasone: randomised double blind multicentre trial. BMJ. 2006; 333(7563):324.
46. Carlisle JB, Stevenson CA. Drugs for preventing postoperative nausea and vomiting. Cochrane Database Syst Rev. 2006;3:CD004125.
47. Jesus EC, Karliczek A, Matos D, Castro AA, Atallah AN. Prophylactic anastomotic drainage for colorectal surgery. Cochrane Database Syst Rev. 2004;4:CD002100.

48. Bretagnol F, Slim K, Faucheron JL. Anterior resection with low colorectal anastomosis. To drain or not? Ann Chir. 2005;130(5):336–9.
49. Verma R, Nelson RL. Prophylactic nasogastric decompression after abdominal surgery. Cochrane Database Syst Rev. 2007;(3):CD004929. Updated 2010.
50. Fitzgerald JE, Ahmed I. Systematic review and meta-analysis of chewing-gum therapy in the reduction of postoperative paralytic ileus following gastrointestinal surgery. World J Surg. 2009;33(12):2557e66.
51. Burton TP, Mittal A, Soop M. Nonsteroidal anti-inflammatory drugs and anastomotic dehiscence in bowel surgery: systematic review and meta-analysis of randomized, controlled trials. Dis Colon Rectum. 2013;56(1):126–34.
52. Klein M, Gögenur I, Rosenberg J. Postoperative use of non-steroidal anti-inflammatory drugs in patients with anastomotic leakage requiring reoperation after colorectal resection: cohort study based on prospective data. BMJ. 2012;26:345.
53. Kehlet H, Wilmore DW. Multimodal strategies to improve surgical outcome. Am J Surg. 2002; 183(6):630–41.
54. Zmora O, Madbouly K, Tulchinsky H, Hussein A, Khaikin M. Urinary bladder catheter drainage following pelvic surgery—is it necessary for that long? Dis Colon Rectum. 2010;53(3):321–6.
55. McPhail MJ, Abu-Hilal M, Johnson CD. A meta-analysis comparing suprapubic and transurethral catheterization for bladder drainage after abdominal surgery. Br J Surg. 2006;93(9):1038–44.
56. Lane JC, Wright S, Burch J, Kennedy RH, Jenkins JT. Early prediction of adverse events in enhanced recovery based upon the host systemic inflammatory response. Color Dis. 2013;15(2):224–30.
57. Scepanovic MS, Kovacevic B, Cijan V, Antic A, Petrovic Z, Asceric R, Krdzic I, Cuk V. C-reactive protein as an early predictor for anastomotic leakage in elective abdominal surgery. Tech Coloproctol. 2013; 17(5):541–7.
58. www.erassociety.org
59. Fearon KC, Ljungqvist O, Von Meyenfeldt M, Revhaug A, Dejong CH, Lassen K, Nygren J, Hausel J, Soop M, Andersen J, Kehlet H. Enhanced recovery after surgery: a consensus review of clinical care for patients undergoing colonic resection. Clin Nutr. 2005;24(3):466–77.

Staging and Evaluation of Rectal Cancer and Pelvic Malignancy

45

Manish Chand, Anita Wale, and Gina Brown

45.1 Introduction

The modern management of rectal cancer and pelvic malignancy relies on accurate and detailed staging information. Clinicians require an increasing amount of information on tumor behavior and characteristics in order to make optimal treatment decisions. A number of these tumor characteristics are not readily detected on tissue biopsy at the time of diagnosis but are being increasingly identified on high quality imaging techniques such as magnetic resonance imaging (MRI). This has placed more emphasis on imaging in the overall management of pelvic malignancy and in particular, rectal cancer. Furthermore, a shift towards neo-adjuvant rather than adjuvant therapy means that it is the *initial* treatment decisions that are most important in terms of clinical outcomes and patient benefit.

The decision as to which imaging modality is the most appropriate to adequately stage the pelvis is equally important. Staging involves assessment of both local and distant disease spread. Cancer is a systemic disease which manifests itself in local disease and symptoms for most patients. Both the local disease or primary malignancy and the potential for systemic disease are interlocked, and features of local spread are important determinants in the likelihood of developing metastatic disease. Whilst there is little debate regarding the most appropriate technique to identify distant metastatic spread—computed tomography (CT) of the chest, abdomen and pelvis; the choice of local staging remains contentious between magnetic resonance imaging (MRI) and endoanal ultrasound (EAUS). In some circumstances where there is uncertainty regarding the presence of metastatic disease, in the liver or lung for example, additional complex imaging in the form of positron emission tomography (PET) may be used to delineate lesions in more detail. Whichever imaging modalities are decided on, it is important to obtain as much information on tumor behavior, spread and characteristics to offer patients the most beneficial treatment and the best clinical outcomes.

We present the important factors that can be identified at staging by imaging techniques that can influence treatment decisions. These prognostic factors may be related to spread of disease as well as tumor behavior. The advantages and disadvantages of the different imaging modalities used in the local staging of rectal cancer and pelvic malignancy are also discussed with particular reference to identification of these prognostic factors.

M. Chand, MBBS, BSc, MRCS (✉)
G. Brown, MBBS, MD, FRCR
Department of Radiology, Royal Mardsen Hospital, Sutton, Surrey, UK
e-mail: mans001@aol.com

A. Wale, BM, BS
Department of Radiology, The Royal Mardsen Hospital NHS Foundation Trust, Sutton, Surrey, UK

H.R.H. Patel et al. (eds.), *Pelvic Cancer Surgery: Modern Breakthroughs and Future Advances*,
DOI 10.1007/978-1-4471-4258-4_45, © Springer-Verlag London 2015

45.2 Assessment of Local Disease Spread

The role of local staging is to provide detailed information early in diagnosis on tumor spread relating to the bowel wall and beyond in addition to behavioral characteristics. Optimal treatment decisions rely on accurate staging information particularly when deciding on the appropriateness of neo-adjuvant therapy. Biopsy material is rarely able to provide such detail in identifying prognostic factors which means imaging is the most reliable method of obtaining this information. Whichever imaging modality is chosen, it must be able to provide information on tumor depth, nodal disease, the relationship of the tumor from the circumferential resection margin (CRM) in addition to adjacent viscera, and vascular invasion. Each is discussed below.

Tumor Depth and Mesorectal Spread

The extent to which tumor penetrates through the bowel wall is an important determinant on whether a patient receives neo-adjuvant treatment and potentially, the type of surgical procedure. It forms part of the American Joint Committee on Cancer (AJCC) TNM staging classification [1] and describes tumor penetration in relation to the layers of the rectal wall. Broadly speaking, tumors that are confined to the bowel wall (T1 and T2) may only require surgery and do not commonly need pre-operative treatment unless they have significant other adverse features [2]. Tumors which penetrate beyond the bowel wall into the surrounding mesorectum and threaten the circumferential resection margin (CRM) are offered neo-adjuvant treatment as there is significant risk of local failure [3]. Both MRI and EAUS can be used to determine tumor depth but selective use of neo-adjuvant treatment depends on more accurate sub-staging of tumor penetration and identification of the mesorectal fascia.

Early T-stage tumors may warrant an alternative surgical approach. For example, T1 lesions may be suitable for a less traumatic local excision such as transanal endoscopic microsurgery (TEMS) rather than total mesorectal excision (TME) [4, 5]. Accurate staging of tumor penetration has implications for over- and under-treatment. Endoanal ultrasound (EAUS) is highly accurate for the local assessment of early rectal cancer. However it is limited by not being able to identify the mesorectal fascia and thus identify whether the circumferential resection margin is threatened [6]. The mesorectal fascia defines the outermost boundary of the mesorectum. Total mesorectal excision (TME) is the gold-standard for oncological clearance of rectal cancer. TME involves excision of the rectum and mesorectum en-bloc [7, 8]. The mesorectal fascia also defines the circumferential resection margin (CRM) of the surgical specimen. Identifying whether the CRM is threatened by tumor is an important component of selective use of chemoradiotherapy (CRT) [3] (Fig. 45.1).

Conversely, MRI is excellent in identifying the CRM [9]. Accuracy for MRI depends on understanding the fields of alignment. Inappropriate technique can lead to under- or over-staging of tumors. Correct field alignment is made in relation to the long axis of the rectum. T2-weighted images are most suitable for distinguishing the layers of the bowel wall [10]. The different layers of the bowel wall are identified from their unique signal characteristic. Disruption through the normal signal characteristic pattern determines the depth of invasion. The depth of spread into the mesorectum is of particular importance. This fatty layer which surrounds the rectum in varying degrees along its length acts as an oncological barrier to tumor spread. Tumor spread which invades the mesorectum is classified as T3. The majority of patients present with T3 tumors, however there is wide variety in survival rates of these patients [11]. Cawthorn reported 5 year survival to be 55 % with tumor penetration less than 4 mm into the mesorectum compared to 25 % when more than 4 mm [12]. Merkel studied patient's survival characteristics with T3 tumors and used a cut-off of 5 mm. Those patients with extramural spread of more than 5 mm had 5 years survival rate of 54 % compared with 85 % for those patients whose tumors had extramural spread of less than 5 mm [13] (Fig. 45.2).

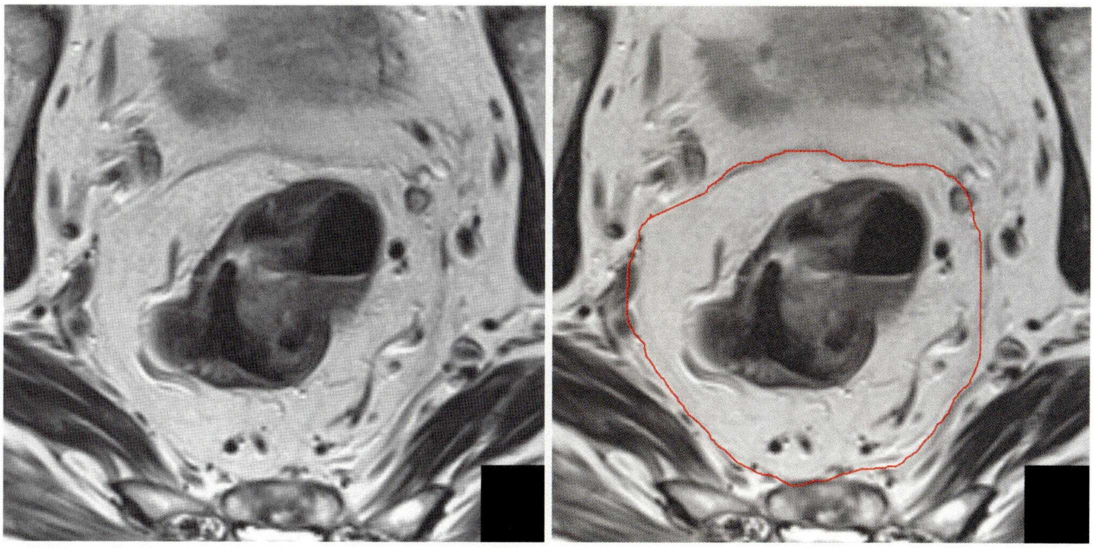

Fig. 45.1 MRI showing circumferential resection margin (see *red line*)

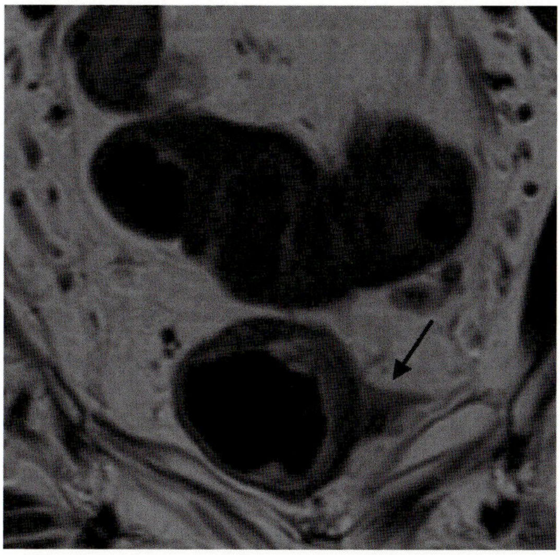

Fig. 45.2 MRI showing tumor penetrating into mesorectum (see *black arrow*)

These early studies highlight the importance of accurate measurement of tumor penetration into the mesorectum and those tumors with a worse prognosis, namely T3c and T3d. Therefore the distinction between T2 and T3 tumors with less than 5 mm mesorectal spread—T3a and T3b; becomes irrelevant as these patients will have minimal benefit from CRT [3]. The accuracy of MRI in delineating the mesorectal fascia and producing comparable results to histological analysis has been shown by the MERCURY Study Group [14, 15]. Two hundred and ninety-five patients who had undergone primary surgery had imaging and histopathological analysis of tumor depth compared. There was correlation between MR and histopathological assessment of tumor spread to within 0.5 mm.

Nodal Disease

Knowledge of tumor spread to locoregional lymph nodes forms part of the local staging of rectal cancer and is an integral component of the AJCC TNM classification [1]. Local lymph node involvement is a known independent marker of poor prognosis [16, 17]. Tumors which exhibit nodal disease independent of depth of tumor penetration (Stage III and Stage IV) are more likely to be offered preoperative radiotherapy although the rationale behind this is becoming less convincing. There is now clear randomized trial evidence that optimal surgical technique is far more important than preoperative radiotherapy in reducing the risk of local disease recurrence [3, 18].

Accurate identification of malignant lymph nodes has been traditionally challenging. As imaging modalities become more accurate in

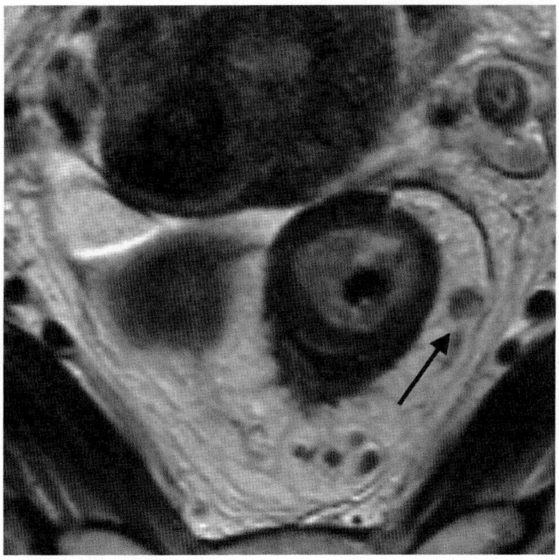

Fig. 45.3 MRI showing a heterogeneous, irregular lymph node in the mesorectum (*black arrow*)

their ability to define adverse features, detailed information on tumor characteristics are expected and influence pre-operative treatment decisions far more. The "gold-standard" for lymph node disease remains histopathological analysis of the resection specimen. However this is only influential in post-surgical setting. Lymph node architecture can be identified on MR. Figure 45.3 demonstrates the anatomical features which can be seen on high resolution images.

Traditionally, lymph nodes size has been a marker of suspicion of malignant disease. This is not the case and has led to incorrect overstaging of nodal disease based solely on size criteria. Although MRI has difficulty in picking up lymph nodes less than 3 mm, however less than 2 % of these are thought to be malignant [19]. In terms of size, and this is maximum diameter, 5 mm may exclude a significant proportion of malignant nodes [19]. In 2003, a study meticulously matching nodes from the in vivo and specimen MRIs with pathology specimens to undertake node for node analysis showed that there was no useful size cut-off for predicting nodal status [19]. This was well supported by existing histological evidence from Dworak—a histological survey of over 12,000 lymph nodes in rectal cancer showed considerable size overlap between normal or reactive nodes and those containing metastases [20].

The outline or border of the node and the signal characteristics demonstrated on MR are important determinants in whether it is benign or malignant. The outline or border of the node alone may help differentiate benign from malignant nodes. A smooth, regular outline is seen in benign nodes. A very small number of lymph nodes with smooth border contour (<6 %) have been shown to be malignant whilst those demonstrating irregular outline are malignant in over 90 % of cases [19]. This characteristic shows the highest levels of sensitivity and specificity. However, when using the signal characteristics and border outline together, the sensitivity is much improved. Signal characteristic is a better and more accurate method of detecting malignant nodes. A universal hypo- or hyper-dense signal is less likely to indicate malignant node involvement compared to a mixed signal characteristic. These nodes show remarkable correlation with histological analysis of nodes. The mixed signal on MR is shown to be areas of necrosis.

EAUS does not predict lymph node involvement any better. Sensitivity and specificity for detection of cancerous lymph nodes in rectal cancer is 73.2 and 75.8 %, respectively [21] although more likely to be accurate in the more proximal parts of the rectum. Swollen reactive nodes, small blood vessels and even local structure such as the seminal vesicles may mimic malignant nodes.

In addition to nodes within the mesorectal envelope, nodes on the lateral pelvic sidewall must be considered. There are differing approaches to how these nodes should be managed between the East and West. Japanese surgeons have traditionally offered patients a more radical operation which involves clearance of these lateral nodes. The argument against this approach is that a significant proportion of patients who will undergo an extensive surgical procedure for little benefit. These nodes are offered neo-adjuvant CRT in the West. It is difficult to visualize these nodes on EAUS in contrast with MRI which is the optimal modality for detection [22]. Studies investigating the identification of lateral wall lymph nodes are almost exclusively limited to Japan. In almost 80 % of cases, the presence of lateral nodes is associated with malignant mesorectal nodes. The incidence of malignant lateral lymph nodes ranges between 8.6 and 24 %, though these rates are mainly from advanced, and often low rectal cancers [23–25] with most studies reporting rates around 10 %. Identification of sidewall lymph nodes remains important as it is a marker for other prognostic factors such as increased mesorectal nodal burden and extramural venous invasion [22]. A mechanism of spread to the pelvic sidewall may well be through the extramural vasculature. Indeed one small randomized trial suggested that CRT and pelvic sidewall dissection resulted in equivalent oncological outcomes [26].

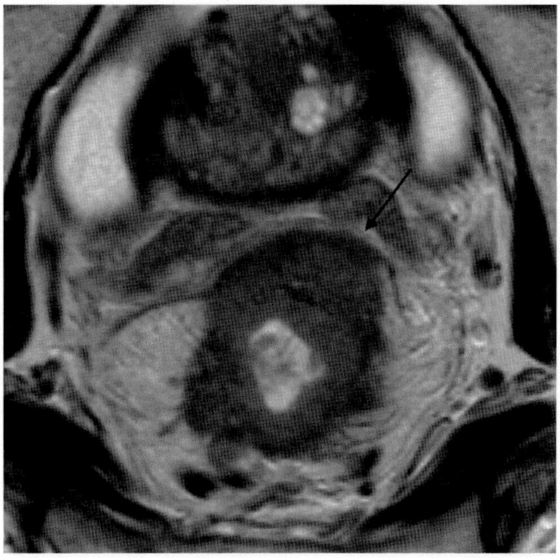

Fig. 45.4 MRI showing tumor at the circumferential resection margin (CRM) anteriorly (*black arrow*)

Circumferential Resection Margin

One of the main advantages of MRI over EAUS is that it can identify the mesorectal fascia that forms the radial margins of excision—the circumferential resection margin (CRM) [9]. Local recurrence of rectal cancer following surgical resection has been dramatically reduced by the introduction of total mesorectal excision (TME). MRI has been shown to accurately predict the relationship between tumor and mesorectal fascia with a high degree of concordance with histology. There is now overwhelming evidence that the tumor spread to involve the CRM is the single-most important determinant of pelvic recurrence and this is not compensated for by the use of radiotherapy [3, 18] (Fig. 45.4).

Tumor spread which threatens the potential CRM has been shown to be a predictive factor of local recurrence [27]. It is now generally accepted that tumor spread within 1 mm of the potential CRM is a strong influence in local recurrence. In fact, one may consider that tumor spread to the CRM is most probably the most important factor in local failure. Recent work by Taylor et al. has shown that rates of local recurrence decreased from 53 % with tumor less than 1 mm from the potential CRM to less than 8 % when the tumor distance from the mesorectal fascia was between 1 and 5 mm [28].

Being able to accurately identify tumor proximity to the mesorectal fascia within a millimeter on MRI has been a challenge. A measured distance of 5 mm on MRI has been shown to strongly correlate with negative CRM on histology, which led to patients being offered chemoradiotherapy when tumors are within 5 mm of the mesorectal fascia. However, this results in substantial overt-treatment of patients with safe margins. The MERCURY Study Group reported that margins could be identified more accurately and reproducibly, using a 1 mm cut-off [28].

Whilst tumor spread to the circumferential margin is well documented to increase the risk of local recurrence [27, 29–31], there is still some confusion regarding the presence of lymph nodes lying close the mesorectal fascia. One suggestion has been that if a lymph node containing tumor cells lies within 1 mm of the CRM thus being staged as a pathologically involved margin, the nodal capsule acts as a barrier to spread and does not lead to tumor recurrence [32]. Shihab et al. analyzed patients from the MERCURY study where there were suspicious nodes within 1 mm of the CRM on MRI. None of these patients had an involved CRM. Thus nodes that are detected by MRI to lie within close proximity of the CRM are unlikely to increase the risk of tumor recurrence [33] (Fig. 45.5).

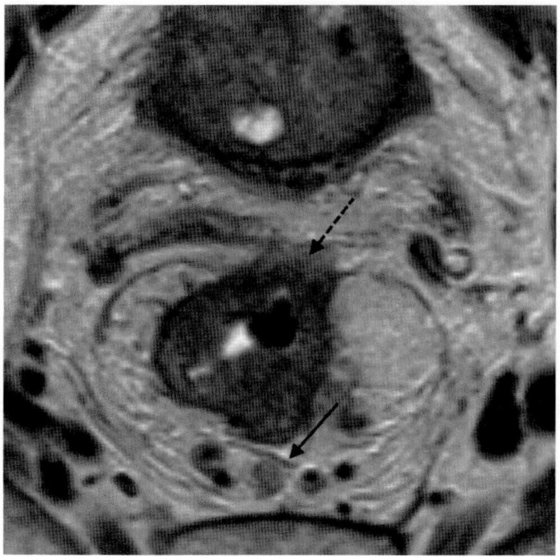

Fig. 45.5 MRI showing a lymph node at the mesorectal fascia. The *solid black arrow* shows the lymph node at the CRM posteriorly and the *dashed black arrow* shows the tumor at the CRM anteriorly

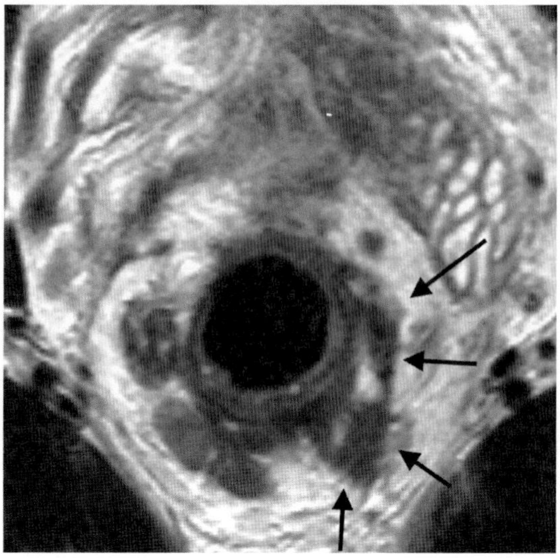

Fig. 45.6 MRI showing characteristics of EMVI, the *black arrows* shows the EMVI as a serpiginous expanded tumor deposit along the path of a vein

Extramural Vascular Invasion

Extramural venous invasion is defined as the presence of tumor cells in the vasculature beyond the muscularis propria. It is known to be associated with poor prognosis and increased rates of local recurrence and distant metastases [34]. It is seen in up to 50 % of rectal cancer patients and almost exclusively associated with more advanced tumors—T3 and T4. EMVI can be identified pre-operatively on MRI with great accuracy [35]. A recent randomized trial comparing neoadjuvant radiotherapy 45Gy plus capecitabine to radiotherapy 50 Gy plus capecitabine and oxaliplatin in patients with resectable T3–4 rectal cancer reported vascular invasion as an independent predictive factor of positive CRM [36] (Fig. 45.6).

Using high spatial resolution MRI, veins are identified as serpiginous or tortuous linear structures on T2-weighted images. Assessment of EMVI using MRI must consider the following components: pattern of tumor margin which gives the appearance of nodularity; location of tumor to relevant vessels which makes tumor invasion more likely; caliber of vessel as tumor infiltration can cause an increase in luminal size; and vessel border if the tumor disrupts the vessel itself. Extension of the primary tumor into a vascular structure indicates EMVI [37].

EUAS is not able to identify this novel prognostic feature. Although the layers of the bowel wall and thus extramural depth may be identified, the spindle-like nature of the vessels and the subtle change in signal is not readily detected. This morphological feature plays more of a role in decision making in the UK and parts of Europe however future reports may lead to increased recognition of EMVI as an important prognostic indicator.

Low Rectal Cancer

Tumors that are defined as "low rectal cancers" have an inherent challenge. This is most likely due to the anatomy of these tumors located in the rigid confines of the pelvis. Traditionally, these tumors were most commonly surgically treated by abdominoperineal resection (APR) compared to anterior resection. There is evidence to show that local recurrence rates for low tumors treated with APR is much higher than low anterior resection [38–41]. The Low Rectal Cancer Study was

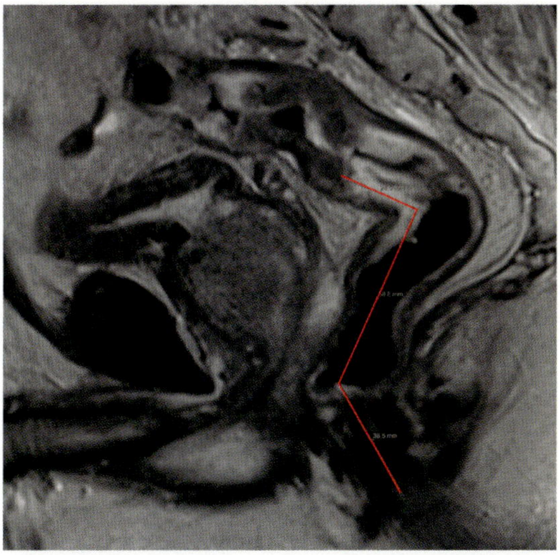

Fig. 45.7 Sagittal section MRI showing tumor height in relation to anal verge

borne out of the need to adequately stage low rectal cancers with MRI to define the surgical planes with accuracy with the aim to reduce the rate of positive circumferential resection margins in APR. Using high resolution MRI, a route map for low tumors is based in anatomical landmarks dividing the rectum into supralevator, intralevator, and infralevator sections. This allows surgeons to make operative decisions accurately based on MRI-predicted planes of excision [42]. A small retrospective study of 33 patients in which MRI was used to predict the plane of excision in order to achieve a negative resection margin reported a positive predictive value of 57 % and negative predictive value of 96 % [43]. Although these results are encouraging there must be appropriate training and education to standardize reporting of these tumors (Fig. 45.7).

45.3 PET/CT

Positron emission tomography (PET) has gained increasing popularity in the last few years. Although it has had limited uses for more than a decade, the combination of PET with CT has shown to be a particularly useful tool. The principle behind PET is the use of radioisotopes with a half-life of around 100 min that through tracers quantify pathological biochemical processes. These biochemical processes are thought to precede physical changes in the anatomy which makes this an exciting field. The most common tracer is fluorine-18-labeled deoxyglucose (FDG). This radioisotope acts as an analog to glucose and identifies cells which have an increased glucose metabolism such as cancer cells (Fig. 45.8).

The role of PET/CT as a combination in staging of rectal cancer is not by any means routine at present. However, it has been shown to have improved accuracy over CT and PET as individual examinations [44]. There remain several questions about the use of PET/CT and where it fits into the repertoire of imaging modalities in the staging of rectal cancer. In the context of preoperative staging, there is little evidence to support its routine use [45]. No direct comparisons have been made in terms of accuracy of preoperative local staging with MRI in large numbers and it is difficult to evaluate the sensitivity and specificity of this technique. However a recent study has shown that MRI and PET/CT may be used in combination for high risk patients (EMVI positive; extramural spread of >5 mm; T4 disease or an involved CRM) as part of a more intensive staging process [46]. In this study, patients were stratified by MRI into whether they were at high or low risk of developing synchronous metastatic disease. Almost 21 % of patients in the high risk group were confirmed to have metastatic disease on PET/CT compared to 4 % in the low risk group. These patients may benefit from a further PET/CT (or liver MRI) in the initial staging process.

Recent interest has been using PET/CT to assess response to neo-adjuvant chemoradiotherapy [47, 48]. Several small studies have been published within the last few years and have indicated positive results in terms of a predictive tool for tumor regression although one of the largest studies of this type has found no benefit in serial scans to assess response and prognosis [49–52]. The general methodology of these studies has been to perform PET/CT before and varying times after neo-adjuvant CRT and measured the

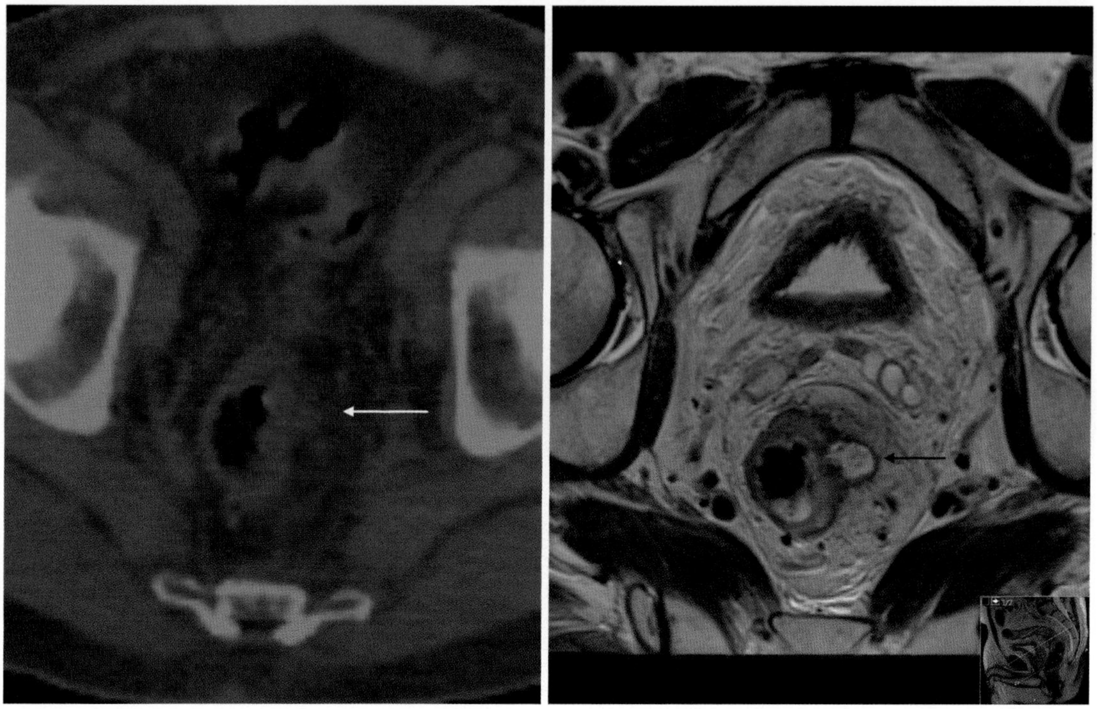

Fig. 45.8 PET/CT of rectum. PET/CT and T2 weighted axial MRI of the rectum in the same patient with recurrent rectal cancer. The *white arrow* shows ill defined uptake in the region of recurrent disease seen clearly on the MRI (*black arrow*)

response in terms of FDG uptake. Further work is necessary before this can be confidently used as a routine modality to assess tumor response. It may be too early to draw comparisons with an established technique like MRI, however the rationale behind using PET/CT as an imaging modality which can not only demonstrate anatomical change but also functional change, is certainly complimentary at a minimum.

45.4 Staging Metastatic Disease

Adequate local staging of disease is mandatory for surgical planning and treatment of the primary tumor. However, it is equally important to assess potential metastatic spread. This may influence the management of the primary tumor in terms of type and timing of treatment. The common sites of metastases of rectal cancer are the liver and lung. This may be related to the site of tumor within the rectum which has a variable lymphatic drainage as well as the influence of venous invasion on tumor behavior. For example, low rectal cancer is more likely to drain to the lateral pelvic sidewall than a tumor of the upper rectum. This lymphatic pathway differs from that of the more common route along the inferior mesenteric vessels. One may expect a different pattern of metastatic spread depending on the location of the tumor within the rectum.

Currently, the optimal imaging modality for assessing metastatic spread is CT of the chest, abdomen and pelvis. This technique is highly accurate to identify lesions to the common sites of metastases and is widely available in most hospitals. Combination of CT with functional imaging techniques such as PET may be more useful if there are ambiguous areas on CT. Alternatively, MRI may be used to image the liver in more detail if there is not adequate evidence of tumor spread on CT (Fig. 45.9).

Liver metastases are commonly identified on CT imaging. However in some cases there may

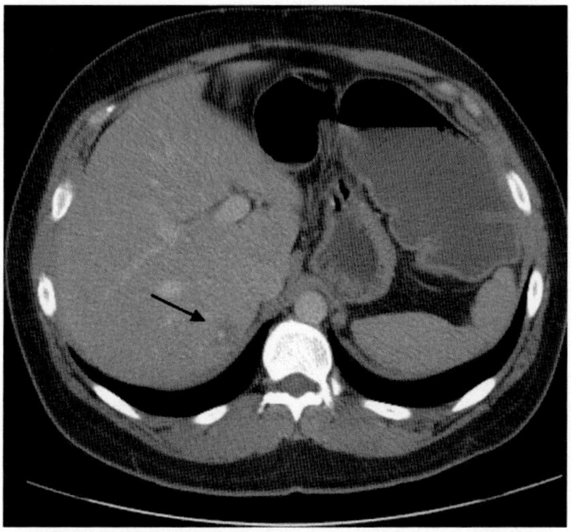

Fig. 45.9 Staging CT of abdomen showing liver lesion (*black arrow*)

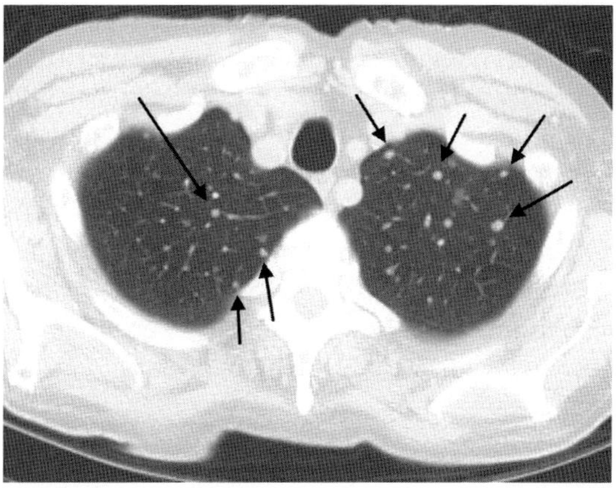

Fig. 45.10 CT showing multiple lung lesions (*black arrows*)

be confusion as to whether a lesion is benign or malignant. Imaging of the liver must be able to accurately characterize the lesion with respect to segmental anatomy and relationship to local vasculature. It must be able to confirm evidence and extent of micro-metastatic disease and discriminate between benign and malignant lesions. CT exploits the relative hypovascularity of hepatic metastases compared with normal liver parenchyma and has accuracy rates of up to 85 % [53]. The use of multi-detector CT can be highly accurate in demonstrating liver lesions. Hypodense lesions with complimentary rim enhancement are indicative of metastatic deposits. Hemangiomas enhance peripherally in a nodular fashion and persistence of enhancement [54]. MRI assessment includes T1 and T2-weighted images with an appropriate contrast agent. Differentiating benign liver lesions from malignant ones is an important ability of MRI. Specific contrast agents are taken up by functioning Kupffer cells and produce characteristic effects on MRI. It is important to be able to distinguish metastases from hemangiomas, fatty infiltration and cysts.

Lung metastases are more common in rectal cancer than colon cancer [55]. CT is routinely performed in the staging of rectal cancer in UK and many places in the USA. However, CT chest may lead to false positive findings [56]. The main advantage of CT over conventional chest radiographs is the detection of smaller lesions [57]. The accuracy in identifying tumor volume is also of benefit when assessing growth rates. PET may be used in conjunction with CT to further evaluate lesions which are not accurately discriminated by CT alone. Relating pulmonary metastases to lung anatomy has a bearing on surgical management. Patients who demonstrate single metastases in one lobe only are much less likely to have unrecognized irresectable disease when compared with those patients with multilobar metastases (Fig. 45.10).

45.5 Summary

Imaging modalities have taken on an increasingly important role in the management of rectal cancer and pelvic malignancy. The ability to identify prognostic features with tremendous accuracy means that imaging influences pre-operative decision making and aids in risk stratification of patients. There is still no universal consensus in the most appropriate imaging technique for local staging and choice is somewhat dictated by the policy on neo-adjuvant therapy.

MRI is the optimal imaging modality in identifying the key prognostic factors such as involvement of circumferential resection margin; extramural venous invasion; nodal disease and tumor depth. By using the most accurate imaging modalities, patients can be offered adjuvant treatment more selectively and not be burdened with the additional morbidity associated with radiotherapy. It is also most useful in assessing treatment response. Distant disease is best staged with CT but when there is diagnostic doubt, additional use of MRI or PET/CT may help.

Key Points

- Imaging is increasingly becoming the central part of pre-operative staging of rectal cancer and pelvic malignancy.
- The common imaging modalities in staging rectal cancer are magnetic resonance imaging (MRI), computed tomography (CT), endoanal ultrasound (EAUS).
- Prognostic factors identified on imaging modalities influence and determine pre-operative oncological therapy.
- The key prognostic factors which determine risk of disease recurrence are tumor spread and depth, nodal disease, vascular invasion, circumferential resection margin involvement, tumor height from the anal verge.
- MRI is the optimal modality in identifying high risk factor for local disease recurrence.
- Circumferential resection margin involvement and tumor spread into the mesorectum are important factors for local disease recurrence.
- CT is the optimal modality in identifying metastatic disease spread.
- Where CT is unable to confidently identify distant metastatic spread, MRI and PET/CT used in combination or alone may be able to clarify.
- PET/CT can be used to assess disease recurrence and response to treatment.
- It is important to choose the most appropriate imaging modality for patients in their circumstance so not to over- or under-stage disease and put patients through unnecessary treatments.

References

1. Edge SB, Compton CC. The American Joint Committee on Cancer: the 7th edition of the AJCC cancer staging manual and the future of TNM. Ann Surg Oncol. 2010;17(6):1471–4.
2. Stamos MJ, Murrell Z. Management of early rectal T1 and T2 cancers. Clin Cancer Res. 2007;13(22 Pt 2): 6885s–9.
3. Taylor FG, Quirke P, Heald RJ, Moran B, Blomqvist L, Swift I, et al. Preoperative high-resolution magnetic resonance imaging can identify good prognosis stage I, II, and III rectal cancer best managed by surgery alone: a prospective, multicenter, European study. Ann Surg. 2011;253(4):711–9.
4. Blackstock W, Russo SM, Suh WW, Cosman BC, Herman J, Mohiuddin M, et al. ACR appropriateness criteria: local excision in early-stage rectal cancer. Curr Probl Cancer. 2010;34(3):193–200.
5. Bretagnol F, Merrie A, George B, Warren BF, Mortensen NJ. Local excision of rectal tumours by transanal endoscopic microsurgery. Br J Surg. 2007; 94(5):627–33.
6. Brown G. Staging rectal cancer: endoscopic ultrasound and pelvic MRI. Cancer Imaging. 2008;8(Spec No A):S43–5.
7. Heald RJ. The 'Holy Plane' of rectal surgery. J R Soc Med. 1988;81(9):503–8.
8. Heald RJ, Husband EM, Ryall RD. The mesorectum in rectal cancer surgery – the clue to pelvic recurrence? Br J Surg. 1982;69(10):613–6.
9. Brown G, Kirkham A, Williams GT, Bourne M, Radcliffe AG, Sayman J, et al. High-resolution MRI of the anatomy important in total mesorectal excision of the rectum. AJR Am J Roentgenol. 2004;182(2):431–9.
10. Taylor FG, Swift RI, Blomqvist L, Brown G. A systematic approach to the interpretation of preoperative staging MRI for rectal cancer. AJR Am J Roentgenol. 2008;191(6):1827–35.
11. Jass JR, Love SB, Northover JM. A new prognostic classification of rectal cancer. Lancet. 1987;1(8545): 1303–6.
12. Cawthorn SJ, Parums DV, Gibbs NM, A'Hern RP, Caffarey SM, Broughton CI, et al. Extent of mesorectal spread and involvement of lateral resection margin as prognostic factors after surgery for rectal cancer. Lancet. 1990;335(8697):1055–9.
13. Merkel S, Mansmann U, Siassi M, Papadopoulos T, Hohenberger W, Hermanek P. The prognostic inhomogeneity in pT3 rectal carcinomas. Int J Colorectal Dis. 2001;16(5):298–304.

14. Shihab OC, Taylor F, Salerno G, Heald RJ, Quirke P, Moran BJ, et al. MRI predictive factors for long-term outcomes of low rectal tumours. Ann Surg Oncol. 2011;18(12):3278–84.
15. Brown G. Extramural depth of tumor invasion at thin-section MR in patients with rectal cancer: results of the MERCURY study. Radiology. 2007;243(1): 132–9.
16. Wolmark N, Fisher B, Wieand HS. The prognostic value of the modifications of the Dukes' C class of colorectal cancer. An analysis of the NSABP clinical trials. Ann Surg. 1986;203(2):115–22.
17. Tang R, Wang JY, Chen JS, Chang-Chien CR, Tang S, Lin SE, et al. Survival impact of lymph node metastasis in TNM stage III carcinoma of the colon and rectum. J Am Coll Surg. 1995;180(6):705–12.
18. Quirke P, Steele R, Monson J, Grieve R, Khanna S, Couture J, et al. Effect of the plane of surgery achieved on local recurrence in patients with operable rectal cancer: a prospective study using data from the MRC CR07 and NCIC-CTG CO16 randomised clinical trial. Lancet. 2009;373(9666):821–8.
19. Brown G, Richards CJ, Bourne MW, Newcombe RG, Radcliffe AG, Dallimore NS, et al. Morphologic predictors of lymph node status in rectal cancer with use of high-spatial-resolution MR imaging with histopathologic comparison. Radiology. 2003;227(2): 371–7.
20. Dworak O. Morphology of lymph nodes in the resected rectum of patients with rectal carcinoma. Pathol Res Pract. 1991;187(8):1020–4.
21. Puli SR, Reddy JB, Bechtold ML, Choudhary A, Antillon MR, Brugge WR. Accuracy of endoscopic ultrasound to diagnose nodal invasion by rectal cancers: a meta-analysis and systematic review. Ann Surg Oncol. 2009;16(5):1255–65.
22. Shihab OC, Taylor F, Bees N, Blake H, Jeyadevan N, Bleehen R, et al. Relevance of magnetic resonance imaging-detected pelvic sidewall lymph node involvement in rectal cancer. Br J Surg. 2011;98(12):1798–804.
23. Takahashi T, Ueno M, Azekura K, Ohta H. Lateral node dissection and total mesorectal excision for rectal cancer. Dis Colon Rectum. 2000;43(10 Suppl):S59–68.
24. Ueno H, Yamauchi C, Hase K, Ichikura T, Mochizuki H. Clinicopathological study of intrapelvic cancer spread to the iliac area in lower rectal adenocarcinoma by serial sectioning. Br J Surg. 1999;86(12):1532–7.
25. Sugihara K, Kobayashi H, Kato T, Mori T, Mochizuki H, Kameoka S, et al. Indication and benefit of pelvic sidewall dissection for rectal cancer. Dis Colon Rectum. 2006;49(11):1663–72.
26. Nagawa H, Muto T, Sunouchi K, Higuchi Y, Tsurita G, Watanabe T, et al. Randomized, controlled trial of lateral node dissection vs. nerve-preserving resection in patients with rectal cancer after preoperative radiotherapy. Dis Colon Rectum. 2001;44(9):1274–80.
27. Adam IJ, Mohamdee MO, Martin IG, Scott N, Finan PJ, Johnston D, et al. Role of circumferential margin involvement in the local recurrence of rectal cancer. Lancet. 1994;344(8924):707–11.
28. Taylor FG, Quirke P, Heald RJ, Moran B, Blomqvist L, Swift I, et al. One millimetre is the safe cut-off for magnetic resonance imaging prediction of surgical margin status in rectal cancer. Br J Surg. 2011;98(6): 872–9.
29. Quirke P, Durdey P, Dixon MF, Williams NS. Local recurrence of rectal adenocarcinoma due to inadequate surgical resection. Histopathological study of lateral tumour spread and surgical excision. Lancet. 1986;2(8514):996–9.
30. Hall NR, Finan PJ, Al-Jaberi T, Tsang CS, Brown SR, Dixon MF, et al. Circumferential margin involvement after mesorectal excision of rectal cancer with curative intent. Predictor of survival but not local recurrence? Dis Colon Rectum. 1998;41(8):979–83.
31. Nagtegaal ID, Quirke P. What is the role for the circumferential margin in the modern treatment of rectal cancer? J Clin Oncol. 2008;26(2):303–12.
32. Cecil TD, Sexton R, Moran BJ, Heald RJ. Total mesorectal excision results in low local recurrence rates in lymph node-positive rectal cancer. Dis Colon Rectum. 2004;47(7):1145–9; discussion 1149–50.
33. Shihab OC, Quirke P, Heald RJ, Moran BJ, Brown G. Magnetic resonance imaging-detected lymph nodes close to the mesorectal fascia are rarely a cause of margin involvement after total mesorectal excision. Br J Surg. 2010;97(9):1431–6.
34. Talbot IC, Ritchie S, Leighton MH, Hughes AO, Bussey HJ, Morson BC. The clinical significance of invasion of veins by rectal cancer. Br J Surg. 1980; 67(6):439–42.
35. Smith NJ, Barbachano Y, Norman AR, Swift RI, Abulafi AM, Brown G. Prognostic significance of magnetic resonance imaging-detected extramural vascular invasion in rectal cancer. Br J Surg. 2008;95(2): 229–36.
36. Rullier A, Gourgou-Bourgade S, Jarlier M, Bibeau F, Chassagne-Clement C, Hennequin C, et al. Predictive factors of positive circumferential resection margin after radiochemotherapy for rectal cancer: the French randomised trial ACCORD12/0405 PRODIGE 2. Eur J Cancer. 2013;49(1):82–9.
37. Smith NJ, Shihab O, Arnaout A, Swift RI, Brown G. MRI for detection of extramural vascular invasion in rectal cancer. AJR Am J Roentgenol. 2008;191(5): 1517–22.
38. MERCURY Study Group. Diagnostic accuracy of preoperative magnetic resonance imaging in predicting curative resection of rectal cancer: prospective observational study. BMJ. 2006;333(7572):779.
39. Marr R, Birbeck K, Garvican J, Macklin CP, Tiffin NJ, Parsons WJ, et al. The modern abdominoperineal excision: the next challenge after total mesorectal excision. Ann Surg. 2005;242(1):74–82.
40. Guillou PJ, Quirke P, Thorpe H, Walker J, Jayne DG, Smith AM, et al. Short-term endpoints of conventional versus laparoscopic-assisted surgery in patients with colorectal cancer (MRC CLASICC trial): multicentre, randomised controlled trial. Lancet. 2005; 365(9472):1718–26.

41. Nagtegaal ID, van de Velde CJ, Marijnen CA, van Krieken JH, Quirke P. Low rectal cancer: a call for a change of approach in abdominoperineal resection. J Clin Oncol. 2005;23(36):9257–64.
42. Shihab OC, Heald RJ, Rullier E, Brown G, Holm T, Quirke P, et al. Defining the surgical planes on MRI improves surgery for cancer of the low rectum. Lancet Oncol. 2009;10(12):1207–11.
43. Shihab OC, How P, West N, George C, Patel U, Quirke P, et al. Can a novel MRI staging system for low rectal cancer aid surgical planning? Dis Colon Rectum. 2011;54(10):1260–4.
44. Cohade C, Osman M, Leal J, Wahl RL. Direct comparison of (18)F-FDG PET and PET/CT in patients with colorectal carcinoma. J Nucl Med. 2003;44(11): 1797–803.
45. Brush J, Boyd K, Chappell F, Crawford F, Dozier M, Fenwick E, et al. The value of FDG positron emission tomography/computerised tomography (PET/CT) in pre-operative staging of colorectal cancer: a systematic review and economic evaluation. Health Technol Assess. 2011;15(35):1–192, iii–iv.
46. Hunter CJ, Garant A, Vuong T, Artho G, Lisbona R, Tekkis P, et al. Adverse features on rectal MRI identify a high-risk group that may benefit from more intensive preoperative staging and treatment. Ann Surg Oncol. 2012;19(4):1199–205.
47. Avallone A, Aloj L, Caraco C, Delrio P, Pecori B, Tatangelo F, et al. Early FDG PET response assessment of preoperative radiochemotherapy in locally advanced rectal cancer: correlation with long-term outcome. Eur J Nucl Med Mol Imaging. 2012;39(12):1848–57.
48. Murcia Durendez MJ, Frutos Esteban L, Lujan J, Frutos MD, Valero G, Navarro Fernandez JL, et al. The value of (18)F-FDG PET/CT for assessing the response to neoadjuvant therapy in locally advanced rectal cancer. Eur J Nucl Med Mol Imaging. 2013;40(1):91–7.
49. Calvo FA, Domper M, Matute R, Martinez-Lazaro R, Arranz JA, Desco M, et al. 18F-FDG positron emission tomography staging and restaging in rectal cancer treated with preoperative chemoradiation. Int J Radiat Oncol Biol Phys. 2004;58(2):528–35.
50. Kalff V, Duong C, Drummond EG, Matthews JP, Hicks RJ. Findings on 18F-FDG PET scans after neoadjuvant chemoradiation provides prognostic stratification in patients with locally advanced rectal carcinoma subsequently treated by radical surgery. J Nucl Med. 2006;47(1):14–22.
51. Martoni AA, Di Fabio F, Pinto C, Castellucci P, Pini S, Ceccarelli C, et al. Prospective study on the FDG-PET/CT predictive and prognostic values in patients treated with neoadjuvant chemoradiation therapy and radical surgery for locally advanced rectal cancer. Ann Oncol. 2011;22(3):650–6.
52. Ruby JA, Leibold T, Akhurst TJ, Shia J, Saltz LB, Mazumdar M, et al. FDG-PET assessment of rectal cancer response to neoadjuvant chemoradiotherapy is not associated with long-term prognosis: a prospective evaluation. Dis Colon Rectum. 2012;55(4): 378–86.
53. Valls C, Andia E, Sanchez A, Guma A, Figueras J, Torras J, et al. Hepatic metastases from colorectal cancer: preoperative detection and assessment of resectability with helical CT. Radiology. 2001;218(1): 55–60.
54. Nino-Murcia M, Olcott EW, Jeffrey Jr RB, Lamm RL, Beaulieu CF, Jain KA. Focal liver lesions: pattern-based classification scheme for enhancement at arterial phase CT. Radiology. 2000;215(3):746–51.
55. Mitry E, Guiu B, Cosconea S, Jooste V, Faivre J, Bouvier AM. Epidemiology, management and prognosis of colorectal cancer with lung metastases: a 30-year population-based study. Gut. 2010;59(10): 1383–8.
56. Grossmann I, Avenarius JK, Mastboom WJ, Klaase JM. Preoperative staging with chest CT in patients with colorectal carcinoma: not as a routine procedure. Ann Surg Oncol. 2010;17(8):2045–50.
57. Davis SD. CT evaluation for pulmonary metastases in patients with extrathoracic malignancy. Radiology. 1991;180(1):1–12.

Radiation Therapy in the Treatment of Rectal Cancer

46

Té Vuong and Tamim Mohammad Niazi

46.1 Introduction

Radiation therapy is a local treatment that was introduced as a mean to improve regional control in conjunction with surgery for patients with locally advanced rectal cancer (RC). Over the last two decades, this treatment modality has evolved significantly, not only through its application in serial randomized clinical trials, but also through the advances in technology along with the introduction of computerized imaging techniques that have allowed accurate evaluation of clinical target volumes. Modern imaging, such as computerized scans (CT) and magnetic resonance imaging (MRI) is now an essential component in determining treatment strategies. Finally, the transition to Total Mesorectal Excision Surgery (TMES) and changes in the pattern of local relapse justify a re-examination of the contemporary radiation practice.

46.2 Rationale for Radiation Therapy

In recent years, the treatment of patients with rectal cancer has seen significant improvements in local control (LC) with the introduction of TME along with new pre-operative therapeutic modalities. Locally advanced RC patients include stage II and III cancers with a range of T2–T4 tumors. These patients are currently treated with similar strategies as per NCCN recommendations (http://www.nccn.org/clinical.asp). In the era of modern tumor imaging, pelvic MRI in particular allows for the precise estimation of the circumferential radial margin (CRM) [1, 2], which represents the most important factor for predicting local recurrence (LR) and systemic disease. The Mercury trial [1] reported that for patients with positive CRM on pre-operative MRI imaging, the risks of LR and systemic spread were significantly higher than for those with negative CRM.

46.3 Radiotherapy Trials

Surgery remains the cornerstone of rectal cancer treatment for locally advanced (T3–4 tumors). To further improve LC in rectal cancer, neoadjuvant (NA) radiotherapy (RT) has been added to surgery. The benefit of NA Short course (SC) RT had first been shown by the Swedish Rectal Cancer Group [3] in the pre TME era. After a median follow-up of 5 years, the LR risk was 11 % in the irradiated group and 27 % in the non-irradiated group and the overall survival (OS) rates were 58 and 48 %, respectively. In spite of these excellent LC results, the role of RT was questioned after the introduction of TME S. In the Dutch TME study [4], the benefit of SCRT

T. Vuong, MD (✉) • T.M. Niazi, MD
Department of Radiation Oncology, Jewish General Hospital, Montreal, QC, Canada
e-mail: tvuong@jgh.mcgill.ca

H.R.H. Patel et al. (eds.), *Pelvic Cancer Surgery: Modern Breakthroughs and Future Advances*,
DOI 10.1007/978-1-4471-4258-4_46, © Springer-Verlag London 2015

followed by immediate TME S was demonstrated, with a 10 year LR rate of 11 % for patients treated with TME S alone vs. 5 % for patients treated with SCRT followed by TME S [5]. In the MRC-CR07 study [6], which has a comparable design, patients with resectable rectal cancer were randomized between NA SCRT followed by immediate S vs. S alone. The S alone patients received postoperative chemotherapy (CT)-long course (LC) RT when the CRM was involved. The LR rate was 5 % in the NA SCRT patients and 12 % in patients undergoing S alone ($p<0.001$), demonstrating that selective postoperative CT-LCRT is not able to provide the same results as preoperative treatment. It has been established that NA RT (either SCRT alone or CT-LCRT) provides significantly better LC than postoperative CT-LCRT, while LR rates are significantly improved in patients receiving NA SCRT. In this study, the benefits of NA SCRT were observed at all tumor levels including the upper third tumor and significant even for patients with specimen obtained within the mesorectal plane. So far no survival benefit has been demonstrated for irradiated patients operated with the TME technique (Table 46.1). In the Dutch TME trial [5], NA SCRT had no effect on OS or cancer-specific survival when all randomized patients were included in the analyses. However, in operated patients with a negative CRM, RT significantly improved cancer-specific survival. Unfortunately, this benefit was offset by an increase in other causes of death, resulting in an equal OS rate compared with S alone group. A subgroup analysis demonstrated that for patients with TNM stage III cancer with a negative CRM, 10-year survival was 50 % in the NA SCRT group vs. 40 % in the S alone group ($p=0.032$). In most studies, the LR rate was reduced from over 10 % for patients treated with S only to 5 % for patients treated with NA RT and S (Table 46.1).

46.4 Role of CRM

In the Dutch TME trial [4] non-irradiated patients with a positive CRM had a LR risk of 23.3 %, whereas those who received radiation showed a drop in LR risk to 15.5 % ($p=0.16$). The MRC-CR07 trial [6] showed a LR rate of 13.8 % in patients receiving NA SCRT with 5×5 Gy and a LR rate of 20.7 % in patients receiving postoperative CT-LCRT.

46.5 Multimodality Treatment Approaches

Several Northern European randomized clinical trials (RCT) studies have demonstrated a significant reduction in the LR rate after SCRT (Table 46.1). There exists a controversy concerning optimal treatment for the different stages of rectal cancer and prioritization of treatment modalities. In Northern Europe, SCRT is the standard of care for most stage II and III rectal cancer patients. CT-LCRT is reserved for more advanced cases with positive CRM. On the other hand, in America and southern Europe, patients are treated with NA LCRT (LCRT, 45–50 Gy) in combination with chemotherapy (CT). Furthermore, as both the EORTC 22921 [7] and FFCD 9203 [8] studies demonstrated that the addition of CT to preoperative LCRT is beneficial to LC in locally advanced tumors (T3–4), patients are now treated with CT-LCRT, followed by TME S.

46.6 Randomized Trials Comparing NA SCRT with CT-LCRT

Two published RCT were conducted comparing SCRT to CT-LCRT: The Polish trial with 312 patients [9] and the Australian trial [10] with 326 patients. Both studies had a similar design and sample size was calculated to demonstrate a difference of 15 % in the rate of sphincter preservation (SPS) and 10 % in LR, respectively. Both trials showed higher rates of early radiation toxicity in the CT-LCRT arm when compared with the SCRT group; grade III to IV acute toxicity rates were 18 % versus 3 % ($P=0.001$) in the Polish trial and 28 % versus 1.9 % ($P=0.001$) in the Australian study. In the Polish trial, the SPS

Table 46.1 Five year local control and overall survival rates results from selected randomized clinical trials

RCT	T/stage (S) status	Number of patients	Median age (years)	Local recurrence rate at 5 years %	OS at 5 years %
German trial: pre op [29]	T1–T4	405	62	6	76
German trial: post op [29]	T1–T4	402	62	13	74
Dutch trial TME S alone [4]	S1–4	908	66	10.9	63.5
Dutch trial NA SCRT + TME [4]	S1–4	897	65	5.6	64.2
MRC CR07 NA SCRT [6]	S1–4	674	65	4.7	70.3
MRC CR07 post OP CT-LCRT [6]	S1–4	676	65	11.5	67.9
Polish trial SCRT [9]	T3–4	155	60	9	67.2 (4 years)
Polish trial CT-LCRT [9]	T3–4	157	59	14.2	66.2 (4 years)
Trans tasman SCRT [10]	T3	163	63	7.5 (3 years)	74
Trans tasman CT-LCRT [10]	T3	163	64	4.4 (3 years)	70
FFCD 9203 NA LCRT [8]	T3–4	367	63	16.5	67.9
FFCD 9203 NA CT-LCRT [8]	T3–4	375	64	8.1	67.4

rate did not differ between the groups: 61 % in the SCRT group and 58 % in the CT-LCRT (P=0.57). In this trial, the LR rate was slightly lower in the SCRT group than in the CT-LCRT group (10.6 % vs. 15.6 % (P=102 .21), whereas the opposite tendency was seen in the Australian study at 7.5 % versus 4.4 % (P=0.24). In this latter trial, a difference was observed in the group of tumors below 5 cm, with 6 out of 48 patients in the CT-LCRT arms. One out of thirty-one patients after SCRT although not statistically significant. Additionally, no increase in late toxicity rates was seen in the SCRT irradiation group compared with the CT-LCRT group. In the Polish study, severe late toxicity was observed in 10.1 % of patients after SCRT and in 7.1 % of patients after CT-LCRT compared to 5.8 % of patients after SCRT vs. 8.2 % of patients after CT-LCRT (p=0.53) in the Australian trial.

There are four out of five contemporary RCT studies testing the oxaliplatin based chemotherapy regimen published: STAR-0145 [11], ACCORD 12/0405-Prodige 246 [12], NSABP R-0447 [13] and the German trial CAO/ARO/AIO-0448 [14], which compared standard NA 5-Fluorouracil (5-FU) based CT and LCRT (CT-RT) to oxaliplatin and 5-FU CT and NA LCRT. Patients with T3 or T4 rectal cancer were recruited sequentially. All but the CAO/ARO/AIO-0448 [14] reported higher morbidity without any improvement in early endpoints such as pathological complete response (pCR) rate.

46.7 Radiation Treatment Volumes

TMES now provides optimal tumor bed resection together with the perirectal nodes within the mesorectal fascia but it is not addressing the pelvic nodes. The Dutch CKVO 95–04 study [4, 5] is unique, having an arm with more than 908 patients treated with TME alone. In this trial, 36 % of patients had positive nodes and the LR rate was 10.9 % after a median follow up of 6 years. Most of the recurrences were located below the S2–3 interspace [15] in patients with negative nodes and negative CRM therefore, consistent with the Swedish experience reporting on the level of S1–S2 interspace [16]. The addition of radiation therapy reduced mostly the perineal, anastomotic leakage as well as the lateral recurrence.

In North America, the definition of clinical target volume for the treatment of rectal cancer has been based on consensus by a panel of experts [17] to include coverage of the tumor bed, entire mesorectum and perirectal, presacraland internal iliac nodes which is supported by the patterns of local recurrence literature. It is imperative to note that the majority of these data were derived before the implementation of quality imaging such as pelvic MRI and the introduction of TMES.

46.8 Radiation Related Toxicities

If the value of radiation therapy is now well-established, cumulative data on long-term toxicities associated with external beam (EBRT) raise concerns. In a meta-analysis, Camma et al. [18] reported an increased risk of septic complications in irradiated patients compared to non-irradiated patients: 21 % vs. 15.2 % ($p \leq 0.001$). Moreover, there was an increased risk of overall complications in the irradiated group: 21 % vs. 5.2 % ($p < 0.003$). Postoperative adverse events were also higher in the radiation treatment group: 57.4 % vs. 42.3 % ($p < 0.02$). Finally, irradiated patients had a 15 % higher risk of death from vascular or infectious causes compared to non-irradiated patients ($p = 0.02$). The Cochrane Database Systematic Review in 2007 by Wong et al. [19], assessing the effect of preoperative RT vs. surgery alone for rectal cancer patients confirmed the benefits of preoperative RT in reducing LR (HR 0.71, 95 % CI 0.64–0.78) with borderline significance with respect to cancer specific and overall survival (OS) (HR 0.93, 95 % CI 0.87–1.0). Late toxicities including pelvic fractures, venothrombosis events, intestinal obstruction, postoperative fistula, cardiovascular death, bowel obstruction, anal sphincter and sexual dysfunction were all increased.

Thus, if neoadjuvant EBRT has been effective in decreasing local recurrence, the number of patients requiring treatment will need to be weighed against the substantial morbidity risks and long-term side effects related to EBRT. Reducing treatment volumes to the level of S1/S2 might be the most effective and simple means to improve therapeutic index.

46.9 Intra Operative Radiation Therapy

The majority of patients with rectal cancer are doing well with current management but there are less favorable cases with positive CRM or recurrent tumors after previous pelvis radiation therapy that remains a clinical management challenge. There are other radiation modalities, apart from EBRT, that could be considered.

The likelihood of achieving tumor down staging and/or R0 improves as a function of dose. Wiltshire et al. [20], who investigated the value of dose escalation with 5-FU CT in a phase II trial for patients with operable rectal cancer. The three dose levels were 40 Gy in 20 fractions, 46 Gy in 23 fractions and 50 Gy in 25 fractions and included 46, 52 and 36 patients, respectively. The pCR rates were 15 %, 23 % and 33 % ($p = 0.07$) respectively and the 2-year relapse free survival was 72, 90 and 89 % respectively ($p = 0.02$). In Lyon RCT study R96–0256 [21] NA RT alone using 39 Gy in 13 fractions was compared to the same RT with boost (85 Gy in 3 fractions) using contact X-ray for 88 patients with low rectal cancer. A significant improvement in pCR rate was seen in the contact X-ray boost arm, (2 % vs. 24 %), along with a complete or near complete sterilization of the operative specimen (34 % vs. 57 %) resulting in a significant increase in SPS in the boost group (44 % vs. 76 %, $p = 0.04$). At a median follow up time of 152 months, although there was no difference in OS and LC, however, the rate of colostomy free survival was 37 % vs. 71 % ($p = 0.001$) in favor of the boost arm. Using modern preoperative staging imaging, Jakobsen et al. [22] conducted a recent RCT trial on T3–4 tumors with dose escalation, comparing CT-LCRT delivering 50.4 Gy in 28 fractions vs. a dose escalation to 60 Gy with the same regimen (50.4 Gy/28) and high dose rate endorectal brachytherapy (HDREBT) as boost modality to deliver 10 Gy. A negative CRM rate of 90 % vs. 99 % respectively was observed ($p = 0.03$) for T3 tumors only in favor of the boost arm.

Intraoperative radiation therapy (IORT) has been developed in order to further optimize local control especially in this unfavorable tumor group.

Most studies have investigated IORT in combination with EBRT. It delivers a higher radiation dose to the CTV at the time of surgical exploration with the advantage of accurate treatment delivery to the area of maximum concern, with adjacent normal structures displaced from the irradiation field. As it is given at the time of surgery, IORT can only be given in a single dose usually varying from 10 to 20 Gy with the peripheral nerve defined as principal dose limiting normal tissue. The benefits of IORT as a means to deliver higher doses and to improve LC have been reported and some data were quite compelling despite being small retrospectives series [23] due to the limited access of IORT equipment worldwide. The results are most beneficial in patients undergoing complete resection. The IORT literature includes a large spectrum of tumors as the selection criteria varied from one center to another, making the evidence of benefits difficult to ascertain. However, Dubois et al. [24] reported on the unique IORT RCT with 142 patients with T3–4 primary and/or recurrent tumors comparing EBRT using 40 Gy alone to the same EBRT with IORT boost (an additional 18 Gy) and did not confirm any disease free survival (DFS) benefits ($p=0.7808$) from the addition of IORT. In this series, the composite population of T3 and T4 tumors did possibly contribute to these negative results.

46.10 Intensity Modulated Radiation Therapy

Radiation therapy was initially based on two-dimensional (2D) planning with standard treatment fields using anatomical bony landmarks. Then, in the early 1990s, three dimensional imaging radiation-planning system (3D planning) were introduced which allowed for 3D definition of the target and normal tissues by using thin section computed tomography (CT) scan. A decade later, the new generation of linear accelerators were equipped with dynamic multileaf collimators (MLC) capable of following the projection of the target as the accelerator gantry arcs around the patient. As a result, MLC delivery and accurate tumor localization of areas at risk, a safe dose to targets in a variety of areas has led to an improvement in local tumor control while reducing the dose to normal structures. This technology has significantly contributed to the therapeutic index of radiation therapy of head and neck cancer. Subsequently, IMRT was tested for treatment of pelvic tumors, in particular with anal canal cancer, and showed to be of value in reducing skin and GI toxicities. However, in rectal cancer, there are few preliminary studies and the benefits of IMRT are lacking. The acute toxicity data from the multi-institutional RTOG study 0822 [25] was not significantly convincing with 51 % of ≥ grade 2 GI toxicity versus 58 % ($p=0.31$) in the conventional 3D based RTOG 0247. Major differences in the clinical target volumes (CTV) contributed to inconsistent results: In gynecological and anal canal cancer, external iliac and inguinal nodes are routinely included whereas in rectal cancer, the CTV is posterior. As presently radiation is presently is given in the context of a NA setting, it is unusual that small bowel loops are closed unlike in the era of adjuvant treatment. Consequently, even with the conventional 3 D technique, the incidence of grave GI toxicity is unusual, especially if the CTV superior limit is adjusted to S1–S2 level.

IMRT had interesting virtues and allowed superior dose conformation within the CTV with the ability to limit normal tissue radiation dose. In our institution, in the less favorable T4 tumors, where optimal tumor downstaging is highly desirable, IMRT was explored as a mean to dose escalation with 60 Gy in 25 fractions during neoadjuvant treatment for 60 patients selected by pelvic MRI with positive CRM [26]. The R0 rate was 90 % and a multivisceral resection rate was 29.5 %. The overall acute toxicity profile was acceptable with a distribution of ≥ grade 3 rate of 16.6 % for GI, 18 % for skin and 10 % for bone marrow.

46.11 High Dose Rate Endorectal Brachytherapy (HDREBT)

In our institution, image guided HDREBT [27, 28] was developed as a highly targeted RT neoadjuvant modality for low T2 and selected T3 rectal cancer.

The treatment consists of 26 Gy in four consecutive fractions prescribed to the deepest aspect of the tumor bed. It is performed in the ambulatory setting, without CT. Acute proctitis was the only toxicity observed with one percent of grade 3. In more than 500 patients treated, at a median follow up time of 5 years, the LR rate was 4.5 %, which compared favorably to NA CT-LCRT. In contrast to EBRT, HDREBT does allow for lower normal tissues exposure to radiation and is given without chemotherapy, thus less costly and toxic. An important observation from this experience remains the excellent LC rate despite the absence of attempt to treat pelvic nodes.

46.12 Summary

In the era of TME, pre-operative RT reduces local recurrence and can be given either with long course RT with 5 Fu based regimen or SCRT. For patients with positive CRM, tumor down staging is highly desirable and SCRT is not as effective to prevent local recurrence. Contemporary pattern of recurrence suggests that it is possible to lower the upper limit of the treatment field level. In an effort to reduce radiation related toxicity, field adjustment along with exploration of new radiation options is desirable.

Key Points

- NA RT, in conjunction with TME improves local control but does not improve OS.
- In patients with positive CRM, NA SCRT is not as effective in reducing LR.
- At present, as no consensus has been reached regarding the superiority of one radiation schedule over the other, standard radiation treatment can be defined as either SCRT or CT-LCRT.
- The 5-Fu based chemotherapy regimen remains standard when long course radiation therapy is used.
- In the era of TME surgery, most recurrences were located below the S2–3 interspace [15] in patients with negative nodes and negative CRM
- Thus, if neoadjuvant EBRT has been effective in decreasing local recurrence, the number of patients requiring treatment will need to be weighed against the substantial morbidity risks and long-term side effects related to EBRT
- Reducing treatment volumes to the level of S1/S2 might be the most effective and simple means to improve therapeutic index.
- The majority of patients with rectal cancer are doing well with current management but there are less favorable cases with positive CRM or recurrent tumors after previous pelvis radiation therapy that remains a clinical management challenge.
- The likelihood of achieving tumor down staging and/or R0 improves as a function of dose.
- The role of IMRT requires further demonstration of meaningful clinical benefits in patient outcomes to further substantiate their routine application in the treatment of rectal cancer.

References

1. Mercury Study Group. Diagnostic accuracy of preoperative magnetic resonance imaging in predicting curative resection of rectal cancer surgery. BMJ. 2006;333(7572):779.
2. Beets-Tan RG, Beets GL, Vliegen RF, Kessels AG, Van Boven H, De Bruine A, von Meyenfeldt MF, Baeten CG, van Engelshoven JM. Accuracy of magnetic resonance imaging in prediction of tumor free resection margin in rectal cancer surgery. Lancet. 2011;357(9255):497–504.
3. Swedish Rectal Cancer Trial. Improved survival with pre-operative radiotherapy radiotherapy in resectable rectal cancer. N Engl J Med. 1997;336(14):980–7.
4. Kapiteijn E, Marijnen CAM, Nagtegaal ID, Putter H, Steup WH, Wiggers T, Rutten HJT, Pahlman L, Glimelius B, Van Krieken J, Han JM, Leer JWH, Van de Velde CJH. Preoperative radiotherapy combined with total mesorectal excision for resectable rectal cancer. N Engl J Med. 2001;345:638–46.

5. van Gijn W, Marijnen CA, Nagtegaal ID, Kranenbarg EM, Putter H, Wiggers T, Rutten HJ, Påhlman L, Glimelius B, van de Velde CJ. Preoperative radiotherapy combined with total mesorectal excision for resectable rectal cancer: 12-year follow-up of the multicentre, randomised controlled TME trial. Lancet Oncol. 2011;12:575–82.
6. Sebag-Montefiore D, Stephens RJ, Steele R, Monson J, Grieve R, Khanna S, Quirke P, Couture J, de Metz C, Myint AS, Bessell E, Griffiths G, Thompson LC, Parmar M. Preoperative radiotherapy versus selective postoperative chemoradiotherapy in patients with rectal cancer (MRC CR07 and NCIC-CTG C016): a multicentre, randomised trial. Lancet. 2009;373:811–20.
7. Bosset JF, Collette L, Calais G, Mineur L, Maingon P, Radosevic-Jelic L, Daban A, Bardet E, Beny A, Ollier JC. Chemotherapy with preoperative radiotherapy in rectal cancer. N Engl J Med. 2006;355:1114–23.
8. Gérard JP, Conroy T, Bonnetain F, Bouché O, Chapet O, Closon-Dejardin MT, Untereiner M, Leduc B, Francois E, Maurel J, Seitz JF, Buecher B, Mackiewicz R, Ducreux M, Bedenne L. Preoperative radiotherapy with or without concurrent fluorouracil and leucovorin in T3–4 rectal cancers: results of FFCD 9203. J Clin Oncol. 2006;24:4620–5.
9. Bujko K, Nowacki MP, Nasierowska-Guttmejer A, Michalski W, Bebenek M, Kryj M. Long-term results of a randomized trial comparing preoperative short-course radiotherapy with preoperative conventionally fractionated chemoradiation for rectal cancer. Br J Surg. 2006;93:1215–23.
10. Ngan SY, Burmeister B, Fisher RJ, Solomon M, Goldstein D, Joseph D, Ackland SP, Schache D, McClure B, McLachlan SA, McKendrick J, Leong T, Hartopeanu C, Zalcberg J, Mackay J. Randomized trial of short-course radiotherapy versus long course chemoradiation comparing rates of local recurrence in patients with T3 rectal cancer: trans-tasman radiation oncology group trial 01.04. J Clin Oncol. 2012; 30:3827–33.
11. Aschele, Cionini L, Lonardi S, Pinto, Cordio S, Rosati G, Artale S, Tagliagambe A, Ambrosini G, Rosetti P, Bonetti A, Negru EM, Maria Chiara Tronconi CM, Luppi G, Silvano G, Cristiano Corsi D, Bochicchio AM, Chiaulon G, Gallo M, Boni L. Primary tumor response to preoperative chemoradiation with or without oxaliplatin in locally advanced rectal cancer: pathologic results of the STAR-01 randomized phase III trial. J Clin Oncol. 2011;29:2773–80.
12. Gérard JP, Azria D, Gourgou-Bourgade S, Martel-Laffay I, Hennequin C, Etienne PL, Vendrely V, François E, de La Roche G, Bouché O, Mirabel X, Denis B, Mineur L, Berdah JF, Mahé MA, Bécouarn Y, Dupuis O, Lledo G, Montoto-Grillot C, Conroy T. Comparison of two neo adjuvant chemoradiotherapy regimens for locally advanced rectal cancer: results of the phase III trial ACCORD 12/0405-Prodige 2. J Clin Oncol. 2010;28:1638–44.
13. Roh MS, Yothers GA, O'Connell MJ, Beart RW, Pitot HC, Shields AF, Parda DS, Sharif S, Allegra CJ, Petrelli NJ, Landry JC, Ryan DP, Arora A, Evans TL, Soori GS, Chu L, Landes RV, Mohiuddin M, Lopa S, Wolmark N. The impact of capecitabine and oxaliplatin in the preoperative multimodality treatment in patients with carci- noma of the rectum: NSABP R-04. ASCO Meet Abstr. 2011;29:3503.
14. Fietkau R, Hohenberger W, Hothorn T, Graeven U, Arnold D, Lang-Welzenbach M, Raab HR, Sülberg H, Wittekind C, Potapov S, Staib L, Hess C, Weigang-Köhler K, Grabenbauer GG, Hoffmanns H, Lindemann F, Schlenska-Lange A, Folprecht G, Sauer R. Preoperative chemoradiotherapy and postoperative chemotherapy with 5-fluorouracil and oxaliplatin versus 5- fluorouracil alone in locally advanced rectal cancer: initial results of the German CAO/ARO/AIO-04 randomized phase III trial. Lancet Oncol. 2012; 13(7):679–87.
15. Nijkamp J, Kusters M, Beets-Tan RG, Martijn H, Beets GL, van de Velde CJ, Marijnen CA. Three-dimensional analysis of recurrence patterns in rectal cancer: the cranial border in hypofractionated preoperative radiotherapy can be lowered. Int J Radiat Oncol Biol Phys. 2011;80(1):103–10.
16. Syk E, Torkzad MR, Blomqvist L, Nilsson PJ, Glimelius B. Local recurrence in rectal cancer: anatomic localization and effect on radiation target. Int J Radiat Oncol Biol Phys. 2008;72(3):658–64.
17. Myerson RJ, Garofalo MC, El Naqa I, Abrams RA, Apte A, Bosch WR, Das P, Gunderson LL, Hong TS, Kim JJ, Willett CG, Kachnic LA. Elective clinical target volumes for conformal therapy in anorectal cancer: a radiation therapy oncology group consensus panel contouring atlas. Int J Radiat Oncol Biol Phys. 2009;74:824–30.
18. Camma C, Giunta M, Fiorica F, Paglioaro L, Craxi A, Cottone M. Preoperative radiotherapy for resectable rectal cancer. J Am Med Assoc. 2000;284:1008–15.
19. Wong RK, Tandan V, De Silva S, Figueredo A. Preoperative radiotherapy and curative surgery for the management of localized rectal carcinoma. Cochrane Database Syst Rev. 2007. (2):CD002102.
20. Wiltshire KL, Ward IG, Swallow C, Oza AM, Cummings B, Pond GR, Catton P, Kim J, Ringash J, Wong CS, Wong R, Siu LL, Moore M, Brierley J. Preoperative radiation with concurrent chemotherapy for resectable rectal cancer: effect of dose escalation on pathologic complete response, local recurrence-free survival, disease-free survival, and overall survival. Int J Radiat Oncol Biol Phys. 2006;64:709–16.
21. Ortholan C, Romestaing P, Chapet O, Gerard JP. Correlation in rectal cancer between clinical tumor response after neoadjuvant radiotherapy and sphincter or organ preservation: 10-year results of the Lyon R 96–02 randomized trial. Int J Radiat Oncol Biol Phys. 2012;83:165–71.
22. Jakobsen A, Ploen J, Vuong T, Appelt A, Lindeberg J, Rafaelsen RS. The dose-effect relationship in chemoradiation of locally advance rectal cancer. A randomized trial comparing two radiation doses. Int J Radiat Oncol Biol Phys. 2012;84(4):950–4.

23. Gunderson L, Willettt C, Calvo FA, Harrison L. Intraoperative irradiation, Current clinical Oncology. 2nd ed. New York: Humana Press; 2011.
24. Dubois J-B, Bussieres E, Richaud P, Rpuanet P, Becouarn Y, Mathoulin-Pélissiers S, Saint-Aubert B, Ychou M. Intra-operative radiotherapy of rectal cancer: results of the French multi-institutional randomized study. Radiother Oncol. 2011;98:298–303.
25. Garofalo M, Moughan J, Hong T, Bendell J, Berger A, Lerma F, Lee R, Anne P, Sharma N, Crane C. RTOG 0822: a phase II study of preoperative (PREOP) chemoradiotherapy (CRT) utilizing IMRT in combination with capecitabine (C) and oxaliplatin (O) for patients with locally advanced rectal cancer. Int J Radiat Oncol Biol Phys. 2011;81(2):S3–4; abstract # 6.
26. Vuong T, Niazi T, Letellier F, Richard C, Liberman S, Faria J, Batist G. A dose escalation phase II study using Intensity Modulated Radiation Therapy (IMRT) and concurrent chemotherapy for patients with advanced rectal cancer and Magnetic Resonant Imaging (MRI) defined positive Circumferential Radial Margins (CRM+). Int J Radiat Oncol Biol Phys. 2011;81(2):S125. Abstract # 252.
27. Vuong T, Belliveau PJ, Michel RP, Moftah BA, Parent J, Trudel JL, Reinhold C, Souhami L. Conformal preoperative endorectal brachytherapy treatment for locally advanced rectal cancer: early results of a phase I/II study. Dis Colon Rectum. 2002;45:1486–93; discussion 1493–5.
28. Vuong T, Richard C, Niazi T, Liberman S, Letellier F, Morin N, Hu K, Anderson D, Devic S. High dose rate endorectal brachytherapy for patients with curable rectal cancer. Semin Colon Rectal Surg. 2010; 21:115–9.
29. Rödel C, Wittekind C, Fietkau R, Martus P, Tschmelitsch J, Hager E, Hess CF, Karstens JH, Liersch T, Schmidberger H, Raab R. Pre operative versus postoperative chemo-radiotherapy for rectal cancer. N Engl J Med. 2004;351:1731–40.

Transanal Approaches to Rectal Cancer Surgery

47

John R.T. Monson and Veerabhadram Garimella

47.1 Introduction

Rectal cancer accounts for a third of colorectal cancer and has been managed by rectal excision for almost 100 years. Radical resection in the form of total mesorectal excision by anterior (AR) or abdominoperineal resection of rectum (APER) remains the standard of care for the overwhelming majority of patients. Despite radical surgery, 30–50 % of patients suffer either local, distant or combined tumor recurrence and of these 34 % die as a result of metastatic disease. Surgery is associated with a 5–8 % rate of mortality and significant complications like wound infection, anastomotic leak, urinary and sexual disturbance and functional disturbance of the bowel occur in upwards of 60 % of patients. In addition, APER results in a perineal wound and associated stoma and psychological complications with attendant increased financial costs.

Radical resection of the rectum came in to vogue in the era where intermediate to late stage cancers were commonest at the time of diagnosis. The fecal occult blood test (FOBT), flexible sigmoidoscopy [1] and colonoscopy based screening for colorectal cancer have resulted in increased diagnosis of early cancers. The first round of FOBT implemented in the United Kingdom has shown 77 % of cancers to be Dukes A and B and 29 % of these in the rectum [2]. Similarly, in the pilot single screening FS trial, 62 % of cancers identified were Dukes A [3]. There also have been improvements in neoadjuvant chemoradiotherapy regimes that help to significantly downstage more advanced rectal tumors that may then be considered for local surgical excision. The combination of these recent developments had resulted in an increased willingness to re-appraise the treatment paradigm for patients with rectal cancer.

47.2 Local Excision vs Tems

Local excision of rectal lesions has been used for many decades. For the most part, such operations were performed using traditional trans-anal surgery in patients with either benign lesions or the very earliest cancers, usually in elderly or infirm patients where radical surgical techniques were considered inappropriate. In more recent years the wider availability of trans-anal endoscopic microsurgery (TEMS) has increased the range of tumors being considered for local resection. TEMS was developed by Buess in 1983 to

J.R.T. Monson, MD, FRCS(Ire,Ed,Eng,Glas), FACS (✉)
Division of Colorectal Surgery, Department of Surgery, University of Rochester Medical Center, Rochester, NY, USA

Department of Colorectal Surgery, University of Rochester Medical Center, Rochester, NY, USA
e-mail: john_monson@urmc.rochester.edu

V. Garimella, MD, FRCS
Department of Colorectal Surgery, University Hospital of North Midlands, Staffordshire, UK

H.R.H. Patel et al. (eds.), *Pelvic Cancer Surgery: Modern Breakthroughs and Future Advances*,
DOI 10.1007/978-1-4471-4258-4_47, © Springer-Verlag London 2015

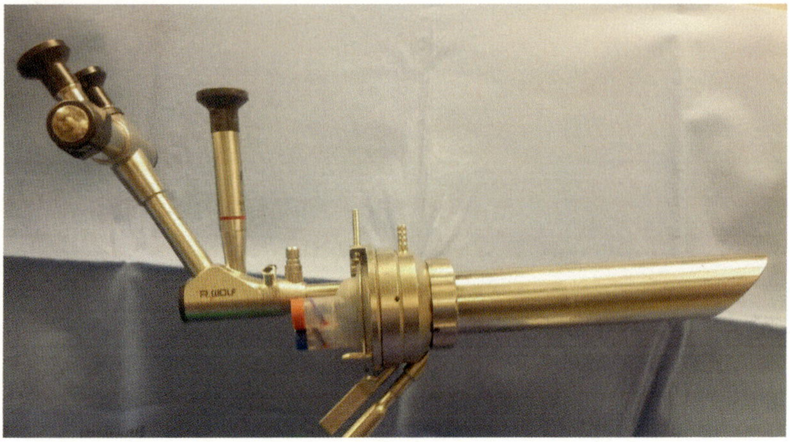

Fig 47.1 TEMS rectoscope with the binocular eye-piece and the instruments in the appropriate ports

overcome the limitations of transanal excision by providing clearer visualization of tumors, the ability to excise more proximal tumors as well as the ability to undertake full thickness excisions with repair of intra-peritoneal defects [4]. In reviews of literature by Maslekar et al. and Sengupta et al. the use of TEMS has been associated with lower local recurrence rates with TEMS. For example, the LR rates using TEMS were 0–6, 14 and 20 % compared to 9.7, 25 and 38 % after traditional trans anal excision for T1, T2 and T3 rectal cancers respectively [5, 6]. A recent meta-analysis of trials comparing local excision (n = 386), TEMS (n = 514) and radical resection has also shown that TEMS was more effective in obtaining clear margins than LE [7].

The instrumentation of TEMS allows true stereoscopic vision thus helping more precise dissection and thereby good circumferential margins (Fig. 47.1). In addition for the majority of patients the excision is full thickness thereby providing good quality tissue specimens for adequate pathological assessment of depth of invasion and on occasions some degree of lymph node sampling. There are now many studies in the literature that demonstrate excellent outcomes in terms of morbidity, mortality and rates of tumor recurrence following TEMS when performed after appropriate case selection based on tumor staging, age and physical fitness of patients, pathological variables of the tumor and technical considerations for TEMS [5, 8–11].

Procedure

The procedure is performed under general anesthetic with full muscle relaxation, as for abdominal surgery. Prior to the procedure, phosphate enemas may be employed to clear the rectum of feces. Full oral bowel preparation is also acceptable but it is essential that the rectum itself is meticulously cleansed so for many surgeons recommend two enemas. A single dose of broad-spectrum antibiotic (Ertapenam or Pipercilin/Tazobactam) is administered. Initially the patient is placed in Lloyd Davies position to assess the position of the tumor. It is essential that when performing TEMS the tumor is in the 6 o'clock position and therefore the patient has to be moved appropriately to achieve this orientation. So, for lateral tumors the patient will be in the decubitus position, reverse Lloyd-Davies for the anterior tumors and remain in the starting Lloyd-Davies position for tumors in a posterior location.

The TEMS rectoscope is inserted and firmly secured to the table using the Martin arm (Fig. 47.1). The tubes are connected for CO_2 insufflation, suction and electro-cautery. The CO_2 insufflation pressure is limited to 20–25 mm of H_2O and uses a specific immediate feedback system for continuous pressure monitoring to maintaining adequate rectal insufflation without excessive proximal colonic distension.

Numerous energy device options have been used for TEMS including Ligasure™, Harmonic

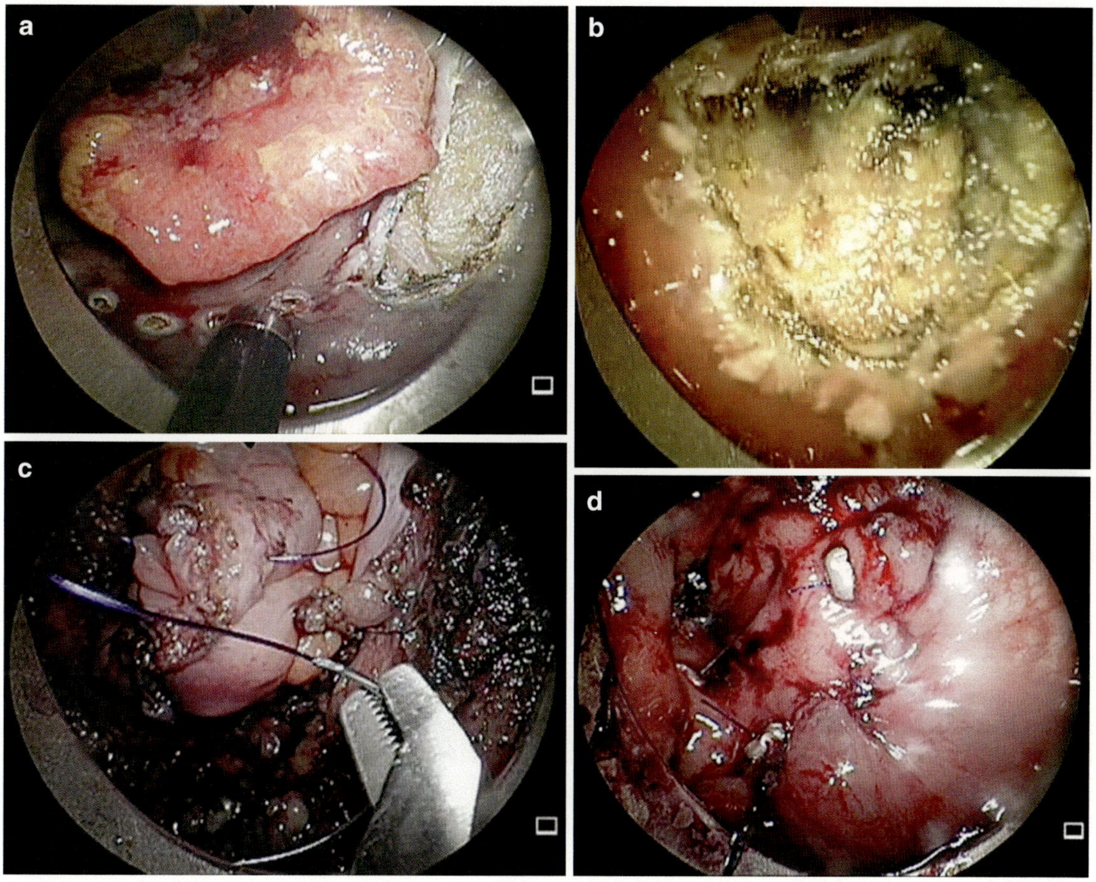

Fig 47.2 (**a**) TEMS Large polypoidal lesion being excised full thickness after marking excision margin with diathermy. (**b**) Mesorectal fat visible at the base after full thickness excision of polyp. (**c**) Suturing of the peritoneal defect after excision of polyp. (**d**) The final appearance of the area after suturing of the defects. The sutures are held in place with beads (seen)

Scalpel™, and water dissection but the commonest option remains traditional electro-cautery using either monopolar or bipolar current via a needle-point instrument. This approach should be used initially to mark out the margins of excision ensuring an adequate cuff of normal tissue (Fig. 47.2a). This step is crucial for adequate excision especially in larger lesions as it helps maintain the correct orientation during resection when the lesion becomes increasingly mobile. In other words it prevents the surgeon wandering off the correct pathway and runs the risk of a positive excision margin. The stereoscopic vision and magnification help in this respect to identify the margins of the tumor. Full thickness excision of the tumor is carried out with coagulation of any bleeding vessels (Fig. 47.2b). Meticulous hemostasis is essential throughout as hemoglobin will absorb the light and make dissection less precise. Identification of areolar tissue and mesorectal fat deep to the muscle layer help confirm the thickness of excision and the aim should be to ensure a vertical dissection through the layers of rectal wall to the depth required—coning of the excision is best avoided (Fig. 47.2b). Routine suturing of the resulting defect was recommended for all lesions in the early days of TEMS. However it is widely recognized as not being necessary assuming there have been no breaches into the peritoneal cavity when careful sutured closure is obviously required (Fig. 47.2c, d). On the other hand routine sutured closure of defects does help to maintain suturing skills for when they are required. Overall, this decision remains a matter of surgeon preference.

For low rectal tumors close to the anal verge maintaining an air seal can present a particular challenge but these lesions can still be excised by wedging the rectoscope up against the anal sphincter thereby permitting adequate rectal insufflation. In addition, when excising these lowest lesions particular care must be taken to avoid excising any significant portion of anal sphincter muscle. This can be challenging at times but is essential if the risks of postoperative incontinence are to be minimized.

Complications

Early post-operative complications are unusual and generally involve mild pain and fever in the first 24 h. Pain is commoner when excision has approached the dentate line and unusual following excision of higher lesions. Post-operative urinary retention is not uncommon in male patients but is rarely a long-term issue. Probably the commonest significant complication is that of a secondary hemorrhage which may occur 5–7 days after surgery. This occurs in less than 3 % of patients but is frightening for the patient because it occurs without warning when the patient is at home. It is therefore useful to at least warn the patient of such a possibility while providing reassurance that the bleeding almost always stops spontaneously and requires no intervention in the overwhelming majority of patients. More unusual complications that have been reported include pelvic sepsis, fistula to the vagina and perineum and intra-peritoneal sepsis. A systematic review of published studies by Middleton et al. showed an overall complication rate 10.3 % for benign adenoma excision and 20 % for carcinoma excision [12] although the majority of these complications are minor in severity.

A review of UK wide TEMS database by Bach et al. showed an overall complication rate of 14.9 % and mortality of 1.4 %. Bleeding was the most common complication (9 %), followed by post op medical complication in 1.9 %, pelvic abscess in 1.7 % and perforation in 0.2 % cases [13]. Perforation in to the peritoneal cavity can be treated either by primary suture (at time of surgery) or conservatively. Morino et al. studied short and long term outcomes of peritoneal perforation after TEMS (n=28) [14]. This study showed that conversion to an abdominal procedure was needed in 10 % (3/28) of patients with a significant peritoneal breach. Long term follow up (48 months) did not show increased peritoneal or liver metastases.

Outcomes for T1 Rectal Cancer

Early rectal cancers with favorable histological features such as SM1 invasion, well to moderate differentiation (G1–2) and no lymphovascular invasion are most suitable for TEM excision. An early study by Blair et al. showed 0 % local recurrence and mortality after local excision in T1 tumors with favorable histological characteristics [15]. However, recurrence rates varying between 0 and 21 % have been reported in the published literature and confirm the importance of appropriate patient selection [13, 16–18]. Bach et al. reviewed 424 rectal cancers of which the majority (253) were T1, and were treated with TEMS [13]. The T1 tumors were further divided in to SM1–3 based on the extent of sub-mucosal invasion. In this the local recurrence rates were 3–4 % and lowest in the Sm1 group [19].

De Graaf et al. compared outcomes in 80 patients undergoing TEMS and 75 patients undergoing TME [20]. TEM was shown to be safer with less blood loss, fewer complications, shorter hospital stay and no mortality. Follow up of more than 5 years showed that overall and cancer specific survival was similar in the two groups although the local recurrence rate after TEMS was shown to be 24 %. The only randomized trial performed to date comparing TEMS alone to radical resection (TME) showed no difference in local recurrence (4 % vs 0 %) or 5 year survival [8]. Heintz et al. studied 103 patients who underwent TEM or TME for T1 rectal cancer [9]. These patients were further stratified into low risk (G1 and 2 with no lympho-vascular invasion) or high risk (G3 and lympho-vascular invasion). The local recurrence and 5 year disease free survival were comparable between TEMS and TME. However, local recurrence rates were higher after TEMS in the high-risk group (33 % vs 18 %). Stipa et al. reviewed 144 patients of whom 86 had T1 cancer. The overall 5 year survival was 83 and 92 % for T1 tumors [21]. Interestingly in this study, of the patients who developed local recurrence the survival was better in those who had radical surgery rather than TEMS excision.

T2–3 Rectal Cancer

Local excision alone for T2–3 rectal cancer leads to an unacceptably high local recurrence rates and the majority of these patients are best served by a radical resection. A review by Tjandra et al. of 22 studies has shown a recurrence of 25 % for T2 and 38 % for T3 rectal cancer [6]. Previous individual case series have shown improved outcomes when local excision/TEMS has been combined with adjuvant chemo-radiotherapy. A phase 2 multi institutional trial performed by CALGB showed 83 % estimated overall survival and 71 % disease free survival in T2 tumors treated with LE and adjuvant therapy [22]. Long term follow up data of the patients in this study group showed overall survival of 42 % and disease free survival of 58 % at 10 years [23]. Guerriri et al. studied 84 T2 and 61 T3 rectal cancers treated with TEMS. These patients were treated with high dose radiotherapy before tumor excision. The rectal cancer specific survival at 97 months in T2 was 90 and 73 % for T3 tumors [17]. In a prospective randomized study Lezoche et al. compared outcomes in patients undergoing TEMS and laparoscopic TME for T2 rectal cancer 6 cm from anal verge [24]. All patients had received neo-adjuvant chemo-radiotherapy. At a median follow up of 84 months the local recurrence was 5.7 % for TEM and 2.8 % for laparoscopic TME group. The survival probability for both the groups was 94 %.

In the last decade another potential role for TEMS has developed for patients thought to have a complete clinical response (CCR) after neoadjuvant chemo-radiotherapy. The pioneering work by Habr-Gama exploring the possibilities of a watch and wait program following CR have resulted in increasing use of TEMS in selected patients to confirm the diagnosis of CR by way of an excisional biopsy. The future will determine the exact role for this approach and longer term follow-up is clearly required before this approach is refined [25, 26].

47.3 Functional Outcomes After TEMS

One of the advantages of TEMS over radical resection of rectum is the maintenance of functionality and preservation of the anal sphincter. However, there have been no direct comparison studies in this regard. TEMS involves dilating the anal canal with a large diameter rectoscope for extended periods of time intuitively raising the possibility of damage to continence and a number of individual studies have addressed these issues [27–31]. Not surprisingly these have shown reduced squeeze pressures and resting tones particularly in relation to the duration of surgery. In addition, the absence of recto anal inhibitory reflex (RAIR) has been reported after TEMS. Despite these findings the majority of case series continue to document no long term problems and have shown adequate function without a change in continence after the initial 6–8 weeks following TEMS.

47.4 Recent Advances in Transanal Surgery

Two recent advances in transanal surgery that look promising are the transanal minimally invasive surgery (TAMIS) and robotic assisted transanal surgery.

TAMIS

In TAMIS, single incision laparoscopic surgery (SILS) port and conventional laparoscopic instrumentation are used to perform transanal surgery [32]. Developed by Atallah et al. the perceived advantages are the readily available equipment and the shorter learning curve as the skills are similar to laparoscopic surgery [32]. The disadvantages as described by the same authors include extreme angles of the instruments that increase external torque resulting in port extrusion. Currently, there is information pertaining to the feasibility of the technique and adequate excision but limited follow up data in rectal cancer excision [33–35]. A variation in the TAMIS technique is the use of a glove port instead of SILS port [36].

Robotic Transanal Surgery

Robotic transanal surgery has been a direct progression to overcome the technical challenges identified in TAMIS. Direct 3D visualization and dexterity of the Da Vinci system could lead to better access to lesions. However, to date only cadaveric studies have been published using the robotic technique [37, 38].

47.5 Summary

There is mounting evidence for the role of local excision of early rectal cancer. TEMS has been shown to achieve better tumor free margins when compared to trans-anal excision. In properly selected cases of T1 rectal cancer, TEMS excision has shown to achieve results comparable to radical resection (TME) while achieving all the benefits of the less invasive approach. Early results of neoadjuvant chemo-radiotherapy to downsize T2/3 rectal cancers followed by TEMS excision look promising and it seems likely that this multi-modality approach to rectal cancer will become more common in the next decade.

Key Points

- Reassessment of surgical practice is required for management of rectal cancer in light of changing cancer trends
- Tumors up to 20 cm from the anal verge can be treated with TEMS
- The stereoscopic magnified view of the tumor along with specially designed instrumentation helps to precisely localize the tumor, achieve full thickness excision with clear margins
- TEMS excision results in better outcomes compared to transanal excision of tumors
- TEMS results shorter procedure time, reduced length of hospital stay and lower complications when compared to TME
- Functional results and continence are not affected by TEMS
- TEMS alone is sufficient for T1 cancer with favorable histological characteristics
- Where possible local recurrences after TEMS excision are best treated with radical resection
- Neo-adjuvant therapy along with TEMS can achieve oncological outcomes comparable to radical resection in T2/3 but with less morbidity, mortality and significantly better quality of life
- The initial results of newer platforms for transanal surgery like TAMIS look promising but comparative studies are required to confirm equipoise with TEMS

References

1. Dafnis G, et al. Transanal endoscopic microsurgery: clinical and functional results. Color Dis. 2004;6(5):336–42.
2. Logan RF, et al. Outcomes of the bowel cancer screening programme (BCSP) in England after the first 1 million tests. Gut. 2012;61(10):1439–46.

3. Atkin WS, et al. Single flexible sigmoidoscopy screening to prevent colorectal cancer: baseline findings of a UK multicentre randomised trial. Lancet. 2002;359(9314):1291–300.
4. Buess G, et al. Transanal endoscopic microsurgery. Leber Magen Darm. 1985;15(6):271–9.
5. Maslekar S, et al. Transanal endoscopic microsurgery: where are we now? Dig Surg. 2006;23(1–2):12–22.
6. Sengupta S, Tjandra JJ. Local excision of rectal cancer: what is the evidence? Dis Colon Rectum. 2001;44(9): 1345–61.
7. Sgourakis G, et al. Transanal endoscopic microsurgery for T1 and T2 rectal cancers: a meta-analysis and meta-regression analysis of outcomes. Am Surg. 2011;77(6):761–72.
8. Winde G, et al. Surgical cure for early rectal carcinomas (T1). Transanal endoscopic microsurgery vs. anterior resection. Dis Colon Rectum. 1996;39(9):969–76.
9. Heintz A, Morschel M, Junginger T. Comparison of results after transanal endoscopic microsurgery and radical resection for T1 carcinoma of the rectum. Surg Endosc. 1998;12(9):1145–8.
10. Buess GF, Raestrup H. Transanal endoscopic microsurgery. Surg Oncol Clin N Am. 2001;10(3):709–31, xi.
11. Palma P, et al. Transanal endoscopic microsurgery: indications and results after 100 cases. Color Dis. 2004;6(5):350–5.
12. Middleton PF, Sutherland LM, Maddern GJ. Transanal endoscopic microsurgery: a systematic review. Dis Colon Rectum. 2005;48(2):270–84.
13. Bach SP, et al. A predictive model for local recurrence after transanal endoscopic microsurgery for rectal cancer. Br J Surg. 2009;96(3):280–90.
14. Morino M, et al. Does peritoneal perforation affect short- and long-term outcomes after transanal endoscopic microsurgery? Surg Endosc. 2013;27(1):181–8.
15. Blair S, Ellenhorn JD. Transanal excision for low rectal cancers is curative in early-stage disease with favorable histology. Am Surg. 2000;66(9):817–20.
16. Lezoche G, et al. Transanal endoscopic microsurgery for 135 patients with small nonadvanced low rectal cancer (iT1-iT2, iN0): short- and long-term results. Surg Endosc. 2011;25(4):1222–9.
17. Guerrieri M, et al. Transanal endoscopic microsurgery for the treatment of selected patients with distal rectal cancer: 15 years experience. Surg Endosc. 2008;22(9):2030–5.
18. Christoforidis D, et al. Transanal endoscopic microsurgery versus conventional transanal excision for patients with early rectal cancer. Ann Surg. 2009;249(5):776–82.
19. Kikuchi R, et al. Management of early invasive colorectal cancer. Risk of recurrence and clinical guidelines. Dis Colon Rectum. 1995;38(12):1286–95.
20. De Graaf EJ, et al. Transanal endoscopic microsurgery versus total mesorectal excision of T1 rectal adenocarcinomas with curative intention. Eur J Surg Oncol. 2009;35(12):1280–5.
21. Stipa F, Giaccaglia V, Burza A. Management and outcome of local recurrence following transanal endoscopic microsurgery for rectal cancer. Dis Colon Rectum. 2012;55(3):262–9.
22. Steele Jr GD, et al. Sphincter-sparing treatment for distal rectal adenocarcinoma. Ann Surg Oncol. 1999;6(5):433–41.
23. Wentworth S, et al. Long-term results of local excision with and without chemoradiation for adenocarcinoma of the rectum. Clin Colorectal Cancer. 2005;4(5):332–5.
24. Lezoche G, et al. A prospective randomized study with a 5-year minimum follow-up evaluation of transanal endoscopic microsurgery versus laparoscopic total mesorectal excision after neoadjuvant therapy. Surg Endosc. 2008;22(2):352–8.
25. Habr-Gama A, Perez RO. The surgical significance of residual mucosal abnormalities in rectal cancer following neoadjuvant chemoradiotherapy. Br J Surg. 2012;99:993–1001. Br J Surg, 2012. 99(11): p. 1601: author reply 1601–2.
26. Habr-Gama A, et al. Complete clinical response after neoadjuvant chemoradiation therapy for distal rectal cancer: characterization of clinical and endoscopic findings for standardization. Dis Colon Rectum. 2010;53(12):1692–8.
27. Cataldo PA, O'Brien S, Osler T. Transanal endoscopic microsurgery: a prospective evaluation of functional results. Dis Colon Rectum. 2005;48(7):1366–71.
28. Kreis ME, et al. Functional results after transanal endoscopic microsurgery. Dis Colon Rectum. 1996;39(10):1116–21.
29. Banerjee AK, et al. Prospective study of the proctographic and functional consequences of transanal endoscopic microsurgery. Br J Surg. 1996;83(2):211–3.
30. Kennedy ML, Lubowski DZ, King DW. Transanal endoscopic microsurgery excision: is anorectal function compromised? Dis Colon Rectum. 2002;45(5): 601–4.
31. Herman RM, et al. Anorectal sphincter function and rectal barostat study in patients following transanal endoscopic microsurgery. Int J Color Dis. 2001; 16(6):370–6.
32. Atallah S, Albert M, Larach S. Transanal minimally invasive surgery: a giant leap forward. Surg Endosc. 2010;24(9):2200–5.
33. Albert MR, et al. Transanal minimally invasive surgery (TAMIS) for local excision of benign neoplasms and early-stage rectal cancer: efficacy and outcomes in the first 50 patients. Dis Colon Rectum. 2013;56(3):301–7.
34. Slack T, Wong S, Muhlmann M. Transanal minimally invasive surgery: an initial experience. ANZ J Surg. 2014;84(3):177–80.
35. Lim SB, et al. Feasibility of transanal minimally invasive surgery for mid-rectal lesions. Surg Endosc. 2012;26(11):3127–32.
36. Hompes R, et al. Transanal glove port is a safe and cost-effective alternative for transanal endoscopic microsurgery. Br J Surg. 2012;99(10):1429–35.
37. Atallah SB, et al. Robotic TransAnal minimally invasive surgery in a cadaveric model. Tech Coloproctol. 2011;15(4):461–4.
38. Hompes R, et al. Preclinical cadaveric study of transanal endoscopic da Vinci(R) surgery. Br J Surg. 2012;99(8):1144–8.

Endoscopic Approaches to Rectal Neoplasia

48

John A. Dumot

Abbreviations

AIN	Anal intraepithelial neoplasia
EMR	Endoscopic mucosal resection
ESD	Endoscopic submucosal dissection
EUS	Endoscopic ultrasound
G	Granular
NG	Nongranular
PP	Pit pattern
TEM	Transanal endoscopic microsurgery

48.1 Introduction

Flexible endoscopic examination of the rectum and colon is quite common and has advantages over the rigid trans-anal endoscopic examination and resection techniques. Flexible endoscopy allows examination of the entire colon and has become the most common gastroenterology procedure in the world. While there remains developed countries that do not promote routine colonoscopy for colorectal cancer screening, the technology is readily available in most medical centers. High definition imaging improves detection and visualization of the lesion margins. The majority of polyps can be easily removed during colonoscopy with routine cold or cautery snares. Removal of larger neoplasia previously referred for surgery is possible with advanced endoscopic techniques discussed in this chapter. An important concept in the endoscopic therapy of advanced colorectal neoplasia is recognition of lesion morphology, and important mucosal characteristics are summarized in this chapter.

Evacuation of the rectum with an enema preparation (tap water, isotonic saline, bisacodyl or sodium phosphate) is recommended before all limited endoscopic procedures to improve visualization for diagnostic purposes. A full bowel preparation and endoscopic evacuation of residue is required before therapy of rectal neoplasia to provide a clear site, reduce the risk of methane gas explosion when using electrocautery and minimize peritoneal soilage in case of perforation. After wide area endoscopic removal of advanced rectal neoplasia, most patients are monitored for a short period and then be discharged home provided there are no significant symptoms suggesting a complication. Limiting oral intake to fluids for the remainder of the day will allow a clear field for endoscopic intervention should delayed bleeding or perforation develop in the interim period. Patients with complicated resections should be monitored closely and receive periprocedural intravenous antibiotics if they experience abdominal pain or the bowel wall was compromised.

J.A. Dumot, DO, FASGE
Division of Gastroenterology and Hepatology, Case Western Reserve University, University Hospitals of Cleveland, Cleveland, OH, USA

Digestive Health Institute, Ahuja Medical Center, Beachwood, OH, USA
e-mail: john.dumot@uhhospitals.org

H.R.H. Patel et al. (eds.), *Pelvic Cancer Surgery: Modern Breakthroughs and Future Advances*,
DOI 10.1007/978-1-4471-4258-4_48, © Springer-Verlag London 2015

48.2 Assessment of Rectal Lesions

Retroflexion of the endoscope to examine the anal verge is an important maneuver during rectal endoscopy. Visualization of the dentate line at the anal verge is accomplished with a fully angulated bending section of the flexible endoscope or colonoscope. Careful inspection of the most distal portion of the rectal vault can reveal hidden lesions and neoplasia at the squamocolumnar anal junction (Fig. 48.1). The technique should be performed with the lumen distended with air or carbon dioxide. The lowest rectal fold or valve is used as a target as the up/down wheel is moved counter clockwise to its fullest extent. Gentle torque is applied to the insertion tube as well as counter clockwise movement of the left/right wheel to complete the maneuver. The operator should gently insert or "give up" approximately 15 cm of the instrument to accomplish the maneuver. The operator should not struggle or force the instrument because perforations of the rectum can occur and do not seem to be related to experience of the physician. Fortunately these perforations are infrequent and rarely need surgical intervention [1]. Retroflexion in difficult situations with a narrow caliber rectum from chronic colitis, radiation therapy or altered surgical anatomy can be avoided and alternatively use careful visualization of the entire mucosa through the anal canal during slow withdrawal of the endoscope in a circular fashion (Fig. 48.1).

Advanced mucosal neoplasia usually refers to lesions with advanced histology (tubulovillous, villous or high grade dysplasia) and are generally ≥10 mm [2]. Large flat lesions or laterally spreading tumors can increase in size and extend over several mucosal folds before becoming invasive. However, smaller lesions can be invasive and the experienced endoscopist takes into account tactile as well as visual features before entertaining endoscopic removal. Mucosal lesion morphology is defined according to the Paris classification of neoplastic lesions [3, 4]. Type 0 lesions are superficial mucosal neoplasia classified as *protruding*, *flat elevated* or *flat* in general terms. Protruding lesions include pedunculated (0-Ip), subpedunculated (0-Isp) or sessile (0-Is). Flat elevated lesions have shoulders less than 2.5 mm and may be flat elevation of the mucosa (0-IIa) or a mixture of flat elevated and central depression (0-IIa + IIc) or flat elevated and raised broad based nodule (0-IIa + Is). Other formations include entirely flat lesions (0-IIb), depressed lesions (0-IIc) and excavated lesions (0-III). Type 1 lesions are polypoid carcinomas usually attached on a wide base. Type 2 lesions are ulcerated carcinomas and raised sharp margins. Type 3 lesions are ulcerated and have no definite limits. Type 4 lesions are non-ulcerated and diffusely infiltrating.

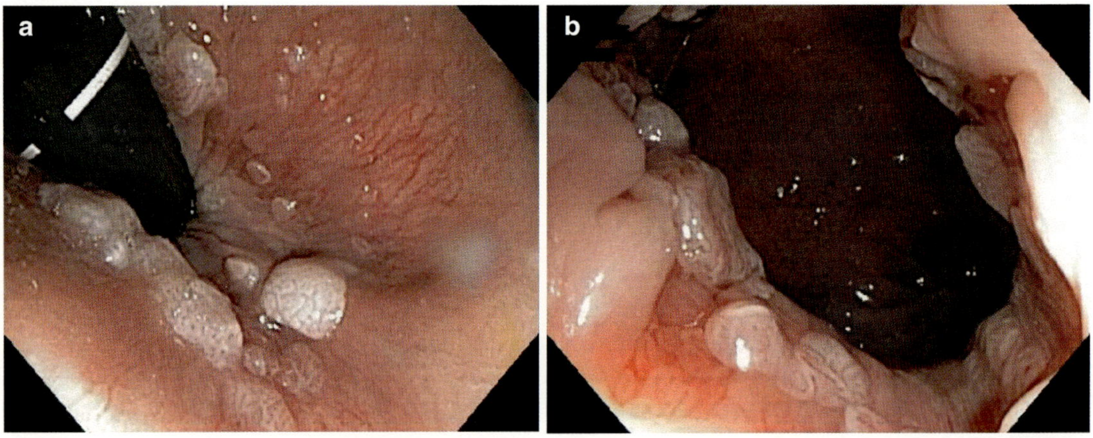

Fig. 48.1 Example of retroflexion view of anal brim. (**a**) Anal Intraepithelial Neoplasia (AIN) 0-IIa grade 2 with immunohistochemical stain for p16 positive favoring an HPV-related pathogenesis. (**b**) AIN lesion on withdrawal of the endoscope

The surface topography of the mucosal lesion is best characterized as granular (G, nodular) nongranular (NG, flat) or mixed. Morphology can be enhanced with dye spraying of indigo carmine 0.4 % or crystal violet 0.05 % solutions, which helps demarcate margins and mucosal patterns. Mucosal morphology is extremely important because it predicts submucosal invasion in advanced lesions. A uniformly 0-IIa G lesion has a very low risk of submucosal invasion (~1 %) compared to the highest risk 0-IIa + c NG lesions with submucosal invasion of 67 % (relative risk, 54; P<0.001) [5]. Depressed areas in neoplastic lesions are clearly associated with an increased risk of submucosal invasion [6, 7]. Other features of colorectal lesions include loss of lobulation within a large protruding nodule, fold convergence, demarcated depressed areas, stalk swelling and fullness should raise a suspicion of submucosal invasion [8].

Mucosal pit pattern (PP) are best described according to the Kudo system [9]. Mucosal PP are highlighted with high definition endoscopes and dye spray chromoendoscopy. Advanced imaging processing with light filters (narrow band imaging, Olympus Medical) or computer modulation of the image (intelligent color enhancement, Fujinon and i-scan, Pentax) can facilitate PP recognition without the dye spray using a virtual chromoendoscopy image. Type IV PP is the most common pattern and corresponds to a tubulovillous adenoma histology. Type III PP is seen with NG lesions and corresponds to tubular adenoma histology. Irregular PP are associated with intramucosal carcinoma or an invasive neoplasm. The Sano mucosal vascular patterns seen with narrow band imaging can further characterize advanced mucosal neoplasia using the capillary arrangements (regular brown mesh networks vs. irregular or complex branching and blind ending) to differentiate noninvasive and invasive lesions [10]. The relationship of PP with submucosal invasion appears to be more significant in sessile and superficial lesions more so than pedunculated lesions [8]. The use of PP recognition and micro vascular features are helpful in determining if a lesion is high risk for invasive disease but no features are uniformly reliable and there is considerable intraobserver variability with inexperienced operators. Therefore, proper tissue handling and histologic evaluation of resected lesions is imperative to guide subsequent care.

48.3 Endoscopic Ultrasound

Endoscopic ultrasound (EUS) is helpful to assess the depth of invasion for mucosal lesions and confirm the presence, size and location of subepithelial lesions. Fine needle aspiration and core biopsy of lesions and lymph nodes are possible with EUS guidance. EUS is not necessary before endoscopic removal of lesions with favorable morphologic features discussed above but can be helpful in large, depressed or ulcerated lesions. Figure 48.2a shows a T1a wide base raised rectal neoplasm measuring 27 mm in width. The wall layers of the rectum are preserved and suggest a lack of invasion. True assessment of invasion is based on pathologic evaluation of the lesion looking for the extent of invasion into the lamina propria, vascular or lymphatic invasion and tumor grade in the resected specimen. Debate on the need to remove lesions en bloc is based on the difficulty assessing lateral margins and cautery artifact of deeper margins with piecemeal resection techniques discussed below and may be avoided with endoscopic submucosal dissection. EUS is very useful for characterizing intramural lesions in the rectum. Figure 48.2b, c shows a large submucosal lesion with a bulky intramural neoplasm of the deep muscularis propria characteristic of a gastrointestinal stromal tumor. Smaller intramural lesions are more commonly rectal carcinoid tumors. EUS is helpful in determining size but endoscopic resection method is a better predictor of complete pathologic response than EUS findings [11].

48.4 Endoscopic Resection Techniques

Most lesions limited to the mucosa and neuroendocrine tumors can be successfully removed with a diagnostic flexible endoscope using a variety of

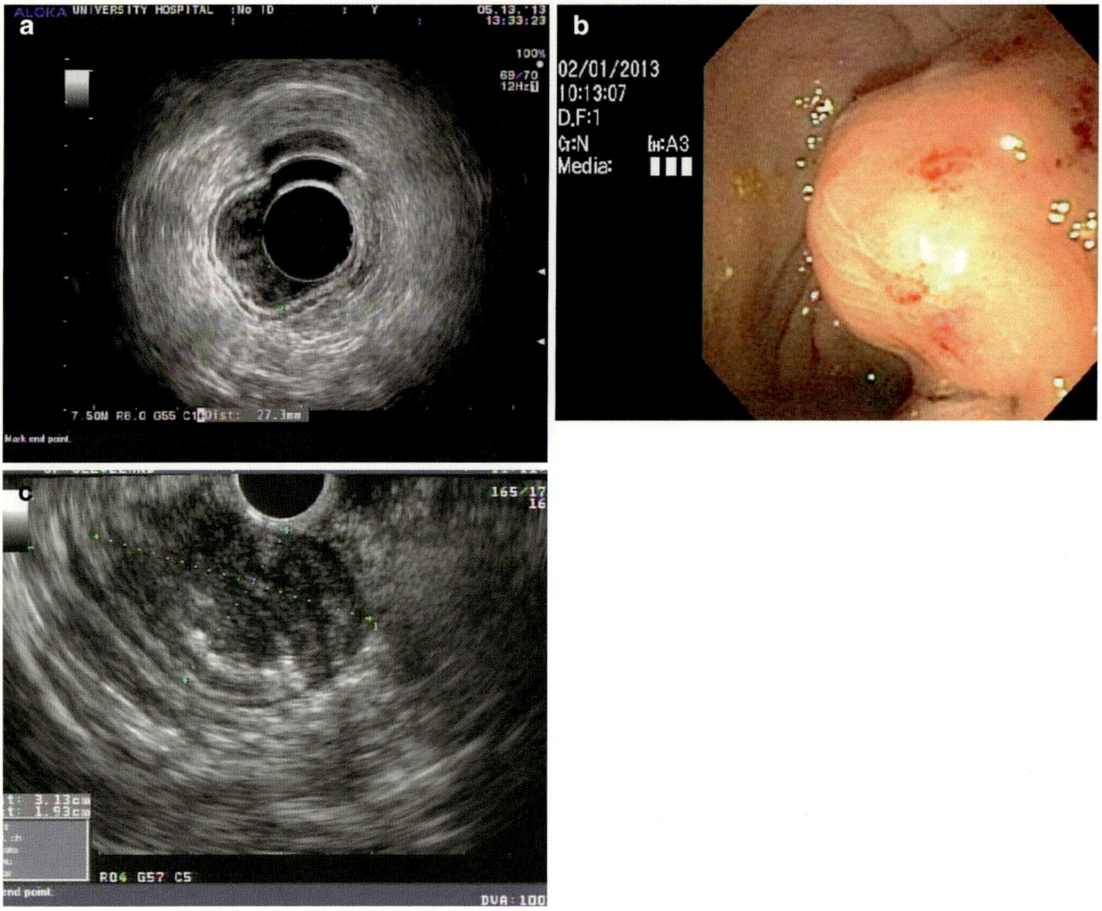

Fig. 48.2 Endoscopic ultrasound images. (**a**) T1a wide base raised rectal neoplasm measuring 27 mm in width. (**b**) A large submucosal lesion seen on routine endoscopy in the rectum. (**c**) The lesion measures 3.1 × 1.9 cm and fine needle aspiration revealed features of a gastrointestinal stromal tumor (GIST) with immunohistochemical stain positive CD 117

devices passed through the accessory channel. Treatment of rectal neoplasms with flexible endoscopes has several advantages over transanal endoscopic microsurgery (TEM). A diagnostic endoscope measures approximately 11 mm in diameter compared to the average operating rectoscope measuring 40 mm. Using the gastroscope provides a shorter device that improves control and reduces time and effort compared to the colonoscope length devices. Most patients having endoscopic resection do well with monitored anesthesia in the deep sedation state compared to general anesthesia for TEM. Candidate lesions for endoscopic resection are listed in Table 48.1. TEM is still the preferred choice for neoplasia with deep submucosal or muscularis propria invasion is suspected if patient characteristics dictate a local excision over traditional anterior resection because TEM allows full thickness resection and

Table 48.1 Rectal neoplasms amenable to endoscopic therapy

Epithelial neoplasms
Adenomatous polyps
Serrated adenomatous polyps
Malignant rectal polyp without stalk or submucosal invasion
Giant hyperplastic polyps
Subepithelial neoplasms
Rectal neuroendocrine (carcinoid) tumors

closure using proven microsurgical techniques. To date, endoscopic closure techniques are limited to smaller defects and are cumbersome to employ. TEM is also preferred for lesions involving a significant portion of the squamocolumnar junction in the anorectal lumen although ESD has been successful for early stage squamous cell carcinoma within the anal canal [12].

Informed consent should outline the decision to pursue endoscopic resection over surgical weighing the risk of incomplete resection and major complications of endoscopic approach to the immediate risks of full thickness surgical resection (leakage, infection, loss of bowel function and general anesthesia). The most common risk of endoscopic resection is delayed bleeding 2–12 days following resection. We schedule complex endoscopic procedures with monitored anesthesia assistance so that the endoscopist can solely focus on the resection task. Dedicated assistance with proper training must demonstrate patience and share the goal of complete resection at the time of the first procedure no matter how long it takes because subsequent sessions will encounter fibrosis at the resection site, which reduces the effect of future resections and increases the risk of perforation.

Conventional Polypectomy

Standard or conventional polypectomy for mucosal lesions using a electrocautery snare is considered the major technical advance since the advent of flexible fiber optic imaging. Progression of the technique into wide area endoscopic mucosal resection (EMR) refers to piecemeal resection with a submucosal injection when the lesion cannot be completely grasped in total by a routine cautery snare. The submucosal injection was first described by Rosenberg before fulguration of rectal and sigmoid polyps with a transanal approach [13]. Injection into the submucosal plane has now become standard of care throughout the gastrointestinal tract with the advent of flexible endoscopic needle-tip catheters making polypectomy safer and easier. A more recent advance includes tinting the saline solution with a pigment such as indigo carmine to color the submucosal layer blue to improve visibility of that tissue plane (Fig. 48.3). Submucosal injection can obscure the peripheral margins of the lesion, therefore, marking the margins with the tip of the closed electrocautery snare can delineate the area to be resected prior to resection. On the other hand, identification of the margins in very subtle flat colorectal neoplasms is often improved after injection of indigo carmine tinted submucosal saline. We find the later to be more common with flat serrated adenomas due to their hyperplastic appearance.

A colloidal additive (succinylated gelatin or hyaluronic acid) can improve the sustainability of the submucosal injection and facilitate wide area piece meal resections compared to saline by reducing the number of injections, resections and procedure time [14]. Other agents such as artificial liquid tears (hypromellose 2.5 % solution) and intravenous volume expanders (hydroxyethyl starch) are more widely available with similar effect. In an excellent review of wide area endoscopic resection techniques of colonic neoplasia, Holt and Bourke recommend intravenous antibiotic prophylaxis and a long acting local anesthetic can be added to the injection solution for resection of advanced neoplasia of the anorectal junction [15].

In piecemeal resection of large polyps, elevate only a portion of the lesion to facilitate capture with the electrocautery snare. Choose the most difficult area first and reposition the patient if needed to achieve a 6 O'clock position with the endoscope. The addition of a friction fit cap to the endoscope tip allows capture of the tissue with application of suction. One cap technique uses a crescent-shaped snare perched at the outer rim and another technique uses a variceal band elastic ligature followed by routine snare cautery. A shorter version of the friction fit cap is commonly utilized to improve visualization during mucosal resection by maintaining a minimum focal length between the mucosa and the endoscope optical lens. Without the cap, positioning of the endoscope is more difficult to maintain endoscopic view especially in angulated and uneven topography. Invasive lesions are difficult to differentiate

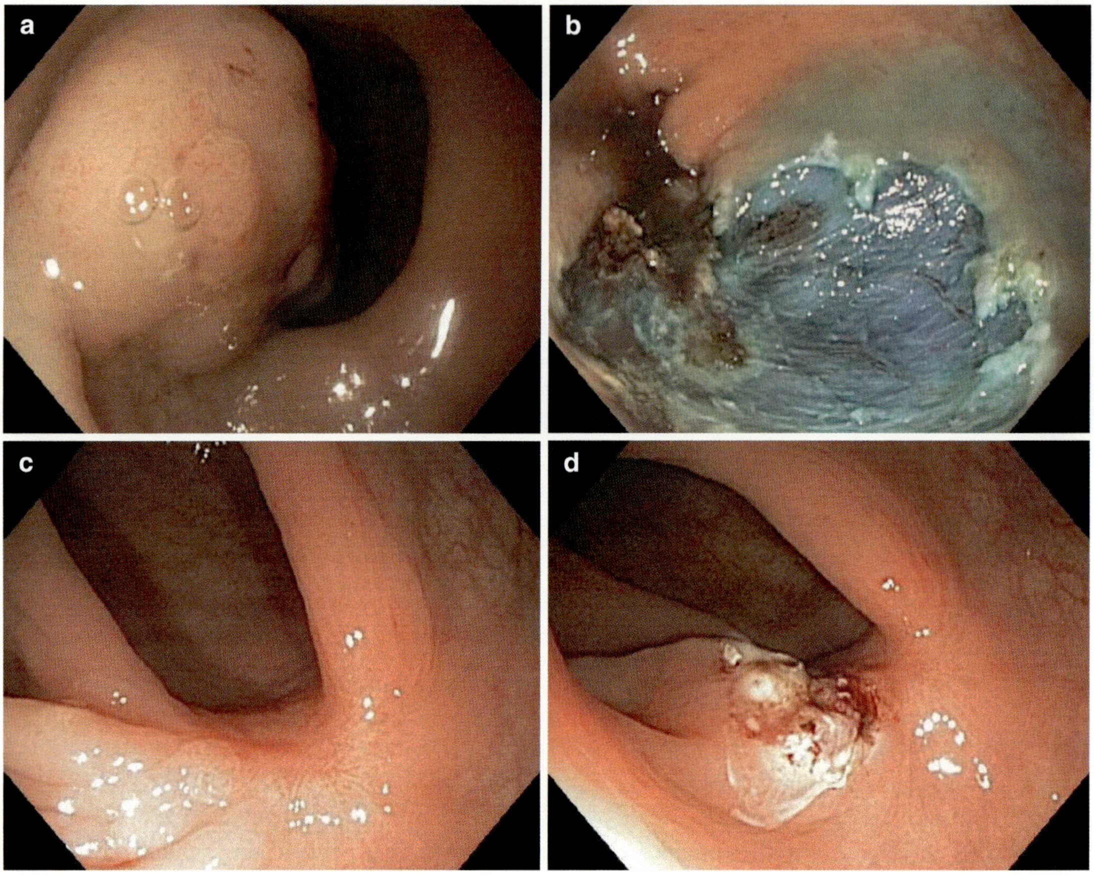

Fig. 48.3 Endoscopic mucosal resection. (**a**) A 40 mm adenoma 0-Isp granular lesion at the rectosigmoid junction. (**b**) EMR site cleared of all neoplasia and reveals blue residual submucosal layer. (**c**) EMR site healed at 3 months with central scar. (**d**) Biopsy and focal electrocautery treatment of any suspected residual adenoma; only hyperplastic change noted on specimens

from fibrous tissue from chronic mucosal prolapsed or prior interventions because both can limit the submucosal injection lift especially at the central portions of the lesion. These clinical situations may be best treated with further advancement in endoscopic submucosal dissection technique.

Endoscopic Submucosal Dissection

Endoscopic submucosal dissection (ESD) is a more tedious technique that utilizes small controlled incisions with the goal of en bloc resection for complete pathologic evaluation. ESD was originally developed for and revolutionized the treatment of early gastric neoplasms. Application of ESD to the colon was temporized by the high rate of perforation however, expert endoscopists were quick to apply those methods to colorectal neoplasms with excellent success using meticulous care. In an early series of 200 patients with laterally spreading tumors with favorable mucosal patterns throughout the colon and rectum treated by expert endoscopists, en bloc resections were achieved in 84 % and tumor free margin achieved in 70 % [16]. The mean size of the tumors was 35 ± 19 mm SD (range, 15–140 mm) and the final pathologic resection specimens revealed 51 adenomas, 99 intramucosal cancers, 22 invasive cancers with minute submucosal penetration T1sm1 (<1,000 μm) and 28 deep submucosal cancers T1sm2 (≥1,000 μm). Of the 180 patients (90 %) with a follow up examination, only one case of local recurrence was found and no lymph node or distant metastasis were found. In a large retrospective study by the same group, EMR was associated with a higher incomplete resection and recurrence rate than ESD [17]. The recurrence rate was 3 of 145 (3 %) lesions treated with ESD compared to 33 of 228 (14 %) treated with EMR ($p<0.0001$). This favorable outcome was noted even though the lesions in the ESD group tended to be significantly larger than those in the EMR group. The rate of perforation was higher in the ESD group (1.3 % vs 6.2 %, p = NS), however all were managed conservatively without surgery. As their experience grew, the endoscopic mucosal pattern dictated their approach. Large laterally spreading G lesions were removed in piecemeal ideally with the largest nodule being resected first. NG lesions required ESD en bloc resection to due a significantly higher rate of submucosal invasion (NG 14 % vs. G 7 %; $P<0.01$) [7]. Unfortunately, even with favorable histologic features after resection and clear early follow up examinations, one case of intramucosal cancer treated with piecemeal resection recurred as a submucosal-like cancer was found 1 cm from the original resection site 2.5 years later.

Equipment and materials for ESD are listed in Table 48.2. ESD characteristically is a two-step process: complete circumferential incision of the lesion followed by submucosal dissection of the plane beneath the lesion using short bursts of electrocautery to coagulate the tissue and blood vessels in the submucosal plane (Fig. 48.4). The peripheral incision is relatively easy and facilitated with injection of saline with indigo carmine blue dye solution (indigo carmine 80 mg per 500 ml saline). Colloid additive is usually not necessary for this step but improves the submucosal dissection process providing a sustained lift of the mucosa. Our unit prefers any commercially available artificial tears solution from the pharmacy. Adding epinephrine (1:100,000) is optional and may improve visualization by reducing intra procedural bleeding.

ESD is effective for removing submucosal lesions of the rectum less than 2 cm. Carcinoid lesions found incidentally on colonoscopy are usually asymptomatic and conventional approach is resection over observation in medically fit patients. Although EMR has been advocated for endoscopic removal with blind snare or band-ligation technique, ESD affords a reliable method for en bloc removal of lesions without invasion of the muscularis propria (Fig. 48.5).

ESD is clearly more technically demanding than EMR but both are associated with bleeding and perforation. Immediate bleeding is routinely encountered during ESD and controlled with a combination of epinephrine injection, hemostatic forceps and endoscopic clips. Factors independently associated with perforations include larger lesions, right sided colon lesions, less experienced endoscopist, and lack of hyaluronic acid in submucosal injection solution [18]. Endoscopic man-

Table 48.2 ESD devices and material

High definition endoscope or colonoscope
CO_2 insufflators—turn air setting to "OFF"
Electrosurgical generator with microprocessor control (ERBE, Tübingen, Germany or Olympus Medical, Tokyo, Japan)
Marginal resection setting—endocut effect 2, duration 1, at 30 W
Submucosal dissection setting—forced or spray coagulation 30 W
Coagulation forceps—soft coagulation effect 5 at 60–80 W
Sclerotherapy needle for injection of solution
Submucosal injection solution drawn up in 10 ml syringe:
Liquid artificial tears—5 ml
Saline—4 ml
Indigo carmine—1 ml
ESD knife options
Dual knife (Olympus KD-650U dual knife)
Insulated tip knife (Olympus KD-611L IT knife2)
Triangle tip knife (Olympus KD-640L TT knife)
Coagulation forceps (Olympus FD-411UR coagrasper)
Friction fit clear cap (e.g. Olympus D-201-type sized for endoscope)
Endoscopic hemostatic clips to control significant bleeding and closure of perforations
Epinephrine solution to control bleeding
Rat-tooth forceps and Roth net to retrieve tissue
Stiff bristle brush to clean knives of chard tissue
Pins and mat material to prepare tissue before fixation

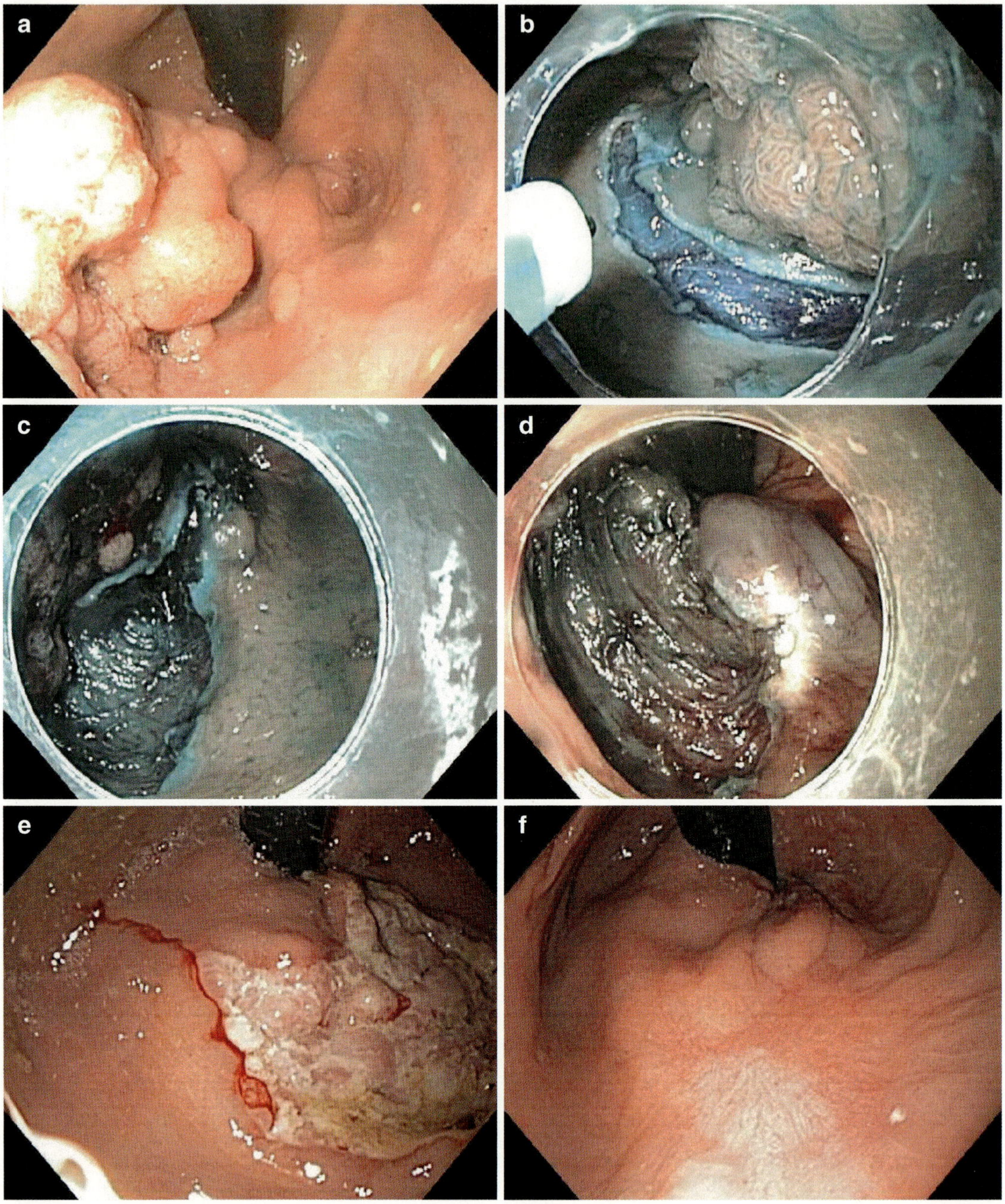

Fig. 48.4 Endoscopic submucosal dissection of a laterally spreading mucosal neoplasia. (**a**) A 50 mm distal rectal adenoma 0-IIa + Is granular lesion seen on retroflexion. (**b**) Circumferential incision of the margins with endoscopic knife after submucosal injection of indigo carmine tinted saline. (**c**) Submucosal layer injection expands layer for endoscopic dissection of the lesion base. (**d**) Final image of muscularis propria of the rectum after ESD. (**e**) Marginal bleeding noted at 10 days after ESD with granulation tissue covering ESD site. (**f**) Complete healing with central depression scar at 6 month follow up exam

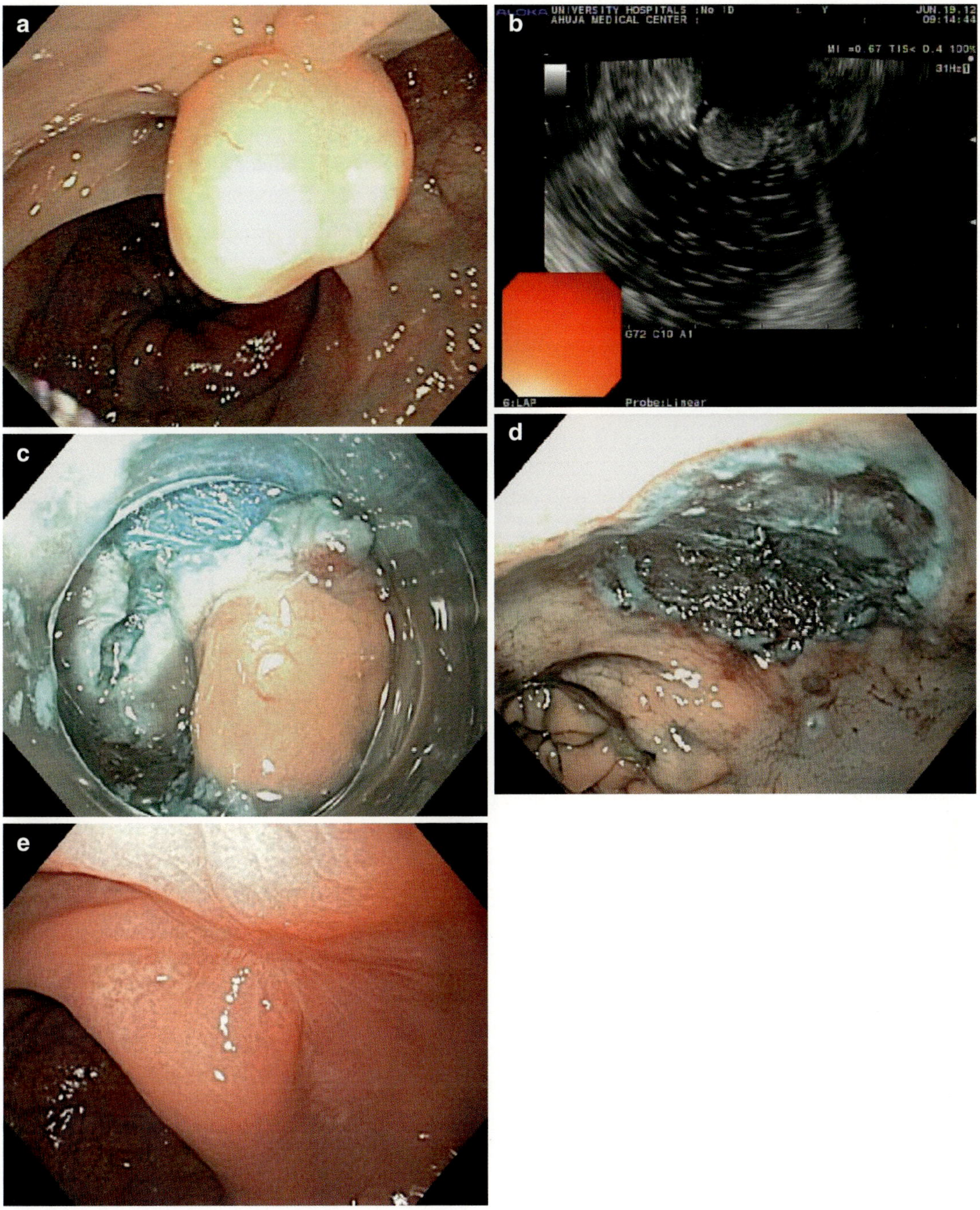

Fig. 48.5 Endoscopic submucosal dissection of a submucosal carcinoid tumor. (**a**) A submucosal lesion protrudes into the lumen at the rectosigmoid junction on the right lateral wall. (**b**) EUS reveals a hyperechoic lesion measuring 11 mm without. (**c**) Circumferential incision after submucosal injection precedes dissection of the deeper margin. (**d**) ESD site immediately following resection of the lesion en bloc. (**e**) ESD site at 3 months shows scar from prior resection

agement of perforations is possible in most cases provided they are recognized early and treated appropriately. Delayed or missed perforations can be devastating and difficult to manage without radiologic or surgical drainage. Recognition begins with inspection of the resection site for defects or penetration through the blue tinted submucosal tissue layer. Insufflation with carbon dioxide during endoscopy reduces the symptoms associated with pneumoperitoneum. Immediate decompression of a pneumoperitoneum with a large bore needle catheter may be necessary when cardiovascular compromise is noted. Attempts at endoscopic closure with hemostatic clips is usually successful with supportive care in a hospital setting. Multidisciplinary approach with administration of intravenous antibiotics, bowel rest and drainage of fluid collections is associated with good outcomes. Frank peritoneal soiling and large defects not amenable to endoscopic closure should be addressed surgically. Most endoscopic perforations of the rectal vault, either during retroflexion or endoscopic therapy can be managed conservatively because they usually occur below the peritoneal reflection.

48.5 Endoscopic Follow Up and Ablation Techniques

Endoscopic follow up exam at 6 weeks if resection is incomplete allows healing of the resected area and treatment of residual neoplasia with repeated applications of the resection techniques discussed above. Patients with lesions containing high grade dysplasia or intraepithelial carcinoma must be examined at 6 months and 12 month intervals due to the higher risk of recurrent and invasive neoplasia. Endoscopic ablation remains a viable option for residual neoplasia after endoscopic resection or when resection is not possible. Ablation without resection is inferior to resection techniques because it does not provide pathologic information and is generally less effective in terms of neoplasia recurrence. Argon plasma coagulation is the most common method of endoscopic ablation in the colon and rectum and most information about its use is based on small case series and limited controlled trials [19–21]. In a large retrospective series of difficult polyps, approximately one of four require ablation with the argon plasma coagulator to areas of non-lifting mucosa due to prior intervention [22]. In general, meticulous resection of lesion margins provides lower recurrence rates than routine use of argon plasma coagulation at the resection margins.

48.6 Summary

Informed consent for endoscopic resection must include delayed bleeding 2–12 days after resection, perforation requiring prolonged hospitalization or surgical intervention and incomplete resection of the neoplasia. In addition, although complete endoscopic en bloc or piecemeal resection of intraepithelial cancers (T1a) with favorable histologic findings is associated with good outcomes, late recurrences of submucosal cancers have been reported infrequently and should be considered in the balance of choosing endoscopic or surgical resection. Advanced endoscopic resection techniques begin with recognition of mucosal features associated with favorable noninvasive lesions compared to those with less favorable features with a higher rate of submucosal and lymph node invasion.

Key Points

- Endoscopists should utilize high definition imaging and dye staining to recognize margins of lesions and characteristic mucosal patterns associated with invasive and noninvasive neoplasms.
- Careful endoscopic examination of the rectal vault and rectosigmoid junction requires an adequate bowel preparation, comfortable patient, and a very flexible endoscope. Addition of a clear friction-fit cap can greatly increase visibility and stability of the endoscope tip for inspection and therapy.
- Endoscopic resection is facilitated by injection of various saline-based dye

containing solution, such as indigo carmine, into the submucosal layer to delineate lesion margins and facilitate endoscopic resection.

- A non-lifting sign found when the submucosal injection does not elevate the lesion and characteristic of neoplastic invasion or scar formation due to prior interventions.
- Advanced endoscopic submucosal dissection resection techniques use colloid laden solutions injected into the submucosal layer for the initial endoscopic circumferential incision followed by submucosal dissection for complete en bloc resection, which improves histologic evaluation and reduces local recurrences.
- Endoscopic submucosal dissection is technically more challenging and associated with higher rates of bleeding and perforation compared to piecemeal endoscopic snare resection.
- Endoscopic submucosal dissection required a dedicated team willing to commit to careful patient selection, prolonged treatment sessions with meticulous attention to intra procedural details.
- Residual neoplasia found at the margins or base of endoscopic resection sites should be ablated using electrocautery such as argon plasma coagulation.
- Careful endoscopic follow-up examination in 6–12 weeks is required to assure complete early remission from neoplasia. Repeated endoscopic examinations are necessary due to late recurrences in and around the endoscopic resection site.
- Proper informed consent should always include the possibility of a surgical alternative and frank discussion of the expected number of endoscopic exams.

References

1. Quallick MR, Brown WR. Rectal perforation during colonoscopic retroflexion: a large, prospective experience in an academic center. Gastrointest Endosc. 2009;69:960–3.
2. Rotondano G, Bianco MA, Buffoli F, et al. The Cooperative Italian FLIN Study Group : prevalence and clinico-pathologic features of colorectal laterally spreading tumors. Endoscopy. 2011;43:856–61.
3. Paris Workshop Participants. The Paris endoscopic classification of superficial neoplastic lesions: esophagus, stomach, and colon. Gastrointest Endosc. 2003;58:S3–S43
4. Endoscopic Classification Review Group. Update on the Paris classification of superficial neoplastic lesions in the digestive tract. Endoscopy. 2005;37:570–8.
5. Moss A, Bourke MJ, Williams SJ, et al. Endoscopic mucosal resection outcomes and prediction of submucosal cancer from advanced colonic mucosal neoplasia. Gastroenterol. 2011;140:1909–18.
6. Hurlstone DP, Sanders DS, Cross SS, et al. Colonoscopic resection of lateral spreading tumours: a prospective analysis of endoscopic mucosal resection. Gut. 2004;53:1334–9.
7. Uraoka T, Saito Y, Matsuda T, et al. Endoscopic indications for endoscopic mucosal resection of laterally spreading tumours in the colorectum. Gut. 2006;55:1592–7.
8. Ikehara H, Saito Y, Matsuda T, et al. Diagnosis of depth of invasion for early colorectal cancer using magnifying colonoscopy. J Gastroenterol Hepatol. 2010;25:905–12.
9. Kudo S, Hirota S, Nakajima T, et al. Colorectal tumours and pit pattern. J Clin Pathol. 1994;47:880–5.
10. Katagiri A, Fu KI, Sano Y, et al. Narrow band imaging with magnifying colonoscopy as diagnostic tool for predicting histology of early colorectal neoplasia. Aliment Pharmacol Ther. 2008;27:1269–74.
11. Son HJ, Sohn DK, Hong CW, et al. Factors associated with complete local excision of small rectal carcinoid tumor. Int J Color Dis. 2013;28:57–61.
12. Chou YP, Saito Y, Matsuda T, et al. Novel diagnostic methods for early-stage squamous cell carcinoma of the anal canal successfully resected by endoscopic submucosal dissection. Endoscopy. 2009;41:E283–5.
13. Rosenberg N. Submucosal saline wheal as a safety factor in fulguration of rectal and sigmoidal polypi. Arch Surg. 1955;70:120–2.
14. Moss A, Bourke MJ, Metz, et al. A randomized double-blind trial of succinylated gelatin submucosal injection for endoscopic resection of large sessile polyps of the colon. Am J Gastroenterol. 2010;105:2375–82.

15. Holt BA, Bourke MJ. Wide field endoscopic resection for advanced colonic mucosal neoplasia: current status and future directions. Clin Gastroenterol Hepatol. 2012;10:969–79.
16. Saito Y, Uraoka T, Matsuda T, et al. Endoscopic treatment of large superficial colorectal tumors: a case series of 200 endoscopic submucosal dissections (with video). Gastrointest Endosc. 2007;66:966–73.
17. Saito Y, Fukuzawa M, Matsuda T, et al. Clinical outcome of endoscopic submucosal dissection versus endoscopic mucosal resection of large colorectal tumors as determined by curative resection. Surg Endosc. 2010;24:343–52.
18. Lee EJ, Lee JB, Choi YS, et al. Clinical risk factors for perforation during endoscopic submucosal dissection (ESD) for large sized, nonpedunculated colorectal tumors. Surg Endosc. 2012;26:1587–94.
19. Brooker JC, Saunders BP, Shah SG, et al. Treatment with argon plasma coagulation reduces recurrence after piecemeal resection of large sessile colon polyps: a randomized trial and recommendations. Gastrointest Endosc. 2002;55:371–5.
20. Regula J, Wronska E, Polkowski M, et al. Argon plasma coagulation after piecemeal polypectomy of sessile colorectal adenomas: long-term follow-up study. Endoscopy. 2003;35:212–8.
21. Mannath J, Subramanian V, Singh R, et al. Polyp recurrence after endoscopic mucosal resection of sessile and flat colonic adenomas. Dig Dis Sci. 2011; 56:2389–95.
22. Buchner AM, Guarner-Argente C, Ginsberg GG. Outcomes of EMR of defiant colorectal lesions directed to an endoscopy referral center. Gastrointest Endosc. 2012;76:255–63.

Open Surgical Management of Rectal Cancer

49

Ahmed Z. Janjua, Brendan J. Moran, and Richard J. Heald

49.1 Introduction

The most significant advance in the treatment of rectal cancer has been the standardization of rectal cancer surgery. A good quality MRI provides a road map for surgical planning and the selective use of neoadjuvant treatment where necessary. These decisions are often difficult in complex scenarios and generally best made in a Multidisciplinary Team (MDT) setting. The Surgeon should meet and examine the patient before discussing treatment planning at the MDT. “Decisions are therefore more important than actual incisions” [1].

The optimal surgical treatment involves Total Mesorectal Excision (TME) with the aim of achieving R0 resection (all margins of the excised specimen free of tumor at Histology). MRI can visualize the mesorectum and can predict if the Circumferential Resection Margin (CRM) is clear of the mesorectal fascia or “threatened” in which case TME alone will not suffice. Challenging decisions have to be made in the low rectum i.e. below the level of the levators where an Abdominoperineal Excision (APE) may be more appropriate if sphincter preservation is not possible or will lead to a poor functional outcome. To achieve an R0 resection in the ultra-low rectal neoplasm where an APE is contemplated it may be necessary to dissect in the intersphincteric plane, or an Extralevator plane-ELAPE for tumors involving the sphincters or levators.

The principles of TME surgery are based on knowledge of the anatomical structures and their relationship within the pelvis, adequate three-dimensional dynamic traction and hemostasis. These principles provide an optimal view so that precise sharp diathermy dissection can be carried out. The principles are the same whether the surgical approach is open, laparoscopic or robotic.

There are two main open operations discussed here for treatment of rectal cancer, namely Anterior Resection and Abdominoperineal Excision.

49.2 Preoperative Measures

The rectal neoplasm should be assessed by the operating surgeon for fixity and tumor height (distance from the lower edge of the tumor to the anal verge) should be measured using a rigid sigmoidoscope. It may be helpful to repeat this under sedation at colonoscopy when biopsies are taken and the rest of the colon assessed as up to 4 % may have a synchronous colonic neoplasm. Occasionally it may be necessary to perform an Examination under Anesthesia (EUA).

A.Z. Janjua, FCS, FRCSI, FRCSI (GENSURG)
B.J. Moran, FRCSI, MCh, FRCS (✉)
Department of Surgery, Hampshire Hospitals Foundation Trust, Basingstoke, Hampshire, UK
e-mail: moran820@btinternet.com

R.J. Heald, CBE, MChir, FRCS
Department of Surgery, Pelican Cancer Foundation, Basingstoke, Hampshire, UK

H.R.H. Patel et al. (eds.), *Pelvic Cancer Surgery: Modern Breakthroughs and Future Advances*,
DOI 10.1007/978-1-4471-4258-4_49, © Springer-Verlag London 2015

Synchronous tumors and polyps should be excluded at Colonoscopy or CT Colonography. A staging CT thorax, abdomen and pelvis and pelvic MRI is mandatory and should be discussed at the MDT.

Co-morbidities such as Diabetes, Hypertension, cardiac and pulmonary conditions should be optimized and appropriate post-operative critical care facilities should be arranged. Informed consent should be obtained for a temporary or a permanent stoma in a patient planned for anterior resection and a permanent stoma and type of reconstruction envisaged in patients in whom an APE is planned. Patient should also be informed of possible complications such as anastomotic leakage, hemorrhage and possibility of sexual and bladder dysfunction. In the female patient the possible need for oophorectomy or en bloc hysterectomy if required, should also be discussed. Our practice is to also consent for appendectomy [2]. It is desirable to have mechanical bowel preparation in patients having restorative rectal surgery especially if a defunctioning ileostomy is being considered as an ileostomy proximal to a loaded colon may not reduce the consequences of an anastomotic leak [3]. Our preferred method for bowel preparation in a patient having a restorative anterior resection is clear fluids orally for 48 h and oral laxatives.

Systemic antibiotic prophylaxis is instituted at induction. DVT prophylaxis is instituted using a combination of pharmacological and mechanical measures.

49.3 Operative Steps

Position

The Lithotomy-Trendelenburg position provides appropriate access to both the abdomen and the perineum and also allows for an assistant to be positioned between the legs. Good light is essential and it may need to be repositioned and refocused from time to time to enlighten the deep recesses of the pelvis. Some surgeons prefer to have a headlight to facilitate adequate visibility.

EUA, Incision and Laparotomy

The patient position is checked and a rectal examination (supplemented with a vaginal examination in a female patient) is performed.

A long vertical midline incision gives adequate exposure. A systematic inspection of the abdominal cavity should then be carried out and the sequence of the operative steps planned. If a low anterior resection is planned it is the authors' preference to mobilize the splenic flexure as a first step and hence reduce the risk of tension or compromise of the anastomotic blood supply [4].

Splenic Flexure Mobilization

The sigmoid colon is lifted forwards, and to the right, by the assistant standing on the patient's right side revealing the white line of Toldt which is divided with diathermy towards the splenic flexure. A plane is then developed in the left upper quadrant between the colon and the gonadal vessels and Gerota's fascia. If the spleen is not adherent to the diaphragm a moist pack placed behind the spleen facilitates splenic flexure mobilization. The omentum is then retracted anteriorly, and to the patients left, and a bloodless plane between the transverse colon and omentum is developed. The dissection continues using diathermy and dynamic traction taking precaution not to avulse any fibrous attachments to the splenic capsule which are best taken down with precise sharp diathermy dissection. Access for this part of the procedure is best while standing in between the patient's legs.

Ligation of the Inferior Mesenteric Artery and Inferior Mesenteric Vein

The key step in left sided colonic mobilization is identifying the fascial covering of the upper part of the mesorectal fascia and the left ureter (usually medial to the gonadal vessels and crossing the iliac bifurcation). This is facilitated by dynamic traction on the sigmoid in an anterior direction and towards the right of the patient taking precautions not to excessively pull on the sigmoid mesentery.

Once a plane has been developed at the pelvic brim, just beyond the midline, a small swab is placed behind the rectal mesentery. The sigmoid traction is then reversed and the peritoneum on the right side is incised over the swab. The swab also helps to protect the autonomic nerves at the level of the pelvic brim by displacing the colonic mesentery anteriorly. The right sided peritoneal dissection is continued in a cranial direction reaching the root of the Inferior Mesenteric Artery (IMA). The operating surgeon standing on the patient's left side then hooks their left index finger behind the IMA pedicle and left thumb in front. The peritoneal attachments are taken down to expose the IMA and to push preaortic nerve tissue off the IMA pedicle. A window is then made by incising over the peritoneum on top of the left index finger which is placed between the aorta, IMA pedicle and Inferior Mesenteric Vein (IMV). The IMA root is displayed freeing any autonomic nerves. The IMA should be clamped, divided and ligated with a transfixion suture about 2 cm from the aorta (high but not flush) to avoid trauma to preaortic autonomic nerves after checking that the ureter has not been lifted forward in this maneuver. For length and mobility of the left colon the IMV needs to be isolated and ligated high up at the inferior border of the pancreas.

Pelvic Posterior, Lateral and Anterior Dissection

Careful pelvic dissection from an oncological perspective is very important with the surgeon being conscious of the circumferential margin bearing in mind the findings of preoperative clinical and radiological assessment. It is convenient to divide the descending colon well above the tumor at this stage, the so called "division of convenience" allowing adequate traction, visibility and packing away of the small bowel. Our preferred technique is to use a large pack to wrap the caecum and small bowel and place a gauze roll inferior to the root of the mesentery. A Finochetti chest retractor with a blade under the gauze roll gives excellent views. The pelvic dissection is a dynamic process which requires three-dimensional traction by an experienced assistant. A second assistant may aid with traction but is guided by the first surgeon in terms of the direction, angle and degree of traction. The apt use of a good sucker is very helpful in pelvic dissection, not only for aspirating fluid and smoke and allowing visibility but is also useful as a retractor in the narrow pelvic spaces.

The easiest place to commence pelvic dissection is in the midline posteriorly with sharp scissors or preferably diathermy dissection identifying the plane between the back of the "Pedicle package" and the gonadal vessels, ureter and pre aortic sympathetic nerves. Dissection within this "Holy plane" will spare autonomic nerves, non-visceral presacral fat pad if present, the parietal fascia of the pelvic side wall, hypogastric plexus, vesicles and the prostate in male patients and vagina in females. The mesorectum looks like a bilobed lipoma and this can be lifted forwards with a St. Mark's (self-illuminated retractor if available) once there is sufficient space to introduce the retractor blade in the correct place behind the mesorectum. Firm traction is applied to display the fine "angel hairs" in the areolar tissue where sharp dissection should proceed in a "below" upwards, "posterior to anterior" and in a "circumferential manner" always commencing in the posterior midline and reverting back to the midline regularly. The inferior hypogastric plexuses curve forward tangentially around the surface of the mesorectum in close proximity, as do the nerves of erection (nervi erigentes) which lie more posteriorly in the same plane, as they emerge from the sacral foramina and converge to join the hypogastric nerves and form the neurovascular bundles of Walsh which should be identified and preserved. Frequent wash out with water is helpful in maintaining good visibility and our preference is water with Proflavine, both of which are cytocidal as well as allowing better views compared with equally effective Povidone-iodine solutions. As the lateral dissection progresses one or two middle rectal vessels may be encountered that will require diathermy or ligation. If bleeding is encountered leaving an adrenaline soaked swab temporarily allows clear visualization. We prefer to develop a plane just in front of Denonvillier's fascia (which lies just behind the seminal vesicles in the male) in the midline anteriorly and then carefully extending laterally to join up with the lateral dissection. The autonomic nerves lie at the outer edges of Denonvillier's fascia and are especially vulnerable at the 10 and 2 o'clock position and deserve attention and precise dissection. Denonvillier's fascia needs to be divided by sharp dissection to access the distal rectum, usually well beyond the distal edge of the tumor at this level. In the female patient it is often helpful to have a "moist swab on a stick" in the vagina to help identify the correct plane behind the vagina to avoid troublesome bleeding from venous plexuses. If bleeding is encountered control is not generally achieved until the vagina is completely mobilized off the rectum but it is worth noting the thin layer of fascia between the middle third of the rectum and vagina. It is important to avoid extending the dissection too far laterally to avoid injury to pelvic side wall vessels and autonomic nerves. The deep posterior and posterolateral dissection is then continued in front of the presacral Waldeyer's fascia avoiding inadvertent trauma to presacral veins which if traumatized may require prolonged pressure and packing to control bleeding. Sharp dissection under good vision at this stage with appropriate retraction is crucial and any attempts at blunt dissection are to be discouraged as they will disrupt the TME specimen. The dissection in the holy plane thus continues laterally and in front on the mesorectal fat surface. The Levator muscles are funnel shaped and in continuity with the external sphincter distally. Careful dissection in the TME "holy plane" leads into the intersphincteric plane (Fig. 49.1). In over 90 % of cases it is possible to extend dissection down to a clean muscle tube where a clamp can be applied beyond the lower edge of the cancer.

Partial Mesorectal Excision (High Anterior Resection and Mesorectal Transection)

Upper rectal tumors (12–15 cm from the anal verge) may not require TME and mesorectal transection 5 cm distal to the lower edge of the tumor is oncologically acceptable and decreases the risk of autonomic nerve injury and allows a higher anastomosis which is less likely to leak than the much lower anastomosis after TME. Generally a neoplasm within 12 cm of the anal verge requires a TME.

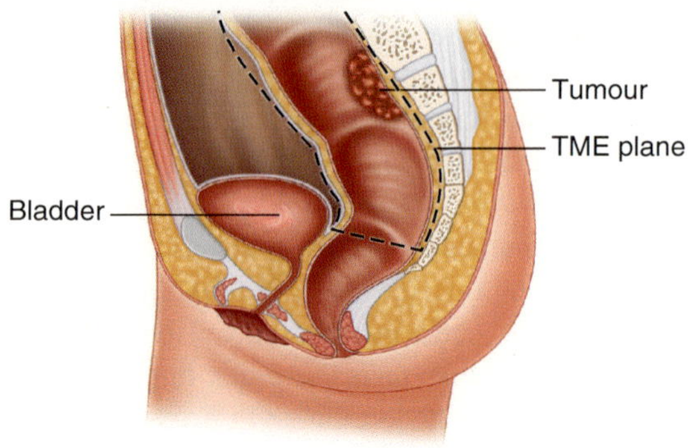

Fig. 49.1 Holy plane of TME dissection

Extended Resections

In order to achieve an R0 resection at times it is necessary to excise en bloc any adherent or involved viscera such as a loop of small bowel, uterus, ovary or the ureter.

Anastomosis

Moran Triple Stapling Technique

Once dissection has been completed well beyond the tumor a linear stapler (TA 30 or 45) is applied well below the tumor and fired but left in place to seal the muscle tube. The ano-rectal tube is then washed with a cytocidal solution such as water and Proflavine or Povidone-Iodine. A second TA 30 or 45 stapler is then placed distal to the first across the washed bowel and fired (see Fig. 49.2). The bowel is then divided with a scalpel between the two staplers. This reduces the risk of incorporating any spilled intraluminal neoplastic cells into the anastomotic staple line [5, 6]. Downward spread of rectal cancer along the muscle tube is usually not an issue and 2 cm distal clear margin beyond the lower edge of palpable cancer is adequate, though a 1 cm margin and the doughnut is acceptable in order to perform a sphincter saving operation. The TME specimen should be assessed for quality and should be a bilobed fatty pedicle package with no tears with a clear naked eye CRM. The cut

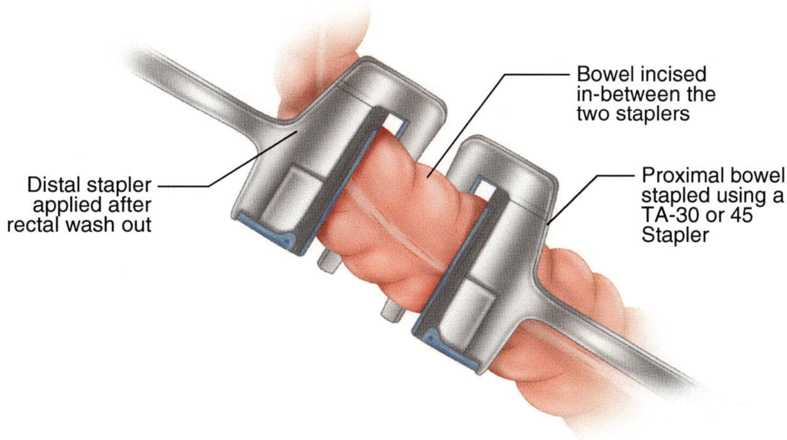

Fig. 49.2 Moran's triple stapling technique

end within the proximal stapler is inspected for clearance and if there is any doubt the staples should be opened and mucosa inspected. The distal stapler should only be taken off after clearance has been confirmed as this allows for possible application of a third stapler below the in situ distal one if the margin is not clear. The pelvic cavity should be washed and inspected for any bleeding and hemostasis secured.

When TME has been performed and a coloanal anastomosis is envisaged a neorectal reservoir has a better functional outcome then a straight end to end coloanal anastomosis. We favor an end to side technique with the side of the distal colon anastomosed to the end of the ano rectum using a circular stapler (28–31 mm head) (see Fig. 49.3). The head is detached and inserted into the lumen of the colon, spike first, after excising part of the staple line on the distal colon. The spike is pushed through the wall on the antimesenteric border, midway between the taenia coli 4–5 cm from the distal colonic end. The staple line defect is closed and the staple line is inverted with interrupted sutures.

The anorectal remnant is gently palpated. The circular staple gun is then gently inserted transanally taking care not to disrupt the transverse staple line. On occasions bimanual placement by the abdominal surgeon is required. Adequate visualization and retraction with a St Marks retractor is vital at this stage. Once happy with this position the spike on the gun is opened ideally just behind the transverse staple line. The head of the gun is brought down and engaged with the gun, the colon is checked for orientation to ensure no twists that would compromise its blood supply. The gun is closed slowly and completely until the green marker is visualized. The closed position is maintained for a minute before firing. The gun is fired and then opened again until a click is heard. The gun is slowly withdrawn without twisting and the doughnuts are checked for integrity and the distal doughnut should be sent for histology if there are concerns about clearance in a low rectal

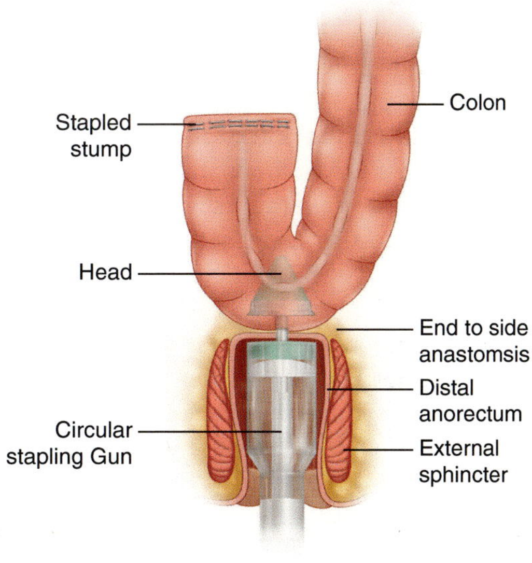

Fig. 49.3 Reconstruction end to side stapled anastomosis

cancer. The anastomosis is tested for air-leaks by filling the pelvis with water, occluding the distal colon with a soft clamp or fingers and insufflating air via the anus. A gross leak may be sutured and this may be possible transanally in very low anastomosis. Two abdominal drains (low suction closed type) are placed in the pelvis and a defunctioning stoma is created.

Defunctioning Stoma

Our practice has been to perform a defunctioning loop ileostomy for anterior resection with TME and coloanal anastomosis. A recent randomized trial reported 28 % leak rate in patients without a defunctioning stoma compared with 10 % in those with a stoma [7]. Loop stoma reduces the consequences of an anastomotic leak and the need for emergency surgery. The defunctioning stoma is reversed at 8–12 weeks postop after a contrast enema confirms no leaks from the anastomotic site.

Abdomino Perineal Excision (APE)

Historically APE was the first attempted major curative rectal resectional operation as popularized by Ernest Miles and Charles Mayo [8]. An APE is necessary if it is not possible to preserve the sphincter complex or the sphincters are of poor functional quality. Traditionally APE has been performed in the Lithotomy-Trendelenburg position with synchronous abdominal and perineal dissection. Recent reports suggest worse outcome in patients having APE compared with anterior resection [9]. This is primarily because of specimen perforation, ‘coning’ or ‘waisting’ at the level of the levators. Availability of high resolution MRI has helped to determine preoperatively if the levators or sphincters are involved [10] and it is now possible to tailor the operation accordingly to obtain an R0 resection. Hence instead of a standard APE (SAPE) an intersphincteric APE (ISAPE) or extra levator APE (ELAPE) may be more appropriate [11].

The abdominal part of an APE is similar to that in an anterior resection with the proviso that abdominal dissection should stop at the level of the origin of the levator ani. There is ongoing controversy as to the optimal position, prone or supine, of the patient for the perineal dissection [1, 10]. The supine position is optimal for Inter Sphincteric APE. The prone position for ELAPE has been popularized by Holm and facilitates better vision and access and is perhaps more suitable for teaching [12]. In ISAPE meticulous dissection is carried out in the intersphincteric plane until it joins up with the abdominal dissection and the specimen is retrieved. It leaves a far smaller defect in the perineum with less healing problems.

In ELAPE, the coccyx is generally excised for ease of access; the dissection is extrasphincteric, and extralevator, and joins up with the abdominal dissection taking the levator muscles as part of the specimen [13]. Optimal healing is achieved by pelvic floor reconstruction using either a biologic mesh or a flap [12] (See Chap. 59).

49.4 Summary

Operative management of rectal cancer is technically challenging. Successful outcome depends upon planning the appropriate operative procedure after thorough preoperative clinical, endoscopic and radiological assessment and optimization of any comorbidities. A CT scan of the thorax, abdomen and pelvis is recommended and a good quality MRI gives valuable information on pelvic anatomy, mesorectum and the potential circumferential resection margin. A thorough knowledge of anatomical structures in the confines of the pelvis, good assistance and dynamic retraction with adequate illumination makes precise sharp dissection with diathermy possible. The focus should be on obtaining a ‘TME package’ which is intact with no tears. The circumferential and longitudinal margins should be clear. For rectal cancers above 12 cm from the anal verge a mesorectal transection 5 cm distal to the lower edge of the tumor is an acceptable operation that reduces the risk of having a stoma and trauma to the autonomic nerves. The authors recommend mobilization of the splenic flexure and high ligation of the inferior mesenteric vein to achieve maximum length and avoid tension on the anastomosis. The Moran Triple stapling technique reduces the risk of tumor cell implantation at the staple line. A defunctioning stoma in patients with TME reduces the consequences of an anastomotic leak. While a majority of patients can be offered a curative anterior resection, an APE may be necessary in patients in whom the sphincters, or levators, are involved or who would prefer a permanent stoma rather than risk poor function.

Key Points

- The single most important development in treatment of Rectal Cancer has been the standardization of TME surgery
- Clinical findings, histology, CT Thorax abdomen and Pelvis and Pelvic MRI should be reviewed at an MDT prior to commencement of treatment
- Careful clinical, endoscopic and radiological assessment is required to select the appropriate procedure of sphincter preserving or Abdominoperineal Excision. Between 80 and 90 % of patients are suitable for a sphincter preserving procedure.
- All patients undergoing anterior resection with TME should be consented and marked for a stoma
- Precise sharp dissection in the "Holy Plane" is recommended
- The Surgeon should be aware of the CRM and aim to resect an intact TME specimen with clear margins
- The Inferior Mesenteric Artery should be ligated high, but not necessarily flush, with aorta
- The Inferior Mesenteric vein should be divided high, just below the inferior pancreatic border, to obtain maximum mobility
- The Moran Triple stapling technique reduces the risk of staple line implantation of cancer cells
- In patients requiring ELAPE some form of reconstruction using either a biologic mesh or a flap should be considered.

References

1. Moore TJ, Moran BJ. Precision surgery, precision terminology: the origins and meaning of ELAPE. Color Dis. 2012;14(10):1173–4.
2. Khan MN, Moran BJ. Four percent of patients undergoing colorectal cancer surgery may have synchronous appendiceal neoplasia. Dis Colon Rectum. 2007;50(11):1856–9.
3. Ulrich AB, Seiler C, Rahbari N, Weitz J, Buchler MW. Diverting stoma after low anterior resection: more arguments in favor. Dis Colon Rectum. 2009;52(3):412–8 [Randomized Controlled Trial].
4. Ludwig KA, Kosinski L. Is splenic flexure mobilization necessary in laparoscopic anterior resection? Another view. Dis Colon Rectum. 2012;55(11): 1198–200. doi:10.097/DCR.0b013e3182688011.
5. Umpleby HC, Fermor B, Symes MO, et al. Viability of exfoliated colorectal carcinoma cells. Br J Surg. 1984;71:659–63.
6. Edwards DP, Sexton R, Heald RJ, Moran BJ. Long-term results show triple stapling facilitates safe low colorectal and coloanal anastomosis and is associated with low rates of local recurrence after anterior resection for rectal cancer. Tech Coloproctol. 2007;11(1): 17–21. Epub 2007 Feb 16.
7. Matthiessen PMDP, Hallbook OMDP, Rutegard JMDP, Simert GMDP, Sjodahl RMDP. Defunctioning stoma reduces symptomatic anastomotic leakage after low anterior resection of the rectum for cancer: a randomized multicenter trial. Ann Surg. 2007;246(2): 207–14.
8. Ernest Miles W. A Method of performing abdomino-perineal excision for carcinoma of the rectum and of the terminal portion of the pelvic colon. Lancet. 1908;172(4451):1812–3.
9. Heald RJ, Chir M, Smedh RK, Kald A, Sexton R, Moran BJ. Abdominoperineal excision of the rectum—an endangered operation. Dis Colon Rectum. 1997;40(7):747–51.
10. Janjua AZ, Moran BJ. Outcomes following surgery without radiotherapy for rectal cancer. Br J Surg. 2012;99(6):878–9 (Br J Surg 2012 99 137–143).
11. English National Low Rectal Cancer Development Programme. www.lorec.nhs.uk.
12. Holm T, Ljung A, Haggmark T, et al. Extended abdominoperineal resection with gluteus maximus flap reconstruction of the pelvic floor for rectal cancer. Br J Surg. 2007;94:232–8.
13. Shihab OC, Heald RJ, Holm T, How PD, Brown G, Quirke P, et al. A pictorial description of extralevator abdominoperineal excision for low rectal cancer. Color Dis. 2012;14(10):e655–60.

50 Laparoscopic Surgical Management of Rectal Cancer

Quentin Denost, Jean-Philippe Adam, and Eric Rullier

50.1 Introduction

Colorectal cancer is the most common intestinal cancer and occurs in the rectum in about 40 % of cases. The rectal cancer incidence was estimated at 40,000 cases in US [1] and 16,000 in France in 2012. There have been significant changes in the management of rectal cancer over the past 10–15 years. A greater understanding of the disease process, more accurate radiological staging, multimodality therapeutic intervention, refined surgical techniques, and more detailed histopathological reporting have all contributed to improvements in the management and survival of patients. For rectal cancer, surgery is the principal treatment leading to cure. With the introduction of total mesorectal excision (TME) involving resection of the fatty tissue around the rectum, local control and survival rates have improved [2]. Moreover, the Dutch rectal cancer trial showed that pelvic radiation before surgery resulted in a statistically significant reduction in local recurrence rate and improvement in overall survival compared with surgery alone [3–5]. In a multidisciplinary approach, input on the surgical management of rectal cancer should occur before beginning any treatment pathway for rectal cancer.

Q. Denost, MD • J.-P. Adam, MD
E. Rullier, MD (✉)
Colorectal Surgery, Sainte-Andre Hospital,
Bordeaux University Hospital, Bordeaux, France
e-mail: eric.rullier@chu-bordeaux.fr

The laparoscopic approach has been widely accepted for colon cancer [6–10] while it is still challenging for rectal cancer due to the difficulties of pelvic exposure and low rectal dissection with the goal of nerves and sphincter preservation [11–14]. A few studies have suggested advantages of the laparoscopic surgery for rectal cancer [8, 15–19]. However, there is currently no professional consensus recommendation on indications for laparoscopic rectal cancer.

50.2 Preoperative Evaluation and Treatment

Patients' Evaluation

History and physical examination remains the cornerstone of the preoperative assessment aiding the clinician in determining the necessary preoperative investigations to assess perioperative risk stratification (ASA score, Possum score). Preoperative radiotherapy, BMI and sex of patient should also be considered by the clinician before laparoscopic rectal excision due to the operative difficulties for pelvic dissection and rectal stapling. The role of laparoscopy has not been clearly defined specifically in cases following neoadjuvant radiochemotherapy and obesity. Firstly, population with preoperative radiotherapy deserves greater attention because an irradiated pelvis results in slightly more

DOI 10.1007/978-1-4471-4258-4_50, © Springer-Verlag London 2015

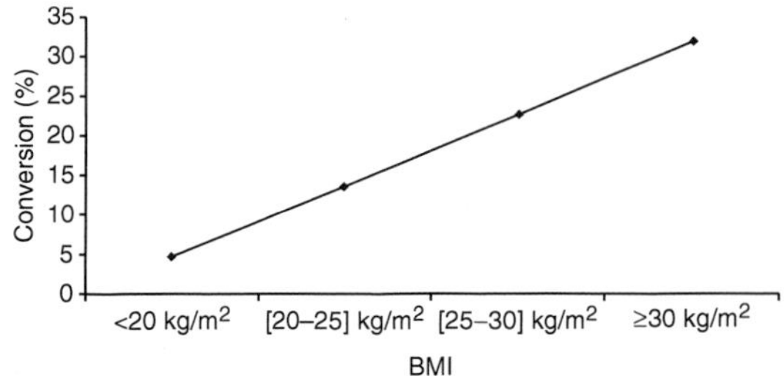

Fig. 50.1 Conversion (%) according to body mass index (From Denost et al. [27]; used with permission

postoperative complications [20, 21] and may induce some technical difficulties to the pelvic dissection. Pelvic fibrosis makes rectal exposure, anatomical landmarks identification and rectal transection more difficult. Our surgical team assessed recently the impact of preoperative radiotherapy on the feasibility of laparoscopic rectal excision with sphincter preservation for rectal cancer. We observed that long course preoperative radiochemotherapy did not modify the risk of conversion and overall and surgical morbidity, especially the rate of anastomotic leakage, after laparoscopic rectal excision for rectal cancer [22]. Secondly, obesity has been associated with increased technical difficulties and perioperative complications in colorectal surgery, both after open and laparoscopic procedures [23–26]. The impact of obesity has been measured mainly for colon resection but not specifically for rectal excision. Our surgical team published recently both short and long term outcomes after laparoscopic rectal cancer excision according to BMI [27]. We observed that BMI affected the technical feasibility of laparoscopic procedure but not the oncologic outcomes. Indeed conversion increased with a higher BMI but without increasing surgical morbidity (Fig. 50.1). Finally, quality of surgery, recurrence and survival were not influenced by BMI after laparoscopic rectal excision. Thus, obesity is not a contra indication of laparoscopic approach for rectal surgery. Patients not suitable for a laparoscopic approach were those with preoperative fixed tumors into adjacent pelvic organ (T4 tumor), or anesthesiologist contra indications.

Tumor Staging

The TNM system, as defined by the American Joint Committee on Cancer, is the most commonly used system and is based on the depth of local tumor invasion (T stage), the extent of regional lymph node involvement (N stage), and the presence of distant metastasis (M stage) [28].

Local Tumor Staging

As part of a full physical examination, rectosigmoidoscopy should be performed in conjunction with a digital rectal examination to determine the length of anal canal, the distance of the lesion from the anal verge and the anal ring, tumor mobility, and to assess tumor position in relation to the sphincter complex.

Clinical staging of the primary tumor by endorectal ultrasound (EUS) or dedicated high resolution rectal MRI should be performed. Circumferential resection margin (CRM), defined as the shortest distance between the rectal tumor (including noncontiguous tumor) and the mesorectal fascia (TME) is considered positive when it is ≤1 mm. EUS and MRI are almost equivalent for accurate measurement of the depth of extramural tumor spread or nodal status involvement. Demonstration of accurate measurement in predicting CRM status with MRI compared with the histopathological reference standard in the MERCURY Study enabled accurate preoperative prognostication [29]. Thus, preoperative MRI are now often preferred to EUS. However, the accuracy of radiological restaging post-CRT is impaired due to the difficulty in differentiating fibrotic or reactive tissue from residual [30]. Endoscopic ultrasonography has been dismissed outright as a restaging [31–33]. Diffusion-weighted MR [34, 35] and fusion positron emission/computed tomography [36] have shown some promising results but larger scale studies are needed.

Distant Metastases Staging

The liver and lungs are the most frequent sites of metastatic disease from rectal cancer [37, 38]. Preoperative chest, abdomen, and pelvis CT scan should be routinely performed before the surgical resection of rectal cancer to detect and assess local

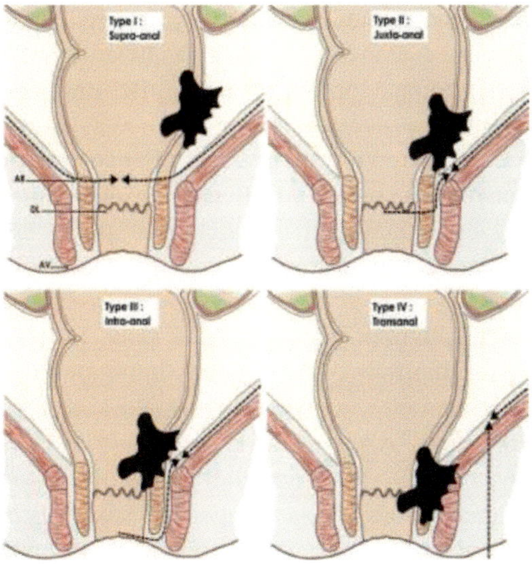

Fig. 50.2 Surgical classification of low rectal cancer (From Rullier et al. [43])

organ penetration or synchronous metastases, which may require a change in the treatment strategy.

Preoperative Treatment

The preoperative management of high rectal cancer is very close to the management of colon cancer. No preoperative treatment is recommended except for T4 tumor. The patients with T3, T4 or N+ mid or low rectal cancer should receive long-course preoperative radiotherapy (45 Gy in 25 fractions during 5 weeks) in association with concomitant chemotherapy in first and fifth weeks [39]. The chemotherapy comprised a continuous infusion of fluorouracil (5FU: 350 mg/m^2/day during 5 days) in association with leucovorin (20 mg/m^2/day in bolus just before the infusion of fluorouracil) [40]. Some T2 lesions close to the anal canal could also receive neoadjuvant treatment in order to facilitate ultralow sphincter preservation [41]. High rectal tumors (>10 cm from the anal verge) do not receive neoadjuvant treatment. Since 2006, patients with mid rectal cancer and a circumferential margin >3 mm at the magnetic resonance imaging could be operated by TME surgery alone [39]. Surgery was performed 6 weeks after the end of radiotherapy. The ongoing French multicenter GRECCAR six trial is evaluating the optimal interval between irradiation and surgery (between 7 and 11 weeks) [42].

Surgical Strategies

Surgical Management of High and Mid Rectal Cancer

For high and mid rectal tumors, the rectum was transected 5 cm below the lower edge of the lesion [20]. Partial mesorectum excision is recommended for high rectal cancer and Total mesorectum excision is recommended for mid rectal cancer with stapled colorectal anastomosis.

Surgical Management of Low Rectal Cancer

Management of low rectal cancer is very different of high and medium rectal cancer. This management is composed by the three following steps: firstly, classification of low rectal cancer in four types [43], secondly, standardization of surgery in four operations, and finally, anticipation of surgery before and decision after neoadjuvant treatment.

The Surgical Classification of low rectal cancer separates patients with rectal cancer below 6 cm from the anal verge in four groups according to the location of the tumor from the anal sphincter (surgical anal canal) (Fig. 50.2):

- Type I: Supra anal tumors: lesions located >1 cm from the anal ring
- Type II: Juxta anal tumors: lesions located ≤1 cm from the anal ring
- Type III: Intra anal tumors: lesions with infiltration of the internal anal sphincter
- Type IV: Trans anal tumors: lesions with infiltration of the external anal sphincter or levator ani muscles

Standardization of surgery defines four surgical procedures, each dedicated to the four types of low rectal cancer:

- Type I: Coloanal anastomosis (CAA), the internal sphincter is preserved
- Type II: Partial intersphincteric resection (pISR)
- Type III: Total intersphincteric resection (tISR)
- Type IV: Abdominoperineal excision (APR)

Classification of low rectal cancer is part of the initial staging of the tumor and is performed by consensus including digital examination by the surgeon, endorectal ultrasound and MRI. It must be performed before neoadjuvant treatment. Rectal palpation is performed with and without voluntary anal contraction to check the exact distance of the tumor from the top of the anal canal. Examination under anesthesia is sometimes necessary, especially when the anal canal is involved or in case of fixed tumors. Rigid rectoscopy informs on tumor location and on distance between the tumor and the dentate line. Endorectal ultrasound and magnetic resonance imaging are necessary for tumor staging and to confirm clinical examination, in term of relation and distance between the tumor and the anal sphincter. Preservation of the intersphincteric plane at MRI is the key point to differentiate types I, II and III low rectal cancers suitable for conservative surgery, from type IV treated by APR.

The advantages of this classification are to facilitate decision making between sphincter preservation and APR in low rectal cancer, in order to propose more sphincter preservation by using techniques of partial and total intersphincteric resection. This classification will allow to assess more homogeneously treatment of low rectal cancer and outcomes between institutions. Finally, it could also be used to convert an APR to a sphincter saving procedure in case of downstaging after irradiation.

Organ Preservation for Rectal Cancer

Rectal excision is the standard treatment of rectal carcinoma. Local excision removing the tumor transanally and leaving in place both the rectum and the mesorectum is a common option at present only in some early rectal cancers. Those are T1 tumors infiltrating the superficial part of the submucosa (Sm1). For the other tumors, i.e. T1Sm2–3, T2, T3 and T4 rectal cancers, rectal excision is conventionally the only chance of cure for the patient. A new concept is to propose local excision in good responders after neoadjuvant chemotherapy in locally advanced rectal cancer. This strategy is called organ preservation. The preliminary results of the ACOSOG US trial suggest feasibility in T2 low rectal cancer with 44 % of pathologic complete response and low surgical morbidity [44]. Long-term results are not yet available. The ongoing French GRECCAR 2 trial (end of inclusion in January 2013) aims to clarify if a T2 tumor could be include in this strategy [45].

50.3 Perioperative Management

Perioperative management involves dieticians, nurses, surgeons and anesthesiologists. All patients had a preoperative bowel preparation. When an ostomy is a consideration, potential site of the ostomy should be marked preoperatively to ensure optimal fitting of the device. Postoperative analgesia was ensured by intravenous morphine chlorhydrate (patient-controlled administration) at a maximum of 4 mg per hour with a single dose of 1 mg and free interval of 10 min for 1–2 days. Postoperative protocol involves nasogastric tube removal at the end of the surgical procedure, fluids intake on postoperative day 1, oral solid food at postoperative day 2, and pelvic drain and catheter removal on postoperative day 3. Postoperative evaluation of C-reactive protein (CRP) is systematically realized at day 3. A CT-scan is performed when abscess or anastomotic leakage is clinically (fever, abdominal pain, anal, vaginal or drain purulent output) or biologically (CRP >100 mg/L) suspected.

50.4 Surgical Technique of Laparoscopic Rectal Surgery

Installation

The patient is positioned in lithotomy position. The surgeon stands to the right of the patient and the monitor is located in his line of vision at the left of the patient. The camera assistant and the scrub nurse stand to the right of the patient, respectively at the left and at the right of the surgeon. A second assistant stands between the legs of the patient. The operative technique was achieved by a five-port procedure (Fig. 50.3). The laparoscopic procedure was standardized:

Step 1: Vascular Ligation

The first step of the procedure consists in grasping the inferior mesenteric vein, which correspond to the first anatomical landmark, and dissecting adhesions between the vein and the proximal jejunum. The primary dissection of the vein from the posterior attachments is particularly useful to identify the plane of dissection of the told fascia, and to dissect the upper border of the inferior mesenteric artery. This step avoids pitfalls during the artery dissection. In order to facilitate the inferior mesenteric artery (IMA) ligation, the second anatomical landmark is the presacral area. Once the vein is completely free, the dissection continues by the exposition of the presacral area using a grasper placed on the sigmoid mesentery giving an optimal view of the promontory. An incision of the peritoneum is performed exactly 2 cm in front of the promontory allowing the beginning of the dissection of the upper part of the mesorectum, which is also the distal part of the IMA. To insure the good plane of dissection, the 'angel hairs' of the mesorectal space are opened and the proximal mesorectum is dissected posteriorly on a few centimeters. The objective is to connect by an horizontal incision the area of the proximal part of the mesorectum and the area located under the vein already dissected. This step allows identifying the artery exactly 2 cm from the aorta in order to preserve the sympathetic nerves and facilitate the end of the dissection of the IMA by using an accurate instrument (Fig. 50.4a). The IMA must be completely free before performing ligation or transection. A various kind of ligation can be used such as clips, suture or modern devices. Thermal fusion can be used in vessels no more than 7 mm without calcification, but requires to stop any tension of the artery before transecting to avoid incomplete sealing. After IMA ligation, the next step is left colonic mobilization.

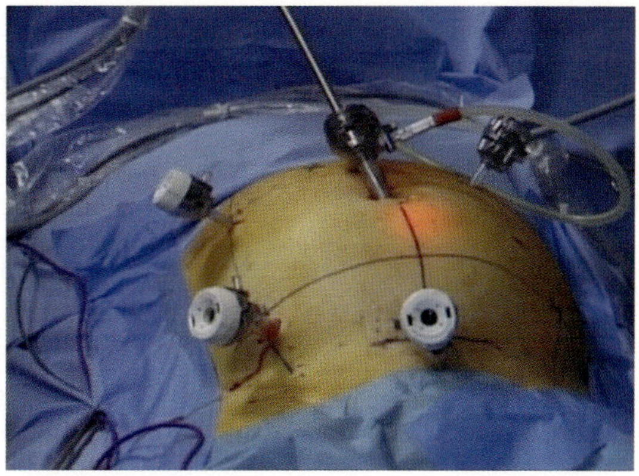

Fig. 50.3 Laparoscopic port sites

Step 2: Mobilization of the Left Colon and the Splenic Flexure

Both surgeon and assistant push up the mesentery to dissect the told fascia via a medial approach. The dissection using scissors begins in the left iliac fossa, preserving the gonadal blood vessels and the left ureter. The advantage of the medial approach is an optimal view and exposure of the planes of dissection. The told fascia dissection is continued as high as possible, especially in front of the Gerota's fascia and close to the splenic flexure. During this step, the IMV is preserved and served as potential landmark to identify the pancreas. By dissecting from the posterior approach, the incision of the transverse mesentery permits to identify the pancreas and to enter in the lesser sac. In some difficult cases, the

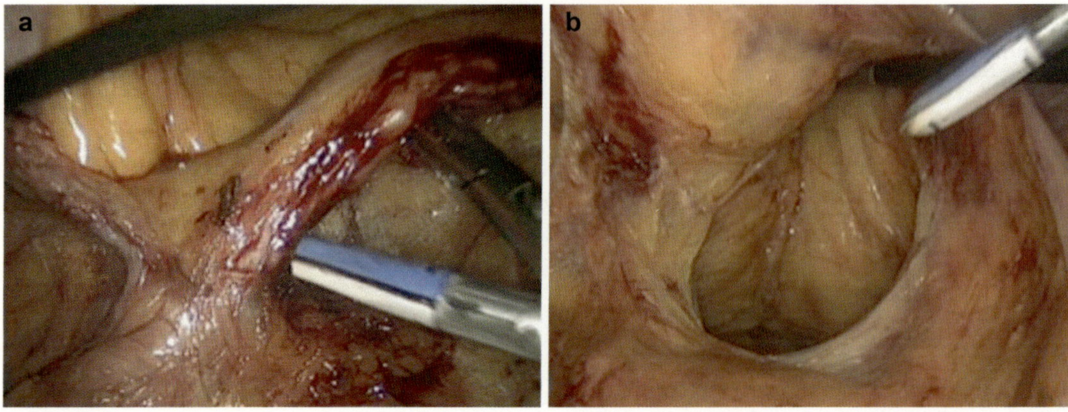

Fig. 50.4 Laparoscopic steps of rectal excision. (**a**) High ligation of the inferior mesenteric artery; (**b**) extra-fascial dissection of the mesorectum

complete dissection of the terminal part of the IMV improves the view of the pancreas giving the plane to open the lesser sac. The complete anterior dissection of the pancreas makes the transverse mesentery totally free and finishes the medial approach. The IMV is then transected close to the pancreas, or 5 cm below if a left transverse colic artery is visualized in this area, to avoid colonic ischemia. The last part of colonic mobilization is the lateral mobilization. By pushing the sigmoid on the right, a peritoneal incision is performed along the left border of the sigmoid, including the rectosigmoid area. The division of the lateral peritoneum continues along the descending colon and finishes at the splenic flexure. In order to avoid splenic decapsulation, adhesions of the greater omentum and the splenocolic ligament must be dissected. The medial approach greatly facilitates this last step of mobilization.

Step 3: Dissection of the Mesorectum

The first step of the dissection of the mesorectum is the high posterior dissection. This extra facial anatomical dissection of the mesorectum can be performed by using scissors and monopolar coagulation, harmonic scalpel (Ultracision^{TM}, Ethicon Endosurgery, Cincinnati, Ohio, USA) or thermal fusion (Ligasure^{TM}, Covidien, Mansfield, Massachusetts, USA). The rectum exposure is achieved by pulling up vertically the rectum using a supra-pubic grasper. The anatomical landmarks are the retrorectal space medially, and the hypogastric nerves laterally. The dissection begins medially 2 cm in front of the sacral promontory and continues caudally and posteriorly at 45 °C along the presacral area, using scissors. The good plane of dissection is located between the mesorectum (yellow tissue) and the presacral fascia (gray tissue). The medial dissection must be stopped 10 cm below the promontory at the level of the retroscral ligament corresponding to the fusion between the presacral and the mesorectal fascias. Adequate tension to the tissues facilitates dissection. Non-traumatic instruments are used without grasping the mesorectum to preserve its integrity. This medial posterior dissection avoids injuries of both superior hypogastric plexus and hypogastric nerves.

The second step is the right lateral dissection after identification of the hypogastric nerves. A cephalic traction of the superior hypogastric plexus at the sacral promontory level induces tension of the hypogastric nerves, which can be visualized as a "fiber" through the soft pelvic tissues or below the peritoneum. An incision of the peritoneum along the right side of the rectum is performed down to the anterior reflection. Lateral pelvic dissection from the hypogastric nerve to the presacral area is then performed connecting the previous medial high posterior dissection. After full right lateral mesorectum mobilization, the same dissection is performed on the left side.

The third step consists in the high anterior dissection. Seminal vesicles in men and cervix in female are the landmarks, which need to be identified. The upper rectum is grasped with cephalic and left lateral traction giving a tension to the opposite anterior and right sides of the rectum. A peritoneal incision is performed anteriorly 2 cm above the Douglass pouch and connects the lateral right incision performed during the previous step. Distal dissection from 1 to 2 cm of right anterior peritoneum allows discovering the right seminal vesicle, which must be completely isolated. In order to preserve both small efferent nerves along the vesicles and the mesorectum which is very thin and fragile at this level, the dissection must be lead close to the seminal vesicles. In female, pelvic exposure is facilitated by uterus fixation to the anterior abdominal wall by using a supra-pubic stitch. The anterior incision of the peritoneum permits to identify the cervix and then to connect the high lateral dissection.

The fourth step is low lateral dissection using the inferior hypogastric plexus as anatomical landmark. The objective is to transect the lateral ligament of the rectum. By following dissection along a virtual line between the seminal vesicle and the hypogastric nerve, the pelvic plexus appears as a 2–3 cm triangle located along the lateral sidewall of the pelvis. To free the mesorectum from the pelvic plexus, some attachments due to vessels and nerves coming from the plexus to the mesorectum have to be cutted. To prevent from plexus injury, perfect hemostasis and adequate traction of the tissue are essential.

Then, the rectum is pulled up for optimal visualization of the low pelvis. After incision of the rectosacral ligament, dissection is continued distally and posteriorly along the levator ani muscle. Presacral nerves (S2–S4) are identified at the mid part of the sacrum and preserved by dissecting close to the mesorectum. For a sphincter saving procedure, the dissection is performed until the top of the anal canal. For an APR, dissection is stopped earlier at the coccyx to avoid disconnection between tumor adhesion and levator ani muscles.

The end of the TME procedure consists in dissecting anteriorly and caudally taking care not to injure Denonvilliers' fascia, the seminal vesicles, the prostate and the vagina. This last step is particularly challenging in men. The oncologic low anterior dissection must be performed in front of the Denonvilliers' fascia, which can be considered as the anterior part of the mesorectum. Care is taken to do an anatomical dissection which preserves both the Denonvilliers' fascia and the anterior mesorectum, which needs to be removed together to achieve a radical oncologic laparoscopic TME excision.

Step 4: Rectal Transection and Reconstruction

For high and mid rectal cancer, the rectum is transected 5 cm below the lower edge of the lesion [20], achieving respectively a partial or a total mesorectal excision. After full mobilization of the rectum, pushing on the perineum facilitates rectal division. Stapler is introduced by the 10 mm supra-pubic port (Fig. 50.5a) [46]. The specimen is then removed from a supra-pubic 6 cm incision. A wound protector is necessary to decrease risks of port-site and local recurrences. Reconstruction with a colonic pouch or a straight colorectal anastomosis is performed laparoscopically (Fig. 50.5b). A colonic pouch is performed if the rectal stump is shorter than 5 cm. The quality of the anastomosis is checked by the completeness of the doughnuts and by a transanal air test.

In low rectal cancer, a low colorectal stapled anastomosis could be very difficult to perform laparoscopically, especially for men, narrow pelvis, and bulky tumors. The alternative is to perform a manual coloanal anastomosis instead of stapled anastomosis which can compromise oncologic margins and anastomosis healing. For very low tumors, intersphincteric resection is used to achieve sphincter preservation with safe distal margin [47]. The low pelvic dissection during the laparoscopic coloanal procedure can be achieved either by the laparoscopic approach or by the perineal approach. In both approaches, rectal transection is performed transanally. The anal canal is exposed by a self-holding retractor (Lone Star Retractor®, Lone Star Medical Products Inc., Houston, TX). The specimen is removed through the anal canal except for thick

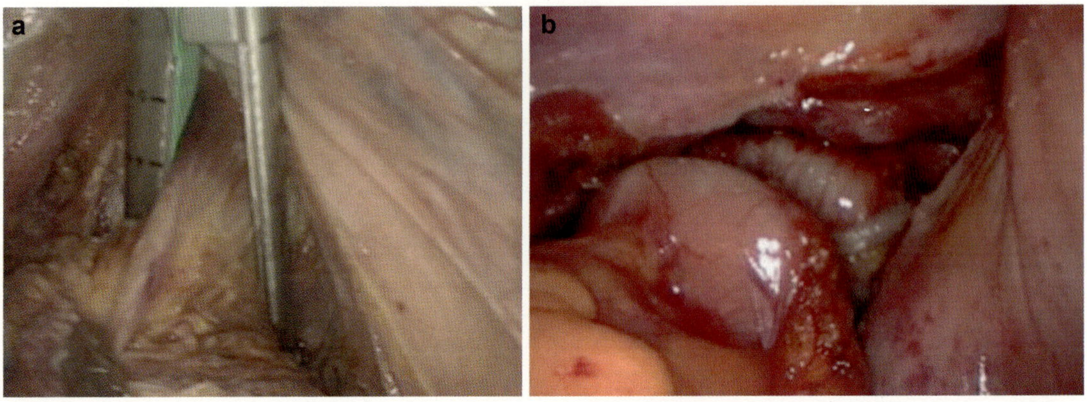

Fig. 50.5 Colorectal anastomosis. (**a**) Supra-pubic stapler; (**b**) circular colorectal anastomosis

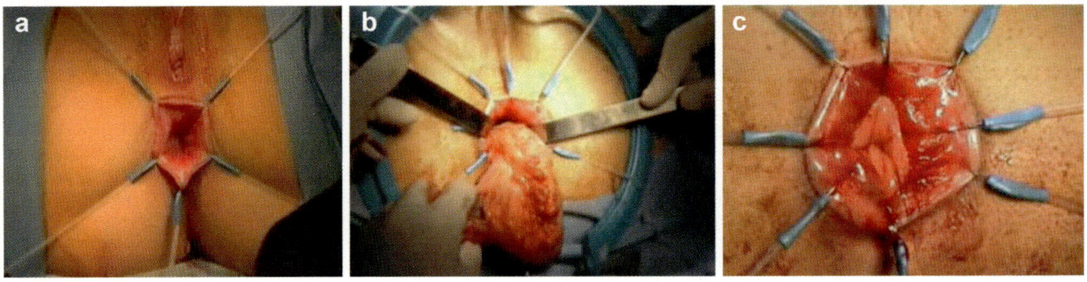

Fig. 50.6 Perineal step. (**a**) Perineal exposure; (**b**) transanal specimen extraction; (**c**) hand-sewn coloanal anastomosis

mesentery or anal stricture, and a hand-sewn side-to-end coloanal anastomosis is performed (Fig. 50.6). For the first laparoscopic approach, surgical procedure was previously described. For the first perineal approach, instead of doing high rectal dissection laparoscopically followed by dissection of the low rectum through the perineum, the procedure begins by a transanal perineal step [48]. A gauze was introduced into the rectum to limit the risk of seeding. The rectum was transected at least 1 cm below the lower edge of the tumor. Then, rectum was closed transanally by suture to avoid intraoperative tumor spillage and facilitate exposure. The perineal dissection of the low rectum was performed transanally along the levator ani muscles. The plane of dissection began into the intersphincteric plane and continued posteriorly to the sheath of the pelvic floor for at least 5 cm. The sheath of the levator ani muscles, which was usually thickened due to irradiation, was then transected to join the plane of the abdominal dissection. Thus, the perineal dissection permitted to dissect as far as possible from the distal rectal wall, where the mesorectum is usually lacking, and therefore to maintain optimal distance between the tumor and surgical resection. The perineal dissection was conducted posteriorly and anteriorly up to 10 cm from the anal verge. It was easier in female than in male due to the shorten length of the anal canal in the former. After the perineal dissection of the distal rectum, a conventional laparoscopic procedure is performed. Surgery is usually easier and faster due to previous low rectal dissection. The primary transanal perineal step represents an interesting surgical alternative option to avoid problems associated with stapling and to decrease the rate of conversion to an open procedure.

A presacral suction drain and a temporary loop ileostomy are used in all TME procedures. The loop ileostomy is closed 8–12 weeks after surgery.

50.5 Quality of Surgery

Criteria of surgical resection quality for rectal cancer included circumferential resection margin [49], number of lymph nodes harvested and Quirke's graded assessment of completeness of mesorectal excision protocol [4].

- Grade 3: Good, intact mesorectum with only minor irregularities of a smooth mesorectal surface and no defect deeper than 5 mm;
- Grade 2: Moderate, moderate bulk to the mesorectum but irregularity of the mesorectal surface, moderate coning of the specimen towards the distal margin;
- Grade 1: Poor, little bulk to the mesorectum with defects down into the muscularis propria and/or very irregular circumferential resection margin.

50.6 Outcomes of Laparoscopic Surgery in Rectal Cancer

For two decades, the outcomes of laparoscopic surgery for rectal cancer have been well documented. Data from high standard of evidence studies are available to validate its feasibility, safety and oncologic validity.

Operative Outcomes

Laparoscopic resection for rectal cancer is more time-consuming than open rectal resection, but associated with lower blood loss based on the main randomized controlled trials (Table 50.1) [17, 18, 50–54]. Conversion to open surgery rates range from 1.2 to 34 % [17, 18, 50–53]. Male sex, higher body mass index, stapled anastomosis and intraoperative rectal fixity are the main factors of conversion [27, 51, 55]. With regard to the results of the CLASICC trial, conversion has a negative impact on postoperative morbidity. In our institution, further analysis revealed that men with a stapled anastomosis had a threefold higher rate of conversion than all other patients (34 % vs 11 %; P<.001) [55]. We recommend not to begin experience in laparoscopic TME in difficult cases i.e. men with high BMI, bulky or fixed tumors, to avoid high risk of conversion to open procedure. Inexperienced surgeons in TME should prefer the laparoscopic approach in favorable cases, i.e. for high rectal cancer, mid rectal cancer in women and low rectal cancer treated by APR. Laparoscopic surgery for mid rectal tumors in men and low rectal cancer treated with sphincter preservation should be reserved for experienced colorectal surgeons.

Postoperative Outcomes

Post operative mortality (from 1 to 5 %) [17, 18, 50, 51, 53] and postoperative morbidity (from 6 to 40 %) [17, 18, 50–55] rates associated with the laparoscopic procedure are similar to those for the open approach. Rates of anastomotic leakage are similar between open and laparoscopic rectal resection [17, 18, 50–54]. However, with regard to the results of the CLASICC trial, conversion has a negative impact on postoperative morbidity. Patients requiring conversion had the highest rate of complications with a doubling of anastomotic leakage, transfusions, hospital mortality and prolonged hospital stay [51]. Therefore, particular attention must be paid in selecting patients for the laparoscopic approach. Regarding the postoperative rehabilitation, most of the studies suggest short-term benefits of the laparoscopic surgery with a reduced length of hospital stay and an improved postoperative comfort with less pain and decreased consumption of analgesics [17, 18, 50–54]. Quality of life following laparoscopic surgery has also been assessed. In the randomized trial of Andresson et al. the health-related quality of life was similar within 12 months after open and laparoscopic procedure [56].

Oncologic Outcomes

The oncologic validity of the laparoscopic approach has been evaluated in the main randomized studies (Table **50.2**). Surgical quality does not differ between open and laparoscopic procedures. The number of lymph nodes resected and

Table 50.1 Main operative and postoperative outcomes from randomized controlled trials comparing laparoscopic versus open surgery for rectal cancer

		Patients	Surgical time		Blood loss		Conversion	Overall morbidity		Anastomotic leakage		Wound infection		Hospital stay	
Study	Year	N	(min)	P value	(ml)	P value	(%)	(%)	P value	(%)	P value	(%)	P value	(Days)	P value
Zhou et al. [54]	2004	L=82	120	0.051	20	<0.050	NA	6.1	0.016	1.1	NA	NA	NA	8.1	0.001
		O=82	106		92			12.4		3.4				13.3	
Guillou et al. [51]	2005	L=253	180	NA	NA		34	18	NA	10	NA	13	NA	11	NA
(CLASICC trial)		O=128	135					14		7		12		13	
Braga et al. [50]	2007	L=83	262	<0.001	150	<0.001	7.2	28.9	0.180	9.6	0.970	7.2	0.170	10.0	0.004
		O=85	209		350			40		10.6		15.3		13.6	
Lujan et al. [17]	2009	L=101	193	0.020	128	<0.001	7.9	33.7	0.956	6	0.237	0	0.243	8.2	0.106
		O=103	172		234			33.0		5		1.9		9.9	
Ng et al. [18]	2009	L=76	213	<0.001	280	0.338	30.3	30.3	NA	1	NA	6.6	NA	8.4	0.013
		O=77	154		337			31.2		3		11.7		10	
Kang et al. [52]	2010	L=170	244	<0.001	200	0.006	1.2	21.2	0.603	1.2	0.499	1.2	0.020	8.0	0.056
(COREAN trial)		O=170	197		217			23.5		0		6.5		9.0	
van der Paas et al. [53]	2013	L=699	240	<0.001	200	<0.001	17	40	0.424	10	0.462	4	0.604	8	0.036
(COLOR II trial)		O=345	188		400			37		13		5		9	

Values are expressed as mean or median as appropriate
L laparoscopic group, *N* number, *NA* not available, *O* open group

Table 50.2 Main oncologic outcomes from randomized controlled trials comparing laparoscopic versus open surgery for rectal cancer

		Patients	Follow-up	Positive CRM		Lymph nodes collected		Local recurrence		OS		DFS	
Study	Year	N	(mo)	(%)	P value	N	P value	(%)	P value	(%)	P value	(%)	P value
Braga et al. [50]	2007	L=83	53.6	1.3	NA	12.7	NA	4 % at 3 years	0.970	NA		NA	
		O=85		2.4		13.6		5.2 % at 3 years					
Lujan et al. [17]	2009	L=101	32.9	4.0	0.422	13.6	0.026	4.8 % at 5 years	NA	72.1 % at 5 years	NA	84.8 % at 5 years	NA
		O=103	34.1	2.9		11.6		5.3 % at 5 years		75.3 % at 5 years		81.0 % at 5 years	
Ng et al. [18]	2009	L=76	87.2	2.6	0.620	11.5	0.700	5	NA	63.9 % at 10 years	0.303	82.9 % at 10 years	0.698
		O=77		1.3		12.0		11		55.1 % at 10 years		80.4 % at 10 years	
Kang et al. [52]	2010	L=170	NA	2.9	0.770	17	0.085	NA		NA		NA	
(COREAN trial)		O=170		4.1		18							
Jayne et al. [8, 69]	2010	L=253	56.3	16.0	0.800	NA		9.4 % at 5 years[a]	0.740	60.3 % at 5 years	0.132	53.2 % at 5 years	0.953
(CLASICC trial)		O=128		14.0				7.6 % at 5 years[a]		52.9 % at 5 years		52.1 % at 5 years	
van der Paas et al. [53]	2013	L=699	NA	10	0.850	13	0.085	NA		NA		NA	
(COLOR II trial)		O=345		10		14							

Values are expressed as mean or median as appropriate
DFS disease-free survival, *L* laparoscopic group, *N* number, *NA* not available, *O* open group, *OS* overall survival
[a]Local recurrence rates in patients undergoing anterior resection

the rate of positive circumferential resection margin are similar whatever the approach [8, 17, 18, 50, 52, 53].

Long-term data available on overall and disease-free survival continue to support the use of laparoscopic surgery for rectal cancer. In the update results of the CLASICC study, the median overall survival was 65.8 and 82.7 months, and the median disease-free survival was 67.1 and 70.8 months in open and laparoscopic groups respectively, without any statistic difference [57]. Definitive results of the ongoing multicenter randomized trials (COLOR II, JCOG, and ACOSOG-Z6051) [58–60] are expected to confirm those of the CLASICC trial [57]. Then, laparoscopic surgery will become the new standard in the treatment of rectal cancer.

Functional Outcomes

With the principles of total mesorectal excision (TME) and autonomic nerve preservation, the incidence of urinary and sexual complications decreased from 40 to 60 % and 10 to 30 % [61–63], to the range of 10–35 % and less than 5 % [64–66], respectively. The magnificence view offered by the laparoscopic approach has brought hope to improve the functional outcomes. For now, no high level of evidence study demonstrates a superiority of laparoscopy for this issue. Sexual function is more frequently impaired in men but the role of laparoscopy is not demonstrated [52, 67, 68].

Key Points

- Laparoscopic approach for rectal cancer excision should be performed in T1, T2 or T3 tumor and by an expert surgeon in both TME and laparoscopic surgery.
- Laparoscopic surgery is contra indicated in patients with preoperative fixed tumors into adjacent pelvic organ (T4).
- High body mass index, male gender, stapled anastomosis and intraoperative rectal fixity are the main risk factors for conversion to an open procedure. Effective selection of the patients is important to minimize the negative impacts of conversion.
- Laparoscopic TME needs to be standardized in progressive steps to insure an optimal oncologic safety and to prevent from intraoperative complications including conversion, hemorrhage, nerve injuries and stapled difficulties.
- Low pelvic dissection can be performed through a prior perineal approach to avoid stapled problems and conversion.
- The oncologic validity of the laparoscopic approach is well established with results of long-term survival and local recurrence that are similar to those reported after open resection.
- Laparoscopic surgery is about to becoming the new standard of care for rectal cancer.
- Perioperative management involves dieticians, nurses, surgeons and anesthesiologists.
- Management of low rectal cancer is composed by the three following steps: firstly, classification of low rectal cancer in four types, secondly, standardization of surgery in four operations.
- For low rectal cancer, restaging after neoadjuvant treatment is mandatory to adapt surgical procedures.

References

1. Siegel R, Naishadham D, Jemal A. Cancer statistics, 2012. CA Cancer J Clin. 2012;62(1):10–29.
2. Heald RJ, Husband EM, Ryall RD. The mesorectum in rectal cancer surgery—the clue to pelvic recurrence? Br J Surg. 1982;69(10):613–6.
3. Kapiteijn E, Putter H, van de Velde CJ. Impact of the introduction and training of total mesorectal excision on recurrence and survival in rectal cancer in The Netherlands. Br J Surg. 2002;89(9):1142–9.
4. Nagtegaal ID, van de Velde CJ, van der Worp E, et al. Macroscopic evaluation of rectal cancer resection

specimen: clinical significance of the pathologist in quality control. J Clin Oncol. 2002;20(7):1729–34.
5. Nagtegaal ID, van Krieken JH. The role of pathologists in the quality control of diagnosis and treatment of rectal cancer-an overview. Eur J Cancer. 2002; 38(7):964–72.
6. Clinical Outcomes of Surgical Therapy Study Group. A comparison of laparoscopically assisted and open colectomy for colon cancer. N Engl J Med. 2004; 350(20):2050–9.
7. Buunen M, Veldkamp R, Hop WC, et al. Survival after laparoscopic surgery versus open surgery for colon cancer: long-term outcome of a randomised clinical trial. Lancet Oncol. 2009;10(1):44–52.
8. Jayne DG, Guillou PJ, Thorpe H, et al. Randomized trial of laparoscopic-assisted resection of colorectal carcinoma: 3-year results of the UK MRC CLASICC Trial Group. J Clin Oncol. 2007;25(21):3061–8.
9. Lacy AM, Garcia-Valdecasas JC, Delgado S, et al. Laparoscopy-assisted colectomy versus open colectomy for treatment of non-metastatic colon cancer: a randomised trial. Lancet. 2002;359(9325):2224–9.
10. Leung KL, Kwok SP, Lam SC, et al. Laparoscopic resection of rectosigmoid carcinoma: prospective randomised trial. Lancet. 2004;363(9416):1187–92.
11. Hartley JE, Mehigan BJ, Qureshi AE, et al. Total mesorectal excision: assessment of the laparoscopic approach. Dis Colon Rectum. 2001;44(3):315–21.
12. Rullier E, Sa Cunha A, Couderc P, et al. Laparoscopic intersphincteric resection with coloplasty and coloanal anastomosis for mid and low rectal cancer. Br J Surg. 2003;90(4):445–51.
13. Scheidbach H, Schneider C, Konradt J, et al. Laparoscopic abdominoperineal resection and anterior resection with curative intent for carcinoma of the rectum. Surg Endosc. 2002;16(1):7–13.
14. Tsang WW, Chung CC, Li MK. Prospective evaluation of laparoscopic total mesorectal excision with colonic J-pouch reconstruction for mid and low rectal cancers. Br J Surg. 2003;90(7):867–71.
15. Bianchi PP, Rosati R, Bona S, et al. Laparoscopic surgery in rectal cancer: a prospective analysis of patient survival and outcomes. Dis Colon Rectum. 2007; 50(12):2047–53.
16. Breukink S, Pierie J, Wiggers T. Laparoscopic versus open total mesorectal excision for rectal cancer. Cochrane Database Syst Rev. 2006(4):CD005200.
17. Lujan J, Valero G, Hernandez Q, et al. Randomized clinical trial comparing laparoscopic and open surgery in patients with rectal cancer. Br J Surg. 2009; 96(9):982–9.
18. Ng SS, Leung KL, Lee JF, et al. Long-term morbidity and oncologic outcomes of laparoscopic-assisted anterior resection for upper rectal cancer: ten-year results of a prospective, randomized trial. Dis Colon Rectum. 2009;52(4):558–66.
19. Pugliese R, Di Lernia S, Sansonna F, et al. Results of laparoscopic anterior resection for rectal adenocarcinoma: retrospective analysis of 157 cases. Am J Surg. 2008;195(2):233–8.
20. Enker WE, Merchant N, Cohen AM, et al. Safety and efficacy of low anterior resection for rectal cancer: 681 consecutive cases from a specialty service. Ann Surg. 1999;230(4):544–52; discussion 552–544.
21. Marijnen CA, Kapiteijn E, van de Velde CJ, et al. Acute side effects and complications after short-term preoperative radiotherapy combined with total mesorectal excision in primary rectal cancer: report of a multicenter randomized trial. J Clin Oncol. 2002; 20(3):817–25.
22. Denost Q, Laurent C, Paumet T, et al. Laparoscopic surgery for rectal cancer: preoperative radiochemotherapy versus surgery alone. Surg Endosc. 2012; 26(7):1878–83.
23. Sarli L, Rollo A, Cecchini S, et al. Impact of obesity on laparoscopic-assisted left colectomy in different stages of the learning curve. Surg Laparosc Endosc Percutan Tech. 2009;19(2):114–7.
24. Scheidbach H, Benedix F, Hugel O, et al. Laparoscopic approach to colorectal procedures in the obese patient: risk factor or benefit? Obes Surg. 2008;18(1):66–70.
25. Gendall KA, Raniga S, Kennedy R, Frizelle FA. The impact of obesity on outcome after major colorectal surgery. Dis Colon Rectum. 2007;50(12):2223–37.
26. Benoist S, Panis Y, Alves A, Valleur P. Impact of obesity on surgical outcomes after colorectal resection. Am J Surg. 2000;179(4):275–81.
27. Denost Q, Quintane L, Buscail E, et al. Short- and long-term impact of body mass index on laparoscopic rectal cancer surgery. Colorectal Dis. 2013;15(4):463–9.
28. Edge SB, Byrd DR, Compton CC, Fritz AG, Greene FL, Trotti A III (eds). AJCC Cancer Staging Manual (7th edn). Springer: New York; 2010.
29. MERCURY Study Group. Extramural depth of tumor invasion at thin-section MR in patients with rectal cancer: results of the MERCURY study. Radiology. 2007;243(1):132–9.
30. Hanly AM, Ryan EM, Rogers AC, et al. Multicenter evaluation of rectal cancer ReImaging pOst Neoadjuvant (MERRION) therapy. Ann Surg. 2014;259:723–7.
31. Evans J, Patel U, Brown G. Rectal cancer: primary staging and assessment after chemoradiotherapy. Semin Radiat Oncol. 2011;21(3):169–77.
32. Vanagunas A, Lin DE, Stryker SJ. Accuracy of endoscopic ultrasound for restaging rectal cancer following neoadjuvant chemoradiation therapy. Am J Gastroenterol. 2004;99(1):109–12.
33. Pastor C, Subtil JC, Sola J, et al. Accuracy of endoscopic ultrasound to assess tumor response after neoadjuvant treatment in rectal cancer: can we trust the findings? Dis Colon Rectum. 2011;54(9):1141–6.
34. Dresen RC, Beets GL, Rutten HJ, et al. Locally advanced rectal cancer: MR imaging for restaging after neoadjuvant radiation therapy with concomitant chemotherapy. Part I. Are we able to predict tumor confined to the rectal wall? Radiology. 2009;252(1):71–80.
35. Kim DJ, Kim JH, Lim JS, et al. Restaging of rectal cancer with MR imaging after concurrent chemotherapy and radiation therapy. Radiographics. 2010;30(2): 503–16.

36. Perez RO, Habr-Gama A, Gama-Rodrigues J, et al. Accuracy of positron emission tomography/computed tomography and clinical assessment in the detection of complete rectal tumor regression after neoadjuvant chemoradiation: long-term results of a prospective trial (National Clinical Trial 00254683). Cancer. 2012;118(14):3501–11.
37. Scheele J, Stang R, Altendorf-Hofmann A, Paul M. Resection of colorectal liver metastases. World J Surg. 1995;19(1):59–71.
38. Mehta S, Johnson RJ, Schofield PF. Staging of colorectal cancer. Clin Radiol. 1994;49(8):515–23.
39. Portier G. Recommendations for clinical practice. Therapeutic choices for rectal cancer. How should neoadjuvant therapies be chosen? Gastroenterol Clin Biol. 2007;31(Spec No 1):1S23–33, 21S89–91.
40. Gerard JP, Conroy T, Bonnetain F, et al. Preoperative radiotherapy with or without concurrent fluorouracil and leucovorin in T3–4 rectal cancers: results of FFCD 9203. J Clin Oncol. 2006;24(28):4620–5.
41. Rullier E, Goffre B, Bonnel C, et al. Preoperative radiochemotherapy and sphincter-saving resection for T3 carcinomas of the lower third of the rectum. Ann Surg. 2001;234(5):633–40.
42. GRECCAR 6: randomized control trial comparing the impact of a lengthening of the interval between the radiochemotherapy and surgery (7 weeks vs. 11 weeks) on complete pathological response in rectal cancer. Available from: http://clinicaltrials.gov/ct2/show/NCT01648894?term=greccar&rank=5.
43. Rullier E, Denost Q, Vendrely V, Rullier A, Laurent C. Low rectal cancer: classification and standardization of surgery. Dis Colon Rectum. 2013;56(5):560–7.
44. Garcia-Aguilar J, Shi Q, Thomas Jr CR, et al. A phase II trial of neoadjuvant chemoradiation and local excision for T2N0 rectal cancer: preliminary results of the ACOSOG Z6041 trial. Ann Surg Oncol. 2012;19(2):384–91.
45. GRECCAR 2: phase III randomized trial of local excision versus total mesorectal excision in downstaged T2T3 low rectal cancer after radiochemotherapy. Available from: http://clinicaltrials.gov/ct2/show/NCT00427375?term=greccar&rank=3.
46. Ito M, Sugito M, Kobayashi A, et al. Relationship between multiple numbers of stapler firings during rectal division and anastomotic leakage after laparoscopic rectal resection. Int J Colorectal Dis. 2008;23(7):703–7.
47. Rullier E, Laurent C, Bretagnol F, et al. Sphincter-saving resection for all rectal carcinomas: the end of the 2-cm distal rule. Ann Surg. 2005;241(3):465–9.
48. Rouanet P, Mourregot A, Azar CC, et al. Transanal endoscopic proctectomy: an innovative procedure for difficult resection of rectal tumors in men with narrow pelvis. Dis Colon Rectum. 2013;56(4):408–15.
49. Nagtegaal ID, Quirke P. What is the role for the circumferential margin in the modern treatment of rectal cancer? J Clin Oncol. 2008;26(2):303–12.
50. Braga M, Frasson M, Vignali A, et al. Laparoscopic resection in rectal cancer patients: outcome and cost-benefit analysis. Dis Colon Rectum. 2007;50(4):464–71.
51. Guillou PJ, Quirke P, Thorpe H, et al. Short-term endpoints of conventional versus laparoscopic-assisted surgery in patients with colorectal cancer (MRC CLASICC trial): multicentre, randomised controlled trial. Lancet. 2005;365(9472):1718–26.
52. Kang SB, Park JW, Jeong SY, et al. Open versus laparoscopic surgery for mid or low rectal cancer after neoadjuvant chemoradiotherapy (COREAN trial): short-term outcomes of an open-label randomised controlled trial. Lancet Oncol. 2010; 11(7):637–45.
53. van der Pas MHGM, Haglind E, Cuesta MA, et al. Laparoscopic versus open surgery for rectal cancer (COLOR II): short-term outcomes of a randomised, phase 3 trial. Lancet Oncol. 2013;14(3):210–8.
54. Zhou ZG, Hu M, Li Y, et al. Laparoscopic versus open total mesorectal excision with anal sphincter preservation for low rectal cancer. Surg Endosc. 2004;18(8): 1211–5.
55. Laurent C, Leblanc F, Gineste C, Saric J, Rullier E. Laparoscopic approach in surgical treatment of rectal cancer. Br J Surg. 2007;94(12):1555–61.
56. Andersson J, Angenete E, Gellerstedt M, et al. Health-related quality of life after laparoscopic and open surgery for rectal cancer in a randomized trial. Br J Surg. 2013;100(7):941–9.
57. Green BL, Marshall HC, Collinson F, et al. Long-term follow-up of the Medical Research Council CLASICC trial of conventional versus laparoscopically assisted resection in colorectal cancer. Br J Surg. 2013;100(1): 75–82.
58. Kitano S, Inomata M, Sato A, Yoshimura K, Moriya Y. Randomized controlled trial to evaluate laparoscopic surgery for colorectal cancer: Japan Clinical Oncology Group Study JCOG 0404. Jpn J Clin Oncol. 2005;35(8):475–7.
59. Fleshman J, American College of Surgeons Oncology Group. (ACOSOG)-Z6051. A phase III prospective randomized trial comparing laparoscopic-assisted resection versus open resection for rectal cancer. Available from: http://clinicaltrials.gov/ct2/show/NCT00726622.
60. COLOR II: a randomized clinical trial comparing laparoscopic and open surgery for rectal cancer. Available from: http://clinicaltrials.gov/ct2/show/NCT00297791?term_color_II&rank_1.
61. Santangelo ML, Romano G, Sassaroli C. Sexual function after resection for rectal cancer. Am J Surg. 1987;154(5):502–4.
62. Kinn AC, Ohman U. Bladder and sexual function after surgery for rectal cancer. Dis Colon Rectum. 1986;29(1):43–8.
63. Chang PL, Fan HA. Urodynamic studies before and/or after abdominoperineal resection of the rectum for carcinoma. J Urol. 1983;130(5):948–51.
64. Havenga K, Enker WE, McDermott K, et al. Male and female sexual and urinary function after total mesorectal excision with autonomic nerve preservation for carcinoma of the rectum. J Am Coll Surg. 1996; 182(6):495–502.

65. Hendren SK, O'Connor BI, Liu M, et al. Prevalence of male and female sexual dysfunction is high following surgery for rectal cancer. Ann Surg. 2005;242(2):212–23.
66. Maurer CA, Z'Graggen K, Renzulli P, et al. Total mesorectal excision preserves male genital function compared with conventional rectal cancer surgery. Br J Surg. 2001;88(11):1501–5.
67. Ohtani H, Tamamori Y, Azuma T, et al. A meta-analysis of the short- and long-term results of randomized controlled trials that compared laparoscopy-assisted and conventional open surgery for rectal cancer. J Gastrointest Surg. 2011;15(8): 1375–85.
68. Jayne DG, Brown JM, Thorpe H, et al. Bladder and sexual function following resection for rectal cancer in a randomized clinical trial of laparoscopic versus open technique. Br J Surg. 2005;92(9):1124–32.
69. Jayne DG, Thorpe HC, Copeland J, et al. Five-year follow-up of the Medical Research Council CLASICC trial of laparoscopically assisted versus open surgery for colorectal cancer. Br J Surg. 2010;97(11):1638–45.

Management of Anal Cancer

51

Burzeen E. Karanjawala and George J. Chang

51.1 Introduction

Anal cancer is a rare type of malignancy of the anus and anal canal, but the incidence has been increasing worldwide. Based on current data, it is estimated that over 7,000 people (incidence of 1.5/100,000 men, 1.9/100,000 women) will be diagnosed with cancer of the anus, anal canal, and anorectum in the United States, and nearly 900 people will die secondary to this diagnosis this year. The median age at diagnosis is 60 years, and diagnosis under 20 years has not been described. With current therapy, 5-year survival rates are approximately 80 % for locally confined disease, 60 % for regional spread, and 31 % for distant metastatic disease [1].

51.2 Etiology

Multiple risk factors for anal cancer have emerged. Behavioral factors, such as lifetime number of sexual partners and high-risk sexual activity such as anal receptive intercourse, may lead to increased risk of HPV and HIV infection. HPV infection, specifically types 16 and 18, has been causally associated with squamous cell carcinoma and anal intraepithelial neoplasia; however, many patients with HPV positive cytology do not develop AIN or anal cancer, suggesting the involvement of additional factors [2–5].

There is also a clear association between immunocompromise, such as HIV/AIDS, and anal cancer. The highest risk is seen in HIV-infected men who have sex with men (MSM) with a demographically adjusted rate ratio of 80.3 versus 26.7 for other HIV-infected men when compared to HIV-uninfected individuals [6]. Because of the increased prevalence of high-grade dysplasia, it is recommended that high-risk individuals with HIV (MSM, history of anogenital warts, women with cervical dysplasia) undergo annual screening with anal cytology and/or high-resolution anoscopy [7, 8].

Transplant recipients have an increased risk of many malignancies, including anal cancer. Based on a cohort study published in 2011, the standardized incidence ratio of anal cancer among patients in the U.S. Scientific Registry of Transplant Recipients was 5.84. The elevated cancer risk in immunosuppressed transplant recipients appears similar to that seen in HIV patients, likely secondary to poor immune control of known oncogenic HPV [9, 10].

Smoking is another risk factor for anal cancer. A large, retrospective cohort study that included

B.E. Karanjawala, MD
Department of General Surgery, University of Texas Medical School at Houston, Houston, TX, USA

G.J. Chang, MD, MS, FACS, FASCRS (✉)
Department of Surgical Oncology, University of Texas MD Anderson Cancer Center, Unit 444, 1400 Pressler Street, 301402, Houston, TX 77230-1402, USA
e-mail: gchang@mdanderson.org

H.R.H. Patel et al. (eds.), *Pelvic Cancer Surgery: Modern Breakthroughs and Future Advances*, DOI 10.1007/978-1-4471-4258-4_51, © Springer-Verlag London 2015

over 336,000 Swedish male construction workers followed from 1971 identified a significantly increased risk for anal cancer among smokers, with a hazard ratio of 2.41 [11]. Other studies have shown similar associations between smoking and anal cancer risk [4, 12].

Despite early case reports raising the concern for associations between anal cancer and benign anorectal disease [13–16], fistulas and fissures do not appear to have a causative relationship with anal cancer [17–19]. Finally, patients with inflammatory bowel disease do not demonstrate an increased risk for anal cancer [19].

51.3 Anorectal Anatomy

The anal canal begins at the level of the puborectalis muscle and extends distally to the anal verge (approximately at the level of the intersphincteric groove). From the anal verge to a distance of 5 cm out is the anal margin. The dentate line defines the boundary of the stratified squamous epithelium of the anoderm with the cuboidal and columnar epithelium of the anorectal transition zone. Tumors that originate above the dentate line may have lymphatic drainage via the inferior mesenteric and internal iliac nodal systems. Whereas, below the dentate line, the drainage is commonly via the superficial inguinal and external iliac lymph nodes [20].

51.4 Precursor Lesions

Like many other cancers, there are preinvasive lesions that may be identified prior the discovery of an anal malignancy. These are briefly described in Table 51.1. Although the natural history of progression of the pre-invasive lesions in invasive cancer has not been fully characterized, in cases such as for anal intraepithelial neoplasia, the natural history may be considered to be analogous to that for progression of cervical dysplasia to cervical cancer [21–28].

Table 51.1 Anal precursor lesions

	Description	Treatment	Special considerations
Anal Intraepithelial Neoplasia (AIN)	Dysplasia of squamous cells of the anal margin/canal; precursor lesion of SCC	Surveillance for low-grade lesions	Common in HIV + HIV treatment can influence progression to SCC
	Low-grade (AIN I)	Topical treatment with Imiquimod or 80 % trichloroacetic acid	Also common in HIV-homosexual men
	Moderate-grade (AIN II) High-grade (AIN III)	Cryotherapy	
Bowen's Disease	Squamous cell carcinoma in situ of the anal margin (high-grade dysplasia)	Unifocal disease: local excision/ablation Multifocal disease: topical treatment with Imiquimod or 80 % trichloroacetic acid	Modern treatment approaches converging with management of AIN
Buschke-Lowenstein tumor	Intermediate lesion between condyloma and invasive SCC; can be very large (up to 30 cm)	Wide-local excision may require APR if there is extensive sphincter involvement	
Paget's disease	Adenocarcinoma in situ of the anal margin; 50–70 % association with other lower GI malignancies	Wide local excision/ablation	Colonoscopy to evaluate for other lower GI lesions

51.5 Anal Margin Malignancies

The vast majority of anal margin cancers are squamous cell in origin. They are similar to SCC of other areas of the body, and, thus, have a similar staging system and treatment. Small tumors that are superficial, such as T1 lesions, may be eligible for treatment with wide local excision. More advanced tumors are typically treated with combined modality chemoradiation therapy regimens. Those that fail this treatment may benefit from surgical therapy. 5-year survival rates range from 70 to 90 % [21].

Basal cell carcinoma of the anal margin is very rare. Like basal cell carcinoma of other parts of the body, wide local excision is the treatment of choice. This tumor often recurs, and re-excision is needed. 5-year survival is nearly 100 % [21].

Perineal Coverage After Resection of Anal Margin Tumors

When wide local excision is performed in the treatment of anal margin tumors, a large defect may remain, and consideration needs to be given to the method of reconstruction of the perineal wound. Split-thickness skin grafts can be used for coverage, especially for superficial wounds [29, 30]. Most cases, however, involve deep wounds, and STSG will result in large defects and poor cosmesis for the patients. Local flaps, such as the V-Y gluteal advancement flap, are commonly used, with generally good results but an approximately 30 % wound dehiscence rate [31].

Rotational myocutaneous flaps, based on a vascular pedicle, can also be used. The gracilis and, when associated with abdominoperineal resection, rectus abdominis flaps are most commonly employed. These flaps can be especially useful in patients with prior pelvic irradiation or those who have failed primary closure of large defects [32, 33].

51.6 Anal Canal Tumors

There are many different types of anal canal tumors, including adenocarcinoma, melanoma, GIST, and epidermoid carcinoma. The histology of epidermoid carcinoma includes squamous cell, basaloid, cloacogenic/transitional cell, and mucoepidermoid types. Squamous cell carcinoma is by far the most common, comprising nearly 80 % of these tumors, but the histologic phenotype may be mixed [34, 35].

Diagnosis

The key to anal cancer management is early diagnosis. The most common presenting complaint is bleeding, occurring in >50 % of patients. Patients may also complain of anal pain, pruritus, tenesmus, change in bowel habits, abnormal discharge, or the sensation of a mass. These complaints are also associated with benign anorectal conditions, and it is important for the clinician to avoid misdiagnosis of anal cancer [34, 35].

Physical examination is important in diagnosis and can help in staging (Table 51.2). The size of the tumor, its appearance, and fixity to surrounding organs or the bony pelvis are important components of preoperative evaluation, as anal SCC often presents at a locally advanced stage. The most common finding is an intraluminal mass that may be exophytic, ulcerated, or flat. On digital rectal exam, anal cancer could be mistaken for a hemorrhoid, so it is important to visualize the lesion with anoscopy/proctoscopy. Colonoscopy is also essential for ruling out more proximal malignancies. For diagnosis, incisional biopsy is recommended. Palpation for inguinal lymphadenopathy should be performed, as approximately one third of anal SCC will demonstrate regional lymph node metastases. Palpable inguinal lymph nodes can be sampled via fine needle aspiration. Sentinel lymph node biopsy has also been investigated, but patients with negative results can later present with inguino-femoral nodal disease [36].

The initial workup and clinical stage assessment should include computed tomography of the abdomen and pelvis to evaluate the primary lesion, regional lymph nodes, and to rule out distant metastatic disease [34, 35]. Endorectal ultrasound and MRI are other modalities that

Table 51.2 Staging of anal canal tumors

Stage	T	N	M
0	Tis	N0	M0
I	T1	N0	M0
II	T2	N0	M0
	T3	N0	M0
IIIA	T1	N1	M0
	T2	N1	M0
	T3	N1	M0
	T4	N0	M0
IIIB	T4	N1	M0
	Any T	N2	M0
	Any T	N3	M0
IV	Any T	Any N	M1
TX	Primary tumor cannot be assessed		
T0	No evidence of primary tumor		
Tis	Carcinoma *in situ* (i.e., Bowen disease, high-grade squamous intraepithelial lesion, and anal intraepithelial neoplasia II–III)		
T1	Tumor ≤2 cm in greatest dimension		
T2	Tumor >2 cm but ≤5 cm in greatest dimension		
T3	Tumor >5 cm in greatest dimension		
T4	Tumor of any size invades adjacent organ(s), e.g., vagina, urethra, and bladder		
NX	Regional lymph nodes cannot be assessed		
N0	No regional lymph node metastasis		
N1	Metastases in perirectal lymph node(s)		
N2	Metastases in unilateral internal iliac and/or inguinal lymph node(s)		
N3	Metastases in perirectal and inguinal lymph nodes and/or bilateral internal iliac and/or inguinal lymph nodes		
M0	No distant metastasis		
M1	Distant metastasis		

AJCC Cancer Staging Manual, 7th ed

can be used for locoregional staging; however, the role for ultrasound may be limited as primary tumor staging is dependent upon tumor size, not depth of penetration in the bowel wall or sphincter complex [37–39]. A chest radiograph or CT of the chest should also be obtained. Fluorodeoxyglucose positron emission tomography with CT has been reported to show utility for staging of anal cancer and may be considered, although its ability to replace conventional contrast-enhanced CT has not been validated [40–45].

51.7 Treatment

Until the 1970s, the primary treatment of anal canal carcinoma was abdominoperineal resection with or without inguinal lymph node dissection. This procedure carried with it high morbidity and had a significant impact on the patient's overall quality of life, while achieving overall survival of only 40–70 %. In 1974, Nigro observed that many patients with locally advanced disease treated with neoadjuvant chemoradiation followed by APR had a complete pathologic response. This led him and other investigators to develop a protocol of radiation therapy with concurrent chemotherapy with 5-fluorouracil and mitomycin-C, and they found overall survival rates in the range of 65–85 % [46, 47]. This discovery has revolutionized the treatment of anal canal carcinoma, and today the primary treatment is combined modality chemoradiation therapy. Since its development, multiple studies have investigated modifications of the Nigro protocol in order to improve treatment response and reduce toxicity.

Radiation Therapy

In 1996, the UK Coordinating Committee on Cancer Research (UKCCCR) reported results from the ACT I trial [48]. This study evaluated the benefit of combined modality therapy versus radiation therapy alone. Radiotherapy had demonstrated 3-year survival rates as high as 75 %, but local control rates around 40–50 %. In this study 585 patients were randomized to receive a total radiation dose of 45 Gy in 20 or 25 fractions over 4–5 weeks or the same radiation therapy dose with the addition of concurrent chemotherapy with 5-FU (1,000 mg/m^2 over 4 days or 750 mg/m^2 over 5 days) during the first and final weeks of radiation. Mitomycin C (12 mg/m^2) was also given on treatment day 1. After a median follow-up of 42 months, local failures occurred in 59 % of the radiotherapy group versus 36 % in the CMT arm, reflecting a 46 % risk reduction for local failure in the group undergoing CMT. The European Organization for Research and Treatment of Cancer (EORTC) study 22,861 confirmed the findings of ACT I, with 5-year local failure rates of 50 and 32 % for radiotherapy alone and CMT, respectively [49]. Two separate studies, RTOG 92–08 and ECOG 4292, examined radiation dose intensification in an effort to improve local control but did not show any improvement compared to standard therapy [50, 51].

Intensity modulated radiation therapy (IMRT) has shown promise in allowing for an increase in dose while sparing surrounding tissues and decreasing toxicity [52]. In a phase II evaluation, RTOG 05–29 demonstrated a reduction of acute grade 2+ hematologic and grade 3+ dermatologic and GI toxicity with IMRT and concurrent chemotherapy with 5-FU and MMC [53]. Brachytherapy is another strategy to optimize local control while limiting pelvic toxicity, but this approach remains investigational [54, 55].

Cisplatin-Based Chemotherapy Regimen

Despite the efficacy of concurrent 5-FU and MMC chemoradiation therapy, it is associated with significant treatment associated toxicity. Early experience with 5-FU and cisplatin-based chemoradiation therapy suggested improved response rates with reduced toxicity [56–58]. Thus, the UKCCCR ACT II trial compared concurrent chemoradiation therapy regimens with 5-FU and MMC or cisplatin. Additionally, the potential for maintenance chemotherapy to improve survival was assessed. In this 2×2 factorial study, 940 patients received either cisplatin-based chemoradiation with (n=222) or without (n=246) maintenance chemotherapy or MMC-based chemoradiation therapy with (n=226) or without (n=246) maintenance chemotherapy. The complete response rate at 26 weeks was 89.6 % versus 90.5 % for the cisplatin vs. MMC groups, respectively. Furthermore, there were no significant differences in the toxicity profiles between the groups. After a median follow-up of 5.1 years, maintenance chemotherapy was not associated with improved 3-year progression-free survival [59].

Induction Chemotherapy

Based on favorable preliminary outcomes with cisplatin-based induction chemotherapy for patients with advanced cancer and the high rates of toxicity associated with MMC based regimens, the strategy of induction chemotherapy was compared to standard MMC chemoradiation in RTOG 98–11 [60–62]. Six hundred forty-four patients were randomized to receive induction chemotherapy with 5-FU and cisplatin followed by 5-FU and cisplatin chemoradiotherapy or to receive standard 5-FU and mitomycin C based chemoradiotherapy. No significant difference was observed in 5-year disease-free (60 % for MMC vs. 54 % for cisplatin) or overall survival (75 % vs. 70 %). Although the rate of severe hematologic toxicity was greater in the MMC arm, the rate of colostomy after treatment was greater in the induction + cisplatin-based chemoradiation arm (19 % vs. 10 %). Thus, the current MMC-based regimen without induction chemotherapy remains the standard of care for anal canal cancer, although cisplatin-based therapy may be acceptable for patients with severe MMC-related toxicity [61, 62].

51.8 Toxicities Associated with Treatment

There are a number of acute and long-term toxicities associated with combined modality treatment of anal cancer. Short-term toxicities are primarily hematologic, particularly with the use of MMC. Severe late toxicities are observed in 10–15 % of patients and are most commonly related to radiation enteritis/proctitis and skin-associated complications. Other toxicities include radiation cystitis and sacral insufficiency fractures

[63–67]. The most common symptom with radiation injury is bleeding, but patients may also complain of diarrhea, urgency, tenesmus, and pain. Patients may also present with fistulas and strictures. Colonoscopy or barium enema should be performed to rule out malignancy as a cause of the patient's symptoms [66, 67].

The primary treatment of radiation-induced toxicity is non-surgical. For radiation-induced proctitis, steroid retention enemas, endoscopic application of formalin, endoscopic argon plasma coagulation, and hyperbaric oxygen therapy have all been tried with varied success. For stricture, endoscopic dilation can be attempted [66].

In patients who have failed medical treatment or those with stenosis, obstruction, refractory pain, perforation, abscess, or fistula, surgical management may be necessary. Options include diversion or resection with or without restoration of intestinal continuity [66]. The choice of operation is dependent upon the patient's presenting problem, with proximal strictures responding well with resection and distal strictures or proctitis requiring permanent diversion [67]. It is also imperative to know the patient's anorectal function in determining the ideal procedure for them.

51.9 Follow-Up After Treatment

As many as 25 % of patients will develop local recurrence within the first 3 years. Patients should be evaluated every 3–6 months for the first 3 years and then every 6–12 months for an additional 2 years. Clinical evaluation with digital rectal exam, palpation of inguinal lymph nodes, and anoscopy is key. Any suspicious lesion should be biopsied to assess for persistence or recurrence of disease. Response to treatment may still be ongoing at 12 weeks after completion of chemoradiation therapy so it is important to correlate post-treatment and pre-treatment findings on clinical examination. Surveillance imaging, such as CT or MRI may help to identify distant or inguinal recurrence; however, the secondary salvage treatment options may be limited.

Patterns of Recurrence

Within 6 months of completion of CRT, evidence of tumor within the anal canal is considered to be persistent disease; whereas, beyond 6 months after complete clinical response, it is recurrent disease. The most common site of recurrence is locoregional—within the anorectal canal, the pelvis, or in the inguinal lymph node basin—and occurs in as much as 30 % of patients. Distant metastatic disease is also seen in as much as 20 % of patients who fail primary therapy. T and N stage of disease have been shown to predict locoregional recurrence, while N stage and basaloid subtype are predictors of distant metastases [68].

51.10 Salvage Therapy for Persistent/Recurrent Disease

Local Recurrence

Historically, surgery was the mainstay of therapy in the treatment of anal canal malignancies, but it is now reserved for patients who demonstrate persistent or recurrent disease after definitive chemoradiotherapy. The goal of surgery is to obtain local control and prevent distant recurrence. Surgical resection should be complete and *en bloc* (R0) to include the perianal skin, involved surrounding organs (e.g., uterus, vagina, prostate), and coccyx or sacrum as the achievement of negative margins is important to prevent locoregional recurrence in these patients (Fig. 51.1). In some cases, pelvic exenteration may be necessary to achieve an R0 resection [69].

Unfortunately, failure of combined modality therapy portends a poorer prognosis and survival may be suboptimal even with salvage surgery. Several studies have demonstrated 5-year survival rates ranging from 25 to 70 % [70–82]. One of the most important factors affecting recurrence and overall and disease-free survival is involvement of the surgical margins. Other factors include lymph node spread, tumor size, and age [78, 80].

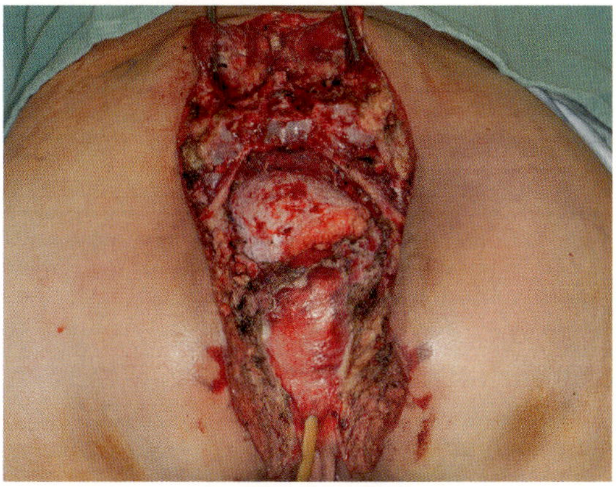

Fig. 51.1 Post-resection photograph showing cut edge of the sacrum, bilateral S3 nerve roots, anterior vaginal wall, and de-epithelialized rectus myocutaneous flap (Copyright held by, and used with permission of, George J. Chang, M.D)

Nodal Recurrence

Regional lymph node recurrence may be identified along the drainage distribution of the anal canal and include mesorectal, inguinal, iliac, or obturator lymph nodes (Fig. 51.2). Mesorectal recurrence often requires proctectomy; whereas inguinal, iliac, or obturator disease may be treated with modified regional lymph node dissection targeting the site of disease without proctectomy. Particularly for intra-pelvic sites of disease, repeat hyper-fractionated chemoradiation therapy may be included prior to salvage surgery as part of the multidisciplinary treatment plan depending on total dose received during initial treatment. Lymph node recurrence, however, occurs more commonly in areas not previously included in the radiation field (e.g., inguinal nodes), and in this case, the treatment of choice is salvage combined modality therapy. Recurrence or persistence following prior definitive radiotherapy may be treated with surgical salvage, including lymph node dissection. Inguinal lymph node dissection carries with it significant morbidity, primarily local wound complications, such as infection, dehiscence, and lymphocele [83, 84]. In cases with prior radiation, coverage with local myocutaneous flaps can help minimize morbidity [85]. Lymphedema is also a potential complication encountered after surgery.

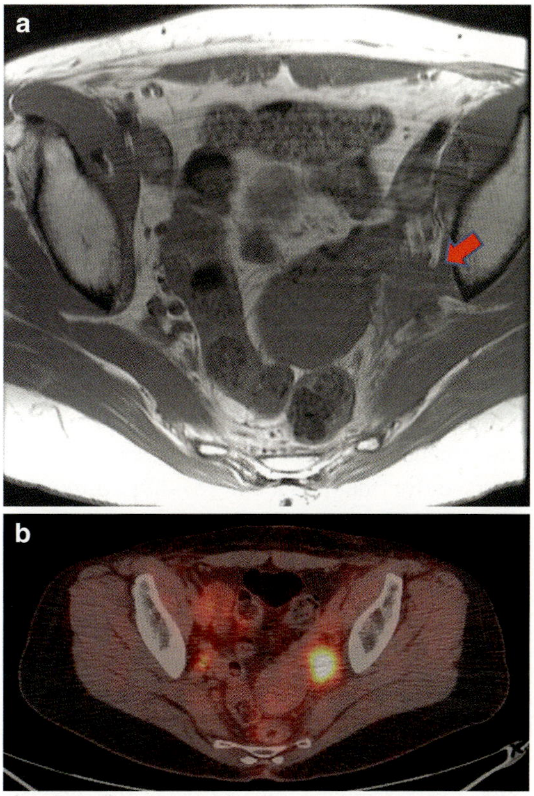

Fig. 51.2 (**a**) Magnetic resonance imaging shows recurrent carcinoma within left obturator space (*red arrow*). (**b**) The same area is shown to be fluoro-deoxy-glucose avid on positron emission tomography (Copyright held by, and used with permission of, George J. Chang, M.D)

Distant Metastatic Recurrence

As many as 20 % of patients can have distant metastatic disease at the time of initial presentation or as evidence of recurrence. The most common site of metastasis is the liver, but spread to the lung, peritoneum, and bone also occurs. The mainstay of therapy is systemic chemotherapy. Surgical resection can be performed in select patients, but prognosis overall is poor [86]. Our preference is to begin with systemic chemotherapy and consider salvage surgical resection only in patients who have demonstrated limited disease responsive to systemic therapy.

51.11 Pelvic Reconstruction

Perineal wound dehiscence occurs in as many as 70–80 % of patients. Prior pelvic radiation is a key contributing factor. There are many reconstructive options developed to facilitate perineal wound healing and decrease the incidence of wound complications. The most commonly used are myocutaneous flaps, such as the vertical rectus abdominis myocutaneous (VRAM) flap, rotational anterolateral thigh flaps, and the gracilis myocutaneous flap (Fig. 51.3). VRAM flaps have the major advantage of providing well vascularized soft-tissue volume with excellent blood supply and associated skin coverage for the perineum [87–89]. Similarly, anterolateral thigh flaps have good blood supply but are more limited by length of the vascular pedicle, particularly in shorter patients. While the gracilis flap can provide good coverage for the perineum, it has little bulk to fill the pelvis [90]. Another option is de-epithelialized gluteal advancement, but it similarly has limited space filling of the true pelvis and may require augmentation with a pedicled omental flap. Several comparative studies of flap reconstruction versus primary closure have demonstrated decreased perineal wound complications with flap reconstruction [87–90]. At MD Anderson Cancer Center, our preferred approach includes routine vertical rectus or anterolateral thigh flap reconstruction after salvage APR.

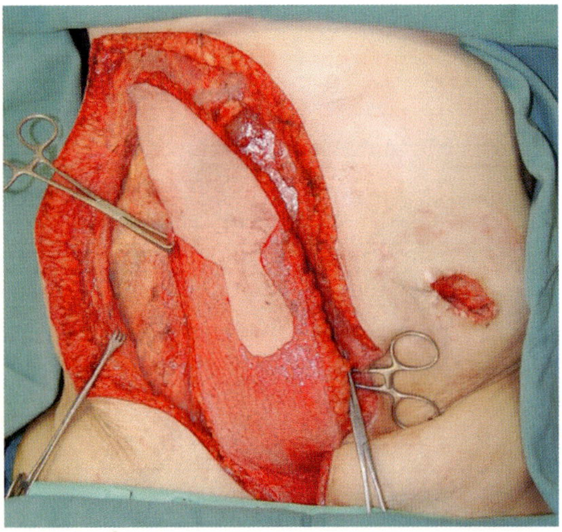

Fig. 51.3 Right rectus abdominus myocutaneous flap has been elevated and partially de-epithelialized. The skin bearing portion will be used to reconstruct the posterior vaginal wall (Copyright held by, and used with permission of, George J. Chang, M.D)

51.12 Summary

The incidence of anal cancer continues to increase worldwide, especially in at-risk populations. Despite advances in treatment, advanced stage disease continues to pose a challenge to clinicians. The mainstay of treatment for primary disease is definitive chemoradiation therapy with salvage surgical resection reserved for persistent or recurrent disease. Newer concurrent chemotherapeutic regimens have been evaluated in an effort to improve treatment outcomes. However, while they have been associated with the potential for reduced toxicity, they have not improved the effectiveness of treatment when compared to MMC therapy. Recurrent or persistent disease should still be approached with surgical salvage observing the principles of radical *en bloc* resection augmented with vascularized soft-tissue reconstruction.

Key Points

- Incidence of anal cancer is increasing
- Associated with HPV infection and immunocompromise
- Surveillance is important in high-risk populations
- Early diagnosis is key to management
- Clinical exam, anoscopy, and biopsy are important for diagnosis and staging
- Local excision is possible for early-stage, small lesions
- Chemoradiation with 5-FU and mitomycin C is the standard of care
- Salvage APR is performed for persistent or recurrent disease
- Recurrence is typically locoregional and occurs in the first 3 years
- Early clinical surveillance is important to assess for persistent/recurrent disease

References

1. Howlader N, Noone AM, Krapcho M, Garshell J, Neyman N, et al., editors. SEER cancer statistics review, 1975–2010. Bethesda: National Cancer Institute. http://seer.cancer.gov/csr/1975_2010/, based on Nov 2012 SEER data submission, posted to the SEER web site, 2013.
2. Daling JR, Sherman KJ, Hislop TG, Maden C, Coates RJ, et al. Sexual practices, sexually transmitted disease, and the incidence of anal cancer. N Engl J Med. 1987;317:973–7.
3. Frisch M, Glimelius B, van den Brule AJC, Wohlfahrt J, Meijer CJ, et al. Sexually transmitted infection as a cause of anal cancer. N Engl J Med. 1997;337(19): 1350–8.
4. Chang GJ, Welton ML. Human papillomavirus, condylomata acuminata, and anal neoplasia. Clin Colon Rectal Surg. 2004;17:221–30.
5. Daling JR, Madeleine MM, Johnson LG, Schwartz SM, Shera KA, et al. Human papillomavirus, smoking, and sexual practices in the etiology of anal cancer. Cancer. 2004;101:270–80.
6. Silverberg MJ, Lau B, Justice AC, Engels E, Gill MJ, et al. Risk of anal cancer in HIV-infected and HIV-uninfected individuals in North America. Clin Infect Dis. 2012;54(7):1026–34.
7. Salit IE, Lytwyn A, Raboud J, Sano M, Chong S, et al. The role of cytology (Pap tests) and human papillomavirus testing in anal cancer screening. AIDS. 2010; 24:1307–13.
8. Berry JM, Palefsky JM, Jay N, Cheng SC, Darragh TM, et al. Performance characteristics of anal cytology and human papillomavirus testing in patients with high-resolution anoscopy-guided biopsy of high-grade anal intraepithelial neoplasia. Dis Colon Rectum. 2009;52:239–47.
9. Ogunbiyi OA, Scholefield JH, Raftery AT, Smith JH, Duffy S, et al. Prevalence of anal human papillomavirus infection and intraepithelial neoplasia in renal allograft recipients. Br J Surg. 1994;81:365–7.
10. Engels EA, Pfeiffer RM, Fraumeni Jr JF, Kasiske BL, Israni AK, et al. Spectrum of cancer risk among US solid organ transplant recipients. JAMA. 2011;306(17): 1891–901.
11. Nordenvall C, Nillson PJ, Ye W, Nyren O. Smoking, snus use, and risk of right- and left-sided colon, rectal, and anal cancer: a 37 year follow-up study. Int J Cancer. 2011;128(1):157–65.
12. Daling JR, Sherman KJ, Hislop TJ, Maden C, Mandelson MT, et al. Cigarette smoking and the risk of anogenital cancer. Am J Epidemiol. 1992;135(2):180–9.
13. Buckwalter JA, Jurayj MN. Relationship of chronic anorectal disease and carcinoma. Arch Surg. 1957; 75:352–61.
14. Holly EA, Whittemore AS, Aston DA, Ahn DK, Nickoloff BJ, Kristiansen JJ. Anal cancer incidence: genital warts, anal fissure or fistula, hemorrhoids, and smoking. J Natl Cancer Inst. 1989;81:726–31.
15. Tseng HF, Morgenstern H, Mack TM, Peters RK. Risk factors for anal cancer: results of a population-based case-control study. Cancer Causes Control. 2003;14: 837–46.
16. Nordenvall C, Nyren O, Ye W. Elevated anal squamous cell carcinoma risk associated with benign inflammatory anal lesions. Gut. 2006;55:703–7.
17. Holmes F, Borek D, Owen-Kummer M, Hassanein R, Fishback J, et al. Anal cancer in women. Gastroenterology. 1988;95:107–11.
18. Frisch M, Olsen JH, Bautz A, Melbye M. Benign anal lesions and the risk of anal cancer. N Engl J Med. 1994;331:300–2.
19. Frisch M, Glimelius B, van den Brule AJ, Wohlfahrt J, Mejier CJ, et al. Benign anal lesions, inflammatory bowel disease and risk for high risk human papillomavirus-positive and–negative anal carcinoma. Br J Cancer. 1998;78(11):1534–8.
20. Barleben A, Mills S. Anorectal anatomy and physiology. Surg Clin N Am. 2010;90:1–15.
21. Garrett K, Kalady MF. Anal neoplasms. Surg Clin N Am. 2010;90:147–61.
22. Martin F, Bower M. Anal intraepithelial neoplasia in HIV positive people. Sex Transm Infect. 2001;77: 327–31.
23. Critchlow CW, Surawicz CM, Holmes KK, Kuypers J, Daling JR, et al. Prospective study of high grade anal squamous intraepithelial neoplasia in a cohort of homosexual men: influence of HIV infection, immunosuppression and human papillomavirus infection. AIDS. 1995;9:1255–62.
24. Chang GJ, Berry JM, Jay N, Palefsky JM, Welton ML. Surgical treatment of high-grade anal squamous intraepithelial lesions: a prospective study. Dis Colon Rectum. 2002;45:453–8.
25. Devaraj B, Cosman BC. Expectant management of anal squamous dysplasia in patients with HIV. Dis Colon Rectum. 2006;49:36–40.
26. Beck DE, Fazio VW. Perianal Paget's disease. Dis Colon Rectum. 1987;30:263–6.
27. Tulchinsky H, Zmora O, Brazowski E, Goldman G, Rabau M. Extramammary Paget's disease of the perianal region. Color Dis. 2004;6:206–9.
28. De Toma G, Cavallaro G, Bitonti A, Polistena A, Onesti MG, Scuderi N. Surgical management of perianal giant condyloma acuminatum (Buschke-Lowenstein tumor). Report of three cases. Eur Surg Res. 2006;38:418–22.
29. Lam DT, Batista O, Weiss EG, Nogueras JJ, Wexner SD. Staged excision and split-thickness skin graft for circumferential perianal Paget disease. Dis Colon Rectum. 2001;44:868–70.
30. Seckel BR, Schoetz DJ, Coller JA. Skin grafts for circumferential coverage and perianal wounds. Surg Clin N Am. 1985;65:365–71.
31. Orkin BA. Perineal reconstruction with local flaps: technique and results. Tech Coloproctol. 2013;17:663–70.
32. Burke TW, Morris M, Roh MS, Levenback C, Gershenson DM. Perineal reconstruction using single

gracilis myocutaneous flaps. Gynecol Oncol. 1995; 57:221–5.
33. Solomon MJ, Atkinson K, Quinn MJ, Eyers AA, Glenn DC. Gracilis myocutaneous flap to reconstruct large perineal defects. Int J Color Dis. 1996;11: 49–51.
34. Fleshner PR, Chalasani S, Chang GJ, Levien DH, Hyman NH, et al. Practice parameters for anal squamous neoplasms. Dis Colon Rectum. 2008;51:2–9.
35. Robb BW, Mutch MG. Epidermoid carcinoma of the anal canal. Clin Colon Rectal Surg. 2006;19:54–60.
36. de Jong JS, Beukema JC, van Dam GM, Slart R, Lemstra C, Wiggers T. Limited value of staging squamous cell carcinoma of the anal margin and canal using the sentinel lymph node procedure: a prospective study with long-term follow-up. Ann Surg Oncol. 2010;17:2656–62.
37. Tarantino D, Bernstein MA. Endoanal ultrasound in the staging and management of squamous-cell carcinoma of the anal canal. Dis Colon Rectum. 2002;45: 16–22.
38. Roach SC, Hulse PA, Moulding FJ, Wilson R, Carrington BM. Magnetic resonance imaging of anal cancer. Clin Radiol. 2005;60:1111–9.
39. Salerno G, Daniels IR, Brown G. Magnetic resonance imaging of the low rectum: defining the radiological anatomy. Color Dis. 2006;8 Suppl 3:10–3.
40. Bannas P, Weber C, Adam G, Frenzel T, Derlin T, et al. Contrast-enhanced [^{18}F]fluorodeoxyglucose-positron emission tomography/computed tomography for staging and radiotherapy planning in patients with anal cancer. Int J Radiat Oncol Biol Phys. 2011;81: 445–51.
41. Mistrangelo M, Pelosi E, Bello M, Ricardi U, Milanesi E, et al. Role of positron emission tomography-computed tomography in the management of anal cancer. Int J Radiat Oncol Biol Phys. 2012;84:66–72.
42. Krengli M, Milia ME, Turri L, Mones E, Bassi MC, et al. FDG-PET/CT imaging for staging and target volume delineation in conformal radiotherapy of anal carcinoma. Radiat Oncol. 2010;5:10.
43. Winton E, Heriot AG, Ng M, Hicks RJ, Hogg A, et al. The impact of 18-fluorodeoxyglucose positron emission tomography on the staging, management and outcome of anal cancer. Br J Cancer. 2009;100: 693–700.
44. Trautmann TG, Zuger JH. Positron emission tomography for pretreatment staging and post-treatment evaluation in cancer of the anal canal. Mol Imaging Biol. 2005;7:309–13.
45. Edge SB, Byrd DR, Compton CC, Fritz AG, Greene FL, Trotti A. AJCC Cancer Staging Manual. 7th ed. New York, NY: Springer, 2009, pp 165–173.
46. Nigro ND, Vaitkevicius VK, Considine Jr B. Combined therapy for cancer of the anal canal: a preliminary report. Dis Colon Rectum. 1974;17: 354–6.
47. Nigro ND. An evaluation of combined therapy for squamous cell cancer of the anal canal. Dis Colon Rectum. 1984;27:763–6.
48. UKCCCR Anal Cancer Trial Working Party. Epidermoid anal cancer: results from the UKCCCR randomized trial of radiotherapy alone versus radiotherapy, 5-fluorouracil, and mitomycin. Lancet. 1996;348:1049–54.
49. Bartelink H, Roelofsen F, Eschwege F, Rougier P, Bosset JF, et al. Concomitant radiotherapy and chemotherapy is superior to radiotherapy alone in the treatment of locally advanced anal cancer: results of a phase III randomized trial of the European Organization for Research and Treatment of Cancer Radiotherapy and Gastrointestinal Cooperative Groups. J Clin Oncol. 1997;15:2040–9.
50. John M, Pajak T, Flam M, Hoffman J, Markoe A, et al. Dose escalation in chemoradiation for anal cancer: preliminary results of RTOG 92–08. Cancer J Sci Am. 1996;2:205–11.
51. Martenson JA, Lipsitz SR, Wagner Jr H, Kaplan EH, Otteman LA, et al. Initial results of a phase II trial of high dose radiation therapy, 5-fluorouracil, and cisplatin for patients with anal cancer (E4292): an Eastern Cooperative Oncology Group study. Int J Radiat Oncol Biol Phys. 1996;35:745–9.
52. Salama JK, Mell LK, Schomas DA, Miller RC, Devisetty K, et al. Concurrent chemotherapy and intensity-modulated radiation therapy for anal canal cancer patients: a multicenter experience. J Clin Oncol. 2007; 25:4581–6.
53. Kachnic LA, Winter K, Myerson RJ, Goodyear MD, Willins J, et al. RTOG 0529: a phase 2 evaluation of dose-painted intensity modulated radiation therapy in combination with 5-flurouracil and mitocycin-C for the reduction of acute morbidity in carcinoma of the anal canal. Int J Radiat Oncol Biol Phys. 2013;86:27–33.
54. Gerard JP, Mauro F, Thomas L, Castelain B, Mazeron JJ, et al. Treatment of squamous cell anal canal carcinoma with pulsed dose rate brachytherapy. Feasibility study of a French cooperation group. Radiother Oncol. 1999;51:129–36.
55. Bruna A, Gastelblum P, Thomas L, Chapet O, Bollet MA, et al. Treatment of squamous cell anal canal carcinoma with pulsed dose rate brachytherapy: a retrospective study. Radiother Oncol. 2006;79:75–9.
56. Rich TA, Ajani JA, Morrison WH, Ota D, Levin B. Chemoradiation therapy for anal cancer: radiation plus continuous infusion of 5-fluorouracil with or without cisplatin. Radiother Oncol. 1993;27:209–15.
57. Doci R, Zucali R, La Monica G, Meroni E, Kenda R, et al. Primary chemoradiation therapy with fluorouracil and cisplatin for cancer of the anus: results in 35 consecutive patients. J Clin Oncol. 1996;14:3121–5.
58. Gerard JP, Ayzac L, Hun D, Romestaing P, Coquard R, et al. Treatment of anal canal carcinoma with high dose radiation therapy and concomitant fluorouracil-cisplatinum. Long-term results in 95 patients. Radiother Oncol. 1998;46:249–56.
59. James RD, Glynne-Jones R, Meadows HM, Cunningham D, Myint AS, et al. Mitomycin or cisplatin chemoradiation with or without maintenance chemotherapy for treatment of squamous-cell carcinoma

of the anus (ACT II): a randomized, phase 3 open-label, 2 × 2 factorial trial. Lancet. 2013;14:516–24.
60. Peiffert D, Giovannini M, Ducreux M, Michel P, Francois E, et al. High-dose radiation therapy and neoadjuvant plus concomitant chemotherapy with 5-fluorouracil and cisplatin in patients with locally advanced squamous-cell anal carcinoma: final results of a phase II study. Ann Oncol. 2001;12:397–404.
61. Ajani JA, Winter KA, Gunderson LL, Pedersen J, Benson 3rd AB, et al. Fluorouracil, mitomycin, and radiotherapy vs fluorouracil, cisplatin, and radiotherapy for carcinoma of the anal canal: a randomized controlled trial. JAMA. 2008;299:1914–21.
62. Gunderson LL, Winter KA, Ajani JA, Pedersen JE, Moughan J, et al. Long-term update of US GI intergroup RTOG 98–11 phase 3 trial for anal carcinoma: survival, relapse, and colostomy failure with concurrent chemoradiation involving fluorouracil/mitomycin versus fluorouracil/cisplatin. J Clin Oncol. 2012; 30:4344–51.
63. Tanum G, Tveit K, Karlsen KO, Hauer-Jensen M. Chemotherapy and radiation therapy for anal carcinoma: survival and late morbidity. Cancer. 1991; 67:2462–6.
64. Broens P, Van Limbergen E, Penninckx F, Kerremans R. Clinical and manometric effects of combined external beam radiation and brachytherapy for anal cancer. Int J Color Dis. 1998;13:68–72.
65. Vordermark D, Sailer M, Flentje M, Thiede A, Kölbl O. Curative-intent radiation therapy in anal carcinoma: quality of life and sphincter function. Radiother Oncol. 1999;52:239–43.
66. Johnston MJ, Robertson GM, Frizelle FA. Management of late complications of pelvic radiation in the rectum and anus. Dis Colon Rectum. 2003; 46:247–59.
67. Turina M, Mulhall AM, Mahid SS, Yashar C, Galandiuk S. Frequency and surgical management of chronic complications related to pelvic radiation. Arch Surg. 2008;143:46–52.
68. Das P, Bhatia S, Eng C, Ajani JA, Skibber JM, et al. Predictors and patterns of recurrence after definitive chemoradiation for anal cancer. Int J Radiat Oncol Biol Phys. 2007;68:794–800.
69. Tan KK, Pal S, Lee PJ, Rodwell L, Solomon MJ. Pelvic exenteration for recurrent squamous cell carcinoma of the pelvic organs arising from the cloaca—a single institution's experience over 16 years. Color Dis. 2013;15:1227–31.
70. Longo WE, Vernava III AM, Wade TP, Coplin MA, Virgo KS, Johnson FE. Recurrent squamous cell carcinoma of the anal canal: predictors of initial treatment failure and results of salvage therapy. Ann Surg. 1994;220:40–9.
71. Ellenhorn JD, Enker WE, Quan SH. Salvage abdominoperineal resection following combined chemotherapy and radiotherapy for epidermoid carcinoma of the anus. Ann Surg Oncol. 1994;1:105–10.
72. Pocard M, Tiret E, Nugent K, Dehni N, Parc R. Results of salvage abdominoperineal resection for anal cancer after radiotherapy. Dis Colon Rectum. 1998;41: 1488–93.
73. Nilsson PJ, Svensson C, Goldman S, Glimelius B. Salvage abdominoperineal resection in anal epidermoid cancer. Br J Surg. 2002;89:1425–9.
74. Akbari RP, Paty PB, Guillem JG, Weiser MR, Temple LK, et al. Oncologic outcomes of salvage surgery for epidermoid carcinoma of the anus initially managed with combined modality therapy. Dis Colon Rectum. 2004;47:1136–44.
75. Ghouti L, Houvenaeghel G, Moutardier V, Giovannini M, Magnin V, et al. Salvage abdominoperineal resection after failure of conservative treatment in anal epidermoid cancer. Dis Colon Rectum. 2005;48:16–22.
76. Ferenschild FT, Vermaas M, Hofer SO, Verhoef C, Eggermont AM, et al. Salvage abdominoperineal resection and perineal wound healing in local recurrent or persistent anal cancer. World J Surg. 2005; 48:16–22.
77. Papaconstantinou HT, Bullard KM, Rothenberger DA, Madoff RD. Salvage abdominoperineal resection after failed Nigro protocol: modest success, major morbidity. Color Dis. 2006;8:124–9.
78. Mullen JT, Rodriguez-Bigas MA, Chang GJ, Barcenas CH, Crane CH, et al. Results of surgical salvage after failed chemoradiation therapy for epidermoid carcinoma of the anal canal. Ann Surg Oncol. 2007;14:478–83.
79. Schiller DE, Cummings BJ, Rai S, Le LW, Last L, et al. Outcomes of salvage surgery for squamous cell carcinoma of the anal canal. Ann Surg Oncol. 2007; 14:2780–9.
80. Stewart D, Yan Y, Kodner IJ, Birnbaum E, Fleshman J, et al. Salvage surgery after failed chemoradiation for anal canal cancer: should the paradigm be changed for high-risk tumors? J Gastrointest Surg. 2007;11: 1744–51.
81. Eeson G, Foo M, Harrow S, McGregor G, Hay J. Outcomes of salvage surgery for epidermoid carcinoma of the anus following failed combined modality treatment. Am J Surg. 2011;201:628–33.
82. Harris DA, Williamson J, Davies M, Evans MD, Drew P, et al. Outcome of salvage surgery for anal squamous cell carcinoma. Color Dis. 2013;15(8):968–73.
83. Tonouchi H, Ohmori Y, Kobayashi M, Konishi N, Tanaka K, et al. Operative morbidity associated with groin dissections. Surg Today. 2004;34:413–8.
84. Soliman AA, Heubner M, Kimmig R, Wimberger P. Morbidity of inguinofemoral lymphadenectomy in vulval cancer. ScientificWorldJournal. 2012;2012:341253.
85. Paley PJ, Johnson PR, Adcock LL, Cosin JA, Chen MD, et al. The effect of Sartorius transposition on wound morbidity following inguinal-femoral lymphadenectomy. Gynecol Oncol. 1997;64:237–41.
86. Pawlik TM, Gleisner AL, Bauer TW, Adams RB, Reddy SK, et al. Liver-directed surgery for metastatic squamous cell carcinoma to the liver: results of a multicenter analysis. Ann Surg Oncol. 2007;14:2807–16.
87. Butler CE, Gundeslioglu AO, Rodriguez-Bigas MA. Outcomes of immediate vertical rectus abdominis myocutaneous flap reconstruction for irradiated

abdominoperineal resection defects. J Am Coll Surg. 2008;206:694–703.
88. Sunesen KG, Buntzen S, Tei T, Lindegaard JC, Nørgaard M, Laurberg S. Perineal healing and survival after anal cancer salvage surgery: 10-year experience with primary perineal reconstruction using the vertical rectus abdominis myocutaneous (VRAM) flap. Ann Surg Oncol. 2009;16:68–77.
89. Tei TM, Stolzenburg T, Buntzen S, Laurberg S, Kjeldsen H. Use of transpelvic rectus abdominis musculocutaneous flap for anal cancer salvage surgery. Br J Surg. 2003;90:575–80.
90. Shibata D, Hyland W, Busse P, Kim HK, Sentovich SM, et al. Immediate reconstruction of the perineal wound with gracilis muscle flaps following abdominoperineal resection and intraoperative radiation therapy for recurrent carcinoma of the rectum. Ann Surg Oncol. 1999;6:33–7.

Management of Locally Advanced and Recurrent Rectal Cancer

52

Cherry E. Koh and Michael J. Solomon

52.1 Introduction

The key principle underpinning the management of locally advanced rectal cancer (LARC) or locally recurrent rectal cancer (LRRC) is that of complete en bloc radical excision with a clear resection margin (R0) [1]. This procedure, also known as pelvic exenteration, is a complex and technically challenging procedure that can be associated with considerable post-operative morbidity. Although pelvic exenteration was first described in 1948, it was not widely accepted until two decades ago because of the high surgical mortality and morbidity [2]. With improved imaging technology, better understanding of pelvic anatomy as well as improved surgical techniques, operative mortality has declined such that most units with the expertise in pelvic exenteration report mortality rates of under 1–2 % [3–5]. Although surgical morbidity remains moderately high, most large contemporary series report an acceptable major complication rate of 24–27 % [3, 4, 6]. Coupled with the numerous case series that have reported good quality of life outcomes in recent years, [7, 8] pelvic exenteration is now accepted as established treatment of LARC or LRRC.

52.2 Magnitude of the Problem

Local recurrence following treatment of primary rectal cancer has declined dramatically since the widespread adoption of total mesorectal excision (TME) and use of neoadjuvant radiotherapy based on pre-operative magnetic resonance (MRI) staging [9–11]. Notwithstanding this, local recurrence can still occur in 5–10 % of patients [12, 13]. Of patients with LRRC, an estimated 50 % will have isolated pelvic recurrence that could be amendable to curative resection [14, 15]. Without treatment, prognosis of LRRC is invariably grim, with a median survival of 6–9 months and patients are typically highly symptomatic particularly with pain [4, 16, 17]. With chemoradiation, median survival can be prolonged to 15 months but patients can remain highly symptomatic [16, 18]. As most patients with LRRC would have previously had radiotherapy, this limits treatment options available at the time of recurrence. Even if re-irradiation is considered, prior radiotherapy limits the amount of additional radiation that can be administered

C.E. Koh, MBBS(Hons), MS(Col Surg), FRACS
M.J. Solomon, MB, BAO, MSc(Clin Epid), FRACS (✉)
Royal Prince Alfred Hospital, Camperdown, NSW, Australia

Surgical Outcomes Research Centre (SOuRCe), Camperdown, NSW, Australia

Discipline of Surgery, University of Sydney, Newtown, NSW, Australia
e-mail: professor.solomon@sydney.edu.au

H.R.H. Patel et al. (eds.), *Pelvic Cancer Surgery: Modern Breakthroughs and Future Advances*,
DOI 10.1007/978-1-4471-4258-4_52, © Springer-Verlag London 2015

[19, 20]. Importantly, chemoradiation alone is not curative even if it does prolong survival [21]. Thus, pelvic exenteration with a clear resection margin (R0) is the only curative option available for these patients [1].

52.3 Presentation

Most patients with LARC or LRRC are symptomatic although a small proportion of patients with LRRC may present with an asymptomatic anastomotic recurrence detectable on routine follow-up. In symptomatic patients, symptoms typically reflect the location of the disease. Common symptoms include pain, rectal bleeding, rectal discharge, tenesmus or altered bowel habits [17, 22]. Of these, pain is the most common symptom and may be the result direct nerve, muscle or bony infiltration, or the result of referred pain. Less commonly, patients may also experience lymphoedema from venous compression, malignant recto-vesical or recto-vaginal fistula or a tumor fungating through the perineum.

52.4 Pre-operative Assessment

The purposes of investigations are to confirm diagnosis and to establish the extent of local disease so as to determine resectability. Although criteria for resectability vary between institutions, several authors have published what they consider resectable (see later). It needs to be emphasized that these constitute recommendations from specialized institutions with an interest in exenterations and as such, the same guidelines are unlikely to apply to all institutions. It is also noteworthy that the goalposts for resectability are constantly changing. With improved surgical technique and experience, what used to constitute absolute contraindication such as pelvic sidewall or proximal sacral involvement have now evolved to become standard surgical practice in selected centers [2, 7, 16].

Clinical Assessment

The utility of clinical assessment depends on the location of the cancer. Cancers involving the anal canal, perineum, low rectum or anastomosis may be readily visible or palpable. However, pain, which frequently accompanies local recurrence may limit the yield of clinical assessment without anesthesia. In patients who have previously undergone an abdomino-perineal excision, clinical assessment is often limited.

Imaging

All patients should be assessed with CT, MRI and positron-emission tomography (PET). PET complement CT in the detection of metastatic disease and have been shown to alter the management in 20–40 % of patients with LARC or LRRC by detecting occult metastasis otherwise undetected on other imaging modalities [23, 24]. As PET detects metabolically active tissue, it is very useful for distinguishing between post-treatment fibrosis and recurrence although false positives can occur with benign post-treatment inflammation. Pitfalls with PET are mucinous tumors and occult peritoneal deposits where PET scans are less accurate. The development of PET-CT by fusion of PET and CT images has partly overcome the problem with small occult metastases [25].

MRI is currently the gold standard for local staging of all rectal cancers whether an early rectal cancer, LARC or LRRC. MRI has revolutionized the assessment of LRRC in that it is most accurate in determining the local extent of the disease and therefore the resectability of LRRC. In doing so, it helps guide patient selection, enables the surgeon to counsel patients appropriately about the magnitude of the anticipated surgery, likely morbidity and facilitates surgical workforce planning on the day of surgery [26]. The accuracy of MRI depends both on the compartment involved as well as the experience of the radiologist interpreting the MR [27, 28]. The major limitation with MRI resides in its inability to accurately diagnose pelvic sidewall involvement [27, 28].

Tissue Diagnosis

Tissue diagnosis is conventionally regarded as gold standard in confirming diagnosis of cancer. While this is true for LARC, tissue diagnosis is not always possible in patients with LRRC. In patients where the tumor is inaccessible via a natural orifice (such as extra-luminal nodal recurrence or previous abdominoperineal excision), one will have to question the utility of a percutaneous biopsy which would violate virginal planes that are unlikely to be included as part of the radical excision thereby posing a small but theoretical risk of tract seeding [29, 30]. Although contentious, in our exenteration practice, a hot PET scan in the presence of a corroborative history, MRI findings and CEA will be accepted as being diagnostic of local recurrence without a biopsy.

Other Investigations

A variety of other investigations are often necessary to confirm diagnosis or assist with surgical planning. They include:

- Colonoscopy
- CEA
- Cystoscopy (with or without ureteric stenting)
- CT angiography
- MR angiography

Colonoscopy and CEA are usually part of routine pre-operative assessment but the need for cystoscopy, CT or MR angiography is selective based on individual circumstances.

52.5 Resectability

The indications and contra-indications for pelvic exenteration vary widely between institutions and continue to evolve with experience. With improved surgical techniques and experience, what used to constitute absolute contraindications such as high sacral or pelvic sidewall involvement are no longer contraindications provided an R0 margin can be achieved safely [2, 5, 31]. There is little doubt that some patients are currently not offered exenteration for what would be considered routine resection in specialized centers [2]. Table **52.1** summarizes published resectability criteria.

Due to the associated surgical morbidity and mortality, pelvic exenteration is generally only offered with a curative intent. Patients with unresectable metastases are therefore not usually considered for pelvic exenteration. However, the presence of synchronous resectable visceral metastases or a history of previously treated metachronous metastases should not preclude consideration for pelvic exenteration provided the patient is medically fit for the procedure [32, 33]. Whether metasectomy and pelvic exenteration should be performed as staged or synchronous procedures and whether a metasectomy first approach is more appropriate is debatable, although synchronous procedures are likely to prolong surgical time and increase surgical morbidity considerably if a major resection is necessary.

Traditionally, pelvic sidewall recurrence was considered a formidable surgical challenge that is incurable [22, 34]. The potential involvement of major neurovascular structures essential for lower limb function coupled with the difficulties in achieving R0 resection margin have contributed to pelvic sidewall recurrence being considered a contraindication for surgical exploration [22, 35–37]. In fact, prior to the advent of MRI, referred pain in the distribution of the sciatic nerve alone was enough to preclude consideration for surgery [38, 39]. However, with improved understanding of pelvic anatomy and surgical technique, pelvic sidewall dissection has become standard practice in many centers [31]. A systematic approach to the pelvic sidewall as described by Austin and Solomon has been shown to achieve R0 resection margins in 53 % of patients with pelvic sidewall involvement, which is comparable to R0 resection rates at other sites of recurrence [6, 31]. Major iliac vessel excision and reconstruction, adopted from allied surgical specialties in the treatment of retroperitoneal soft tissue sarcomas has demonstrated that en bloc iliac vessel excision and reconstruction can improve R0 rates with acceptable morbidity and

Table 52.1 Resectability of locally recurrent rectal cancer

Institution/country	Authors year	Relative contraindication	Absolute contraindication
Leeds United Kingdom	Mirnezami et al. 2010 [26]	Distant metastasis	Encasement of external iliac vessels
		Primary stage IV disease	Extension of tumor through sciatic notch
		Extensive pelvic sidewall involvement	Presence of lower limb oedema from venous or lymphatic obstruction
		Predicted R1 or R2 resection	Poor performance status
		Sacral invasion above S2-S3 junction	
	Boyle et al. 2005[a] [5]		Presence of extensive abdominal or thoracic metastases
			Encasement of external iliac vessels
			Extension of tumor through sciatic notch
			Sacral invasion above the level of S2–3 junction
Lund Sweden	Zoucas et al. 2010[a] [35]		Adherence or invasion of sacrum at or above S2 level
			Extensive lateral or circumferential pelvic wall involvement
			Encasement of sciatic notch or external iliac vessels
			Presence of unresectable distant metastasis
Texas United States	Gannon et al. 2007 [37] and Pawlik et al. 2006[a] [36]	Ureteral obstruction	Distant metastases
		Poor candidate for surgery because of medical comorbidities	Involvement of common or external iliac vessels
		Poor candidate for surgery because of inability to care for stomas or senility	Metastasis to para-aortic nodes
			Involvement of the sacrum proximal to S1 (note: some consider S2 involvement to an absolute contraindication)
			Tumor extension through sciatic foramen
			Pelvic sidewall involvement
Washington United States	Ogunbiyi et al. 1997 [22][a]	*The authors defined resectable disease as*	Midline posterior tumors adherent or invading the distal sacrum below S2
		Isolated perianastomotic or perineal recurrence	
		Tumors invading adjacent pelvic structures such as bladder, prostate or vagina	
		Absence of invasion of lateral pelvic sidewalls, upper sacrum and pelvic nerves (ad indicated by neurologic signs and symptoms)	
		No involvement of ureters as indicated by absence of hydronephrosis on imaging	

Ogunbiyi et al. defined resectability more by what was resectable rather than what was non-resectable
[a]Authors do not distinguish between relative versus absolute contraindication

graft patency rates [40, 41]. En bloc excision of sciatic nerve, where necessary to achieve R0 resection margins is a well established practice in the sarcoma literature with better than anticipated functional outcomes [42–44]. Patients typically require a foot brace to prevent foot drop but mobility is acceptable. Although patients report mild to moderate physical impairment, most prefer some degree of disability over amputation [42].

To enable even more radical resections of the pelvic sidewall for tumors extending through the sciatic notch, Nielsen et al. recently reported on their initial experience with external hemi-pelvectomy (hind quarter amputation) on eight highly selected patients with a variety of locally advanced or recurrent pelvic malignancies [45]. External hemi-pelvectomy is highly morbid procedure that is generally reserved for malignant sarcomas of the pelvis but where possible, a limb preserving form of hemi-pelvectomy (internal hemipelvectomy) with bony reconstruction is favored [46]. Although hemi-pelvectomy has been reported sporadically for carcinomas of the pelvis, unlike sarcomas, its role in carcinomas remains unclear [45, 47–50]. Oncological outcomes following hemi-pelvectomy in general are poor and longer term follow up data is scant [45, 47]. In the absence of long term oncological and quality of life data, these procedures should only be offered in expert centers on an individual basis where lesser surgical interventions are not possible. Patients need to be counseled appropriately and ideally, surgical, oncological and longitudinal quality of life outcomes in these patients should be assessed to further define the role of hemi-pelvectomy in LARC or LRRC.

En bloc sacrectomy may be required in 9–24 % of all pelvic exenterations in order to achieve R0 resection margins [3–6]. Sacrectomies at or below S3 are generally classed as low sacrectomies whereas high sacrectomies involves sacral transection at the level of S1 or 2. High sacrectomies are associated with increased intra-operative blood loss, surgical morbidity and post-surgical neurological deficit [4, 51–53]. Although oncological and functional outcomes following sacrectomies for a range of skeletal and soft tissue tumors are well described, literature on sacrectomy for LARC or LRRC is much more limited [51]. While low sacrectomies are widely accepted because of comparable R0, survival and morbidity rates as those who do not require en bloc sacrectomy, [54–57] high sacrectomies were traditionally considered a contraindication for surgery [5, 22]. However, as with the paradigm shift with pelvic sidewall involvement, high sacrectomies are no longer a contraindication for surgery [53, 58, 59]. In a recent study by Milne et al. which included 21 patients who underwent en bloc S1/S2 sacrectomy for LRRC, R0, median and 5 year survivals of 74 %, 59 months and 38 % were reported respectively [53]. In another study by Dozois et al. on high sacrectomy for LRRC, an R0 rate of 100 % and a 5 year survival of 30 % were reported [58]. Importantly, post-operative function seemed good with the former study reporting no difference in neurological deficits between low and high sacrectomy patients and the latter reporting acceptable post-operative ambulation, function and improved pain control [53, 58]. Although more studies are needed, favorable oncologic outcomes coupled with an acceptable morbidity profile and functional outcome necessarily means that high sacrectomy should no longer constitute a contraindication for surgery.

Rarely, pelvic exenteration may be considered for palliative purposes. These are typically patients with symptoms that cannot be adequately palliated using alternative treatment options such as uncontrolled enterovaginal or vesical fistulae, offensive fungating tumors or patients with intractable pain [22, 60]. Several small and highly selected case series have reported dramatically improved symptom control [17, 60, 61]. Naturally, such radical approach to palliation carries the risk of bringing forth the patient's demise but this also highlights the importance of quality of life and patient choice in decision making.

52.6 Treatment

Multi-disciplinary Team Approach

Treatment decision for LARC or LRRC patients should be made in a multi-disciplinary setting. These meetings should include all relevant surgical and medical specialties as well as allied health specialists such as cancer coordinator, stomal therapists and psych-oncologists. These meetings are also useful for work force planning to ensure the necessary specialties are available on the designated operation day.

Pre-operative Chemoradiation

Patients who are radiotherapy naïve should undergo pre-operative long course chemoradiation [62]. The role of re-irradiation in patients previously irradiated patients is currently unclear [19]. Re-irradiation options include external beam radiotherapy, intensity modulated radiotherapy (IMRT) or intra-operative radiotherapy (IORT). IMRT is a relatively new radiotherapy technique that delivers differential radiation doses precisely to better conform to the three-dimensional shape of the tumor. In doing so, parts of the tumor can receive higher doses while protecting surrounding critical structures [63]. IORT can deliver a much higher biological dose directly to the tumor bed without increasing tissue toxicity but requires purpose built operating theaters to do so [19]. This seems useful where resection margins may have been compromised but this simply underscores the importance of an R0 resection margin [19, 64, 65].

The role of re-staging after chemoradiation is currently unclear although the consensus from an international collaboration, the Beyond TME collaboration, recommends restaging with MRI and PET to assess treatment response prior to exenteration (manuscript in preparation).

Compartments of the Pelvis and Dissection Planes

Conceptually, the pelvis can be divided into five compartments (Fig. 52.1). They are the central, anterior, posterior and the two lateral compartments. Each compartment overlaps at their periphery and are each centered on a different structure. The central compartment is centered on the tip of the coccyx, while the anterior, posterior and lateral compartments are centered on the urethra, the third sacral vertebra and the ischial spines respectively. The contents of each compartment are listed in Table 52.2. Within each compartment are different extra-TME dissection planes and this is illustrated in Fig. 52.2. With these in mind, the surgeon can then conceptualize the three-dimensional anatomy of the cancer so as to formulate a surgical plan when the pelvic MRI is reviewed with an experienced MR radiologist.

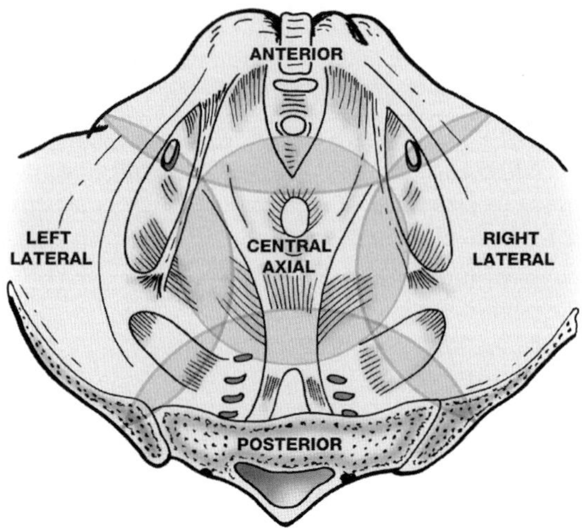

Fig. 52.1 Diagram of the pelvis illustrating the five pelvic compartments, each overlapping at their periphery. Each compartment is centered on a different structure with the anterior, central, posterior and lateral compartments centered on the urethra, the tip of the coccyx, the third sacral vertebra and the ischial spines respectively

Surgical Technique

Pelvic exenteration is a heterogeneous group of operations where the specific procedure will vary depending on the location and the extent of the tumor. Because of this, there is no standardized surgical approach although broad principles can be applied. Of note, there is no universally accepted terminology for types of exenteration. Terms such as central, visceral, complete and total exenteration are often used interchangeably while others would use composite resection or abdominosacral resection to imply en bloc sacral resection. For clarity, exenteration is best defined

Table 52.2 Contents within the compartments

Compartment	Viscera	Muscle	Bone	Others
Anterior	Bladder	Obturator internus	Pubic symphysis	Dorsal venous complex
	Urethra	Obturator externus	Superior pubic ramus	
	Males: prostate, seminal vesicles, vas deferens	Anterior pelvic floor (pubococcygeus, puborectalis part of levator)	Inferior pubic ramus	
	Females: anterior vagina			
Central	Females: posterior half of vagina, uterus, cervix, ovaries, fallopian tubes, broad ligament, round ligament	Pelvic floor muscles (iliococcygeus part o levator ani)	S4 and 5 sacral vertebra	
	Rectum		Coccyx	
Posterior	Rectum	Pelvic floor muscles (coccygeus)	Sacrum (S1-S5)	Branches and tributaries of the internal iliac vessels
		Piriformis	Coccyx	Sacral nerve roots (S1–S4)
				Anterior sacroccocygeal ligament
				Medial sacrotuberous ligament
				Sacrospinous ligament
Lateral	Ureter	Piriformis	Ischial spine	Internal iliac artery and vein
		Obturator internus	Ischial tuberosity	External iliac artery and vein
		Coccygeus		Obturator artery and vein
				Lateral sacrotuberous ligament
				Sacrospinous ligament
				Lumbosacral trunk
				Sciatic nerve distal to ischial spine
				Obturator nerve

Because the compartments overlap at their periphery, some structures appear more than once within the table

as complete or partial based on the number of compartments excised.

All procedures can be subdivided into an exploratory phase, a dissection phase and a reconstructive phase. All procedures begin with an exploratory phase where the aim is to rule out occult metastatic disease that may preclude curative resection and to isolate the pelvic cancer from all small bowel loops by meticulous adhesiolysis, en bloc excision of contiguously involved small bowel loops and dividing the colon along its anatomical planes.

The aim of the dissection is to achieve a clear microscopic margin (R0). As a general principle, a compartmental approach is adopted whereby involvement of a compartment would necessitate

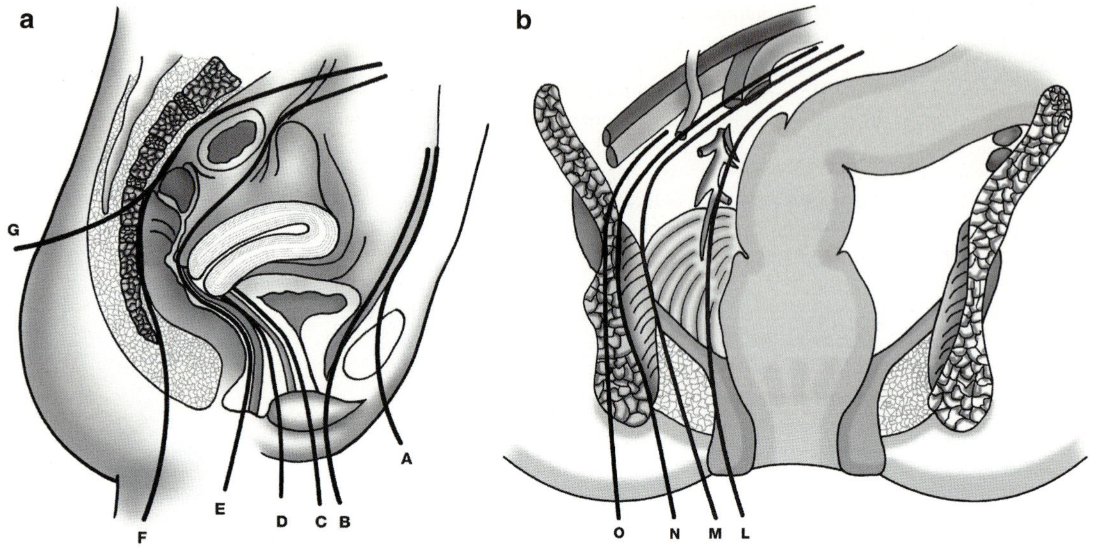

Fig. 52.2 (**a**) Sagittal section of a female pelvis demonstrating possible dissection planes. *Plane A–G* are the surgical dissection planes available. (**b**) Coronal section of a pelvis demonstrating possible dissection planes. *Plane L* is the TME plane; *plane M* is the extra-vascular plane which would involve excision of iliac vasculature; *plane N* is the plane that involves en bloc excision of obturator internus; *plane O* involves en bloc excision of ischial spine or ischial tuberosity

complete excision of the compartment at its soft tissue bony junction or if the tumor extends very close to this margin, en bloc excision of the adjacent bone. Attempting to obtain a soft tissue margin in the former is likely to result in an unacceptably high rate of involved margins. In LRRC, the dissection planes are often poorly defined due to fibrosis from previous radiotherapy and total mesorectal excision. While detailed technical description of each exenteration procedure is beyond the scope of this chapter, it is important to highlight the modern breakthroughs in exenteration techniques.

Lateral Neurovascular Approach

Central to pelvic sidewall dissection is the appreciation that key neurovascular structures are organized in a "layered" manner where the ureter lies superficial to iliac arteries, iliac veins, lumbosacral trunk and obturator internus (Fig. 52.3). To gain access to a deeper structure, the superficial lying structure is dissected out so as to "float" it off the pelvic sidewall (Fig. 52.3). Lateral compartment dissection begins with ureterolysis and pelvic lymphadenectomy which facilitates vascular dissection and exposes the sacral plexus. The appropriate dissection plane is usually predetermined by the staging MRI (Fig. 52.2). Where possible, the internal iliac artery should be ligated distal to the gluteal branches so as to

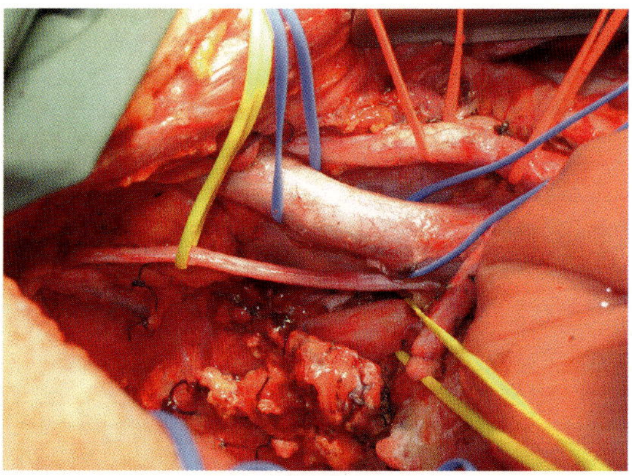

Fig. 52.3 Intra-operative photo of pelvic sidewall demonstrating the right common, external and ligated internal iliac arteries (*red* vessel loops); the right common, external and ligated internal iliac veins (*blue* vessel loops); obturator nerve and lumbosacral trunk (*yellow* vessel loops). This photo demonstrates the "layered" organization of the lateral compartment neurovascular structures. Ligation of internal iliac artery and vein allows and common and external iliac systems to be "floated" off the pelvic sidewall

reduce the likelihood of buttock claudication and to preserve the option of a gluteal artery based flap. Even where formal excision of the internal iliac vasculature is not necessary, in situ ligation of these vessels can help limit blood loss when a distal sacrectomy is planned.

Dissection of the iliac veins is much more challenging due to the variable anatomy and thin walled veins. Loss of venous control is more commonly the cause of catastrophic bleeding in exenterative surgery. The surgeon can usually expect at least a visceral, spinal (or presacral) branch and a gluteal tributary at each level. Pre-emptive suture ligation after dissection of an appropriate venous cuff will ensure vascular control and progressively devascularize the pelvis. In LRRC, the extra-vascular plane is often virginal compared to the TME plane and may be comparatively easier to dissect even if vascular excision is not required.

Identification of the lumbosacral trunk is a key step in lateral compartment dissection as it leads to obturator internus muscle and ischial spine. Preserving the lumbosacral trunk for lower limb motor function is generally possible even if a distal sacrectomy is necessary. To completely excise the lateral compartment, obturator internus can be excised at its origin with or without en bloc excision of ischial spine or ischial tuberosity.

Anterior Compartment Dissection

Conventionally, the anterior dissection plane is the retro-pubic plane at the junction between bladder and pubic bone. As with the principles of en bloc bony excision in the lateral and posterior compartments to improve R0 resection, the same can be applied to the anterior compartment. In LRRC where there is extensive prostatic involvement or involvement of the membranous urethra following previous abdomino-perineal excision in men, en bloc pubic bone excision and excision of proximal penile urethra may be required to achieve a clear resection margin. In a study by Solomon et al. patients with LRRC who underwent en bloc cystectomy had a R0 rate of 64 % but this contrasts with an R0 rate of 100 % in patients who underwent en bloc cystectomy and pubic bone excision (pubic symphysis or bilateral inferior pubic ramus excision) when the membranous urethra was involved (manuscript in preparation). Although long term oncological data from pubic bone excision is not yet available, this demonstrates technique modification can further improve R0 resection rates. Of note, even if central pubic excision is performed, internal fixation is typically not required. Mesh reconstruction to the divided ends of pubic rami with overlying flap reconstruction is generally all that is required.

Posterior Compartment Dissection

The surgical approach for high versus low sacrectomy differ in that a high (S1/S2) sacrectomy generally requires a prone approach whereas a low sacrectomy (S3 and distal) can be performed via an abdominolithotomy approach. High sacrectomies can be highly morbid because division of proximal sacral nerve roots which can cause considerable lower limb motor and sensory deficits. Division of distal sacral nerve roots can result in an atonic bladder. Therefore, patients should be counseled appropriately about en bloc cystectomy even if it is not required oncologically. In patients where there is central involvement of L5 or S1, a central anterior table excision can be performed for L5 and S1 leaving the remainder of the sacrum intact thus preserving pelvic stability and sacral nerve roots.

Sacrectomy is usually the final step after completion of both the abdominal (lateral, anterior and other posterior dissections) and perineal phases of the procedure. This includes abdominal and perineal reconstruction where a prone sacrectomy is required. Posterior dissection begins in the TME plane but stops about 2 cm above the point where tumor adheres to sacrum. For distal sacrectomy, piriformis and sacral nerve roots are divided. After completion of the remainder of perineal dissection, the perineal surgeon disconnects gluteus maximus and tunnels immediately posterior to the coccyx and sacrum to the level of intended sacral division. A malleable retractor is then inserted to protect natal cleft tissue as the abdominal surgeon performs the sacrectomy using a 20 mm osteotome and mallet (Fig. 52.4).

Where a prone sacrectomy is to be performed, to ensure that sacral transection is performed at

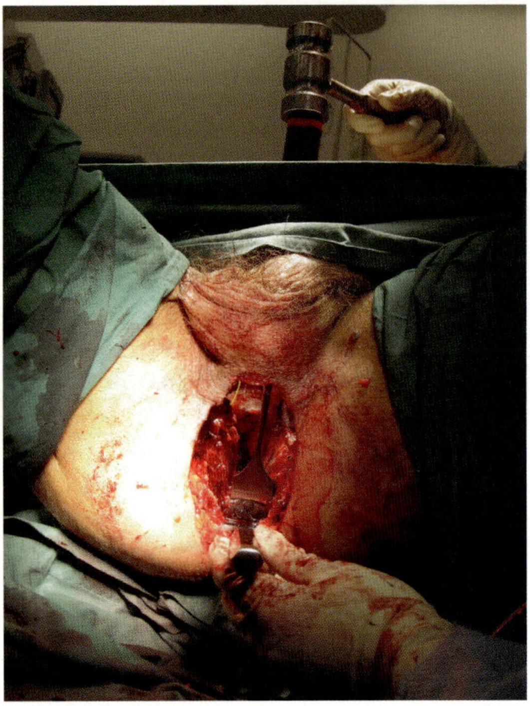

Fig. 52.4 Distal sacrectomy performed via an abdomino-lithotomy approach using a 20 mm osteotome. Natal cleft tissues are protected with a malleable retractor

the appropriate level, an orthopedic staple is secured into the sacrum 2 cm above the desired point of transection. The position of this staple is checked with intra-operative x-ray to confirm the point of sacral transection. It is also useful in these cases to have both lumbosacral trunks marked with a yellow vessel loop and a suture to orientate the rectus abdominis myocutaneous flap to avoid flap malrotation. Abdominal sponges are also left in the pelvis anterior to the sacrum to prevent small bowel from coming into contact with the anterior aspect of sacrum which may be inadvertently injured as the sacrum is being divided from the prone approach using an oscillating saw. Dural sac should be ligated in high sacrectomies to prevent ongoing cerebro-spinal fluid leakage.

Reconstruction

Consideration has to be given to visceral, abdominal and perineal reconstruction. Where cystectomy is performed, an ileal or colonic conduit will be required. Although ileal conduits are preferred, it may not be advisable in patients where small bowel loops have been heavily irradiated. A colonic conduit out of the radiation field may be associated with less complications in this setting [66]. The use of orthotopic neobladder reconstruction is popular within gynae-oncology literature [67, 68] but few are considering the technique in LARC or LRRC [69]. Where a segmental ureteric excision was performed, options include an end-to-end ureteric anastomosis, bladder re-implantation with a psoas hitch or nephrectomy. Re-implanting the ureter into the contralateral ureter or the use of a gastric or jejunal interposition graft are alternatives but the former is avoided if possible to prevent potential repercussions on both kidneys should surgical complications ensue.

In patients where a wide perineal excision or high sacrectomy has been performed, consideration needs to be given to reconstruction using a myocutaneous flap [70]. A rectus abdominis myocutaneous flap is the workhorse for this reconstruction as flap harvest can be incorporated to the laparotomy incision in addition to providing a bulky and well-vascularized tissue with a skin paddle for reconstruction. In patients with previous bilateral stomas, assessing patency of the inferior epigastric artery is recommended. Alternative tissue flaps include gluteal V-Y advancement flaps, inferior gluteal artery perforator based flaps or anterior thigh flaps [71–74]. It is important that skin paddle harvested is not excessive as this will only introduce donor site morbidity. If a rectus abdominis myocutaneous flap is harvested, mesh reconstruction of the abdominal wall will be necessary.

52.7 Outcomes and Prognosis

Reported surgical mortality rates range between 0.3 and 8 % although larger series in recent years have tended to report mortality rates of under 1 % [3, 4, 75]. Published complication rates vary even

Table 52.3 Common complications experienced in exenteration patients

Septic	
	Urinary tract infection
	Wound infection
	Pneumonia
	Deep seated intra-abdominal/pelvic collections
	Osteomyelitis
	Gastrointestinal complications
	Prolonged ileus
	Small bowel obstruction
	Enterocutaneous fistula
	Anastomotic leak
	Colo-vaginal fistula
Cardiorespiratory	
	Atrial fibrillation or other cardiac arrthymias
	Myocardial infarction
	Pulmonary embolism (deep venous thrombosis)
	Wound complications
	Wound dehiscence
	Persistent perineal sinus
	Perineal flap necrosis
	Infected prosthetic mesh
	Hematomas
Urological	
	Urinary retention
	Urological leak
	Colovesical fistula
Neurological	
	Sciatic nerve palsy
Stomal complications	
	Stomal dehiscence
	Ischemia

more widely between 21 and over 70 % [3, 38, 76, 77]. The widely disparate complication rates reflect the lack of consistency in reporting. While some authors only report major complications, other report all documented complications. However, major complication rates of about 25 % are generally reported by the larger and more recent studies. Common complications are listed in Table 52.3.

The main aim of surgery is to achieve an R0 margin [1]. Many studies have now demonstrated the survival difference between patients who have R0, R1 and R2 resection margins [3–5]. R0 rates within the literature vary between 38 and 85 % depending on the type of exenteration offered and the experience of the institution [3, 5, 34, 76, 78, 79]. Table 52.4 summarizes R0 and survival data from the larger case series published in the last 5 years.

Numerous other studies have attempted to characterize prognostic indicators for LRRC. Wanebo et al. and Yamada et al. reported that an elevated CEA conferred a worse prognosis compared to patients with normal CEA [34, 59]. Hahnloser et al. and Suzuki et al. found that patients with symptomatic recurrence, particularly when the symptom was pain was associated with a worse prognosis [4, 38]. In the large study by Hahnloser et al. from the Mayo clinic, the number of points of fixation within the pelvis was also found to be predictive of survival [4].

Quality of life in patients following pelvic exenteration is an area that remains understudied [80]. A meta-analysis by Thaysen et al. reported found only seven studies that evaluated quality of life in exenteration patients [80]. Based on existing studies, what is known is that quality of life in exenteration patients can be comparable with patients after TME for primary rectal cancer and that bony resection, the need for double stomas, gender or age do not influence quality of life [7, 8]. The issue of chronic pain in this group of patients is even more under-studied. In a recent study by You et al. pain is predictive of poorer quality of life and is associated with reduced survival [81]. More prospective studies with longer follow ups are required. However, within the confines of current knowledge, it would appear that the quality of life of patients are not worse than that of patients with primary rectal cancer [7].

In the only study that evaluated the cost effectiveness of pelvic exenteration, the authors concluded that surgery is cost effective particularly when calculated using utilities derived from patient preferences [82].

Table 52.4 R0 and survival data from the larger series in the last 5 years

Authors/year	N	R0 (%)	5 year survival (%)	R1/R2 survival	Comments
Heriot et al. 2008 [3]	160	98 (61)	49	25 % for R1 9 % for R2	
Kusters et al. 2009 [83]	170	92 (54)	40		Anastomotic and presacral recurrences had the best and the worst outcomes respectively
Jiang et al. 2011 [84]	187	87 (47)	31	17.2 % for R1 0 % for R2	Patients with lymph node metastases had worse survival
Rahbari et al. 2011 [6]	92	54 (59)	47	26 % 3 year OS for R1 11 % 3 year OS for R2	Exenteration in the setting of metastatic disease can lead to good outcomes if clear margins for pelvic disease can be achieved
Neilsen et al. 2012 [85]	40	15 (38)	17		LARC had better survival than LRRC even when both had R0
Zoucas et al. 2010 [35]	33	19 (64)	Not reported		2 year survival of 75 %

LARC Locally Advanced Rectal Cancer, *LRRC* Locally Recurrent Rectal Cancer

Conclusions

Pelvic exenteration is a complex procedure that requires meticulous pre-operative planning and specialized post-operative care. The boundaries of resectability are constantly being challenged. Improved surgical technique has reduced surgical mortality and morbidity to an acceptable level. Increased surgical radicality over the years has also improved R0 rates thereby increasing the prospects of long term survival. As with oncological results with many other cancers, best results with exenteration is most likely from high volume centers. Smaller centers are therefore encouraged to consider onward referral and to collaborate with larger centers for best outcomes.

Key Points

- Locally advanced primary rectal cancer and locally recurrent rectal cancer require the same meticulous surgical planning, intra-operative surgical approach and post-operative care
- Criteria for resectability continue to evolve. Boundaries are constantly being pushed and smaller centers are encouraged to collaborate with more experienced centers and to consider onward referral if appropriate. The most important determinant for resectability is the ability to achieve a clear resection margin.
- The single most important factor predicting long term survival is a clear resection margin (R0). Others include an elevated CEA (>10), symptomatic presentation (especially pain) and number of points of fixation in the pelvis
- Patient selection for surgery is based on a high quality pelvic MRI and PET scan. MRI determines the extent of local disease so as to determine resectability and the latter rules out distant metastasis.
- All patients require input from a multidisciplinary team including allied health specialists (cancer coordinator, stomal therapy, psychologists, physiotherapists and dieticians)

- A major breakthrough in the surgical approach to locally recurrent rectal cancer is the compartmental approach adopted from sarcoma surgery
- Anatomically, the pelvis can be divided into five compartments including the anterior, central, posterior and two lateral compartments. Within each compartment are different possible dissection planes.
- With improved surgical technique and better understanding of pelvic anatomy, surgical mortality and major complications in large contemporary series are usually under 1 % and about 25 % respectively.
- Quality of life studies following pelvic exenteration are relatively scant but based on available data, global quality of life seems acceptable. The need for bony resection or double stomas does not appear to affect quality of life. The impact of pain on quality of life and survival needs further evaluation.
- Follow up after pelvic exenteration is currently not well defined.

References

1. Bhangu A, Ali S, Darzi A, Brown G, Tekkis P. Meta-analysis of survival based on resection margin status following surgery for recurrent rectal cancer. Colorectal Dis. 2012;14(12):1457–66.
2. Solomon M. Re-exenteration for recurrent rectal cancer. Dis Colon Rectum. 2013;56(1):4–5.
3. Heriot A, Byrne C, Lee P, Dobbs B, Tilney H, Solomon M, et al. Extended radical resection: the choice for locally recurrent rectal cancer. Dis Colon Rectum. 2008;51:284–91.
4. Hahnloser D, Nelson H, Gunderson L, Hassan I, Haddock M, O'Connell M, et al. Curative potential of multimodality therapy for locally recurrent rectal cancer. Ann Surg. 2003;237:502–8.
5. Boyle K, Sagar P, Chalmers A, Sebag-Montefiore D, Cairns A, Eardley I. Surgery for locally recurrent rectal cancer. Dis Colon Rectum. 2005;48(5):929–37.
6. Rahbari N, Ulrich A, Bruckner T, Münter M, Nickles A, Contin P, et al. Surgery for locally recurrent rectal cancer in the era of total mesorectal excision: is there still a chance for cure? Ann Surg. 2011;253(3):522–33.
7. Austin K, Young J, Solomon M. Quality of life of survivors after pelvic exenteration for rectal cancer. Dis Colon Rectum. 2010;53(8):1121–6.
8. Esnaola N, Cantor S, Johnson M, Mirza A, Miller A, Curley S, et al. Pain and quality of life after treatment in patients with locally recurrent rectal cancer. J Clin Oncol. 2002;20(21):4361–7.
9. Heald R, Ryall R. Recurrence and survival after total mesorectal excision for rectal cancer. Lancet. 1986;327(8496):1479–82.
10. Al-Sukhni E, Milot L, Fruitman M, Beyene J, Victor J, Schmocker S, et al. Diagnostic accuracy of MRI for assessment of T category, lymph node metastases, and circumferential resection margin involvement in patients with rectal cancer: a systematic review and meta-analysis. Ann Surg Oncol. 2012;19(7):2212–23.
11. Taylor F, Mangat N, Swift I, Brown G. Proforma-based reporting in rectal cancer. Cancer Imaging. 2010;10(1A):S142–50.
12. Peeters K, Marijnen C, Nagtegaal I, Kranenbarg E, Putter H, Wiggers T, et al. The TME trial after a median follow-up of 6 years: increased local control but no survival benefit in irradiated patients with resectable rectal carcinoma. Ann Surg. 2007;246(5): 693–701.
13. Ngan S, Burmeister B, Fisher R, Solomon M, Goldstein D, Joseph D, et al. Randomized trial of short-course radiotherapy versus long-course chemoradiation comparing rates of local recurrence in patients with T3 rectal cancer: Trans-Tasman Radiation Oncology Group trial 01.04. J Clin Oncol. 2012;30(31):3827–33.
14. McDermott F, Hughes E, Pihl E, Johnson W, Price A. Local recurrence after potentially curative resection for rectal cancer in a series of 1008 patients. Br J Surg. 1985;72:34–7.
15. Rao A, Kagan A, Chan P, Gilbert H, Nussbaum H, Hintz B. Patterns of recurrence following curative resection alone for adenocarcinoma of the rectum and sigmoid colon. Cancer. 1981;48(6):1492–5.
16. Sagar P, Pemberton J. Surgical management of locally recurrent rectal cancer. Br J Surg. 1996;83(3): 293–304.
17. Miner T, Jaques D, Paty P, Guillem J, Wong W. Symptom control in patients with locally recurrent rectal cancer. Ann Surg Oncol. 2003;10(1):72–9.
18. Pacini P, Cionini L, Pirtoli L, Ciatto S, Tucci E, Sebaste L. Symptomatic recurrences of carcinoma of the rectum and sigmoid. The influence of radiotherapy on the quality of life. Dis Colon Rectum. 1986;29(12):865–8.
19. Konski A, Suh W, Herman J, Blackstock AJ, Hong T, Poggi M, et al. ACR Appropriateness Criteria®-recurrent rectal cancer. Gastrointest Cancer Res. 2012;5(1):3–12.
20. Heriot A, Tekkis P, Darzi A, Mackay J. Surgery for local recurrence of rectal cancer. Colorectal Dis. 2006;8:733–47.
21. Lopez-Kostner F, Fazio V, Vignali A, Rybicki L, Lavery I. Locally recurrent rectal cancer predictors

and success of salvage surgery. Dis Colon Rectum. 2001;44:173–8.
22. Ogunbiyi O, Mckenna K, Birnhaum E, Fleshman J, Kodner I. Aggressive management of recurrent rectal cancer—is it worthwhile? Dis Colon Rectum. 1997; 40:150–5.
23. Watson A, Lolohea S, Robertson G, Frizelle F. The role of positron emission tomography in the management of recurrent colorectal cancer: a review. Dis Colon Rectum. 2007;50(1):102–14.
24. Davey K, Heriot A, Mackay J, Drummond E, Hogg A, Ngan S, et al. The impact of 18-fluorodeoxyglucose positron emission tomography-computed tomography on the staging and management of primary rectal cancer. Dis Colon Rectum. 2008;51(7):997–1003.
25. Vogel W, Wiering B, Corstens F, Ruers T, Oyen W. Colorectal cancer: the role of PET/CT in recurrence. Cancer Imaging. 2005;5:S143–9.
26. Mirnezami A, Sagar P, Kavanagh D, Witherspoon P, Lee P, Winter D. Clinical algorithms for the surgical management of locally recurrent rectal cancer. Dis Colon Rectum. 2010;53(9):1248–7.
27. Messiou C, Chalmers A, Boyle K, Wilson D, Sagar P. Pre-operative MR assessment of recurrent rectal cancer. Br J Radiol. 2008;81:468–73.
28. Dresen R, Kusters M, Daniels-Gooszen A, Cappendijk V, Nieuwenhuijzen G, Kessels A, et al. Absence of tumor invasion into pelvic structures in locally recurrent rectal cancer: prediction with preoperative MR imaging. Radiology. 2010;256(1):143–50.
29. Lundstedt C, Stridbeck H, Andersson R, Tranberg K, Andren-Sandberg A. Tumor seeding occurring after fine needle biopsy of abdominal malignancies. Acta Radiol. 1991;32(6):518–20.
30. Smith E. Complications of percutaneous abdominal fine-needle biopsy. Review. Radiology. 1991;178(1): 253–8.
31. Austin K, Solomon M. Pelvic exenteration with en bloc iliac resection for lateral wall involvement. Dis Colon Rectum. 2009;52(7):1223–33.
32. Hartley J, Lopez R, Paty P, Wong W, Cohen A, Guillem J. Resection of locally recurrent colorectal cancer in the presence of distant metastases: can it be justified? Ann Surg Oncol. 2003;3:22–33.
33. Maetani S, Onodera H, Nishikawa T, Morimoto H, Ida K, Kitamura O, et al. Significance of local recurrence of rectal cancer as a local or disseminated disease. Br J Surg. 1998;85:521–5.
34. Yamada K, Ishizawa T, Niwa K, Chuman Y, Akiba S, Aikou T. Patterns of pelvic invasion are prognostic in the treatment of locally recurrent rectal cancer. Br J Surg. 2001;88:988–93.
35. Zoucas E, Frederiksen S, Lydrup M, Månsson W, Gustafson P, Alberius P. Pelvic exenteration for advanced and recurrent malignancy. World J Surg. 2010;34(9):2177–84.
36. Pawlik T, Skibber J, Rodriguez-Bigas M. Educational review pelvic exenteration for advanced pelvic malignancies. Ann Surg Oncol. 2006;13(5):612–23.
37. Gannon C, Zager J, Chang G, Feig B, Wood C, Skibber J, et al. Pelvic exenteration affords safe and durable treatment for locally advanced rectal carcinoma. Ann Surg Oncol. 2007;14(6):1870–7.
38. Suzuki K, Dozois R, Devine R, Nelson H, Weaver A, Gunderson L, et al. Curative reoperations for locally recurrent rectal cancer. Dis Colon Rectum. 1996;39(7):730–6.
39. Attiyeh F, Ellis H, Killingback M, Oates G, Schofield P, Staab H, et al. Symposium: the management of recurrent colorectal cancer. Int J Colorectal Dis. 1986;1(3):133–51.
40. Schwarzbach M, Hormann Y, Hinz U, Leowardi C, Böckler D, Mechtersheimer G, et al. Clinical results of surgery for retroperitoneal sarcoma with major blood vessel involvement. J Vasc Surg. 2006;44(1): 46–55.
41. Song T, Harris EJ, Raghavan S, Norton J. Major blood vessel reconstruction during sarcoma surgery. Arch Surg. 2009;144:817–22.
42. Brooks A, Gold J, Graham D, Boland P, Lewis J, Brennan M, et al. Resection of the sciatic, peroneal, or tibial nerves: assessment of functional status. Ann Surg Oncol. 2002;9(1):41–7.
43. Fuchs B, Davis A, Wunder J, Bell R, Masri B, Isler M, et al. Sciatic nerve resection in the thigh: a functional evaluation. Clin Orthop Relat Res. 2001;382:34–41.
44. Bickels J, Wittig J, Kollender Y, Kellar-Graney K, Malawer M, Meller I. Sciatic nerve resection: is that truly an indication for amputation? Clin Orthop Relat Res. 2002;399:201–4.
45. Nielsen M, Rasmussen P, Keller J, Laurberg S. Preliminary experience with external hemipelvectomy for locally advanced and recurrent pelvic carcinoma. Colorectal Dis. 2011;14:152–6.
46. Wedemeyer C, Kauthe M. Hemipelvectomy- only a salvage therapy? Orthop Rev. 2011;3(e4):12–9.
47. Baliski C, Schachar N, McKinnon J, Stuart G, Temple W. Hemipelvectomy: a changing perspective for a rare procedure. Can J Surg. 2004;47:99–103.
48. Hamanishi J, Higuchi T, Mandai M, Fukuhara K, An M, Nakayama T, et al. Intractable recurrent cervical cancer with pelvic bone involvement successfully treated with external hemipelvectomy. J Obstet Gynaecol Res. 2008;34(1):112–6.
49. Apffelstaedt J, Driscoll D, Spellman J, Velez A, Gibbs J, Karakousis C. Complications and outcome of external hemipelvectomy in the management of pelvic tumors. Ann Surg Oncol. 1996;3(3):304–9.
50. Wanebo H, Whitehill R, Gaker D, Wang G, Morgan R, Constable W. Composite pelvic resection. Arch Surg. 1987;122:1401–6.
51. Harji D, Griffiths B, McArthur D, Sagar P. Surgery for recurrent rectal cancer: higher and wider? Colorectal Dis. 2012;15:139–45.
52. Fourney D, Rhines L, Hentschel S, Skibber J, Wolinsky J, Weber K, et al. En bloc resection of primary sacral tumors: classification of surgical approaches and outcome. J Neurosurg Spine. 2005;3(2):111–22.

53. Milne T, Solomon M, Lee P, Young J, Stalley P, Harrison J. Assessing the impact of a sacral resection on morbidity and survival after extended radical surgery for locally recurrent rectal cancer. Ann Surg. 2013;258:1007–13.
54. Moriya Y, Akasu T, Fujita S, Yamamoto S. Total pelvic exenteration with distal sacrectomy for fixed recurrent rectal cancer in the pelvis. Dis Colon Rectum. 2004;47:2047–53.
55. Melton G, Paty P, Boland P, Healey J, Savatta S, Casas-Ganem J, et al. Sacral resection for recurrent rectal cancer: analysis of morbidity and treatment results. Dis Colon Rectum. 2006;49(8):1099–107.
56. Mannaerts G, Rutten H, Martijn H, Groen G, Hanssens P, Wiggers T. Abdominosacral resection for primary irresectable and locally recurrent rectal cancer. Dis Colon Rectum. 2001;44(6):806–14.
57. Sagar P, Gonsalves S, Heath R, Phillips N, Chalmers A. Composite abdominosacral resection for recurrent rectal cancer. Br J Surg. 2009;96(2):191–6.
58. Dozois E, Privitera A, Holubar S, Aldrete J, Sim F, Rose P, et al. High sacrectomy for locally recurrent rectal cancer: can long-term survival be achieved? J Surg Oncol. 2011;103:105–9.
59. Wanebo H, Antoniuk P, Koness R, Levy A, Vezeridis M, Cohen S, et al. Pelvic resection of recurrent rectal cancer. Technical considerations and outcomes. Dis Colon Rectum. 1999;42(11):1438–8.
60. Yeung R, Moffat F, Falk R. Pelvic exenteration for recurrent and extensive primary colorectal adenocarcinoma. Cancer. 1993;72:1853.
61. Finlayson C, Eisenberg B. Palliative pelvic exenteration: patient selection and results. Oncology. 1996;10(4):479–84.
62. Vermaas M, Ferenschild F, Nuyttens J, Marinelli A, Wiggers T, van der Sijp J, et al. Preoperative radiotherapy improves outcome in recurrent rectal cancer. Dis Colon Rectum. 2005;48:918–28.
63. Veldeman L, Madani I, Hulstaert F, De Meerleer G, Mareel M, De Neve W. Evidence behind use of intensity-modulated radiotherapy: a systematic review of comparative clinical studies. Lancet Oncol. 2008;9(4):367–75.
64. Dresen R, Gosen M, Martijn H, Nieuwenhuijzen G, Creemers G, Daniels-Gooszen A, et al. Radical resection after IORT-containing multimodality treatment is the most important determinant for outcome in patients treated for locally recurrent rectal cancer. Ann Surg Oncol. 2008;15(7):1937–47.
65. Ferenschild F, Vermaas M, Verhoef C, Dwarkasing R, Eggermont A, de Wilt J. Abdominosacral resection for locally advanced and recurrent rectal cancer. Br J Surg. 2009;96(11):1341–7.
66. Teixeira S, Ferenschild F, Solomon M, Rodwell L, Harrison J, Young J, et al. Urological leaks after pelvic exenterations comparing formation of colonic and ileal conduits. Eur J Surg Oncol. 2011;38(4):361–6.
67. Angioli R, Panici P, Mirhashemi R, Mendez L, Cantuaria G, Basile S, et al. Continent urinary diversion and low colorectal anastomosis after pelvic exenteration. Quality of life and complication risk. Crit Rev Oncol Hematol. 2003;48(3):281–5.
68. Husain A, Curtin J, Brown C, Chi D, Hoskins W, Poynor E, et al. Continent urinary diversion and low-rectal anastomosis in patients undergoing exenterative procedures for recurrent gynecologic malignancies. Gynecol Oncol. 2000;78(2):208–11.
69. Koda K, Tobe T, Takiguchi N, Oda K, Ito H, Miyazaki M. Pelvic exenteration for advanced colorectal cancer with reconstruction of urinary and sphincter functions. Br J Surg. 2002;89(10):1286–9.
70. Jacombs A, Rome P, Harrison JD, Solomon M. Assessment of the selection process for myocutaneous flap repair and surgical complications in pelvic exenteration surgery. Br J Surg. 2013;100(4): 561–7.
71. Boccola M, Rozena W, Ek E, Teh B, Croxford M, Grinsell D. Inferior gluteal artery myocutaneous island transposition flap reconstruction of irradiated perineal defects. J Plas Reconst Aesthet Surg. 2010;63(7):1169–75.
72. Di Mauro D, D'Hoore A, Penninckx F, De Wever I, Vergote I, Hierner R. V-Y Bilateral gluteus maximus myocutaneous advancement flap in the reconstruction of large perineal defects after resection of pelvic malignancies. Colorectal Dis. 2009;11(5):508–12.
73. Hainsworth A, Al Akash M, Roblin P, Mohanna P, Ross D, George M. Perineal reconstruction after abdominoperineal excision using inferior gluteal artery perforator flaps. Br J Surg. 2012;99(4):584–8.
74. Luo S, Raffoul W, Piaget F, Egloff D. Anterolateral thigh fasciocutaneous flap in the difficult perineogenital reconstruction. Plast Reconstr Surg. 2000;105(1):171–3.
75. Ferenschild F, Vermaas M, Verhoef C, Ansink A, Kirkels W, Eggermont A, et al. Total pelvic exenteration for primary and recurrent malignancies. World J Surg. 2009;33(7):1502–8.
76. Harris D, Davies M, Lucas M, Drew P, Carr N, Beynon J, et al. Multivisceral resection for primary locally advanced rectal carcinoma. Br J Surg. 2011;98:582–8.
77. Jimenez R, Shoup M, Cohen A, Paty P, Guillem J, Wong W. Contemporary outcomes of total pelvic exenteration in the treatment of colorectal cancer. Dis Colon Rectum. 2003;46(12):1619–25.
78. Bell S, Dehni N, Chaouat M. Primary rectus abdominis myocutaneous flap for repair of perineal and vaginal defects after extended abdominoperineal resection. Br J Surg. 2005;92:482–6.
79. López-Basave H, Morales-Vásquez F, Herrera-Gómez A, Rosciano A, Meneses-García A, Ruiz-Molina J. Pelvic exenteration for colorectal cancer: oncologic outcome in 59 patients at a single institution. Cancer Manag Res. 2012;4:351–6.
80. Thaysen H, Jess P, Laurberg S. Health-related quality of life after surgery for primary advanced rectal cancer and recurrent rectal cancer: a review. Colorectal Dis. 2012;14(7):797–803.
81. You Y, Habiba H, Chang G, Rodriguez-bigas M, Skibber J. Prognostic value of quality of life and pain in patients with locally recurrent rectal cancer. Ann Surg Oncol. 2011;18(4):989–96.
82. Miller A, Cantor S, Peoples G, Pearlstone D, Skibber J. Quality of life and cost effectiveness analysis of

therapy for locally recurrent rectal cancer. Dis Colon Rectum. 2000;43(12):1695–701.
83. Kusters M, Dresen R, Martijn H, Nieuwenhuijzen G, van de Velde C, van den Berg H, et al. Radicality of resection and survival after multimodality treatment is influenced by subsite of locally recurrent rectal cancer. Int J Radiat Oncol Biol Phys. 2009;75(5):1444–9.
84. Jiang Y, Wan Y, Liu Y, Wang X, Pan Y, Wu T, et al. Surgical outcomes for 187 patients with locally recurrent rectal cancer and analysis of prognostic factors. Zhonghua Wei Chang Wai Ke Za Zhi. 2011;14(8):582–5.
85. Nielsen M, Rasmussen P, Lindegaard J, Laurberg S. A 10-year experience of total pelvic exenteration for primary advanced and locally recurrent rectal cancer based on a prospective database. Colorectal Dis. 2012;14(9):1076–83.

Dealing with Complications of Rectal Surgery

53

Mia DeBarros and Scott R. Steele

53.1 Introduction

Background

Colorectal cancer remains a major healthcare concern worldwide. In 2009, it was the second leading cause of death for both men and women in the United States alone, and accounted for an estimated 49,920 deaths; while globally, it is the fourth leading cause of cancer-related death [1, 2]. By location, one-third of colorectal cancer cases occur in the rectum [3]. It is estimated that 40,290 men and women (23,500 men and 16,790 women) will be diagnosed with rectal cancer and 51,690 men and women will die of cancer of the colon and rectum in 2012 [4]. The mainstay of treatment for this disease is surgical excision with appropriate tumor-specific mesorectal excision. Over time this has evolved to incorporate transanal and minimally invasive approaches that have resulted in minimizing the overall morbidity. Yet, as the surgical management of rectal cancer becomes more complex, the associated complications are also more varied. This chapter seeks to describe the presentation, prevention and management of complications associated with current procedures available for the surgical management of rectal cancer.

Principles of Oncologic Rectal Surgery

Although other sections of this text are devoted to an in-depth discussion regarding this topic, a few points are worth highlighting. First, the overriding oncologic principle of rectal cancer resection involves achieving negative proximal, distal and radial margins. Appropriate radial (i.e., circumferential resection) margins are best aided by performing a total mesorectal excision (TME) [5]. The use of TME is based on the hypothesis that the local field of rectal cancer spread is primarily limited to the mesorectal envelope; if this is removed en bloc, then all tumor satellite can be removed as well. Previous studies have demonstrated a reduction in positive radial margins and local failure rates in stage II and III cancers following TME, with an improvement in overall survival to 68–78 % [6]. Currently, a 1–2 cm distal margin (pending tumor height) and a

Disclaimers The views expressed are those of the author(s) and do not reflect the official policy of the Department of the Army, the Department of Defense or the U.S. Government

Financial Disclosures None

M. DeBarros, MD
Department of General Surgery, Madigan Army Medical Center, Fort Lewis, WA, USA

S.R. Steele, MD (✉)
Department of Surgery, Madigan Healthcare System, 9040a Fitzsimmons Dr, Tacoma, WA 98431, USA

Colon and Rectal Surgery, Madigan Army Medical Center, Tacoma, WA, USA
e-mail: harkersteele@me.com

H.R.H. Patel et al. (eds.), *Pelvic Cancer Surgery: Modern Breakthroughs and Future Advances*,
DOI 10.1007/978-1-4471-4258-4_53, © Springer-Verlag London 2015

proximal margin of at least 5 cm are recommended. However, the radial margin remains critical when determining prognosis, and is one potential factor in the surgeon's control. On the other hand, simply adhering to the oncologic principles of rectal cancer surgery (i.e. complete TME) is not without consequences, as this requires a distal resection and anastomosis, resulting in potential increases in operative time, anastomotic leak rates, chronic wounds and functional disorders related to the dissection itself or to adjunct treatments.

53.2 Surgical Approaches for Rectal Cancer Surgery

Surgical management of rectal cancer has become more varied and complex, especially as new modalities are developed. With the advent of minimally invasive excision and adjuvant therapy, small distal rectal cancers can be treated with lower morbidity and mortality of a more invasive procedure. Newer modalities such as robotic surgery are also finding a place in the armament of rectal cancer surgery. Each modality has its own indications, contraindications and associated complications. Current surgical approaches are described here only briefly, as they are beyond the scope of this chapter and covered more thoroughly elsewhere in this text.

Local Excision

The earliest form of surgical management for rectal cancer involved local excision alone, until the advent of anesthesia and blood transfusions, which allowed for the rise of the abdominal-perineal resection (APR) for rectal cancer. The APR subsequently lowered recurrence and improved cure rates, but was also associated with a higher morbidity. Local excision was then relegated to palliative procedures, but has resurfaced again for use in the treatment of T1N0 and select T2N0 rectal tumors when paired with adjuvant chemoradiation [7]. Modalities include the traditional transanal excision (TAE), along with transanal endoscopic microsurgery (TEM), and more recently, transanal minimally invasive surgery (TAMIS). TEM was developed in the 1980s to remove large rectal polyps beyond the reach of TAE. It is now widely available, utilizes specialized optics and equipment, allows excision of early stage rectal cancers with improved oncologic margins, and access to more proximal lesions with decreased morbidity and mortality compared to TAE [8–10]. TAMIS was first reported in 2009 and is a hybrid between TEM and single-port laparoscopy, utilizing many of the same instruments [11].

Radical Excision

The APR was first described in 1908. Current indications include tumors that are close to or extending into the anal sphincter complex, such that a safe distal margin cannot be achieved, or the presence of a mid-rectal tumor in a patient with poor continence. Tumors that do not involve the sphincter and allow for a 1–2 cm distal margin are eligible for a low-anterior resection (LAR). While definitions vary slightly, the ultra-low LAR is variation of standard LAR made possible by a colo-anal anastomosis for distal rectal cancers. Contra-indications to LAR include baseline fecal incontinence, tumor invasion of the anal sphincter musculature or rectovaginal septum, tenesmus and technical factors such as body habitus, tumor location and tumor size [12].

Laparoscopy is now a widely practiced approach in most in oncologic procedures, including the resection of colorectal cancers. Laparoscopic LAR involves the exploration and mobilization of the colon and rectum, with improved optics to aid in rectal dissection, followed by a bowel resection and anastomosis creation completed either intra- or extra-corporeally [13]. Robotic surgery was introduced as a way to overcome the limitations of laparoscopy and is gaining traction as more colorectal surgeons become familiar with the technique [14]. Whether performed open or via a minimally invasive approach, the principles of proper oncologic surgery are maintained.

53.3 Complications Associated with Rectal Cancer Surgery

Intra-operative Complications

Bleeding

Significant intra-operative bleeding in the pelvis is a commonly feared, but relatively uncommon complication—with a reported incidence ranging from 3 to 9.4 %. The most common location is the presacral venous plexus, which communicates with the internal vertebral system. In the lithotomy position, the hydrostatic pressure increases to two to three times that of the inferior vena cava, making bleeding from this location very difficult to control with standard electrocautery, suture ligation or clipping. Traditional control methods include pelvic packing and sterile metallic or titanium thumbtacks. Other reported methods are local hemostatic agents (i.e., thrombin and gelfoam) or sponges with endoscopic helical tackers, absorbable hemostats, bone wax, tamponading tissue expanders or saline bags, indirect coagulation via muscle fragmentation and rectus abdominus muscle autotransplant.

While all methods have a wide range of various reports of success in the literature, each are also subject to limitations and drawbacks [15]. Packing often requires return to the operating room for removal. Tack use is subject to availability and limitations on placement (contraindicated near ureters and the sacral foramina) with associated complications of chronic pain, anastomotic leaks and fistula formation. Hemostatic agents need a dry field to prevent washout, which is often a formidable task during brisk bleeding. The tamponade effect with the use of sponges, tissue expanders and saline bags is not a reliable option with low anastomosis, secondary to ischemia and breakdown, though can be used in the dissection phase. Muscle transplant is a difficult and time-consuming process in a deep and narrow pelvis and should not be attempted as first-line management. The use of indirect coagulation on a muscle fragment to form a coagulum patch is more difficult in deeper pelvic sources and lateral locations.

A special note should be made of lateral pelvic bleeds, as the origin may be from the iliac system, especially in re-operative pelvic cases. Indiscriminant use of electrocautery most often results in worsening the situation. Rather, initial packing and localization of the source is imperative to avoid further injury. Caution should be performed to avoid excessive suction use, as blood loss can be severe and swift. Rather, direct pressure with isolation of the injury, achieving proximal and distal control (where possible), and suture repair is preferable. This may involve dissecting out the common iliac artery and vein at the pelvic inlet. Recalling the typical course of the left common iliac vein carries it under the right iliac artery is important to avoid further injury. In extreme cases, successful ligation of the pelvic inflow and outflow has been described. While this maneuver carries a theoretical risk of central pelvic necrosis, this is often only employed in the direst of situations for otherwise uncontrollable bleeding [16, 17]. Finally, angiographic embolization and (increasingly) endovascular techniques may also be considered, though require technical expertise and/or temporary stabilization of the patient in cases where their use would require transportation out of the operating room, which may not be feasible [18, 19].

Another more frequently encountered source of bleeding is anastomotic bleeding, for both anterior resections and following local excisions. In stapled anastomosis, there is a reported incidence of 1–45 %. This bleeding is often relatively minor with the passing of dark blood at the first bowel movement, and will cease without any intervention [14]. If there is continued or refractory bleeding, control is initially attempted with sutures or clips rather than electrocautery to prevent thermal injury and possible delayed leak. A circular-stapled anastomotic bleed has been reported to be more commonly associated with a delay in presentation. Conservative management may be attempted with a rectal tube placement and a normal saline with 1:100,000 epinephrine instillation, though not as commonly employed. Patients who fail this treatment or become hypotensive should return to the operating room for an exam under anesthesia and more definitive control [20–24]. Endoscopy can be extremely useful in this situation, as direct visualization of the source along with a working channel in the scope will allow commonly used means to identify and control the bleeding vessel (i.e., endoscopic clips, injection, coagulation).

Genitourinary Injuries

The iatrogenic genitourinary injury is a rare, but feared complication in pelvic surgery. The ureters are frequently subjected to damage because of their anatomical location, crossing over the bifurcation of the common iliac artery before descending into the pelvis in a lateral to medial course. While ureteral injury occurs in ~1 % of colorectal procedures, colorectal surgery accounts for 5–15 % of all ureteral injuries and APR is one of the most commonly associated procedures [25]. Risk factors for injury include a history of prior pelvic operations, radiation therapy, inflammatory bowel disease, and extensive neoplasm causing distortion of surgical planes and unrecognized congenital anomalies. Prevention of injury is possible by direct visualization or knowledge of critical steps in which the ureter is in close proximity. However, prior pelvic surgery may result in an aberrant location of the ureters, often following a more medial course, or cause the ureters to make sudden turns instead of their more gradual arching path. The placement of prophylactic ureteral stents does not prevent injury to the ureters; however, they do allow for early identification of injuries [25–28]. Mechanisms of injury include laceration, ligation, devascularization and indirect burns from stray energy. Ureteral injuries that are discovered intra-operatively should be repaired immediately. Delayed presentation can occasionally be managed conservatively, although there are case series that report favorable outcomes with operative intervention upon presentation [29]. Diagnosis of ureteral injury can be achieved intraoperatively via an on-table intravenous pyelogram or the retrograde instillation of methylene blue solution or radiographic contrast through ureteral catheters [25]. The principles of repair involve the use of absorbable sutures to prevent stone formation, a tension-free repair over a stent and placement of closed-suction drain in proximity of repair. The type of repair depends mainly on the location of injury [25]. Transections at the level of the high ligation of the inferior mesenteric artery are most often repaired primarily, with proximal and distal mobilization of the two ends, and a spatulated end-to-end anastomosis performed over a double-J stent. Injuries at the iliac bifurcation are either repaired primarily or ligated at the distal stump with a Boari flap or psoas hitch repair [25, 30, 31]. Injuries from anterolateral or perineal dissection are repaired by creation of ureterneocystostomy.

Bladder injuries may occur during placement of laparoscopic trocars or during open or laparoscopic dissection. Similar to ureteral injuries, risk factors include a history of prior radiation, inflammatory bowel disease, malignant infiltration and chronic infection. Iatrogenic injuries are graded from 1 to 5 for severity [32, 33]. Injuries discovered intraoperatively are repaired at that time depending on the grade. In general, almost all bladder injuries can be successfully managed with direct repair and Foley catheter drainage. Care must be taken to ensure there is no damage to the trigone area, where urological expertise is typically warranted. Grades I or 2 may require a Foley catheter placement for 7–14 days while grades 3–5 are repaired in multiple layers using absorbable suture and placement of closed-suction drains, along with catheter drainage. Bladder injuries missed intraoperatively present early in the post-operative period with increased output from drains, drainage from the surgical incision or vagina, ileus, oliguria and the presence of ascites with elevated BUN and creatinine. Diagnosis is made via CT cystogram [34, 35]. The extent of the injury and clinical stability of patient will most often dictate the subsequent management, with options ranging from catheter drainage alone, percutaneous drainage, or surgical exploration. In general, injury grades 3–5 require operative repair.

Urethral injury is extremely rare and is more often associated with traumatic Foley catheter placement. Intraoperative iatrogenic injury may occur during the perineal dissection portion of an APR or transanal dissection of an LAR at the membranous or prostatic portion, particularly if there is a large, penetrating anterior tumor or extensive scarring. Other risks include obliteration of anatomical planes due to tumor desmoplastic reaction or edema from neoadjuvant radiation therapy. Prevention is accomplished with placement of a large diameter Foley catheter, and frequent evaluation to ensure the correct surgical plane is being followed during the anterior portion of the dissection. Intraoperative diagnosis is often made when the Foley catheter is visualized. A suspected injury can be visualized by retrograde instillation of methylene blue via the catheter or urethral meatus. Intraoperative injuries that are small are repaired with absorbable suture and Foley catheter left in place for approximately 2–4 weeks. It is often advisable to upsize the catheter (i.e., 20 Fr) in attempt to minimize stricture formation. Unfortunately, most urethral injuries are delayed presentations commonly diagnosed as a fistula. These fistulas rarely close with conservative management and usually require urinary diversion followed by repair and reconstruction. If there is a large injury or delay in diagnosis, proximal urinary diversion via a suprapubic catheter should be placed and a delayed repair performed by an urologist [25].

Complications Associated with TAMIS/TEM-Perforation into the Peritoneum

With the increasing use of local excision modalities of TEM and TAMIS, it is important to recognize the intraoperative complications that may occur. Overall, the reported complication rate for these modalities is 6–31 % [36–47]. Especially when resecting higher lesions, or in anterior lesions with a deep pelvic cul-de-sac, full thickness excision may result in perforation into the peritoneum. This has been reported in 0–9 % [39, 42, 47–49]. Although perforation may require a conversion to laparotomy, surgeons performing these approaches should be facile with primary closure via transanal suture repair as the first option [49]. Admission, bowel rest, and empiric intravenous antibiotics are often employed for known peritoneal entry, or cases of postoperative pneumoperitoneum in an otherwise clinically well and stable patient. Any signs of clinical deterioration should warrant emergent evaluation and often requires abdominal exploration and diversion.

Early Postoperative Complications

Anastomotic Leak

Incidence and Risk Factors

Anastomotic leak is one of the most feared complications in rectal cancer surgery. A review of the literature reveals an incidence ranging from 1 to 19 %, with more recent studies reporting a less than 10 % incidence [50–54]. The risk factors associated with leak are numerous and can be classified according to patient factors, disease factors and intraoperative factors (Table 53.1). The literature regarding these risk factors is considerable and varies in the strength of associated with leak; however, ASA classification, malnutrition and weight loss have shown consistently stronger

Table 53.1 Risk factors associated with anastomotic leak

Patient risk factors
Tobacco use
Alcohol use
Obesity
Age >65
ASA > 3
Malnutrition <3.0
Weight >10 % TBW
Disease factors
Emergent surgery
Steroid or immunomodulator use
Malignancy
Level of tumor (rectal lesion below peritoneal reflection
Anastomotic height
Preoperative radiation therapy
Intraoperative factors
Poor perfusion to conduit and anastomosis
Anastomosis or conduit under tension
Sigmoid colon conduit
Prolonged operative time
Excessive blood loss
Blood transfusion

associations with leak occurrence, while factors such as obesity, age, smoking, and alcohol usage have weaker associations [52, 55–79].

Prevention of Anastomotic Leaks: Techniques and Adjuncts

Prevention and reduction of risk of anastomotic leaks requires recognition and mitigation of risk factors pre-operatively and intra-operatively as well as the use of adjuncts. Intra-operatively, meticulous technique to prevent excessive blood loss, undue tension on the anastomosis and ensuring a good blood supply are vital to ensuring a quality anastomosis. Multiple intraoperative and postoperative adjuncts are utilized with varying degrees of success. Intra-operative adjuncts include the use of buttressing materials, air leak testing the anastomosis and a restrictive resuscitation strategy. In the post-operative period, supplemental oxygen therapy, the use of protective diverting stomas and pelvic drains are also reported.

Intervening on modifiable patient risk factors such as obesity, smoking and alcohol use should be attempted, though not often feasible in the setting of malignancy where more prompt surgical intervention is performed. Patients with known pre-operative malnutrition should receive supplemental nutrition in the form of enteral nutrition or TPN prior to undertaking operative intervention. Preoperative prophylaxis in the form of bowel preparation or IV and PO antibiotics, while decreasing the rate of surgical site infections, has not been shown to decrease the rate of leak on colorectal anastomosis [68, 80], and is left to the discretion of the surgeon.

Intra-operatively, adequate perfusion to the conduit and anastomosis can be difficult to ascertain and clinical judgment is needed as there are no reliable or accurate devices that are widely available [52]. Indicators of perfusion include the color of the mucosa and bleeding from the staple line. The prevention of tension on the anastomosis will also ensure perfusion. This is achieved by high ligation of the inferior mesenteric vein at the level of the duodenum and artery pedicle. Although this can compromise blood supply, this is usually not typical when collateral circulation is intact and care is taken to avoid resection of the mesentery too close to the bowel. A bulldog or vascular clamp may be placed initially on the pedicle prior to formal ligation to temporarily stop blood flow and evaluate for collateral supply. Additionally, proper mobilization of the splenic flexure will assist in achieving adequate length for the proximal bowel to reach the pelvis. Sigmoid colon conduits are generally not recommended because of tenuous blood supply after high ligation. One of the most difficult anastomosis with regards to blood supply and tension occurs in the setting of preoperative XRT and the need for a colo-anal anastomosis. Meticulous technique in creation of the anastomosis cannot be overemphasized. The use of hand-sewn versus stapled technique has been extensively studied in the literature with the most recent Cochrane meta-analysis finding both techniques are equivalent [52, 81, 82]. Single versus double-layer sutures have also been studied with randomized data reporting no adverse outcomes in either suture group [83]. Yet, in mid-to-low pelvic anastomosis, the decision of which to perform is often a moot point, as stapled anastomoses are technically easier and are predominately performed.

Buttressing materials (i.e., fibrin glue, SEAMGUARD® (W.L. Gore & Associates, Newark, DE] along the staple line or omentoplasty have had mixed reports of success in preventing leaks [84–91]. The air leak test is supported throughout the literature as a simple method of determining the integrity of a fresh anastomosis prior to closure and helps identify any problems with the anastomosis that can be addressed intraoperatively or suggest proximal diversion may be required [92–95]. While clinical leaks may still develop, testing for air leaks is not known to be harmful, and positive tests have been associated with higher rates of subsequent clinical leaks [52]. Restrictive fluid strategy is reported in the literature to decrease overall post-operative complications, however its role in prevention of leak is less clear. Most studies demonstrate a good safety profile when compared to usual care and its use can be considered good practice [96–102].

Post-operative adjuncts include the use of supplemental oxygen, pelvic drains and a protective, diverting stoma. While most of the supplemental oxygen studies focus on the prevention of surgical site infections, there are several studies regarding the use of supplemental O2 in prevention of anastomotic leak [103, 104]. By increasing the O2 saturation in arterial blood, it is believed to increase the mucosal O2 tension at the site of bleeding and prevent ischemia. This was initially demonstrated in a rat model that demonstrated a higher bursting pressure and hydroxyproline content (a marker of collagen content) after hyperbaric chamber treatment [90]. Following this, a Spanish study used 80 % FiO2 in 45 patients undergoing LAR and found better tissue oxygen levels at the anastomosis compared to controls with no complications in either test group. In a recent randomized control trial, patients were randomized to a control arm of 30 % Fi02 or experimental arm of 80 % FiO2 for 6 h post rectal cancer resection. In this study, there was 46 % reduction in anastomotic complications ($p < 0.05$) [103].

Protective stomas are utilized to divert fecal flow away from the fresh anastomosis; however, there is ongoing debate as to whether or not the presence of a diverting stoma merely decreases the severity of the leak or actually prevents it [60, 70, 75, 105–111]. A recent Cochrane review reported the decreased incidence of anastomotic leak and the need for urgent return to the OR for leak (RR = 0.33, 95 % CI 0.21–0.53) [110]. The placement of pelvic drains is also under debate and several authors have found a decrease in leak incidence while others studies found it to be an independent risk factor for leak [112–119]. Unfortunately, drain use remains largely dogmatic and is most often performed at the discretion of the surgeon.

Presentation and Management

Anastomotic leak presentation depends largely on what level the leak occurs: intraperitoneal or extraperitoneal. Intraperitoneal leaks often present with generalized peritoneal signs, while extraperitoneal leaks are often insidious in presentation due to lack of an innervated peritoneal surface. Patients may only present with symptoms associated with the location such as urinary dysfunction. Leaks can further be broken down into free and contained leaks. A free leak occurs when fecal contents spread freely throughout the peritoneal cavity. A contained leak occurs when fecal contents leak into the pelvis and become walled off, resulting in a pelvic abscess. Free leaks present with signs of sepsis and diffuse peritonitis or feculent fluid from the incision or drains. Contained leaks can present with sepsis, but symptoms such as chronic pelvic pain or fistula or more indicative of a contained leak. Management of intraperitoneal and extraperitoneal leaks is summarized in Figs. 53.1 and 53.2.

Hemodynamically unstable patients need immediate fluid resuscitation, IV antibiotics and operative intervention to assess the size, site, accessibility, viability of the bowel ends, and fecal load of the proximal colon. If there is a major defect in the anastomosis (Fig. 53.3), it can be resected and re-done with proximal diversion, drain placement and on-table colonic lavage. If the anastomosis is high or mid-rectal, there are several options. Minor defects can occasionally undergo repair with proximal diversion and drain placement if there is no fecal load in the proximal colon, and the patient is stable with a reasonable nutrition status. However, this is likely only possible when the leak is identified very early and there is a paucity of inflammation in the abdomen and the bowel wall remains supple. Finally if the patient is too unstable and damage control surgery is planned, then a takedown of the anastomosis with creation of a colostomy and Hartman's stump is the quickest and safest option. All repairs or re-do attempts should have thorough washout of the abdominal cavity and omental flap over the repair to prevent fistula formation. If a defect cannot be defined and phlegmon is present, minimal pelvic dissection is undertaken to prevent the liberation of sepsis, minimize the injury to ureters or the iliac vessels or to the bowel. The pelvis should be washed out, an omentoplasty performed and pelvic drains placed.

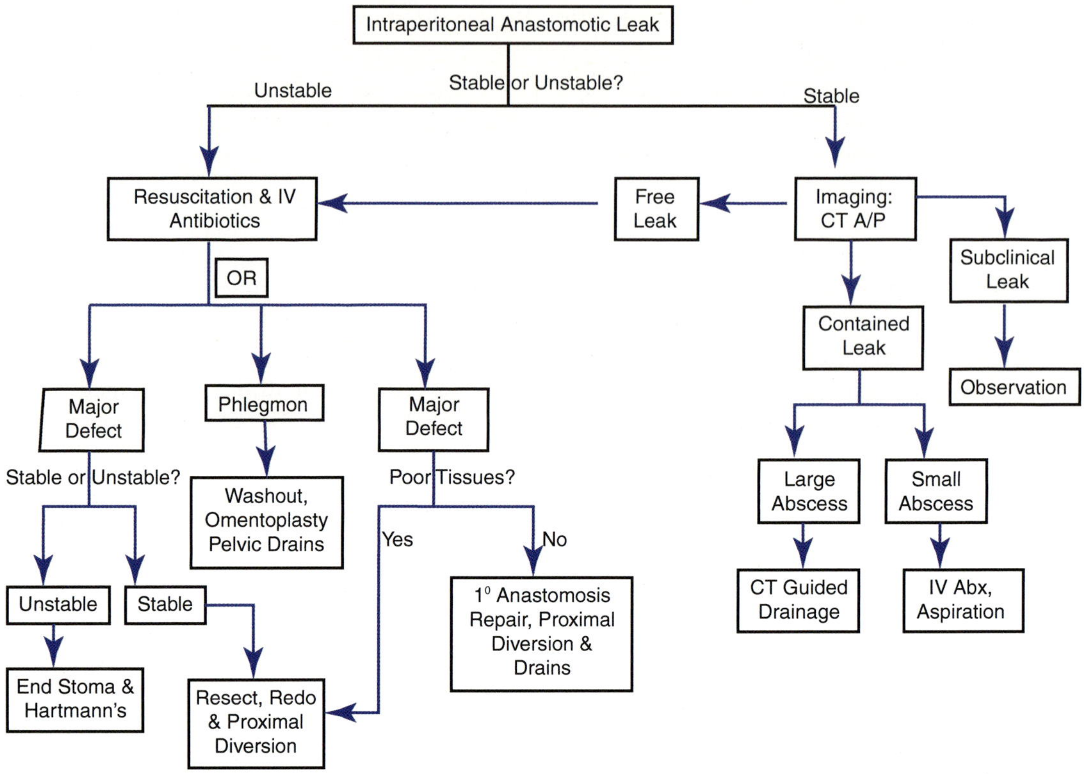

Fig. 53.1 Intraperitoneal leak management algorithm

Hemodynamically stable patients need a triple phase CT to delineate location and size of the leak or abscess. Intraperitoneal abscess or contained leaks are eligible for non-operative management. This consists of drainage, antibiotics, bowel rest and TPN or a low residual diet. For upper pelvis abscess or contained leak in colorectal anastomosis, CT-guided percutaneous drainage can be undertaken with transabdominal route preferred over the transgluteal. Lower pelvic abscess are managed to according to their location: anterior or posterior. Anterior abscess with intraperitoneal sepsis require operative intervention. Posterior abscess require a water-soluble contrast enema (WCSE) to determine if is in continuity or contained. Abscess that is not in continuity should undergo EUA and transanal drainage. For those in continuity, IV antibiotics and CT-guided drainage is first-line therapy. Anterior abscess without intraperitoneal sepsis are managed in a similar fashion to posterior abscess. Colo-anal contained anastomosis leaks benefit from early EUA with frequent reassessment and trans-anastomotic drainage. While endoluminal stents have been described, their use remains largely anecdotal and recommendations await further experience. Long-term sequelae of anastomotic leaks include fistula formation, stricture, chronic presacral cavity, pain and the need for a permanent stoma [51, 120].

Infection and Wound Complications

Incidence

Surgical Site Infection (SSI) is one of the most common nosocomial infections among surgical patients, occurring in approximately 2 % of surgical procedures and accounting for 20 % of health care-associated infections [121]. Colorectal surgery is associated with an even higher rate of SSI (up to 30 %), secondary to high bacterial load in the distal gastrointestinal tract [122,

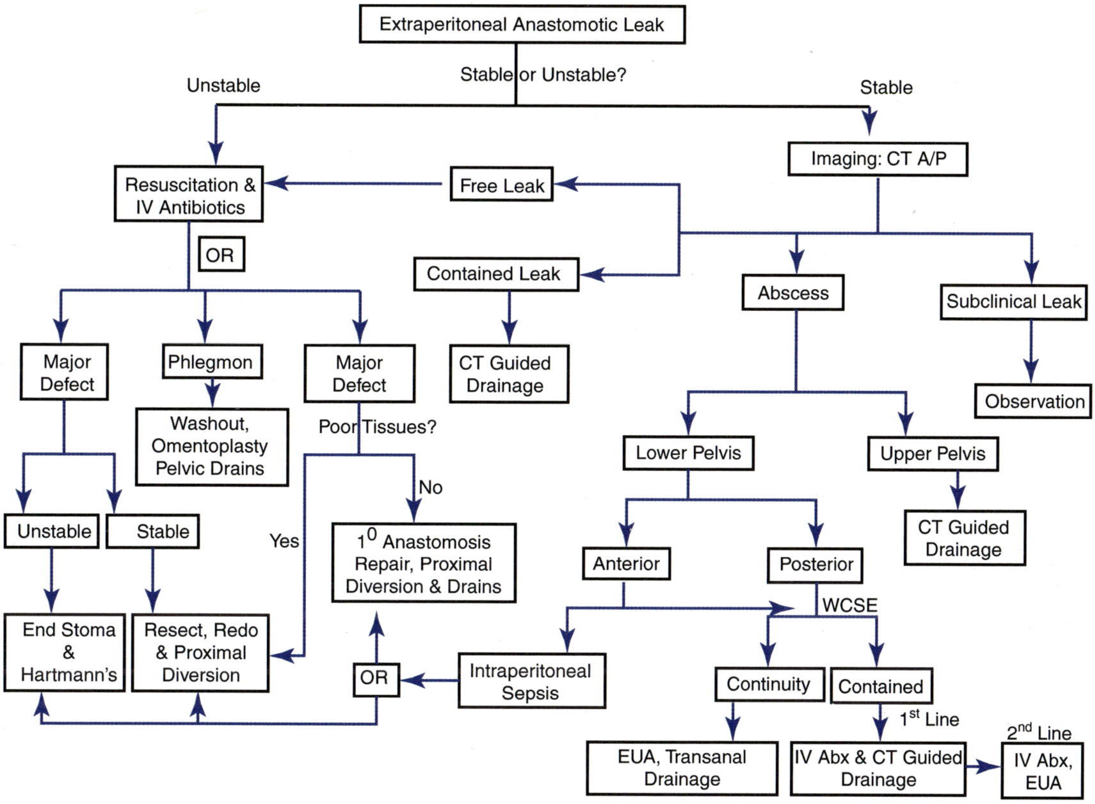

Fig. 53.2 Extraperitoneal leak management algorithm

123]. Within colorectal surgery, procedures on the rectum carry a higher risk of SSI compared to other sites within in the colon. A prospective study of patients undergoing elective colorectal surgery stratified the data from colon and rectal cases separately. SSI was documented in 18 % in rectal cases compared to 9.4 % in colon cases. Italian investigators further stratified the location of surgery to right and left colon and rectum as well as site of infection (incisional or deep space). Again, rectal surgery was associated with a higher rate of SSI compared to the right colon (17.6 % vs. 8 %), while left colon surgery had a similar rate of SSI (18.4 %, p=0.022). Rectal surgery and left-side colon surgery also had a higher rate of deep space and organ infections compared to right-side colon surgery (p=0.029) [122, 124]. Risk factors for all surgery and specific to rectal surgery are summarized in Table 53.2 [103, 104, 122, 124–129].

Prevention

Prevention involves modification of general risk factors as well as the use of adjuncts when appropriate, also summarized in Table 53.2 [103, 104, 122, 124–129]. Mechanical bowel preparation is believed to prevent SSI by reducing the fecal content and thus bacterial load, but multiple studies demonstrate no benefit in prevention of SSI. Furthermore, a recent meta-analysis suggests that anastomotic leak rate might actually be increased. In this study the use of rectal enemas in both colonic and rectal surgery was also examined. An overall leak rate of 4.4 % in the enema group was comparable to 3.4 % in the no enema group (OR=1.32, 0.74–2.36). Specifically in rectal surgery, leaks were present 7.4 % in the enema group and 7.9 % in the no enema group (OR=0.93, 0.34–2.52). SSI was present 9.9 % in the enema group and 8.0 % in the no enema group (OR=1.26, 0.85–1.88) [130]. Oral

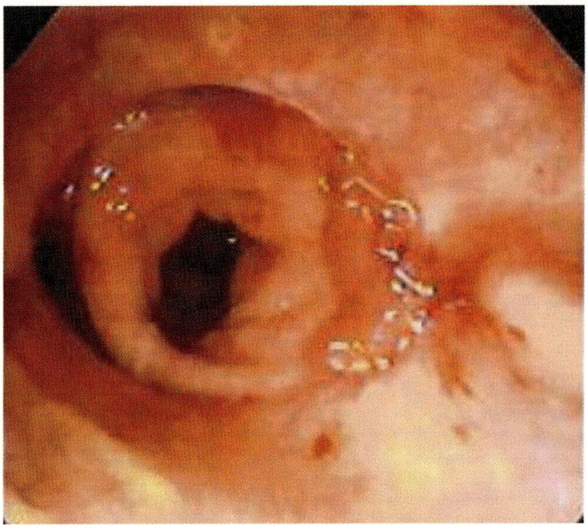

Fig. 53.3 Anastomotic disruption in a diverted patient viewed endoscopically

antibiotics have also been examined as a preventive measure. While studies show there is a reduction with use of non-absorbable oral and parenteral antibiotics in colorectal surgery, there is also a higher rate of nausea and vomiting in these patients which predisposes them to aspiration so use can be considered in carefully selected patients [131].

Management

SSI typically present on the fifth to seventh postoperative day unless *Clostridium perfringens* or beta-hemolytic *Streptococcus* is the etiological agent, in which case infection manifests as early as postoperative day 1 or 2. Surgical wounds appearing infected require the standard wound treatment of drainage and debridement. Antibiotic should be given only if cellulitis is present, or in patients with underlying immunosuppression. Deep wound infections of the fascia or muscle require return to the operating room for exam under anesthesia, debridement and washout with packing and closure by secondary intention. Larger wounds may benefit from use of vacuum-assisted device, which allow for easier wound care and faster closure of the wound. Patients with suspected intra-abdominal abscess should undergo CT scan with intravenous, oral and rectal contrast. The findings of a rim-enhancing fluid collection and surrounding inflammatory stranding are diagnostic. Treatment is drainage of abscess with most amenable to percutaneous catheter drainage. Success rates range from 65 to 90 % and depend on size, complexity, etiology and microbial flora [65, 132–134].

Table 53.2 Risk factors and prevention for SSI

General risk factors	General prevention measures
Malnutrition	Tobacco cessation
Diabetes mellitus	Alcohol cessation
Immunosuppression	Improved nutrition status
Age >60	Prophylactic antibiotics with appropriate gram-negative and anaerobic coverage with appropriate timing of dosing and discontinuation within 24 h of surgery
ASA >2	Hair removal using clippers
Increased preoperative hospital stay	Meticulous technique and dissection
Extensive surgery	Avoidance of excessive intraoperative blood loss Normothermia maintenance
Independent risk factors in rectal surgery	**Specific prevention measures**
Multiple co-morbidities	Combined non-absorbable oral and parenteral antibiotics
Preoperative use of steroids	Postoperative oxygen therapy
Ostomy creation	Silver-impregnated dressings
Preoperative radiation	Intra-operative antibiotic peritoneal lavage Antibiotic impregnated beads for APR sacral cavity

Wound Issues in APR

Wound issues in APR are a well-known complication and can range from minor wound separation to a chronically infected cavity, fistula or sinus. The rates of wound complications range from 11 to 50 % [135]. Risk factors vary and the importance of one over the other has not been determined, although some factors such as preoperative radiation are consistently a risk factor for delayed wound healing, with rates of 2–3 times to that of no radiation treatment. Other factors such as diabetes, smoking, gender, steroid use and malnutrition have differed from study to study [135–143]. Prevention of wound complications is aimed at modifiable risk factors such as nutritional status and tobacco cessation, prevention of intra-operative fecal or purulent contamination and excessive intraoperative bleeding. The use of pelvic drains is also felt to be beneficial by eliminating the dead space; however, benefit did not extend beyond 1 month. The drain(s) should brought out through a separate incision, because of higher rates of non-healing when exiting through the incision [144, 145] . With preoperative radiation or extensive resection, the transposition of healthy tissue such as omentum or gracilis or rectus abdominus muscle was reported in some studies to improve wound healing, but a systematic review did not show benefit with use of omentoplasty [146–149]. In recalcitrant chronic wounds, a search for other etiology such as fistula or recurrence of malignancy should be initiated. Imaging is utilized to determine the presence of a chronic sinus or fistula. Treatment should be based on standard principles of fistula management, depending on the source, output and clinical condition of the patient. Chronic draining sinus is managed in a similar fashion to pilonidal disease with curettage and excision of chronic granulation tissue, hair follicles and skin bridges. Large wounds may require the use of vacuum-assisted closure or myocutaneous flaps such as the gracilis muscle for closure and healing [135, 150–153] .

Functional Issues

With improvement in surgical technique and increasing use of multi-modality treatment, overall survival from rectal cancer has improved drastically. This produces a double-edge sword in which patients have longer life expectancy but have the potential for with functional disturbances such as incontinence and fecal, urinary and sexual dysfunction. Table 53.3 summarizes the risks associated with functional issues.

Table 53.3 Risk factors with functional issues

Fecal incontinence
Preoperative radiation therapy
Anastomotic height
Tumor height
Intra-operative blood loss >1400 mL
Pudendal or levator ani nerve damage
Urinary dysfunction
Low rectal cancer, <5 cm from anal verge
Lymph node involvement
History of urinary dysfunction
Anastomotic leak
Suture entrapment
Preoperative radiation therapy
Electrocautery injury
Sexual dysfunction
Patient age
Preoperative libido dysfunction
Preoperative radiation therapy
Low rectal tumor requiring APR
Low anterior resection syndrome
Anastomotic leak
Preoperative radiation therapy
Poor trans-anal stapling technique
Excessive circumferential margins in TME

Fecal Incontinence

Normal continence is a complex process requiring integration between sphincters, pelvic floor muscles, stool volume and consistency, rectal compliance and intact peripheral and central nervous systems. The inferior hypogastric plexus supplies autonomic function of the rectum, organs of the genitourinary tract, bladder and urethra. This coarse, flat meshwork of nerves contains sympathetic and parasympathetic nerve fibers. Parasympathetic fibers are supplied by pelvic splanchnic nerves (nervi erigentes) originating from sacral nerves S2 to S4. The hypogastric nerves supply the sympathetic fibers of the plexus [154–157]. During dissection of lateral planes in deep portions of the pelvis, both inferior hypogastric plexus and pelvic splanchnic nerves are at risk for injury. To preserve autonomic nerve function, autonomic nerve preserving TME (ANP-TME) was described in the mid-1970s by Tsuchiya and colleagues [158, 159]. However, the prevalence of fecal incontinence still remains high, with reports of up to 40 %, and preoperative radiation therapy (PRT) increasing the rate up to 60 % [160–162]. There is no general consensus for the most influential independent risk factors, however, PRT, anastomotic and tumor height, excessive intra-operative blood loss and damage to pudendal or levator ani nerves are all implicated [154, 161–171].

Work up of fecal incontinence begins with a thorough history including preoperative level of fecal and urinary continence. Physical exam involves visual inspection of the perianal area and digital rectal exam to assess anal sphincter tone. Diagnostic studies include endoscopic anal ultrasound, anorectal manometry, pudendal nerve terminal motor latency, electromyography and defecography [172]. Treatment depends on etiology, but should begin with conservative medical management measures first. Bulking and constipating agents such as fiber, laxatives and loperimide are all recommended but there is actual little evidence of efficacy in functional incontinence [173]. Retrograde transanal irrigation is reported as a means to relieve incontinence difficulties. This is achieved by instilling lukewarm water in the anal canal and washing out the fecal contents [173]. In a small series of rectal cancer patients, this was effective in 79 % of patients; however, the technique is time and resource consuming with fecal soiling still occurring after correct performance of technique. [174–177] For incontinence from sphincter or neuronal injury, sacral nerve simulation provides marked improvement in function in up to 80 % patients. Several studies evaluated the use of SNS in rectal cancer patients and the results have been positive [178–182].

Urinary Dysfunction

The incidence of urinary dysfunction is also high and ranges from 30 to 70 %. It is the most common early post-operative complication in APR [183–186]. Urinary dysfunction includes retention, stress incontinence and urgency, with retention as one of the more common forms of dysfunction. Bladder contractility is under control of parasympathetic fibers via pelvic branches of inferior hypogastric plexus. Damage to these nerves results in denervation of the detrusor muscle, causing a partial paralysis. This manifests as a hypo- or acontractile bladder with decreased sensation resulting in retention [187, 188]. Damage to the hypogastric nerves results in stress incontinence and urgency in female patients. Predictive factors for bladder dysfunction include a low rectal cancer (<5 cm from the anal verge), lymph node involvement and a history of urinary dysfunction prior to surgery [154, 189, 190]. Extensive work-up is not required and treatment consists of bladder decompression for 5–7 days post-operatively. While most patients experience resolution of symptoms within 3 months post-operatively, persistent symptoms benefit from urologic consultation for further work-up [191]. Continued difficulties 6 months postoperatively are likely to have permanent problems requiring management via intermittent self-catheterization [191, 192].

Sexual Dysfunction

The incidence of sexual dysfunction in males undergoing APR is reported as 15–50 %, while those undergoing anterior resection and TME report impotence ~20–46 % and ejaculation failure 20–60 % [184, 193]. In women, underreporting obscures incidence, but may be 10–20 % [194, 195]. Postoperative dysfunction is usually the result of nerve damage, but can be dependent on multiple factors to include: patient age, preoperative libido, preoperative radiation therapy, lack of a standard definition for sexual dysfunction, and social and cultural barriers to discussing sexual complaints. Overall, the type of dysfunction is related to pattern of nerve injury. In males, damage to superior hypogastric plexus or hypogastric nerve results in ejaculatory difficulties such as retrograde ejaculation. Damage to inferior hypogastric plexus, pelvic splanchnic or cavernous nerves result in erectile dysfunction. In females, damage to parasympathetic and sympathetic nerve fibers results inability to produce vaginal and vulvar lubrication. Dyspareunia occurs with injury to the cavernous fibers and inferior hypogastric resulting in denervation of the vaginal wall, decreased lubrication and loss of suppleness [155, 184, 196].

Management is tailored to the patient and involves a frank discussion preoperatively and post-operatively to effectively manage patient expectations. For males, treatment of erectile dysfunction should be multi-modal with use of medications such as phosphodiesterase-5 inhibitors (i.e., Viagra) and psychotherapy to enhance pharmacological treatment [193, 197]. Penile prosthesis are also effective, but extremely invasive and irreversible, and normally are a consideration as a last resort after other measures have failed [193]. In females, treatment is based primarily on psychotherapy particularly for libido disorders. The use of systemic estrogen therapy is reported but only for short-term courses given increased risk of thromboembolic events and endometrial cancer [198]. Topical estrogen therapy is given to improve vaginal lubrication and vulvar atrophy [68, 199]. Phosphodiesterase inhibitors are an option for refractory vaginal dryness and vulvar atrophy. Improved clitoral sensitivity is also reported [200]. Dyspareunia or vaginumus is managed with pelvic floor rehabilitation using Kegel exercises and biofeedback with good results. There are no standard surgical treatments for these conditions although vestibulectomy or perineoplasty has been reported [193].

Low Anterior Resection Syndrome

Low anterior resection syndrome (ARS) is severe bowel dysfunction resulting in incontinence of flatus, feces, urgency and frequency that occurs after low anterior resection. Reported incidence is 10–20 % and apparently related to location of anastomosis in proximity to the anal verge. Anastomoses within 3 cm of the anal verge have increased severity of ARS compared to an anastomosis within 6 cm of the anal verge [165, 201–204]. Ultra-LAR has higher incidence of ARS with one case series reporting 30 % [205]. ARS is thought to occur by one or more of several pathophysiologic mechanisms: rectal reservoir dysfunction, colonic dysmotility or anal sphincter damage [205–207]. Prevention is somewhat achieved by limiting the amount of radiation delivered to the sphincter when possible. 3DXRT with full or partial sphincter blocking reduces the amount of radiation delivered to the sphincter complex [208]. Similarly, technical considerations with avoidance of undue pelvic trauma to surrounding tissues and the sphincter mechanism.

Signs and symptoms of ARS include a mix of high bowel frequency per day with liquid stools, multiple evacuations within a limited amount of time period, urgency and fecal incontinence. Most patients undergoing LAR initially experience this constellation of symptoms and most recover within 6 months of surgery. Work-up begins in those with continued symptoms several months postoperatively [205]. Diagnosis includes documentation of symptoms, number and type of bowel movements per day and objective testing utilized in a standard fecal incontinence work-up. Findings suggestive of ARS are low volume in the neorectum, low evacuation, a wide anorectal posterior angle greater than 110° along with a barium shadow in the anal canal at rest.

Treatment is multi-modal with medical therapy, rehabilitation and surgery, reflecting the multifactorial pathophysiology associated with this syndrome. There is no gold standard algorithm; however, the general consensus is that conservative management should be attempted first with surgical treatment being reserved for a last line therapy [205]. Treatment begins with medical therapy including bulking agents, high fiber diet, valproate sodium, diazepam, topical phenylephrine, amitriptyline and loperimide [209]. Loperamide is usually first line medical therapy for anti-motility effect and increase in anal sphincter tone [210]. Rehabilitative therapy involves biofeedback with improved success when combined with medical therapy. High-risk patients that classically fail biofeedback include history of XRT, previous anal or pelvic surgery or pelvic organ prolapse. Sacral neuromodulation is available, however more randomized control trials and long-term follow-up are needed [211, 212]. In intractable ARS, surgical management should be sought. Procedures such as sphincteroplasty or sphincteric substitution with gracilis or gluteus transposition or artificial sphincter have been described, though many patients ultimately require a definitive stoma [205].

Late Postoperative Complications

Stricture

Anastomotic strictures are well known to colorectal surgeons, but poorly defined in the literature [52, 213]. One definition is a "chronic narrowing or obstruction to the flow of intestinal contents resulting in clinical signs and symptoms of complete or partial bowel obstruction" [214]. Some define stricture by symptoms such as inability to evacuate stool, while others use the inability to pass a rigid proctoscope or index finger on DRE [215–217]. Stricture is found on screening endoscopy or by patient presentation. There are reports of up to 20 % incidence, but the actual incidence is difficult to determine because of reports of spontaneous resolving "silent strictures" [52, 213]. Strictures may be the result of benign disease, malignancy, radiotherapy, IUDs or iatrogenic with colorectal anastomosis as the most common cause [214, 218]. Risk factors associated with stricture formation are anastomotic leak or ischemia, PRT to the area, stapled anastomosis and lower rectal lesions [52, 216, 217]. A smaller series also reported mucin-producing tumors as a risk factor [217]. A Cochrane review analyzed nine randomized control trials for complications related to stapled versus hand-sewn anastomosis but did not find any differences in evaluated metrics, however stricture was more common in stapled anastomosis with a risk difference of 4.6 % (95 % CI 1.2–8.1 %) and number needed to treat of 17 (95 % CI 12–31) [82]. Treatment of benign strictures is managed by non-operative means with stool-bulking agents to gradually dilate the anastomosis. Other options include use of DRE and Hegar dilators for distal strictures [52]. The use of endoscopic Savary dilation with bougies of increasing diameter has been reported with good success in the literature, although patients who required more than three dilations were not able to achieve normal defecation [219]. Another option is use of pneumatic balloon dilation in symptomatic patients [220]. Predictors of poor response to conservative management include previous radiation therapy, local recurrence of malignancy and prior large anastomotic dehiscence [221].

For those that fail first line treatment, both expanding metallic stents (SEMS) and endoscopic trans-anal resection of strictures (ETARS) have been reported with good results. Complications include bleeding requiring reoperation, asymptomatic anastomotic perforation and technical failure in acutely angled strictures [222]. Other options include biodegradable stents, which have similar efficacy to SEMS, electroincision to produce radial incisions in the scar with balloon dilation, circular/linear stapler resection of the stricture and dilation with concomitant corticosteroid injection [223–225].

Chronic Perineal Pain

Perineal pain is common after anorectal surgery, but is also prevalent following Ultra-LAR for malignancy. Pain is thought to be the result of pelvic floor muscle spasms or levator ani syndrome. The pain usually resolves 2–3 week, but pain continuing beyond a month is considered chronic and an etiology should be sought, as pain may be the result of anastomotic leak or recurrent or residual disease. Work-up to determine etiology, starts with exam under anesthesia. Adjunct diagnostic tools involve imaging such as CT scan or EUS.

Treatment begins with a work-up to exclude local complications or recurrent disease, with directed therapy accordingly. Outside of this, conservative management beginning with warm Sitz Baths and non-steroidal inflammatory medication is warranted. Pelvic floor muscle spasms can benefit from the addition of anti-spasmodics such as diazepam or cyclobenzaprine [135]. Electrogalvanic muscle stimulation is utilized in severe spasms with reported success [226]. Patients with severe spasm also require such adjuncts as Botulinum toxin [227]. For patients that fail all other treatment modalities, APR may be considered. Despite this radical treatment, this procedure has been reported to provide good pain relief to unfortunate patients that are refractory to other measures [135].

Perineal Hernia

Perineal hernia is a rare complication of pelvic surgeries, specifically APR, pelvic exenterations and cystourethrectomy. The incidence is estimated to be 0.2–0.62 %, though historically rates are cited as high as 7 % [228, 229]. Associated risk factors include tobacco use, chemoradiation, malnutrition, wound infection and chronic wound [228–230]. Patients report a "vague dragging sensation" and discomfort upon standing. More rarely, they present with bowel obstruction, urinary symptoms, perineal wound breakdown or pain [226, 230, 231]. When found, this hernia is repaired from either the perineum or the abdomen or a combined approach. Typically the abdominal approach allows superior visualization, avoidance of iatrogenic bowel or vascular injury and ease of mesh placement; however some groups have reported success with the perineal approach [228, 230]. Repair involves reduction, excision of the sac and closure of defect. Defect closure is accomplished with either mesh or autologous tissue, such as gracilis flaps or omentum [135, 226, 228].

53.4 Summary and Conclusion

In summary, while the development of multimodal therapy for rectal cancer has led to better outcomes and survival, several complications and functional issues can occur. The colorectal surgeon must be well versed in the presentation, work-up and diagnosis of these to allow patients to have a better quality of life after their treatment of rectal cancer.

Key Points

- The most common location of bleeding is the presacral venous plexus. Control is difficult to achieve with electrocautery, suture ligation or clipping. Pelvic packing, metallic or titanium thumbtacks are more effective. Other methods include bone wax, endoscopic helical tackers, hemostatic sponges or local agents, tamponading saline bags or indirect coagulation with muscle fragmentation. Anastomotic bleeding is more commonly encountered and should be treated initially with conservative management, followed by endoscopic management.
- Genitourinary complications occur infrequently, but are catastrophic if missed. The ureters are the most frequently damaged because of their anatomical location. Ureteral stents do not prevent injury but they do allow for early identification of injuries. Intraoperative injury requires immediate repair. The principles of repair are the use of absorbable sutures to prevent stone formation, a tension-free repair over a stent and placement of closed-suction drain in proximity of repair. The type of repair depends on the location of injury.
- In transanal approaches such TAMIS and TEMS, perforation into the peritoneum can occur. This may be successfully repaired transanally, although formal laparotomy may be required. Diversion is typically only required with delayed presentation.
- Anastomotic leak is a devastating complication. Principles of prevention include mitigation of modifiable patient risk and intraoperative factors, along with the use of adjuncts. Intra-operative adjuncts include the use of buttressing materials, air leak testing the anastomosis and a restrictive resuscitation strategy. In the post-operative period, supplemental oxygen therapy, the use of protective diverting stomas and pelvic drains are also reported.
- Management of an anastomotic leak depends on whether it is contained or free. Contained leaks in hemodynamically stable patients should undergo CT scan imaging and can be managed with conservatively with percutaneous drainage, antibiotics and bowel rest. Hemodynamically, unstable patients and free leaks should undergo resusci-

tation with intravenous fluids, broad spectrum IV antibiotics and return to the operating room for operative intervention to assess the size, site, accessibility, viability of the bowel ends, and fecal load of the proximal colon. Anastomotic location and the status of the patient determine the procedure to be performed, but generally involve diversion or repair (in select cases).

- Surgical site infections are common following colorectal surgery with proctectomies having a higher rate of SSI. Oral and systemic antibiotics have shown to reduce the rate of SSI in rectal cases, but the use of mechanical bowel preparation has not. Intravenous antibiotics should have appropriate gram negative and anaerobic coverage and be dosed appropriately. Aggressive wound infection management should be undertaken to prevent further spread.
- Functional issues such as low anterior resection syndrome, urinary dysfunction and sexual dysfunction are relatively common occurrences after rectal cancer surgery. Patients should be counseled preoperatively regarding these matters. Most will resolve several months after surgery and can be managed conservatively, but appropriate work-up is required to determine cause and course of management to be taken.
- Fecal incontinence following proctectomy is multi-factorial, but can usually be managed with medical management with bulking or constipating medications. Evaluation involves physical examination and objective testing such as endoscopic anal ultrasound, anorectal manometry, pudendal nerve terminal motor latency, electromyography and defecography. Sacral nerve modulation has shown promise. Surgery is reserved for failures and may require permanent diversion.
- Anastomotic stricture following restorative procedures may occur, though the true incidence is difficult to determine. Strictures may be found on screening endoscopy or by patient symptoms. Causes include recurrent, malignancy, radiotherapy, or ischemia at the anastomosis. Treatment of benign strictures is managed by non-operative means with stool-bulking agents to gradually dilate the anastomosis or endoscopic serial dilation. Other options include biodegradable stents, which have similar efficacy to SEMS, electroincision to produce radial incisions in the scar with balloon dilation, circular/linear stapler resection of the stricture and dilation with concomitant corticosteroid injection. Recurrent disease should have a complete oncological work-up and then resected accordingly.
- Perineal pain is common after surgery, especially ultra-LAR. Pain is thought to be the result of pelvic floor muscle spasms or levator ani syndrome. The pain usually resolves in 2–3 week, but pain continuing beyond a month is considered chronic and an etiology should be sought. Work-up to determine etiology includes an exam under anesthesia, along with adjunct diagnostic tools such as CT scan or EUS. Treatment includes conservative management with warm Sitz Baths, non-steroidal inflammatory medication, bulking agents, and antispasmodics for pelvic floor muscle spasms. Diversion may be required in rare cases.

References

1. Parkin DM, Bray F, Ferlay J, et al. Global cancer statistics, 2002. CA Cancer J Clin. 2005;55(2):74–108.
2. US Cancer Statistics Working Group. United States Cancer Statistics (USCS): 1999—2007 incidence and mortality data. Atlanta: U.S. Department of Health and Human Services, CDC, National Cancer Institute. 2010 [cited 10 July 2012]. Available from: http://www.cdc.gov/uscs.
3. Jemal A, Murray T, Samuels A, et al. Cancer statistics, 2003. CA Cancer J Clin. 2003;53:5–26.
4. Howlader N, Noone AM, Krapcho M, Neyman N, Aminou R, Altekruse SF et al. SEER cancer statitics review 1975–2009 (Vintage 2009 Populations). Estimated new cancer cases and deaths for 2012 all races by sex, Table 11. [serial on the Internet]. 2012. Available from: http://seer.cancer.gov/csr/1975_2009_pops09/results_single/sect_01_table.01.pdf.
5. Heald RJ. The holy plane of rectal surgery. J R Soc Med. 1988;81(9):503–8.
6. Adam IJ, Mohamdee MO, Martin IG, et al. Role of circumferential margin involvement in the local recurrence of rectal cancer. Lancet. 1994;344(8924):707–11.
7. Benson ABI, Arnoletti JP, Bekali-Saab T et al. NCCN guideline panel members NCCN clinical practice guidelines in oncology: rectal cancer version 3. 2012. NCCN Clinical Practice Guidelines in Oncology (NCCN Guidelines) Rectal Cancer. Version 1.2015. Available at http://www.nccn.org/professionals/physician_gls/pdf/rectal.pdf. Accessed 12 Nov 2015.
8. Moore JS, Cataldo PA, Osler T, Hyman NH. Transanal endoscopic microsurgery is more effective than traditional transanal excision for resection of rectal masses. Dis Colon Rectum. 2008;51(7):1026–30.
9. Papagrigoriadis S. Trans-anal endoscopic microsurgery for the management of large or sessile rectal adenomas: a review of the technique and indications. Int Semin Surg Oncol. 2006;3:313.
10. Christoforidis D, Cho HM, Dixon MR, et al. Transanal endoscopic microsurgery versus conventional transanal excision for patients with early rectal cancer. Ann Surg. 2009;249(5):776–82.
11. Atallah S, Albert M, Larach S. Transanal minimally invasive surgery: a giant leap forward. Surg Endosc. 2010;24:2200–5.
12. Bleday R, Brindezi N. Surgical treatment of rectal cancer. In: Beck DE, Roberts PL, Saclarides TJ, Senagore AJ, Stamos MJ, Wexner SD, editors. The ASCRS textbook of colon and rectal surgery. 2nd edn. New York: Springer; 2011. p. 743–56.
13. Braga M, Frasson M, Vignali A. Laparoscopic resection in rectal cancer patients: outcome and cost-benefit analysis. Dis Colon Rectum. 2007;50(7):464–71.
14. Lim TR, Mahesh V, Singh S, Tan BH, Elsadig M, Radhakrishnan N, et al. Endoscopic mucosal resection of colorectal polyps in typical UK hospitals. World J Gastroenterol. 2010;16(42):5324–8.
15. Germanos S, Bolanis I, Saedon M, Baratsis S. Control of presacral venous bleeding during rectal surgery. Am J Surg. 2010;200:e33–5.
16. Sadahiro S, Ishida H, Suzuki T, Ishikawa K, Tajima T, Makuuchi H. Vesicular blood flow after ligation of the internal iliac arteries in Low anterior resection or abdominoperineal resection. Dis Colon Rectum. 1999;42(11):1475–9.
17. Oderich GS, Panneton JM, Hofer J, Bower TC, Cherry Jr KJ, Sullivan T, et al. Iatrogenic operative injuries of abdominal and pelvic veins: a potentially lethal complication. J Vasc Surg. 2004;39(5):931–6.
18. Arthurs ZM, Sohn VY, Starnes BW. Vascular trauma: endovascular management and techniques. Surg Clin N Am. 2007;87(5):1179–92.
19. Zhou W, Bush RL, Terramani TT, Lin PH, Lumsden AB. Treatment options of iatrogenic pelvic vein injuries: conventional operative versus endovascular approach—case reports. Vasc Endovasc Surg. 2004;38(6):569–73.
20. Martinez-Serrano MA, Pares D, Pera M, Pascual M, Courtier R, Egea MJ, et al. Managment of lower gastrointestinal bleeding after colorectal resection and stapled anastomosis. Tech Coloproctol. 2009;13(1):49–53.
21. Perez RO, Sousa Jr A, Bresciani C, Proscurshim I, Coser R, Kiss D, et al. Endoscopic management of postoperative stapled colorectal anastomosis hemorrhage. Tech Coloproctol. 2007;11(1):64–6.
22. Baron TH, Norton ID, Herman L. Endoscopic hemoclip placement for post-sphincterotomy bleeding. Gastrointest Endosc. 2000;52(5):662–7.
23. Prakash C, Chokshi H, Walden DT, Aliperti G. Endoscopic hemostasis in acute diverticular bleeding. Endoscopy. 1999;31(6):460–3.
24. Linn TY, Moran BJ, Cecil TD. Staple line hemorrhage following laparoscopic left-sided colorectal resections may be more common when the inferior mesenteric artery is preserved. Tech Coloproctol. 2008;12(4):289–93.
25. Delacroix Jr SE, Winters JC. Urinary tract injures: recognition and management. Clin Colon Rectal Surg. 2010;23(2):104–12.
26. Nam YS, Wexner SD. Clinical value of prophylactic ureteral stent indwelling during laparoscopic colorectal surgery. J Korean Med Sci. 2002;17(5):633–5.

27. Pokala N, Delaney CP, Kiran RP, Bast J, Angermeir K, Fazio VW. A randomized-control trial comparing intraoperative versus sequential prophylactic ureteric catheter insertion in Re-operative and complicated colorectal surgery. Int J Color Dis. 2007;22(6):683–7.
28. Chahin F, Dwivedi A, Paramesh A. Implications of lighted stenting in laparoscopic colectomy. J Soc Laparoendosc Surg. 2002;6(1):49–62.
29. Mahendran HA, Singam P, Ho C, Hong GE, Hee TG, Zainuddin ZM. Iatrogenic ureter injuries: eleven years experience in a tertiary hospital. Med J Malaysia. 2012;67(2):169–72.
30. Delacroix Jr SE, Winters JC. Urologic complications of colorectal surgery. In: Whitlow CB, Beck DE, Margolin DA, Hicks TC, editors. Improved outcomes in colon and rectal surgery. New York: Informa Healthcare Communications; 2009.
31. Warkwick RT, Worth PH. The psoas bladder hitch procedure for the replacement of the lower third of the ureter. Br J Urol. 1969;41(6):701–9.
32. Turkeri NL. Bladder trauma. In: Hohenfellner M, Santucci RA, editors. Emergencies in urology. Berlin: Springer; 2007. p. 249.
33. Corriere Jr JN, Sandler CM. Management of the ruptured bladder: seven years of experience with 111 cases. J Trauma. 1986;26(9):830–3.
34. Deck AJ, Shaves S, Talner L, Porter JR. Computerized tomography cystography for the diagnosis of traumatic bladder rupture. J Urol. 2000;164(1):43–6.
35. Jarrett TW, Vaughan Jr ED. Accuracy of computerized tomography in the diagnosis of colovesical fistula secondary to diverticular disease. J Urol. 1995;153(1):44–6.
36. Guerrieri M, Baldarelli M, Organetti L, et al. Transanal endoscopic microsurgery for the treatment of selected patients with distal rectal cancer: 15 years experience. Surg Endosc. 2008; 22(9):2030–5.
37. Floyd ND, Saclarides TJ. Transanal endoscopic microsurgical resection of pT1 rectal tumors. Dis Colon Rectum. 2006;49(2):164–8.
38. Bach SP, Hill J, Monson JR, et al. Association of coloproctology of great Britain & Ireland Transanal Endoscopic Microsurgery (TEM) collaboration. A predictive model for local recurrence after transanal endoscopic microsurgery for rectal cancer. Br J Surg. 2009;96(3):280–90.
39. Endreseth BH, Wibe A, Svinsås M, Mårvik R, Myrvold HE. Postoperative morbidity and recurrence after local excision of rectal adenomas and rectal cancer by transanal endoscopic microsurgery. Color Dis. 2005;7(2):133–7.
40. Baatrup G, Elbrønd H, Hesselfeldt P, et al. Rectal adenocarcinoma and transanal endoscopic microsurgery. Diagnostic challenges, indications and short-term results in 142 consecutive patients. Int J Color Dis. 2007;22(11):1347–52.
41. Kreissler-Haag D, Schuld J, Lindemann W, König J, Hildebrandt U, Schilling M. Complications after transanal endoscopic microsurgical resection correlate with location of rectal neoplasms. Surg Endosc. 2008;22(3):612–6.
42. Stipa F, Burza A, Lucandri G, et al. Outcomes for early rectal cancer managed with transanal endoscopic microsurgery: a 5-year follow-up study. Surg Endosc. 2006;20(4):541–5.
43. Maslekar S, Pillinger SH, Monson JR. Transanal endoscopic microsurgery for carcinoma of the rectum. Surg Endosc. 2007;21(1):97–102.
44. Lezoche E, Guerrieri M, Paganini AM, Feliciotti F. Transanal endoscopic microsurgical excision of irradiated and nonirradiated rectal cancer. Surg Laparosc Endosc. 1998;8(4):249–56.
45. Serra-Aracil X, Vallverdú H, Bombardó-Junca J, Pericay-Pijaume C, Urgellés-Bosch J, Navarro-Soto S. Long-term follow-up of local rectal cancer surgery by transanal endoscopic microsurgery. World J Surg. 2008;32(6):1162–7.
46. Lezoche E, Guerrieri M, Paganini AM, Baldarelli M, De Sanctis A, Lezoche G. Long-term results in patient with T2–3 N0 distal rectal cancer undergoing radiotherapy before transanal endoscopic microsurgery. Br J Surg. 2005;92(12):1546–52.
47. Dafnis G, Påhlman L, Raab Y, Gustafsson UM, Graf W. Transanal endoscopic microsurgery: clinical and functional results. Color Dis. 2004;6(5):336–42.
48. Guerrieri M, Baldarelli M, Morino M, et al. Transanal endoscopic micro-surgery in rectal adenomas: experience of six Italian centres. Dig Liver Dis. 2006;38(3):202–7.
49. Ganai S, Kanumuri P, Rao RS, Alexander AI. Local recurrence after transanal endoscopic microsurgery for rectal polyps and early cancers. Ann Surg Oncol. 2006;13(4):547–56.
50. Wong NY, Eu KW. A defunctioning ileostomy does not prevent clinical anastomotic leak after a Low anterior resection: a prospective comparative study. Dis Colon Rectum. 2005;48(11):2076–9.
51. Phitayakorn R, Delaney CP, Reynolds HL, et al. Standardized algorithms for management of anastomotic leaks and related abdominal and pelvic abscess after colorectal surgery world. J Surg. 2008;32:1147–56.
52. Davis B, Rivadeneira DE. Complications of colorectal anastomoses: leaks, strictures, and bleeding. Surg Clin North Am. 2013;93(1):61–87.
53. Branagan G, Finnis D. Prognosis after anastomotic leak in colorectal surgery. Dis Colon Rectum. 2005;48(5):1021–6.
54. Platell C, Barwood N, Dorfmann G, Makin G. The incidence of anastomotic leaks in patients undergoing colorectal surgery. Color Dis. 2007;9(1):71–9.
55. Buchs NC, Gervaz P, Secic M. Incidence, consequences, and risk factors for anastomotic dehiscence after colorectal surgery: a prospective monocentric study. Int J Color Dis. 2008;23(3):265–70.
56. Jestin P, Pahlman L, Gunnarsson U. Risk factors for anastomotic leakage after rectal cancer surgery: a case-control study. Color Dis. 2008;10(7):715–21.
57. Makela JT, Kiviniemi H, Laitinen S. Risk factors for anastomotic leakage after left-sided colorectal resec-

tion with rectal anastomosis. Dis Colon Rectum. 2003;46(5):653–60.
58. Golub R, Golub RW, Cantu Jr R, Stein HD. A multivariate analysis of factors contributing to leakage of intestinal anastomoses. J Am Coll Surg. 1997;184(4):364–72.
59. Suding P, Jensen E, Abramson MA, et al. Definitive risk factors for anastomotic leaks in elective open colorectal resection. Arch Surg. 2008;143(9):907–11; discussion 11–12.
60. Bertelsen CA, Andreasen AH, Jørgensen T, et al. Anastomotic leakage after anterior resection for rectal cancer: risk factors. Color Dis. 2010;12(1):37–43.
61. Choi HK, Law WL, Ho JW. Leakage after resection and intraperitoneal anastomosis for colorectal malignancy: analysis of risk factors. Dis Colon Rectum. 2006;49(11):1719–25.
62. Jung SH, Yu CS, Choi PW, et al. Risk factors and oncologic impact of anastomotic leakage after rectal cancer surgery. Dis Colon Rectum. 2008;51(6): 902–8.
63. Asteria CR, Gagliardi G, Pucciarelli S. Anastomotic leaks after anterior resection for mid and low rectal cancer: survey of the Italian society of colorectal surgery. Tech Coloproctol. 2008;12(2):103–10.
64. Nesbakken A, Nygaard K, Westerheim O, et al. Audit of intraoperative and early postoperative complications after introduction of mesorectal excision for rectal cancer. Eur J Surg. 2002;168(4):229–35.
65. Benoist S, Panis Y, Alves A, Valleur P. Impact of obesity on surgical outcomes after colorectal resection. Am J Surg. 2000;179(4):275–81.
66. Rullier E, Laurent C, Garrelon JL. Risk factors for anastomotic leakage after resection of rectal cancer. Br J Surg. 1998;85(3):355–8.
67. Gendall KA, Raniga S, Kennedy R, et al. The impact of obesity on outcome after major colorectal surgery. Dis Colon Rectum. 2007;50(12):2223–37.
68. Basson R, Althof S, Davis S, Fugl-Meyer K, Goldstein I, Leiblum S, et al. Summary of the recommendations on sexual dysfunctions in women. J Sex Med. 2004;1(1):24–34.
69. Lee MR, Hong CW, Yoon SN, et al. Risk factors for anastomotic leakage after resection for rectal cancer. Hepatogastroenterology. 2006;53(71):682–6.
70. Eberl T, Jagoditsch M, Klingler A. Risk factors for anastomotic leakage after resection for rectal cancer. Am J Surg. 2008;196(4):592–8.
71. Schrock TR, Deveney CW, Dunphy JE. Factor contributing to leakage of colonic anastomoses. Ann Surg. 1973;177(5):513–8.
72. Kim MJ, Shin R, Oh HK, et al. The impact of heavy smoking on anastomotic leakage and stricture after low anterior resection in rectal cancer patients. World J Surg. 2011;35(12):2806–10.
73. Altomare DF, Binda G, Ganio E, et al. Long-term outcome of Altemeier's procedure for rectal prolapse. Dis Colon Rectum. 2009;52(4):698–703.
74. Law WL, Chu KW. Anterior resection for rectal cancer with mesorectal excision: a prospective evaluation of 622 patients. Ann Surg. 2004;240(2):260–8.
75. Matthiessen P, Hallböök O, Andersson M, Rutegård J, Sjödahl R. Risk factors for anastomotic leakage after anterior resection of the rectum. Color Dis. 2004;6(6):462–9.
76. Alves A, Panis Y, Trancart D, et al. Factors associated with clinically significant anastomotic leakage after large bowel resection: multivariate analysis of 707 patients. World J Surg. 2002;26(4):499–502.
77. Locke R, Hauser CJ, Shoemaker WC. The use of surface oximetry to assess bowel viability. Arch Surg. 1984;119(111):1252–6. Arch Surg, 1984. 119(11): 1252–1256.
78. Attard JA, Raval MJ, Martin GR, Kolb J, Afrouzian M, Buie WD, et al. The effects of systemic hypoxia on colon anastomotic healing: an animal model. Dis Colon Rectum. 2005;48(7):1460–70.
79. Sheridan WG, Lowndes RH, Young HL. Tissue oxygen tension as a predictor of colonic anastomotic healing. Dis Colon Rectum. 1987;30(11):867–71.
80. Millan M, García-Granero E, Flor B, García-Botello S, Lledo S. Early prediction of anastomotic leak in colorectal cancer surgery by intramucosal pH. Dis Colon Rectum. 2006;49(5):595–601.
81. Stapled versus handsewn methods for colorectal anastomosis surgery [database on the Internet] 2001.
82. Stapled versus handsewn methods for colorectal anastomosis surgery. Cochrane Database Syst Rev. 2012;(2):CD003144 [database on the Internet] 2012 [cited June 2012].
83. Burch JM, Franciose RJ, Moore EE, et al. Single-layer continuous versus two-layer interrupted intestinal anastomosis: a prospective randomized trial. Ann Surg. 2000;231(6):832–7.
84. Gaertner WB, Hagerman G, Potter MJ, et al. Experimental evaluation of a bovine pericardium-derived collagen matrix buttress in ileocolic and colon anastomoses. J Biomed Mater Res B Appl Biomater. 2010;92(1):48–54.
85. Hagerman GF, Gaertner WB, Ruth GR, et al. Bovine pericardium buttress reinforces colorectal anastomoses in a canine model. Dis Colon Rectum. 2007;50(7):1053–6.
86. Hoeppner J, Willa K, Timme S, et al. Reinforcement of colonic anastomoses with a collagenous double-layer matrix extracted from porcine dermis. Eur Surg. 2010;45(2):68–76.
87. Fajardo AD, Chun J, Stewart D, et al. 1.5:1 meshed AlloDerm bolsters for stapled rectal anastomoses does not provide any advantage in anastomotic strength in a porcine model. Surg Innov. 2011;18(1):21–8.
88. Goldsmith HS. Protection of low rectal anastomosis with intact omentum. Surg Gynecol Obstet. 1977;144(4):584–6.
89. Lanter B, Mason RA. Use of omental pedicle graft to protect low anterior colonic anastomosis. Dis Colon Rectum. 1979;22(7):448–51.
90. Agnifili A, Schietroma M, Carloni A. Omentoplasty is effective in lowering the complications of ano-rectal resections. Minerva Chir. 2004;59(4):363–8.

91. Agnifili A, Schietroma M, Carloni A, et al. The value of omentoplasty in protecting colorectal anastomosis from leakage. A prospective randomized study in 126 patients. Hepatogastroenterology. 2004;51(60):1694–7.
92. Beard JD, Nicholson ML, Sayers RD, et al. Intraoperative air testing of colorectal anastomoses: a prospective, randomized trial. Br J Surg. 1990;77(10):1095–7.
93. Yalin R, Aktan AO, Yeğen C, et al. Importance of testing stapled rectal anastomoses with air. Eur J Surg. 1993;159(1):49–51.
94. Ricciardi R, Roberts PL, Marcello PW, et al. Anastomotic leak testing after colorectal resection: what are the data? Arch Surg. 2009;144(5):407–11.
95. Schmidt O, Merkel S, Hohenberger W. Anastomotic leakage after low rectal stapler anastomosis: significance of intraoperative anastomotic testing. Eur J Surg Oncol. 2003;29(3):239–43.
96. Noblett SE, Snowden CP, Shenton BK, et al. Randomized clinical trial assessing the effect of Doppler-optimized fluid management on outcome after elective colorectal resection. Br J Surg. 2006;93(9):1069–76.
97. Rahbari NN, Zimmermann JB, Schmidt T, et al. Meta-analysis of standard, restrictive and supplemental fluid administration in colorectal surgery. Br J Surg. 2009;96(4):331–41.
98. Donati A, Loggi S, Preiser JC, et al. Goal-directed intraoperative therapy reduces morbidity and length of hospital stay in high-risk surgical patients. Chest. 2007;132(6):1817–24.
99. Kimberger O, Arnberger M, Brandt S, et al. Goal-directed colloid administration improves the microcirculation of healthy and perianastomotic colon. Anesthesiology. 2009;110(3):496–504.
100. Brandstrup B, Tønnesen H, Beier-Holgersen R, et al. Effects of intravenous fluid restriction on postoperative complications: comparison of two perioperative fluid regimens: a randomized assessor-blinded multicenter trial. Ann Surg. 2003; 238(5):641–8.
101. Abraham-Nordling M, Hjern F, Pollack J, et al. Randomized clinical trial of fluid restriction in colorectal surgery. Br J Surg. 2012;99(2):186–91.
102. Futier E, Constantin JM, Petit A, Chanques G. Conservative vs restrictive individualized goal-directed fluid replacement strategy in major abdominal surgery: a prospective randomized trial. Arch Surg. 2010;145(12):1193–200.
103. García-Botello SA, García-Granero E, Lillo R, et al. Randomized clinical trial to evaluate the effects of perioperative supplemental oxygen administration on the colorectal anastomosis. Br J Surg. 2006;93(6):698–706.
104. Schietroma M, Carlei F, Cecilia EM. Colorectal infraperitoneal anastomosis: the effects of perioperative supplemental oxygen administration on the anastomotic dehiscence. J Gastrointest Surg. 2012;16(2):427–34.
105. Peeters KC, Tollenaar RA, Marijnen CA. Risk factors for anastomotic failure after total mesorectal excision of rectal cancer. Br J Surg. 2005;92(2):211–6.
106. Boccola MA, Lin J, Rozen WM, et al. Reducing anastomotic leakage in oncologic colorectal surgery: an evidence-based review. Anticancer Res. 2010;2(30):2, review Raliocsae-b.
107. Matthiessen P, Hallböök O, Rutegård J, et al. Defunctioning stoma reduces symptomatic anastomotic leakage after low anterior resection of the rectum for cancer: a randomized multicenter trial. Ann Surg. 2007;246(2):207–14.
108. Hüser N, Michalski CW, Erkan M. Systematic review and meta-analysis of the role of defunctioning stoma in low rectal cancer surgery. Ann Surg. 2008;248(1):52–60.
109. Tan WS, Tang CL, Shi L. Meta-analysis of defunctioning stomas in low anterior resection for rectal cancer. Br J Surg. 2009;96(5):462–72.
110. Covering ileo- or colostomy in anterior resection for rectal carcinoma. [database on the Internet] 2010.
111. Chude GG, Rayate NV, Patris V, et al. Defunctioning loop ileostomy with low anterior resection for distal rectal cancer: should we make an ileostomy as a routine procedure? A prospective randomized study. Hepatogastroenterology. 2008;55(86–87):1562–7.
112. Gerber A. Editorial: the anastomosis should be made without tension. Surg Gynecol Obstet. 1976; 142(1):75–6.
113. Tsujinaka S, Kawamura YJ, Konishi F, et al. Pelvic drainage for anterior resection revisited: use of drains in anastomotic leaks. ANZ J Surg. 2008;78(6):461–5.
114. Yeh CY, Changchien CR, Wang JY, et al. Pelvic drainage and other risk factors for leakage after elective anterior resection in rectal cancer patients: a prospective study of 978 patients. Ann Surg. 2005;241(1): 9–13.
115. Galandiuk S, Fazio VW. Postoperative irrigation-suction drainage after pelvic colonic surgery. A prospective randomized trial. Dis Colon Rectum. 1991;34(3):223–8.
116. Prophylactic anastomotic drainage for colorectal surgery [database on the Internet] 2004.
117. Merad F, Hay JM, Fingerhut A, et al. Is prophylactic pelvic drainage useful after elective rectal or anal anastomosis? A multicenter controlled randomized trial. French Association for Surgical Research. Surgery. 1999;125(5):529–35.
118. Berliner SD, Burson LC, Lear PE. Use and abuse of intraperitoneal drains in colon surgery. Arch Surg. 1964;89:686–9.
119. Smith SR, Connolly JC, Crane PW. The effect of surgical drainage materials on colonic healing. Br J Surg. 1982;69(3):153–5.
120. Nicksa GA, Dring RV, Johnson KH, Sardella WV, Vignati PV, Cohen JL. Anastomotic leaks: what is the best diagnostic imaging study? Dis Colon Rectum. 2007;50(2):197–203.

121. de Lissovoy G, Fraeman K, Hutchins V, et al. Surgical site infection: incidence and impact on hospital utilization and treatment costs. Am J Infect Control. 2009;37(5):387–97.
122. Konishi T, Watanabe T, Kishimoto J. Elective colon and rectal surgery differ in risk factors for wound infection: results for prospective surveillance. Ann Surg. 2006;244:758–63.
123. Mai V, Morris Jr J. Colonic bacterial flora: changing understandings in the molecular age. J Nutr. 2004;134:459–64.
124. Degrate L, Garancini M, Misani M, et al. Right colon, left colon, and rectal surgeries are not similar for surgical site infection development. Analysis of 277 elective and urgent colorectal resections. Int J Color Dis. 2011;26:61–9.
125. Gruessner U, Clemens M, Pahlpatz PV, et al. Improvement of perineal wound healing by local administration of gentamicin-imprenated collagen fleeces after abdominoperineal excision for rectal cancer. Am J Surg. 2001;182(5):502–9.
126. Ruiz-Tovar J, Santos J, Arroyo A. Effect of peritoneal lavage with clindamycin-gentamicin solution on infections after elective colorectal cancer surgery. J Am Coll Surg. 2012;214(2):202–7.
127. Kreiger BR, Davis DM, Sanchez JE. The use of silver nylon in preventing surgical site infections following colon and rectal surgery. Dis Colon Rectum. 2011;54:1014–9.
128. Bratzler DW, Hunt DR. The surgical infection prevention and surgical care improvement projects: national initiatives to improve outcomes for patients having surgery. Clin Infect Dis. 2006;43:322–30.
129. Fry DE. Surigcal site infections and the Surgical Care Improvement Project (SCIP): evolution of national quality measures. Surg Infect. 2008;9: 579–84.
130. Mechanical bowel preparation for elective colorectal surgery [database on the Internet] 2011.
131. Bellows CF, Mills KT, Kelly TN, et al. Combination of oral non-absorbable and intravenous antibiotics versus intravenous antibiotics alone in the prevention of surgical site infections after colorectal surgery: a meta-analysis of randomized controlled trials. Tech Coloproctol. 2011;15(4):385–95.
132. Khurrum BM, Hua ZR, Bautista O. Percutaneous postoperative intra-abdominal abscess drainage after elective colorectal surgery. Tech Coloproctol. 2006;6(3):159–64.
133. Scheter S, Eisenstat TE, Oliver GC. Computerized tomographic scan-guided drainage of intra-abdominal abscesses. Preoperative and postoperative modalities in colon and rectal surgery. Dis Colon Rectum. 1994;37(10):984–8.
134. Cinat ME, Wilson SE, Din AM. Determinants for successful percutaneous image-guided drainage of intra-abdominal abscess. Arch Surg. 2002;137(7):845–9.
135. Ogilvie JW, Ricciardi R. Complications of perineal surgery. Clin Colon Rectal Surg. 2009;22(1):51–9.
136. Rosen L, Veidenheimer MC, Coller JA, et al. Mortality, morbidity and patterns of recurrence after abdominoperineal resection for cancer of the rectum. Dis Colon Rectum. 1982;25(3):202–8.
137. Rothenberger DA, Wong WD. Abdominoperineal resection for adenocarcinoma of the low rectum. World J Surg. 1992;16(3):478–85.
138. Chadwick MA, Vieten D, Pettitt E. Short course preoperative radiotherapy is the single most important risk factor for perineal wound complication after abdominoperineal excision of the rectum. Color Dis. 2008;8(9):756–61.
139. Nissan A, Guillem JG, Paty PB. Abdominoperineal resection for rectal cancer at a specialty center. Dis Colon Rectum. 2001;44(1):27–35.
140. Group SCCS. Randomized study on preoperative radiotherapy in rectal carcinoma. Ann Surg Oncol. 1996;3(5):423–30.
141. Trial SRC. Intial report from a swedish multicentre study examining the role of preoperative irradiation in the treatment of patients with resectable rectal carcinoma. Br J Surg. 1993;80(10):1333–6.
142. Horn A, Halvorsen JF, Dahl O. Preoperative radiotherapy in operable rectal cancer. Dis Colon Rectum. 1990;33(10):832–28.
143. Party MRCRCW. Randomized trial of surgery alone versus radiotherapy followed by surgery for potentially operable locally advanced. Lancet. 1996;348(9042):1605–10.
144. Hartz RS, Poticha SM, Shields TW. Healing of the perineal wound. Arch Surg. 1980;115(4):471–4.
145. Waits JO, Dozios RR, Kelly KA. Primary closure and continuous irrigation of the perineal wound after proctectomy. Mayo Clin Proc. 1982;57(3):185–8.
146. Shibata D, Hyland W, Busse P. Immediate reconstruction of the perineal wound with gracilis muscle flaps following abdominoperineal resection and intraoperative radiation therapy for recurrent carcinoma of the rectum. Ann Surg Oncol. 1999;6(1):33–7.
147. Radice E, Nelson H, Mercill S. Primary myocutaneous flap closure following resection of locally advanced pelvic malignancies. Br J Surg. 1999;86(3):349–54.
148. De Broux E, Parc Y, Rondelli F. Sutured perineal omentoplasty after abdominoperineal resection for adenocarcinoma of the lower rectum. Dis Colon Rectum. 2005;48(3):476–81.
149. Nilsson PJ. Omentoplasty in abdominoperineal resection: a reivew of the literature using a systematic approach. Dis Colon Rectum. 2006;49(9): 1354–61.
150. Del Pino A, Abcarian H. The difficult perineal wound. Surg Clin N Am. 1997;77(1):155–74.
151. Pemberton JH. How to treat persistent perineal sinus after rectal excision. Color Dis. 2003;5(5):486–9.
152. Yousaf M, Witherow A, Gardiner KR. Use of vacuum-assisted closure for healing a persistent perianal sinus following panproctocolectomy: report of a case. Dis Colon Rectum. 2004;47(8):1403–8.

153. Hyman NH. Unhealed perineal wound. In: Fazio VW, Church JM, Delaney CP, editors. Current therapy in colon and rectal surgery. 2nd ed. Philadelphia: Elsevier/Mosby; 2005. p. 241–3.
154. Wallner C, Lange MM, Bonsing BA. Causes of fecal and urinary incontinence after total mesorectal excision for rectal cancer based on cadaveric surgery: a study from the cooperative clinical investigators of the Dutch total mesorectal excision trial. J Clin Oncol. 2008;26(27):4466–72.
155. Havenga K, Enker WE. Autonomic nerve preserving total mesorectal excision. Surg Clin N Am. 2002;82(5):1008–18.
156. Maas CP, De Ruiter MC, Kenter GG, Trimbos JB. The inferior hypogastric plexus in gynecologic surgery. Gynecol Tech. 1999;5:55–62.
157. Ali M, Johnson IP, Hobson J, Mohammadi B, Khan FA. Anatomy of the pelvic plexus and innervation of the prostate gland. Clin Anat. 2004;17(2):123–9.
158. Tsuchiya S, Ohki S. Radical surgery for rectal cancer with preservation of pelvic autonomic nerves. Taipei: Republic of China Surgical Society; 1992.
159. Enker WE, Thaler HT, Cranor ML, Polyak T. Total mesorectal excision in the operative treatment of carcinoma of the rectum. J Am Coll Surg. 1995;181(4):355–46.
160. Bretagnol F, Troubat H, Laurent C. Long-term functional results after rectal cancer treatment. Gastroenterol Clin Biol. 2004;28(2):155–9.
161. Lange MM, den Dulk M, Bossema ER. Risk factors for fecal incontinence after rectal cancer treatment. Br J Surg. 2007;94(10):1278–84.
162. Peeters KC, van de Velde CJ, Leer JW, et al. Late side effects of short-course preoperative radiotherapy combined with total mesorectal excision for rectal cancer: increased bowel dysfunction in irradiated patients—a Dutch colorectal cancer group study. J Clin Oncol. 2005;23(25):6199–206.
163. Welsh FK, McFall M, Mitchell G. Preoperative short-course radiotherapy is associated with faecal incontinence after anterior resection. Color Dis. 2003;5(6):563–8.
164. Amin AI, Hallbook O, Lee AJ, et al. A 5 cm colonic pouch coloanal reconstruction following anterior resection for Low rectal cancer results in acceptable evacuation and continence in the long term. Color Dis. 2003;5(1):33–7.
165. Karanja ND, Schache DJ, Heald RJ. Function of the distal rectum after low anterior resection for carcinoma. Br J Surg. 1992;79(2):114–6.
166. Gotzinger P, Wamser P, Herbst F. Colo-anal anastomosis: improvement of early function outcome by reconstruction with the colonic pouch. Chirurg. 2001;72(1):49–53.
167. Putta S, Andreyev HJ. Faecal incontinence: a late side-effect of pelvic radiotherapy. Clin Oncol R Coll Radiol. 2005;17(6):469–77.
168. Pollack J, Holm T, Cedermark B. Long term effect of preoperative radiation therapy on anorectal function. Dis Colon Rectum. 2006;49(3):345–52.
169. Hayne D, Vaizey CJ, Boulos PB. Anorectal injury following pelvic radiotherapy. Br J Surg. 2001;88(8):1037–48.
170. Wallner C, Maas CP, Dabhoiwala NF, et al. Innervation of the pelvic floor muscles: a reappraisal for the levator Ani nerve. Obstet Gynecol. 2006;108(3 Pt 1):529–34.
171. Koda K, Saito N, Seike K. Dennervaton of the neorectum as a potential cause of defecatory disorder following low anterior resection for rectal cancer. Dis Colon Rectum. 2005;48:210–7.
172. Sands DR, Madsen MA. Fecal incontinence. In: Beck DE, Roberts PL, Saclarides TJ, Senagore AJ, Stamos MJ, Wexner SD, editors. The ACRS textbook of colon and rectal surgery. 2nd ed. New York: Springer; 2011.
173. Emmertsen KJ, Laurberg S. Bowel dysfunction after treatment for rectal cancer. Acta Oncol. 2008;47(6):994–1003.
174. Christensen P, Bazzocchi G, Coggrave M, Abel R, Hultling C, Krogh K, et al. A randomized controlled trial of transanal irrigation versus conservative bowel management in spinal cord injured patients. Gastroenterology. 2006;131(3):738–41.
175. Christensen P, Olsen N, Krogh K, Bacher T, Laurberg S. Schintergraphic assessment of retrograde colonic washout in fecal incontinence and constipation. Dis Colon Rectum. 2003;46(1):68–76.
176. Gosselink MP, Darby M, Zimmerman DD, Smits AA, van Kessel I, Hop WC, et al. Long term follow-up of retrograde colonic irrigation for defecation disturbances. Color Dis. 2005;7(1):65–9.
177. Iwama T, Imajo M, Yaegashi K, Mishima Y. Self washout method for defecational complaints following low anterior rectal resection. Jpn J Surg. 1989;19(2):251–3.
178. Rasmussen OO, Buntzen S, Sorenson M, Laurberg S, Christiansen J. Sacral nerve stimulation in fecal incontinence. Dis Colon Rectum. 2004;47(7):1158–62; discussion 62–3.
179. Pillinger SH, Gardiner A, Duthie GS. Sacral nerve stimulation for fecal incontinence. Dig Surg. 2005;22(1–2):1–5.
180. Matzel KE, Stadelmaier U, Bittorf B, Hohenfellner M, Hohenberger WH. Bilateral sacral nerve stimulation for fecal incontinence after low anterior resection. Int J Color Dis. 2002;17(6):430–4.
181. Ratto C, Grillo E, Parello A, Petrolino M, Costamagna G, Doglietto GB. Sacral neuromodulation in treatment of fecal incontinence following anterior resection and chemoradiation for rectal cancer. Dis Colon Rectum. 2005;48(5):1027–36.
182. Lim JT, Hastie IA, Hiscock RJ, Shedda SM. Sacral nerve stimulation for fecal incontinence: long term outcomes. Dis Colon Rectum. 2011; 54(8):969–74.
183. Hollabaugh RSJ, Stiener MS, Sellers KD, Samm BJ, Dmochowski RR. Neuroanatomy of the pelvis: implications for colonic and rectal resections. Dis Colon Rectum. 2000;43(10):1390–7.

184. Moriya Y. Function preservation in rectal cancer surgery. Int J Clin Oncol. 2006;11(5):339–43.
185. Vironen JH, Kairaluoma M, Aalto AM, Kellokumpu IH. Impact of functional results on quality of life after rectal cancer surgery. Dis Colon Rectum. 2006;49(5):568–78.
186. Junginger T, Kneist W, Heintz A. Influence of identification and preservation of pelvic autonomic nerves in rectal cancer on bladder dysfunction after total mesorectal excision. Dis Colon Rectum. 2003;46(5):621–8.
187. Havenga K, Enker WE, McDermott K, Cohen AM, Minsky BD, Guillem J. Male and female sexual and urinary function after total mesorectal excision with autonomic nerve preservation for carcinoma of the rectum. J Am Coll Surg. 1996;182(6):495–502.
188. Kim JH, Noh TI, Oh MM, Park J, Lee JG, Um JW, et al. Voiding dysfunction after total mesorectal excision in rectal cancer. Int Neurourol J. 2011;15(3):166–71.
189. Benoist S, Panis Y, Denet C, Mauvais F, Mariani P, Valleur P. Optimal duration of urinary drainage after rectal resection: a randomized controlled trial. Surgery. 1999;125(2):135–41.
190. Grigsby PW, Russell A, Bruner D, Eifel P, Koh WJ, Spanos W, et al. Late injury of cancer therapy on the female reproductive tract. Int J Radiat Oncol Biol Phys. 1995;31(5):1281–99.
191. Lange MM, Maas CP, Marijnen CA, Wiggers T, Rutten HJ, Kranenbarg EK, et al. Urinary dysfunction after rectal cancer treatment is mainly caused by surgery. Br J Surg. 2008;95(8):1020–8.
192. Sterk P, Shekarriz B, Gunter S, Nolde J, Keller R, Bruch HP, et al. Voiding and sexual dysfunction after deep rectal resection and total mesorectal excision: prospective study on 52 patients. Int J Color Dis. 2005;20(7):423–7.
193. Eveno C, Lamblin A, Mariette C, Pocard M. Sexual and urinary dysfunction after protectomy for rectal cancer. J Visceral Surg. 2010;147(1):e21–30.
194. Walsh PC, Schlegal PN. Radical pelvic surgery with preservation of sexual function. Ann Surg. 1988;208(4):391–400.
195. Lindsey I, Mortensen NJ. Iatrogenic impotence and rectal dissection. Br J Surg. 2002;89(12):1493–4.
196. Lindsey I, Guy RJ, Warren BF, Mortensen NJ. Anatomy of Denonvilliers' fascia and pelvic nerves, impotence and implications for the colorectal surgeon. Br J Surg. 2000;87(10):1288–99.
197. Lindsey I, George B, Kettlewell M, et al. Randomized, double-blind, placebo-controlled trial of sildenafil (Viagra) for erectile dysfunction after rectal excision for cancer and inflammatory bowel disease. Dis Colon Rectum. 2002;45(6):727–32.
198. da Silva GM, Hull T, Roberts PL, et al. The effect of colorectal surgery in female sexual function, body image, self esteem and general health: a prospective study. Ann Surg. 2008;248(2):266–72.
199. Zippe CD, Nandipati KC, Agarwal A, Raina R. Female sexual dysfunction after pelvic surgery: the impact of surgical modifications. BJU Int. 2005;96(7):959–63.
200. Kaplan SA, Reis RB, Kohn IJ, Ikeguchi EF, Laor E, Te AE, et al. Safety and efficacy of sildenafil in postmenopausal women with sexual dysfunction. Urology. 1999;53(3):481–6.
201. Emmertsen KJ, Laurberg S. Low anterior resection syndrome score: development and validation of a symptom-based scoring system for bowel dysfunction after Low anterior resection for rectal cancer. Ann Surg. 2012;255(5):922–8.
202. Pucciani F. Low anterior resection syndrome. Societa Italiana di Chirugia ColoRettale. 2009;24:211–7.
203. Pucciani F, Bologna A, Chianchi F, Cortesini C. Anorectal physiology following sphincter saving operations for rectal cancer. Dig Surg. 1993;10:33–8.
204. Allgayer H, Christoph FD, Rohde W, Koch GH, Tuschoff T. Prospective comparison of short-and long-term effects of pelvic floor exercise/biofeedback training in patient with fecal incontinence after surgery plus irradiation versus surgery alone for rectal cancer: clinical, functional and endoscopic/endosonographic findings. Scand J Gastroenterol. 2005;40(10):1168–75.
205. Seow-Choen F, Goh HS. Prospective randomized trial comparing J colonic pouch-anal anastomosis and straight coloanal reconstruction. Br J Surg. 1995;82(5):608–10.
206. Farouk R, Duthie GS, Lee PW, Monson JR. Endosonographic evidence of injury to the internal anal sphincter after low anterior resection: long term follow-up. Dis Colon Rectum. 1998;41(7):888–91.
207. Nakahara S, Itoh H, Mibu R, Ikeda S, Oohata Y, Kitano K, et al. Clinical and manometric evaluation of anorectal function following low anterior resection with low anastomotic line using EEA stapler for rectal cancer. Dis Colon Rectum. 1988;31(10):762–6.
208. Gervaz P, Lavertu S, Kazemba B, Pemberton JH, Haddock MG, Gunderson LL. Sphincter-preserving radiation therapy for rectal cancer: a simulation study using three-dimensional computerized technology. Color Dis. 2006;8(7):570–4.
209. Ehrenpreis ED, Chang D, Eichenwald E. Pharmcotherapy for fecal incontinence: a review. Dis Colon Rectum. 2007;50(5):641–9.
210. Hanauer SB. The role of loperimide in gastrointestinal disorders. Rev Gastroenterol Disord. 2008;8(1):15–20.
211. Ho YH, Chiang GM, Tan M, Low JY. Biofeedback therapy for excessive stool frequency and incontinence following anterior resection or total colectomy. Dis Colon Rectum. 1996;39(11):1289–92.
212. Pucciani F, Ringressi MN, Redditi S, Masi A, Giani I. Rehabilitation of fecal incontinence after sphincter saving surgery for rectal cancer: encouraging results. Dis Colon Rectum. 2008;51(10):1552–8.
213. Garcea G, Sutton CDF, Lloyd TD, et al. Management of benign rectal strictures: a review of

present therapeutic procedures. Dis Colon Rectum. 2003;46(11):1451–60.
214. Schlegel RD, Dehni N, Parc R. Results of reoperations in colorectal anastomotic strictures. Dis Colon Rectum. 2001;44(10):1464–8.
215. Ambrosetti P, Francis K, De Peyer R, et al. Colorectal anastomotic stenosis after elective laparoscopic sigmoidectomy for diverticular disease: a prospective evaluation of 68 patients. Dis Colon Rectum. 2008;51(9):1345–9.
216. Bannura GC, Cumsille MA, Barrera AE, et al. Predictive factors of stenosis after stapled colorectal anastomosis: prospective analysis of 179 consecutive patients. World J Surg. 2004;28(9):921–5.
217. Kumar A, Daga R, Vijayaragavan P, et al. Anterior resection for rectal carcinoma—risk factors for anastomotic leaks and strictures. World J Gastroenterol. 2011;17(11):1475–9.
218. Luchtefeld MA, Milsom JW, Senagore AJ, Surrell JA, Mazier WP. Colorectal anastomotic stenosis: results of a survey of the ASCRS membership. Dis Colon Rectum. 1989;32(9):733–6.
219. Werre A, Mulder C, van Heteren C, et al. Dilation of benign strictures following low anterior resection using savary-gilliard bougies. Endoscopy. 2000;32(5):385–58.
220. Araujo SE, Costa AF. Efficacy and safety of endoscopic balloon dilation of benign anastomotic strictures after oncologic anterior rectal resection: report on 24 cases. Surg Laparosc Endosc Percutan Tech. 2008;18(6):565–8.
221. Pucciarelli S, Toppan P, Pilati PL, et al. Efficacy of dilatations for anastomotic colorectal stenoses: prognostic factors. Int J Color Dis. 1994;9(3):149–52.
222. Forshaw MJ, Maphosa G, Sankararajah D, et al. Endoscopic alternatives in managing anastomotic strictures of the colon and rectum. Tech Coloproctol. 2006;10(1):21–7.
223. Janík V, Horák L, Hnaníček J, et al. Biodegradable polydioxanone stents: a new option for therapy-resistant anastomotic strictures of the colon. Eur Radiol. 2011;21(9):1956–61.
224. Nissotakis C, Sakorafas GH, Vugiouklakis D, Kostopoulos P, Peros G. Transanal circular stapler technique: a simple and highly effective method for the management of high-grade stenosis of low colorectal anastomoses. Surg Laparosc Endosc Percutan Tech. 2008;18(4):375–85.
225. Lucha Jr PA, Fticsar JE, Francis MJ. The strictured anastomosis: successful treatment by corticosteroid injections—report of three cases and review of the literature. Dis Colon Rectum. 2005;48(4):862–5.
226. Hull TI, Milsom JW, Church J, Oakley J, Lavery I, Fazio V. Electrogalvanic stimulation for levator Ani syndrome: how effective is it in the long term? Dis Colon Rectum. 1993;36(8):731–3.
227. Joo IS, Agachan F, Wolff B, Nogueras JJ, Wexner SD. Initial north american experience with botulinum toxin type a for treatment of anismus. Dis Colon Rectum. 1996;39(10):1107–11.
228. So JB, Palmer MT, Shellito PC. Postoperative perineal hernia. Dis Colon Rectum. 1997;40(8):954–7.
229. Aboian E, Winter DC, Metcalf DR, Wolff BG. Perineal hernia after protectomy: prevalence, risks and management. Dis Colon Rectum. 2006;49(10):1564–8.
230. Skipworth RJ, Smith GH, Anderson DN. Secondary perineal hernia following open abdominoperineal excision of the rectum: a case report and review of the literature. Hernia. 2007;11(6):541–5.
231. Beck DE, Fazio VW, Jagelman DG, Lavery JC, McGronagle BA. Postoperative perineal hernia. Dis Colon Rectum. 1987;30(1):21–4.

Pre-sacral Tumors

54

Amit Merchea and Eric J. Dozois

54.1 Introduction

Tumors of the presacral or retrorectal space are rare and demonstrate indolent growth. Numerous tumor types may be encountered as the presacral space may contain totipotential cells that differentiate into the three germ cell layers. Often patients have nonspecific clinical symptoms. Diagnosis and treatment planning is accomplished by a combination of physical examination, advanced imaging techniques, and possibly percutaneous biopsy. Diagnosis is often delayed and surgical treatment can be complicated—frequently necessitating a multidisciplinary approach, with the potential for neoadjuvant chemoradiotherapy, for safe and appropriate treatment.

Presacral tumors have a published incidence of <1 % but the true incidence is likely higher. A series by Jao et al. [1] reported 120 patients with presacral tumors over a 19-year period who underwent surgery. Other reports have described an incidence between 0.003 and 0.014 % [2, 3]. Uhlig and Johnson [4] have previously developed a comprehensive classification system for presacral tumors and divides them into congenital, neurogenic, osseous, or miscellaneous groups. A modification of this classification further subcategorizes these tumors based on their malignant or benign nature—which may significantly impact treatment (Table 54.1).

A. Merchea, MD
Department of Colon and Rectal Surgery, Mayo Clinic, Jacksonville, FL, USA

E.J. Dozois, MD (✉)
Department of Colon and Rectal Surgery, Mayo Clinic, Rochester, MN, USA
e-mail: Dozois.Eric@mayo.edu

54.2 Anatomy

A complete understanding of the anatomy of the presacral space is essential in the management of these tumors. The presacral space is a potential space bounded superiorly by the peritoneal reflection and inferiorly by the retrosacral fascia (which extends from the S4 vertebra to the rectum a few centimeters cephalad to the anorectal junction). The mesorectum is the anterior border and the posterior border is composed of the presacral fascia. Laterally, the space is defined by the ureters, the iliac vasculature, and sacral nerve roots (Fig. 54.1).

Presacral tumors may arise from or locally invade pelvic structures (Fig. 54.2). In malignant cases, these structures may need to be sacrificed at the time of resection if an oncologically appropriate operation is done. Due to the high risk of injury and resection of local-regional structures, it is important to counsel patients on the potential for anorectal, sexual, or physical debility following surgery. Loss of bilateral S3 nerve roots will result in incontinence and mandates an end colostomy. If all sacral nerve roots on either side are sacrificed, but one side is preserved, normal function will be maintained [5]. High ligation of the inferior mesenteric artery,

H.R.H. Patel et al. (eds.), *Pelvic Cancer Surgery: Modern Breakthroughs and Future Advances*,
DOI 10.1007/978-1-4471-4258-4_54,

Table 54.1 Classification of presacral tumors

Congenital	**Osseuos**
Benign	*Benign*
Developmental cysts	Giant cell tumor
Rectal duplication	Osteoblastoma
Anterior sacral meningocele	Aneurysmal bone cyst
Adrenal rest tumor	*Malignant*
Malignant	Osteogenic sarcoma
Chordoma	Ewing sarcoma
Teratocarcinoma	Myeloma
Neurogenic	Chondrosarcoma
Benign	**Miscellaneous**
Neurofibroma	*Benign*
Schwanomma	Lipoma
Ganglioneuroma	Fibroma
Malignant	Leiomyoma
Neuroblastoma	Hemangioma
Ganglioneuroblastoma	Endothelioma
Ependymoma	Desmoid
Malignant peripheral nerve sheath tumors	*Malignant*
	Liposarcoma
	Fibrosarcoma/malignant fibrous histiosarcoma
	Leiomyosarcoma
	Metastatic carcinoma
	Other

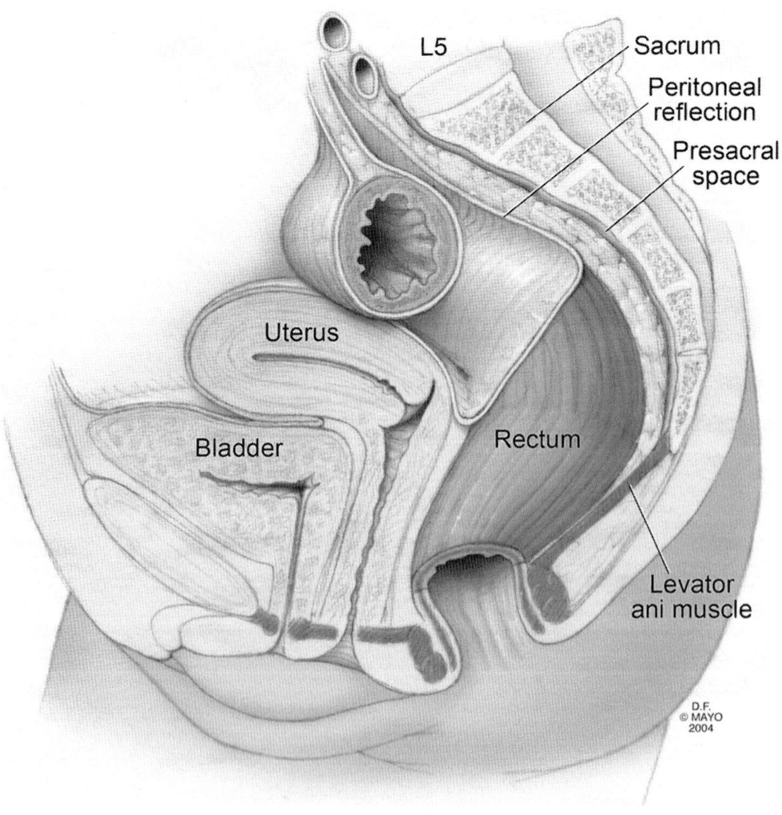

Fig. 54.1 The presacral space (By permission of Mayo Foundation for Medical Education and Research. All rights reserved)

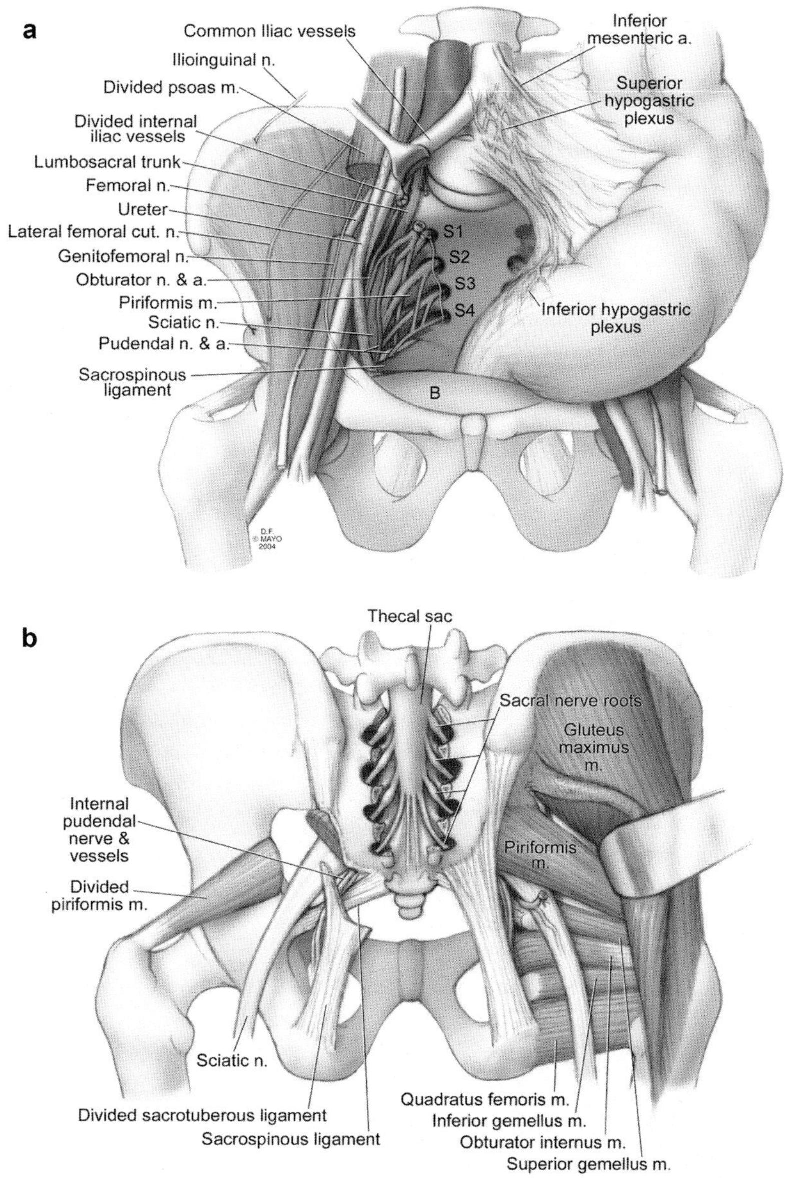

Fig. 54.2 Neurovascular relationships of the pelvis. (**a**) Anterior view. (**b**) Posterior view (By permission of Mayo Foundation for Medical Education and Research. All rights reserved)

or during mobilization of the rectum near the sacral promontory, may result in injury to the hypogastric nerves resulting in retrograde ejaculation and/or bladder dysfunction [6]. Injury to the Nervi erigentes (parasympathetic fibers from S2 to S4), which course anteriorly in the lateral stalks, may result in erectile dysfunction. The pudendal nerve (S2–S4) courses inferiorly to the perineum—a sensory branch carries fibers to the skin of the penis and glans and a motor branch innervates the external anal sphincter. A unilateral pudendal nerve injury does not generally result in incontinence because there is cross innervation of the fibers between the right and left pudendal nerves at the level of the spinal cord [7].

If adequate resection necessitates sacrectomy, our practice utilizes the skills of an oncologic orthopedic and spine surgeon to assist. Familiarity of the bony pelvis, spinal nerve roots, and pelvic ligaments and musculature is imperative for safe conduct of the operation. The majority of the sacrum can be safely removed with stability maintained in non-irradiated patients if more than half of the S1 vertebral body is preserved.

54.3 Diagnosis

Presacral tumors are often found incidentally and diagnosis requires a high degree of clinical acumen. Symptoms, when present, are often vague and non-specific [8]. Those patients that complain of pain (pelvic, perineal) more often present with malignant tumors, and those with neurologic dysfunction (urinary/fecal incontinence, sexual dysfunction), also often have more advanced tumors [1, 9]. Some patients complain of perineal drainage or posterior midline dimpling—leading to a misdiagnosis of pilonidal disease or perianal fistula [10].

A comprehensive neurologic examination must be completed to define any deficits and to document function preoperatively. In a series from the Mayo Clinic, 97 % of presacral tumors could be palpated on digital rectal examination [1]. Digital rectal examination aides in defining the proximal extent of the lesion, and tumor fixation to pelvic structures. Endoscopic evaluation should be completed to evaluate for penetration into the rectal lumen or other synchronous colorectal lesions.

Evaluation of presacral lesions is greatly enhanced by computed tomography (CT) and/or magnetic resonance imaging (MRI) with interpretation by a radiologist specializing in musculoskeletal disease. These imaging modalities are complimentary and aid in operative planning. MRI has superior soft-tissue contrast resolution which may provide improved determination of the anatomic extent of the tumor [11]. MRI is also more sensitive than CT in spinal imaging—demonstrating cord abnormalities (meningocele, nerve root or thecal sac involvement) [12]. CT has a superior ability to evaluate cortical bone destruction. Imaging will determine more accurately than physical exam whether a lesion is cystic, solid, or heterogeneous and whether adjacent pelvic structures are involved.

Some patients who present with a presacral tumor will have a rare congenital disorder called Currarino Syndrome. Currarino Syndrome is an autosomal dominant disorder characterized by: (1) sacral anomalies, (2) presacral masses (such as an anterior sacral meningocele or teratoma, sometimes more than one), and (3) anorectal malformations [13, 14] (Fig. 54.3). Taking a detailed family history will often reveal a consistent autosomal dominant pattern of these anomalies.

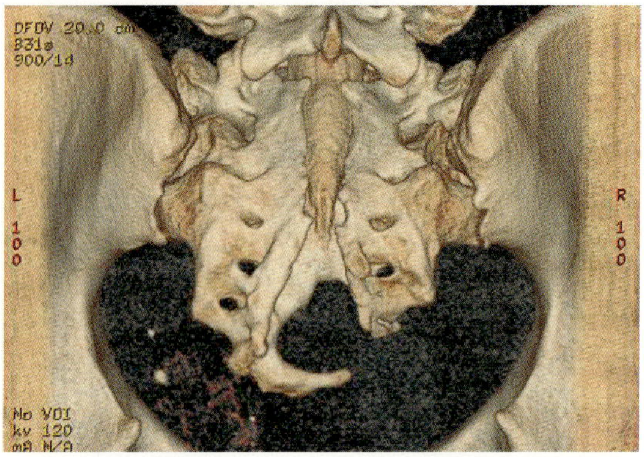

Fig. 54.3 Three-dimensional CT reconstruction of the posterior sacrum demonstrating scimitar anomaly, commonly seen in Currarino syndrome (By permission of Mayo Foundation for Medical Education and Research. All rights reserved)

Preoperative determination of benign versus malignant status of presacral tumors is critical to make decisions on use of adjuvant therapy and plan lines of surgical resection. Advancements in modern imaging techniques have improved the ability to identify malignant lesions without a biopsy. Some authors, in fact, believe that biopsy of presacral lesions is contraindicated and unnecessary in tumors deemed resectable [1, 9, 15, 16]. In a recent review by the Mayo Clinic, preoperative biopsy of solid or heterogeneous tumors demonstrated a high concordance with post-operative pathology compared to imaging alone (91 % vs. 36 %) with a low complication rate. Moreover, almost half of patients could not be given a definitive diagnosis based on imaging alone and of those over one-third were found to be malignant tumors [17]. Simple cystic lesions are usually not biopsied as management is generally not altered by biopsy results. Patients with malignant tumors responsive to neoadjuvant chemoradiation (Ewing sarcoma, osteogenic sarcoma, neurofibrosarcoma, etc.) will have tissue confirmation of their disease prior to initiating therapy. Additionally, biopsy results will provide information regarding the need for wide en-bloc oncologic resection verses

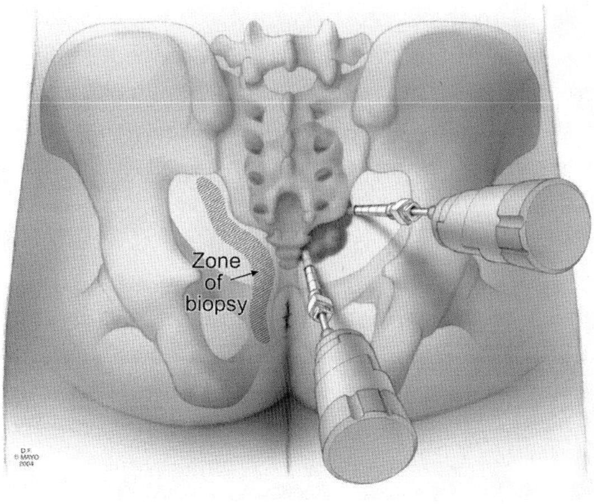

Fig. 54.4 Zones of suggested CT guided biopsy, within the field of proposed resection (By permission of Mayo Foundation for Medical Education and Research. All rights reserved)

a potentially limited, nerve- or function-sparing intralesional resection. In our practice, all solid or heterogeneous tumors undergo pre-operative percutaneous (most often either trans-sacral or trans-perineal) biopsy and no tumor is biopsied trans-rectally or trans-vaginally. Route of biopsy should be planned to be within the field of proposed resection so that the tract may be excised if necessary (Fig. 54.4).

54.4 Surgical Treatment

The primary treatment modality of presacral tumors is operative removal. Reasons for an aggressive approach are obvious for malignant tumors. For benign lesions, there exists a known risk of malignant transformation with certain tumors [18]. Some lesions may obstruct the vaginal canal and lead to complicated vaginal delivery [19]. An untreated anterior sacral meningocele may become infected resulting in potentially life-threatening meningitis.

Operative intervention should occur at tertiary care referral centers by a multidisciplinary team experienced in the surgical management of complex pelvic tumors. Additionally, surgeons specializing in pelvic tumor resection may be more likely to be successful in preservation of function and the ability to achieve a complete resection [20, 21].

Technically, there are three general approaches to the resection of presacral tumors: (1) transabdominal only, (2) perineal or parasacral only, or (3) a combined anterior-posterior approach. The approach utilized is determined based on the sacral level of the tumor, as demonstrated on pre-operative imaging studies. Low tumors (below S3) can generally be resected via a posterior-only approach if en-bloc resection is not necessary, whereas high lesions (above S3) require a transabdominal (anterior) approach. Tumors located at the mid-sacral region will often require a combined approach, especially when en-bloc sacral resection is necessary.

Posterior Approach (Tumors Below S3)

The posterior approach was initially described by Kraske in 1886 [22]. The patient is placed in the prone-jackknife position with the buttock spread. An incision is made over the lower portion of the sacrum and coccyx and carried down to the anus, protecting the external anal sphincter. Transection of the anococcygeal ligament and entry into the deep post-anal space, or coccygectomy, may facilitate exposure and resection of the tumor. The lesion can often be dissected in a plane between the mesorectal fat and the tumor. A finger inserted into the anal canal and rectum that pushes the tumor into the wound, may improve exposure and aid in dissection of the lesion. If necessary, a portion of the posterior rectal wall may be excised with the tumor and subsequently closed in two layers with suture. The need for routine coccygectomy for congenital cystic lesions remains debated [10, 23].

Anterior and Combined Anterior-Posterior Approach (Mid Sacral and Higher Tumors)

This technique involves positioning the patient in the lithotomy position, followed by transferring the patient to the prone position once the transabdominal mobilization and creation of end colostomy (if necessary) is complete. Alternatively, a modified lateral position can be used so that synchronous abdominal and parasacral incisions can be made.

Once the initial incision is made, one must first evaluate for any distant metastatic disease. The sigmoid colon and rectum are then mobilized and the presacral space entered. Just below the sacral promontory. The ureters and hypogastric nerves should be identified and protected throughout the dissection. In some circumstances, the tumor may be mobilized from the posterior wall of the rectum or mesorectum without the need for rectal resection. However, the oncologic principles of en-bloc, wide margin resection should not be compromised.

Operative Strategy

The lateral sacral arteries and veins may be ligated to limit blood loss from large, vascular tumors. Additionally, internal iliac artery ligation may by necessary, especially in cases where there is a high risk of pelvic hemorrhage. This decreases the mean blood flow, mean arterial pressure, and overall pulse pressure within the pelvis [24, 25]. One must avoid accidental ligation of the common or external iliac artery branches, or injury to the hypogastric vein which is deep and lateral to the artery. Preoperative involvement of a vascular surgeon is suitable if major vascular structures appear involved on imaging.

If a wide perineal/sacral excision is expected, we often use a myocutaneous flap from the rectus abdominus to close the perineum. The posterior dissection is started in a similar manner to what has been previously described. When a sacrectomy is required, we employ the skills of an orthopedic surgeon to assist in the dissection. The sacrospinous and sacrotuberous ligaments are transected, along with the piriformis muscle to expose the sciatic nerves. An osteotomy is then performed at the S3 level (effort should be made to preserve at least one S3 nerve root). The neural sac may require ligation. Once the sacrum is divided, it can be removed en-bloc with the tumor.

54.5 Results and Prognosis

Among the primary determinants of prognosis after surgical resection of presacral lesions are tumor biology and completeness of resection. Wide margin, en-bloc resection is mandated in the case of malignant tumors, however a nerve and function sparing, intralesional or marginal resection may be employed in benign lesions. Incomplete resection, or violation of the tumor margins, portends a worse prognosis and increases the risk of locoregional recurrence [1, 20, 26]. A report of 21 patients with malignant presacral tumors by Lev-Chelouche et al. demonstrated that complete resection was achieved in 15 patients and that most recurrences were seen in patients with incomplete resection—of these patients, 50 % ultimately died of their disease [15].

Sacrococcygeal chordomas are the most common malignant presacral tumors and the quality of surgical resection predicts outcome. Fuchs et al. reported on 52 patients over 21-years who underwent surgical treatment and found that at a mean follow-up of 7.8 years, 23 patients were alive with no evidence of disease. The local recurrence rate was 44 %. Overall survival at 5, 10, and 15 years was 74, 52, and 47 % respectively. The most significant predictor of survival was a wide margin resection [13].

Neurogenic tumors, both benign and malignant, account for a large number of presacral tumors. A comprehensive study by Dozois et al. aimed to characterize the clinical and pathologic features of these tumors. Over a nearly 50 year period, 89 patients were identified, of which 48 % were found to have malignant lesions (most commonly, malignant peripheral nerve sheath tumors). The most common benign lesion was schwanomma. There were no post-operative deaths and morbidity was seen in 13 % of patients. Survival in patients with malignant lesions was 48 % at 5 years. In the experience described, most of these tumors underwent a suboptimal (<2 cm margin) dissection despite the presence of malignancy. This was often justified by a need to preserve neurologic function in the setting of an unknown primary and concern for intraoperative hemorrhage associated with more aggressive approaches. The later experience demonstrated improved results when adjuvant treatment is administered and en-bloc resection was done [20]. More recently, nerve-sparing intra-lesional resections have been reported for pre-operatively confirmed benign neurogenic tumors with good results [23].

Surgical outcomes of presacral cystic lesions depend highly on the benign or malignant status of the lesion. However, few data exist on malignant cystic lesions. Tailgut cysts are the most common cystic lesion reported. In a study from the Mayo Clinic [27], 31 patients underwent complete surgical resection via a posterior (n=20), anterior (n=9), or combined (n=2) approach. Malignant transformation of the cyst was noted in 13 % of patients (adenocarcinoma in three patients, carcinoid in one), one benign recurrence was identified at last follow-up and mortality was nil.

54.6 Summary

Presacral tumors are rare and demonstrate indolent growth. The clinician must maintain a high index of suspicion to identify these lesions. Surgical management of these tumors is often recommended, regardless of their malignant status due to the almost universal risk of malignant transformation. Biopsy is highly recommended in patients with solid or heterogeneous tumors to rule out malignancy, guide neoadjuvant treatment, and plan for the extent of resection. Purely cystic lesions can most often proceed directly to resection. These tumors are best evaluated and treated by an experienced multidisciplinary team.

Key Points

- Presacral tumors are rare, demonstrate indolent growth and have a varied differential diagnosis.
- >95 % of lesions are palpable on digital rectal examination.
- Advanced imaging studies (CT/MRI) are complementary and should be considered in all patients.
- Percutaneous biopsy of solid or heterogeneous lesions should be undertaken to guide potential neoadjuvant therapy, and to help define the margins of resection. Purely cystic lesions do not need percutaneous biopsy.
- Biopsies should never be done transrectally or transvaginally.
- There are three approaches to resection: anterior only, posterior only, combined (anterior-posterior)
- A multidisciplinary team, including a colorectal, orthopedic, spine, vascular, and/or plastic surgeon should be employed as needed.
- Tumor biology and completeness of resection have the most significant impact on prognosis.

References

1. Jao SW, Beart Jr RW, Spencer RJ, Reiman HM, Ilstrup DM. Retrorectal tumors. Mayo Clinic experience, 1960–1979. Dis Colon Rectum. 1985;28(9): 644–52.
2. Spencer RJ, Jackman RJ. Surgical management of precoccygeal cysts. Surg Gynecol Obstet. 1962;115: 449–52.
3. Whittaker LD, Pemberton JD. Tumors ventral to the sacrum. Ann Surg. 1938;107(1):96–106.
4. Uhlig BE, Johnson RL. Presacral tumors and cysts in adults. Dis Colon Rectum. 1975;18(7):581–9.
5. Gunterberg B, Kewenter J, Petersen I, Stener B. Anorectal function after major resections of the sacrum with bilateral or unilateral sacrifice of sacral nerves. Br J Surg. 1976;63(7):546–54.

6. Bauer JJ, Gelernt IM, Salky B, Kreel I. Sexual dysfunction following proctocolectomy for benign disease of the colon and rectum. Ann Surg. 1983; 197(3):363–7.
7. Bernstein WC, Bernstein EF. Sexual dysfunction following radical surgery for cancer of the rectum. Dis Colon Rectum. 1966;9(5):328–32.
8. Glasgow SC, Birnbaum EH, Lowney JK, Fleshman JW, Kodner IJ, Mutch DG, et al. Retrorectal tumors: a diagnostic and therapeutic challenge. Dis Colon Rectum. 2005;48(8):1581–7.
9. Hobson KG, Ghaemmaghami V, Roe JP, Goodnight JE, Khatri VP. Tumors of the retrorectal space. Dis Colon Rectum. 2005;48(10):1964–74.
10. Singer MA, Cintron JR, Martz JE, Schoetz DJ, Abcarian H. Retrorectal cyst: a rare tumor frequently misdiagnosed. J Am Coll Surg. 2003;196(6):880–6.
11. Yang BL, Gu YF, Shao WJ, Chen HJ, Sun GD, Jin HY, et al. Retrorectal tumors in adults: magnetic resonance imaging findings. World J Gastroenterol. 2010;16(46):5822–9.
12. Lee KS, Gower DJ, McWhorter JM, Albertson DA. The role of MR imaging in the diagnosis and treatment of anterior sacral meningocele. Report of two cases. J Neurosurg. 1988;69(4):628–31.
13. Pendlimari R, Leonard D, Dozois EJ. Rare malignant neuroendocrine transformation of a presacral teratoma in patient with Currarino syndrome. Int J Color Dis. 2010;25(11):1383–4. Case Reports [Letter].
14. Leonard D, Pendlimari R, Larson DW, Dozois EJ. Currarino syndrome: typical images of a rare condition. Tech Coloproctol. 2010;14(3):289–90.
15. Lev-Chelouche D, Gutman M, Goldman G, Even-Sapir E, Meller I, Issakov J, et al. Presacral tumors: a practical classification and treatment of a unique and heterogeneous group of diseases. Surgery. 2003;133(5):473–8.
16. Macafee DA, Sagar PM, El-Khoury T, Hyland R. Retrorectal tumours: optimization of surgical approach and outcome. Colorectal Dis. 2012;14(11):1411–7.
17. Merchea A, Larson DW, Hubner M, Wenger DE, Rose PS, Dozois EJ. The value of preoperative biopsy in the management of solid presacral tumors. Dis Colon Rectum. 2013;56:756–60.
18. Waldhausen JA, Kolman JW, Vellios F, Battersby JS. Sacrococcygeal teratoma. Surgery. 1963;54: 933–49.
19. Sobrado CW, Mester M, Simonsen OS, Justo CR, deAbreu JN, Habr-Gama A. Retrorectal tumors complicating pregnancy. Report of two cases. Dis Colon Rectum. 1996;39(10):1176–9.
20. Dozois EJ, Wall JC, Spinner RJ, Jacofsky DJ, Yaszemski MJ, Sim FH, et al. Neurogenic tumors of the pelvis: clinicopathologic features and surgical outcomes using a multidisciplinary team. Ann Surg Oncol. 2009;16(4):1010–6.
21. Dozois EJ, Jacofsky DJ, Billings BJ, Privitera A, Cima RR, Rose PS, et al. Surgical approach and oncologic outcomes following multidisciplinary management of retrorectal sarcomas. Ann Surg Oncol. 2011;18(4):983–8.
22. Kraske P, Perry EG, Hinrichs B. A new translation of professor Dr P. Kraske's Zur Exstirpation Hochsitzender Mastdarmkrebse. 1885. Aust N Z J Surg. 1989;59(5):421–4.
23. Sullivan P, Merchea A, Leonard D, Hebert-Blouin M, Spinner R, Dozois E. Does neurological function improve following resection of benign pre-sacral neurogenic tumors? Dis Colon Rectum. 2012;55(5):e214. Abstract.
24. Burchell RC. Physiology of internal iliac artery ligation. J Obstet Gynaecol Br Common w. 1968;75(6): 642–51.
25. Tomacruz RS, Bristow RE, Montz FJ. Management of pelvic hemorrhage. Surg Clin North Am. 2001;81(4):925–48.
26. Kaiser TE, Pritchard DJ, Unni KK. Clinicopathologic study of sacrococcygeal chordoma. Cancer. 1984;53(11): 2574–8.
27. Mathis KL, Dozois EJ, Grewal MS, Metzger P, Larson DW, Devine RM. Malignant risk and surgical outcomes of presacral tailgut cysts. Br J Surg. 2010; 97(4):575–9.

Treatment of Rectal Cancer with Synchronous Liver Metastasis

55

Terence Jackson and Christopher Thomas Siegel

55.1 Introduction

The introduction of Oxaliplatin and Irinotecan based chemotherapeutic regimens for the treatment of metastatic rectal cancer has sparked new interest in the multidisciplinary treatment of metastatic rectal cancer to the liver. Since 2003, the introduction of multiple new chemotherapeutic and biologic agents for the treatment of metastatic rectal cancer in conjunction with improved techniques in liver surgery have resulted in significant improvements in overall and disease-free survival for patients with metachronous and synchronous metastatic rectal cancer in the liver. A synchronous liver metastasis (SLM) is defined as liver metastasis diagnosed during diagnostic work-up or at the time of operation for the primary tumor [1]. Some authors also include under this definition liver lesions diagnosed within 3 months of resection of the primary tumor [2]. However it may be defined, the presence of liver metastasis is thought to be one of the most important determinants of survival in patients with rectal cancer [3].

The liver represents 75.7 % of all synchronous metastases [1]. SLM are identified in 20 % of all patients who have a resection for colorectal cancer (CRC) either preoperatively or at the time of laparotomy [4] and 30–45 % of all patients with CRC are found to have liver metastasis at autopsy [5]. Compared to metachronous liver metastasis, patients with synchronous liver metastasis in rectal cancer (RC-SLM) present at a younger age group and more often have bilobar liver involvement [1, 6]. The prognosis for patients with SLM is worse than those with metachronous liver metastasis [6–9]. Although, it is believed that rectal cancer with synchronous liver metastases (RC-SLM) represents a more disseminated form of the primary disease, advancements in chemotherapy and surgical techniques have enabled us to effectively deal with even multiple, bilobar liver metastatic lesions.

Liver resections offer long term survival in patients with RC-SLM. They are currently performed with low mortality and morbidity. There is a significant difference in survival between patients with resected versus non-resected liver metastasis [10]. Survival is less than 30 % in patients with untreated metastases after 1 year and less than 5 % after 5 years [1]. Finlay et al., estimated the mean doubling time for liver metastasis from rectal cancer to be 155 days [11]; a relatively slow growth rate. Hence, not only is

T. Jackson, MD
Department of General Surgery, University Hospital Case Medical Center, Case Western Reserve University, Cleveland, OH, USA

C.T. Siegel, MD, PhD (✉)
Department of Surgery, Division of Hepatobiliary and Transplant Surgery, Liver Center of Excellence, UH Digestive Health Institute, Cleveland, OH, USA

Department of Surgery, University Hospital Case Medical Center, Case Western Reserve University, Cleveland, OH, USA
e-mail: christopher.siegel@uhhospitals.org

H.R.H. Patel et al. (eds.), *Pelvic Cancer Surgery: Modern Breakthroughs and Future Advances*,
DOI 10.1007/978-1-4471-4258-4_55, © Springer-Verlag London 2015

definitive treatment of RC-SLM imperative but needs to be managed aggressively to maximize potential patient survival benefit.

55.2 Prognostic Factors

Survival is directly related to the extent of liver metastases. In a study about survival in patients with colorectal liver metastasis, Hotta et al., found survival to be longer in patients with ≤10 liver metastasis [12]. Fong et al., and Nagashima et al., studied and presented scoring systems for the factors affecting survival after liver resection for colorectal metastasis [13, 14]. K-RAS and BRAF gene testing is recommended as a part of workup for RC-SLM, as they influence the choice of chemoimmunotherapy. Lymph node status and depth of invasion of the primary tumor, metastatic tumor size, number and palpability on clinical examination, pre liver resection CEA and pathological margin of hepatic resection, are all determinants of survival [13–15]. Preoperative tumor marker (CEA) levels serve as a baseline for detection of postoperative recurrent lesions and are prognostic of survival after liver surgery. Histologically, the presence of severe focal dedifferentiation and expression of sialylLe^x protein in the primary tumor have been associated with a significantly greater incidence of synchronous liver metastasis [16].

Apart from the above mentioned factors, symptoms at presentation of RC-SLM, the possibility of resection with adequate margins and response to chemotherapy also play a role in determining the optimal plan of management of a case of RC-SLM.

55.3 Multidisciplinary Treatment Planning

According to the NCCN guidelines for the treatment of stage IV rectal cancer with resectable metastatic lesions, primary tumor treatment options include combination chemotherapy, staged or synchronous resection of metastasis and rectal lesion, or infusional 5-FU/leucovorin and radiation to the pelvis. These treatment options differ significantly in terms of which facet of tumor burden is the priority for initial treatment. The choice of initial starting treatment modality is based upon whether the patient presents with symptoms or obstruction, the extent of tumor burden in the rectum, the extent of tumor burden in the liver, and the concern for extrahepatic spread (Fig. 55.1). A complete history and physical is performed to determine whether the patient is symptomatic or obstructed. Imaging studies including a contrast enhanced chest CT is performed to evaluate for lung metastasis or mediastinal adenopathy. Imaging studies obtained to evaluate the liver are often center specific and may include a triple phase CT of the liver with arterial and venous phase imaging or a contrast-enhanced MRI scan. Benefits of contrast enhanced CT include ease of acquisition, relatively standardized protocols, and high sensitivity and specificity for detecting liver metastases [17, 18]. Approval of the 3-Tesla MRI by the FDA in 2001 for body imaging, as well as the introduction of several new MRI contrast agents, has improved the sensitivity of MRI in identifying metastatic lesions in the liver. Benefits of MRI scan include lack of radiation, ability to differentiate metastatic disease from underlying benign liver tumors, and high sensitivity. MRI of the pelvis and endorectal ultrasound are used to evaluate the rectal primary tumor in relation to T staging and lymph node involvement. PET or PET-CT may be obtained to identify occult extrahepatic metastatic disease such as lymphatic spread along the aortic, iliac or portal lymph node chain. The use of PET imaging has been shown to identify patients with a better prognosis for survival after liver resection [19] and can be useful to help determine which primary treatment algorithm the patient should undergo, although a recent review of the literature did not support routine use of PET/CT in preoperative staging [20]. Using PET selectively when MRI or CT raises questions on nodal involvement or extrahepatic spread may be a more judicious and cost effective way to guide the surgical management of these patients. CT scans have a high negative predictive value for assessment of lymph node involvement, however,

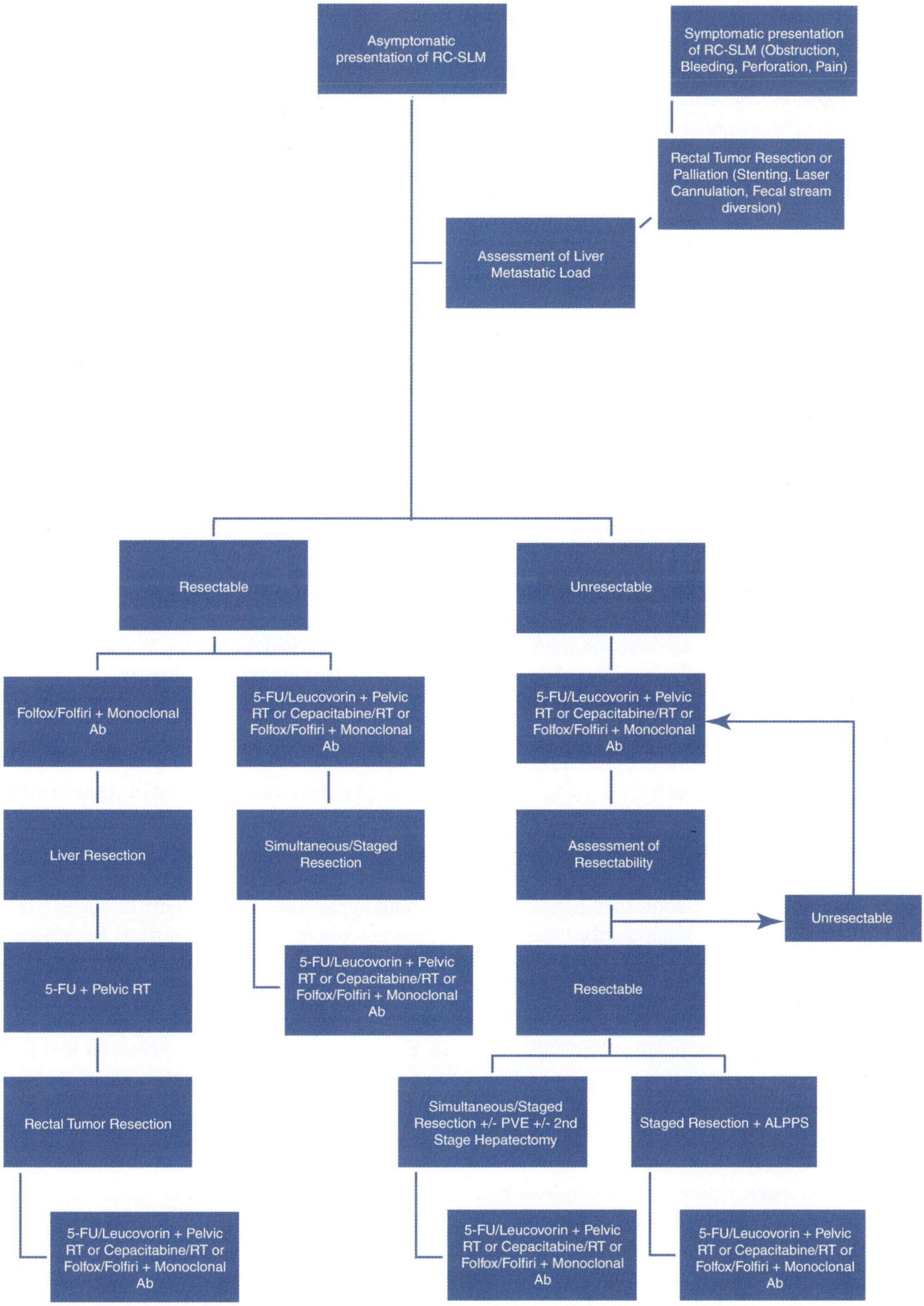

Fig. 55.1 Treatment algorithm

they are known to have a low positive predictive value. Intraoperatively, unless a positive lymph node is identified early during dissection and confirmed by frozen section, a more extensive dissection of the portocaval, hepatic artery or pancreatoduodenal lymph nodes based on CT findings, is not recommended.

As is evidenced by the NCCN guidelines for the treatment of rectal cancer with resectable liver metastasis, there is no defined algorithm for the initial treatment of patients. A useful starting point is to determine whether the patient is symptomatic from the primary tumor in terms of pain, bleeding, obstruction or perforation. If the patient has symptoms then staging studies should be performed to document the extent of liver metastases, whether the rectal primary tumor can be resected with adequate margins and whether extrahepatic spread is present. In these patients surgery is often performed as the initial treatment with either resection of the primary tumor or diversion of the fecal stream. If the patient presents for emergent or urgent operation then liver resection should not be performed at this time due to increased morbidity and mortality [21]. If the patient is stable and undergoes a more elective operation then resection can be considered for patients with limited disease, i.e., less than a formal lobectomy with the intent of not delaying the start of chemotherapy.

The initial treatment of asymptomatic patients should be discussed in the context of a multidisciplinary tumor board with input from medical oncology, radiation oncology, colorectal surgery and hepatobiliary surgery. The decision to begin with a multidrug systemic chemotherapy regimen versus 5-FU/leucovorin and pelvic radiation often is determined by the extent of disease in the pelvis as well as the extent of disease in the liver and whether the planned surgical approach is simultaneous resection, staged resection or a "liver first" approach. Controversy exists over the optimal initial treatment regimen and there are no randomized trials that evaluate outcome.

Advocates of systemic chemotherapy as the initial treatment regimen argue that response to treatment allows for evaluation of tumor biology and helps to select patients that will do best with aggressive surgical therapy [22]. Downsizing large tumors is often possible due to the high response rates with current chemotherapeutic options, and chemotherapy can be interrupted after 2–3 months for a short course of pelvic radiation in patients ultimately undergoing resection [23]. Advocates of 5-FU/leucovorin and radiation as the initial treatment regimen argue this treatment reduces pelvic recurrences, reduces overall morbidity and shortens the length of time required for the patient to reach surgical therapy. In general, only a minority of patients who present with rectal cancer and synchronous liver metastasis are eligible to undergo surgery as their initial treatment modality. Those patients should have disease in the rectum which can be resected with adequate margins, no signs of extrahepatic metastasis and limited liver involvement.

55.4 Management of the Primary Tumor

Resection of the primary tumor is the gold standard treatment for patients rectal cancer. The development and improvement of chemotherapeutic agents and metallic stents have helped spare patients with rectal cancer the morbidity of extensive perineal/pelvic resections. Neoadjuvant chemotherapy can help control metastases, reduce the volume and number of SLM and thus modify the type of hepatic resection required. For patients with uncontrollable hepatic disease, in whom surgery poses high risk of mortality and morbidity, chemotherapy can serve as a first line treatment modality. Combination chemotherapy regimens, combined with agents targeted to vascular endothelial growth factor (VEGF) or epithelial growth factor (EGF) receptor can downstage patients for resection [24].

Radiotherapy is also a crucial part of preoperative combined modality therapy for RC-SLM. Pelvic radiotherapy is needed to downstage a non-resectable primary tumor and achieve R0 resection. The German trial CAO/ARO/AIO-94, published in 2003 proved the efficacy of neoadjuvant chemoradiotherapy. Preoperative combined modality therapy (chemoradiotherapy/chemoimmunotherapy) has been widely accepted and mentioned in the National Comprehensive Cancer Network (NCCN) guidelines as the standard treatment for locally advanced rectal cancer [25–27]. Radiation doses used are 45–50 Gy in 25–28 fractions. 5-FU based chemotherapy is used concurrently as a radiosensitizer. Recommended preoperative primary treatment includes 2–3 months of (1) (FOLFIRI or FOLFOX or CapeOX) ± bevacizumab or (2) (FOLFIRI OR FOLFOX) ± panitumumab or cetuximab [KRAS wild-type gene only] or (3) Infusional IV 5-FU/pelvic RT or (4) bolus 5-FU/leukovorin/pelvic RT or (5) capecitabine/RT can also be used [26].

It is very important to accurately assess the patient's response to combined modality therapy (CMT). An unresected primary tumor poses a risk of distressing symptoms or complications and morbidity due to emergency procedures. Patients with a good response to CMT may also have problems with vanishing hepatic metastasis [28]. Re-evaluation for resection should be considered, in otherwise unresectable patients after 2 months of preoperative chemotherapy and every 2 months thereafter [26].

Following removal of the primary tumor, adjuvant systemic therapy contributes to improved survival [29]. Six months of perioperative treatment is preferred. NCCN guidelines suggest the use of infusional IV 5-FU/pelvic RT or bolus 5-FU/leucovorin/pelvic RT or cepacitabine/RT or 5-FU ± leucovorin or FOLFOX or cepecitabine ± oxaliplatin, then infusional 5-FU/RT or bolus 5-FU/leucovorin/RT or capecitabine/RT, then 5-FU ± leucovorin or FOLFOX or capecitabine ± oxaliplatin [26]. In Patients who did not receive preoperative radiotherapy, postoperative pelvic radiotherapy results in a lower rate of pelvic recurrence in patients with RC-SLM when compared with patients that undergo surgery alone [2]. However, increased morbidity in patients receiving adjuvant radiotherapy compared to those receiving neoadjuvant therapy makes treatment prior to surgery preferable.

55.5 Management of Synchronous Liver Metastases

Surgical resection for cure is the only possibility to obtain long-term survival and must be considered even if patients have poor prognostic factors [15]. When surgery isn't possible or in the neoadjuvant setting, chemotherapy plays a major role in reducing the metastatic load on the liver and changing the type of hepatic resection required. Chemotherapy for liver metastasis may be administered systemically or regionally. Trans-arterial chemo-embolization has been effectively used for localized liver lesions. For extensive liver metastasis, systemic chemotherapy or regional chemotherapy by hepatic arterial infusion (HAI) of cytotoxic agents such as floxuridine, fluorouracil, oxaliplatin or irinotecan can be useful [24]. In the neoadjuvant setting, HAI provides significant tumor response but similar or even higher response rates may be obtained by systemic chemotherapy [30]. A trend towards better long term outcomes has been seem with HAI. Following chemotherapy, resectability is determined by location of the lesions, extent of disease and adequate hepatic function [2].

Optimal surgical strategy for RC-SLM patients that present as possible resection candidates, is still debatable. Traditionally, patients have undergone a two-staged procedure with resection of the primary tumor followed by chemotherapy and subsequent liver resection [3]. In this strategy various treatment regimens of chemotherapy can be employed. NCCN guidelines suggest 2–3 months of preoperative chemoradiotherapy or chemoimmunotherapy. Another standard of care is chemoradiotherapy using 5-FU and leucovorin given concurrently with radiation over 5 weeks, and then 6–10 weeks after the last dose of radiotherapy, patients undergo rectal surgery. If no complications occur, SLM is treated as early as 3 months after rectal surgery. However, the mean delay between resection of the primary tumor and subsequent resection of the liver metastasis is 6 months [31]. Sauer et al., demonstrated that up to 50 % of patients do not receive optimal treatment after rectal surgery because of postoperative complications [27]. Some patients may be undertreated because postoperative morbidity doesn't allow achievement of the complete treatment, and because of the psychological effect of long-term of treatment, leading some patients to refuse complete management [4]. A staged procedure is sometime required due to complications of the primary neoplasm such as bowel obstruction or colonic perforation, and the need for extensive hepatic resection. Staged resection may also be required due to late referral after the primary tumor was resected [15].

Advancement in anesthesia and operative techniques have made it possible to simultaneously resect the primary tumor and liver secondaries in RC-SLM, with low mortality and acceptable morbidity. Similar surgical outcomes have been reported after two-staged and simultaneous resections, that included major hepatectomies or requiring resection of multiple hepatic segments [32]. It also has potential benefits in terms of quality of life and cost [33–35]. Until recently, the eligibility for simultaneous resection was restricted to right colon tumors or a limited number of metastases [36, 37]. Criteria for selection used in a recent publication included fitness for anesthesia, expected R0 resection of the primary tumor, no unresectable extrahepatic disease and adequate predicted volume of hepatic remnant post resection [3].

Groups have also reported simultaneous laparoscopic resection (SLR) of rectal carcinoma and SLM [38, 39]. Such a procedure is considered after discussion with colorectal and liver surgeons for R0 resection and adequate laparoscopic exposure of metastatic liver lesions [39]. The inclusion criteria for such a procedure includes a rectal tumor fit for anterior resection with end-to-end anastomosis, number of liver lesions ≤ 2 and absence of a history of abdominal operations [38]. A complicated or advanced rectal lesion, liver lesions adjacent to major vessels or in the caudate lobe would exclude SLR [39]. Preservation of abdominal wall, better compliance, shorter hospitalization, early resumption of social activities, good cosmetic results are some of the advantages of a totally laparoscopic procedure. Another important role of such a technique is in the context of a two-staged hepatectomy in case of rectal cancer with bilobar or extensive SLM. The second stage hepatectomy may be easier owing to less adhesions from the totally laparoscopic first surgery [40–42]. During a simultaneous laparoscopic resection, the colorectal resection is usually done first but if there is a large blood loss during liver surgery or if Pringle's maneuver is anticipated, then liver resection may be performed first. This will be less harmful to the anastomosis because it will be made after the possibility of high mesenteric pressure, lowered intestinal perfusion and the possibility of major blood loss has passed [39].

Mentha et al., first described the "liver first" approach in patients with colon and rectal cancers with advanced SLM [42]. This approach has also been used in patients with advanced rectal cancer with SLM [31]. De Jong et al., described their 5 year experience with "liver first" procedures and found that it was feasible in approximately four-fifths of their patients [43]. In the Liver first approach, patients are primarily treated with neoadjuvant systemic chemotherapy. If there is no progressive disease, a laparotomy is performed with the intention of performing resection of liver metastases. After successful resection of liver metastases, patients are treated with neoadjuvant radiotherapy (with or without chemotherapy) for the primary rectal tumor. Four weeks after the end of neoadjuvant radiotherapy, imaging is performed to check for unresectable metastases. If none are found, rectal resection is performed 8–10 weeks after the last radiotherapy dose [31].

The rationale behind the "liver first" approach is to control the SLM at the same time as the rectal primary and allow unhurried chemotherapy before rectal surgery when indicated. Removing all known liver metastases at the first surgical intervention protects the patients from progression of liver metastases when the patient is receiving radiotherapy for the rectal primary tumor and may improve the patient's state of mind when dealing with long term treatment of cancer. However, with this approach, response to chemotherapy cannot be assumed to persist. There is a possibility of progression after initial response and an intervention in the rectum as early as 2–4 weeks from chemotherapy may be required. In addition, the use of Irinotecan and Oxaliplatin as neoadjuvant systemic chemotherapy may produce chemotherapy associated steatosis and venous outflow problems which can render liver surgery more difficult and hazardous [42].

In the presence of extensive liver tumor burden, future liver remnant becomes a major factor in the planning for a hepatectomy. Historically, portal vein embolization has been used to assist with growth of the future liver remnant. The procedure involves either ligation of the portal vein in segments planned for resection or coil embolization performed by interventional radiologists. In patients with high likelihood of low future liver remnant, PVE results in hypertrophy of the unresected segment, thus resulting in better functional hepatic reserve. Traditionally, portal vein embolization served as a bridge between resections in a two-staged hepatectomy. Portal vein embolization (PVE) is also a useful tool to achieve resectability in extensive or bilobed lesions. The patient undergoes preoperative PVE of the segments to be resected. One month after PVE, repeat imaging is done to assess hypertrophy and surgery is performed.

Baumgart et al., described a new two-step technique for obtaining adequate parenchymal hypertrophy in patients requiring extended hepatic resection with limited functional reserve [44] (Fig. 55.2). Known as the ALPPS (Associating Liver Partition and Portal Vein Ligation for Staged Hepatectomy) approach, this two-step procedure consists of ligation of portal veins to the segment planned to be removed. In order to ligate intrahepatic portal collaterals, the liver parenchyma is divided in situ. This induces accelerated hypertrophy in the remaining segment. Devascularization of segments prevents neovascularization and interlobar perfusion. This induces a median hypertrophy of 74 % in a very short time frame. After an interval of 6–12 days (median 9 days), the resection is completed [44–46]. Recently, this entire procedure has also been completed laparoscopically [47].

55.6 Follow Up

Surveillance for a patient with RC-SLM includes history and physicals every 3–6 months for 2 years, then every 6 months for a total of 5 years; CEA levels every 3–6 months for 2 years, then every 6 months for a total of 5 years; chest/abdominal/pelvic CT annually for up to 5 years; colonoscopy in 1 year with a repeat in 1, 3, 5 years [26]. The most common site of recurrence is the liver remaining after the resection [5]. Adjuvant systemic therapy contributes to improved survival. All patients undergoing liver resection should receive intense follow-up and adjuvant chemotherapy [6]. Recent studies suggest follow up for 10 years for late recurrences [48].

55.7 Discussion

It is obvious that a multidisciplinary approach is required for adequate management of RC-SLM. Planning and cooperation between specialists in hepatobiliary and colorectal surgery, and oncology is required to maximize patient survival benefit. Optimal treatment regimen for combined disease has yet to be determined. Infusional 5-FU with pelvic RT as neoadjuvant therapy may not provide the best treatment for liver metastases with potential for progression systemically. Liver metastasis and other systemic secondaries have been found to respond well with newer chemotherapy agents e.g. FOLFOX, FOLFIRI and monoclonal antibodies e.g. Bevacizimab, panitumumab, cetuximab. Due to combined toxicity it usually is not possible to use FOLFOX/FOLFIRI with RT. Potential problems with this approach relates to rectal tumor extent and risk of pelvic recurrence without the use of neoadjuvant radiation. More recently short course radiation after full systemic chemotherapy has been described and demonstrated promising outcomes [4].

Recent advancement in the approach to hepatic metastasis have allowed for patient with more extensive disease to undergo surgery with improvement in overall survival. Newer procedures such as two-step liver resections, laparoscopic resection, PVE with resection and

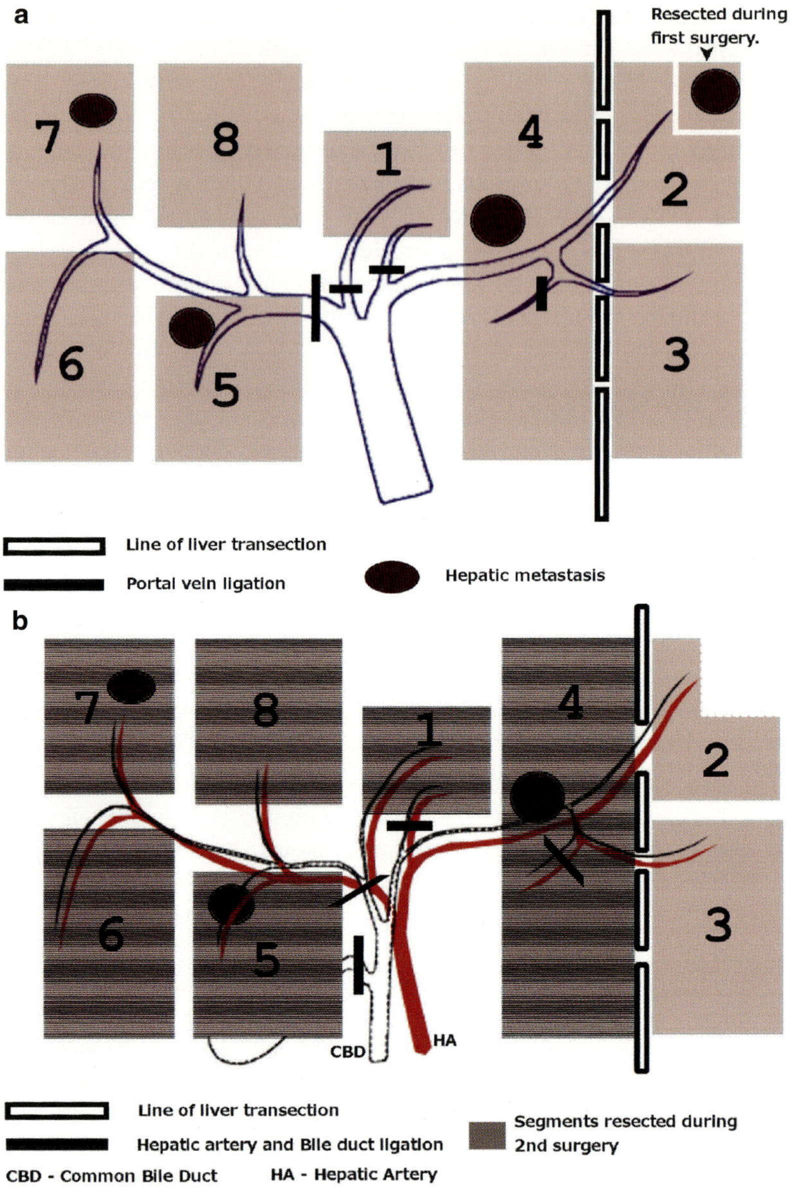

Fig. 55.2 (**a**) ALPPS—step 1, (**b**) ALPPS—step 2

the ALPPS procedure increase our ability to offer patients options for cure. However, the optimal strategy still needs to be determined, hopefully by a randomized clinical trial.

References

1. Sylvain Manfredi MD, Come Lepage MD, Cyril Hatem MD, Olivier Coatmeur MD, Jean Faivre PD, Anne-Marie Bouvier PD. Epidemiology and management of liver metastases from colorectal cancer. Ann Surg. 2006;244:254–9.
2. Kim JW, Kim YB, Kim NK, Min BS, Shin SJ, Ahn JB, Koom WS, Seong J, Keum KC. The role of adjuvant pelvic radiotherapy in rectal cancer with synchronous liver metastasis: a retrospective study. Radiat Oncol. 2010;5:75. doi:10.1186/1748-717X-5-75.
3. Roxburgh CS, Richards CH, MougSJ FAK, McMillan DC, Horgan PG. Determinants of short- and long-term outcome in patients undergoing simultaneous resection of colorectal cancer and synchronous colorectal liver metastases. Int J Colorectal Dis. 2012;27(3):363–9. doi:10.1007/s00384-011-1339-9. Epub 2011 Nov 17.
4. Turrini O, Viret F, Guiramand J, Lelong B, Be'ge T, Delpero JR. Strategies for the treatment of synchronous liver metastasis. Eur J Surg Oncol. 2007;33: 735–40.

5. Phillips SF, Pemberton JH, Shorter RG. The large intestine: physiology, pathophysiology, and disease. New York: Raven Press, Ltd; 1991, 1991528.
6. Tsai MS, Su YH, Ho MC, Liang JT, Chen TP, Lai HS, Lee PH. Clinicopathological features and prognosis in resectable synchronous and metachronous colorectal liver metastasis. Ann Surg Oncol. 2007;14(2):786–94. Epub 2006 Nov 14.
7. Sugihara K, Hojo K, Moriya Y, Yamasaki S, Kosuge T. Takayama pattern of recurrence after hepatic resection for colorectal metastases. Br J Surg. 1993;80(8): 1032–5.
8. Scheele J, Stang R, Altendorf-Hofmann A, Paul M. Resection of colorectal liver metastases. World J Surg. 1995;19(1):59–71.
9. Fong Y, Cohen AM, Fortner JG, Enker WE, Turnbull AD, Coit DG, Marrero AM, Prasad M, Blumgart LH, Brennan MF. Liver resection for colorectal metastases. J Clin Oncol. 1997;15(3):938–46.
10. Wanebo HJ, Semoglou C, Attiyeh F, Stearns Jr MJ. Surgical management of patients with primary operable colorectal cancer and synchronous liver metastases. Am J Surg. 1978;135(1):81–5.
11. Finlay IG, Meek D, Brunton F, McArdle CS. Growth rate of hepatic metastases in colorectal carcinoma. Br J Surg. 1988;75:641–4.
12. Hotta T, Takifuji K, Uchiyama K, Yokoyama S, Matsuda K, Higashiguchi T, Tominaga T, Oku Y, Nasu T, Yamaue H. Potential predictors of survival after surgery for colorectal cancer patients with synchronous unresectable liver metastases. Oncol Rep. 2006;16(6):1369–74.
13. Fong Y, Fortner J, Sun RL, Brennan MF, Blumgart LH. Clinical score for predicting recurrence after hepatic resection for metastatic colorectal cancer: analysis of 1001 consecutive cases. Ann Surg. 1999; 230(3):309–18.
14. Nagashima I, Takada T, Matsuda K, Adachi M, Nagawa H, Muto T, Okinaga K. A new scoring system to classify patients with colorectal liver metastases: proposal of criteria to select candidates for hepatic resection. J Hepatobiliary Pancreat Surg. 2004;11(2):79–83.
15. Fujita S, Akasu T, Moriya Y. Resection of synchronous liver metastases from colorectal cancer. Jpn J Clin Oncol. 2000;30(1):7–11.
16. Ono M, Sakamoto M, Ino Y, Moriya Y, Sugihara K, Muto T, Hirohashi S. Cancer cell morphology at the invasive front and expression of cell adhesion-related carbohydrate in the primary lesion of patients with colorectal carcinoma with liver metastasis. Cancer. 1996;78(6):1179–86.
17. ChezmarJL RWM, Megibow AJ, Hulnick DH, Nelson RC, Bernardino ME. Liver and abdominal screening in patients with cancer: CT versus MR imaging. Radiology. 1988;168:43–7.
18. Oliva MR, Saini S. Liver cancer imaging: role of CT, MRI, US and PET. Cancer Imaging. 2004;4 Spec No A:S42–6.
19. Strasberg SM, Dehdashti F, Siegel BA, Drebin JA, Linehan D. Survival of patients evaluated by FDG-PET before hepatic resection for metastatic colorectal carcinoma: a Prospective Database Study. Ann Surg. 2001;233(3):293–9.
20. Brush J, Boyd K, Chappell F, Crawford F, Dozier M, Fenwick E, Glanville J, McIntosh H, Renehan A, Weller D, Dunlop M. The value of FDG positron emission tomography/computerised tomography (PET/CT) in pre-operative staging of colorectal cancer: a systematic review and economic evaluation. Health Technol Assess. 2011;15(35):1–192, iii–iv.
21. Savage AP, Malt RA. Elective and emergency hepatic resection. Determinants of operative mortality and morbidity. Ann Surg. 1991;214(6):689–95.
22. Brouquet A, Zimmitti G, Kopetz S, Stift J, Julié C, Lemaistre AI, Agarwal A, Patel V, Benoist S, Nordlinger B, Gandini A, Rivoire M, Stremitzer S, Gruenberger T, Vauthey JN, Maru DM. Multicenter validation study of pathologic response and tumor thickness at the tumor-normal liver interface as independent predictors of disease-free survival after preoperative chemotherapy and surgery for colorectal liver metastases. Cancer. 2013;119(15):2778–88.
23. Shin, et al. Upfront systemic chemotherapy and preoperative short-course radiotherapy with delayed surgery for locally advanced rectal cancer with distant metastases. Radiat Oncol. 2011;6:99.
24. Coppa GF, Eng K, Ranson JH, Gouge TH, Localio SA. Hepatic resection for metastatic colon and rectal cancer. An evaluation of preoperative and postoperative factors. Ann Surg. 1985;202(2):203–8.
25. Nahas CS, Akhurst T, Yeung H, Leibold T, Riedel E, Markowitz AJ, Minsky BD, PatyPB WMR, Temple LK, Wong WD, Larson SM, Guillem JG. Positron emission tomography detection of distant metastatic or synchronous disease in patients with locally advanced rectal cancer receiving preoperative chemoradiation. Ann Surg Oncol. 2008;15(3):704–11. Epub 2007 Sep 20.
26. NCCN clinical practice guidelines in oncology (NCCN Guidelines) Version 4.2013. NCCN.org.
27. Sauer R, Becker H, Hohenberger W, et al. Preoperative versus postoperative chemo radiotherapy for rectal cancer. N Engl J Med. 2004;351:1731–40.
28. Elias D, Youssef O, Sideris L, Dromain C, Baton O, Boige V, Ducreux M. Evolution of missing colorectal liver metastases following inductive chemotherapy and hepatectomy. J Surg Oncol. 2004;86(1):4–9.
29. Okuyama K, Onoda S, Tohnosu N, Yamamoto Y, Koide Y, Hanaoka A, Seki Y, Hara T, Nishijima H, Isono K. The prognostic significance of resection of primary tumor in gastric and colorectal cancer patients with synchronous liver metastasis. Jpn J Surg. 1988; 18(1):7–17.
30. Mocellin S, Pilati P, Lise M, Nitti D. Meta-analysis of hepatic arterial infusion for unresectable liver metastases from colorectal cancer: the end of an era? J Clin Oncol. 2007;25(35):5649–54.
31. Ayez N, Burger JW, van der Pool AE, Eggermont AM, Grunhagen DJ, de Wilt JH, Verhoef C. Long-term results of the "liver first" approach in patients with locally advanced rectal cancer and synchronous

liver metastases. Dis Colon Rectum. 2013;56(3):281–7. doi:10.1097/DCR.0b013e318279b743.
32. Capussotti L, Ferrero A, Viganò L, Ribero D, Lo Tesoriere R, Polastri R. Major liver resections synchronous with colorectal surgery. Ann Surg Oncol. 2007;14(1):195–201.
33. Chua HK, Sondenaa K, Tsiotos GG, Larson DR, Wolff BG, Nagorney DM. Concurrent vs. staged colectomy and hepatectomy for primary colorectal cancer with synchronous hepatic metastases. Dis Colon Rectum. 2004;47(8):1310–6.
34. Reddy SK, Pawlik TM, Zorzi D, Gleisner AL, Ribero D, Assumpcao L, Barbas AS, AbdallaEK CMA, VautheyJN LKA, Mantyh CR, Morse MA, Clary BM. Simultaneous resections of colorectal cancer and synchronous liver metastases: a multi-institutional analysis. Ann Surg Oncol. 2007;14(12):3481–91. Epub 2007 Sep 1.
35. Hillingsø JG, Wille-Jørgensen P. Staged or simultaneous resection of synchronous liver metastases from colorectal cancer—a systematic review. Colorectal Dis. 2009;11(1):3–10. doi:10.1111/j.1463–1318.2008.01625.x. Epub 2008 Jul 11.
36. Weber JC, Bachellier P, Oussoultzoglou E, Jaeck D. Simultaneous resection of colorectal primary tumour and synchronous liver metastases. Br J Surg. 2003;90(8):956–62.
37. Lyass S, Zamir G, Matot I, Goitein D, Eid A, Jurim O. Combined colon and hepatic resection for synchronous colorectal liver metastases. J Surg Oncol. 2001;78(1):17–21.
38. Chen KY, Xiang GA, Wang HN, Xiao FL. Simultaneous laparoscopic excision for the treatment of rectal carcinoma and the synchronous hepatic metastasis. Zhonghua Zhong Liu Za Zhi. 2009;31(1):69–71.
39. Lee JS, Hong HT, Kim JH, Lee IK, Lee KH, Park IY, Oh ST, Kim JG, Lee YS. Simultaneous laparoscopic resection of primary colorectal cancer and metastatic liver tumor: initial experience of single institute. J Laparoendosc Adv Surg Tech A. 2010;20(8):683–7. doi:10.1089/lap.2010.0039.
40. Bretagnol F, Hatwell C, Farges O, Alves A, Belghiti J, Panis Y. Benefit of laparoscopy for rectal resection in patients operated simultaneously for synchronous liver metastases: preliminary experience. Surgery. 2008;144:436–41.
41. Pessaux P, Panaro F. Advantages of the first-step totally laparoscopic approach in 2-staged hepatectomy for colorectal synchronous liver metastasis. Surgery. 2009;145(4):453. doi:10.1016/j.surg.2008.09.016.
42. Mentha G, Roth AD, Terraz S, Giostra E, Gervaz P, Andres A, Morel P, Rubbia-Brandt L, Majno PE. 'Liver first' approach in the treatment of colorectal cancer with synchronous liver metastases. Dig Surg. 2008;25(6):430–5.
43. de Jong MC, van Dam RM, Maas M, Bemelmans MH, OldeDamink SW, Beets GL, Dejong CH. The liver-first approach for synchronous colorectal liver metastasis: a 5-year single-centre experience. HPB (Oxf). 2011;13(10):745–52. doi:10.1111/j.1477–2574.2011.00372.x. Epub 2011 Sep 5.
44. Schnitzbauer AA, Lang SA, Goessmann H, Nadalin S, Baumgart J, Farkas SA, Fichtner-Feigl S, Lorf T, Goralcyk A, Hörbelt R, Kroemer A, Loss M, Rümmele P, Scherer MN, Padberg W, Königsrainer A, Lang H, Obed A, Schlitt HJ. Right portal vein ligation combined with in situ splitting induces rapid left lateral liver lobe hypertrophy enabling 2-staged extended right hepatic resection in small-for-size settings. Ann Surg. 2012;255(3):405–14.
45. Torres OJ, Moraes-Junior JM, Lima NC L, Moraes AM. Associating liver partition and portal vein ligation for staged hepatectomy (ALPPS): a new approach in liver resections. Arq Bras Cir Dig. 2012;25(4):290–2.
46. Baumgart J, Lang S, Lang H. A new method for induction of liver hypertrophy prior to right trisectionectomy: a report of three cases. HPB. 2011;13:71–2.
47. Machado MA, Makdissi FF, Surjan RC. Totally laparoscopic ALPPS is feasible and may be worthwhile. Ann Surg. 2012;256(3):e13.
48. Vigano L, Ferrero A, Lo Tesoriere R, Capussotti L. Liver surgery for colorectal metastases: results after 10 years of follow-up. Long-term survivors, late recurrences, and prognostic role of morbidity. Ann Surg Oncol. 2008;15(9):2458–64.

56 Selective Non-operative Treatment in Rectal Cancer After Neoadjuvant Chemoradiation: Lessons Learned from the "Watch-and-Wait" Approach

Angelita Habr-Gama, Patricio Bernardo Lynn, and Rodrigo Oliva Perez

56.1 Introduction, Rationale for Selective Non-operative Treatment

Neoadjuvant chemoradiation (NCR) is one of the preferred treatment strategies for locally advanced distal rectal cancer. The greatest advantage of this approach has been the lower risk of local failures observed in many studies using different regimens of RT with or without concomitant chemotherapy followed by radical surgery [1–4]. In addition, this approach is associated with lower toxicity rates and better functional results when compared to adjuvant CRT, even though no differences in survival have been observed [4].

The use of radiation with or without chemotherapy may lead to significant tumor cell death both in the primary tumor and perirectal nodes. The effects on the primary tumor may result in a shift towards earlier T stage classification, smaller tumor size (downsizing) and variable degrees of replacement of cancer cells by fibrotic tissue (tumor regression grade). The perirectal nodes may also be affected by treatment eventually resulting in nodal sterilization and fewer recovered nodes after proper total mesorectal excision. Even though the effects of neoadjuvant therapy in tumor downsizing and downstaging have been suggested to increase the possibility of sphincter preservation, none of the available randomized trials have been able to demonstrate higher rates of sphincter preserving operations among experimental arms when compared to control arms [5].

In some cases tumor regression is so significant that no residual cancer is found in the pathological specimen, a phenomenon known as Complete Pathological Response (pCR). Many studies have shown that oncological outcome is associated with tumor response to neoadjuvant therapy (final pathological stage) and those patients that present pCR have the best oncological outcomes [6–10].

On the other hand, radical surgery (TME) is still the cornerstone of the treatment of rectal cancer. However, surgical resection is associated with significant immediate morbidity and even mortality. Anastomotic leak, probably the most dreaded complication is reported in up to 12 % of cases [11]. Perioperative mortality may reach 3 % and is significantly higher, reaching up to 13 % when an anastomotic leak is present among patients who do not undergo temporary diversion [12, 13]. It should also be considered that a temporary stoma is frequently required, with additional morbidity or even mortality related to stoma creation and takedown that must also be taken into account [14].

A. Habr-Gama, MD, PhD • P.B. Lynn, MD
Department of Colorectal Surgery, Angelita and Joaquim Gama Institute, São Paulo, Brazil

R.O. Perez, MD, PhD (✉)
Colorectal Surgery Division, Department of Gastroenterology, Angelita and Joaquim Gama Institute, University of São Paulo School of Medicine, São Paulo, Brazil
e-mail: rodrigo.operez@gmail.com

H.R.H. Patel et al. (eds.), *Pelvic Cancer Surgery: Modern Breakthroughs and Future Advances*,
DOI 10.1007/978-1-4471-4258-4_56, © Springer-Verlag London 2015

Furthermore, despite the standardization of nerve sparing techniques, the rates of urinary and sexual dysfunctions are still significant. Finally, even though sphincteric function and quality of life among patients undergoing ultra-low anterior resections are acceptable, results are far from perfect. In a report of patients undergoing ultra-low anterior resections, the median fecal incontinence score rate was 11 with nearly half of patients with significant fecal incontinence [15].

With all these considerations, one could argue: *Is it justified to treat patients with significantly morbid and sometimes mutilating procedure when not a single cancer cell is present*?

For these reasons, it has been suggested a non-operative approach (also known as the "Watch and Wait" approach) in selected low rectal cancer patients that present specific features after NCR that suggests the presence of complete pathological response without having to perform a radical operation exclusively to confirm the absence of residual cancer.

56.2 Response Assessment: How?

The identification of patients that harbor no residual disease is one of the greatest challenges in rectal cancer management. Unfortunately, up to date, there is no perfect tool for this purpose. Instead, assessment of tumor response is performed with a combination of different modalities that decrease the possibility of missing residual undetected tumor.

Patients with a high suspicion of pathological response according to clinical and radiological criteria are considered Complete Clinical Responders (cCR). These are the candidates for this selective non-operative treatment. The role of each modality will be discussed with special emphasis on clinical assessment.

56.3 Clinical Assessment

Absence of symptoms after NCR should not be considered as a reliable method of assessment of tumor response. Most patients experience improvements in symptoms after treatment but active assessment is still required to rule out persistent disease.

Clinical assessment performed by an experienced colorectal surgeon including digital rectal examination and proctoscopy is definitely one of the most useful tools. Although studies have reported disappointing results regarding sensitivity and specificity of this modality in identifying pCR patients, a few considerations may be worthwhile mentioning. First, standardization of what a is complete clinical response was unavailable when published. Also, patients were assessed using rather short intervals from CRT completion, a well-known factor that may considerably affect response rates (as will be discussed later). Finally, examinations were performed by different surgeons with different levels of expertise what could also have influenced results [16].

In an effort to provide standardization of clinical and endoscopic findings consistent with complete clinical response, a recent study has reported commonly observed features among these patients as well as findings that should warrant prompt surgical action. Not only these findings may aid surgeons in identifying individual patients that are likely to present complete tumor regression, they also may provide a basis for standardization of cCR to allow future studies investigating the role of alternative treatment strategies in such patients [17].

According to the stringent criteria provided in that study, patients with the following findings at digital rectal examination and proctoscopy (rigid or flexible) may be considered as complete clinical responders:

1. Whitening of the mucosa in the area previously occupied by the tumor (Fig. 56.1).
2. A subtle loss of pliability of the rectal wall harboring the scar; usually observed during manual insufflations at proctoscopy with light stiffness of the wall. In the context of no additional positive findings of residual cancer, this may also be considered as a feature of cCR.
3. Telangiectasia (small derogative blood vessels seen on the rectal mucosa at the area previously harboring the primary cancer) is also

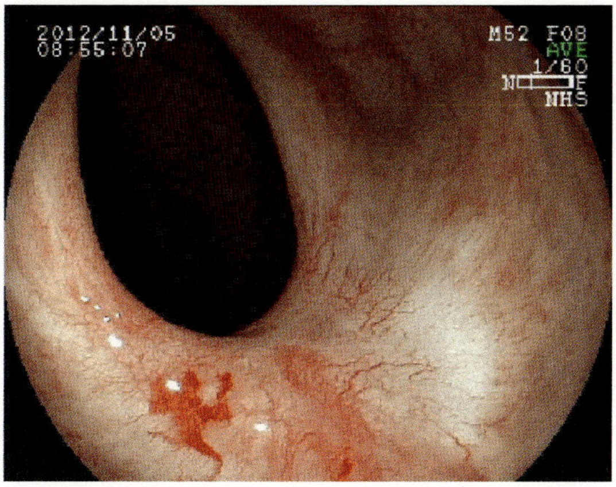

Fig. 56.1 Endoscopic view of a complete clinical response

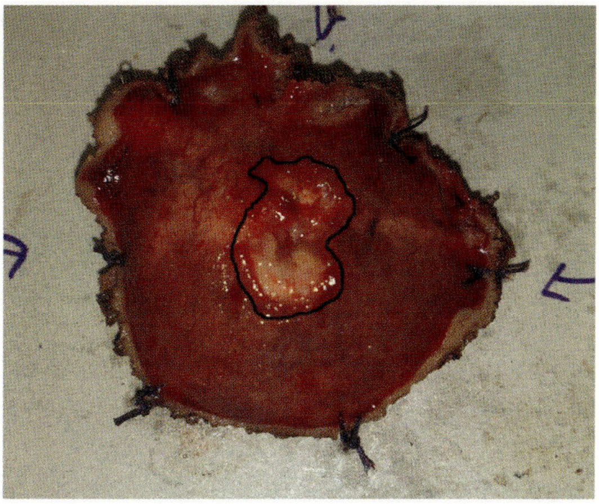

Fig. 56.2 Surgical specimen resected with TEM (Transanal Endoscopic Microsurgery) showing an incomplete response

frequently observed in complete clinical responders, even in long-term follow-up.

4. Whenever a tumor cannot be felt or seen, patients should be considered as complete clinical responders.

Alternatively, the following findings should be considered as incomplete clinical response and therefore warrant immediate surgical resection. Even though this may lead to a proportion of patients with pCR despite clinical findings of persistent cancer, it seems to be the safest procedure.

1. Any residual deep ulceration with or without a necrotic center.
2. Any superficial ulcer, irregularity, even in the presence of only mucosal ulceration.
3. Any palpable nodule, defined by digital rectal examination, even in the presence of mucosal complete integrity.

In any of these situations, a surgical action is warranted, at least for diagnostic purposes. A non-surgical approach in this scenario is not recommended (Fig. 56.2).

One recent study has investigated the impact of the use of these stringent criteria in selecting patients likely to have a complete pathological response. In this study, simply by looking at specimen photographs, surgeons were asked to indicate complete pathological responders. Curiously, these criteria led to positive and negative predictive values ≥90 % for the identification of complete responders without any tactile information obtained from DRE, biopsies or radiological imaging [18].

56.4 Imaging Studies

Radiological assessment of response is of paramount importance for the appropriate selection of patients for an alternative treatment strategy such as the "Watch & Wait" approach following a complete clinical response. Not only they provide assessment of the primary tumor (within the rectal wall) but also of the mesorectal lymph nodes that are not accessible to clinical examination alone and a possible site for metastatic disease even in the presence of complete primary tumor regression (ypT0).

Basically, the same imaging modalities used for initial staging can be used for tumor response assessment. Endorectal Ultrasound (ERUS), has been studied for this purpose and in a recent report with 60 patients, the overall accuracy of the method for T staging was less than 40 % when assessment was performed after 45 days from CRT completion [19]. Assessment at 6–8 weeks may have improved accuracy to 75 %. However, identification of ypT0 was particularly poor [20].

Magnetic resonance imaging (MRI) is now considered standard for primary tumor staging

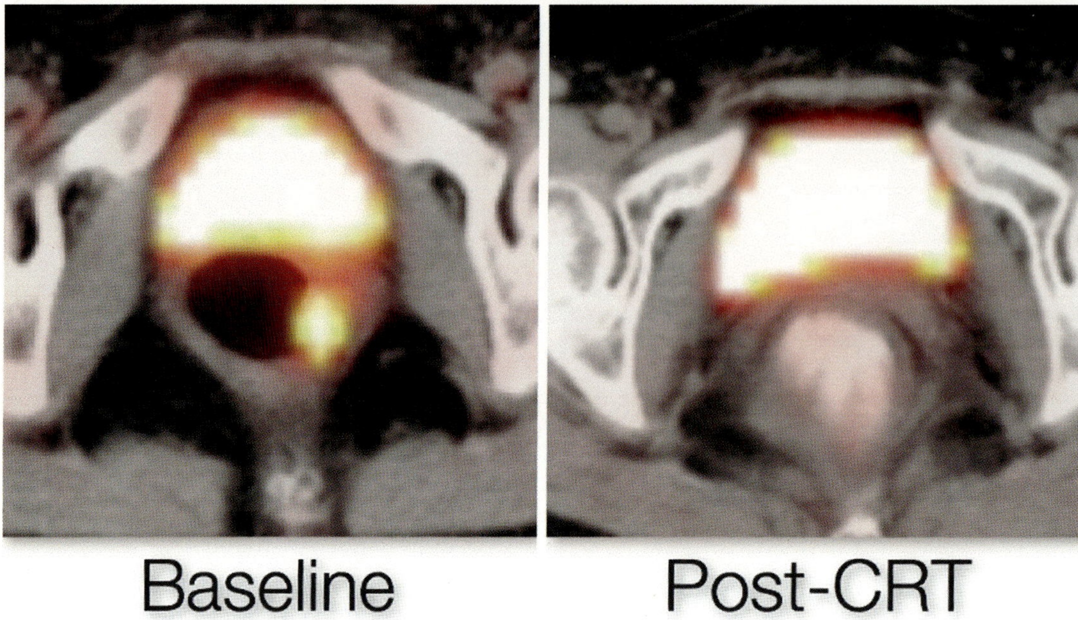

Fig. 56.3 PET/CT of a complete clinical response patient before and after CRT

and assessment of response after CRT. Findings of areas with low signal intensity replacing the area of the previous tumor or even no detectable abnormalities in MRI are consistent with radiological features of a complete clinical response. Three different patterns of low-signal intensity have been described in patients with complete clinical response: minimal fibrosis, transmural fibrosis and irregular fibrosis [21]. Also, histological tumor regression is currently estimated by MRI imaging with a classification inspired by tumor regression grading systems. This MRI "tumor regression grade" classification proved to correlate well with survival [22].

Diffusion-weighted MRI (DWI) is a functional MR imaging technique that uses differences in the extracellular movement of water protons to discriminate between tissues of varying cellularity. In tissues with increased cellularity (neoplasia), the diffusion of water is restricted, resulting in remaining high signal intensity on DWI-MR. In recent studies, the diagnostic performance for predicting a pathologic complete tumor response was improved with DWI MRI compared with standard MRI in nearly 20 %, reaching ≥90 % overall accuracy [23].

Positron-emission tomography (PET) with computed tomography (CT) may provide additional information regarding metabolic activity in tumors after neoadjuvant CRT. In addition to the visual identification of FDG uptake within the area of the rectal wall harboring the tumor or within the mesorectum, PET/CT allows the estimation of the metabolism profile. Standard uptake values (SUV) are direct estimations of tissue metabolism and may be used for the distinction of residual inflammatory changes and residual cancer. Measurement of SUV in two different intervals from FDG injection is routinely performed (1 and 3 h) and allows two distinct patterns (dual time) of metabolism. Increase in SUV (between 1 and 3 h) suggests the presence of residual cancer whereas decrease suggests inflammatory or fibrotic changes [24].

Several studies have suggested the use of PET/CT in assessing tumor response to CRT with conflicting results.[25–28]. In our experience, PET/CT when performed 12 weeks after chemoradiation completion was able to predict Complete Response with an accuracy of 85 % [29] (Fig. 56.3).

56.5 CEA

The determination of CEA levels before and after CRT may be useful during assessment of tumor response. In one retrospective report of patients undergoing different CRT regimens it was showed that a pre treatment CEA level <2.5 ng/dl was predictor of ypCR [30].

An increase in CEA levels or persistence of at least 70 % from baseline has been suggested as predictor of worse outcome in patients with CEA levels >6 ng/ml at baseline [31]. Also, different cutoff values have been considered for patients undergoing CRT when compared to standard colorectal cancer patients. A retrospective analysis of 109 patients undergoing neoadjuvant therapy, identified a cutoff value for CEA <2.7 ng/ml at 4 weeks from RT completion to be predictor of tumor regression [32].

In our experience, no correlation with both pre-treatment CEA and variation between pre and post treatment CEA levels and tumor response or oncological outcomes was detected. On the other hand, a post-CRT level <5 ng/ml after at least 8 weeks from CRT completion was associated with increased rates of earlier disease stage and complete tumor regression [33].

56.6 Endoscopic Biopsies After CRT

During endoscopic evaluation of a residual lesion, forcep's biopsies are frequently performed and considered by many to be useful in assessment of tumor response. Even though a positive result implies obvious persistence of residual tumor, negative results may warrant cautious interpretation.

In a retrospective review of patients undergoing neoadjuvant CRT and significant tumor downsizing, post-CRT biopsies resulted in a negative predictive value of 21 %. In other words, a negative biopsy truly identified a pCR in only 21 % of cases [34].

Nevertheless, endoscopic biopsies may have a role in the management of these patients since a positive biopsy is sometimes a useful argument to convince patients who refuse radical surgery to accept treatment in the presence of residual cancer despite significant symptom relief.

56.7 Factors Associated with Tumor Response After CRT

Tumor response to CRT is not uniform and many factors may play a role. The specific CRT regimen and interval between CRT completion and assessment of response seem to be as important as tumor and patient-related characteristics.

56.8 Chemoradiation Regimen

Fractionated long course chemoradiation followed by surgery after 6–8 weeks or pelvic short-course irradiation with 25 Gy in five fractions followed by immediate surgery are the two most used regimens in the preoperative treatment of patients with resectable T3–4 rectal cancer. Benefits in local disease control seem to be equivalent between them, but there are significant differences in terms of tumor downstaging [35].

The rates of pCR are significantly lower in patients undergoing short-course RT, when compared with those undergoing long-course. At first glance, the long-course regimen includes chemotherapy and this could be determinant for that difference. It should also be considered that damaged cancer cells need time to undergo necrosis after radiotherapy and usually patients undergoing short-course RT, surgery is performed 1 week after RT completion whereas long-course CRT is followed by radical surgery after at least 6–8 weeks. In fact, one randomized study has demonstrated that pathological regression is more pronounced in the presence of combination of chemo and radiation therapy when compared to radiation therapy alone [36]. A very recent systematic revision from Cochrane, including five randomized controlled trials comparing CRT vs RT alone for resectable stage II or III rectal cancer, showed that the first approach was associated with a higher rates of ypCR [37].

A review of phase II and III studies using different neoadjuvant CRT regimens for rectal cancer including >4,000 patients in 71 studies with different regimens, reported a ypT0 rate that varied from 0 to 42 %. In this review, pCR was significantly associated with the delivery of radiation doses higher than 45-Gy, 5-FU regimens with continuous infusion and the use of a second drug (being oxaliplatin the most frequent additional drug) [38].

The association of higher rates of pCR and the addition oxaliplatin to the traditional scheme of 5-FU has been strongly questioned in light of the results of a recent prospective randomized trial that showed that this addition was not associated with better rates of pCR. Instead, patients treated with oxaliplatin experienced significantly more treatment-related toxicities [39].

Targeted biological drugs used for metastatic disease, such as bevazicumab and cetuximab, were included in phase I and II studies in combination with other drugs aiming to increase response rates. Results, however, were disappointing. A review of these trials also suggested a sub-additive interaction between capecitabine, oxaliplatin, and cetuximab as reflected by decreased rate of pCR (9 vs. 16 %) and significant decrease in tumor regression grades (more than 50 % of tumor regression) among surgical specimens from these patients when compared with patients undergoing treatment with capecitabine and oxaliplatin alone CRT regimens [40]. It is not clear whether the inclusion of patients according to the K-ras status could have any influence in response to neoadjuvant CRT with this triple approach [41].

56.9 Timing for Tumor Response Assessment

The optimal interval between CRT and surgery has not yet been identified for rectal cancer. The Lyon R90–01 study is so far the only randomized trial that evaluated the time interval between the completion of CRT therapy and surgery (2 weeks vs 6 weeks), and demonstrated improved T and N downshift with the longer interval (6 weeks) [42]. In addition, retrospective studies echo the finding that a longer interval to surgery may actually increase pCR rates [43]. In a recent review of the Cleveland Clinic experience, there was a steep increase in the pCR rate after 7 weeks from CRT completion; this increase reached a plateau only after 12 weeks [7].

A longer interval to surgery may confer another benefit. A review of patients treated with different intervals after neoadjuvant therapy suggested that delayed surgical resection was associated with decreased perioperative morbidity and no oncologic compromise [44]. In fact, preliminary results from a prospective non-randomized trial showed that in presence of tumor response to CRT (5FU + RT) the addition of two cycles of FOLFOX-6 scheme and delaying surgery for 12 weeks resulted in a modest increase of ypT0 rate without increasing postoperative complications [45]. Altogether, these results may suggest that 12-week intervals are perhaps ideal prior to assessment of tumor response following CRT completion. There are currently ongoing randomized trials addressing the question of 6 or 12-week intervals following CRT completion in rectal cancer that are likely to lead to more definitive conclusions in the near future [46].

Still, there is a possibility that not all patients would benefit from waiting more than 6 weeks, as suggested by a recent study using PET/CT to evaluate tumor metabolism [47]. Some patients may actually develop increase in tumor metabolism between 6 and 12 weeks suggesting no actual benefit. However, it is not clear whether this increment in metabolism is detrimental and that interruption (surgery) at 6 weeks provides any benefit for these patients.

56.10 Tumor Features and Biology

Several aspects of the primary rectal cancer such as tumor height, extension and initial disease staging, have been considered to be predictors of tumor response or complete pathological response to neoadjuvant treatment. Even though very few studies have included patients with cT2N0 rectal cancer treated by neoadjuvant CRT, these tumors seem to be more likely to develop complete clinical response [29]. The ACOSOG trial that included cT2N0 for neoadjuvant CRT followed by local excision resulted in a surprisingly high pCR (ypT0) rate of 44 % [48].

In one retrospective study of over 500 patients tumor extension was an independent predictive factor of pCR after neoadjuvant CRT. In this study, circumferential tumor extent of <60 % was a significant predictor of pCR. Even though tumor distance from the anal verge was not a predictor of pCR, tumors located in the distal 5 cm of the rectum were more likely to develop greater tumor downstaging [49]. More recently, another study identified that high pre-treatment CEA levels and tumors located in the distal 5 cm of the rectum were less likely to develop pCR [50].

In the near future, molecular biology will help the identification of tumors that will respond completely to CRT. Currently available studies in this regard however have failed to demonstrate a useful gene signature capable of predicting response to CRT and significant limitations have been identified. First, studies have used different endpoints of response (complete response in some and "good" response in others). Second, different platforms for gene expression are currently available and were actually used. Finally, there was no overlap in terms of genes predicting response in each of these studies [51–54].

56.11 The Watch-and-Wait Protocol

Patients with complete tumor regression, either after clinical assessment (cCR) or after transanal local excision (ypT0), have been enrolled in a strict follow-up program with no immediate surgery (Fig. 56.4). It is critical the adherence to the program because distinguishing between complete and near-complete responses may be difficult in some situations and final decision is only possible after a few follow-up visits. This is why an empirical 12-month probation period has been suggested where only patients that sustain a complete clinical response are considered as true cCR's [55].

The algorithm includes monthly follow-up visits with digital rectal examination and rigid proctoscopy in every visit for the first 3 months and every 2–3 months during the rest of the first year. CEA levels are determined every 2 months. Radiological studies, including MRI or PET/CT are performed at the time of initial tumor response assessment and every 6 months if there are no signs of tumor recurrence. Patients are aware that complete clinical regression of their primary tumor may be temporary and tumor regrowth may occur at any time during follow-up. Small nodules or scars may develop over time and can be managed by full-thickness transanal excision (either by standard or Transanal Endoscopic Microsurgery techniques), primarily as a diagnostic approach. Patients with complete primary tumor response after FTLE (ypT0) are also considered as cCR and are not recommended to further resection.

In the case of obvious recurrence, radical surgery is strongly recommended.

After 1 year of sustained, complete clinical response, patients are recommended for follow-up visits every 3 months.

This treatment strategy has evolved since the beginning of our experience in 1991. Our accuracy in clinical assessment of tumor response has probably improved significantly with growing experience. At the beginning, patients were more frequently followed without immediate surgery when a near-complete clinical response was considered and expecting that time would lead to a complete clinical response. More recently, these patients have been more frequently assessed using full-thickness local excision (FTLE) as a diagnostic procedure, and according to the pathologic report managed by strict observation or referred to immediate radical surgery.

56.12 Results

In order to understand if there was any oncological benefit of radical surgery in the setting of complete tumor regression, a retrospective study was carried out at our Institution where patients with complete pathological response (pCR) managed by radical surgery were compared to

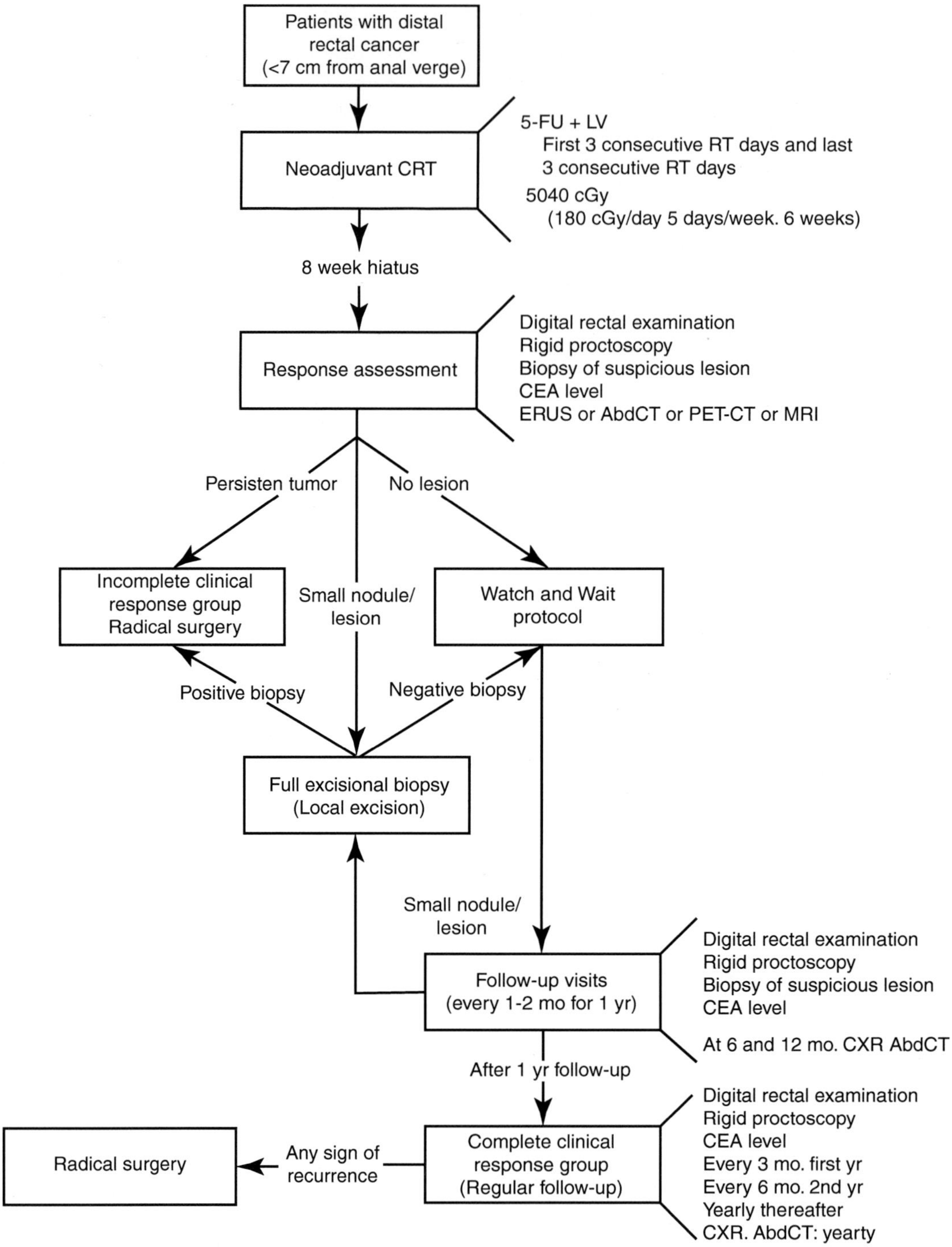

Fig. 56.4 The watch-and-wait algorithm

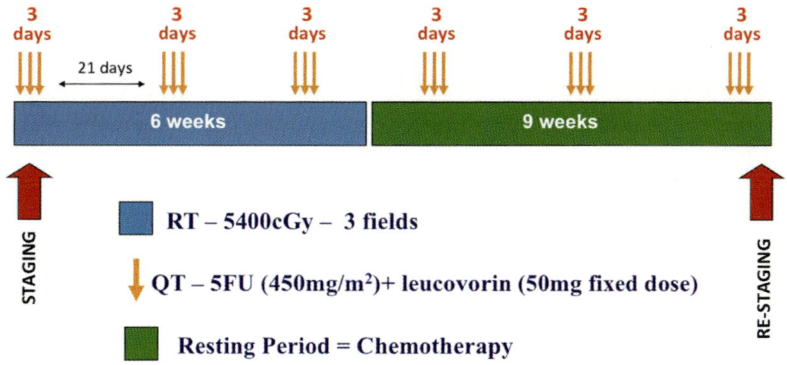

Fig. 56.5 The extended protocol

patients with cCR managed non-operatively [56]. Patients managed by observation alone had similar outcomes to those managed by radical surgery in terms of long-term survival. Local recurrences were higher in the observation group. However, all recurrences were confined to the rectal wall and amenable to surgical salvage [57]. No exclusive pelvic relapses without endorectal component was observed.

A very similar study has recently been reported from another Institution revealing identical oncological outcomes with no survival benefit among patients with pCR managed by radical TME over patients with cCR managed by observation alone. Curiously, this study suggested a worse functional outcome among patients in the resection group (pCR) when compared to the "watch and wait" group [58].

Up to now, most of local recurrences in patients with cCR after neoadjuvant CRT were amenable to salvage therapy [59]. These recurrences and their salvage procedures were performed at considerably long intervals after CRT completion (mean >50 months). In almost half of the cases an abdominoperineal resection (APR) was performed. Also, a third of these patients presented with low and superficial recurrences, amenable to full thickness transanal excision [57].

A significant subgroup of patients presented early tumor regrowth (within 12 months from CRT completion). These patients were most commonly misdiagnosed as cCR and had their definitive surgical treatment postponed for variable periods of time. This raised the question whether these patients could have been harmed from an oncologic point of view by delaying definitive surgical treatment. Long-term data revealed that they fared no worse than patients with incomplete clinical response managed by radical surgery after 8 weeks from CRT completion. Noteworthy, final pathology in this group revealed significant tumor downstaging and even lower rates of lymph node metastases, supporting the idea that downstaging is a time-dependent phenomenon [60].

In an effort to increase the rates of tumor response, the delivery of chemotherapy during the waiting or resting period between radiation completion and tumor response assessment has been implemented in our Institution (Fig. 56.5). In a preliminary report of our series including T2/T3 distal rectal cancers, the sustained complete clinical response rate (>12 months) was 51 % with no significant increase in chemotherapy-related toxicity rates [61, 62]. It should be noticed that only 8 % of our series required APR, allowing a sphincter preserving strategy in 92 % of the series.

Conclusions

Complete clinical response may be observed in up to 50 % of patients with rectal cancer following neoadjuvant chemoradiation. The actual percentage of patients that will develop complete response may vary according to baseline staging, type of chemoradiation regimen and timing of assessment of response. Specific clinical, endoscopic and radiological features may identify patients likely to have a complete pathological response. Management of these highly selected patients without immediate radical surgery and strict surveillance ("Watch & Wait") may provide an interesting alternative avoiding significant morbidity and mortality associated with radical surgery without compromising oncological outcomes. As understanding of molecular biology aspects associated with these tumors grow and additional tools may further improve selection of appropriate candidates for this organ-sparing procedure in patients with distal rectal cancer.

Key Points

- Neoadjuvant CRT may lead to tumor downstaging and downsizing
- Complete pathological response (pCR) is associated with best oncological outcomes.
- Chemoradiation regimen may ultimately affect pCR rates
- Interval between CRT and assessment may influence pCR rates
- cCR is a defined by stringent criteria based on clinical and radiological studies.
- There seems to be no oncological benefit in radical surgery after pCR over observation alone after cCR.
- Salvage is nearly always possible provided there is strict follow-up adherence

References

1. Cedermark B, Johansson H, Rutqvist LE, Wilking N, Stockholm Colorectal Cancer Study Group. The Stockholm I trial of preoperative short term radiotherapy in operable rectal carcinoma. A prospective randomized trial. Cancer. 1995;75(9):2269–75.
2. Martling A, Holm T, Johansson H, Rutqvist LE, Cedermark B, Stockholm Colorectal Cancer Study Group. The Stockholm II trial on preoperative radiotherapy in rectal carcinoma: long-term follow-up of a population-based study. Cancer. 2001;92(4): 896–902.
3. Kapiteijn E, Marijnen CA, Nagtegaal ID, Putter H, Steup WH, Wiggers T, et al. Preoperative radiotherapy combined with total mesorectal excision for resectable rectal cancer. N Engl J Med. 2001;345(9): 638–46.
4. Sauer R, Becker H, Hohenberger W, Rödel C, Wittekind C, Fietkau R, et al. Preoperative versus postoperative chemoradiotherapy for rectal cancer. N Engl J Med. 2004;351(17):1731–40.
5. Gérard J-P, Rostom Y, Gal J, Benchimol D, Ortholan C, Aschele C, et al. Can we increase the chance of sphincter saving surgery in rectal cancer with neoadjuvant treatments: lessons from a systematic review of recent randomized trials. Crit Rev Oncol Hematol. 2012;81(1):21–8.
6. Quah H-M, Chou JF, Gonen M, Shia J, Schrag D, Saltz LB, et al. Pathologic stage is most prognostic of disease-free survival in locally advanced rectal cancer patients after preoperative chemoradiation. Cancer. 2008;113(1):57–64.
7. Kalady MF, de Campos-Lobato LF, Stocchi L, Geisler DP, Dietz D, Lavery IC, et al. Predictive factors of pathologic complete response after neoadjuvant chemoradiation for rectal cancer. Ann Surg. 2009; 250(4):582–9.
8. Maas M, Nelemans PJ, Valentini V, Das P, Rödel C, Kuo L-J, et al. Long-term outcome in patients with a pathological complete response after chemoradiation for rectal cancer: a pooled analysis of individual patient data. Lancet Oncol. 2010;11(9): 835–44.
9. Chan AKP, Wong A, Jenken D, Heine J, Buie D, Johnson D. Posttreatment TNM staging is a prognostic indicator of survival and recurrence in tethered or fixed rectal carcinoma after preoperative chemotherapy and radiotherapy. Int J Radiat Oncol Biol Phys. 2005;61(3):665–77.
10. Habr-Gama A, Perez RO, Nadalin W, Nahas SC, Ribeiro U, Sousa AH S, et al. Long-term results of preoperative chemoradiation for distal rectal cancer correlation between final stage and survival. J Gastrointest Surg. 2005;9(1):90–9; discussion 99–101.
11. Chessin DB, Enker W, Cohen AM, Paty PB, Weiser MR, Saltz L, et al. Complications after preoperative combined modality therapy and radical resection of locally advanced rectal cancer: a 14-year experience from a specialty service. J Am Coll Surg. 2005;200(6):876–82; discussion 882–4.
12. Eriksen MT, Wibe A, Norstein J, Haffner J, Wiig JN, Norwegian Rectal Cancer Group. Anastomotic leakage following routine mesorectal excision for rectal cancer in a national cohort of patients. Color Dis. 2005;7(1):51–7.
13. Matthiessen P, Hallböök O, Rutegård J, Simert G, Sjödahl R. Defunctioning stoma reduces symptomatic anastomotic leakage after low anterior resection of the rectum for cancer: a randomized multicenter trial. Ann Surg. 2007;246(2):207–14.
14. Perez R, Habr-Gama A, Seid V. Loop ileostomy morbidity: timing of closure matters. Dis Colon Rectum. 2006;49:1539–45.
15. Denost QQ, Laurent CC, Capdepont MM, Zerbib FF, Rullier EE. Risk factors for fecal incontinence after intersphincteric resection for rectal cancer. Dis Colon Rectum. 2011;54(8):963–8.

16. Hiotis SP, Weber SM, Cohen AM, Minsky BD, Paty PB, Guillem JG, et al. Assessing the predictive value of clinical complete response to neoadjuvant therapy for rectal cancer: an analysis of 488 patients. J Am Coll Surg. 2002;194(5):131; discussion 135–6.
17. Habr-Gama A, Perez RO, Wynn G, Marks J, Kessler H, Gama-Rodrigues J. Complete clinical response after neoadjuvant chemoradiation therapy for distal rectal cancer: characterization of clinical and endoscopic findings for standardization. Dis Colon Rectum. 2010;53(12):1692–8.
18. Smith FM, Chang KH, Sheahan K, Hyland J, O'Connell PR, Winter DC. The surgical significance of residual mucosal abnormalities in rectal cancer following neoadjuvant chemoradiotherapy. Br J Surg. 2012;99(7):993–1001.
19. Huh JW, Park Y-A, Jung EJ, Lee KY, Sohn SK. Accuracy of endorectal ultrasonography and computed tomography for restaging rectal cancer after preoperative chemoradiation. J Am Coll Surg. 2008;207(1):7–12.
20. Radovanovic Z, Breberina M, Petrovic T, Golubovic A, Radovanovic D. Accuracy of endorectal ultrasonography in staging locally advanced rectal cancer after preoperative chemoradiation. Surg Endosc. 2008;22(11):2412–5.
21. Lambregts DMJ, Maas M, Bakers FCH, Cappendijk VC, Lammering G, Beets GL, et al. Long-term follow-up features on rectal MRI during a wait-and-see approach after a clinical complete response in patients with rectal cancer treated with chemoradiotherapy. Dis Colon Rectum. 2011;54(12):1521–8.
22. Patel UB, Brown G, Rutten H, West N, Sebag-Montefiore D, Glynne-Jones R, et al. Comparison of magnetic resonance imaging and histopathological response to chemoradiotherapy in locally advanced rectal cancer. Ann Surg Oncol. 2012;19:2842–52.
23. Lambregts DMJ, Vandecaveye V, Barbaro B, Bakers FCH, Lambrecht M, Maas M, et al. Diffusion-weighted MRI for selection of complete responders after chemoradiation for locally advanced rectal cancer: a multicenter study. Ann Surg Oncol. 2011;18(8):2224–31.
24. Zhuang H, Pourdehnad M, Lambright ES, Yamamoto AJ, Lanuti M, Li P, et al. Dual time point 18F-FDG PET imaging for differenciating malignant from inflammatory processes. J Nucl Med. 2001;42(9):1412–7.
25. Huh JW, Min JJ, Lee JH, Kim HR, Kim YJ. The predictive role of sequential FDG-PET/CT in response of locally advanced rectal cancer to neoadjuvant chemoradiation. Am J Clin Oncol. 2012;35(4):340–4.
26. Yoon MS, Ahn S-J, Nah B-S, Chung W-K, Song J-Y, Jeong J-U, et al. The metabolic response using 18F-fluorodeoxyglucose-positron emission tomography/computed tomography and the change in the carcinoembryonic antigen level for predicting response to pre-operative chemoradiotherapy in patients with rectal cancer. Radiother Oncol. 2011;98(1):134–8. Elsevier Ireland Ltd.
27. Chennupati SK, Quon A, Kamaya A, Pai RK, La T, Krakow TE, et al. Positron emission tomography for predicting pathologic response after neoadjuvant chemoradiotherapy for locally advanced rectal cancer. Am J Clin Oncol. 2012;35(4):334–9.
28. Shanmugan S, Arrangoiz R, Nitzkorski JR, Yu JQ, Li T, Cooper H, et al. Predicting pathological response to neoadjuvant chemoradiotherapy in locally advanced rectal cancer using 18FDG-PET/CT. Ann Surg Oncol. 2012;19(7):2178–85.
29. Perez RO, Habr-Gama A, Gama-Rodrigues J, Proscurshim I, Julião GPS, Lynn P, et al. Accuracy of positron emission tomography/computed tomography and clinical assessment in the detection of complete rectal tumor regression after neoadjuvant chemoradiation: long-term results of a prospective trial (National Clinical Trial 00254683). Cancer. 2011;15.
30. Moreno García V, Cejas P, Blanco Codesido M, Feliu Batlle J, de Castro CJ, Belda-Iniesta C, et al. Prognostic value of carcinoembryonic antigen level in rectal cancer treated with neoadjuvant chemoradiotherapy. Int J Color Dis. 2009;24(7):741–8.
31. Kim CW, Yu CS, Yang S-S, Kim KH, Yoon YS, Yoon SN, et al. Clinical significance of pre- to post-chemoradiotherapy s-CEA reduction ratio in rectal cancer patients treated with preoperative chemoradiotherapy and curative resection. Ann Surg Oncol. 2011;18(12):3271–7.
32. Jang NY, Kang S-B, Kim D-W, Kim JH, Lee K-W, Kim IA, et al. The role of carcinoembryonic antigen after neoadjuvant chemoradiotherapy in patients with rectal cancer. Dis Colon Rectum. 2011;54(2):245–52.
33. Perez RO, São Julião GP, Habr-Gama A, Kiss D, Proscurshim I, Campos FG, et al. The role of carcinoembriogenic antigen in predicting response and survival to neoadjuvant chemoradiotherapy for distal rectal cancer. Dis Colon Rectum. 2009;52(6):1137–43.
34. Perez RO, Habr-Gama A, Pereira GV, Lynn PB, Alves PA, Proscurshim I, et al. Role of biopsies in patients with residual rectal cancer following neoadjuvant chemoradiation after downsizing: can they rule out persisting cancer? Color Dis. 2012;14(6):714–20.
35. Bujko K, Nowacki MP, Nasierowska-Guttmejer A, Michalski W, Bebenek M, Kryj M. Long-term results of a randomized trial comparing preoperative short-course radiotherapy with preoperative conventionally fractionated chemoradiation for rectal cancer. Br J Surg. 2006;93(10):1215–23.
36. Bosset J-F, Calais G, Mineur L, Maingon P, Radosevic-Jelic L, Daban A, et al. Enhanced tumorocidal effect of chemotherapy with preoperative radiotherapy for rectal cancer: preliminary results—EORTC 22921. J Clin Oncol. 2005;23(24):5620–7.
37. De Caluwé L, Van Nieuwenhove Y, Ceelen WP. Preoperative chemoradiation versus radiation alone for stage II and III resectable rectal cancer. Cochrane Database Syst Rev. 2013;(2):CD006041.
38. Sanghera P, Wong DWY, McConkey CC, Geh JI, Hartley A. Chemoradiotherapy for rectal cancer: an updated analysis of factors affecting pathological response. Clin Oncol (R Coll Radiol). 2008;20(2):176–83.
39. Gérard J-P, Azria D, Gourgou-Bourgade S, Martel-Laffay I, Hennequin C, Etienne P-L, et al. Comparison of two neoadjuvant chemoradiotherapy regimens for

locally advanced rectal cancer: results of the phase III trial ACCORD 12/0405-Prodige 2. J Clin Oncol. 2010;28(10):1638–44.
40. Weiss C, Arnold D, Dellas K, Liersch T, Hipp M, Fietkau R, et al. Preoperative radiotherapy of advanced rectal cancer with capecitabine and oxaliplatin with or without cetuximab: a pooled analysis of three prospective phase I-II trials. Int J Radiat Oncol Biol Phys. 2010;78(2):472–8.
41. Glynne-Jones R, Mawdsley S, Harrison M. Cetuximab and chemoradiation for rectal cancer—is the water getting muddy? Acta Oncol. 2010;49(3):278–86.
42. Francois Y, Nemoz CJ, Baulieux J, Vignal J, Grandjean JP, Partensky C, et al. Influence of the interval between preoperative radiation therapy and surgery on downstaging and on the rate of sphincter-sparing surgery for rectal cancer: the Lyon R90–01 randomized trial. J Clin Oncol. 1999;17(8):2396.
43. Tulchinsky H, Shmueli E, Figer A, Klausner JM, Rabau M. An interval >7 weeks between neoadjuvant therapy and surgery improves pathologic complete response and disease-free survival in patients with locally advanced rectal cancer. Ann Surg Oncol. 2008;15(10):2661–7.
44. Kerr SF, Norton S, Glynne-Jones R. Delaying surgery after neoadjuvant chemoradiotherapy for rectal cancer may reduce postoperative morbidity without compromising prognosis. Br J Surg. 2008;95(12):1534–40.
45. Garcia-Aguilar JJ, Smith DDD, Avila KK, Bergsland EKE, Chu PP, Krieg RMR. Optimal timing of surgery after chemoradiation for advanced rectal cancer: preliminary results of a multicenter, nonrandomized phase II prospective trial. Ann Surg. 2011;254(1):97–102.
46. Evans J, Tait D, Swift I, Pennert K, Tekkis P, Wotherspoon A, et al. Timing of surgery following preoperative therapy in rectal cancer: the need for a prospective randomized trial? Dis Colon Rectum. 2011;54(10):1251–9.
47. Perez RO, Habr-Gama A, São Julião GP, Gama-Rodrigues J, Sousa AHS, Campos FG, et al. Optimal timing for assessment of tumor response to neoadjuvant chemoradiation in patients with rectal cancer: do all patients benefit from waiting longer than 6 weeks? Int J Radiat Oncol Biol Phys. 2012;84(5):1159–65.
48. Garcia-Aguilar J, Shi Q, Thomas CR, Chan E, Cataldo P, Marcet J, et al. A phase II trial of neoadjuvant chemoradiation and local excision for T2N0 rectal cancer: preliminary results of the ACOSOG Z6041 Trial. Ann Surg Oncol. 2012;19(2):384–91.
49. Das P, Skibber JM, Rodriguez-Bigas MA, Feig BW, Chang GJ, Wolff RA, et al. Predictors of tumor response and downstaging in patients who receive preoperative chemoradiation for rectal cancer. Cancer. 2007;109(9):1750–5.
50. Restivo A, Zorcolo L, Cocco IMF, Manunza R, Margiani C, Marongiu L, et al. Elevated CEA levels and low distance of the tumor from the anal verge are predictors of incomplete response to chemoradiation in patients with rectal cancer. Ann Surg Oncol. 2013;20(3):864–71.
51. Watanabe T, Komuro Y, Kiyomatsu T, Kanazawa T, Kazama Y, Tanaka J, et al. Prediction of sensitivity of rectal cancer cells in response to preoperative radiotherapy by DNA microarray analysis of gene expression profiles. Cancer Res. 2006;66(7):3370–4.
52. Ghadimi BM, Grade M, Difilippantonio MJ, Varma S, Simon R, Montagna C, et al. Effectiveness of gene expression profiling for response prediction of rectal adenocarcinomas to preoperative chemoradiotherapy. J Clin Oncol. 2005;23(9):1826–38.
53. Kim I-J, Lim S-B, Kang HC, Chang HJ, Ahn S-A, Park H-W, et al. Microarray gene expression profiling for predicting complete response to preoperative chemoradiotherapy in patients with advanced rectal cancer. Dis Colon Rectum. 2007;50(9):1342–53.
54. Rimkus C, Friederichs J, Boulesteix A-L, Theisen J, Mages J, Becker K, et al. Microarray-based prediction of tumor response to neoadjuvant radiochemotherapy of patients with locally advanced rectal cancer. Clin Gastroenterol Hepatol. 2008;6(1):53–61.
55. Habr-Gama A, de Souza PM, Ribeiro U, Nadalin W, Gansl R, Sousa AH, et al. Low rectal cancer: impact of radiation and chemotherapy on surgical treatment. Dis Colon Rectum. 1998;41(9):1087–96.
56. Habr-Gama A, Perez RO, Nadalin W, Sabbaga J, Ribeiro U, Sousa AH S, et al. Operative versus nonoperative treatment for stage 0 distal rectal cancer following chemoradiation therapy: long-term results. Ann Surg. 2004;240(4):711–7; Discussion 717–8.
57. Habr-Gama A, Perez RO, Proscurshim I, Campos FG, Nadalin W, Kiss D, et al. Patterns of failure and survival for nonoperative treatment of stage c0 distal rectal cancer following neoadjuvant chemoradiation therapy. J Gastrointest Surg. 2006;10(10):1319–28; discussion 1328–9.
58. Maas M, Beets-Tan RGH, Lambregts DMJ, Lammering G, Nelemans PJ, Engelen SME, et al. Wait-and-see policy for clinical complete responders after chemoradiation for rectal cancer. J Clin Oncol. 2011;29(35):4633–40.
59. Habr-Gama A, Gama-Rodrigues J, Sao Juliao GP, Proscurshim I, Sabbagh C, Lynn PB, et al. Local recurrence after complete clinical response and watch and wait in rectal cancer after neoadjuvant chemoradiation: impact of salvage therapy on local disease control. Int J Radiat Oncol Biol Phys. 2014;88:822–8.
60. Habr-Gama A, Perez RO, Proscurshim I, Dos Santos Nunes RM, Kiss D, Gama-Rodrigues J, et al. Interval between surgery and neoadjuvant chemoradiation therapy for distal rectal cancer: does delayed surgery have an impact on outcome? Int J Radiat Oncol Biol Phys. 2008;71(4):1181–8.
61. Habr-Gama A, Perez RO, Sabbaga J, Nadalin W, São Julião GP, Gama-Rodrigues J. Increasing the rates of complete response to neoadjuvant chemoradiotherapy for distal rectal cancer: results of a prospective study using additional chemotherapy during the resting period. Dis Colon Rectum. 2009;52(12):1927–34.
62. Habr-Gama A, Sabbaga J, Gama-Rodrigues J, Sao Juliao GP, Proscurshim I, Bailao Aguilar P, et al. Watch and wait approach following extended neoadjuvant chemoradiation for distal rectal cancer: are we getting closer to anal cancer management? Dis Colon Rectum 2013;56:1109–17.

Considerations for Management of Hereditary Rectal Cancer and Desmoid Tumors

57

James M. Church

57.1 Introduction

As part of the large intestine, the rectum is inevitably involved in all the syndromes of hereditary colorectal cancer. As part of the mechanism for defecation and continence, it is also inevitably involved in considerations of bowel function, quality of life and body image. The drive to minimize the threat of colorectal cancer in these syndromes has led to the frequent replacement of the rectum by an ileal pouch, especially in familial adenomatous polyposis. However retaining the natural rectum offers several advantages including simpler index surgery, a significantly lower rate of surgical complications, avoidance of a temporary stoma, and better bowel function. A debate has ensued and continues to this day regarding the fate of the rectum in patients with syndromes of hereditary colorectal cancer. In this chapter the threat and the management of the rectum in the two major syndromes will be discussed and a balanced consideration of each side of the argument presented. Finally, desmoid disease, a biologically benign but sometimes clinically malignant manifestation of the germline *APC* mutation of familial adenomatous polyposis will be discussed in as much as it influences surgical strategy in affected patients.

J.M. Church, MD, MBChB, MMedSci, FRACS
Department of Colorectal Surgery, Digestive Disease Institute, Cleveland Clinic, Cleveland, OH, USA
e-mail: church@ccf.org

57.2 The Syndromes

There are three relatively common syndromes of hereditary colorectal cancer that call for surgical decisions affecting the rectum: Lynch syndrome (LS), familial adenomatous polyposis (FAP) and *MYH*-associated polyposis (MAP).

Lynch Syndrome

Lynch syndrome is a dominantly inherited syndrome of colorectal cancer predisposition due to a germline mutation in a gene involved with DNA mismatch repair. There are five genes that could be mutated in LS, in descending order of frequency *MSH2, MLH1, MSH6, PMS2* and *EPCAM*. The effect of an inactivating germline mutation any one of these genes is to produce a "mutator phenotype", where errors occurring during DNA replication go unrepaired and produce mutations in other susceptible genes [1]. This is seen in tumor tissue from LS patients, manifest as microsatellite instability (MSI-H). When affected tumor is stained for the proteins produced by the mismatch repair genes (immunohistochemistry, IHC), the absent protein indicates which is the mutated gene. Germline testing can then be focused accordingly.

Clinically, patients affected with LS can be suspected based on family history [2–4] and also by various appearances in tumor histology (tumor infiltrating lymphocytes, Crohn's-like reaction,

H.R.H. Patel et al. (eds.), *Pelvic Cancer Surgery: Modern Breakthroughs and Future Advances*,
DOI 10.1007/978-1-4471-4258-4_57, © Springer-Verlag London 2015

Table 57.1 Amsterdam criteria for defining HNPCC [2–4]

	Amsterdam I	Amsterdam II	Amsterdam-like
Family history	3 relatives with colorectal cancer	3 relatives with LS associated cancers	2 relatives with LS associated cancers and one with an advanced adenoma
Age of onset	One cancer under age 50	One cancer under age 50	One cancer under age 50
Relationships	2 relatives are first degree of the third	2 relatives are first degree of the third	2 relatives are first degree of the third
Excluding	FAP/MAP	FAP/MAP	FAP/MAP

mucinous differentiation and signet ring cells) [5]. Sixty percent of LS cancers are right sided but 20 % are in the rectum. There is overlap between LS and hereditary non-polyposis colorectal cancer (HNPCC), defined clinically by the Amsterdam Criteria (Table 57.1).

About 50 % of LS families meet Amsterdam Criteria [6], but the combination of a MSI-H tumor in a patient with an Amsterdam positive family is quite compelling. Amsterdam positive families should be referred for genetic counseling and testing. Amsterdam positive families with a patient who has a microsatellite stable tumor are said to be Familial Colon Cancer Type X, and have not been genetically characterized [7]. Thus, not all Amsterdam positive families have LS, and not all LS families fulfill Amsterdam criteria. Clinicians must be alert to a strong family history and a suggestive tumor phenotype, use genetic testing of tumors where this is available, and have a low threshold for referral for genetic counseling.

One caveat has arisen regarding IHC in rectal cancers. Some staining may be weaker as a result of neo-adjuvant radiation, especially for MSH6. This can confuse interpretation of the result. In addition some tumors disappear altogether after neo-adjuvant therapy, so that biopsies should be taken before chemoradiation begins [8].

Familial Adenomatous Polyposis (FAP)

FAP is an autosomal dominantly inherited syndrome of tumor predisposition due to a germline mutation in the tumor suppressor gene *APC*. *APC* is a key "gatekeeper" gene that controls **β[beta]** catenin degradation and so the activation status of multiple genes stimulating cell growth and differentiation. It is one of the first genes inactivated in the chromosomal instability mechanism leading to sporadic colorectal cancer and in FAP loss of APC from a germline mutation and a second sporadic "hit" leads to extensive tumor formation in multiple organs. The large bowel is primarily affected and multiple adenomas start to form, usually in the second decade of life. Untreated, colorectal cancer develops usually about age 39. The severity of the expression of the germline mutation varies from one patient and one family to another, with the locus of the mutation being one determinant. Extracolonic manifestations of FAP include gastroduodenal polyps and desmoid disease [9]. Desmoid disease is the second most common cause of death in patients with FAP. It is a proliferations of fibroblasts with a spectrum of presentations, either as tumors or sheets, often within the abdomen where they kink and distort bowel [10]. Desmoid disease sometimes affects operative strategy in FAP, in particular plans for the rectum.

Myh-Associated Polyposis (MAP)

MAP is an autosomal recessively inherited syndrome of colorectal cancer predisposition due to biallelic inheritance of mutations in *MYH,* a gene involved in DNA base excision repair. Loss of MYH means that oxidized DNA replicates falsely. Oxidized guanine will bond with thymine instead of cytosine, creating a G=C to T=A transversion in the next generation of cells. This transversion is a mutation that can alter the function of susceptible genes. Both *APC* and *KRAS* are susceptible genes, and adenomas as well as serrated polyps are part of the MAP phenotype. Clinically MAP most often presents as a sort of "mini" FAP. The family history is often different however, reflecting recessive inheritance, but MAP can mimic LS, classical FAP, sporadic colorectal cancer, young age of onset colorectal cancer and even serrated polyposis [11].

57.3 The Rectum, the Pouch, and the Patient

The Rectum

The rectum is a unique organ anatomically and physiologically. This uniqueness demands careful consideration when planning a surgical strategy in patients with syndromes of hereditary colorectal cancer. Anatomically, the rectum lies within the bony pelvis, surrounded by critical vascular, neural, urinary and reproductive structures. Resection is often complicated, and demands a high level of appreciation of the anatomy and physiology and the likely effects of surgery on them. Technical excellence in surgery is demanded so that good outcomes may be achieved. Secondly the function of the rectum is as a conduit for defecation. Its ability to accommodate allows for deferment of the call to stool, while the integrity of the anal sphincters and their reflex arcs provides for discrimination of gas from liquid and solid, and control of passage of stool and gas. Removal of part of the rectum decreases accommodation and increases stool frequency while replacement of the rectum completely introduces a new physiology to the patient: the ileal pouch [12].

The Ileal Pouch

An ileal pouch works because a pro-peristaltic limb is stapled to an anti-peristaltic limb, creating an a-peristaltic segment of bowel. This allows the pouch to act as a reservoir and minimizes urgency, but in practical terms increases frequency of defecation. Frequency of defecation depends on the efficiency of pouch emptying, and because the a-peristaltic pouch empties by gravity, patients have to sit for longer. Because the stool empties best when it is liquid, seepage can be an issue. A hand-sewn pouch-anal anastomosis removes the anal transition zone but promotes more seepage, anastomotic stenosis, and can be more difficult to survey. All these considerations play into strategies for dealing with colorectal cancer risk secondary to a hereditary colorectal cancer syndrome [13, 14].

The Patient

Patients coming to surgery for a syndrome of hereditary colorectal cancer are often young, and at least in the polyposis syndromes are often asymptomatic. Prophylactic colectomy or proctocolectomy is routine in FAP, while colectomy in LS is often at least partially prophylactic. Balanced against the desire to minimize cancer risk must be the need to preserve the lifestyle of these asymptomatic or minimally symptomatic patients. Teenage patients are at the start of their social, academic and physical lives. To create disabling diarrhea, incontinence, anal irritation, let alone a permanent ileostomy, retrograde ejaculation, impotence and female sterility is disastrous. The effects of serious complications of prophylactic surgery in patients with hereditary colorectal cancer are not limited to the patient. The repercussions ripple throughout the family as at-risk siblings and children become apprehensive about their own fate. Compliance may suffer as they defer testing, surveillance and treatment, and leave themselves open to developing cancer. There are so many issues involved in the surgical strategy for patients with hereditary colorectal cancer that a center of excellence featuring an experienced, multidisciplinary team is the optimal environment for care [15].

Patients with LS are different to those with FAP in that they are older at time of surgery and consequently have more co-morbidities and less functional reserve. Complications of surgery tend to be more consequential and functional outcomes worse. The surgical strategies used in FAP do not necessarily apply to LS.

57.4 The Rectum and Lynch Syndrome

LS syndrome presents with a primary rectal cancer about 20 % of the time; slightly more often when there is a germline *MSH6* mutation. A MSI-H rectal cancer is very likely to be associated with LS, as sporadic, hypermethylation MSI-H tumors are almost never found there [16]. Biopsy of a rectal cancer for microsatellite instability and immunohistochemistry is a good way of screening for LS, as long as it is done prior to neo-adjuvant chemoradiation.

One of the hallmarks of LS is a high incidence of both synchronous and metachronous colon neoplasia. It is essential that LS patients with a rectal cancer undergo high quality colonoscopy. Proximal neoplasms must be removed and if they are advanced, total proctocolectomy with ileal pouch-anal anastomosis or end ileostomy is indicated. If there is no synchronous proximal neoplasm, consideration turns to the chances of a metachronous neoplasm. There are few data addressing the risk of a metachronous colon cancer in a patient whose rectum has been removed for a primary cancer. Kalady et al. reported on 33 patients with HNPCC who underwent rectal resection for cancer [17]. Thirteen patients (39.4 %) developed a metachronous high-risk colonic adenoma and five patients (15.2 %) developed metachronous colonic cancer, three of them advanced. In all, 17 of 33 patients (51.5 %) developed high-risk adenoma or cancer, over a 6 year follow-up after proctectomy. Whether this risk is high enough to indicate routine proctocolectomy is questionable. These patients were an average of 61 years old, an age where pouch function may not be good [18]. The increased magnitude of the surgery and the need for a temporary stoma in patients with co-morbidities is also daunting and finally the use of neo-adjuvant radiation and chemotherapy is another cause for pause in taking up the radical option. If a standard anterior resection is done however, then prevention of metachronous neoplasia falls on colonoscopists' shoulders.

Colonoscopic surveillance after anterior resection in a patient with LS must be meticulous and uncompromising. Stoffel et al. reported an adenoma miss rate in HNPCC of 55 % [19], and interval cancers can develop in a 1 year from a "negative" examination [20]. Good compliance with surveillance recommendations is essential and should be emphasized during the decision-making process at initial presentation.

Oncologic results after resection of rectal cancers in patients with LS are not well documented in the literature. Samowitz et al. reported on 990 rectal cancers and found that survival was significantly worse in MSI-H tumors [21]. This was surprising as sporadic MSI-H colorectal cancers and LS colon cancers have a better than expected prognosis. In the Samowitz et al. series there were 22 MSI-H rectal cancers, 1 with a BRAF mutation, 2 with MLH1 promoter methylation and 4 expressing CIMP. Most, therefore, were likely LS. Approximately half of their patients received neo-adjuvant therapy, which may have affected prognosis adversely, although the influence of 5 flouroacil-based chemotherapy on prognosis in MSI-H colorectal cancer is controversial. In the absence of firm data indicating that LS rectal cancers should be managed differently to sporadic MSI-H tumors or MSS tumors, standard approaches to staging, neo-adjuvant therapy and resection should be followed.

57.5 The Rectum and Familial Adenomatous Polyposis

Patients with FAP are almost guaranteed to develop colorectal cancer if the colorectal polyps are not removed. In general there are too many adenomas to be managed endoscopically and so prophylactic colectomy has become routine. The issues are the timing of the surgery and the extent of the resection.

Timing generally revolves around the risk of cancer, which is determined by the number, size, histology (presence of high grade dysplasia) and rapidity of growth of the adenomas. Patients with symptoms attributable to the polyps are operated without delay, as are those with large, severely dysplastic or rapidly developing adenomas. In patients with small, infrequent and stable adenomas without high-grade dysplasia, surgery may be deferred until convenient.

The extent of surgery in patients with FAP comes down to a choice between colectomy and ileorectal anastomosis and proctocolectomy with ileostomy or ileal pouch-anal anastomosis. This is a choice between keeping the rectum or removing the rectum; keeping the organ of defecation with the associated risk of metachronous rectal cancer but a definite advantage in bowel function, or losing the organ of defecation and making do with a non-physiological replacement in the interest of minimizing cancer risk. Some centers recommend universal pouch anal anastomosis for all patients with FAP [22], while others triage patients according to rectal cancer risk. Data show quite conclusively that rectal cancer risk is determined by the colorectal polyp counts [23]. When there are <5 rectal adenomas and <1,000 colonic adenomas, proctectomy for rectal cancer or advanced neoplasia is extremely uncommon. With 5–20 rectal adenomas at colectomy, proctectomy may be required in about a third of patients but when there are >20 rectal adenomas, later proctectomy is likely in over half of cases. In many studies describing rectal cancer risk after IRA, data were at least partially derived from a time prior to 1983, when the ileal pouch anastomosis became widely adopted as an alternative to IRA and ileostomy in patients with FAP. In this "pre pouch" era, rectums severely affected by polyposis that would now be resected were retained, leading to artificially raised rectal cancer rates in subsequent years [24]. Current management triages patients into IRA or IPAA depending on the rectal polyp count. Such a policy has resulted in very low rates of proctectomy and cancer.

Technical Considerations: Ileorectal Anastomosis

Length of Rectum

For optimal function, a 15 cm length of rectum should be retained. If less than 10 cm of rectum is left, stool frequency may be disabling, even in the young. For more elderly patients, the rectosigmoid junction may be included and an ileosigmoid anastomosis performed. This may minimize stool frequency and incontinence in patients with tiring sphincters.

Anastomosis

The ileorectal anastomosis has a bad reputation for leaking and stenosing. It involves union of two ends of bowel of different sizes and thicknesses, and has been approached in many ways. The author, using a Cheatle slit if necessary, prefers a handsewn end-to-end anastomosis. Others have used an end of rectum to side of ileum, an end of ileum to side of rectum, or a side of ileum to side of rectum anastomosis. The more distorted and complex the anastomosis, the higher the chance of suboptimal function, stenosis and leak. Crossing staple lines, different bowel thickness and blood supply are also concerns. Blood supply must be preserved in the face of a potential gap between the last sigmoid branch of the inferior mesenteric artery and the upper branch of the superior rectal artery.

Mesenteric Defect

The mesenteric defect created by the ileorectal anastomosis is a potential site for small bowel torsion through the internal hernia. In my practice it is closed.

Surveillance

Yearly proctoscopy is important after IRA. The examination is usually performed in the office without sedation. Two sodium phosphate enemas are enough for preparation but should be given within 30 min of the examination. A flexible endoscope gives a much better view of all the mucosa than a rigid proctoscope. The terminal ileum is checked for about 10–15 cm, the anastomosis itself is viewed and then the rectum is checked systematically. Polyps less than 5 mm diameter can be counted but not removed. Larger polyps are all removed. If the patient is taking a non-steroidal anti-inflammatory drug, adenomas may be suppressed, although the outline of polyps (polyp ghosts) can often be seen. If it has been a long time since the original colectomy, and especially if the rectal mucosa is scarred from prior polypectomies, cancer can be very subtle. Any flat, erythematous area should be biopsied. Doubtful areas can be re-examined in 6 months.

Technical Considerations: Proctectomy and IPAA

Rectal Dissection

Preoperative evaluation should try to exclude rectal cancer. Large rectal polyps should be excised or biopsied because if there is a rectal cancer staging must be done and neo-adjuvant chemoradiation may be indicated. A total mesorectal excision is performed with close attention to planes, minimizing the chance of damage to nervi erigentes in men. Rectal dissection may be difficult in patients who have had an ileorectal anastomosis, as repeated fulguration of rectal polyps promotes perirectal fibrosis that destroys planes.

The Anastomosis

Choices are a stapled pouch anal anastomosis or a handsewn anastomosis. The stapled anastomosis allows better function and is easier to examine and survey. A handsewn anastomosis creates a little more mesenteric tension, sometimes stenosis, and is associated with worse anal control of mucus or stool. It clears most of the anal transition zone but does not guarantee freedom from cancer. It is more difficult to survey [25].

If a patient presents with profuse polyposis and adenomas exist in the anal transition zone, mucosal stripping and handsewn anastomosis is needed. If the anal transition zone is free a stapled anastomosis is preferred.

Keep It Straight

Twists in the IPAA may occur if the pouch is allowed to slide around the stapler anvil. While this may seem minor at the time it can create shelves in the pouch that interfere with emptying and disturb pouch function.

Pelvic Adhesions

Pelvic adhesions may be promoted by the pelvic dissection preceding pouch anal anastomosis. There is a suspicion that FAP patients are more prone to severe adhesions than usual, because of the *APC* mutation and its effect on fibroblasts already evident in desmoid disease. Pelvic adhesions affect the neo terminal ileum, which can be kinked into the presacral space causing an afferent loop syndrome. They also affect the ovaries and tubes, reducing fecundity. Options to minimize adhesions include performance of clean, technically precise surgery, the use of anti-adhesion sheets and the use of minimally invasive surgical approaches.

Surveillance

Yearly surveillance of an ileal pouch anastomosed to the anus is a crucial part of cancer prevention. First the pouch is prepared with two sodium phosphate enemas. Then inspection is performed with a flexible endoscope. This is usually easily done in the office in patients with a stapled IPAA but those with a handsewn IPAA may have a tender, excoriated anus. Lidocaine jelly may help minimize discomfort during the examination, as does the use of a pediatric gastroscope. The pouch is then systematically examined, beginning with the afferent limb. The oversewn blind end of the J pouch is also inspected and then the body of the pouch. Superficial ulcerations along suture lines, especially around the entrance of the afferent limb of the pouch, are common and clinically insignificant. Polyps should be biopsied and small excrescences are often lymphoid follicles. The anal transition zone and pouch anal anastomosis is closely examined, by retroflexion if possible. Sometimes the only opportunity to see this area is when the scope slowly exits the anus. Anal transition zone polyps are best dealt with in the operating room with the patient anesthetized [26].

57.6 Rectal Cancer in FAP

We have analyzed rectal cancers in FAP and found that they present in three ways: symptomatic rectal cancers at presentation; asymptomatic, unsuspected rectal cancers found at proctocolectomy: rectal cancers found after IRA, during surveillance or by symptoms [27]. Table 57.2 shows unpublished data about these three presentations

Table 57.2 Rectal cancer in patients with familial adenomatous polyposis

	Primary rectal cancer (n=34)	Incidental rectal cancer (n=5)	Rectal cancer on surveillance (n=19)	Total (n=58)
AJCC stage				
I	12	4	8	24
II	5	0	4	9
III	13	1	5	19
IV	3	0	1	4
Surgery				
IPAA	14	2	6	22
Ileostomy	15	0	12	27
Ileo-rectal anastomosis	3	3	1	7
Chemoradiation				
Pre-op	0	0	2	2
Post-op	5	1	2	8
Both	2	0	2	4
Total	7	1	6	14

of rectal cancer in FAP. The majority of patients presented with rectal cancer at diagnosis, and most of these were diagnosed before surgery; only 5/39 were not. The 19 rectal cancers diagnosed during surveillance of an IRA were mostly early stage although poor compliance led to some advanced lesions. Data on surgery performed show that some patients with upper rectal cancer can still have an ileorectal anastomosis. Some of the cases of proctocolectomy and ileostomy were due to an ultra-low rectal cancer that required an abdomino-perineal resection, and some were due to the timing of the surgery being before the pouch era. Overall, 5 year survival of patients with primary rectal cancer was 72.4 %, with incidental cancer was 100 % and with secondary rectal cancer was 69.7 %.

57.7 The Rectum and Desmoid Disease

Desmoid disease is an extracolonic manifestation of a germline mutation in *APC* that is due to uncontrolled growth of fibroblasts. This produces a spectrum of lesions ranging from white sheets on the mesentery of the small bowel, to three-dimensional tumors in the abdomen or abdominal wall. These tumors can grow rapidly, necrose, and erode into the bowel causing abscess and fistula [28, 29]. Desmoid sheets (desmoid reaction) tend to pucker and distort adjacent tissue and can cause intestinal and ureteric obstruction. Desmoid disease can force a change in surgical strategy in FAP by making IPAA impossible [30]. The fistulas and obstructions it causes can require more surgery and lead to stomas and total parenteral nutrition. Desmoid disease is the second most common cause of death in FAP [31]. It is much better to avoid desmoid disease than to have to treat it, as there is no predictably effective agent that acts against it, and resection is fraught with complications and beset with a high recurrence rate. The exceptions are abdominal wall desmoids (45 % of all desmoids in FAP), which can usually be resected without difficulty and for which the recurrence rate is a little over 1 in 3. As desmoid disease is usually precipitated by abdominal surgery, avoiding surgery in a high risk patient is a reasonable strategy to pursue. Risk factors include gender (women > men), a family history of desmoid disease, other extracolonic manifestations of Gardner's syndrome and an APC mutation 3′ of codon 1400 [32].

While some small studies did not show any relationship between type of surgery and occurrence of desmoid disease, the Cleveland Clinic has data incriminating pouch surgery [33]. Table 57.3 shows that IRA is less "desmoidogenic" than IPAA. It also shows that for an

Table 57.3 Postoperative desmoid incidence according to type of surgery and technique

	Open IRA	Laparoscopic IRA	Open IPAA	Laparoscopic IPAA	Total
N	44	66	69	19	198
N Patients with desmoids tumors	4	5	10	8	27
%	9.1	7.6	15.9	42.1*	14

IRA ileorectal anastomosis, *IPAA* ileal pouch anal anastomosis

*P<0.01, open IPAA vs. Laparoscopic IPAA

Table 57.4 Treatment for intra-abdominal fap-associated desmoid disease according to stage

Stage	No treatment	Sulindac 150–200 mg bid	Tamoxifen (120 mg daily) or raloxifene, (120–240 mg daily)	Methotrexate and vinorelbine	Adriamycin/ doxorubicin	Resection[a]
I	++	+	–	–	–	±
II		+++	+	–	–	+
III		+	++	+++		++
IV			+	+	+++	+++

[a]If this can be accomplished without resection of a functionally significant length of small bowel

IRA, laparoscopic surgery seems to minimize desmoid disease but for an IPAA, laparoscopy magnifies desmoid risk. This seems counter-intuitive but may be related to increased tension in the small bowel mesentery in pouches done laparoscopically. A defined etiology remains unclear.

A patient who's proposed surgery is most affected by desmoid disease is the one undergoing secondary proctectomy with plans for an IPAA. In our experience, 39 % of such patients had desmoid disease and in 19 % of patients it influenced surgical plans. In 13 % it prevented an IPAA [34]. However in no patient did it prevent proctectomy, minimizing a concern that had been raised by others and that had formed the rationale for prophylactic proctectomy in patients at risk for desmoid disease [35]. Such a strategy is unnecessary. Treatment of patients with intra-abdominal desmoid disease can be based on a desmoid staging system published by the Collaborative Group of the Americas on Inherited Colorectal Cancer [36]. Table 57.4 gives details of suggested treatment bases on stage. Desmoid disease can be monitored by physical examination, abdominal CT or MRI. It tends to be more benign as patients age.

Conclusion

This chapter has covered the main ways in which hereditary colorectal cancer affects the rectum. Syndromes of hereditary colorectal cancer make management of the patient and family crucial, but the principles established to maximize cure of any rectal cancer apply just as much in patients with a hereditary syndrome as in patients with sporadic disease.

Key Points

- The rectum is potentially involved in all syndromes of hereditary colorectal cancer
- Rectal polyp counts in FAP are used to triage patients to the operative alternatives: <5 ileorectal anastomosis, >20, ileal pouch anal anastomosis, 5–20, either
- Lynch syndrome patients with a rectal cancer can be offered either total proctocolectomy and ileal pouch anal anastomosis, or anterior resection, depending on age and comorbidity.
- When performing an IRA, 15 cm of rectum are needed for optima, function

- A retained rectum requires annual surveillance, as does an ileal pouch anal anastomosis
- Ileal Pouch anal anastomosis seems to result in an increased tendency to form desmoid tumors
- Desmoid tumors occur in 15 % of patients with FAP, and desmoid reaction in another 15 %
- Most follow abdominal surgery, 50 % of intraabdominal/mesenteric,
- The most severe desmoids occur in young women. Other risk factors are the presence of extracolonic manifestations of Gardner's syndrome, a family history of desmoids, and an *APC* mutation 3′ of codon 1400.
- Desmoid tumors should be staged and treated according to Stage

References

1. Schneider R, Schneider C, Kloor M, Fürst A, Möslein G. Lynch syndrome: clinical, pathological, and genetic insights. Langenbecks Arch Surg. 2012;397: 513–25.
2. Vasen HF, Mecklin JP, Khan PM, Lynch HT. The International Collaborative Group on Hereditary Non-Polyposis Colorectal Cancer (ICG-HNPCC). Dis Colon Rectum. 1991;34(5):424–5.
3. Vasen HF, Watson P, Mecklin JP, Lynch HT. New clinical criteria for hereditary nonpolyposis colorectal cancer (HNPCC, Lynch syndrome) proposed by the International Collaborative group on HNPCC. Gastroenterology. 1999;116(6):1453–6.
4. Kalady MF, McGannon E, Vogel JD, Manilich E, Fazio VW, Church JM. Risk of colorectal adenoma and carcinoma after colectomy for colorectal cancer in patients meeting Amsterdam criteria. Ann Surg. 2010;252:507–11.
5. Shia J, Ellis NA, Paty PB, Nash GM, Qin J, Offit K, Zhang XM, Markowitz AJ, Nafa K, Guillem JG, Wong WD, Gerald WL, Klimstra DS. Value of histopathology in predicting microsatellite instability in hereditary nonpolyposis colorectal cancer and sporadic colorectal cancer. Am J Surg Pathol. 2003; 27(11):1407–17.
6. Hampel H, Frankel WL, Martin E, Arnold M, Khanduja K, Kuebler P, Nakagawa H, Sotamaa K, Prior TW, Westman J, Panescu J, Fix D, Lockman J, Comeras I, de la Chapelle A. Screening for the Lynch syndrome (hereditary nonpolyposis colorectal cancer). N Engl J Med. 2005;352(18):1851–60.
7. Lindor NM, Rabe K, Petersen GM, et al. Lower cancer incidence in Amsterdam-I criteria families without mismatch repair deficiency: familial colorectal cancer type X. JAMA. 2005;293(16):1979–85.
8. Klarskov L, Holck S, Bernstein I, Okkels H, Rambech E, Baldetorp B, Nilbert M. Challenges in the identification of MSH6-associated colorectal cancer: rectal location, less typical histology, and a subset with retained mismatch repair function. Am J Surg Pathol. 2011;35(9):1391–9.
9. Church J. Familial adenomatous polyposis. Surg Oncol Clin N Am. 2009;18:585–98.
10. Quintini C, Ward G, Shatnawei A, Xhaja X, Hashimoto K, Steiger E, Hammel J, Diago Uso T, Burke CA, Church JM. Mortality of intra-abdominal desmoid tumors in patients with familial adenomatous polyposis: a single center review of 154 patients. Ann Surg. 2012;255(3):511–6.
11. Church J, Heald B, Burke C, Kalady M. Understanding MYH-associated neoplasia. Dis Colon Rectum. 2012;55(3):359–62.
12. Bryant CL, Lunniss PJ, Knowles CH, Thaha MA, Chan CL. Anterior resection syndrome. Lancet Oncol. 2012;13(9):e403–8. doi:10.1016/S1470-2045(12)70236-X.
13. Navaneethan U, Shen B. Diagnosis and management of pouchitis and ileoanal pouch dysfunction. Curr Gastroenterol Rep. 2010;12(6):485–94.
14. McGuire BB, Brannigan AE, O'Connell PR. Ileal pouch-anal anastomosis. Br J Surg. 2007;94(7):812–23.
15. Mallinson EK, Newton KF, Bowen J, Lalloo F, Clancy T, Hill J, Evans DG. The impact of screening and genetic registration on mortality and colorectal cancer incidence in familial adenomatous polyposis. Gut. 2010;59(10):1378–82.
16. Kalady MF, Sanchez JA, Manilich E, Hammel J, Casey G, Church JM. Divergent oncogenic changes influence survival differences between colon and rectal adenocarcinomas. Dis Colon Rectum. 2009;52(6): 1039–45.
17. Kalady MF, Lipman J, McGannon E, Church JM. Risk of colonic neoplasia after proctectomy for rectal cancer in hereditary nonpolyposis colorectal cancer. Ann Surg. 2012;255(6):1121–5.
18. Delaney CP, Fazio VW, Remzi FH, Hammel J, Church JM, Hull TL, Senagore AJ, Strong SA, Lavery IC. Prospective, age-related analysis of surgical results, functional outcome, and quality of life after ileal pouch-anal anastomosis. Ann Surg. 2003;238(2):221–8.
19. Stoffel EM, Turgeon DK, Stockwell DH, Zhao L, Normolle DP, Tuck MK, Bresalier RS, Marcon NE, Baron JA, Ruffin MT, Brenner DE, Syngal S, Great Lakes-New England Clinical Epidemiology and Validation Center of the Early Detection Research Network. Missed adenomas during colonoscopic surveillance in individuals with Lynch Syndrome (hereditary nonpolyposis colorectal cancer). Cancer Prev Res (Phila). 2008;1(6):470–5.

20. Vasen HF, Nagengast FM, Khan PM. Interval cancers in hereditary non-polyposis colorectal cancer (Lynch syndrome). Lancet. 1995;345(8958):1183–4.
21. Samowitz WS, Curtin K, Wolff RK, Tripp SR, Caan BJ, Slattery ML. Microsatellite instability and survival in rectal cancer. Cancer Causes Control. 2009;20(9):1763–8.
22. Kartheuser AH, Parc R, Penna CP, Tiret E, Frileux P, Hannoun L, Nordlinger B, Loygue J. Ileal pouch-anal anastomosis as the first choice operation in patients with familial adenomatous polyposis: a ten-year experience. Surgery. 1996;119(6):615–23.
23. Church J, Burke C, McGannon E, Pastean O, Clark B. Predicting polyposis severity by proctoscopy: how reliable is it? Dis Colon Rectum. 2001;44:1249–54.
24. Church J, Burke C, McGannon E, Pastean O, Clark B. Risk of rectal cancer in patients after colectomy and ileorectal anastomosis for familial adenomatous polyposis: a function of available surgical options. Dis Colon Rectum. 2003;46:1175–81.
25. von Roon AC, Will OC, Man RF, Neale KF, Phillips RK, Nicholls RJ, Clark SK, Tekkis PP. Mucosectomy with handsewn anastomosis reduces the risk of adenoma formation in the anorectal segment after restorative proctocolectomy for familial adenomatous polyposis. Ann Surg. 2011;253(2):314–7.
26. Hurlstone DP, Saunders BP, Church JM. Endoscopic surveillance of the ileoanal pouch following restorative proctocolectomy for familial adenomatous polyposis. Endoscopy. 2008;40(5):437–42.
27. Liang J, Church J. Rectal cancers in patients with familial adenomatous polyposis. Fam Cancer. 2013;12(4):749–54.
28. Soravia C, Berk T, McLeod RS, Cohen Z. Desmoid disease in patients with familial adenomatous polyposis. Dis Colon Rectum. 2000;43(3):363–9.
29. Sagar PM, Möslein G, Dozois RR. Management of desmoid tumors in patients after ileal pouch-anal anastomosis for familial adenomatous polyposis. Dis Colon Rectum. 1998;41(11):1350–5.
30. Penna C, Tiret E, Parc R, Sfairi A, Kartheuser A, Hannoun L, Nordlinger B. Operation and abdominal desmoid tumors in familial adenomatous polyposis. Surg Gynecol Obstet. 1993;177(3):263–8.
31. Arvanitis ML, Jagelman DG, Fazio VW, Lavery IC, McGannon E. Mortality in patients with familial adenomatous polyposis. Dis Colon Rectum. 1990;33:639–42.
32. Elayi E, Manilich E, Church J. Polishing the crystal ball: knowing genotype improves ability to predict desmoid disease in patients with familial adenomatous polyposis. Dis Colon Rectum. 2009;52(10):1762–6.
33. Church J, Vogel J. Minimally invasive pouch surgery predisposes to desmoid tumor formation in patients with familial adenomatous polyposis. Familial Cancer. 2005;4:49.
34. Church J, Xhaja X, Warrier S, LaGuardia L, O'Malley M, Kalady M. Desmoid tumors do not prevent proctectomy following abdominal colectomy and ileorectal anastomosis in patients with familial adenomatous polyposis. Dis Colon Rectum. 2014;57(3):343–7.
35. Vasen HF, Möslein G, Alonso A, Aretz S, Bernstein I, Bertario L, et al. Guidelines for the clinical management of familial adenomatous polyposis (FAP). Gut. 2008;57:704–13.
36. Church J, Berk T, Boman BM, Guillem J, Lynch C, Lynch P, Rodriguez-Bigas M, Rusin L, Weber T. Staging intra-abdominal desmoid tumors in familial adenomatous polyposis: a search for a uniform approach to a troubling disease. Dis Colon Rectum. 2005;48(8):1528–34.

Cost of Medical Care: Whose Money Are We Talking About?

58

Anthony J. Senagore

58.1 Introduction

In a typical economic system, there are relationships between multiple stakeholders who alternately play the role of vendor and customer. The future of US healthcare under the Affordable Care Act remains to be defined, however under any reasonable set of assumptions clinical performance of an Accountable Care Entity will require far greater attention to both clinical outcomes and cost of care delivery. This new beast will replace the highly fragmented economic structure in the US where: individuals purchase insurance but play little role as consumers of their health care; insurers have little stake in quality outcomes and chose to purchase services as a commodity for their beneficiaries; hospitals and physicians are generally reimbursed by separate pools of capital; and physicians are asked to be the gatekeepers in resource consumption only to experience no reward but all the risks associated with denying access. This discussion will attempt to define the opportunities to understand cost of care and variances in resource consumption by providers during the episode of care for the patient undergoing colorectal resection. The specific costs around oncologic staging, adjuvant treatment, and oncologic specific outcome will not be addressed as this discussion is worthy of its own independent analysis.

58.2 Episode of Care

The Medicare prospective payment system (PPS) was implemented in 1983 for the purpose of insuring access to care for the beneficiaries and to provide some means of cost control, under the assumption that clinicians would employ medically appropriate treatment across a bell shaped spectrum of disease complexity. This program has been managed by the Centers for Medicare and Medicaid Services (CMS). Since the original implementation of this program the current definition of the episode of care has evolved into the 30 day period beginning with the day of surgery. The resources consumed during this classic time frame includes any preoperative testing within 72 h of admission, OR costs (types and numbers of instrumentation, consumables, operative duration), hospital days (includes nursing time, room use, etc.), postoperative diagnostics, and pharmaceuticals. These costs have historically been bundled" into Diagnosis Related Groups (DRG) under CMS. The assumption has been that current CMS (MS-DRG) methodology accurately adjusts for both preoperative and procedural specific risks for colectomy. The current system

A.J. Senagore, MD, MS, MBA
Department of Surgery, University Hospitals/Case Western Reserve University, Cleveland, OH, USA
e-mail: anthony.senagore@uhhospitals.org

H.R.H. Patel et al. (eds.), *Pelvic Cancer Surgery: Modern Breakthroughs and Future Advances*,
DOI 10.1007/978-1-4471-4258-4_58, © Springer-Verlag London 2015

for colectomy consists of MS-DRG 331 ($9,275), MS-DRG 330 ($14,587), and MS-DRG 329 ($29,819) based upon the data published for 2013. This system however potentially rewards certain hospital-acquired complications of surgical care, while simultaneously punishing certain costs associated with processes of care that actually reduce complications [1]. Ideally, this process should be refined using evidence based definitions of the optimal cost structure of the "perfect outcome" (i.e. short length of stay, appropriate resource consumption, and no complications or readmission), and define statistically achievable results and true outlier definition. This refined risk adjustment should provide specific definitions of complications and the related cost structure for both cost effective mitigation and treatment strategies, including the impact of readmission. This level of detail does not currently exist in the actual or ACA proposed world of reimbursement leaving the provider to survive by more fully understanding their own unique circumstances of resource consumption and reimbursement. Unfortunately, an additional limitation of the current system is a complete absence of a specific and consistent methodology for intra-institutional and cross institution cost and quality comparisons [2, 3]. Reports comparing the ACS-NSQIP system to either the University Health Consortium or the Solucient® risk adjustment methodologies have demonstrated potentially different assessments within the same institution [2, 3]. Despite all of these limitations, the current discussion will attempt to define processes of care that appear capable of supporting cost efficient care of the colorectal surgical patient.

58.3 Preoperative Testing

The preoperative assessment for colorectal surgery should be patient-centric based upon an accurate history and physical examination, with particular emphasis of the risk of cardiac, pulmonary and infectious complications. Because so many more patients are elderly today it is also wise to consider the functional capacity of the patient determined by pre-admission activity level. The Duke Activity Status Index (Table 58.1) is one example of a tool to define physical vigor [4].

Table 58.1 Functional Status Assessment

Functional class	Metabolic equivalents	Activity
I	>8	Run, swim, play tennis, ski
II	4–5	Yardwork, climb stairs, walk up a hill
III	<4	Light housework, grocery shopping, walking
IV	<4	Bebound, limited activities of daily living

From Hlatky et al. [13]. Reprinted with permission from Elsevier

An alternative approach is the 6 min walk, which has been suggested as both an assessment of preoperative activity of daily living as well as a standard postoperative recovery score [5].

Aside for a complete blood count and complete metabolic profile, routine laboratory studies are rarely useful in the absence of specific patient risk factors [6]. There is considerable data supporting the contention that preoperative testing is expensive, with current estimates suggesting that this area alone accounts for 10 % of the more than $30 billion spent on laboratory testing annually [7]. Korvin et al. 13 reviewed the screening test results of almost 20,000 tests performed on 1,000 and determined that of the almost 20,000 tests 2,223 abnormal results were identified [8]. However, 675 had been predicted on clinical assessment, 1,325 abnormalities did not yield new diagnoses, and 223 led to 83 new diagnoses in 77 patients (none of which were deemed clinically significant) [8]. A similar analysis of 2,000 patients selected randomly from a database of patients screened for elective surgery determined that of 2,785 preoperative admissions tests studied (1,828 not indicated), only 96 were abnormal (10 unanticipated; 4 clinically significant) [9]. The same concern exists regarding the role of screening chest x-rays in patients without cancer or clinical risk factors. Rucker et al. assessed 872 patients with screen chest x-ray, and found serious abnormalities in only 1/368 patients without risk factors compared to 22 % of patients with risk factors (all predicted based on history) [10]. Michota, recommended a patient-centric strategy for additional testing and this reference is strongly recommended to the reader [11]. The available data suggests that each institution assess its cost-effective strategy for assessing patient risk and potential preoperative risk reduction to avoid unnecessary cost.

58.4 Preoperative Prophylaxis Strategies

The two complications following colectomy currently addressed by mandated prophylaxis strategies are surgical site infection (SSI) and deep venous thrombosis/pulmonary embolus (DVT). The complications have been associated with significantly increased risk of cost of care and therefore have been deemed to be largely avoidable complications. As a result, CMS mandated implementation of the Surgical Care Improvement Program consisting of strategies designed to reduce the rate of SSI after colectomy [12, 13]. These SSI related strategies include: administration of antibiotics within 60 min of incision; specifically recommended antibiotics; termination of prophylaxis within 24 h; use of clippers for hair removal; prophylaxis strategies has shown mixed results, particularly in relation to colectomy [12, 13]. Hawn et al. assessed the temporal relationship between SCIP implementation and surgical site infection rates and failed to identify any change in infection rates (11.3 %) for colectomy despite significant improvement in the adoption of care components [14]. Stulberg et al. performed a similar analysis of the Premiere Database which represents an all-payers US dataset and determined that a high level of adoption of all the components of SCIP was associated with a lower institutional risk of SSI. However, no individual component of the care plan could be identified as individually important to the outcome [15].

The two additional SCIP measures are related to the timely administration of DVT prophylaxis with the principal support being provided by the Canadian multicenter trial which demonstrated equal efficacy for standard or low molecular weight heparin [16]. A comprehensive analysis of the Michigan Surgical Quality Consortium Database suggested similar benefit for any combination of DVT prophylaxis for colectomy patients with either open or laparoscopic resection [17].

Surgical Technique and Perioperative Care

The body of data is clearly supportive of the multiple benefits associated with the implementation of laparoscopic colectomy versus open colectomy [18–22]. The benefits include reduced length of stay, reduced complication rates, and superior performance with regards to discharge to home rather than subacute care facilities [18–22]. In addition to the short term clinical benefits, the data also strongly support a reduced total cost of care when the procedure is performed by trained laparoscopic surgeons [23–27]. Review of all of these data demonstrates consistent benefits related to reduction in both hotel cost and nursing costs related directly to the shortened length of stay. In addition, the faster return to normal diet creates less need for parenteral support with fluids and medication further reducing the cost. Finally, the reduction in complications reduces the burden of both length of stay and diagnostics and therapeutics required to manage the complications. Therefore, it would be very difficult for a completely open team to compete with a team appropriately utilizing laparoscopic techniques for both quality and cost.

The data also clearly support the adoption of enhanced recovery protocols for the optimal management of the colectomy patient. In the four armed trial by the LAFA group, it was clear that implementation of an enhanced recovery protocol could improve the outcomes with open colectomy compared to standard care [27]. However, the addition of laparoscopic surgery dramatically improved the outcome still further [27].

While the various components of the plans may vary, the consistent variables seem to be effective multi-modal analgesia to reduce narcotic exposure, early ambulation, and early feeding [28–31]. The data are also helpful in demonstrating that breaching the care plan by either failure of the patient to progress as scheduled or from deviations of the care team can predictably lead to failure to achieve the important outcomes of ERAS [28, 32, 33]. Finally, two separate analyses of 1,000 consecutive cases performed at two separate facilities but sharing a very similar care plan confirmed consistent outcomes related to OR duration, length stay, complications, and readmission rates [34, 35]. Therefore, the care plan can be consistently applied across facilities if the care team is dedicated to full implementation. demonstrated significant advantages in favor of the former.

Conclusions

The data clearly demonstrate that costs related to the performance of colorectal resections can be effectively managed if the care team is fully aware of the current state of resource consumption and outcomes. An outline for attacking and successfully reducing the cost of care has been outlined with attention across the continuum of care from preadmission to discharge. While in the case of laparoscopic surgery there is the need for specific surgical skills, much of the remaining quality improvement and reduction in cost of care is related to the adoption of a structured care plan with minimal variation. There will need to be enhancements to the risk adjustment tools before effective and fair comparisons can be drawn between providers, however almost any system can achieve significant improvement in their cost structure by simple introspection and adoption of evidence based strategies of care. The continued implementation of the Affordable Care Act will drive greater degrees of innovation of care as the system demands higher quality at a lower cost. As the ancient Chinese proverb states "may you live in interesting times"; well I think we have collectively fulfilled the charge.

Key Points

- Understand cost structure of surgical care.
- Quantifying practice expense is essential.
- The Affordable Care Act will drive handled payments in the United States.
- Understand how surgeon behavior drives hospital costs.
- Understand key components of ERAS.
- Define patient-centered preoperative evaluation.
- Understand sources of waste in your delivery system.

References

1. Steinberg SM, Popa MR, Bethel MJ, Michalek JA, Ellison EC. Comparison of risk adjustment methodologies in surgical quality improvement. Surgery. 2008;144(4):662–7; discussion 662–7.
2. Senagore AJ, Brannigan A, Kiran RP, Brady K, Delaney CP. Diagnosis-related group assignment in laparoscopic and open colectomy: financial implications for payer and provider. Dis Colon Rectum. 2005;48(5):1016–20.
3. Hall BL, Hirbe M, Waterman B, Boslaugh S, Dunagan WC. Comparison of mortality risk adjustment using a clinical data algorithm (American College of Surgeons National Surgical Quality Improvement Program) and an administrative data algorithm (solucient) at the case level within a single institution. J Am Coll Surg. 2007;205(6):767–77.
4. Hlatky MA, Boineau RE, Higginbotham MB, et al. A brief self administered questionnaire to determine functional capacity (the Duke activity status index). Am J Cardiol. 1989;64:651–4. Reprinted with permission from Elsevier.
5. Moriello C, Mayo NE, Feldman L, Carli F. Validating the 6 minute walk test as a measure of recovery after elective colon resection surgery. Arch Phys Med Rehabil. 2008;89:1083–9.
6. Michota FA, Frost SD. The preoperative evaluation: use the history and physical rather than routine testing. Cleve Clin J Med. 2004;71:63–70.
7. Kaplan EB, Sheiner LB, Boeckmann AJ, et al. The usefulness of preoperative laboratory screening. JAMA. 1985;253:3576–81.
8. Korvin CC, Pearce RH, Stanley J. Admissions screening: clinical benefits. Ann Intern Med. 1975;83:197–203.
9. Turnbull JM, Buck C. The value of preoperative screening investigations in otherwise healthy individuals. Arch Intern Med. 1987;147:1101–5.

10. Rucker L, Frye EB, Staten MA. Usefulness of screening chest roentgenograms in preoperative patients. JAMA. 1983;250:3209–11.
11. Michota FA. The preoperative evaluation and use of laboratory testing. Cleve Clin J Med. 2006;73 Suppl 1:S4–7.
12. Jones RS, Brown C, Opelka F. Surgeon compensation: "pay for performance", the American College of Surgeons National Surgical Quality Improvement Program, the Surgical Care Improvement Program, and other considerations. Surgery. 2005;138:829–36.
13. Griffin FA. Reducing surgical complications: five million lives campaign. JCAHO J Qual Patient Saf. 2007;33:660–5.
14. Hawn MT, Vick CC, Richman J, Holman W, Deierhoi RJ, Graham LA, Henderson WG, Itani KM. Surgical site infection prevention: time to move beyond the surgical care improvement program. Ann Surg. 2011;254(3):494–9; discussion 499–501.
15. Stulberg JJ, Delaney CP, Neuhauser DV, Aron DC, Fu P, Koroukian SM. Adherence to surgical care improvement project measures and the association with postoperative infections. JAMA. 2010;303(24):2479–85.
16. McLeod RS, Geerts WH, Sniderman KW, Greenwood C, Canadian Colorectal Surgery DVT Prophylaxis Trial investigators, et al. Subcutaneous heparin versus low-molecular-weight heparin as thromboprophylaxis in patients undergoing colorectal surgery: results of the canadian colorectal DVT prophylaxis trial: a randomized, double-blind trial. Ann Surg. 2001;233(3): 438–44.
17. Henke PK, Arya S, Pannucci C, Hendren S, Kubus J, Engelsbe M, Campbell D. Procedure-specific venous thromboembolism prophylaxis: a paradigm from colectomy surgery. Surgery. 2012;152(4):528–34; discussion 534–6.
18. Shaligram A, Smith L, Pallati P, Simorov A, Meza J, Oleynikov D. Can laparoscopy for colon resection reduce the need for discharge to skilled care facility? Surg Endosc. 2013;27(11):4038–43.
19. Owen RM, Perez SD, Lytle N, Patel A, Davis SS, Lin E, Sweeney JF. Impact of operative duration on postoperative pulmonary complications in laparoscopic versus open colectomy. Surg Endosc. 2013;27(10): 3555–63.
20. Patel SS, Patel MS, Mahanti S, Ortega A, Ault GT, Kaiser AM, Senagore AJ. Laparoscopic versus open colon resections in California: a cross-sectional analysis. Am Surg. 2012;78(10):1063–5.
21. Kakarla VR, Nurkin SJ, Sharma S, Ruiz DE, Tiszenkel H. Elective laparoscopic versus open colectomy for diverticulosis: an analysis of ACS-NSQIP database. Surg Endosc. 2012;26(7):1837–42.
22. McKay GD, Morgan MJ, Wong SK, Gatenby AH, Fulham SB, Ahmed KW, Toh JW, Hanna M, Hitos K, South Western Sydney Colorectal Tumor Group. Improved short-term outcomes of laparoscopic versus open resection for colon and rectal cancer in an area health service: a multicenter study. Dis Colon Rectum. 2012;55(1):42–50.
23. Vaid S, Tucker J, Bell T, Grim R, Ahuja V. Cost analysis of laparoscopic versus open colectomy in patients with colon cancer: results from a large nationwide population database. Am Surg. 2012;78(6):635–41.
24. Alkhamesi NA, Martin J, Schlachta CM. Cost-efficiency of laparoscopic versus open colon surgery in a tertiary care center. Surg Endosc. 2011;25(11): 3597–604.
25. Eisenberg DP, Wey J, Bao PQ, Saul M, Watson AR, Schraut WH, Lee KK, James Moser A, Hughes SJ. Short- and long-term costs of laparoscopic colectomy are significantly less than open colectomy. Surg Endosc. 2010;24(9):2128–34.
26. Bosio RM, Smith BM, Aybar PS, Senagore AJ. Implementation of laparoscopic colectomy with fast-track care in an academic medical center: benefits of a fully ascended learning curve and specialty expertise. Am J Surg. 2007;193(3):413–5.
27. Wind J, Hofland J, Preckel B, Hollmann MW, Bossuyt PM, Gouma DJ, van Berge Henegouwen MI, Fuhring JW, Dejong CH, van Dam RM, Cuesta MA, Noordhuis A, de Jong D, van Zalingen E, Engel AF, Goei TH, de Stoppelaar IE, van Tets WF, van Wagensveld BA, Swart A, van den Elsen MJ, Gerhards MF, de Wit LT, Siepel MA, van Geloven AA, Juttmann JW, Clevers W, Bemelman WA. Perioperative strategy in colonic surgery; LAparoscopy and/or FAst track multimodal management versus standard care (LAFA trial). BMC Surg. 2006;6:16.
28. Lawrence JK, Keller DS, Samia H, Ermlich B, Brady KM, Nobel T, Stein SL, Delaney CP. Discharge within 24 to 72 hours of colorectal surgery is associated with low readmission rates when using enhanced recovery pathways. J Am Coll Surg. 2013;216(3):390–4.
29. Fierens J, Wolthuis AM, Penninckx F, D'Hoore A. Enhanced recovery after surgery (ERAS) protocol: prospective study of outcome in colorectal surgery. Acta Chir Belg. 2012;5:355–8.
30. Al Chalabi H, Kavanagh DO, Hassan L, Donnell KO, Nugent E, Andrews E, Keane FB, O'Riordain DS, Miller A, Neary P. The benefit of an enhanced recovery programme following elective laparoscopic sigmoid colectomy. Int J Colorectal Dis. 2010;25(6):761–6.
31. Senagore AJ, Emery T, Luchtefeld M, Kim D, Dujovny N, Hoedema R. Fluid management for laparoscopic colectomy: a prospective, randomized assessment of goal-directed administration of balanced salt solution or hetastarch coupled with an enhanced recovery program. Dis Colon Rectum. 2009;52(12):1935–40.
32. Al Chalabi H, Kavanagh DO, Hassan L, Donnell KO, Nugent E, Andrews E, Keane FB, O'Riordain DS, Miller A, Smart NJ, White P, Allison AS, Ockrim JB, Kennedy RH, Francis NK. Deviation and failure of enhanced recovery after surgery following laparoscopic colorectal surgery: early prediction model. Colorectal Dis. 2012;14(10):e727–34.
33. Gash KJ, Greenslade GL, Dixon AR. Enhanced recovery after laparoscopic colorectal resection with primary anastomosis: accelerated discharge is safe

and does not give rise to increased readmission rates. Colorectal Dis. 2012;14(10):1287–90.
34. Delaney CP, Brady K, Woconish D, Parmar SP, Champagne BJ. Towards optimizing perioperative colorectal care: outcomes for 1,000 consecutive laparoscopic colon procedures using enhanced recovery pathways. Am J Surg. 2012;203(3):353–5; discussion 355–6.
35. Senagore AJ, Delaney CP. A critical analysis of laparoscopic colectomy at a single institution: lessons learned after 1000 cases. Am J Surg. 2006;191(3): 377–80.

Approaches to Management of Fecal Incontinence

59

Michael A. Valente and Tracy L. Hull

59.1 Introduction

Fecal incontinence (FI) after pelvic surgery is a poorly understood phenomenon that occurs in a large, heterogeneous populations of patients undergoing both surgical resection and pelvic radiotherapy. FI can be a disabling complication that may or may not improve over time and has a profoundly negative effect on a patient's quality of life. Colorectal surgery, especially rectal resection for carcinoma, urological surgery for bladder and prostate cancer, and gynecological surgery, including hysterectomy, all have the potential to cause variable degrees of FI and rectal urgency in the postoperative period and beyond. Despite the fact that FI is a well known possibility after pelvic surgery leading to several studies to evaluate the pathophysiology of the disorder, no unified theory as to the exact etiology is agreed upon. Furthermore, the treatment of FI after pelvic surgery is purely empirical in nature with little or no randomized controlled trials to support any one treatment over another. This chapter will focus on the many possible etiologies of FI after pelvic cancer surgery and discuss the current and future treatment options available.

M.A. Valente, DO, FACS, FASCRS (✉)
T.L. Hull, MD
Department of Colon and Rectal Surgery, Cleveland Clinic, Cleveland, OH, USA
e-mail: valentm2@ccf.org

59.2 Incidence, Prevalence, and Quality of Life

Fecal incontinence after pelvic surgery is difficult to quantify as there as many facets included in the term FI. These include urgency, leakage of mucous, leakage of liquid stool, difficulty with control of solid stool and frank loss of an entire bowel motion. Additionally disturbances in frequency of defecation including multiple small stools in a short span of time are sometimes included in this definition by researchers. This lack of clarity leads to the wide range reported in the literature. FI after rectal cancer resection is reported to range from 0 to 71 % [1–4]. This also includes patients that have undergone radiotherapy, and the contribution for that element of the treatment plan also is unclear. FI has also been reported in a significant number of gynecological and urological cancer patients after they have undergone pelvic surgery with or without radiation.

Previously, it was believed that FI after pelvic surgery, especially after rectal cancer resection, was a transient phenomenon, where patients reverted back to "normal" or at least acceptable defecation by 6–12 months after surgery [5–7]. However, several long-term studies have reported the sustained presence of FI and other disabling defecatory symptoms well beyond 12 months [1–3]. This data supports the concept that FI after pelvic surgery likely results from permanent changes rather than just temporary dysfunction in the early postoperative period.

H.R.H. Patel et al. (eds.), *Pelvic Cancer Surgery: Modern Breakthroughs and Future Advances*,
DOI 10.1007/978-1-4471-4258-4_59, © Springer-Verlag London 2015

Permanent defecation dysfunction imparts a profoundly negative impact on patient's lives with a significant decrease in measures of quality of life and overall mental health status [4, 8]. Initially research efforts focused on cancer cure without appreciable attention to quality of life factors. With the widespread availability of validated tools to quantify and document effects of surgical treatment on quality of life, these tools should be routinely administered and incorporated into the treatment regime of these complex surgical patients [4, 9].

59.3 Etiologies

As awareness grew that FI could be a permanent problem after surgical treatment of pelvic malignancies, considerable investigational research to elicit the mechanism leading to this problem have been conducted over the past several decades [1–7]. Several anatomical and physiological abnormalities have been defined. However since the act of defecation is so complex, in-depth understanding of the multifactorial nature of this problems is not completely understood [4, 10]. Many factors have been shown to contribute to FI such as anal sphincter damage, loss of a rectal reservoir, damage to the autonomic nerves, as well as the possible negative consequences of radiotherapy. As a result of this multifaceted etiological picture, no single treatment exists to manage and treat FI after pelvic cancer surgery and thus, a tailored approach for each patient is mandated.

59.4 Rectal Resection

Over the past several decades, the technical ability to perform sphincter-saving operations has become increasingly utilized for treating low rectal cancers. It has been estimated that approximately 80 % of rectal cancer patients can undergo a sphincter-sparing operation [4]. Advances in surgical technique such as awareness of the importance of total mesorectal excision (TME) for low rectal cancers have helped improve survival from rectal cancer. Improvement in survival has also been aided by factors beyond surgical technique such as campaigns targeting earlier diagnosis along with advances in radiotherapy. However, with the increased ability to perform very low colorectal or coloanal anastomoses coupled with increased survival, the risk of FI after surgery is increasingly evident. It is now accepted that up to 90 % of these patients will subsequently have a change in bowel habits, ranging from increased bowel frequency and evacuatory dysfunction to FI [4, 11–13]. These dysfunctional symptoms after low rectal resection vary considerably between patients and have been collectively termed the *anterior resection syndrome*. The anterior resection syndrome can be characterized by increased bowel frequency, erratic defecatory patterns, rectal urgency, clustering of stools (multiple small stools in a short span of time), tenesmus, obstructed defecation and FI [3, 6, 11]. More simply stated—anterior resection syndrome is disordered bowel function after rectal resection leading to a decreased quality of life [4]. This syndrome is incompletely understood, and is attributed to a loss of the rectal reservoir. There may also be additional effects from direct damage to the anal sphincters and injury to the autonomic nerves. For example, neurological or direct physical damage to internal anal sphincter can result in decreased anal resting pressure, which may or may not recover over time [2, 8] with a resultant loss of the rectoanal inhibitory reflex (RAIR) in over 60 % of patients [14]. It is speculated that this could contribute to passive incontinence of stool. Damage to the striated external sphincter muscle can be manifested by decreased squeeze pressures and this could be mediated by nerve plexus injury during pelvic dissection and rectal mobilization. Additionally, during mobilization of the sigmoid and rectum, especially when dissecting around the inferior mesenteric artery, the parasympathetic pelvic splanchnic nerves may become damaged. This could result in a denervated colonic segment with an increased transit time and a greater number of nonpropagating contractions. This combination could lead to increased transit of the fecal bolus in the remaining left colon with in turn could cause severe fecal urgency and possibly incontinence [15].

By definition, various amounts of rectum are removed during a low anterior resection with a subsequent loss of rectal capacity. There is an intuitive belief that the more rectum left in situ, the better the postoperative bowel function. Studies have been designed to look at the resultant effect that rectal stump length has on function. Many have shown that a low anastomosis, 6–8 cm from the anal verge, gives patients significantly more problems with FI postoperatively [16, 17]. Not all studies found this conclusion. Jehle et al. reported on a series of 55 patients where they found that the level of the colorectal or coloanal anastomosis had no correlation with post operative continence. Their data showed that FI was directly related to sphincter damage and autonomic nerve injury [18].

However there are still surgeons who feel that a decreased rectal reservoir is an important contributing factor for rectal urgency and incontinence. This has led these researchers to examine ways to develop an alternative neorectal construction, such as the colonic J pouch, transverse coloplasty, and a side-to-end anastomosis. Studies looking at the colonic J pouch have shown that it decreases bowel frequency up to 1 year after surgery. However comparing this to a traditional straight anastomosis, at 2 years stool frequency was the same in both groups [19–22]. A natural further question is whether the anticipated improvement in quality of life for the first and possibly 2 years after reconstruction with a colonic J pouch should make surgeons consider constructing a colonic J pouch when feasible for all low pelvic anastomosis. This also remains an unsettled question.

Construction of a colonic J pouch can lead to new problems with expulsion of stool. The only settled controversy is that the limbs of the colonic J pouch should be from 6 to 8 cm. Outside of this, the effect that volume of the neorectum has on influencing fecal continence and urgency and the way it should be constructed remains unclear. No overwhelming benefit between colonic J pouch and a side-to-end (side of proximal colon to end of rectal stump) anastomosis has shown superior results [4, 23]. Our institution currently has ongoing studies to determine if either the colonic J or side-to -end anastomosis is superior. We know that about 25 % of patients cannot have a colonic J pouch due to problems with reach or a fatty pouch that will not fit into a narrow (particularly male) pelvis [24]. We still feel there is benefit to a neo reservoir and therefore attempt to construct either a colonic J pouch or side-to-end anastomosis when feasible in patients not enrolled in this study.

In conclusion, any of these changes mentioned above either in combination or as a sole contributor could lead to significant defecatory dysfunction. The exact role played by nerve disturbance, sphincter damage, or decreased rectal reservoir will require further study.

59.5 Gynecological Surgery

Hysterectomy for both benign and malignant conditions is the most widely performed major gynecological operation in the United States with up to 40 % of the female population undergoing this operation by the sixth decade of life [25]. Both bladder and bowel abnormalities have been reported after this operation with long-term bladder impairment occurring in 30–75 % of patients [26, 27]. Bowel dysfunction, on the other hand, has mostly been reported to be constipation and irritable bowel-like symptoms [25, 28–33]. The bladder and bowel dysfunction after hysterectomy may be related to the disruption of the autonomic nerve fibers that are carried in the pelvic plexus. These sympathetic and parasympathetic nerve fibers run in the cardinal and uterosacral ligaments. During dissection of parametrial tissue and division of the uterosacral ligaments, injury may occur.

Very few studies have looked at FI and anorectal dysfunction after hysterectomy [28, 34]. Sood et al. studied anorectal dysfunction after radial hysterectomy for cervical cancer in 11 patients [34]. They performed manometry, balloon defecation, and pudendal nerve latency testing in both the preoperative period and 6-months postoperatively. They found significantly lower resting and squeeze pressures at 6 months after surgery, bilaterally impaired pudendal nerve latency as well as decreased self reported quality of life. Similarly, Altman and colleagues reported on 76 patients undergoing hysterectomy and concluded that patients had an increased risk of mild to moderate anal incontinence after hysterectomy and that adding a bilateral salpingo-oophorectomy substantially increased such risk [28]. Therefore, gynecological surgeons should be mindful of this possibility when counseling patients for both benign and cancer related hysterectomy.

59.6 Urological Surgery

Prostatectomy, whether performed though the perineum or through a retropubic approach, carries a risk of bowel-related symptoms, including FI, as shown in several studies [35–38]. Bishoff and colleagues [35] reported on their experience with perineal and retropubic prostatectomy and found FI rates between 15 and 18 %. Likewise, Ruiz-Deya et al. [38] reported a 7 % rate of new FI after perineal prostatectomy. The etiology of FI from a perineal approach may include direct damage to the rectum and anal sphincters while the retropubic approach likely causes damage to the autonomic nerves. Again urological surgeons need to be aware of this possible postoperative problem in order to give accurate preoperative counseling.

59.7 Pelvic Radiotherapy

Radiotherapy for anal, rectal, cervical, uterine, bladder and prostate cancers is often used as primary or adjuvant therapy. Whether the delivery method is internal or external beam or brachytherapy, all radiation has possible destructive effects on anorectal structures as well as the potential to cause neuropathy to the autonomic pelvic nerves. Multiple studies have demonstrated direct anorectal dysfunction from radiation therapy which in turn leads to the possibility of FI, especially if administered after a low anterior resection [39–44]. In a cadaveric study, Wallner and colleagues studied the effects of radiation after low anterior resection with TME and found that radiation decreased the compliance of the residual rectal remnant due to fibrosis. There also was likely disruption of the myenteric plexus of the internal anal sphincter, compromising the RAIR and affecting anal pressures [40].

Currently there is limited modern prospective data on the effect radiation therapy may have on FI, especially in regards to rectal resection. Interestingly, most of the published series use data from previous decades when enhanced radiotherapy techniques were not available/utilized. Further research utilizing modern radiation therapy techniques is needed. Ideally these studies would utilize tools to evaluate bowel and anal function before and after radiation is administered. The additive effects of rectal resection would also need to be factored into a study such as this.

59.8 Treatment

Currently, there are no standard treatment algorithms for helping patients that suffer with FI after pelvic cancer surgery. Any therapeutic approach should be based on the suspicion of a sphincter lesion, confirmed or suspected nerve lesions, or the influence of any radiotherapy. Concurrent urinary incontinence should also be taken into consideration as well. All treatments that are currently available are purely empirical and symptom-based [4]. These various therapies are similar to the existing treatments that are utilized for fecal incontinence and other rectal evacuatory disorders. Treatments modalities can be broadly divided into nonoperative and operative management. Treatment should be individualized and based on the severity of the patient's symptoms, the patient's overall condition, history of radiotherapy and the degree to which the incontinence is affecting the patient's quality of life [44]. It should be emphasized again that most of these treatments are lacking any randomized, placebo-controlled trials and are still investigational with needed and anticipated ongoing research.

59.9 Nonoperative Management

Medical Therapy

Fiber supplementation, which focuses on optimizing stool frequency and consistency, has long been a cornerstone in the treatment of minor FI. Whether synthetic or natural, fiber has the capacity to absorb fluid and add bulk, which solidifies the stool in the presence of diarrhea and FI. In a study by Bliss et al. a 50 % reduction in incontinence episodes were demonstrated with addition of daily fiber supplementation versus placebo in all patients with incontinence to liquid or loose stool [45]. Increasing dietary and adding supplemental fiber is an inexpensive an easy maneuver and should be considered as a first line therapy. It should be remembered that many forms of natural fiber such as fruits and vegetables may augment FI if stools become looser with consumption of these foods. At our institution we focus on exogenous fiber such as Metamucil®, Citracel®, and other similar products. We find that this also must be individualized as some products may not improve stool consistency while others may work better for the individual patient. We start with a teaspoon usually at night and gradually increase the amount to 1–3 teaspoons, two to three times daily over several weeks. Gradual increases are required to lessen the side effects of increased gas and bloating. Also pectin which is used to thicken jelly can be purchased at the grocery store and is another agent that can be used to thicken stool.

The judicial use of constipating agents in patients with loose stools and FI has been used for several decades. These "bowel stopping" medications include drugs such as loperamide (Imodium®), diphenoxylate with atropine (Lomotil®), codeine, tincture of opium, paregoric, and amitriptyline. Loperamide, a synthetic opioid, elicits its effect by inhibiting large and small bowel motility through activation of the Mu receptors of the circular and longitudinal muscles in the bowel wall. Loperamide solidifies the stool and increases rectal compliance, therefore theoretically decreasing urgency. Specifically to controlling FI after restorative proctectomy, Hallgren et al. showed that loperamide increased resting anal pressures and thus improved anal sphincter function and continence [46]. Loperamide has also been shown to improve rectal sensation, retention of fluid load, and also increases the rectal anal inhibitory reflex [47].

The anticholinergic drug atropine is a potent inhibitor of gastrointestinal motility and works very effectively to control loose stools but may have some disconcerning side effects, such as dry mucous membranes and drowsiness [48]. Similarly, the opioid derivatives (codeine, tincture of opium, paregoric) also work extremely well in inhibiting intestinal motility. They are considered as a treatment options typically if all other bowel stoppers have failed to improve a symptomatic patient.

Amitriptyline, a tricyclic antidepressant that has anticholinergic properties, has also been studied as treatment for FI and bowel dysfunction. Santoro et al. [47] showed an 89 % decrease in fecal incontinence symptoms in patients with idiopathic FI and a reduction in the frequency and amplitude of rectal motor complexes. Its effect on patients that have had pelvic cancer surgery has not been studied.

The use of rectal irrigation and enemas has been advocated in patient's that suffer from fecal incontinence, rectal urgency, and constipation with generally good results [49]. Koch and colleagues reported on their use of retrograde colonic irrigation to treat fecal incontinence after low anterior resection [50]. In their study of 26 patients, they reported a decrease in episodes of incontinence, improvement in overall incontinence scores, along with improvement in quality of life scores after low rectal resection.

At our institution, we carefully evaluate the symptoms that distress patients. For patients with multiple small stools in a short period of time (typically in the morning) we advise they use a tap water enema to clean out the left colon, attempting to administer the enema at the same time each morning after breakfast. The goal is to expel stool in the entire left colon at one time in order to decrease the trips to the bathroom. We also use loperamide and advise patients to start with one pill (2 mg) each morning if they have soft stools. If this amount leads to constipation, the liquid form can be used to decrease the dosage. Sometimes one dose every other morning is sufficient to improve their defecation issues. Typically a combination of medical treatments with or without enemas is recommended. We keep in regular contact with patients in an effort to individualize their treatment to improve their bowel issues.

Biofeedback

Biofeedback therapy is a long established treatment for FI since Engel et al. pioneered the technique in 1974 [51]. Biofeedback's utilizes a combination of auditory, visual, and other sensory information to improve patient's awareness of rectal sensation and reinforce appropriate synchronized anal sphincter contractions to improve both FI and constipation [52].

Several studies, including randomized controlled trials, have demonstrated that biofeedback improves FI in 44–100 % of patients [53, 54]. In a recent retrospective review of 513 patients, Byrne, et al. demonstrated that biofeedback for non-surgical related FI had a 70 % improvement in incontinence scores, maximum sphincter pressures, and subsequent improvement in quality of life variables [55].

The use of biofeedback to treat FI for anterior resection syndrome has also been studied [56, 57]. In a retrospective, non-randomized review of 70 patients, Kim et al. showed a significant improvement in bowel frequency and FI scores, and a decrease in the use of antidiarrheal medications [57].

Despite the multiple studies showing biofeedback's utility in FI, an analysis of 11 randomized studies on biofeedback to treat FI concluded that biofeedback is not more efficacious than conservative measures [58] but this was focusing on FI not associated overall with pelvic cancer surgery. Regardless of this data, biofeedback should still be strongly considered as a non-invasive therapy for highly motivated patients [51]. It can be used in combination with medical therapy as a "multimodal rehabilitation program" to treat the negative effects of anterior resection syndrome [59–61]. Pucciani et al. [60] established such a program for patients with bowel dysfunction from all types of etiologies that consisted of pelviperineal kinesiology, biofeedback, volumetric rehabilitation, and anal electostimulation. The authors studied 88 patients after low rectal resection with pre-treatment and post-treatment incontinence scoring tools. They concluded that after a mean of 121 days of treatment, 24 % of the patients became symptom free and 34 % experienced improvement in their symptoms. They reported that patients with pelvic floor prolapse, a history of radiotherapy, and previous anorectal or pelvic surgery have the worst outcomes. Again with the significant negative effect on quality of life resulting from anterior resection syndrome, any improvement is welcome and should be pursued.

Injectables

The injection of biocompatible intra-anal bulking agents has increasingly gained acceptance and recent FDA approval to treat FI. The main indication for these agents is minor FI due to anal sphincter dysfunction [61, 62]. This would be a possible option for the treatment of minor FI in patients after low anterior resection [21]. Clinical studies with appropriate long-term follow-up are needed before any recommendations can be firmly endorsed.

59.10 Operative Management

Sacral Nerve Stimulation

Neuromodulation of the sacral nerves was first developed for the management of urinary incontinence over two decades ago. Subsequently, sacral nerve stimulation (SNS) for urinary incontinence was noted to also improve concurrent FI in many of these patients. Over the last decade, SNS has become FDA approved and a widely accepted option for patients plagued with fecal incontinence secondary to both neurogenic and/or sphincter muscle abnormalities. SNS has subsequently been validated in multiple studies over this time period as well [63–65] and the range of indications for SNS in FI is steadily evolving [66]. Initially, the mechanism of directly stimulating the sacral nerves to recruit inactive motor units was thought to have a direct effect on the anal sphincters by improving muscle strength (resting and squeeze pressures) [67, 68]. Subsequent investigations have included studies which demonstrate that SNS results in improved rectal sensory threshold and balloon expulsion time [69] and also decreasing antegrade and increasing retrograde colonic activity [70].

There has been promising results in a small number of patients undergoing SNS for FI after rectal resection for cancer [10, 14, 15, 71]. Matzel and colleagues reported the first attempt using SNS for FI after low anterior resection with a straight coloanal anastomosis, after all conservative measures failed. After bilateral sacral lead placement, the patient experienced perfect anal continence and greatly improved quality of life scores [71]. Subsequent work has shown similar promising results in a limited number of additional patients [10, 14, 72]. The concept of SNS to treat FI after pelvic cancer surgery is attractive. Its place in the overall treatment algorithm will be the focus of future research.

Recently, percutaneous tibial nerve stimulation has been used successfully for urinary incontinence and has shown improvement for a limited number of patients with FI as well [73–75]. It is speculated to work in a similar manner to SNS via retrograde stimulation of the pelvic nerves through the posterior tibial nerve [73]. Tibial nerve stimulation is not approved for FI in the US. Many facets of this treatment remain unknown even for mainstream FI patients. Therefore further research is needed in patients with FI *not* associated with pelvic cancer surgery before it can be translated into treatment for the group of patients we are focusing on in this chapter.

Anterior Overlapping Sphincter Repair

The overlapping sphincter repair (OSR) is a traditional treatment for FI in patients with a known external sphincter defect. Initial results after repair are quite satisfactory [76, 77], but several studies have shown decreasing efficacy over time [78–80]. There are no reports of OSR performed for FI after pelvic surgery in the literature. It is conceivable that after a low anterior resection in a patient with an occult preoperative external sphincter injury, repair may improve FI. If patients had radiation therapy, the condition of the anal skin would need to be carefully assessed as healing may be negatively affected and a non-healing wound could result. Overall however, the place of OSR in the era of increased use of SNS is being debated for all patients with FI. Therefore, it seems unlikely, except in very limited circumstances, that OSR would be used to treat patients with FI after pelvic cancer surgery.

Postanal Sphincter Repair

Historically, for patients with FI due to neurogenic or idiopathic reasons, the Park's postanal repair was devised as a treatment. The goal was to lengthen the anal canal and correct the anorectal angle [81]. In the United States, the posterior repair has not gained widespread support, likely due to the poor long-term continence rates of 33 % at 5 years [82]. However, FI after rectal resection for cancer has been treated successfully by postanal sphincter repair in a small series of patients [83]. Ho and colleagues used endoanal ultrasound and manometry while evaluating FI in patients after low anterior resection. They found mostly internal anal sphincter injuries, presumably due to the transanal insertion of the stapling instrument, which can occur in up to 18 % of patients [21, 83, 84]. Treating patients with a postanal sphincter repair in this group, they showed a decrease in overall incontinence episodes and stool frequency after mean follow-up of 3.2 years.

Neosphincter Techniques

The artificial bowel sphincter (ABS) and dynamic stimulated graciloplasty (DG) are treatment modalities that may be beneficial in some patients with FI, and could be considered before fecal diversion is undertaken. There is currently minimal data on either of these two modalities to treat FI after pelvic surgery. Since the stimulator is no longer available in the US, the DG is typically not considered as a treatment option for any patient with FI. Melenhorst and colleagues reported successfully using an ABS in 43 patients, where one had FI after a low anterior resection for an early stage rectal cancer [85]. We have used the ABS to treat patients after rectal resection led to FI. Again caution is advised if there has been radiation therapy administered to the anal skin as healing is typically compromised. Problems with healing even in patients with nonradiated skin are significant, so again caution in assessing the anal skin is advised. Additionally, the plane around the distal rectum is breeched with rectal mobilization for a low anastomosis. Development of the plane to place the ABS can be extremely difficult in these patients and lead to inadvertent colostomies which may not heal or fistulize. While ABS is an option, it should only be performed by centers with sizeable experience that will be alert to all these possible pitfalls.

Fecal Diversion

When all other reasonable therapeutic options have been exhausted, diversion of the fecal stream with either a colostomy or ileostomy can be performed. Despite the construction of a stoma, a patient's quality of life may be significantly improved versus their pre-stoma defecatory situation. With fecal diversion, an uncontrolled perineal colostomy can essentially be turned into a more predictable and manageable situation for the patient. In a study by Otto and colleagues, they reported that up to 5 % of patients after a low anterior resection will need a subsequent second operation for a colostomy due to severe FI [86]. A colostomy for FI will continue to remain a good alternative for the severely incontinent patient that has failed all standard and salvage therapies. A word of caution in performing a distal colostomy after a rectal resection and anastomosis. The marginal artery which will supply the distal colon must be respected. Any injury will lead to ischemia of the distal segment. That bowel is located deep in the pelvis and extraction will be difficult.

59.11 Summary

Fecal incontinence after pelvic cancer surgery is a poorly understood condition potentially affecting large numbers of patients with resultant negative effects on quality of life. The true overall incidence and severity of symptoms is largely underreported in the literature. Knowledge of the etiological factors is still evolving but this is largely a multifactorial problem. With an increased understanding of the possible mechanisms that cause FI after pelvic cancer surgery, potential targeted therapies for treatment are emerging. Ongoing, prospective research protocols with standardized fecal incontinence scoring systems are warranted.

Key Points

- Fecal incontinence (FI) after pelvic surgery for colorectal, gynecological and urologic cancers is common
- The symptoms of FI after pelvic surgery may partially or fully recover over time or may be permanent
- The precise mechanism of FI after pelvic surgery is not completely understood and is thought to be multifactorial
- Potential etiological factors include: disruption to the pelvic autonomic nerves, loss of rectal reservoir, anal sphincter damage, and effects of radiotherapy
- FI after pelvic surgery has a profound negative impact on quality of life and mental health status
- Treatment modalities are currently empirical and largely symptom-based and lack prospective, randomized controlled trials to support any one treatment over another
- Treatments consist of nonoperative, conservative therapy versus operative interventions

- Conservative measures include dietary modifications, pharmacological agents, rectal irrigation, biofeedback, and pelvic floor rehabilitation
- Operative interventions have minimal data supporting their use and include: neuromodulation of sacral and tibial nerves, direct sphincter repair, neosphincter construction, and fecal diversion
- Ongoing investigations to better understand the etiologies of FI after pelvic surgery coupled with standardization of FI scoring systems are essential for developing targeted therapies and possible prevention.

References

1. van Duijvendijk P, Slors JF, Taat CW, van Tets WF, van Tienhoven G, Obertop H, et al. Prospective evaluation of anorectal function after total mesorectal excision for rectal carcinoma with or without preoperative radiotherapy. Am J Gastroenterol. 2002;97:2282–9.
2. Williamson ME, Lewis WG, Finan PJ, Miller AS, Holdsworth PJ, Johnston D. Recovery of physiologic and clinical function after low anterior resection of the rectum for carcinoma: myth or reality? Dis Colon Rectum. 1995;38:411–8.
3. Ortiz H, Armendariz P. Anterior resection: do the patients perceive any clinical benefit? Int J Color Dis. 1996;11:191–5.
4. Bryant CL, Lunniss PJ, Knowles CH, Thaha MA, Chan CL. Anterior resection syndrome. Lancet Oncol. 2012;13:e403–8. doi:10.1016/S1470-2045(12)70236-X.
5. Pedersen IK, Christiansen J, Hint K, Jensen P, Olsen J, Mortensen PE. Anorectal function after low anterior resection for carcinoma. Ann Surg. 1986;204:133–5.
6. Paty PB, Enker WE, Cohen AM, Minsky BD, Friedlander-Klar H. Long-term functional results for coloanal anastomosis for rectal cancer. Am J Surg. 1994;167:90–5.
7. Carmona JA, Ortiz H, Perez-Cabanas I. Alterations in anorectal function after anterior resection for cancer of the rectum. Int J Color Dis. 1991;6:108–10.
8. Pucciarelli S, Del Bianco P, Efficace F, Toppan P, Serpentini S, Friso ML, et al. Health-related quality of life, faecal continence and bowel function in rectal cancer patients after chemoradiotherapy followed by radical surgery. Support Care Cancer. 2010;18:601–8.
9. Sprangers M, Te Velde A, Aaronson N. The construction and testing of the EORTC colorectal cancer-specific quality of life questionnaire module, (QLQ-CR38). Eur J Cancer. 1999;35:238–47.
10. Holzer B, Rosen HR, Zaglmaier W, Klug R, Beer B, Novi G, et al. Sacral nerve stimulation in patients after rectal resection-preliminary report. J Gastrointest Surg. 2008;12:921–5.
11. Williamson ME, Lewis WG, Holdsworth PJ, Finan PJ, Johnston D. Decrease in the anorectal pressure gradient after low anterior resection of the rectum. A study using continuous ambulatory manometry. Dis Colon Rectum. 1994;37:1228–31.
12. Ho YH, Low D, Goh HS. Bowel function survey after segmental colorectal resections. Dis Colon Rectum. 1995;38:259–63.
13. Lee WY, Takahashi T, Pappas T, Mantyh CR, Ludwig KA. Surgical autonomic denervation results in altered colonic motility: an explanation for low anterior resection syndrome? Surgery. 2008;143:778–83.
14. Jarrett ME, Matzel KE, Stosser M, et al. Sacral nerve stimulation for faecal incontinence following a rectosigmoid resection for colorectal cancer. Int J Color Dis. 2005;20:446–51.
15. Szmulowicz UM, Hull TL. Colonic physiology. In: Beck DE, Roberts PL, Saclarides TJ, Senagore AJ, Stamos MJ, Wexner SD, editors. The ASCRS textbook of colon and rectal surgery. 2nd ed. New York: Springer; 2011. p. 23–39.
16. Ho YH, Wong J, Goh HS. Level of anastomosis and anorectal manometry in predicting function following anterior resection for adenocarcinoma. Int J Color Dis. 1993;8:170–4.
17. McDonald PJ, Heald RJ. A survey of postoperative function after rectal anastomosis with circular stapling devices. Br J Surg. 1983;70:727–9.
18. Jehle EC, Haehnel T, Starlinger MJ, Becker HD. Level of the anastomosis does not influence functional outcome after anterior rectal resection for rectal cancer. Am J Surg. 1995;169:147–52.
19. Lazorthes F, Chiotasso P, Gamagami RA, Istvan G, Chevreau P. Late clinical outcome in a randomized prospective comparison of colonic J pouch and straight coloanal anastomosis. Br J Surg. 1997;84:1449–51.
20. Ho YH, Tan M, Seow-Choen F. Prospective randomized controlled study of clinical function and anorectal physiology after low anterior resection: comparison of straight and colonic J pouch anastomoses. Br J Surg. 1996;83:978–80.
21. Ho YH, Seow-Choen F, Tan M. Colonic J-pouch function at six months versus straight coloanal anastomosis at two years: randomized controlled trial. World J Surg. 2001;25:876–81.
22. Remzi FH, Fazio VW, Gorgun E, Zutshi M, Church JM, Lavery IC, Hull TL. Quality of life, functional outcome, and complications of coloplasty pouch after low anterior resection. Dis Colon Rectum. 2005;48:735–43.
23. Brown CJ, Fenech DS, McLeod RS. Reconstructive techniques after rectal resection for rectal cancer. Cochrane Database Syst Rev. 2008;(16):CD006040.

24. Fazio VW, Zutshi M, Remzi FH, Parc Y, Ruppert R, Fürst A, et al. A randomized multicenter trial to compare long-term functional outcome, quality of life, and complications of surgical procedures for low rectal cancers. Ann Surg. 2007;246:481–8.
25. Altman D, Zetterstrom J, Lopez A, Polack J, Nordenstam J, Mellgre A. Effect of hysterectomy on bowel function. Dis Colon Rectum. 2004;47:502–9.
26. Chen GD, Lin LY, Wang PH, Lee HS. Urinary tract dysfunction after radical hysterectomy for cervical cancer. Gynecol Oncol. 2002;85:292–7.
27. Brooks RA, Wright JD, Powell MA, Rader JS, Gao F, Mutch DG, Wall LL. Long-term assessment of bladder and bowel dysfunction after radical hysterectomy. Gynecol Oncol. 2009;114:75–9.
28. Richards DH. A post-hysterectomy syndrome. Lancet. 1974;2:983–5.
29. Roovers JP, van der Bom JG, Huub van der Vaart C, Fousert DM, Heintz AP. Does mode of hysterectomy influence micturition and defecation? Acta Obstet Gynecol Scand. 2001;80:945–51.
30. Heaton KW, Parker D, Cripps H. Bowel function and irritable bowel symptoms after hysterectomy and cholecystectomy—a population based study. Gut. 1993;34:1108–11.
31. van Dam JH, Gosselink MJ, Drogendijk AC, Hop WC, Schouten WR. Changes in bowel function after hysterectomy. Dis Colon Rectum. 1997;40:1342–7.
32. Taylor T, Smith AN, Fulton M. Effects of hysterectomy on bowel and bladder function. Int J Color Dis. 1990;5:228–31.
33. Gurnari M, Mazziotti F, Corazziari E, Badiali D, Alessandrini A, Carenza L, et al. Chronic constipation after gynaecological surgery: a retrospective study. Ital J Gastroenterol. 1988;20:183–6.
34. Sood AK, Nygaard I, Shahin MS, Sorosky JI, Lutgendorf SK, Rao SS. Anorectal dysfunction after surgical treatment for cervical cancer. J Am Coll Surg. 2002;195:513–9.
35. Bishoff JT, Motley G, Optenberg SA, Stein CR, Moon KA, Browning SM, et al. Incidence of fecal and urinary incontinence following radical peritoneal and retropubic prostatectomy in a national population. J Urol. 1998;160:454–8.
36. Dahm P, Silverstein AD, Weizer AZ, Young MD, Vieweg J, Albala DM, et al. A longitudinal assessment of bowel related symptoms and fecal incontinence following radical perineal prostatectomy. J Urol. 2003;169:2220–4.
37. Korman HJ, Mulholland TL, Huang R. Preservation of fecal continence and bowel function after radical perineal and retropubic prostatectomy: a questionnaire-based outcomes study. Prostate Cancer Prostatic Dis. 2004;7:249–52.
38. Ruiz-Deya G, Davis R, Srivastav SK, Wise AM, Thomas R. Outpatient radical prostatectomy: impact of standard perineal approach on patient outcome. J Urol. 2001;166:581–6.
39. Putta S, Andreyev HJ. Faecal incontinence: a late side-effect of pelvic radiotherapy. Clin Oncol. 2005; 17:469–77.
40. Wallner C, Lange MM, Bonsing BA, Maas CP, Wallace CN, Dabhoiwala NF, et al. Causes of fecal and urinary incontinence after total mesorectal excision for rectal cancer based on cadaveric surgery: a study from the cooperative clinical investigations of the Dutch total mesorectal excision trial. J Clin Oncol. 2008;26:4466–72.
41. Peeters KC, van de Velde CJ, Leer JW, Martijn K, Junggeburt JM, Kranenbarg EK, et al. Late side effects of short-course preoperative radiotherapy combined with total mesorectal excision for rectal cancer: increased bowel dysfunction in irradiated patients—a Dutch colorectal cancer group study. J Clin Oncol. 2005;23:6199–206.
42. Pollack J, Holm T, Cedermark B, Holmstrom B, Mellgren A. Long-term effect of preoperative radiation therapy on anorectal function. Dis Colon Rectum. 2006;49:345–52.
43. Welsh FK, McFall M, Mitchell G, Miles WF, Woods WG. Preoperative short-course radiotherapy is associated with faecal incontinence after anterior resection. Colorectal Dis. 2003;5:563–8.
44. Counihan TC, Madoff RD. Fecal incontinence. In: Fazio VW, Church JM, Delaney CP, editors. Current therapy in colon and rectal surgery. 2nd ed. Philadelphia: Elsevier Mosby; 2005. p. 105–12.
45. Bliss DZ, Jung HJ, Savik K, Lowry A, LeMoine M, Jensen L, et al. Supplementation with dietary fiber improves fecal incontinence. Nurse Res. 2001;50:203–13.
46. Halgren T, Fasth S, Delbro DS, Nordgren S, Oresland T, Hulten L. Loperamide improves anal sphincter function and continence after restorative proctocolectomy. Dig Dis Sci. 1994;39:2612–8.
47. Santoro GA, Eitan BZ, Pryde A, Bartolo DC. Open study of low-dose amitriptyline in the treatment of patients with idiopathic fecal incontinence. Dis Colon Rectum. 2000;43:1676–82.
48. Gordon PH, Schouten WR. In: Gordon PH, Nivatvongs S, editors. Principles and practice of surgery for the colon, rectum, and anus. 3rd ed. New York: Informa Healthcare; 2007. p. 293–331.
49. Christensen P, Krogh K, Buntzen S, Payandeh F, Laurberg S. Long-term outcome and safety of transanal irrigation for constipation and fecal incontinence. Dis Colon Rectum. 2009;52:286–92.
50. Koch SM, Rietveld MP, Govaert B, van Gemert WG, Baeten CG. Retrograde colonic irrigation for faecal incontinence after low anterior resection. Int J Color Dis. 2009;24:1019–22.
51. Engel BT, Nikoomanesh P, Schuster MN. Operant conditioning of rectosphincteric responses in the treatment of fecal incontinence. N Engl J Med. 1974;29:646–9.
52. Sands D, Madsen MA. Fecal incontinence. In: Beck DE, Roberts PL, Saclarides TJ, Senagore AJ, Stamos MJ, Wexner SD, editors. The ASCRS textbook of colon and rectal surgery. 2nd ed. New York: Springer; 2011. p. 309–22.
53. Heymen S, Scarlett Y, Jones K, Ringel Y, Drossman D, Whitehead WE. Randomized controlled trial

shows biofeedback to be superior to pelvic floor exercises for fecal incontinence. Dis Colon Rectum. 2009;52:1730–7.
54. Solomon MJ, Pager CK, Rex J, Roberts R, Manning J. Randomized, controlled trial of biofeedback with anal manometry transanal ultrasound, or pelvic floor retraining with digital guidance alone in the treatment of mild to moderate fecal incontinence. Dis Colon Rectum. 2003;46:703–10.
55. Byrne CM, Solomon MJ, Young JM, Rex J, Merlino CL. Biofeedback for fecal incontinence: short-term outcomes of 513 consecutive patients and predictors of successful treatment. Dis Colon Rectum. 2007;50: 417–27.
56. Dubovy VA. Biofeedback training in the treatment of anterior resection syndrome. Lik Sprava. 2006;5–6: 55–60.
57. Kim KH, Yu CS, Yoon YS, Yoon SN, Lim SB, Kim JC. Effectiveness of biofeedback therapy in the treatment of anterior resection syndrome after rectal cancer surgery. Dis Colon Rectum. 2011;54:1107–13.
58. Norton C, Cody JD. Biofeedback and/or sphincter exercises for the treatment of faecal incontinence in adults. Cochrane Database Syst Rev. 2012;(7): CD002111.
59. Pucciani F, Iozzi L, Masi A, Cianchi F, Cortesini C. Multimodal rehabilitation for faecal incontinence: experience of an Italian centre devoted to faecal disorder rehabilitation. Tech Coloproctol. 2008;7:139–47.
60. Pucciani F, Ringressi MN, Redditi S, Masi A, Giani I. Rehabilitation of fecal incontinence after sphinctersaving surgery for rectal cancer: encouraging results. Dis Colon Rectum. 2008;51:1552–8.
61. Maeda Y, Laurberg S, Norton C. Perianal injectable bulking agents as treatment for faecal incontinence in adults. Cochrane Database Syst Rev. 2010;(5): CD007959.
62. Tjandra JJ, Dykes SL, Kumar RR, Ellis CN, Gregorcyk SG, Hyman NH, Buie WD. Practice parameters for the treatment of fecal incontinence. Dis Colon Rectum. 2007;50:1497–507.
63. Wexner SD, Coller JA, Devroede G, Hull T, McCallum R, Chan M, et al. Sacral nerve stimulation for fecal incontinence: results of a 120-patient prospective multicenter study. Ann Surg. 2010;251:441–9.
64. Mellgren A, Wexner SD, Coller JA, Devroede G, Lerew DR, Madoff RD, Hull T. Long-term efficacy and safety of sacral nerve stimulation for fecal incontinence. Dis Colon Rectum. 2011;54:1065–75.
65. Altomare DF, Ratto C, Ganio E, Lolli P, Masin A, Villani RD. Long-term outcome of sacral nerve stimulation for fecal incontinence. Dis Colon Rectum. 2009;52:11–7.
66. Matzel K. Sacral nerve stimulation. In: Wexner SD, Fleshman JW, editors. Colon and rectal surgery: anorectal operations. Philadelphia: Lippincott Williams & Wilkins; 2012. p. 153–148.
67. Michelsen HB, Buntzen S, Krogh K, Laurberg S. Rectal volume tolerability and anal pressures in patients with fecal incontinence treated with sacral nerve stimulation. Dis Colon Rectum. 2006;49: 1039–44.
68. Kenefick NJ, Vaizey CJ, Cohen RC, Nicholls RJ, Kamm MA. Medium-term results of permanent sacral nerve stimulation for faecal incontinence. Br J Surg. 2002;89:896–901.
69. Ganio E, Luc AR, Clerico G, Trompetto M. Sacral nerve stimulation for treatment of fecal incontinence: a novel approach for intractable fecal incontinence. Dis Colon Rectum. 2001;44:619–29.
70. Michelsen HB, Christensen P, Krogh K, Rosenkilde M, Buntzen S, Theil J, et al. Sacral nerve stimulation for faecal incontinence alters colorectal transport. Br J Surg. 2008;95:779–84.
71. Matzel KE, Stadelmaier U, Bittorf B, Hohenfellner M, Hohenberger W. Bilateral sacral spinal nerve stimulation for fecal incontinence after low anterior rectum resection. Int J Color Dis. 2002;17:430–4.
72. Ratto C, Grillo E, Parello A, Petrolino M, Costamagna G, Doglietto GB. Sacral neuromodulation in treatment of fecal incontinence following anterior resection and chemoradiation for rectal cancer. Dis Colon Rectum. 2005;48:1027–36.
73. Hotouras A, Thaha MA, Boyle DJ, Allison ME, Currie A, Knowles CH, et al. Short-term outcome following percutaneous tibial nerve stimulation for faecal incontinence: a single centre prospective study. Colorectal Dis. 2012;14:1101–5.
74. Cooperberg MR, Stoller LM. Percutaneous neuromodulation. Urol Clin North Am. 2005;32:71–8.
75. Boyle DJ, Prosser K, Allison ME, Williams NS, Chan CL. Percutaneous tibial nerve stimulation for the treatment of urge fecal incontinence. Dis Colon Rectum. 2010;53:432–7.
76. Karoui S, Leroi AM, Koning E, Menard JF, Michot F, Denis P. Results of sphincteroplasty in 86 patients with anal incontinence. Dis Colon Rectum. 2000;43: 813–20.
77. Grey BR, Sheldon RR, Telford KJ, Kiff ES. Anterior anal sphincter repair can be of long term benefit: a 12-year case cohort from a single surgeon. BMC Surg. 2007;7:1.
78. Zutshi M, Tracey TH, Bast J, Halverson A, Na J. Ten-year outcome after anal sphincter repair for fecal incontinence. Dis Colon Rectum. 2009;52:1089–94.
79. Bravo Gutierrez A, Madoff RD, Lowry AC, Parker SC, Buie WD, Baxter NN. Long-term results of anterior sphincteroplasty. Dis Colon Rectum. 2004;47:727–31.
80. Halverson AL, Hull TL. Long-term outcome of overlapping anal sphincter repair. Dis Colon Rectum. 2002;45:345–8.
81. Browning GG, Parks AG. Postanal repair for neuropathic faecal incontinence: correlation of clinical result and anal canal pressures. Br J Surg. 1983;70:101–4.
82. Carraro PS, Kamm MA, Nichols RJ. Longterm results of postanal repair for neurogenic fecal incontinence. Br J Surg. 1994;81:140–4.
83. Ho YH. Postanal sphincter repair for anterior resection anal sphincter injuries: report of three cases. Dis Colon Rectum. 2001;44:1218–20.

84. Farouk R, Duthie GS, Lee PW, Monson JR. Endosonographic evidence of injury to the internal anal sphincter after low anterior resection: long-term follow-up. Dis Colon Rectum. 1998;41:888–91.
85. Melenhorst J, Koch SM, van Gemert WG, Baeten CG. The artificial bowel sphincter for faecal incontinence: a single centre study. Int J Color Dis. 2008;23:107–11.
86. Otto IC, Ito K, Ye C, Hibi K, Kasai Y, Akiyama S, Takagi H. Causes of rectal incontinence after sphincter-preserving operations for rectal cancer. Dis Colon Rectum. 1996;39:1423–7.

Index

H.R.H. Patel et al. (eds.), *Pelvic Cancer Surgery: Modern Breakthroughs and Future Advances*,
DOI 10.1007/978-1-4471-4258-4, © Springer-Verlag London 2015

R

U

Printed by Printforce, the Netherlands